GERIATRIC
EMERGENCY
MEDICINE

GERIATRIC EMERGENCY MEDICINE

Gideon Bosker, M.D., F.A.C.E.P.
Editor-in-Chief
Clinical Assistant Professor,
Oregon Health Sciences University;
Director, Continuing Medical Education,
Department of Emergency Medicine,
Good Samaritan Hospital & Medical Center,
Portland, Oregon

George R. Schwartz, M.D., F.A.C.E.P.
Editor
Consultant in Family, Community and Emergency Medicine,
Healing Research, Inc.,
Santa Fe;
Emergency Medicine, Los Alamos Medical Center;
Medical Director, The Bridge Centers,
Los Alamos, New Mexico

Jeffrey S. Jones, M.D.
Editor
Research Director and Staff Physician,
Department of Emergency Medicine,
Butterworth Hospital, Grand Rapids;
Assistant Professor of Emergency Medicine,
Michigan State University College of Human Medicine,
Grand Rapids, Michigan

Michael Sequeira, M.D., F.A.C.E.P.
Associate Editor
Assistant Clinical Professor,
Oregon Health Sciences University;
Associate Director, Department of Emergency Medicine,
Good Samaritan Hospital and Medical Center,
Portland, Oregon

with 107 *illustrations*

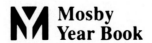

**Mosby
Year Book**

St. Louis   Baltimore   Boston   Chicago   London   Philadelphia   Sydney   Toronto

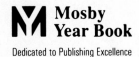

Mosby
Year Book
Dedicated to Publishing Excellence

Editor: Richard Weimer
Editorial assistant: Rina Steinhauer

Copyright © 1990 by Mosby–Year Book, Inc.
A Mosby imprint of Mosby–Year Book, Inc.

Printed in the United States of America

The C.V. Mosby Company
11830 Westline Industrial Drive, St. Louis, Missouri 63146

Library of Congress Cataloging in Publication Data
Geriatric emergency medicine / Gideon Bosker, editor-in-chief ; George
　Schwartz, editor ; Jeffrey S. Jones, editor ; Michael Sequeira,
　associate editor.
　　　p.　　cm.
　　ISBN 0-8016-1808-8 : $65.00 (est.)
　　1. Geriatrics.　2. Emergency medicine.　I. Bosker, Gideon.
　　[DNLM: 1. Emergencies––in old age.　WB 105 G3694]
　RC952.5.G438　1990
　618.97'025––dc20
　DNLM/DLC
　for Library of Congress　　　　　　　　　　　89-13337
　　　　　　　　　　　　　　　　　　　　　　　　　　　CIP

PH/VH/VH　9　8　7　6　5　4　3　2　1

In loving memory of
Martin Bosker and Milton Schwartz

Contributors

J. Michael Albrich, M.D., F.A.C.E.P., F.A.C.P.

Department of Emergency Medicine, Good Samaritan Hospital, Oregon Health Sciences University, Portland, Oregon

Steven A. Baum, M.D.

Clinical Assistant Professor of Medicine, Geriatric Research, Education and Clinical Center, Sepulveda VA Medical Center, Sepulveda, California

Bruce Blank, M.D.

Department of Urology, Good Samaritan Hospital & Medical Center, Portland, Oregon

Gideon Bosker, M.D., F.A.C.E.P.

Clinical Assistant Professor, Oregon Health Sciences University; Director, Continuing Medical Education, Department of Emergency Medicine, Good Samaritan Hospital & Medical Center, Portland, Oregon

Richard Caesar, M.D., F.A.C.E.P.

Department of Emergency Medicine, Good Samaritan Hospital & Medical Center, Portland, Oregon

Louis A. Cannon, M.D.

Cardiology Fellow, Department of Cardiovascular Disease, University Hospital, Cincinnati, Ohio

Marjorie Chevrier, R.N., C.E.N.

Department of Emergency Medicine, Akron General Medical Center, Akron, Ohio

Clark Chipman, M.D., F.A.C.E.P.

Chief, Emergency Services, Emanuel Hospital; Associate Clinical Professor, University of Oregon Health Science Center, Portland, Oregon

William Cook, M.D.

Chairman, Department of Obstetrics and Gynecology, Akron General Medical Center; Assistant Professor of Obstetrics and Gynecology, Northeastern Ohio Universities College of Medicine, Rootstown, Ohio

Edward M. Cordasco, M.D., F.A.C.P.

Director, Occupational Respiratory Clinic, Cleveland Clinic Foundation, Cleveland, Ohio

Mohamud Daya, M.D., F.A.C.E.P.

Assistant Professor, Department of Emergency Medicine, Oregon Health Sciences University, Portland, Oregon

Gerald B. Demarest, M.D.

Associate Professor of Surgery and Director, Burn and Trauma Service, University of New Mexico Medical Center, Albuquerque, New Mexico

Lewis DeMent, M.D., F.A.C.E.P.

Department of Emergency Medicine, Good Samaritan Hospital & Medical Center, Portland, Oregon

Stephen L. Demeter, M.D., F.A.C.P., F.C.C.P.

Professor and Head, Division of Pulmonary Medicine, Northwestern Ohio Universities College of Medicine, Rootstown, Ohio

James Dougherty, M.D., F.A.C.E.P.

Research Director and Staff Physician, Department of Emergency Medicine, Akron General Medical Center; Assistant Clinical Professor of Emergency Medicine, Northeastern Ohio Universities College of Medicine, Rootstown, Ohio

Knut Eie, EMT-IV

Paramedic, Coeur de Lane, Idaho

Boni E. Elewski, M.D.

Assistant Professor of Dermatology, Case Western Reserve University, University Hospital of Cleveland, Cleveland, Ohio

Michael L. Freedman, M.D.

Professor, Department of Medicine; Director, Division of Geriatrics, New York University, Bellevue Medical Center, New York, New York

Sally Shaw Garrigan, M.S.W.

Good Samaritan Hospital & Medical Center, Department of Social Work, Portland, Oregon

Steven E. Gentry, M.D., F.A.C.E.P.

Assistant Professor of Medicine, University of Pittsburgh School of Medicine; Pulmonary Unit, Montefiore Hospital, Pittsburgh, Pennsylvania

John W. Grigsby, M.D., F.A.C.E.P.

Chief, Department of Emergency Medicine, Good Samaritan Hospital & Medical Center, Portland, Oregon

Robert J. Grimm, M.D., F.A.C.P.

Department of Neurology, Neurological Sciences Center, Portland, Oregon

Stephen Hamburger, M.D.

Professor and Chairman, Department of Medicine, University of Missouri, Kansas City, Missouri

David M. Igdaloff, M.D.

Clinical Assistant Professor, University of California, Davis; Private Practice, Walnut Creek, California

William L. Isley, M.D.

Assistant Professor, Department of Medicine, University of Missouri, Kansas City, Missouri

Jeffrey S. Jones, M.D.

Research Director and Staff Physician, Department of Emergency Medicine, Butterworth Hospital, Grand Rapids; Assistant Professor of Emergency Medicine, Michigan State University College of Human Medicine, Grand Rapids, Michigan

Stephen R. Jones, M.D., F.A.C.P.

Chief of Medicine; Associate Professor of Medicine, Oregon Health Sciences University; Good Samaritan Hospital & Medical Center, Portland, Oregon

Michael Kaempf, M.D.

Department of Urology, Good Samaritan Hospital & Medical Center, Portland, Oregon

Elizabeth Hatfield Keller, R.N., B.S.N., C.E.N., EMT-P

Paramedic, Private Practice

Diana Koin, M.D.

Private Practice

Wendy Levinson, M.D.

Director, Primary Care Clinic, Good Samaritan Hospital & Medical Center, Portland, Oregon

Daniel K. Lowe, M.D.

Professor of Surgery, Oregon Health Sciences University, Portland, Oregon

Sally E. Martin, M.A.S.N., R.N.C., G.N.P.

Associate Chief, Nursing Service for Nursing Home Care, Sepulveda Veterans Administration Medical Center; Assistant Clinical Professor, UCLA School of Nursing, Los Angeles, California

M. J. McMullen, M.D., F.A.C.E.P.

Staff Physician, Department of Emergency Medicine, Akron General Medical Center; Assistant Clinical Professor of Emergency Medicine, Northeastern Ohio Universities College of Medicine, Rootstown, Ohio

Sue Mendelsohn, M.N., R.N.C., G.N.P.

Lecturer/Clinical Instructor, UCLA School of Nursing, Los Angeles, California

Matthew Montgomery, M.D.

Department of Obstetrics and Gynecology, Raleigh General Hospital, Beckley, West Virginia

Joseph G. Ouslander, M.D.

Medical Director, Jewish Homes for the Aging of Greater Los Angeles, Victory Campus, Multicampus Division of Geriatric Medicine, UCLA School of Medicine, Los Angeles, California

Louis J. Perretta, M.D., F.A.C.E.P.

Department of Emergency Medicine, Good Samaritan Hospital & Medical Center, Portland, Oregon

Dennis P. Price, M.D., F.A.C.E.P.

Attending Physician, Clinical Assistant Professor of Medicine, Department of Emergency Medicine, Bellevue Hospital Center, New York; Staff Physician, The Medical Center at Princeton, Princeton, New Jersey

Robert Rafal, M.D.

Attending Neurologist, Private Practice, La Jolla, California

Elizabeth London Rogers, M.D.

Chief of Staff, Baltimore VA Medical Center; Associate Professor of Medicine, University of Maryland Medical School, Baltimore, Maryland

Steven Romisher, M.D.

Staff Physician, Department of Emergency Medicine, Akron General Medicine Center, Akron, Ohio

Laurence Z. Rubenstein, M.D., M.P.H.

Associate Professor of Medicine; Clinical Director, Geriatric Research, Education and Clinical Center, Sepulveda VA Medical Center, Sepulveda, California

David Rush, Pharm. D.

Professor of Pharmacy and Medicine, University of Missouri Schools of Medicine and Pharmacy, Kansas City, Missouri

Sandra M. Schneider, M.D., F.A.C.E.P.

Associate Professor of Medicine, University of Pittsburgh School of Medicine; Director, Emergency Medical Services, Montefiore Hospital, Pittsburgh, Pennsylvania

George R. Schwartz, M.D., F.A.C.E.P.

Consultant in Family, Community and Emergency Medicine, Healing Research, Inc., Santa Fe; Emergency Medicine, Los Alamos Medical Center; Medical Director, The Bridge Centers, Los Alamos, New Mexico

Michael Sequeira, M.D., F.A.C.E.P.

Assistant Clinical Professor, Oregon Health Sciences University; Associate Director, Department of Emergency Medicine, Good Samaritan Hospital & Medical Center, Portland, Oregon

Dan Tandberg, M.D.

Associate Professor of Emergency Medicine, Division of Emergency Medicine, University of New Mexico School of Medicine; Medical Director, New Mexico Poison Control Center, University of New Mexico Hospital, Albuquerque, New Mexico

Rein Tideiksaar, Ph.D.

Director, Falls and Immobility Program, Gerald and Mary Ellen Ritter Department of Geriatrics and Adult Development, Mount Sinai Medical Center; The Jewish Home and Hospital for the Aged, New York, New York

Donald D. Trunkey, M.D.

Chairman and Professor, Department of Surgery, Oregon Health Sciences University, Portland, Oregon

Carole L. Turner, M.N., R.N.C., G.N.P.

Jewish Homes for the Aging of Greater Los Angeles; Assistant Clinical Professor, UCLA School of Nursing, Los Angeles, California

Richard C. U'Ren, M.D.

Associate Professor, Department of Psychiatry, Oregon Health Sciences University, Portland, Oregon

Pam Wheeler, R.N.

Geriatric Nurse Coordinator, Division of Gerontology, Good Samaritan Hospital & Medical Center, Portland, Oregon

Donald A. Wiens, M.D., F.A.C.E.P.

Staff Physician, Department of Emergency Medicine, Good Samaritan Hospital & Medical Center, Portland, Oregon

Richard A. Yeager, M.D.

Assistant Professor of Surgery, Oregon Health Sciences University; Veteran's Administration Hospital, Portland, Oregon

Gary Young, M.D., F.A.C.E.P.

Director, Department of Emergency Medicine; Assistant Professor of Emergency Medicine, VA Medical Center, Oregon Health Sciences University, Portland, Oregon

Preface

Geriatric emergency medicine has evolved into a bona fide — and increasingly fashionable — clinical discipline, if for no other reason than because the United States has become a graying nation. At present, 38 million individuals over the age of 65 constitute 12% of our population and more than 32% of total hospital admissions in America. By the year 2012, one in every five Americans will be over 65, and there will be more than 16 million people over the age of 85.

At present, the average American who attains the age of 80 has a life expectancy of approximately 7 to 10 years. The average life expectancy for a woman in this country reaching adulthood is estimated to be about 84 years, and for a man it is 72. Although only 5% of these elderly people live in nursing homes, such chronic conditions as coronary artery disease, cancer, cerebrovascular disease, and diabetes are common in the geriatric population. Because these afflictions are frequently characterized by acute exacerbations or sudden deterioration, the elderly tend to be significant clients of outpatient services, especially emergency departments. This is particularly true of the 27% of elderly people living alone who must also cope with multiple medical problems and who function poorly both mentally and physically.

As a result of these demographic patterns, hospital emergency departments are encountering an increasing number of medical and surgical disorders unique to the elderly population. In many respects, geriatric emergencies are similar to those that occur in younger patients. The elderly, however, tend to have multiple problems, and their symptoms frequently do not fit classic patterns. Hence, diagnosis, assessment, and triage of these patients can be difficult and problematic. Emergency care for the elderly is characterized by many unique aspects. For example, nearly one in four emergency department admissions for the elderly is caused by a drug-related adverse patient event (DRAPE). The Department of Health and Human Services reported that in 1988 there were 240,000 hospital admissions for adverse drug reactions and 40% of these befell individuals 65 years or older, the majority of whom were diagnosed or managed initially in the emergency department setting. A review of cardiovascular disease compliance studies attributes an annual 125,000 death toll at the doorstep of medication noncompliance or drug toxicity. With respect to traumatic injuries in the geriatric age group, falls rather than motor vehicle accidents constitute the most important cause of morbidity and mortality in this age group; again, it is primarily in the emergency department, where intrinsic versus extrinsic etiologies of syncopal episodes must be diciphered, where the initial assessment and management of hip fractures transpire, and where the subdural hematoma must be suspected and appropriately evaluated.

Over the past decade, the geriatric medical imperative has made a profound and lasting impact on American health care; the field of emergency medicine is no exception. There is simply no escape from the fact that as emergency medicine and related disciplines — critical care, prehospital medicine, geriatric nursing, and such geriatric-oriented subspecialties as cardiology and neurology — evolve, our attention, by necessity, increasingly will be directed at older Americans. Those of us in emergency medicine who have gained experience in managing elderly patients have become poignantly aware, first, of the unique manner in which the elderly respond to nonurgent medical and surgical problems and, second, of the ways in which their signs and symptoms differ in such life-threatening disorders as myocardial infarction, sepsis, and myxedema coma. For example, we now know that geriatric patients over the age of 85 are more likely to present with shortness of breath than with chest pain as the initial manifestation of acute myocardial infarction. Syncope in the elderly carries a vast array of possibilities for differential diagnosis, from autonomic neuropathy and cardiac bradydysrhythmias to drug-induced orthostatic hypotension and vasovagal syncope, entities that must frequently be sorted out in the emergency setting. This variable display of symptoms in older patients underscores the importance of recent investigations indicating that elderly patients spend more time in emergency departments, undergo more diagnostic tests, and are more likely to be misdiagnosed than their younger counterparts. Finally, the "return visit" or "bounce-back" rate for geriatric patients is higher than it is for any other subpopulation seen in the acute setting.

Complicating the complex, often elusive nature of acute illnesses in the elderly is the necessity of rapidly initiating lifesaving measures and instituting precise interventions, which must frequently be accomplished with only a limited data base. There is also the pitfall of inappropriate triage, which may be characterized by either unnecessary hospitalization of an elderly patient with a minor illness who is better left in the familiar surroundings of the home environment, or failing to hospitalize an older patient whose serious illness produces little in the way of conspicuous signs or symptoms. Such decisions are complicated by the fact that clinical conditions that are not life threatening may produce exaggerated symptoms in the elderly, while such life-threatening disorders as myocardial infarction may produce minimal clinical symptoms, an irony that requires the clinician to maintain an unusually high index of suspicion.

Because elderly Americans and the diseases they suffer from now constitute an ever-increasing percentage of emergency department visits, the time has come for a comprehensive book that specifically addresses assessment and intervention strategies in this patient population. The purpose of this reference is to serve as a clinically oriented resource for the care of elderly patients in a modern hospital emergency department or in any facility that treats older patients. Much to the credit of this group of contributors and editors, this book attempts to reflect a recognition of unique medical needs of geriatric patients in regard to emergency diagnosis, management, and triage. Spanning a diverse range of acute care specialties, from cardiology, neurology, and endocrinology to clinical pharmacology, toxicology, and surgical diseases, these authors have recognized the geriatric imperative in emergency medicine, and they have tried to bring both sensitivity and clinical rigor to the emergency needs of older Americans. Of particular note is the section on acute geriatric nursing, because more than in perhaps any other area of medicine, the out-of-hospital nursing link is critical for good patient care.

If this book succeeds in heightening the emergency practitioner's awareness of the clinical and social issues surrounding the care of acutely ill geriatric patients, it will have served its purpose.

Gideon Bosker
Editor-in-Chief

Acknowledgments

Geriatric Emergency Medicine would not have come to fruition without the commitment and creative talents of many individuals who, over the past four years, have devoted their time and energy to this project. In this regard, we gratefully acknowledge David Culverwell, Publisher, and Richard Weimer, Executive Editor, who must be credited with having the vision and intelligence to recognize that geriatric emergency medicine would one day take root as a critical subspecialty within the general field of emergency medicine. Without their commitment and expansive view of medical publishing, this book would not exist.

In this vein, the editor-in-chief also wishes to thank John W. Grigsby, M.D., F.A.C.E.P., Chief of Emergency Services at Good Samaritan Hospital, Portland, Oregon, for his ongoing commitment and support of educational programs devoted to geriatric emergency medicine since 1982. Dr. Grigsby's insights into the future of emergency medicine have inspired much of this project, and his invaluable editorial contributions and responsibilities for the previous edition of this book are sincerely appreciated by the editorial team.

The original manuscript was meticulously organized and catalogued according to subject headings by Rina Steinhauer, whose valuable insights and editorial dissection have been retained in the outlines that appear at the beginning of each chapter. Her organizational skills and conceptual insights are sincerely appreciated. The design of the book evolved through many different stages; its final crystalline form can be credited to Liz Fett, whose comments, sketches, and designs were inspired and carefully wrought throughout the book's development. The cover logo, in which an hourglass also reveals the near-mirror images of two elderly faces, is an original contribution by Elise Stimac, and we wish to express our thanks for her graphic panache and visual illumination.

Dr. Schwartz would particularly like to acknowledge the enormous help in manuscript organization and preparation by his wife Kathleen Schwartz, who has been deeply committed to this project throughout the years of its development.

And finally, the bottom line. As all editors and academicians know in their hearts, every book has its guiding light. The guiding light steering this book to its ultimate completion has been Karen Edwards, Senior Project Manager, without whom this book would not have the editorial polish it has achieved in its finished form. We sincerely express our appreciation to Ms. Edwards, who has been an editorial pillar of strength and policeman throughout the later stages of the book and who has had the enormous responsibility of correcting and conceptually tightening a massive volume of material within a relatively short amount of time. She is a silent hero behind the scenes of this project, and we thank her for her outstanding talent and commitment.

The Editors

Contents

Introduction

Geriatric Emergency Medicine

George R. Schwartz, M.D., F.A.C.E.P.

Our older population represents a substantial (12%) and ever-increasing portion of the patients who present in emergency departments. Even in 1976 elderly patients used one third of hospital beds and almost one third of each health care dollar.[1] This number has now increased and is closer to 40%. Sensitivity to the problems and needs of older people is vital as we witness an increasingly vigorous longevity and the general aging of our population. It is amazing that emergency medical units still are often planned without the elderly as a prime consideration despite the projections that within 50 years one of every five persons will be over the age of 65. Even now, more than 11% of the population is 65 or older, up from 4% in 1900. Of the 65 and older group, those aged 75 or greater rose from 29% in 1900 to 38% in 1970; it is expected to reach over 40% by the year 2000.[2]

Care of elderly patients in the emergency department requires changes in emphasis. A particular pitfall is focusing too closely on the patient's presenting problem without exercising sufficient vigilance in identifying possible underlying conditions, both social and medical, that may have caused the acute medical problem or injury. Elderly persons in particular require this type of attention. For example, falls are a major source of morbidity and mortality in the elderly and often have treatable causes, both medical (e.g., underlying diseases) and environmental (e.g., clothing, rugs, poor lighting, etc.).[3]

As with persons of any age group, elderly individuals frequently need active medical intervention that must be based on very limited information. Lifesaving actions might have to be taken even before a patient's identity is known: bleeding stopped, shock treated, fractures diagnosed and splinted, respiratory arrests or obstructions immediately alleviated, and lacerations sutured. Often the patient is not known by the staff, and there is little history on which to proceed, but prompt medical decisions must be made with attention to the known physiologic differences and response to trauma.

However, for a physician to stop treatment after the life-threatening problem has been controlled or the obvious presenting symptom cared for is to lose a substantial opportunity to evaluate problems that may have precipitated the accident or illness. Such considerations often directly influence the responses to treatment. Nutrition, drugs, and underlying medical problems are important factors in the development of emergency medical problems and are discussed in the sections that follow.

FOOD AND NUTRITION

Many older people live alone and are on fixed, low incomes. Loneliness, decreased sensitivity to taste, physical infirmity, and decreased vision all act to reduce the motivation to shop for fresh food items. Thus, there is a tendency to rely on processed foods and food that will keep on the shelf. Numerous studies have demonstrated that elderly patients frequently consume less than the minimum daily requirement of most vitamins. In addition, malabsorption can cause or compound nutritional deficiencies. Poor dentition reduces mastication, and frequent hypochlorhydria as well as decreased intestinal secretions further tend to reduce absorption.[4] Additionally, many processed and prepackaged foods have sufficient doses of monosodium glutamate (MSG) to produce or add to symptoms of dizziness, edema, and depression.

The use of supplemental vitamins does not solve what is usually an overall problem with diet, not just insufficient intake of vitamins. Overall nutritional inadequacy is more prevalent than is usually appreciated. Vitamin deficiencies may result in weakness and a tendency to being accident prone. In fact, there is a likelihood that we are not diagnosing underlying nutritional conditions by recognizing early presenting symptoms. Symptoms of early niacin deficiency, for example, include incapacity for mental and physical effort, loss of appetite, poor sleeping patterns, dizziness, syncope, paresthesias, palpitations, and depression. These symptoms will appear well before the classic symptoms of diarrhea, dermatitis, and dementia. Also, mental changes caused by vitamin B_2 deficiency may appear before anemia.

Early scurvy represents another example of vitamin insufficiency. Vitamin C in food deteriorates when kept for a prolonged period of time, when stored without refrigeration, or when exposed to light. Scurvy does not just suddenly appear; there is a slow and insidious progression of subtle signs and symptoms before the classic clinical manifestations occur. Infection or other stress may precipitate rapid development of signs and symptoms.

Common symptoms in early scurvy include joint pains, stiffness and pain with motion, unsteadiness of gait, and signs of confusion. Later, of course, there are problems of bleeding gums, skin changes, hair changes, overall depression and lassitude, and eventually death. The point, again, is not to promote supplemental vitamin use but to emphasize that emergency problems in the elderly can appear against a background that may include nutritional inadequacy.

Another example of vitamin insufficiency may be seen in older people who have intermittently used alcohol to excess. When seen in an emergency department, these individuals might not have used alcohol for weeks; however, a chronic thiamine deficiency might cause or aggravate dizziness, memory lapses, or syncope, which could be related to the acute problem.

Poor nutrition over a period of months can lead to anemia with confusion and weakness.[5] In addition, osteoporosis is a frequently encountered problem that may lead to an increase in fractures. Hip fractures in women are particularly serious in mortality and morbidity and may be reduced through diet and estrogens.[6]

PHYSIOLOGIC CONSIDERATIONS

Clinically, evaluation of elderly persons is affected by the "normal" changes of aging. However, studies have shown that there are no changes in hemoglobin and hematocrit and few changes in fasting blood glucose, serum electrolyte concentration, and blood gas values in the absence of disease. Further, in this book we will explore age-related functional reduction in renal, pulmonary, and immune functions as well as reduced ability to maintain homeostasis after trauma. However, suffice it to say at this point that physiologic changes should not be ascribed to "normal aging" until a thorough investigation or suitable referral is made.

MEDICATION PROBLEMS

It is not always possible to obtain a detailed history of medications that the patient is taking, but it may be these medications that have resulted in acute injury. Examples of such medications are phenothiazines, diuretics (with inadequate potassium replacement), tranquilizers, and antihypertensive medications (which can cause orthostatic hypotension). Falls may also be associated with weakness due to anorexia or dehydration. Syncope may result from digitalis or diuretic use. In addition, drug interactions with nutritional factors are just beginning to be understood. Isoniazid-type drugs can result in symptoms of vitamin B_6 deficiency, Dilantin can precipitate folic acid deficiency anemia, and colchicine may reduce vitamin B_{12} absorption.

Older people tend to suffer from degenerative disorders, are more susceptible to various diseases, and frequently are taking several medications. Confusion, vision impairment, and forgetfulness can add to a medication problem.

About 3% of all hospital admissions are related to drug-induced illnesses. Of the drugs implicated in adverse reactions by Caranosus and colleagues,[7] four drugs led the list and accounted for 75% of these problems: aspirin, digoxin, coumarin, and diuretics. Of hospital admissions for drug reaction, more than 35 to 40% are usually for people older than 60 years.

It is also possible that reactions to medications are more easily overlooked in elderly persons because of the overall increase in medical disorders in this age group and the common habit of ascribing unclassifiable symptoms to aging in general.

Thus, a general principle of geriatric medicine as practiced in the emergency department is to be highly aware of medication problems as a cause of disease. In prescribing any medications, those with the fewest side effects should be given priority. In addition, if family members or friends are available, they should be made aware of the treatment plans.

Absorption dynamics and renal and hepatic metabolism may be impaired in elderly persons, leading to decreased excretion and metabolism. Drug distribution is altered because of changes in body composition (lean mass decreases, fat increases), and plasma binding through lowered albumin may cause increased free-drug actions. Thus, the concept of "standard doses" has to be reevaluated, and doses must be more individualized for people over the age of 60.

A fall, resulting in lacerations or other injuries, may be due to syncope caused by cardiac disease or various drugs (e.g., antihypertensives, vasodilators, tranquilizers, antiarrhythmic agents, antidepressants, aminophylline, beta-adrenergic agents, nitroglycerin, calcium antagonists) that can also cause syncope.

In an emergency department geriatric practice, overall emphasis has to be on detecting treatable problems or disorders that may underlie the acute presenting symptoms.

SYMPTOMS IN THE ELDERLY

Although a usual approach is to focus on diagnosis, it is worthwhile to consider overlooked diagnoses so as to alert the emergency practitioner to frequently unrecognized disorders. One such study[8] points out the need to evaluate for anemia, tuberculosis, and thyroid disease with myxedema coma and sensory alterations. A majority of cases of myxedema coma are in those over 70. Also, psychiatric conditions may often be undiagnosed, particularly depressive states. The possibility of AIDS should not be overlooked. It may present a confusing clinical picture, with dementia and pneumonia, as well as malignancies. Cases in the elderly usually result from blood transfusions (generally from transfusions before 1985, when blood bank testing was instituted), although sexual transmission is also possible.

Experienced clinicians recognize atypical presentations as being common in elderly persons (e.g., painless myocardial infarction, sepsis without fever, asymptomatic bacteriuria, or pneumonia presenting as confusion). Thyrotoxicosis in the elderly often presents not as a hyperkinetic syndrome but as a nonspecific clinical picture with weight loss, constipation, apathy, and other mental changes. Another example is hyponatremia, probably caused by oversecretion of antidiuretic hormone. This syndrome can result in marked mental status changes and is much more common in elderly individuals.

A further important consideration must be "sleep apnea," which can result in life-threatening cardiovascular and respiratory disorders.[9] This condition, present to some extent in one third of all elderly persons, is another reason to exercise particular care with medications.

DIAGNOSTIC CONSIDERATIONS

A study of diagnoses in people over 60 in one emergency department over a 6-month period is presented in Table 1–1. A comparison with the most common diagnoses in general practice (Table 1–2) shows the tremendous difference in the nature of conditions seen on an emergency basis from those treated in general office practice. For example, hypertension was the basis for 15% of visits in one large study; however, it was involved on an emergency basis with less than 2% of emergency department admissions. On the other hand, pulmonary/respiratory symptoms accounted for 2% or less of office visits. Putting all respiratory tract diagnoses together, there are 65/517 or 13%. When bronchitis, influenza, and upper respiratory infections (URIs) are added to this total, almost 17% of the emergency diagnoses refer to disorders within the respiratory system.

Table 1–1 Emergency Department Diagnoses in Patients over 60: 6-Month Retrospective Compilation

Diagnosis	No. of patients
Abdominal pain	24
Alzheimer's disease, dementia, confusion	12
Anal or rectal hemorrhoids (nonbleeding)	3
Anemia	11
Arrhythmia	14
Asthma	7
Back pain	7
Bronchitis	10
Cancer complications	6
Cardiopulmonary arrest	2
Chest pain (myocardial infarction)	11
R/O (myocardial infarction)	46
Angina	18
Chronic obstructive pulmonary disease	9
Congestive heart failure (CHF)	33
Diabetes mellitus	13
Diverticulitis	5
Dizziness/weakness	6
Drug overdose	2
Electrolyte imbalance/dehydration	21
Epididymitis or prostatitis	4
Fever (to be worked up)	6
Gallbladder (specific Dx)	5
Gastroenteritis	6
Gastrointestinal bleeding	10
Hypertension	8
Influenza	6
Infection, soft tissue	6
Intestinal obstruction	10
Liver disease	2
Musculoskeletal pain	6
Parkinson's disease	6
Pleural effusion	4
Pneumonia	40
Pyelonephritis/urinary tract infection	9
Pulmonary edema	5
Pulmonary embolus	3
Psychiatric diagnosis	4
Renal impairment	3
Renal stone/colic	5
Respiratory failure	4
Rheumatic heart disease	3
Sepsis or R/O	12
Stroke	16
Syncope	9
Trauma	43
Ulcer	4
Urinary retention	4
Upper respiratory infection	5
Vomiting	3
Miscellaneous (dermatologic, neurologic, zoster, etc.)	8
Total	519

Table 1–2   Most Common Diagnoses in the Elderly (65 Years and Over)

U.S. California study (1977)	% of all diagnoses	Wisconsin study (1978)	% of all diagnoses
Hypertension	15.1	All cardiovascular disorders	14.4
Ischemic heart disease	9.8	Hypertension	8.9
General medical examination	8.1	Diabetes	5.5
Degenerative joint disease	6.5	Arthritis of all types	4.8
Diabetes	5.0	General medical examinations	3.1
Depression/anxiety	2.9	Surgical aftercare	2.8
Soft tissue injuries	2.3	Neuroses, etc.	2.0
Urinary tract infection	2.2	Obesity	1.8
Emphysema	2.0	Emphysema	1.3
Acute upper respiratory infection	1.9	Cerebrovascular disorders	1.3
Fractures/dislocations	1.5		
Acute sprains/strains	1.3		
Dermatitis/eczema	1.2		
Acute lower respiratory infections	1.0		
Bursitis, etc.	1.0		
Total	61.8%	Total	45.9%

POST–EMERGENCY DEPARTMENT CARE

Elderly patients often need posttreatment care that may require wheelchairs, aids, special diets, physical therapists, or medical-surgical devices. Return for care by a primary physician may be delayed in a patient with such immediate needs. Emergency units that serve older patients must have resource information and personnel to arrange for the special care for the patient (e.g., home care, visiting nurses). Such care is often available, at least on a short-term basis, but requires experienced personnel to circumnavigate what is to the uninitiated a bewildering maze of bureaucracy.

HOME HEALTH CARE

The emphasis in the provision of health care to the elderly must be on maintaining functional capability. In the rush to diagnose and "work up" some conditions, this goal is occasionally forgotten. A prolonged hospitalization and subsequent intermediate care facility stay for an elderly person may render them unable to return home. The defects in home health care add to this dilemma. These latter issues are in the early stages of review through the U.S. Congress,[10] but currently there are marked deficiencies in our ability to offer home care after an acute episode.

A review of Table 1–1 shows many groups seen in emergency facilities who could benefit from long-term home health care (e.g., those with Parkinson's disease, Alzheimer's disease and other states of dementia, stroke victims, and some of those disabled from trauma). At least 15 to 20% of those seen in emergency facilities would benefit from home health care. Katz and his colleagues[11] demonstrated that for independent people living in a community between the ages of 65 and 69 years, the total life expectancy was 16.5 years, but, for 6.5 of these years the elderly person required assistance due to substantial major functional impairment. Over the age of 85, 60% of the remaining years require substantial assistance.

An important issue for emergency health workers is to help provide medical and social care to maximize independent life. Sometimes, a small intervention (e.g., restoring electrolyte balance or helping to provide a visiting nurse) can result in major functional improvement. As our aging population gains more political power, we will see an increase in our ability as health care providers to offer needed home care services.

We are seeing not only an increase in the longevity of our population, but an increase in elderly citizens who are vocal and politically active. Aided by the substantial financial base of many pensioners, organizations of senior citizens and retired people are exerting unprecedented political and economic power.

GERIATRIC EVALUATION UNITS

With the complex array of social factors, physical impairments, nutritional considerations, polymedications, as well as an increased need for rehabilitation and follow-up care, a specialized focus on older patients is needed. Such an approach is demonstrably superior.

The patients in one geriatric evaluation unit had markedly lower mortality and were less likely to be in a nursing home after hospitalization. Moreover, the control group patients underwent substantially more acute hospitalization. Mental improvement in the geriatric units was superior, as was functional status.[12-14]

The results from this randomized trial of effectiveness were so conclusive that the geriatric evaluation unit should be considered a superior manner of caring for our acutely ill elderly and, overall, a financially responsible method for so doing. Initial investment in personnel, facilities, and equipment "pays off" in overall savings.

The problem arises when federal Medicare, which pays for the hospitalization, cannot provide the financial assistance to reduce hospitalization in the future. The development of health maintenance organizations (HMOs) is one answer to this dilemma, although strong profit motives have put this into question. Long-term solutions are probably governmental and political.

Although the advances in geriatric evaluation units have primarily been in patient facilities with intensive multidisciplinary efforts, the following basic lessons can be applied to emergency facilities.

1. Impaired elderly patients can respond dramatically to treatment.
2. Specific attention to problems peculiar to, or found more frequently in, elderly populations is the simplest and least expensive approach (e.g., nutrition, physical therapy and rehabilitation, polypharmacy, social and living conditions).
3. The first step in focusing on such problems requires a basic check list to be used with all patients over the age of 65 that can be readily implemented in an emergency department. Such a check list could uncover areas of need that can be addressed by home health care services, visiting nurses, and senior centers.* For example:

> Living conditions
> Meals, nutrition
> Sensory changes (e.g., eyes, ears, touch)
> Medications — total (i.e., over-the-counter, herbal cures, and related types)
> Past medication problems (e.g., falls, dizziness, low potassium)
> Husband's or wife's health (If not living, when did he or she die?)
> Presence of depression or sleep disorders
> Home care needed

THE VERY OLD

The human life span is close to 115 years, although it is still extremely rare to find a person older than 105. As the geriatric population increases, there must be clearer distinctions between disease and disability — that is, some disease conditions (e.g., arthritis) account for much more disability than others (e.g., chronic lung disease or high blood pressure).

One study evaluated disability[15] and discovered that arthritis/rheumatism accounted for 34% of the total disability, followed by stroke, visual impairment, heart disease, and dementia.

The continued focus of *Geriatric Emergency Medicine* is to learn to treat the acute disease or acute manifestation

---

*This is not meant to substitute for a regular history and physical examination. It is an attempt to highlight particular, often overlooked areas.

of a chronic disease process with concern for minimizing the concurrent disability. This is most relevant with the very old who may have a diagnostic listing of many diseases of which only one results in substantial disability.

We have tended to consider the field of geriatrics as a whole rather than paying attention to the special problems of each subgroup. Clear delineations such as neonate, adolescent, etc., which are found in the field of pediatrics, are not readily forthcoming in the older population. As the geriatric population becomes larger and the old and very old are studied more closely, it is likely that we will see clearer physiologic subgroups.

Ethical Considerations

Already there are many new concerns when treating the very old, ranging from the philosophical (what is human) to more specific concerns about quality of life.[16] For example, the heightened concerns about "dying with dignity" relate to the advent of machines and procedures for sustaining organs and prolonging life. This increases the pressure felt by physicians and caregivers, whose role must be fervently prolife. One actual case illustrates what can happen when this orientation is not maintained.

An 81-year-old man was brought into the hospital after being discovered comatose at home. He had been depressed and living alone and had a history of cirrhosis and hypertension. Upon physical exam he had no response to pain and showed persistent hypotension with dilated, nonreactive pupils. His respirations were poor, and he needed ventilatory support. The working diagnosis was "acute stroke" with the mechanism being central nervous system bleeding. When he did not improve and, in fact, deteriorated after 12 hours, the family was advised of his serious preterminal state. The decision was made to follow his wishes — that his life not be prolonged through extraordinary means. He was disconnected from his life support systems after a little more than 12 hours of hospitalization so that he could die with dignity. Subsequently, a blood test revealed toxic levels of Doriden. In the rush to assist the elderly in dying, the presence of very treatable acute problems can be overlooked. The pressures of prepaid health plans and competition for resources such as hospitals and nursing homes have added to this dilemma.[17]

On the other hand, there is a rational place for withholding treatment in some cases, particularly when the decision has been made well before the acute episode. For example, a 74-year-old man with rapidly progressive amyotrophic lateral sclerosis, weighing less than 90 pounds, reached the point where he could only move his eyes. While on board an airplane, he stopped breathing shortly after he had been given supplemental oxygen in an effort to improve his comfort. His respiratory arrest was probably due to the fact that his oxygen level was suddenly raised in the presence of long-standing hypercarbia and hypoxia. This caused a loss of his hypoxic stimulus to respiration.

Few, if any, could argue that intubation, ventilation, and tracheostomy would have been suitable at that time. There, indeed, comes a time to die.

The decision to withhold possible lifesaving treatment (e.g., intravenous fluids, ventilators, adrenaline, cardiopulmonary resuscitation) is very difficult to make in the emergency setting. In almost all cases, treatment should be given to avoid making the more serious error of not acting, which can result in the patient's death; after treatment, the patient's status can be reviewed.

In the field of geriatric medicine, the number of issues concerning biomedical ethics has grown rapidly. Analysis of ethical dilemmas, however, requires factual data, clarity, and examination of motives and consequences in addition to application of established rules and principles.

With this level of complexity, the acute care physician or nurse is rarely in any position to assess such issues adequately unless the situation has been previously reviewed and a decision made.[18]

"The Geriatric Demographic Imperative," as described by the gerontologist John Rowe, is leading to increasing attention to the myriad problems of the aging population. This includes not only needed research and treatments but an enhanced focus on early detection and prevention. To some extent this imperative leads to increased awareness of health issues such as cholesterol in all age groups.

Geriatric emergency medicine has the additional mission of rapidly assessing and treating acute medical or surgical emergency conditions and restoring patients to their former level of stability, or providing the needed treatment and referral to enhance their functional abilities. The ultimate goal: to increase an individual's life expectancy with the least disability.

REFERENCES

1. Butler RN: Testimony before the U.S. Senate Special Committee on Aging, October 1, 1976.
2. Ford AB: The aged and their physicians: the practice of geriatrics, Philadelphia, 1986, WB Saunders Co.
3. Tinetti ME and Speechly M: Prevention of falls among the elderly, N Engl J Med 320:1055, 1989.
4. Gupta KL, Dworkin B, and Gambert SR: Common nutritional disorders in the elderly: atypical manifestations, Geriatrics 43:87–97, 1988.
5. Morgan AG et al: National survey in the elderly, Int J Vitam Nutr Res 43:465, 1973.
6. Dequeker J and Geusens P: Contributions of aging and estrogen deficiency to postmenopausal bone loss, N Engl J Med 313:453, 1985.
7. Caranosus GJ: Drug reactions. In Schwartz G et al: Principles and practice of emergency medicine, ed 2, Philadelphia, 1986, WB Saunders Co.
8. Geboes K, Hellemans S, and Bossaert H: Is the elderly patient accurately diagnosed? Geriatrics 34:91, 1979.
9. Shepard JW: Cardiorespiratory changes in obstructive sleep apnea. In Kruger MH, Roth T, and Dement WC, editors: Principles and practice of sleep medicine, Philadelphia, 1989, WB Saunders Co, p 537.
10. House Bill 3436: The Medicare Long-Term Care Catastrophic Protection Act, 1988.
11. Katz S et al: Active life expectancy, N Engl J Med 309:1218–1224, 1983.
12. Rubenstein LZ, Abrass IB, and Kane RL: Improved care for patients on a new geriatric evaluation unit, J Am Geriatr Soc 29:531, 1981.
13. Rubenstein LZ et al: Effectiveness of a geriatric evaluation unit: a randomized clinical trial, N Engl J Med 311:1664, 1984.
14. Rubenstein LZ et al: The Sepulveda VA geriatric evaluation unit: data on 4-year outcomes and predictors of improved patient outcomes, J Am Geriatr Soc 32:503, 1984.
15. Ford AB et al: Health and function in the old and very old, J Am Geriatr Soc 36:187–197, 1988.
16. Thomas JE: Indicators of humanhood and the care of aging, chronically ill patients, Clin Geriatr Med 2:3–16, 1986.
17. Thomasma DC: Quality-of-life judgements, treatment decisions, and medical ethics, Clin Geriatr Med 2:17–28, 1986.
18. Wanzer SH et al: The physician's responsibility toward hopelessly ill patients, N Engl J Med 320:844, 1989.

Detecting Acute Disease

Michael L. Freedman, M.D.

A decline in physiologic systems

Painless, silent myocardial infarction

Pulmonary embolism: more common than suspected

Pneumonia: a late diagnosis

Cancer: a major cause of death

Masquerade of the acute abdomen

"Masked" hyperthyroidism and "apathetic" thyrotoxicosis

The insidious onset of hypothyroidism

Elderly alcoholism: a hidden problem

Depression and the risk of suicide

Drug reactions and polypharmacy

Intervening appropriately

Due to the atypical presentation of many diseases in the elderly, these patients often pose a diagnostic enigma. As a result, physicians encountering geriatric illnesses face the possibility of making inaccurate assessments, prescribing inadequate therapies, and, worst of all, allowing preventable morbidity and mortality to pass unseen and unchecked.

It is axiomatic that "classic" signs and symptoms of diseases in the elderly are either delayed, altered, or absent. Indeed, physical disease may present as a psychiatric disturbance, or, conversely, emotional problems may manifest as a physical problem.[1] (See Table 2–1.) In addition, the cumulative effect of life's normal stresses and various environmental influences, added to a typical background of multisystem disease, exacerbates the task of evaluating patient signs and symptoms. (See Table 2–2.) Finally, given the increased sensitivity of the elderly to drug therapy and the likelihood of multiple drug usage, the clinician may be further bewildered in the attempt to differentiate an organic entity from an adverse drug reaction.

Many physicians prove unprepared clinically to deal with acute disease in the elderly.[2,4] On the one hand, physicians in training often avoid geriatric care, since they regard it as tedious and unexciting. On the other, nonspecific complaints in the elderly — particularly those relating to anorexia, weight loss, acute confusion, incontinence, and dizziness — are frequently dismissed as symptoms of old age. In other cases, physicians interpret these complaints as evidence of dementia or neurosis and miss the physical problem entirely. Perhaps an even more fundamental cause of neglect, though, is that the majority of medical schools and other teaching institutions fail to provide physicians with an integrated education in geriatric medicine.[2,4]

The result of this combination of confusing clinical presentation and deficient training is inadequate care of the elderly patients. To better arm those physicians called on to provide acute treatment to our geriatric population, this review focuses on the basic characteristics of aging, as well as 10 clinical situations that threaten the aged, including myocardial infarction, pulmonary embolism, pneumonia, cancer, the acute abdomen, hyperthyroidism, alcoholism, depression, and drug therapy.

Table 2–1 Clinical Situations with Atypical Presentations in the Elderly

Acute myocardial infarction
Pulmonary embolism
Pneumonia
Cancer
Acute abdomen
Hyperthyroidism
Hypothyroidism
Alcoholism
Depression
Drug therapy

Table 2–2   Characteristics of Aging Patients

Physiologic functions diminished

Accumulation of life's stresses, diseases, and environmental hazards

"Classic" signs and symptoms of disease possibly absent, delayed, or altered

Physical disease may present as psychiatric syndrome

Psychiatric illness may present as a medical complaint

Multiple medical, psychiatric, and social problems in the same patient

Drug effects more pronounced and adverse reactions more common

A DECLINE IN PHYSIOLOGIC SYSTEMS

The first key to providing proper care to elderly patients is a realization that the increasing geriatric population stands to strikingly affect the patient mix in nearly every primary care practice.[2,5] Second, practitioners must have close knowledge of the fundamental changes that the body undergoes with the aging process.

More than 11% of the U.S. population is over 65 years of age today. This age group increases by some 1,000 people daily and will account for approximately 20% of the population by the year 2030.[6] The significance of this growth assumes perspective when one realizes that even today our relatively small geriatric group utilizes over 33% of acute hospital beds and buys fully one-quarter of all drugs. Considering that these patients are presently responsible for some 30% of total health care expenses and an astounding 50% of the federal health care budget, we can expect a strong change of medical priorities over the next 50 years. Clearly, a medical understanding of geriatric disorders will be of paramount value as these changes occur.

Throughout life, the body adjusts to environmental stresses in order to maintain an internal homeostasis. While in youth the functional capacity of most human organs exceeds that which is necessary for normal operations by 4 to 10 times, organ reserve declines over time in a linear fashion beginning at about age 30.[5,7] After this time, the body's ability to exert homeostatic control and to respond to the stress of illness wanes. From the clinical perspective, it is the weakening of the renal, hepatic, immunologic, pulmonary, cardiac, and intellectual functions that cause greatest concern.[8]

In the kidney, both structural and functional changes occur.[9,10] Glomerular filtration, for example, falls an average of 50% between the ages of 20 and 90.[11] In fact, an 80-year-old person possesses only about half of the renal blood flow, glomerular filtration rate, and number of intact nephrons of a 40-year-old person.[12] Despite these changes, however, creatinine levels often appear normal due to a decline in creatinine production, based on the decrease in lean body mass. Similarly, blood urea nitrogen (BUN) usually remains normal secondary to diminished protein intake.[12]

Although liver function tests reveal no consistent abnormalities in the elderly, hepatic metabolism diminishes with age for two reasons. First, hepatic blood flow decreases, making first-pass hepatic extraction and metabolism less efficient.[13] And, second, the ability of environmental stresses — such as tobacco smoke, alcohol, and drugs — to induce metabolizing enzymes fades with age.[14,16]

Immunologically, aging causes a decrease in primary antibody response and cellular immunity, as well as elevations in the amount of abnormal immunoglobulins and immune complexes.[17] These changes create increased risk for infection, autoimmunity, and, perhaps, neoplasm.[18]

Pulmonary function also worsens with age due to anatomic, physiologic, and environmental factors. From an anatomic standpoint, some 68% of elderly patients will show some degree of kyphosis and have both a decrease in alveolar surface area and an increase in small airway closing volume due to diminished lung elasticity.[19,20] Physiologically, vital capacity and the FEV_1 decrease and residual volume increases with age. In addition, the alveolar-arterial oxygen difference $(A\text{-}a)O_2$ widens with age due mainly to a fall in arterial oxygen partial pressure from unventilated alveoli and the increase in closing volume. In a young patient, the $(A\text{-}a)O_2$ measures about 8 mm Hg, but an 80-year-old patient has an $(A\text{-}a)O_2$ of nearly 24 mm Hg.[21] Lastly, depending on the elderly patient's environmental exposure to cigarette smoke, other inhalational toxins, and substances which can produce pneumoconiosis, pulmonary function will lessen accordingly.

Cardiac function declines with age consequent to both physiologic changes and the high incidence of atherosclerotic coronary artery disease in senescence. The physiologic changes encompass a decrease in heart rate, especially during exercise, and a fall in the cardiac output secondary to a lowered stroke volume.[22] Coronary artery disease, on the other hand, affects some 40 to 50% of the elderly.[23-27] Although its severity varies widely among patients, ischemic heart disease accounts for over 33% of all deaths in persons over 65 years of age.

Finally, the intellectual function of elderly people deteriorates selectively. Some intellectual capacities — such as the synthesis of new information, visual-motor coordination, and some nonverbal processes — begin faltering as early as the third decade.[29] Most often, patients will reflect this as changes rather than deterioration in cognitive performance, since other indices actually improve with age, such as vocabulary and "crystallized" intelligence. In fact, even linguistic learning is efficient in healthy individuals at high ages; a familiar index for this is the number of people over 65 years of age who learn Morse code to obtain amateur radio licenses. Also, familiar response patterns and verbal mental processes generally show little change — barring other causes of brain dysfunction, such as senile dementia — and learning capabilities often relate more to the circumstances, pace, and the presence of central nervous system disease than to age itself.[30] Nevertheless, it is also true that cognition worsens faster in elderly patients with problems like decreased visual or auditory acuity and changes in sleep patterns.[2]

PAINLESS, SILENT MYOCARDIAL INFARCTION

The majority of elderly patients with acute myocardial infarction (AMI) show signs and symptoms that vary significantly from those seen in middle-aged patients. In fact, some one third of elderly AMI patients fail to complain of any symptoms. This may be due to a reduction in cerebral blood flow and oxygenation from myocardial dysfunction or a higher incidence of mental deterioration in this age group.[28,31] In those who are symptomatic, the most frequent single initial symptom is dyspnea that rapidly increases in severity. AMI also frequently manifests in this age group with acute confusion, syncopal episodes, renal failure, hemiplegia (from cerebral infarction secondary to hypotension or embolism), peripheral emboli, vomiting, and extreme weakness. About 20% of elderly patients with AMI do show the classic symptoms of chest pain at onset; a quarter of these patients, however, also have a prior history of angina.

Note, too, that the physical and laboratory changes noted with AMI in younger patients are virtually the same in the elderly. Arrhythmias, hypotension, an increase in venous pressure, and a gallop rhythm usually occur. By the same token, electrocardiographic and cardiac enzyme changes in the elderly match those of the young. In fact, these abnormalities are sometimes the only way to detect AMI in the elderly.

PULMONARY EMBOLISM: MORE COMMON THAN SUSPECTED

Pulmonary embolism occurs in a large number of elderly, as evidenced by the finding of this lesion in as many as 30% of autopsies. Patients particularly vulnerable include those with congestive heart failure, femoral fractures, atrial fibrillation, chronic venous disease, and hemiplegia. However, any elderly, sedentary person risks developing a pulmonary embolism as a result of an increased likelihood of incurring a peripheral venous thrombosis. Indeed, most pulmonary emboli in the geriatric age group arise indirectly from the leg veins with propagation to the iliofemoral veins.

Unfortunately, the clinical presentation of pulmonary embolism in any age group often deceives physicians. However, it may be even more difficult in the elderly.

While arterial blood gas changes in a young patient, for example, may incite physician suspicion of a pulmonary embolism, the physiologic increase in $(A-a)O_2$ in the elderly, translating to a lowered PaO_2, may prove confusing.[37] Also, a small pulmonary embolism in a geriatric patient may simulate left ventricular failure by causing sudden tachypnea, an inexplicable tachycardia, increased venous pressure, and atrial fibrillation. In addition, geriatric patients sometimes present with only minimal signs and symptoms of venous thrombosis in close proximity to the embolic event. These include calf discomfort without tenderness, slight calf or ankle edema, increased warmth, and dilatation of the superficial veins in one foot or leg.

PNEUMONIA: A LATE DIAGNOSIS

Both the incidence and the mortality of lower respiratory tract infections increase with age.[18] However, the usual clinical picture of pyrexia, a productive cough of sudden onset, pleurisy, and signs of pulmonary consolidation commonly fail to present early in the course of an elderly patient's pneumonia. Although any of these elements may be present, their onset is insidious and their effect less dramatic.

In general, geriatric patients demonstrate a nonspecific deterioration in health, and approximately 30% fail to mount a febrile response. Indeed, it usually takes from 7 to 9 days from the onset of symptoms to the diagnosis of sepsis and pneumonia in the elderly as compared to 2 to 3 days in younger patients. Also, an increase in respiratory rate, tachycardia, and rales may prove helpful to the diagnosis, but these are not specific findings and can be part of any number of other diagnoses.

Recent studies do indicate that two laboratory studies may aid physicians in diagnosing pneumonia. First, the height of the leukocyte response appears nearly equal in older and younger patients. One study shows a white blood cell count of $15,300/\mu L^3$ for the elderly and $13,900/\mu L^3$ for younger patients. Also, the erythrocyte sedimentation rate is higher in the elderly — 80 mm/hour versus 58. 6 mm/hour for younger persons.[38]

CANCER: A MAJOR CAUSE OF DEATH

Currently, about 1 in 8 deaths in the elderly results from cancer, and the probability of developing it within five years of any age increases from 1 in 700 for a 25-year-old to 1 in 14 for a 65-year-old.[39]

In a younger person, cancer is usually the main or only disease process. Alternatively, cancer in the elderly often presents in the face of multiple disease processes and disabilities. This makes new symptoms due to malignancy easy for physicians to overlook. For instance, physicians may not heed patient complaints of a change in bowel habits, mild rectal bleeding, bony or "arthritic" pain, weakness, malaise, fatigue, weight loss, anorexia, or peripheral neurologic deficits. Physicians may also discount the significance of some findings — such as hypercalcemia, anemia, or mental confusion — in an older patient. Without a doubt, these abnormalities in a young patient would raise a "red flag" in the physician's mind and spark a search for multiple myeloma, leukemia, or rectal, colon, prostatic, gastric, breast, or lung cancer. Indeed, it is precisely these six carcinomas which account for two thirds of all cancer mortality in old age.[40] Hence, physicians must take seriously new signs and symptoms in the elderly, no matter how nonspecific, and cautiously rule out cancer as their cause.

MASQUERADE OF THE ACUTE ABDOMEN

To the diagnostician's chagrin, elderly patients with an acute abdomen often fail to exhibit the usual signs, symptoms, and findings of guarding, rigidity, localized pain, and an elevated white blood cell count. Instead, this diagnosis frequently requires physician observation of more subtle clues.[41] In the first place, many geriatric patients are unable to communicate fully due to deafness, mental deterioration, or the inability to articulate. Also, this age group has both an increased tolerance to pain in many cases and an inability to localize or describe the pain adequately. As an example, the patient with intestinal obstruction and colicky pain may not report pain at all but instead display periods of restlessness alternating with periods of comfort. Some physicians may erroneously interpret these episodes as hysteria or acting out.[42,43]

Examination of the elderly may be both difficult and deceptive in this setting. On the one hand, kyphosis can limit physician access to abdominal structures. On the other, the elderly patient's inability to cooperate or to relax the abdominal muscles during examination may confuse the clinical picture. Also, physicians may note hypothermia rather than the usual temperature elevation as generalized sepsis ensues. Likewise, the expected finding of an elevated white blood cell count may never occur despite diffuse or long-standing peritonitis.

Because these patients often reach the advanced stages of an acute abdomen with sepsis and shock before the diagnosis is apparent, the mortality rate for this problem is high. In fact, diffuse peritonitis causes fatality in over 12% of patients over 60 years old and in over 30% of those past age 70.[41] These difficulties in detection make it imperative that physicians observe closely elderly patients with any abdominal complaints and maintain vigilance for even the slightest hint of acute abdominal disease.

"MASKED" HYPERTHYROIDISM AND "APATHETIC" THYROTOXICOSIS

The hyperactivity, restlessness, irritability, eye signs, goiter, and thyroid bruit, which are common in younger patients with hyperthyroidism or thyrotoxicosis, present in only about 25% of elderly patients.[44] In geriatric patients, hyperthyroidism frequently occurs with few symptoms attributable directly to thyroid disease. Instead, these patients often have primary symptoms or findings linked to another organ system, most commonly the heart ("masked" hyperthyroidism).[44,49] Some patients develop congestive heart failure (which is poorly responsive to therapy), paroxysmal or fixed cardiac arrhythmia, and cardiomegaly. Others report psychiatric complaints that may encompass depression, confusion, symptoms of chronic brain syndrome, and psychomotor retardation. Gastrointestinal manifestations, on the other hand, frequently include anorexia or constipation, and physicians may find evidence of increased bone calcium turnover in the form of hypercalcemia, osteoporosis, and fractures.[50]

In addition, some 10 to 15% of elderly patients with hyperthyroidism develop "apathetic" thyrotoxicosis.[36] Here, the major symptoms prove to be tremendous apathy and inactivity.[45,51] Most of these patients look extremely old and wrinkled but not particularly ill. Unfortunately, when exposed to physiologic stress, they may develop coma and die. Eight clinical characteristics can aid physicians in making this diagnosis:

1. Placid, apathetic facies
2. Signs of depression or lethargy
3. The absence of exophthalmos and the presence of blepharoptosis
4. Muscle wasting
5. Cardiovascular dysfunction, especially atrial fibrillation
6. Weight loss
7. A small goiter
8. Abnormal, but sometimes only slightly elevated, thyroid function tests

Thyrotoxic elderly patients may possess all or any combination of these characteristics.

THE INSIDIOUS ONSET OF HYPOTHYROIDISM

Physicians see relatively few elderly patients with overt myxedema. Indeed, up to two thirds of patients diagnosed as hypothyroid present with only impaired mobility and general health, as well as apathy and depression.[52] Also, some geriatric patients have very mild or absent symptoms. The slow, gradual onset of this disease combined with the attendant physical and mental slowness, cold intolerance, and deafness make it almost impossible to distinguish this problem from natural aging.[53] In essence, if the physician fails to consider this diagnosis when the patient enters the examination room, it probably will be missed. The fact that it generally takes from 3 to 5 years from the onset of the disease for the diagnosis to become apparent underscores this problem of detection.[48] Additionally, the presence of concomitant multiple pathology in the elderly compounds the diagnostic task.

In general, the physical examination proves more crucial toward making the diagnosis than the historical complaints noted above. Physicians should search primarily for skin changes, such as dry, coarse, nonsebaceous skin with swelling and puffiness of the face, ankles, neck, and wrist. These patients also develop baggy eyelids, a gruff voice, defects in taste and smell, limb pains with signs of neuropathy, arthralgias, ataxia, cardiomegaly, and hypothermia, in addition to the classic delayed relaxation of the ankle jerk. Also, the elderly person with hypothyroidism may show weight gain or loss. Often patients gain weight consequent to the metabolic slowdown associated with hypothyroidism, but if they also have anorexia, they may uncharacteristically lose weight. Finally, when advanced, hypothyroidism can cause coma, just as it does in younger patients.

ELDERLY ALCOHOLISM: A HIDDEN PROBLEM

Alcoholism in the elderly oftentimes remains hidden from physicians by both the patient and family. It has an incidence of approximately 2.2% in persons over 65 in the United States, and women make up fully two thirds of all elderly alcoholics.[54,55]

In one third of elderly alcoholics, however, the alcohol problem stems from illness, bereavement, or psychologic and environmental stress late in life. These patients usually make excuses for their drinking, citing alcohol's benefit for a number of their perceived but actually hypochondriacal ailments. They tend to keep their problem from the family when possible. When discovered, they sometimes use the family's embarrassment over their problem as blackmail. Families usually succumb to this pressure, and, to avoid gossip or scandal, they readily supply their elderly relative with alcohol.[55]

Generally, physicians come in contact with geriatric alcoholics after their increasing alcohol intake and decreasing food intake result in an illness or mishap. Another potential problem with alcohol-induced malnourishment is the development of central nervous system problems, such as the Wernicke-Korsakoff syndrome.[56] If unrecognized by a physician and, therefore, untreated, thiamine deficiency results in permanent neurologic damage. In fact, 40% of all psychiatric admissions in this age group relate to alcoholism or its cerebral sequelae. Recent studies[73] have emphasized alcohol-related myopathy, particularly cardiomyopathy. If the alcohol connection is not identified, treatment may focus on the cardiac symptoms (e.g., CHF, pulmonary edema) and miss the treatable alcoholism.

To discover alcoholism in the elderly, physicians must search for the problem and not be misled by the patient's age, especially in those with neurotic symptoms. It is important to question the patient as well as the family and indicate a compassionate willingness to help. In addition, physicians should rule out alcoholism as an inciting factor in any patient with cerebral symptoms.

DEPRESSION AND THE RISK OF SUICIDE

In the elderly, psychiatric symptomatology shifts from outwardly directed manifestations, such as conversion symptoms and anxiety states, to inwardly directed symptomatology, including anxious ruminations, depression, and hypochondriasis. Of these, depression proves not only the most common, but also the most devastating.[57,58]

Depression begins insidiously and frequently in relation to ill health.[59] In most cases, depression is the method of adjustment for elderly patients with excessive physical complaints and limited resources for coping. It appears to stem from a lack of resiliency when stressed by multiple chronic illnesses, environmental changes, bereavement, and social rejection, as well as changing catecholamine levels. Since elderly patients may somaticize their depression, physicians and relatives often miss the usual markers of depression, such as anhedonia, lack of energy, loss of appetite and libido, early morning awakening, ideas of worthlessness, and negativistic body feelings. Too frequently, the family and physician view these characteristics as appropriate in an older person.

When the depression becomes severe enough, suicide and suicide attempts are great risks.[60] Primary care physicians need to develop familiarity with the danger signals for suicide, particularly since the elderly rarely frequent mental health clinics or visit psychiatrists.[61] Physicians should realize that white geriatric males have the highest rate of successful suicide of any group.[60] Other potential clues to the suicidal elderly patient include recent changes in sleep or appetite patterns, increasing agitation, bizarreness of hypochondriacal symptomatology, the presence of medically uncontrollable or importuning complaints, severe physical deterioration, or any other change in long-standing symptomatology.[62] Noting these signs, physicians should consider taking action to prevent the elderly patients from taking their lives. Depending on the severity of the patient's depression, this can range from psychiatric hospitalization or frequent office visits to family counseling and close contact with social workers.

DRUG REACTIONS AND POLYPHARMACY

Elderly patients have twice the risk for an adverse drug reaction, in or out of the hospital, as a younger person.[63,65] This stems partially from 1) age-related alterations in body composition and drug distribution, metabolism, and excretion and 2) the multiple pharmaceuticals commonly prescribed to geriatric patients.

With age, lean body mass and body water decrease and body fat increases. This results in more drug per weight of metabolically active tissue and a smaller volume of distribution for the drug. In addition to these changes, a decrease in serum albumin to bind or inactivate drugs, combined with decreases in renal or hepatic function, makes it more likely that the elderly patient will accumulate toxic levels of drugs.[66-68] In the case of some hypnotics and tranquilizers, an inappropriate dose may cause the frail but functioning geriatric to become confused and incontinent.[62]

As the number of disease states and prescriptions multiply with age, tolerance decreases sharply not only to individual drugs but also to drug interactions. For instance, a patient receiving both methyldopa and haloperidol may develop signs of dementia in about a week, and it may take as long as 2 to 3 days after withdrawal to reverse these effects.[69] To check for polypharmacy as a problem, review all medications prescribed, purchased over the counter, or obtained from friends or relatives. Frequently, discontinuance of an often-used sleeping pill or tranquilizer rapidly reverses mental and physical symptoms. In addition, physicians may discover that the patient is using several medications which interact adversely.[70-72]

INTERVENING APPROPRIATELY

Physicians faced with elderly patients must anticipate possible problems and neither overlook nonspecific symptoms or signs nor attribute them solely to the aging process. As shown, cavalier response to geriatric patients can lead tragically to misdiagnosis and inappropriate therapy. Dealing effectively with aged patients, then, requires knowledge of 1) the pathophysiologic changes occurring during aging, 2) differential diagnosis as it applies to the geriatric population, and 3) the limits and subtleties of drug therapy in this group. In fact, the increasing number of elderly patients makes this information imperative for all primary care physicians. Its assimilation into modern medical practice will inevitably result in improved care for geriatric patients and decrease the present level of morbidity and mortality among them.

REFERENCES

1. Barsky AJ: Hidden reasons some people visit doctors. Ann Intern Med 94:492, 1981.
2. Dans PE and Kerr MR: Gerontology and geriatrics in medical education, N Engl J Med 300:228, 1979.
3. Reichel W: Family practice and care of the elderly. Am Fam Phys 20:85, 1979.
4. Williamson J: Geriatric medicine: whose specialty? Ann Intern Med 91:774, 1979.
5. Fries JF: Aging, natural death and the compression of morbidity, N Engl J Med 303:130, 1980.
6. Bedtine RW: Geriatric medicine, an overview. In Eisdorfer C, editor: Annual review of gerontology and geriatrics, New York, 1980, Springer Publishing Co.
7. Shock NW: Mortality and measurment of aging. In Strehler BE et al, editors: The biology of aging, Washington DC, 1960, American Institute of Biological Sciences.
8. Masoro EJ et al: Analysis and exploration of age-related changes in mammalian structure and function, Fed Proc 38:1956, 1979.
9. Ouslander JG: Drug prescribing for the elderly, West J Med 135:455, 1981.
10. Epstein M: Effects of aging on the kidney, Fed Proc 38:168, 1979.
11. Rowe JW et al: The effect of age on creatinine clearance in man: a cross-sectional and longitudinal study, J Geront 31:155, 1976.
12. Rowe JW: Aging and renal function, Ann Rev Gerontol Geriatrics 1:161, 1980.
13. Bender AD: The effect of increasing age on the distribution of peripheral blood flow in man, J Am Geriatr Soc 13:192, 1965.
14. Adelman RC: Age-dependent effect in enzyme induction — a biochemical expression of aging, Exp Gerontol 6:75, 1971.
15. Vestal RE et al: Effects of age and cigarette smoking on propranolol disposition, Clin Pharm Ther 26:8, 1979.
16. Wood AJ et al: Effect of aging and cigarette smoking on antipyrine and indocyanine green elimination, Clin Pharm Ther 26:16, 1979.
17. Makinodon T: Immunity and aging. In Finch JCE and Hayflick L, editors: Handbook of the biology of aging, New York, 1977, Van Nostrand Reinhold.
18. Roberts-Thompson IC, Whittingham S, and Youngchairyud U: Aging, immune response, and mortality, Lancet 2:368, 1974.
19. Edge JR et al: The radiographic appearance of the chest in persons of advanced age, Br J Radiol 37:769, 1964.
20. Wright RR: Elastic tissue of normal and emphysematous lungs. A tridimensional histologic study, Am J Pathol 39:355, 1961.
21. Rahn H and Fern WO: A graphical analysis of the respiratory gas exchange. The O_2–CO_2 diagram, Washington DC, 1955, American Physics Society.
22. Strandell T: Cardiac output in old age. In Caird FI, Dall JLC, and Kennedy RD, editors: Cardiology in old age, New York, 1976, Plenum Press.
23. Kennedy RD and Caird FI: Application of the Minnesota code to population studies of the electrocardiogram in the elderly, Gerontol Clin 14:5, 1972.
24. Webb CR: Myocardial infarction, Geriatrics 41(2):89, 1986.
25. Olbrich O and Woodford-Williams E: The normal precordial electrocardiogram in the aged, J Gerontol, 510, 1985.
26. Stark ME and Vacek JL: The initial electrocardiogram during admission for myocardial infarction. Use as a predictor of clinical course and facility utilization, Arch Intern Med 147(5):843, 1987.
27. Camm AJ and Ward DE: Clinical electrocardiography. In Martin A and Camm AJ, editors: Heart disease in the elderly, New York, 1984, John Wiley & Sons.
28. Caird FI and Dall JLC: The cardiovascular system. In Brocklehurst JC, editor: Textbook of geriatric medicine and gerontology, ed 2, New York, 1978, Churchill Livingstone.
29. Eisdorfer C: Intelligence and cognition in the aged. In Busse EW and Pfeiffer E, editors: Behavior and adaptation in late life, ed 2, Boston, 1977, Little Brown.
30. Bennett R and Eisdorfer C: The institutional environment and behavior change. In Sherwood S, editor: Long-term care: a handbook for researchers, planners and providers, New York, 1975, Spectrum.
31. Rodstein M: The characteristics of non-fatal myocardial infarction in the aged, Arch Intern Med 98:84, 1956.
32. Pathy MS: Clinical presentation of myocardial infarction in the elderly, Br Heart J 29:190, 1967.
33. Presentation of myocardial infarction in the elderly (Editorial), Lancet 2(8515):1077, 1986.
34. Bayer AJ et al: Changing presentation of myocardial infarction with increasing old age, J Am Geriatr Soc 34:263, 1986.
35. Reference deleted in proofs.
36. Goldman L: Acute chest pain: emergency room evaluation, Hosp Pract 21(7):94A, 1986.
37. Glassroth J and Make B: A disciplined approach to hypoxemia, ER Reports 1:13, 1980.
38. Finkelstein MS et al: Differences in presentation of pneumococcal bacteremia based on age of patient, Clin Res 29:444a, 1981.
39. Editorial: Aging and cancer, Lancet 1:131, 1976.

40. Hodkinson HM: Cancer in the aged. In Brocklehurst JC, editor: Textbook of geriatric medicine and gerontology, ed 2, New York, 1978, Churchill Livingstone.
41. Charlesworth D and Baker RH: Surgery in old age. In Brocklehurst JC, editor: Textbook of geriatric medicine and gerontology, ed 2, New York, 1978, Churchill Livingstone.
42. Rosen P, Marx JA, and Pons PT: Intestinal obstruction: the great masquerader. Part I, ER Reports 1:21, 1980.
43. Wangensteen OH: Understanding the bowel obstruction problem, Am J Surg 135(2):131, 1978.
44. Thomas FB, Mazzaferri EL, and Skillman TG: Apathetic thyrotoxicosis: a distinctive clinical and laboratory entity, Ann Intern Med 72:679, 1970.
45. Mazzaferri EL: Coping with thyroid emergencies. Part I: Thyroid storm, ER Reports 1:123, 1980.
46. Davis PJ and Davis FB: Hyperthyroidism in patients over the age of 60 years, Medicine 53:161, 1974.
47. Gilbert PD: Thyroid function and disease. In Libbow LS and Sherman FT, editors: The core of geriatric medicine, St. Louis, 1981, CV Mosby.
48. Irvine RE and Hodkinson HM: Thyroid disease in old age. In Brocklehurst JC, editor: Textbook of geriatric medicine and gerontology, ed 2, New York, 1978, Churchill Livingstone.
49. Levine SA and Sturges CC: Hyperthyroidism masked as heart disease, Boston Med Surg J 190:233, 1924.
50. Bartels EC: Hyperthyroidism in patients over 65, Geriatrics 20:459, 1965.
51. Serri O et al: Coma secondary to apathetic thyrotoxicosis, Can Med Assoc J 119:605, 1978.
52. McKeron CG: Hyperthyroidism, Update Plus 1:727, 1971.
53. Billewicz WZ et al: Statistical methods applied to the diagnosis of hypothyroidism, Quart J Med 38:255, 1969.
54. Rosin AJ and Glatt MM: Alcohol excess in the elderly, Quart J Med 32:53, 1971.
55. Droller H: Some aspects of alcoholism in the elderly, Lancet 2:137, 1964.
56. Marx JA and Rosen P: Increasing detection of the Wernicke-Korsakoff syndrome, ER Reports 2:121, 1981.
57. Comfort A: Dementia in the elderly, treatable or untreatable, ER Reports 2:19, 1981.
58. Comfort A: A practice of geriatric psychiatry, New York, 1980, American Elsevier.
59. Post F: The functional psychoses. In Isaacs AD and Post F, editors: Studies in geriatric psychiatry, Chichester, 1978, John Wiley.
60. Kreitman N: Age and "parasuicide" (attempted suicide), Psychol Med 6:113, 1976.
61. Charaton FB, Sherman FT, and Libow LS: Geriatric psychiatry. In Libow LS and Sherman FT, editors: The core of geriatric medicine, St Louis, 1981, CV Mosby.
62. Post F: Psychiatric disorders. In Brocklehurst JC, editors: Textbook of geriatrics and gerontology, ed 2, New York, 1978, Churchill Livingstone.
63. Seidl LG et al: Studies on the epidemiology of adverse drug reactions. III. Reactions in patients on a general medical service, Bull Johns Hopkins Hosp 119:299, 1966.
64. Schwartz G, Bosker G, and Grigsby JW: Geriatric emergencies, Bowie, MD, 1985, Robert J Brady Co.
65. Ray WA: Psychotropic drug use and the risk of hip fracture. N Engl J Med 316(7):363, 1987.
66. Greenblatt DJ et al: Drug disposition in old age, N Engl J Med 306(18):1081–1088, 1985.
67. Symposium: Managing medication in an aging population: physician, pharmacist, and patient perspectives, J Am Geriatr Soc 30(11 suppl), 1985.
68. Downs GE, Linkewich JA, and DiPalma JR: Drug interactions in elderly diabetics, Geriatrics 36(7):45, 1986.
69. Thorton WE: Dementia induced by methyldopa and haloperidol, N Engl J Med 294:1222, 1976.
70. Leach S and Roy SS: Adverse drug reactions: an investigation on an acute geriatric ward, Age Aging 15:241, 1986.
71. Pickles H and Fuller S: Prescriptions, adverse reactions, and the elderly, Lancet 2(8497):40, 1986.
72. Ouslander JG: Drug therapy in the elderly, Ann Intern Med 97:711, 1981.
73. Urbano-Marquez A et al: The effects of alcoholism on skeletal and cardiac muscle, N Engl J Med 320:409, 1989.

Emergency Care
of the Elderly

Age-Related Differences in Emergency Department Use and Care

Steven A. Baum, M.D., **and Laurence Z. Rubenstein**, M.D., M.P.H.

Utilization of emergency care

Evaluation of patient population

Characteristics of elderly patients coming to emergency departments

Clinical approaches in geriatric emergency care

Little is known about how the care received in emergency departments by the elderly population differs from that received by younger people. We prospectively abstracted emergency department (ED) records of 1,620 consecutive patients visiting a large community hospital ED over a 22-day period in 1984 for demographic and medical variables. The charts of patients presenting with five specific complaints (dyspnea, chest pain, abdominal pain, syncope, and conditions resulting from motor vehicle accidents) were also analyzed for process of care variables and, for hospitalized patients, the accuracy of the ED diagnosis.

UTILIZATION OF EMERGENCY CARE

Older people (i.e., age 65 and over) do not seem to be overutilizers of the ED for minor complaints — in fact, they tend to be more acutely ill on presentation than younger people. Older people were more likely to be hospitalized (46% versus 10%, p < .001), to arrive by ambulance (35% versus 10%, p < .001), and to have an identified source of primary care (95% versus 64%, p < .01). Older people stayed longer in the ED than younger people if they were eventually released home but shorter if admitted to the hospital. Test ordering patterns for specific complaints varied by patient age (e.g., older patients had more electrocardiograms [ECGs] performed for chest pain and fewer urinalyses for abdominal pain than younger patients). Therapy for specific complaints showed less age ef-

fect. Although generally more diagnostic tests were performed on older patients, the ED diagnosis tended to be more accurate for younger patients. Our data indicate that ED care may be substantially different for the elderly, with implications for future planning and financing of medical care.

As is well known, the elderly use a disproportionate share of the total health care budget. Though only 11.3% of the U.S. population is age 65 and over, this segment currently accounts for 38% of all hospital inpatient days, with Medicare bearing about 74% of these costs. The government pays 64% of the health care bill for the elderly, which currently is approaching $100 billion.[1] With the elderly growing both in absolute number and as a percentage of the population, there is increasing pressure to distribute the limited federal medical care funds in a fair and cost-effective manner. Information concerning utilization of health services by the elderly is essential in planning new health care strategies. One area that has not yet been adequately studied is care of the elderly in EDs.

EDs represent an important interface between the acute hospital and the community. About one sixth of hospital admissions originate in the ED, and 10 to 30% of ED visits result in hospital admission at most urban medical centers with EDs.[2] For patients hospitalized from the ED, the ED physician often formulates the diagnostic impression and determines the initial stages of hospital evaluation and treatment of admitted patients. EDs also provide a substantial amount of primary care for people not hospitalized, especially for those without established relationships to community physicians or with chronic physical disabilities and for people falling ill at night.[3-7]

Although demographic data exist on ED patients, few have been analyzed by age.[4,6,8-13] Furthermore, few data are available on the process of care given patients in the ED and how care given to elderly patients differs from that given to younger people. This study confirms previously noted demographic patterns and describes age-related differences in some measures of the care process occurring in a large community hospital ED. As well, process of care for patients with some specific common and serious presenting complaints is analyzed in more detail by age group. The accuracy of the ED diagnostic impression as it relates to the patient's age is also examined.

EVALUATION OF PATIENT POPULATION

The population studied included all patients coming to the ED of St. Joseph's Medical Center in Burbank, California, during a 22-day period in February, 1984. This facility, a 498-bed voluntary community hospital, receives about 80 ED visits per day. It serves a community that has 15.3% of its population 65 years and older, based on U.S. Census data, which compares to 11% for Los Angeles County as a whole. Physicians trained in emergency medicine are on duty 24 hours a day, and private physicians may see their patients in the ED as well. In this period, 1,947 patients entered the ED. Excluded from further study were patients arriving in cardiac arrest (N = 19), people who left without being seen by a physician (N = 32), and worker's compensation cases (N = 173), whose records were sequestered in a special file and were unavailable. Charts for 1,620 (94%) of the remaining 1,723 patient visits were available for examination by the primary investigator within 24 hours of the visit. Demographic information abstracted included age, sex, marital status, insurance status, identification with a regular source of medical care, and arrival time in the ED. The category of the presenting complaint (traumatic versus nontraumatic), the length of time spent in the ED, whether the ED physician or a personal physician initially saw the patient, and the final ED disposition were also recorded. Additional data were collected on those patients with the specific chief complaints of abdominal pain (AP, N = 156), chest pain (CP, N = 117), shortness of breath (SOB, N = 113), motor vehicle accident (MVA, N = 84), and falls associated with loss of consciousness (LOC, N = 21). These data included information on diagnostic tests and procedures ordered, medications prescribed or administered,

and therapeutic procedures performed. Specific presenting complaints were selected for analysis in order to provide stratified complaint-specific data. Close comparison of the care process for old and young patients needs such stratification by complaint because proportions of presenting complaints vary by age. These five were chosen because they were easily identified on the chart and because they were among the most common presenting complaints for both young and old patients.

Of the 491 patients with these five complaints, 203 (41%) were admitted to the acute hospital. We were able to obtain the hospital discharge summaries of 171 of these patients (84%) for review to determine the final diagnoses, which were then compared to the diagnostic impression on the ED record. The relationship between the ED diagnosis and final hospital diagnosis was rated as being "same diagnosis" (the final diagnosis was the same diagnosis stated on the ED record), "related diagnosis" (different specific diagnoses but with similar pathophysiologic mechanisms), or "different diagnosis" (diagnoses with different pathophysiologic mechanisms).

Statistical methods used included chi-square tests for comparing categorical data and Student's t-test for comparing means and standard errors of the mean. Two-tailed confidence intervals were used for calculating significance levels.

CHARACTERISTICS OF ELDERLY PATIENTS COMING TO EMERGENCY DEPARTMENTS

Table 3-1 describes characteristics of patients presenting to the ED by age group. The age and sex distributions for ED patients mirror the catchment area characteristics as determined in the 1980 census, as did marital status. The only notable difference was in the 75 and over age range where patients came to the ED at twice their proportion in the community (12% versus 6%). Patients presenting to the ED were likely to have some form of medical insurance, with only 4.2% of patients overall not having any insurance. Not unexpectedly, only 0.6% of patients age 65 and older were uninsured versus 12.4%

Table 3-1   Characteristics of Patients Presenting to the Emergency Department, by Age Group

Characteristic	0–16 yrs	17–44 yrs	45–54 yrs	55–64 yrs	65–74 yrs	≥ 75 yrs	All ages
N (%)	274 (16.9)	748 (46.1)	117 (7.2)	146 (9.2)	140 (8.6)	195 (12.0)	1,620 (100.0)
% Female	44.2	50.4	45.3	50.7	58.6	67.7	51.8
% With PMD*	75.2	55.1	70.1	83.6	95.7	94.9	70.4
% Uninsured	9.5	14.6	10.3	8.2	0.7	0.5	4.2
% Arriving by ambulance	3.6	9.8	12.0	22.6	23.6	41.0	15.0
% With traumatic complaint	46.0	42.1	35.9	28.8	25.2	22.6	37.3
% Admitted to hospital	4.0	8.0	15.4	28.8	33.6	54.9	18.0
Mean LOS,* Min ± SE*	90.6 ± 3.1	104.4 ± 2.8	105.6 ± 6.4	102.9 ± 5.2	125.9 ± 6.7	131.2 ± 5.6	107.0 ± 1.8

*PMD = usual private source of primary medical care; LOS = length of stay; SE = standard of error.

of patients under 65 years old (p < .001). Of patients with Medicare coverage, 40.7% carried supplemental insurance. The proportion of patients able to identify a personal physician or other regular source of medical care increased progressively with age among adults, from 55% of people under 45 years old to 95% of those over 75 years old. Ambulance use was also markedly age related. Overall, 15% of ED visits came by ambulance, but over 35% of those 65 and older used ambulance transportation versus 12% for those under 65 years old (p < .001). The time of day seemed to have little bearing on ambulance use in that the percentage of each age group arriving by ambulance did not significantly vary between the time periods examined. The proportion of patients with a trauma-induced primary complaint decreased steadily with age. Among people presenting with traumatic problems, there was no significant age difference in ambulance use — thus most of the age difference in ambulance use occurred among patients with nontraumatic complaints. Virtually all patients, old and young, were living in their own homes prior to the ED visit — less than 3% of the older patients were living in nursing homes. The mean length of stay in the ED was significantly longer for patients 65 and older than for younger patients (129.0 ± 4.2 minutes versus 104.4 ± 2.3 minutes, p < .001).

The probability of being admitted to the hospital increased progressively with age. Of patients 65 and older, 46.3% were admitted versus 10.2% of patients under 65 (p < .001). Admitted patients had almost twice the mean age of patients discharged home (61.1 ± 1.6 years versus 34.6 ± 0.6 years, p < .001). Among patients not hospitalized, mean patient age was higher during the workday hours. The pattern indicated that for less serious problems younger patients tend to use EDs more after working hours while older patients use them fairly evenly around the clock.

Table 3–2 also shows some additional data on length of time spent in the ED. Overall, admitted patients stayed longer in the ED than patients not admitted (145.9 ± 5.6 minutes versus 96.9 ± 1.7 minutes, p < .001). Among admitted patients, those 65 years and older stayed the shortest mean time in the ED. Conversely, of those discharged home, older patients stayed the longest. Patients with nontraumatic complaints (N = 975) tended to stay longer in the ED than those with traumatic ones (N = 576) (112.4 ± 2.4 minutes versus 97.8 ± 2.5 minutes, p < .001); however, this difference was confounded by the fact that traumatic complaints were more common among younger patients.

Table 3–2 provides process of care data by patient age for the three most common specific presenting complaints studied: shortness of breath (SOB), chest pain (CP), and abdominal pain (AP). Data on these complaints show much more age dependency than was the case for patients as a whole. For all three complaints, older patients

were over twice as likely to be admitted to the hospital than younger patients. Among admitted patients, younger patients with all three complaints stayed significantly longer in the ED.

Ordering patterns for several diagnostic tests had a significant relationship to patient age, while others did not. For example, among patients with SOB, age was positively related to the ordering of chest x-rays, ECGs, and blood gas analyses. For patients presenting with CP, however, age was not significantly related to the frequency of ordering ECGs or blood gas analyses and was inversely related to ordering chest x-rays — though this was confounded by the higher admission rate of older patients and the fact that chest x-rays were often planned to be taken after admission. Among patients with AP, ECGs and abdominal x-rays were obtained significantly more often among older patients, but urinalyses were obtained significantly more often among younger patients. Older patients had significantly more blood tests performed for all three complaints. Also for all three complaints, older patients were more likely to have intravenous catheters inserted.

Tables 3–3 and 3–4 list additional process of care data by age for all five studied presenting complaints combined. Intravenous lines and parenteral therapies were used significantly more frequently in older patients, although this was confounded by admission status. For those sent home, fewer prescriptions were written for patients aged 65 and older compared with younger patients. On the other hand, documentation on the ED record of recommending over-the-counter medicine was more common in the older age ranges. For both hospitalized and nonhospitalized patients, physicians ordered significantly more blood tests for older patients. Significantly more tests were ordered in the ED for patients who were admitted to the hospital than for those discharged home (p < .001). Overall, ED physicians ordered significantly more blood tests than private physicians (p < .01) — a trend particularly apparent among older patients.

For hospitalized patients with the five studied complaints, accuracy of ED diagnostic impressions was compared with final diagnoses of hospital discharge summaries. Overall, older patients were somewhat less likely to be diagnosed accurately by the ED physician than younger patients (74% versus 79%). Although not statistically significant, this trend occurred in spite of the fact that significantly more diagnostic tests were performed in the ED on the elderly. Older patients had significantly longer hospital stays (9.1 + 0.6 days versus 5.6 ± 0.6 days, p < .001).

CLINICAL APPROACHES IN GERIATRIC EMERGENCY CARE

Our study population and research design place some limits on the generalizability of the collected data. First,

Table 3–2   Process of Care Parameters for Three Presenting Complaints in Young versus Old Patients

Parameter	Young (16–64 yrs)	Old (≥ 65 yrs)	p value
Shortness of Breath			
N	65	48	
% Admitted to hospital	20.0	69.0	< .001
Mean LOS* of admitted patients (min ± SE*)	194.5 ± 12.8	142.9 ± 14.8	< .001
Mean LOS of discharged patients (min ± SE)	83.8 ± 6.3	116.7 ± 16.7	< .001
Mean number of blood tests or panels (± SE)	0.60 ± 0.15	1.65 ± 0.66	< .001
% Chest x-ray	65.9	87.3	< .05
% Electrocardiogram	20.2	62.6	< .001
% Blood gas	21.6	50.0	< .01
% Respiratory therapy	26.2	35.4	< .01
% Intravenous access	15.4	64.6	< .001
% Parenteral therapy	33.8	56.2	< .05
Chest Pain			
N	77	40	
% Admitted to hospital	35.1	77.5	< .001
Mean LOS of admitted patients (min ± SE)	176.2 ± 11.6	154.3 ± 10.5	< .001
Mean LOS of discharged patients (min ± SE)	115.5 ± 8.8	113.4 ± 12.7	NS*
Mean number of blood tests or panels (± SE)	0.70 ± 0.23	2.32 ± 0.35	< .001
% Chest x-ray	26.0	17.5	NS
% Electrocardiogram	80.5	92.5	NS
% Blood gas	11.7	12.5	NS
% Intravenous access	42.9	67.5	< .05
% Parenteral therapy	28.6	40.0	NS
Abdominal Pain			
N	123	33	
% Admitted to hospital	23.6	54.5	< .01
Mean LOS of admitted patients (min ± SE)	154.9 ± 12.4	125.1 ± 14.0	< .01
Mean LOS of discharged patients (min ± SE)	130.8 ± 10.8	142.2 ± 12.4	NS
Mean number of blood tests or panels (± SE)	1.54 ± 0.13	2.25 ± 0.37	< .01
% Plain abdominal x-rays	29.3	66.7	< .001
% Complex abdominal imaging studies†	10.6	6.0	NS
% Electrocardiogram	15.4	33.3	< .05
% Urinalysis	68.3	39.4	< .05
% Intravenous access	21.1	36.4	NS
% Parenteral therapy	37.4	39.4	NS

*LOS = length of stay; NS = not significant; SE = standard of error.

†Complex abdominal imaging studies include x-rays with contrast, computerized tomography, and ultrasonography.

Burbank has a rather large working force of younger people who do not live in the area. We do not know how this might affect the comparisons of demographic data between the catchment area and the ED population. Large differences have been noted in ED care between facilities in different areas of the same city based on the characteristics of the local population.[4,8-15] Second, our population had higher rates of insurance coverage than many other EDs. Third, while most previous ED studies have been done in EDs that utilize physicians in training for some or all medical coverage, our ED instead utilizes only full-time, experienced physicians trained in emergency medicine. As house staff have different patterns of test ordering than more experienced physicians, our data may not be directly comparable to these studies. Some relatively minor seasonal variations in why patients come to EDs have been documented,[12,19] whereas our data were all collected in one month. Because our data collection relied on chart review, the urgency of each visit and other subtle factors could not be accurately addressed. One other limitation is the nature of the hospital and the type of medical plan. For example, enrollment in an HMO may affect patient visits.[23] Finally, the degree of completeness of the ED charts was not determined. Despite these limitations, our findings shed light on important aspects of ED care which may be important in planning improved care for the elderly.

Our data reveal several aspects of ED care of the elderly not described before. Though older patients make more visits to physicians per year on the average than younger people, our study confirms previous studies indicating that older people do not visit EDs much more often than younger people.[4,6,8-13] However, the overrepresentation of the very elderly (age 75 and over) in an

Table 3–3 Process of Care Parameters for All Five Examined Presenting Complaints Combined, Comparing Young versus Old Patients

Parameter	Young (17–64 yrs)	Old (≥ 65 yrs)	p
N	355	136	
% Admitted to hospital	21.1	66.9	< .001
% Intravenous access	22.8	54.4	< .001
% Oral or rectal medicines given in emergency department	19.4	21.3	NS*
% Parenteral medicines given in emergency department	31.0	44.8	< .02
% Of patients discharged home given prescriptions	44.2	25.0	< .001
% Of patients discharged home with recommendation of OTC* preparation	25.3	41.9	< .01

*NS = not significant; OTC = over the counter.

ED population has not been previously reported. The relative increase of ED visits found in the age 75 and over category almost certainly relates to the greater frequency and severity of disease in this age group, which is further reflected in the extremely high proportion of ED visits resulting in hospital admission among this age group. Another study found that patients older than 60 years have the lowest percentage of nonemergent ED visits when ED visits were examined and classified for "true emergency" versus "primary care."[6] All of these observations run counter to the popular perception that older people overutilize emergency services for minor complaints in response to anxiety or so that ambulances may be used for transportation. In fact, quite the opposite seems to be the case. Although not specifically measured, it was our impression that even though most older people have private physicians, they use EDs for care, for several reasons, including severity or acuity of illness, convenience, and lack of availability of their private physicians.

Our data concerning sex distribution, time of day, presence of a primary physician or other regular source of care, and proportion of traumatic complaints with respect to age are similar to those in other studies. Of additional note in our study was the progressively increasing use of ambulance services with age, particularly by the very elderly. This confirms another study that found that 25% of all ambulance services were used by

11% of those people 65 and older,[14] and it presumably reflects older people's decreased mobility when sick as well as the more severe nature of their illnesses.

We found that time actually spent in the ED was a function of both age and discharge disposition. We interpret these data to mean that, since the elderly present with more diffuse and nonspecific complaints, more time is needed to gather data before the treating physician is comfortable releasing the elderly patient home. Once the decision to hospitalize the patient is made, however, the ED staff transports older patients to the ward faster than younger patients. This trend is opposite to that found by Wilson and Simson (1983) in a large inner-city ED where older patients waited longer to be admitted.[15] Unfortunately, actual physician time spent with patients was not assessed in either study, and it must be acknowledged that some of the time spent in the ED results from administrative delay, such as waiting for test results or transportation. We were unable to document whether such administrative delay varied by age, but no such trend was obvious.

In the ED studied, care given to the elderly did not conform to the dictum "older adults are underinvestigated and overtreated." For the presenting complaints studied, the fact that older patients in general had more diagnostic tests ordered may relate to the higher likelihood of serious disease possibilities in the differential diagnosis in the older age ranges. This could prompt physicians

Table 3–4 Mean Number of Blood Tests or Panels Ordered per Patient by Type of Physician Seeing Patient and by Disposition, Comparing Young and Old Patients

	Young (17–64 yrs)	Old (≥ 65 yrs)	p value (young vs. old)
Patients seen by EMD*	2.29 ± 0.14	3.86 ± 0.23	< .001
Patients seen by PMD*	1.88 ± 0.29	2.86 ± 0.26	< .001
Patients admitted to hospital	1.88 ± 0.10	3.49 ± 0.16	< .001
Patients discharged home	0.68 ± 0.02	1.17 ± 0.18	< .001

*EMD = emergency department staff doctor; PMD = private physician or consultant.

to investigate more thoroughly older patients before releasing them home. In addition, the elderly are characterized as frequently presenting with symptoms that are vague and nonspecific,[16] which may also encourage the ordering of extra tests before a final disposition is made. Other investigators[17] have shown that the absolute number of tests ordered does not necessarily reflect the quality of care or improve diagnostic accuracy. Furthermore, some authors feel that the ordering of diagnostic tests, ECGs, and simple x-rays is the major contributing factor in the escalation of health care costs.[18] While we were not able to determine what proportion of diagnostic tests for older and younger patients were actually useful, it was our impression that tests are not overordered for the elderly vis-á-vis younger patients. Further, tests seem to be somewhat more useful among the elderly who frequently present atypically with disease.[16]

Until recently, ED visits were the most rapidly increasing segment of hospital use.[20] Clearly, emergency medical service networks have improved morbidity and mortality statistics in some classes of disease. It has been estimated that 75,000 deaths per year would be preventable by instituting a universal effective emergency medical system.[21] However, comprehensive regionalized emergency services are expensive, can be inefficient, and funding is unlikely.[20] Indeed, strategies are being proposed to triage nonurgent patients to less labor-intensive, and presumably cheaper, sources of medical care. These include requiring a higher copayment for care received in an ED,[22] reducing reimbursement rates for visits deemed "not emergent," and creating a separate emergency care system for diagnosis-related groups (DRGs). The implementation of DRGs' reimbursement by Medicare conceivably might lead to the triaging of ED patients presenting with low reimbursement complaints differently if they are older and have Medicare than if they are younger.

Clearly, cost containment efforts are essential to the continued stability of the medical care system. However, they should not come in ways that will have adverse impacts on health outcomes nor unfairly single out a group of high-risk individuals — particularly the elderly. If it were true that elderly overutilize emergency services, then these efforts to target Medicare might be appropriate. However, our and other data cited previously suggest that elderly patients do not use EDs substantially more frequently than other age segments of society and, in fact, tend to be more severely ill when entering the ED. Furthermore, elderly patients require significantly more ED services per visit than younger patients. Thus, efforts to limit ED expenditures, unless carefully directed, would probably affect the health care of the elderly more than that of younger individuals and might have selectively adverse impacts on this frail segment of society. To truly address this question, further studies are needed to define the determinates of ED quality of care and how variations in quality affect outcomes of old versus young patients.

ACKNOWLEDGMENTS

The authors wish to acknowledge Nada Cugalj, M.S., for statistical assistance, and Beverley Philbrook for secretarial assistance.

This paper was presented at the 1985 Annual Meeting of the American Geriatrics Society, New York.

REFERENCES

1. Health Care Finance Administration: Reported in U.S. Senate Special Committee on Aging, Developments in Aging, Volume 1, 1982.
2. Gibson G: Patterns and trends of utilization of emergency medical services. In Schwartz et al, editors: Emergency medicine, Philadelphia, 1978, WB Saunders, pp 1513–1518.
3. Fleming NS and Jones HC: The impact of outpatient department and emergency room use on costs in the Texas Medicaid program, Med Care 21:892–910, 1983.
4. Huntley H: Emergency department visits: a statewide survey, J Am Coll Emerg Phys 6:296–299, 1977.
5. Magnusson G: The hospital emergency department as the primary source of medical care, Scand J Soc Med 8:149–156, 1980.
6. Parker S: Emergency room utilization at Hermann Hospital, Tex Med 74:62–70, 1978.
7. Walker LL: Why do patients use the emergency room? Hosp Topic 53:19–21, 45, 1975.
8. Agisim E: The nature of visits to Wisconsin's emergency departments, Wisc Med J 74:131–134, 1975.
9. Magnusson G: Utilization of a hospital emergency department in Stockholm: the effects of age, sex, and marital status, Scand J Soc Med 8:141–148, 1980.
10. Pearson DA, Bernacki EJ, and Meigs JW: An emergency medical care facility: program characteristics and patient attributes, J Am Coll Emerg Phys 5:174–179, 1976.
11. Walker LL: Inpatient and emergency department utilization: the effects of distance, social class, age, sex, and marital status, J Am Coll Emerg Phys 5:105–110, 1976.
12. Weinerman ER et al: Yale studies in ambulatory care: V. Determinants of use of hospital emergency services, Am J Public Health 56:1037–1056, 1976.
13. White HA and O'Connor PA: Use of the emergency room in a community hospital, Public Health Rep 85:163–168, 1970.
14. Gerson LW: Emergency medical service utilization by the elderly, Ann Emerg Med 11:610–612, 1980.
15. Wilson LB and Simson S: Black elderly use of emergency services, Penn Med 86:48–50, 52, 54, 1983.
16. Kane RA, Ouslander JG, and Abrass IB: Essentials of clinical geriatrics, New York, 1984, McGraw-Hill.
17. Schroeder SA, Schliftman A, and Piemme TE: Variation among physicians in use of laboratory tests: relationship to quality of care, Med Care 12:709–713, 1974.
18. Schroeder SA and Martin AR: Will changing how physicians order tests reduce medical costs? (editorial), Ann Intern Med 94:534–535, 1981 (pt. 1).
19. Torrens PR and Yedvab DG: Variations among emergency room populations: a comparison of four hospitals in New York City, Med Care 8:60–75, 1979.
20. Crippen DW: Emergency medicine redux: the rise and fall of a community medical specialty, Ann Emerg Med 12:539–540, 1984.
21. Committee on Public Policy of the American College of Emergency Physicians: Emergency medical services: problems, programs, and policies, J Am Coll Emerg Phys 3:176, 1974.
22. O'Grady KF, Manning WG, Newhouse JP, and Brook RH: The impact of cost sharing on emergency department use, N Engl J Med 313:484–490, 1985.
23. Hosfield G and Ryan M: HMOs and utilization of emergency medical services: a metropolitan survey, Ann Emerg Med 18:374, 1989.

Teaching Geriatric Emergency Medicine

Jeffrey S. Jones, M.D.

The diseases of the aged are worthy of the most careful study: an old man may
be of more value to the community than a hundred infants. Let us not dismiss
his ailments with the facile diagnosis: You are old.
                                          IL NASCHER,[1] 1917

Educational objectives

Instructional methods

In 1909, when Dr. Nascher coined the term "geriatrics," a newborn child could expect to live about 48 years.[2] Today, 25 million Americans, or 11% of the population, are over 65.[3] By the year 2030, that figure is predicted to reach 20%.[4] The significance of this growth assumes perspective when one realizes that even today our relatively small geriatric population accounts for more than 33% of a physician's time, 25% of medications, and 40% of acute hospital admissions.[5]

This growing geriatric population will result in increased demands for health care services, particularly emergency medical care. As changes come about in public funding of health care, the elderly will turn to the emergency department for primary as well as crisis care. These centers offer 24-hour availability, accessibility without regard to cost, community and social service referral, entry into the long-term health care system, and are intimately involved in prehospital geriatric care. Better trained professional and support personnel will be needed to provide these services effectively and economically. During the past 10 years, the American Geriatrics Society, the Institute of Medicine, and the Association of American Medical Colleges have recommended that appropriate actions be taken for better preparation of future practitioners to render health care to the growing elderly population.[2]

Despite these calls for the introduction of geriatrics and gerontology into the medical education system, most primary care physicians prove unprepared clinically to deal with acute disease in the elderly.[6-8] A review of the emergency medicine core content developed by the Graduate Education Committee of the American College of Emergency Physicians[9] reveals no specific requirements for geriatric care skills. In 1987, Tintinalli emphasized the importance of adding geriatrics to the emergency medicine curriculum to improve the understanding and management of the ill or injured older patient.[10]

An educational program in geriatric medicine should include an emphasis on the physiology of normal aging, the pathophysiology of associated diseases, functional assessment, and concepts of treatment and management, both in the acute and intensive care setting. Attention should be directed as well to the behavioral aspects of illness, socioeconomic factors, and ethical and legal considerations that may impinge on medical management.[11] Opportunities for investigation related to the elderly in the basic sciences, clinical medicine, or health services are essential. This chapter presents an integrated geriatrics curriculum designed to operate within a three-year emergency medicine residency program.

EDUCATIONAL OBJECTIVES

In 1986, the Akron General Emergency Medicine Program and Geriatric Assessment Center began developing training in geriatric medicine as an integral part of the emergency medicine residency.[12] The first step in preparing a comprehensive geriatrics curriculum was a review of more than 40 articles from existing family practice and internal medicine programs. However, few of those programs attempted to reflect the skills and knowledge of acute geriatric care. Joint planning sessions were organized between a group of experienced teachers of emergency medicine and emergency medicine residents to identify those educational objectives necessary for training in geriatric emergencies (Table 4–1).

The first three objectives concern the clinical aspects of aging: physiologic changes, diagnostic testing, and altered pharmacokinetics. The remaining objectives deal with disease states in the elderly. These six objectives then were further defined using a framework of specific topics or subject areas (Table 4–2). Topics were chosen because they reflected a survey of needs perceived by the residents and faculty members and dealt with subject areas not adequately covered by other aspects of the training program.

The first objective focused on the physical impairments and functional disorders common with aging. The clinician should have the knowledge and skills to distinguish between aging and the diseases associated with aging.[6] By recognizing the changes expected with aging, the physician can avoid chasing phantom diseases[5] or neglecting important signs that indicate disease. Physiologic changes associated with growing old become apparent after age 30 and have a direct bearing on the patient's lifestyle, the diagnosis of disease, and the patient's response to the stress of illness.[6] From the clinical standpoint, it is the weakening of the renal, hepatic, immunologic, pulmonary, cardiac, and intellectual functions that cause greatest concern.[13] Loss of function with consequent loss of independence is the most dreaded possibility faced by older persons. Thus, history taking and physical examination should include not only the detection of disease but also functional assessment.[6]

Second only to the history and physical examination in detection of illness, the routine laboratory evaluation aids the clinician in management of the elderly patient. The laboratory exam is particularly useful because of the high chance of multiple diseases, each looking clinically similar. However, appropriate use of diagnostic testing, including electrocardiograms and radiographs, requires an understanding of how physiological changes in aging affect normal standards (objective 2).

Another area requiring special emphasis is the altered pharmacokinetics in aged patients (objective 3). Poor patient compliance, multiple drug regimens, communication problems, and changes in enzyme and organ function combine to make drug therapy more difficult.[14] The sum of these difficulties is that elderly patients have twice the risk for an adverse drug reaction as younger persons.[14] Although poisoning in this age group is uncommon, older persons are more likely to develop serious symptoms and may require a longer detoxification time because of impaired elimination of the toxin from the body.[15]

The pathologic changes associated with aging (objective 4) have been known since Hippocrates listed them as "dyspnea, catarrh accompanied by cough, dysuria, pains in the joints, vertigo, apoplexy, cachexia, pruritis of the whole body, insomlency, defluxions of the bowel, of the eyes, and of the nose, glaucoma, and dullness of hearing."[16] Besides the symptoms and signs of age-associated disease, however, the clinician must be aware of those diseases that present atypically in the elderly patient (objective 5). It is well known that the classic signs and symptoms of diseases in older patients may be delayed, altered, or absent.[4] Recent clinical studies of acute poisonings,[15] trauma,[17] burns,[18] head injuries,[19] battered elderly,[20] and other medical and surgical conditions emphasize the subtle signs of illness and adverse prognosis of injury in the aged. Other diseases and problems should be given repeated emphasis in a geriatrics curriculum because they require a diagnostic and therapeutic approach different from that used for the younger patient. Examples of these include syncope, acute dementia, pulmonary embolism, and the acute abdomen.

The final objective deals with common psychiatric and behavioral disorders. In the elderly population, physical disease may manifest as a psychiatric disorder, or, conversely, emotional problems may present as physical problems.[13] Most of the psychiatric syndromes manifested by elderly patients are amenable to early treatment.[13] Prompt recognition and intervention are therefore imperative. Untoward responses to aging include alcoholism and drug abuse. Alcoholism is the second most frequent cause for admitting elderly patients to a psychiatric facility.[6] Since many elders use psychotropic drugs, clinicians need to be alert to unintentional as well as intentional misuse. The elderly account for approximately 25% of reported suicides, many of which might be prevented by early recognition and treatment of depression.[6] The emergency physician should expect to see more social and adaptational problems in elderly patients and learn efficient utilization of available social services.

Table 4–1 Educational Objectives

1. Identify and assess physical and functional impairments common with aging (3 hours).*

2. Understand how physiologic changes in aging affect diagnostic testing (2 hours).

3. Knowledge of the altered pharmacokinetics in elderly patients and its role in toxicology (3 hours).

4. Understand and treat the group of diseases peculiar to the elderly (6 hours).

5. Recognize certain diseases and injuries that present a different clinical picture in old age (10 hours).

6. Differentiate and treat common psychosocial emergencies in the elderly (4 hours).

*Approximate conference time necessary to adequately cover the educational objective.

Table 4–2   The Emergency Geriatrics Curriculum

Objective I.   Identify and assess physical and functional impairments common with aging.

Specific topics	Instructional methods			
	Didactic lectures	Case conferences	Journal clubs	Learning activity
Physiology of aging	X			Lecture by retired physician
History and physical exam in elderly	X			History-taking forms
Common signs and symptoms	X		X	
Evaluation of functional ability		X		Functional assessment test
Health maintenance in the elderly		X		Charts audit review

Objective II.   Understand how physiologic changes in aging affect diagnostic testing.

Specific topics	Instructional methods			
	Didactic lectures	Case conferences	Journal clubs	Learning activity
Effects of age on common lab tests	X			Lecture by pathologist
ECG* changes in the elderly		X		ECG review, CCU* rotation
Radiologic changes with aging	X			Radiology teaching files, radiology rotation

Objective III.   Gain a knowledge of the altered pharmacokinetics in elderly patients.

Specific topics	Instructional methods			
	Didactic lectures	Case conferences	Journal clubs	Learning activity
Age-related pharmacokinetics	X			
Prescribing for the elderly	X	X		Methods to simplify pill counting
Common drug reactions	X	X	X	
Poisoning in the elderly		X	X	Poison control presentation, toxicology cases
Cardiovascular drug therapy	X			Lecture by cardiologist
OTC* medications		X		
Psychotropic drug use	X		X	Lecture by psychiatrist

Objective IV.   Understand and treat those diseases peculiar to the elderly.

Specific topics	Instructional methods			
	Didactic lectures	Case conferences	Journal clubs	Learning activity
Geriatric dermatoses	X			Lecture by dermatologist, slides
Failure to thrive in elderly		X		Medicine rotation
Gynecology in the aged female	X	X	X	Lecture by gynecologist, gynecology rotation
Thyroid disease in the elderly	X	X		
Geriatric ophthalmology — cataracts, glaucoma, macular degeneration	X	X		Lecture by ophthalmologist, discuss exam of the aging eye
Parkinsonism		X		Videotape of patient, differential diagnosis of tremor
Metabolic bone disease	X	X		Radiology teaching file
Rheumatic diseases and their complications	X		X	Lecture by rheumatologist
Temporal arteritis, polymyalgia		X		
Common foot disorders	X		X	Orthopedic clinic, radiographs, lecture by podiatrist

*ECG = electrocardiogram; CCU = coronary care unit; OTC = over the counter; CHF = congestive heart failure; MI = myocardial infarction; ICU = intensive care unit; DRGs = diagnosis-related groups.

NOTE: The curriculum emphasizes those emergency medicine problems and diseases that require a diagnostic and therapeutic approach different from that used in the younger patient and that are not customarily covered in other sections of the emergency medicine curriculum.

Continued.

Table 4–2   The Emergency Geriatrics Curriculum — cont'd

Objective IV. (Continued).

Specific topics	Instructional methods			
	Didactic lectures	Case conferences	Journal clubs	Learning activity
Anemia and hematologic emergencies in the elderly	X			Medicine rotation
Urinary retention		X		Demonstrate suprapubic catheter
Tuberculosis	X	X		

Objective V.   Recognize certain disorders presenting a different clinical picture in old age.

Specific topics	Instructional methods			
	Didactic lectures	Case conferences	Journal clubs	Learning activity
Thermoregulation — hypothermia and heat-related problems		X		
Infection and antibiotic therapy	X	X	X	Review of chart audit
Injuries/common fractures in late life	X			Lecture by orthopedic surgeon, trauma conference, radiographs
Cardiovascular disease in aging (CHF,* MI,* arrhythmias)	X	X	X	CCU* rotation, ECG* review, Mega code scenario
Endocarditis in geriatrics		X		
Hypertension in the elderly	X	X		Discuss modes of therapy
Silent pulmonary embolism		X		Ventilation-perfusion scan review
Respiratory problems in the aged	X	X	X	ICU* rotation
Evaluation of acute abdomen in the elderly	X			Surgery rotation, abdominal radiographs
Constipation in the aged		X		
Pain syndromes (chest, back, abdominal)		X		
Hypercalcemia, hyperparathyroidism		X		
Complications of diabetes in elderly	X	X	X	
Oncologic emergencies	X		X	Lecture by oncologist
Evaluation of syncope in elderly	X	X		
The weak and dizzy patient	X	X		
Bedside diagnosis of cerebrovascular accident	X			Videotape of patient

Objective VI.   Differentiate and treat common psychosocial disorders in the elderly.

Specific topics	Instructional methods			
	Didactic lectures	Case conferences	Journal clubs	Learning activity
Organic brain syndrome	X		X	Mental status exam, videotape
Acute dementia/confusion	X			Review of chart audit
Depression in the elderly, suicide	X	X	X	Lecture by psychiatrist
Alcoholism, drug abuse in elderly	X	X		
Social problems and community service programs	X	X		Lecture by social worker, visiting nurse service
Economic resources (Medicaid, Medicare)	X			Discuss cost containment, DRGs* coordinator
Abuse and neglect in the aged		X	X	Videotape of patient
Doctor-patient relationship	X	X		Lecture by retired physician, discuss ethical considerations

INSTRUCTIONAL METHODS

The six objectives and subject topics listed in Table 4–2 are not order dependent and can be completed during the 36 months of residency. This curriculum is not intended to create a geriatric block rotation; it is designed to be integrated into an existing curriculum of an established program and still achieve the primary goal of exposing the residents to more intensive training in geriatric emergencies. Because residents respond differently to various methods of instruction, a variety of instructional methods, including didactic lectures, individual readings, journal clubs, clinical case conferences, audits, and supervised patient care, are used and can be individualized by each program.

Resident conferences, workshops, and grand rounds should include four to eight hours per year on geriatric topics (Table 4–2). This is significantly less than the 38 hours of pediatric conference time suggested by the Task Force on Length of Training in Emergency Medicine.[21] The presentations may be made by guest speakers, geriatrics faculty, or emergency medicine faculty and residents. One staff physician should maintain liaison with faculty members of other departments with similar interests and expertise in the problems of aging. In addition, there may be local community agencies that show interest and abilities in addressing the special needs of the elderly that can be utilized for guest lectures.

The content offered in lectures was supplemented by a bibliography of current articles relating to geriatric emergencies with reference to particular subject areas (curriculum syllabus). Articles were selected from a recent bibliography published by the American Geriatrics Society[22] and from a review of the geriatric literature by staff physicians. Preference was given to recent publications; almost all of the references are from the past five years.

Much of the teaching can be done on a case-by-case basis. Clinical case conferences should specify history taking and examination techniques needed to properly evaluate an aged patient. This discussion should include references to the general aspects of aging and its effect on diagnostic testing as well as such neglected topics as clinical pharmacology and ethical and legal issues. In addition, journal clubs are a useful and popular forum for teaching geriatric skills. Our sessions are 90 minutes in length, take place monthly, and are devoted to the critical review of four to six papers chosen by an attending physician. The seminars should follow a relatively standard format and may be oriented to specific geriatric topics, such as oncologic emergencies, infections, or rheumatic diseases.

Frequent chart audits may be used to evaluate patient management skills.[23] The auditor reviews patient charts and provides feedback to the resident to help identify areas of strength and weakness. Other standard educational tools and forums also may be used to supplement and expand the knowledge and skills of trainees and staff. They include library resources, slide presentations, audiovisual teaching skills, special symposia on aging, and research forums. It is not necessary to adhere rigidly to suggested methods of instruction. Flexibility and creativity in the delivery of information is a necessary part of any successful curriculum.

To give residents adequate opportunity to practice clinical skills, these objectives may be emphasized during the training program, such as the off-service rotations in orthopedics, internal medicine, cardiology, and general surgery. In the emergency department, there should be considerable emphasis on the geriatric aspects of the patient's illness, including social problems, mental status examination, appropriate diagnostic testing, and health maintenance.

A number of formal and informal methods provide feedback to residents. All residents should review their evaluations from each clinical rotation and from the yearly in-training examination. In addition, a modified "Palmore Facts on Aging Quiz"[24] is given to all residents and students each year. The test consists of 25 true/false statements covering the basic physical, mental, and social facts about aging. The purpose of this test is to stimulate group discussions, measure and compare different groups' levels of information, identify common misconceptions about aging, and study attitudes toward the aged.

The curriculum has been implemented at Akron General Medical Center with favorable response from house staff and students. The variety of specific topics offered has assisted residents in realizing their deficits in the area of acute geriatrics and has inspired further individual study. When used in combination with enthusiastic faculty, the program may strengthen positive attitudes toward geriatric medicine and improve medical care.

REFERENCES

1. Freeman JR: Aging: its history and literature, New York, 1979, Human Sciences Press, p 130.
2. Panneton PE, Mortisugu KP, and Miller AM: Training health professionals in the care of the elderly, J Am Geriatr Soc 30:144–149, 1982.
3. Judd RL: Demographics of the elderly, EMS Management Advisor 1:1–6, 1986.
4. Bedtine RW: Geriatric medicine, an overview, Ann Rev Gerontol Geriatrics 1:200–215, 1980.
5. National Institute on Aging, Public Health Service, Department of Health and Human Services: Report on education and training in geriatrics and gerontology, Bethesda, Md, February 1984, Public Health Service (adminstrative document).
6. Dans PE and Kerr MR: Gerontology and geriatrics in medical education, N Engl J Med 300:228–231, 1979.
7. Reichel W: Family practice and care of the elderly, Am Fam Physician 20:85–89, 1979.
8. Williamson J: Geriatric medicine: whose speciality? Ann Intern Med 91:774–780, 1979.
9. Special Committee on the Core Content Revision: Emergency medicine core content, Ann Emerg Med 15:853–862, 1986.
10. Tintinalli JE: The importance of a geriatrics curriculum, Ann Emerg

Med 15:1366, 1986.

11. American Geriatrics Society: Guidelines for fellowship training programs in geriatric medicine, May 1986.

12. Jones J et al: A geriatrics curriculum for emergency medicine training programs, Ann Emerg Med 15:1275–1281, 1986.

13. Freedman ML: Problems in detecting acute disease in the elderly, ER Reports 3:49–53, 1982.

14. Ouslander JG, Brenner B, and Sinkinson CA: Prescribing drugs for the elderly patients, ER Reports 5:93–100, 1984.

15. Klein-Schwartz W, Oderda GM, and Booze L: Poisoning in the elderly, J Am Geriatr Soc 31:195–199, 1983.

16. Freiden R and Walshe TM: Physical changes associated with aging. In Walshe TM, editor: Manual of clinical problems in geriatric medicine, Boston, 1985, Little, Brown & Co Inc.

17. Oreskovich MR et al: Geriatric trauma: injury patterns and outcome, J Trauma 24:565–572, 1984.

18. Feller I, Flora JD, and Bawol R: Baseline results of therapy for burned patients, JAMA 236:1943–1947, 1976.

19. Klauber MR et al: Epidemiology of head injury: a prospective study of an entire community—San Diego County, California, 1978, J Epidemiol 113:500–509, 1981.

20. Rathbone-McCuan E and Voyles B: Case detection of abused elderly parents, Am J Psychiatry 139:189–192, 1982.

21. Asch SM and Weigand JV: A pediatric curriculum for emergency medicine training programs, Ann Emerg Med 15:19–27, 1986.

22. Rosenthal M: Geriatrics: an updated bibliography. J Am Geriatr Soc 34:148–171, 1986.

23. Shannon RP: Attitudes towards the elderly: the role of medical education. In Human values in the health care of the elderly, Philadelphia, 1978, Society for Health and Human Values.

24. Miller RB and Dodder RA: A revision of Palmore's Facts on Aging quiz, Gerontologist 20:673–675, 1980.

Geriatric Pharmacology and Toxicology

Drug Therapy
Drug Prescribing and Systematic Detection of Adverse Drug Reactions

J. Michael Albrich, M.D., F.A.C.E.P., F.A.C.P., **and Gideon Bosker**, M.D., F.A.C.E.P.

As the United States enters the twenty-first century, a large fraction of its population will approach old age. Mean survival has increased over 60% since the turn of the last century so that elderly Americans 65 years and older will constitute 20% of the population by the year 2010. Moreover, by the year 2000, there will be 15 million Americans over the age of 85 which, at present, is the fastest growing segment of the geriatric population.

With advancing age, individuals become susceptible to a number of clinical disorders. Current approaches to most geriatric disorders use drug therapy. Thus, the elderly find themselves burdened not only by diseases of old age, but with the consumption — for therapeutic purposes — of an ever-increasing number of potent drugs, many of which can precipitate adverse side effects and compromise quality of life.[1-10]

Treatment with medications is associated with a wide variety of adverse drug reactions (ADRs) including adverse drug interactions (ADIs). While there is fierce debate regarding the risks and benefits of drug therapy in many disorders endemic to the elderly population, one thing remains clear: Adverse drug reactions and interactions are directly related to *the number of drugs* taken concurrently.[4]

Regardless of whether drug therapy is provided in the acute hospital setting, the ambulatory environment, or the chronic care institution, no other risk factor or group of risk factors compares with polypharmacy as a cause of adverse drug reactions and interactions in the geriatric population. A number of British and American studies have corroborated that persons over 65 years of age living independently take an average of 2.8 drugs per day.[3] In nursing homes the number increases to an average of 3.4, while about 9 drugs per day are prescribed for the hospitalized elderly (Table 5–1).

Table 5–1   Medications for Hospitalized Elderly

Country	Average drugs per hospitalized patient
United States	9.1
Canada	7.1
Israel	6.3
New Zealand	5.8
Scotland	4.6

One recent study conducted by Larsen at the University of Washington[4] has demonstrated that there is a ninefold increased risk of having an adverse drug reaction when four or more drugs are taken simultaneously. Not surprisingly, 3 to 5% of all hospital admissions are related to adverse drug reactions, and of all hospital admissions for the elderly, 15 to 25% are complicated by an adverse drug reaction. Some of these reactions are life threatening, and it is estimated that adverse drug reactions in the United States may account for up to 30,000 deaths each year.

The potential toxicity of drugs in the elderly is exacerbated by the burgeoning pharmaceutical landscape. At present, 8,000 prescription drugs are available in the United States, including 9 beta-blockers, 15 cephalosporins, 12 nonsteroidal anti-inflammatory drugs (NSAIDs), 8 oral sulfonylureas, 13 diuretic preparations, 3 ACE inhibitors, 15 penicillins, and 4 calcium channel blockers. A new entity is approved for human use every 2 to 3 weeks and two thirds of all physician visits culminate in a prescription for a drug. In 1981, American physicians wrote 1.8 billion prescriptions, an average of 6.2 prescriptions for every woman, man, and child in the country. Over the past 8 years, it is estimated that the total number of prescriptions and pills have increased by 27% and 35%, respectively.[11]

As the number of geriatric patients receiving pharmacologic treatment continues to rise, physicians are increasingly challenged with the diagnosis, identification, and management of adverse drug reactions among the elderly.

Inaccurate diagnoses of adverse drug reactions in elderly patients are common. Patients often experience multiple, nonspecific symptoms — a problem further complicated because many elderly patients on potent drug regimens suffer from dementia, depression, or other psychiatric disturbances. In addition, because in this age group drug toxicity usually affects the central nervous system, its symptoms are frequently attributed to other underlying causes, such as sepsis, neurologic disease, and metabolic derangements. Finally, because medical illnesses in the elderly may be difficult to recognize, drugs may be prescribed for the incorrect diagnosis, thereby confusing the clinical picture even more. This exposes the patient to the risk of taking unnecessary medications, while neglecting the underlying condition.[12]

Table 5–2   Causes of Unintentional Drug Toxicity Among the Elderly

- Duplications
- Self-selection of drugs
- Taking p.r.n. drugs too frequently
- Automatic refills
- Omissions
- Pharmacy error
- Drug-induced confusion
- Recreational misuse

Complicating assessment of drug-related toxicity is poor drug compliance, which is frequent among the elderly (Table 5–2). In addition to not taking their medications, some elderly patients make unauthorized changes in their dosing intervals. Up to 70% of the geriatric population take over-the-counter (OTC) drugs that may interfere with, inhibit, or potentiate prescribed medications. Complex regimens can confuse the geriatric patient, particularly if the patient has cognitive impairments. Physical limitations may also hinder drug compliance.

Pharmacologic therapy of the elderly, therefore, requires knowledge not only of appropriate drug dosages, potential side effects, and altered pharmacokinetics of outpatient drugs, but an increased awareness of potential interactions between chronic and acute medications.[13]

Although it is generally assumed that the elderly are more susceptible to adverse drug reactions, some investigators argue that no good evidence exists in the medical literature to support this contention. Rather, these experts suggest that drug treatment of the elderly is complicated by the presence of coexisting diseases, multiple medications, self-selection of drugs, inappropriate dosing, multiple doctors, difficulty with compliance, and other factors inherent to the geriatric age group (Table 5–3).

Based on numerous reports and clinical reviews, it is clear that in order to reduce the risks of drug therapy in the elderly, it is useful to categorize precipitating factors into physician-, patient-, and drug-related groups.[14]

PHYSICIAN-RELATED RISK FACTORS FOR ADVERSE DRUG REACTIONS (Table 5–4)

The majority of adverse drug reactions in the elderly are difficult to detect because symptoms are vague and nonspecific and, not infrequently, mimic symptoms of illnesses common to the geriatric age group. As a result, manifestations of many drug reactions and side effects are often overlooked or ignored by the physician. Difficulty

Table 5–3   Risk Factors for Adverse Drug Reactions

- Multiple drug regimens
- Incorrect diagnosis
- Lack of compliance
- Poor OTC drug history
- Changes in drug metabolism
- Changes in drug effect (cardiac)
- Multiple physicians
- Generic versus trade names

Table 5–4   Causes of Adverse Drug Reactions in the Elderly

Physician Factors

- Physician prescribes a high-risk drug to vulnerable host (i.e., ASA for patient with peptic ulcer disease)

- Physician prescribes highly interactive drug to "pharmacologically vulnerable" patient (i.e., captopril to patient on potassium-sparing agent, diphenhydramine to patient on anticholinergics, etc.)

- Physician prescribes inappropriate compensatory drug for unrecognized drug effect (i.e., tricyclic antidepressant to treat beta-blocker depression, major tranquilizer to treat benzodiazepine agitation, etc.)

- Automatic drug prescribing (i.e., standard orders for ICU, CCU, or chronic care facilities)

- Lack of follow-up on drug effects or poor longitudinal monitoring of drug interactions

in obtaining a history in this age group, the lack of specific physical findings, and the inability to alter the progression of disease can lull the clinician into unsafe prescribing habits and poor case detection patterns.[15]

For example, physicians who prescribe drugs primarily in response to symptoms may fail to detect adverse drug reactions and interactions which, in many cases, obscure the underlying medical condition that prompted initial drug therapy. In these cases, the clinician is at risk for prescribing a compensatory drug which, unwittingly, has been added to treat an adverse reaction caused by *another drug* rather than the primary illness against which the physician thinks the treatment is being directed.

Two common — and potentially harmful — patterns that have emerged include prescribing a cyclic antidepressant (CA) to treat the clinical depression induced by a lipophilic (e.g., propranolol) beta-blocker and the addition of a major tranquilizer to the drug regimen of patients with Alzheimer's disease to treat unrecognized benzodiazepine agitation. Another well-described pitfall is the propensity of the subspecialist to focus on a single organ system and institute treatment that neglects drug effects on other organ systems as well as the patient's global pharmacologic landscape.

Noncompliance with prescription medications contributes significantly to the incidence of adverse drug reactions and interactions in the geriatric age group. Rates of noncompliance with prescribed medications have been shown to be substantially higher if the patient is unaware of the purpose for which the drug is prescribed.[2-4] Interestingly, studies show that elderly patients are more likely to understand the use of OTC drugs when the medication is given to them by a friend or family member than when it is prescribed by a physician. In this regard, *physician instructions for drug use,* complemented by written information, have been shown to be integral to a patient's understanding of the purpose of prescribed medication; this approach is associated with increased compliance rates.

Prescribing new drugs that are touted to be effective in the elderly but whose clinical safety and efficacy has been proven primarily in only younger, otherwise well patients is a particularly insidious problem. Most large pharmaceutical studies tend to exclude the very old and extremely ill patient because of the difficulty in evaluating drug efficacy and side effects. And, almost without exception, pharmaceutical trials are short term, and rarely exceed four months in duration. Consequently, in all but the most unusual and urgent circumstances, the clinician is on safer ground waiting until careful trials with older patients appear in the literature so that the risks of adverse reactions, drug interaction, and the long-term effects of newer drugs can be fully assessed in this vulnerable patient population.

Perhaps the first — and simplest — step toward eliminating the most important risk factor (i.e., the total number of drugs consumed) burdening the elderly is to recognize and combat the physician's *compulsion to prescribe* drugs for this age group (Table 5–5). It is estimated that 75% of all geriatric patient-physician contacts result in the addition of a prescription drug to the patient's therapeutic regimen. Part of the problem appears to be a discrepancy between physician and patient expectations regarding the necessity for drug administration. One large study has shown that up to 80 to 90% of physicians are under the impression that their patients expect a prescription drug as part of their outpatient therapy.[16]

However, when patients are interviewed regarding their desires for drug intake, they indicate the need primarily for a thorough examination, consultation, and reassurance and for a prescription in only 30 to 50% of physician contacts. This proclivity for drug use has been instilled into the general population by the pharmaceutical industry and, perhaps more importantly, by their own experiences with physicians who prescribe with such great avidity. Thus, it appears that the unfounded expectations of both physicians and patients contribute to excessive prescribing of medications.

The pharmaceutical industry has long recognized the pivotal role of the physician in sales of their products. To this end, the medical community is the target of a multibillion dollar annual drug promotion and continuing education campaign. Some studies suggest that these

Table 5–5   Physician Prescribing Behavior: Patterns and Pitfalls

- Two thirds of all physician visits lead to prescription for drug.
- American patients receive about four times more medication for a specific complaint than patients in Scotland.
- In one study, 60% of physicians prescribed antibiotics for common cold.
- Duke University study suggested 64% of antibiotic usage in hospitalized patients was either unnecessary or inappropriately dosed.

efforts are the most important external influence on physician prescribing habits. For example, 85% of all prescriptions written by practitioners graduating in 1960 are for medications introduced after graduation about which they have had no formal education. It is not surprising, then, that the date of graduation from medical school has been shown to be a critical factor affecting physician choice of therapeutic agents.

Until recently, physician prescribing knowledge in geriatric therapeutics had not been examined in a systematic way. Early studies documented significant misuse of psychotropic drugs in nursing homes and suggested that the physician's knowledge base in geriatric clinical therapeutics may be inadequate. Ferry and his associates devised a questionnaire to test the prescribing knowledge of primary care physicians in Pennsylvania.[7] They concluded that less than 30% of responding doctors "exhibited adequate knowledge of prescribing for the elderly." They also identified physician variables positively and negatively associated with an adequate knowledge of geriatric pharmacotherapy. Positive associations included the importance of professional meetings, perception of the need for continuing medical education, board eligibility or certification, group (rather than solo) practice, and a practice which had at least 25 to 50% geriatric patients. Negative associations were the number of years since licensure and the belief that drug advertisements are an important source of drug information. These associations speak eloquently for themselves. It is generally assumed by the lay public that physicians continually update their prescribing knowledge. Most doctors do attend conferences, read literature, and discuss topics in therapeutics with colleagues and pharmaceutical representatives. But this and other studies question the adequacy of these methods for staying current with geriatric drug prescribing.[3-6]

Physician supervision of medications for the elderly, particularly in the nursing home environment, has been judged inadequate by several authors in England who reviewed repeat prescriptions for psychotropic drugs without a physician visit. These studies demonstrated a strong association between the number of times a prescription was refilled without seeing a physician and the age of the patient. In a large general practice in England, 70% of patients taking psychotropic and/or cardiovascular drugs had not contacted their physician in more than a month, and, of these, half had not been in contact with their physicians for a 6-month period.[8] Inasmuch as psychotropics are capable of producing a variety of adverse reactions, their use demands constant vigilance. Ironically, those patients least able to monitor their own medications (i.e., the oldest and most frail elderly) were most likely to be taking these drugs without supervision. Attitude surveys of these older patients found them very receptive to physician intervention aimed at withdrawing drugs judged detrimental or no longer useful.

Medication surveillance is one of several areas in geriatric medicine well suited to the use of computer technology. This area has been pioneered by pharmacists maintaining records for nursing homes in California. Currently, it is feasible to modify computer software designed for medical offices to facilitate drug surveillance. *The Medical Letter* publishes IBM-based software and a handbook that allows the physician to anticipate and avoid adverse drug interactions.

PATIENT-RELATED RISK FACTORS FOR ADVERSE DRUG REACTIONS

The two major patient-related risk factors associated with adverse drug reactions are compliance and age-associated changes in drug distribution and metabolism.

If compliance is defined as taking prescribed medications in a specified manner, then the elderly as a group are noncompliant at least 50% of the time in the community setting. The complexity of a three-drug regimen, for example, is sufficiently great so that even patients under age 45 demonstrate noncompliance rates equal to those of the elderly. Patient noncompliance is a diverse category that includes errors of omission and commission. In a group of elderly diabetics with heart failure, analysis of noncompliance rates found a number of factors that, interestingly enough, were *not* associated with altered or inappropriate drug intake. These include age, number of associated diseases, functional impairment of the patient, and frequency of hospitalization. Only one factor clearly correlated with both errors of omission and commission: *the number of drugs* in the patients' regimen.[4] Level of confusion and dementia were not assessed in this study, but other investigations have suggested that compliance suffers even with the limited forgetfulness so common in this age group.

Compliance errors of *commission* include mixing of *alcohol* or *over-the-counter drugs* with prescribed drugs. It is estimated that alcoholism is present in up to 10% of the elderly population. Alcohol interacts adversely with all sedative drugs (e.g., benzodiazepines, antipsychotics, and some antihypertensives) while such OTC drugs as the antihistamines may add to the anticholinergic effects of prescribed antipsychotics, antidepressants, and antiparkinsonian medications. *Laxative abuse* is thought to increase with age, and this may result in fluid and electrolyte disorders. Self-overmedication by *repeat dosing* or overuse also represents errors of commission, although their prevalence is unknown.

Environmental limitations are a major obstacle to compliance and play a major role in inappropriate drug intake in the elderly. For example, the elderly patient with arthritis may be unable to open childproof bottles or split pills to obtain a fractional dose, whereas the patient with limited mobility may have difficulty getting to the bathroom and, therefore, discontinue or disrupt regular use of diuretics. Retinopathy and peripheral neuropathy may make use of insulin impossible for the older patient who lives alone.

Changes in drug effect and metabolism with aging vary widely among individuals in old age. The greater the age the greater the divergence between chronologic and biologic aging; said another way, not everyone's biologic functions decline at the same rate. Thus, the "appropriate dose" will usually follow the maxim, "Start low, go slow" in order to accommodate wide patient variability in the elderly.

PATHOPHYSIOLOGY AND PHARMACOKINETICS

A number of age-related changes in pharmacokinetics affect drugs commonly prescribed for the elderly. Alterations in absorption, distribution, metabolism, and elimination can precipitate adverse reactions or potentiate drug toxicity.

Because drugs are taken up passively and are not transported in active forms, absorption generally does not change with increasing age. However, distribution may be altered because the fat/muscle ratio increases with age. The fat portion of body weight increases from midlife averages of about 18% for men and 33% for women to 36% and 48% respectively for individuals aged 65 or over. As a result, the volume of distribution for water-soluble drugs decreases with age, whereas that for fat-soluble drugs increases with age.[7]

Relatively water-soluble drugs include acetaminophen (Tylenol) and alcohol. Diazepam (Valium) and lidocaine are examples of fat-soluble drugs. In the elderly, acetaminophen and other water-soluble drugs will attain higher plasma levels. On the other hand, diazepam and lidocaine will be distributed across a greater volume of fat, causing markedly delayed metabolism and a prolonged half-life elimination.

Serum albumin also decreases with age. This alteration is important for highly protein-bound drugs, such as sulfonylureas, for which effective concentrations depend upon the amount of unbound drug. Thus, drug interactions that decrease protein binding for such drugs as chlorpropamide (Diabinese) and tolbutamide (Orinase) may lead to toxicity in the elderly patient.[17]

Renal and hepatic clearance of drugs may also be affected by the aging process. Liver blood flow is decreased 40 to 50% in the elderly. But hepatic drug metabolism varies widely with individuals, and there are no predictable age-related alterations.

The glomerular filtration rate (GFR), however, is reduced by approximately 35% in the geriatric age group. Unlike hepatic clearance, the GFR reduction leads to predictable, directly proportional decreases in the clearance of drugs dependent on the kidney for excretion. Examples of such drugs include lithium, digoxin, cimetidine

Table 5–6   Assessment of Adverse Drug Reactions

Primary Drug Reaction
  Single drug causing single target organ side effect

Secondary Drug Reaction
  Two drugs interact: one potentiates or negates the effect of the other through competition at metabolic breakdown sites, displacement from protein-binding sites, or some other mechanism

Drug Withdrawal
  Narcotics, benzodiazepines, beta-blockers

Tertiary Drug Reaction
  "Falling drugs," psychometric changes, etc.

(Tagamet), procainamide (Pronestyl), most commonly used antimicrobials, and chlorpropamide (Diabinese).[18]

Age-related changes in pharmacodynamics affect the use of a number of drugs. For example, the number of beta-adrenergic receptors is markedly reduced on lymphocytes of elderly patients. Therefore, plasma levels of propranolol (Inderal) and metoprolol (Lopressor) are higher and can cause marked hypotension, bradycardia, or central nervous system depression in the susceptible elderly patient.

TYPES OF ADVERSE DRUG REACTIONS

When evaluating and identifying potential drug reactions in the ambulatory setting, classifying adverse geriatric pharmacologic events into four groups is helpful (Tables 5–6 and 5–7):

1. Primary drug reactions
2. Secondary drug interactions
3. Drug withdrawal syndromes
4. Tertiary extrapharmacologic drug effects

Primary drug reactions.   These occur when a single medication, usually one with a narrow toxic-to-therapeutic ratio, is responsible for the patient's symptoms. Common examples include cimetidine psychosis, theophylline-induced seizures, propranolol depression, and digitalis toxicity. Other primary reactions are narcotic-induced respiratory depression, chronic salicylism, and lidocaine psychosis.

Table 5–7   Evaluation of Drug Toxicity in the Elderly

Toxic/therapeutic ratio: A time-honored concept that is valuable primarily when measuring dose-related adverse effects of a single drug in a patient with uncomplicated disease pattern

Interdrug toxicity: Much more applicable concept in the elderly, where there is a ninefold increase in adverse drug toxicity with consumption of four or more drugs

Extrapharmacologic toxicity: Tertiary clinical pathology (falls, hip fractures) not included in classic categories of drug toxicity and measurable only through large-scale epidemiologic surveys; not included as "adverse" drug reaction in package insert (i.e., propensity to cause falling)

Secondary drug interactions. These toxic reactions result from the interaction between two medications, one causing an increased plasma level of the other drug. Common examples include the interaction between first-generation sulfonylurea agents (chlorpropamide, tolbutamide) and sulfonamide antibiotics. The sulfonamides impair hepatic metabolism of sulfonylureas, thus causing elevated plasma levels, which may lead to increased insulin release and symptomatic hypoglycemia. Salicylates, phenylbutazone, and nonsteroidal anti-inflammatory drugs (NSAIDs) can also displace sulfonylurea from its serum protein binding sites, causing hyperinsulinemia and hypoglycemia.[18]

Because it is a potent inhibitor of the P-450 cytochrome oxidase system in the liver, cimetidine (Tagamet) has the potential for increasing the effective plasma concentration of a number of important drugs that undergo hepatic metabolism. These drugs include lidocaine, phenytoin (Dilantin), aminophylline, benzodiazepines (Valium, Dalmane), propranolol (Inderal), and warfarin (Coumadin). Thus, any elderly patient who is taking cimetidine in addition to one of these medications is at high risk for developing a secondary drug interaction.

Erythromycin and ciprofloxacin inhibit hepatic breakdown of aminophylline and theophylline compounds — as well as carbamazepine — and can induce elevations of these bronchodilators into the toxic range. Other examples of secondary drug interactions include blunted beta-receptor site sensitivity to propranolol caused by indomethacin (Indocin) and the mutual inhibition of cyclic antidepressants and centrally acting alpha-sympatholytic antihypertensives such as alpha-methyldopa (Aldomet) and clonidine (Catapres).[18]

Drug withdrawal syndromes. In the elderly, traditional drug withdrawal syndromes caused by addicting medications such as phenobarbital, benzodiazepine, and alcohol usually do not differ in their clinical presentations from those seen in younger patients. However, older patients carry an additional risk of drug withdrawal syndromes from nonaddicting medications such as beta-blockers or other antihypertensives.

Sudden cessation of beta-blockers or calcium channel blockers, for example, can produce angina and rebound hypertension in susceptible elderly patients. The two classes of agents are not cross-protective with respect to their antianginal properties. In fact, myocardial infarction is precipitated in 2 to 3% of patients when propranolol is abruptly withdrawn, usually in elderly patients at high cardiovascular risk. The proposed mechanism for rebound symptoms is an extended period of beta-receptor supersensitivity to endogenous catecholamine stimulation.

Extrapharmacologic effects. Finally, tertiary extrapharmacologic effects are a consideration for elderly patients taking a large number of medications. Recent studies have reported that the elderly have a 50% to 150% increased risk of falling and sustaining a hip fracture when taking cyclics, long-acting anxiolytics, or antipsychotic medications (Table 5–8).[20]

GENERAL PRINCIPLES AND PATIENT EVALUATION

Although clinical manifestations of drug toxicity are legion, they may be particularly subtle in the elderly (Table 5–9). In the case of digoxin or insulin toxicity, the nature of the drug reaction can frequently be diagnosed from the history, physical examination, and laboratory data base alone.[21] However, when a drug reaction is expressed as a minimal alteration in mental status or mood, fatigue, focal neurologic lesion, coma, seizure disorder, cardiac arrest, myopathy, or nonspecific symptoms complex, the diagnosis may be much more elusive. In such cases, if the clinician does not use a systematic approach to drug evaluation, the disease may go undiagnosed in the ambulatory setting and, hence, may go untreated.

To ensure rapid recognition of adverse drug reactions and the institution of appropriate therapy, familiarity with common medications and the ability to assess drug toxicity with little quickly available historical, physical, and laboratory data are essential.

Table 5–8   Types of Adverse Drug Reactions in the Elderly

Primary Drug Reactions
(One drug — one side effect)
- Cimetidine psychosis
- Narcotic-induced respiratory depression
- Lidocaine psychosis
- Theophylline seizures
- Insulin reaction
- Chronic salicylism

Secondary Drug Interactions
(Requires at least two drugs to cause interaction)
- Sulfonylurea/sulfonamide
- Cimetidine/lidocaine
- Erythromycin/theophylline
- Indomethacin/propranolol
- Tricyclic antidepressant/alpha-sympatholytic

Drug Withdrawal Syndromes
(Addictive and nonaddictive withdrawal)
- Beta-blocker withdrawal (angina)
- Calcium channel-blocker withdrawal (angina, hypertension)
- "Addictive drug" withdrawal syndromes (benzodiazepines, narcotics, etc.)

Tertiary "Extrapharmacologic" Effects
(Measurable only by epidemiologic studies)
- Falls caused by tricyclics, anxiolytics, and antipsychotics (short half-life versus long half-life agents)
- Traumatic injuries caused by drug-induced orthostatic hypotension

Table 5–9 Some Presenting Symptoms of Drug Toxicity and Adverse Drug Reactions in the Elderly

- Acute delirium
- Akathisia
- Altered vision
- Bradycardia
- Cardiac arrhythmias
- Chorea
- Coma
- Confusion
- Constipation
- Fatigue
- Glaucoma
- Hypokalemia
- Orthostatic hypotension
- Paresthesias
- Psychic disturbance
- Pulmonary edema
- Severe bleeding
- Tardive dyskinesia
- Urinary hesitancy

History. To evaluate the possibility of drug toxicity, the physician should obtain a complete drug history, noting recent medication changes, including deletions, additions, and adjustments in dosages. Inquiry should be made about OTC drug use, especially formulations containing salicylates, antihistamines, and sympathomimetics. Aspirin-containing compounds can lead to gastritis in addition to chronic salicylism. Moreover, antihistamines such as diphenhydramine (Benadryl) can produce anticholinergic symptoms that may be potentiated by other commonly prescribed medications, such as cyclic antidepressants and antipsychotics. Finally, sympathomimetics such as pseudoephedrine (Sudafed) and phenylpropanolamine-containing compounds can precipitate hypertension, angina, or even myocardial infarction.[22]

Physical examination. A thorough physical exam and vital signs can help detect abnormalities frequently associated with adverse drug reactions and toxicity. Such alterations in body temperature as hypothermia are associated with drug-induced hypoglycemia, whereas temperature elevations may be caused by anticholinergic drugs. Elevated blood pressure may reflect abrupt withdrawal from beta-blockers or clonidine. Increases in resting heart rate may indicate not only beta-blocker withdrawal, but occult toxicity due to cyclic antidepressants or aminophylline. Profound, symptomatic bradycardia may be the first manifestation of beta-blocker toxicity, which is potentiated by concomitant use of calcium channel blockers such as diltiazem.

Hyperventilation, especially when associated with respiratory alkalosis, is a nonspecific finding but may be the first manifestation of chronic salicylism in the elderly patient. An irregular or rapid pulse may reflect digoxin, aminophylline, or cyclic antidepressant toxicity. Neurologic findings, such as nystagmus, may suggest sedative (phenobarbital, benzodiazepine) intoxication, while constricted pupils may reflect opiate intoxication. Wheezing may be the first sign of beta-blocker or salicylate toxicity.

The physical exam should assess abnormalities in the skin, mucous membranes, and pupillary size. Dry mouth, hypertension, and mydriasis suggest anticholinergic toxicity. A recent history of mental fatigue, depression, or altered thought processes may indicate beta-blocker toxicity or exaggerated effects from anxiolytic drugs of the benzodiazepine group.[22]

Laboratory evaluation. The laboratory exam is invaluable and may reveal metabolic and electrolyte abnormalities associated with drug toxicity. Thiazide and loop diuretics may cause hyponatremia and hypokalemia, the former sometimes severe enough to induce coma and seizures. A decreased serum bicarbonate level may indicate chronic salicylism or an anion gap acidosis. Azotemia may reflect not only excessive diuretic use but also renal failure precipitated by NSAIDs of the propionic acid group.

In the geriatric patient, any alterations in mental status that cannot be explained by sepsis, myocardial infarction, hypotension, or metabolic abnormalities should be evaluated for the possiblity of drug toxicity. Blood levels of phenytoin, digoxin, phenobarbitol, aminophylline, and salicylates are frequently helpful to detect adverse drug reactions caused by these agents. Ultimately, accurate assessment and diagnosis of drug toxicity depends on the association of recent changes in the drug dosage or frequency with the recent onset of central nervous system (CNS), gastrointestinal, cardiac, or metabolic derangements.

IMPORTANT ADVERSE REACTIONS ENCOUNTERED IN THE AMBULATORY SETTING

A British study of nearly 2,000 geriatric patients admitted to the hospital examined the drugs most often associated with adverse reactions (Table 5–10). Diuretics were responsible for the greatest absolute number of side effects, but they were also the most frequently used medications. Drug groups with the highest risk of adverse reactions were antihypertensives and antiparkinsonian drugs (13%), diuretics (11%), psychotropic drugs (12%), and digitalis (11.5%). Smaller studies in both the extended care and home setting have confirmed these findings.[1-7]

Cardiovascular Medication — Beta-Blocking Agents

Toxicity from beta-blockers primarily affects the cardiovascular and central nervous systems. The most common cardiovascular side effects include hypotension, congestive heart failure, bradycardia, and high-degree heart block. The most common respiratory manifestation is bronchoconstriction. Central nervous system alterations — associated primarily with beta-blockers of the lipophilic class (e.g., propranolol) — include depression, altered mental status, and decreased libido. Some of the newer hydrophilic agents, such as atenolol, are associated with less CNS toxicity.

Table 5–10   Indicators of Possible Toxicity

Selected drugs	Reactions
Chlorpropamide (Diabinese)	Hepatic changes, signs of congestive heart failure, bone marrow depression, seizures
Digitalis	Anorexia, nausea, vomiting, arrhythmias, blurred vision, other visual disturbances (colored halos around objects)
Furosemide (Lasix)	Severe electrolyte imbalance, impaired hearing and/or balance (ototoxicity), hepatic changes, pancreatitis, leukopenia, thrombocytopenia
Ibuprofen (Advil, Motrin, Nuprin)	Nephrotic syndrome, fluid retention, ototoxicity, blood dyscrasias
Lithium	Diarrhea, drowsiness, anorexia, vomiting, slurred speech, tremors, blurred vision, unsteadiness, polyuria, seizures
Methyldopa (Aldomet)	Hepatic changes, mental depression, nightmares, dyspnea, fever, tachycardia, tremors
Phenothiazine tranquilizers	Tachycardia, arrhythmias, dyspnea, hyperthermia, excessive anticholinergic effects
Procainamide (Pronestyl, Procan, others)	Arrhythmias, mental depression, leukopenia, agranulocytosis, thrombocytopenia, joint pain, fever, dyspnea, skin rash
Theophylline (Bronkodyl, Elixophyllin, others)	Anorexia, nausea, vomiting, GI bleeding, tachycardia, arrhythmias, irritability, insomnia, muscle twitching, seizures
Tricyclic antidepressants	Arrhythmias, congestive heart failure, seizures, hallucinations, jaundice, hyperthermia, excessive anticholinergic effects

A number of medications, including cimetidine, oral contraceptives, furosemide, and hydralazine, increase beta-blocker effects and may produce clinical symptoms. Concomitant use of intravenous verapamil and propranolol is contraindicated, because the combination may produce irreversible hypotension and profound bradycardia.

Beta-blockers may also abolish symptoms of hypoglycemia and should be avoided in patients with diabetes mellitus. Diabetics who are taking a concomitant beta-blocker should be treated with $D_{50}W$ intravenously if they present with focal deficits or any mental status changes.

In addition to supportive treatment, glucagon is recommended for severe beta-blocker overdose. Glucagon directly activates adenyl cyclase and mimics beta-agonist activity. Treatment with an IV bolus (50 μg/kg), an IV infusion (1 to 5 μg/hr), or a combination of the two has been successful in several cases. Severe overdoses unresponsive to glucagon may require administration of epinephrine or a pacemaker.[19,23]

For a variety of reasons, outpatients with heart disease frequently require adjustments — as well as additions and subtractions — in their antianginal regimen. Dramatic cardiac events, however, including unstable angina, rebound hypertension, and myocardial infarction have been described following abrupt cessation of beta-adrenoceptor blocking agents, such as propranolol. While such observable — and relatively uncommon — clinical events are sufficient to argue persuasively against the abrupt withdrawal of antianginal agents in patients with chronic stable angina, the association and frequency of silent myocardial ischemia from beta-blockade withdrawal has been less well studied. Furthermore, given the steadily increasing number of outpatients taking calcium antagonists alone and in combination with beta-blockers for treatment of chronic angina, two important questions regarding pharmacologic manipulation of these patient have surfaced: 1) does the presence of calcium blockers in individuals also taking beta-blockers protect against the beta-blockade withdrawal syndrome, and 2) what is the frequency of transient myocardial ischemia from abrupt cessation of calcium antagonist monotherapy?

In an attempt to answer these questions, a study from Denmark investigated the occurrence of transient myocardial ischemia as detected by ambulatory electrocardiographic monitoring. In 47 patients with chronic stable angina and proven coronary artery disease, abrupt withdrawal of beta-blockers, either as monotherapy or in combination with calcium antagonists (group 1, n = 25), was compared with abrupt cessation of calcium antagonist monotherapy (group 2, n = 22) as regards the occurrence of symptomatic cardiac events and total ischemic activity as measured by ambulatory monitoring. The first two monitorings were performed in the hospital (at entry into study and at 48 hours after withdrawal of drugs) and the third monitoring, 5 days after withdrawal, was performed out of the hospital and during daily activity (monitoring occasions 1, 2, and 3).

The investigators found that in group 1, the frequency of total ischemia increased by 64% and 148% from monitoring occasions 1 and 2 and 1 to 3, respectively, and *silent* ischemia increased by 100% and 129%, respectively. However, no significant change in transient myocardial ischemia following cessation of drug was noted in group 2 (calcium monotherapy). The heart rate at onset of ischemia increased significantly in group 1 in contrast to group 2, which had significant increases only during out-of-hospital monitoring periods. Based on these results, the researchers concluded that a rebound in ischemic activity — predominantly *silent* — occurs after abrupt withdrawal of beta-blockers and that angina does not, in itself, seem to be a reliable parameter for assessing ischemic activity. Furthermore, it seems that combined therapy with calcium antagonists neither protects against the effects of beta-blocker withdrawal nor increases ischemic activity.

The results of this investigation make it clear that abrupt withdrawal from beta-blockade may result in transient myocardial ischemia whether or not patients manifest clinical symptoms (e.g., angina). In fact, the finding of predominantly *silent* ischemia with beta-blocker cessation suggests that all patients should be considered at risk for potential morbid cardiac events when such therapy is abruptly discontinued. Put another way, this study suggests that relying exclusively on clinical symptomatology to indicate adverse effects of antianginal drug withdrawal may lead to a serious underestimation of ischemic phenomena as measured by ST-segment depression on ambulatory electrocardiogram (ECG). Unfortunately, this study did not address the question as to whether gradual withdrawal of beta-receptor blockade is preferable to sudden cessation.

The role of calcium antagonists has also been clarified. Based on this study, it appears as if abrupt withdrawal of this class of antianginal agents is not associated with significant transient myocardial ischemia. And, finally, the presence of calcium antagonists does not protect against ischemic events produced by beta-blocker withdrawal.

Calcium Channel Blockers

Patients with calcium channel blocker toxicity usually present with an accentuation of the drug's desired clinical effects, i.e., high degree of atrioventricular (AV) block, hypotension, and, on occasion, CNS changes or congestive heart failure.

Hypotension results from the drug's direct effect on ventricular and vascular smooth muscle and has been reported in 3.4 to 6% of patients taking nifedipine and in 5 to 10% of patients treated with verapamil for supraventricular tachycardia. Although most cases of hypotension are mild, some patients will require aggressive treatment. Infusion of IV calcium appears to be the best available treatment for such overdoses. The initial dose of 10 to 20 ml of a 10% calcium gluconate solution may be repeated every 8 hours. For cases refractory to IV calcium, fluids and vasopressors may be necessary.

Bradycardia and a high degree of AV block may also occur, and they are most often associated with verapamil or diltiazem use, because of their potent, negative inotropic effect on the sinus and AV nodes. In such cases, temporary pacing may be required. Because of its potent, negative inotropic effect on the ventricle, verapamil or diltiazem can precipitate congestive heart failure in patients with depressed myocardial contractility. Headache is a common side effect and is most commonly seen in patients taking nifedipine. Other CNS side effects include dizziness, sleep disturbance, and mood changes.

The variability of action among calcium antagonists is so pronounced that interchanging one calcium channel blocker for another sometimes proves impossible. In contrast to the case of beta-blockers or theophylline derivatives, in which differences among agents basically involve such minor factors as duration of action, appearance of CNS side effects, or receptor subselectivity, the various calcium channel blockers often cannot treat the same disease process.

Such differences in clinical effect do offer distinct advances in terms of individualizing therapy, however. A patient with angina, AV node conduction disturbance, and mild congestive heart failure, for instance, would benefit most from nifedipine. In this patient, nifedipine 1) relaxes coronary artery tone, which helps the angina, 2) does not change directly SA or AV node conduction, which leaves the conduction disturbance unaffected, and 3) dilates peripheral vessels (decreasing afterload and, thereby, myocardial oxygen demand), which aids the congestive heart failure. Using either diltiazem or verapamil in the same patient would primarily treat the anginal symptoms, may possibly exacerbate the conduction disturbance, would probably not affect the congestive heart failure significantly, and may even make it worse.

In contrast to verapamil and diltiazem, which should not be prescribed to patients with sinoatrial disease, atrioventricular block, congestive heart failure, or severe ventricular dysfunction (and only cautiously to those on a beta-blocker), nifedipine does not affect electrical conduction anywhere in the heart and can be used safely in patients with the aforementioned conditions. The net physiologic effects of nifedipine's actions are 1) increased coronary blood flow, 2) decreased afterload, 3) reduced myocardial oxygen consumption, and 4) increased cardiac output.

Because nifedipine is the most potent peripheral and coronary vasodilator among the calcium channel blockers and because it decreases systemic vascular resistance — thus decreasing afterload and improving cardiac output — it is more suitable for combined therapy with a beta-blocker or digitalis. Its pharmacologic advantages make nifedipine the initial drug of choice in elderly patients who have marginal cardiac output, are prone to episodes of congestive heart failure, are taking beta-blockers or digitalis, or have a history of conduction disturbances. Nifedipine has also been used as monotherapy in elderly patients and seems to be very effective. Of clinical importance is the fact that the reflex tachycardia sometimes reported with nifedipine tends to be less of a problem for the elderly, because baroreceptor sensitivity is often reduced in this population.

Several studies have concluded that combined treatment with beta-blockers and nifedipine increases antianginal efficacy compared with monotherapies, without increasing adverse effects. Moreover, nifedipine rarely precipitates congestive heart failure or profound bradycardia, two adverse consequences that have been observed with the other calcium channel blockers.

In one large study designed to measure the safety of combined intravenous diltiazem and propranolol therapy for angina, cardiac output was lowered in all patients, and because of the additive negative dromotropic activities of these two drugs, the researchers concluded that ECG monitoring was warranted. Frequent episodes of profound asymptomatic bradycardia (rates less than 50) have also been observed with combined oral therapy of diltiazem and beta-blockers.

There has been considerable controversy regarding the appropriate use of the different calcium channel blockers (nifedipine, verapamil, and diltiazem) in patients with coronary artery disease. Some experts have argued that because of its depressive effect on sinoatrial node automaticity, increase in AV node conduction time, and decrease in cardiac muscle contractility, diltiazem (Cardizem) should not be used in patients with left ventricular dysfunction. The calcium blocker, nifedipine (Procardia), on the other hand, does not suppress sinus node rate, decreases afterload, and increases cardiac output, which has prompted some cardiologists to recommend its use as an angina agent in the subpopulation of cardiac patients with left ventricular dysfunction.

The potential wisdom of these approaches is now somewhat clearer. According to a 5-year multicenter trial, there is now strong evidence to suggest that postinfarction patients with left ventricular dysfunction (i.e., ejection fraction less than 40%) should not be given the calcium antagonist diltiazem. The 23-center study with 2,466 patients who had isoenzyme-proven Q-wave or non-Q-wave myocardial infarction were randomized to 60 mg of diltiazem 4 times a day or placebo and then followed for 12 to 52 months. Although total cardiac mortality appeared to be equal for placebo and diltiazem-treated groups, when investigators began to look at results in specific patient subgroups, they found marked differences between diltiazem and placebo.

When ejection fraction fell below 40%, diltiazem was associated with significantly increased risk represented by a 1.31 hazard ratio as compared to the control group (hazard ratio = 1.0). Moreover, the risk of adverse cardiac consequences increased as the ejection fraction fell. Although a deleterious effect of diltiazem (1.41 hazard ratio) was also observed in those patients who had x-ray manifestations of pulmonary congestion upon admission, the drug seemed to benefit those patients without congestion and ejection fractions greater than 40%.

Investigators cited left ventricular dysfunction as the principal factor determining the potential benefits versus drawbacks of diltiazem therapy. Based on this multicenter trial, it seems prudent to withhold therapy with the calcium antagonist diltiazem in those postinfarction patients with either 1) an ejection fraction less than 40%, 2) x-ray proven pulmonary congestion upon admission, or 3) chronic congestive heart failure. Although, at present, no comparative data are available for the calcium antagonist nifedipine, it may be that its potent vasodilatory effects and capacity for increasing cardiac output will make it the calcium channel blocker of choice in this prespecified patient population.

Antiarrhythmics

Appropriate therapy for ventricular arrhythmias remains a dilemma for the practicing clinician. While a host of potent antiarrhythmic agents are now available that can ameliorate or eradicate most serious rhythm disturbances, the long-term survival benefit of such therapy is unproven. Furthermore, these agents have numerous adverse effects well known to primary care practitioners, ranging from benign problems, such as rash or gastrointestinal intolerance, to serious hematologic or immunologic derangements.

In recent years, the paradoxical tendency for these drugs to induce rather than control arrhythmias has become more widely recognized and a cause for great concern. Drug-associated arrhythmias, or proarrhythmias, have ranged from an increase in premature ventricular contractions to life-threatening phenomena, such as refractory ventricular tachycardia, torsades de pointes ventricular tachycardia associated with marked prolongation of the QT interval, and ventricular fibrillation.

The purpose of one retrospective study was to evaluate the clinical and electrocardiographic features of drug-associated ventricular fibrillation in a large group of patients seen at a referral center over a 5-year period. In particular, the investigators sought to define the time between the initiation of therapy and the onset of fibrillation, and to identify clinical or laboratory parameters that predicted this occurrence.[24]

The study group consisted of 28 patients, from among 603 referred for evaluation, who had 38 episodes of drug-associated ventricular fibrillation. Data on each patient were obtained from review of available medical records, including age, sex, type of heart disease, functional class, and left ventricular ejection fraction when available. For each episode of fibrillation, dosage of antiarrhythmic and duration of therapy prior to the event, serum drug and potassium levels on the day fibrillation occurred, and electrocardiograms after fibrillation, as well as in the control of drug-free state, were obtained. In addition, a subgroup of 26 patients receiving quinidine, procainamide, or disopyramide as a single antiarrhythmic agent who developed fibrillation was compared to a control group of 62 patients who received these same agents but did not develop fibrillation.

The most striking finding from this review was that the interval between the initiation of antiarrhythmic therapy and onset of ventricular fibrillation was usually very short. For the whole study group, the median duration of therapy before fibrillation onset was 4 days, while, for the group receiving quinidine, procainamide, or disopyramide, the median duration was only 3 days. Over 70% of drug-induced fibrillation occurred within 10 days of the onset of therapy.

In comparing the study group that developed fibrillation versus the control group that did not, the left ventricular ejection fraction was significantly lower in the study group (0.28 versus 0.43). These individuals were also more likely to have received concomitant therapy with digitalis, diuretics, and potassium supplements, although there was no clinical or laboratory evidence of digitalis toxicity in any of these cases and the serum potassium level was less than 3.5 mEq/L in only eight of the fibrillation episodes. The QT interval before drug therapy was slightly longer in the study group, but there was no significant difference between the groups in the degree of QT prolongation while receiving antiarrhythmics.[24]

Primary care practitioners need to recognize the significant potential hazards of antiarrhythmic drug therapy. In particular, the proarrhythmic potential of these agents can be life threatening. Left ventricular dysfunction and concomitant treatment with digitalis and diuretics predispose patients to the development of ventricular fibrillation during antiarrhythmic therapy. Drug-induced ventricular fibrillation seems to be a very early event, frequently occurring within 3 days of initiating treatment and most often by 10 days.

Based on these findings, it seems prudent to initiate antiarrhythmic therapy in a monitored inpatient setting whenever possible, especially in those at increased risk for ventricular fibrillation (i.e., those on digitalis therapy or the presence of low left ventricular ejection fraction). Furthermore, until more data are available regarding the long-term survival benefit of antiarrhythmic therapy, these agents should be used very judiciously and reserved for those with malignant and symptomatic ventricular arrhythmias. Finally, with respect to assessment and triage of patients on antiarrhythmic therapy, physicians should maintain a high index of suspicion in those patients complaining of syncopal symptoms, palpitations, or other manifestations of cerebral hypoperfusion within a few days of initiation of such therapy.

Lidocaine. Occurring either in a prehospital or an ED setting, lidocaine toxicity alters conduction (high degree of atrioventricular block, asystole, and widened QRS complex) and impairs myocardial contractility. It most often affects the central nervous system and usually occurs during rapid IV infusion. CNS effects include lightheadedness, somnolence, coma, and seizures. Supportive care and discontinuation of lidocaine infusion are generally sufficient treatment in the emergency setting.

Fluid repletion or pharmacologic cardiac acceleration may be necessary for hypotension due to heart block or negative inotropic actions. Treat seizures with benzodiazepines (Valium, 5 to 10 mg IV) rather than phenytoin.[22]

Quinidine. Quinidine toxicity may be either acute or chronic. Many of the gastrointestinal, CNS, ECG, and other findings (headache, flushed skin, blurred vision with mydriasis) are similar to findings seen in anticholinergic stimulation. This correspondence suggests that quinidine and other anticholinergic drugs, such as cyclic antidepressants and antipsychotics, may produce an additive effect.

The ECG changes, which consist primarily of conduction delays including PR, QRS, and QT prolongation, correlate closely with the severity of the clinical course. Quinidine toxicity may also cause severe hypotension and severe systemic acidosis.

In addition to supportive treatment, studies suggest that alkalinization may be appropriate for quinidine toxicity since alkaline serum decreases the free levels of the highly protein-bound drug.[22]

The newer antiarrhythmic oral agents, tocainide, mexiletine, and flecainide, produce a number of CNS and gastrointestinal side effects, some of which may necessitate discontinuing the drug in an elderly patient. Approximately 20% of all elderly patients taking tocainide stop the drug because of dizziness, confusion, nightmares, coma, or seizures. Gastrointestinal side effects that precipitate discontinuance include nausea, vomiting, and constipation. Mexiletine produces the same CNS and GI symptomatology as tocainide, and discontinuance rates as high as 40% have been reported.

Digitalis

Geriatric patients are at high risk for developing toxicity from digitalis glycosides. Several factors lead to increased risk, including concurrent administration of other drugs such as quinidine or disopyramide and metabolic abnormalities such as hypokalemia, hypomagnesemia, and renal failure. Toxicity should be suspected in any patient taking digoxin who develops new gastrointestinal, ocular, or central nervous system complaints, or in whom sinus bradycardia, AV conduction defects, junctional tachycardia, or premature ventricular contractions (PVCs) develop without an underlying cause.

Anorexia, confusion, and depression are the most common symptoms of digoxin intoxication, while nausea, vomiting, and visual changes, so common in young patients, are frequently absent in the elderly. However, elderly patients may develop CNS symptoms of digoxin toxicity even with normal plasma digoxin levels.

Geriatric patients' complaints are nonspecific and include anorexia, abdominal pain, fatigue, malaise, headache, and visual disturbances. Cardiac toxicity may be present, with increased vagal tone or enhanced automaticity producing sinus bradycardia, variable degrees of AV conduction block, or ventricular ectopy. Ventricular arrhythmias are the most common dysrhythmic derangements, but atrial and junctional tachycardias with variable nodal conduction blocks also occur in 2 to 6% of patients.[25]

Serum digoxin levels should be obtained whenever you suspect underdigitalization or overdigitalization, or when progressive cardiac or renal failure occurs. Levels above 2 ng/ml are associated with increased risk of toxic effects.

The clinical pharmacology of digoxin depends on various parameters, including absorption, distribution, metabolism, and elimination. Increasing age seems to be associated with delayed absorption of digoxin. Other medications, including kaolin pectate, cholestyramine, neomycin, and metoclopramide may also delay absorption when given concurrently.

Drug interactions further complicate digoxin therapy. Disopyramide and quinidine reduce digoxin clearance by nearly 50%. Spironolactone and calcium channel blockers may also increase the serum digoxin level. Therefore, levels should be obtained to anticipate toxicity when these drugs are part of the patient's regimen. Hypokalemia associated with concurrent diuretic therapy augments digitalis cardiotoxicity.

Management consists of stopping digoxin therapy, cardiac monitoring, maintaining normal to high-normal serum potassium levels, and, when toxicity is life threatening, initiating appropriate antiarrhythmic therapy (phenytoin 50 mg/min until a loading dose of 1,000 mg is achieved) in combination with antidigoxin antibodies.

Although digitalis has been the cornerstone of therapy for congestive heart failure for more than two centuries, the use of digoxin in such patients remains controversial. Some studies have shown that digoxin may be discontinued without adverse consequences in up to 75% of patients with stable heart failure and sinus rhythm, while other experts consider atrial fibrillation with a rapid ventricular response to be the only absolute indication for digoxin therapy. Additional debate over the potential CNS depressive effects of the drug (especially in the postmyocardial infarction [MI] period), its potential proarrhythmic properties, and controversy regarding the effect of digoxin on the long-term survival of patients with ischemic heart disease have induced the Captopril-Digoxin Multicenter Research Group to examine the comparative efficacy and safety of digoxin versus captopril therapy in patients with mild to moderate heart failure.

The principal objective of their randomized, double-blind multicenter trial was: 1) to determine whether treatment with captopril or digoxin, in addition to diuretic maintenance therapy, was associated with improved exercise tolerance during a period of 6 months and 2) to assess the relative proportions of patients on each drug requiring hospitalization or emergency department visits for exacerbations of congestive heart failure.[25]

Entry criteria included patients younger than age 75 years who had a left ventricular ejection fraction less than 40%, a treadmill exercise time (greater than 4 minutes, but less than the age- and sex-predicted average maximum) limited by dyspnea or fatigue, and sinus rhythm and heart failure secondary to ischemic heart disease or primary myocardial disease. The investigators concluded that compared with placebo, captopril therapy resulted in significantly improved treadmill exercise time (mean increase 82 s versus 35 s) and improved New York Heart Association class (41% versus 22%), but digoxin therapy did not. Although digoxin treatment increased ejection fraction (4.4% increase) compared with captopril (1.8% increase) and placebo (0.9% increase), the number of ventricular premature beats (VPBs) decreased 45% in the captopril group and increased 4% in the digoxin group in those patients whose baseline ambulatory electrocardiogram revealed more than 10 premature beats per hour.

With respect to treatment failures, the requirements for stepped-up diuretic therapy, hospitalization, and emergency visits were significantly more in the patients receiving placebo compared with those receiving either active drug. A greater number of possible adverse side effects such as transitory hypotension, dizziness, or lightheadedness were attributable to captopril (44.2% of patients) during the blinded portion of the study than to either digoxin (30.2%) or placebo, even though the rate of discontinuation was lower in the captopril (2.9%) versus digoxin group (4.2%). Based on this study, the authors conclude that captopril treatment is significantly more effective than placebo and is an alternative to digoxin therapy in patients with mild to moderate heart failure who are receiving diuretic maintenance therapy.

A recent study of outpatient prescribing practices in the elderly suggests that most physicians prescribe diuretics alone or in combination with digoxin for the initial pharmacologic maintenance of patients with mild to moderate heart failure and sinus rhythm. Despite the widespread use of digoxin, controversy remains concerning the wisdom, side effects, and overall efficacy (i.e., improvement in functional status) of using digoxin in patients with heart failure and sinus rhythm.

Based on the results of this first placebo-controlled trial comparing the effects of digoxin and captopril treatment, in which exercise time and functional class improved significantly in the captopril but not digoxin group, it now appears reasonable for physicians to prescribe captopril (25 mg t.i.d. for the first week, and then increase to 50 mg t.i.d., if tolerated) as a first-line adjunct to diuretic therapy in the patient *with mild to moderate* heart failure. Although this group of patients can be expected to have both a diminished mean VPB and lower treatment failure rate, the physician should still observe for potential side effects attributable to captopril therapy.

This trial included primarily patients in NYHA functional class II. It is important to note, however, that 34 patients with major cardiac symptoms, including 30 with increased heart failure, were excluded from the study and, therefore, no recommendations can be made at present regarding the safety or efficacy of captropril in subgroups with higher degrees of functional impairment. Finally, the fact that 58% of the captopril group studied were previously on digoxin therapy (before being assigned randomly to the captopril therapy) suggests that captopril might be efficacious in patients who fail to respond to digoxin therapy (treatment failures) or cannot tolerate the drug due to adverse side effects.

Antihypertensive Drug Toxicity

Seventy percent of the elderly individuals treated with antihypertensive medications show symptoms of sadness, fatigue, apathy, agitation, or insomnia. Reserpine, propranolol, and methyldopa are the worse offenders, but clonidine, guanethidine, and hydralazine are also capable of producing symptoms of mental depression. Other nonantihypertensive agents with similar effects include neuroleptics, tranquilizers, hypnotics, digoxin, antiparkinsonian drugs, anticancer agents, corticosteroids, and nonsteroidal anti-inflammatory agents (NSAIDs). (See Table 5–11.)

Used both in the management of congestive heart failure and hypertension, *diuretics* are associated with

Table 5–11   Evolution of Antihypertensive Drug Therapy

Step	1970	1980	Current
I	Diuretic	Beta-blocker/diuretic	Vasodilator, alpha-blocker, angiotensin converting enzyme (ACE) inhibitor, calcium antagonist
II	Sympatholytic, methyldopa, beta-blocker, reserpine, etc.	Diuretic/beta-blocker	Diuretic/beta-blocker
III	Vasodilator hydralazine, minoxidil	Vasodilator hydralazine, minoxidil, alpha-blocker, ACE inhibitor, calcium antagonist	Beta-blocker/diuretic
IV	Others	Others	Others

more adverse reactions than any other drug. They are also among the most commonly prescribed drugs for the elderly. Hypovolemia and postural hypotension, electrolyte imbalances (hyponatremia, hypercalcemia, and hypokalemia), glucose intolerance, and hyperuricemia are the most common adverse reactions (Table 5–12).

Hypokalemia may induce or augment digoxin toxicity, while severe hyponatremia may produce stupor, seizures, and coma. Mild hyperuricemia is common but rarely induces an acute gouty attack. Serum uric acid levels, however, can be helpful when the patient presents with a monoarticular arthritis.

Finally, loop diuretics can induce painful urinary retention and symptoms of prostatism in elderly men with gland enlargement. Spironolactone and triamterene may induce hyperkalemia in patients with reduced renal failure or those taking ACE inhibitors.

The *centrally acting sympatholytic drugs,* clonidine and methyldopa, can cause postural hypotension, CNS depression, and sexual dysfunction (Table 5–13). The CNS depression associated with clonidine decreases mental acuity so that patients can appear "senile" or demented in addition to feeling tired or drowsy. Moreover, sudden discontinuation of clonidine can cause a withdrawal syndrome of headache, sweating, and rebound hypertension. If a patient on clonidine therapy presents with symptoms of rebound hypertension, insomnia, headache, or arrhythmias, suspect that the patient may have discontinued the drug abruptly.

All antihypertensives, including thiazide diuretics and spironolactone, may cause sexual dysfunction. Patients may complain of depression and fatigue in an attempt to mask underlying sexual dysfunction. Methyldopa and clonidine can also cause gynecomastia.

Peripheral vasodilators used to treat hypertension may produce symptoms that induce the elderly to seek emergency care. Hydralazine (Apresoline) and prazosin (Minipress) are useful for either hypertension alone or in association with congestive heart failure. Enalapril, lisinopril, and captopril are also vasodilators that block the formation of angiotensin II (Table 5–14).[1,7]

Elderly patients may experience sudden syncope after taking the first dose of prazosin or report some combination of dizziness, headache, or lethargy. Usually, these symptoms will clear after 2 or 3 days of therapy. The concomitant intake of beta-blockers or diuretics may enhance this first-dose side effect (Table 5–15).

Hydralazine, which is contraindicated in coronary artery or valvular disease, can produce CNS manifestations, such as headache or depression. Reflex tachycardia, angina, lupus syndrome, and fluid retention have also been reported.

Although it is associated with fewer side effects and is increasingly popular in treating hypertension, ACE inhibitors can produce a number of symptoms and side effects including hyperkalemia. Captopril (Capoten) may

Table 5–12   Side Effects of Commonly Used Diuretics

Diuretic	Hypo-kalemia	Hyper-kalemia	Acidosis	Alkalosis	Hyper-uricemia	Hyper-calcemia	Hyper-glycemia	Hypertri-glyceridemia	Hypo-natremia	Hypo-magnesemia
Thiazide	+	−	−	+	+	+	+	+	+	+
Loop diuretics	+	−	−	+	+	−	+	+	+	+
Potassium-sparing	−	+	+	−	−	−	−	−	−	+

Table 5–13   Adverse Side Effects of Antihypertensive Drugs

	Impotence	Ejaculation difficulties	Decreased libido	Gyneco-mastia
Thiazides	?	−	+	−
Spironolactone	+	−	+	+
Methyldopa	+	+	+	+
Clonidine	+	+	−	+
Propranolol	+	−	+	−
Hydralazine	?	−	−	−
Prazosin	+	−	−	−

Table 5–14   Antihypertensive Drug and Disease Interaction Profiles

	Alpha-blockers	ACE inhibitors	Beta-blockers	Calcium antagonists	Diuretics
Effects of antihypertensive agents on coexisting disease					
Angina	No effect	Beneficial (?)	Beneficial	Beneficial	No effect
CHF	± Beneficial	Beneficial	Worsen	± Beneficial	Beneficial
Arrhythmias	No effect	No effect	± Beneficial	Beneficial	May worsen
COPD	No effect	No effect	Worsen	Beneficial (?)	No effect
Effects of antihypertensive agents on concomitant metabolic disorders					
Hyperlipidemia	Improve	No effect	Worsen	No effect	Worsen
Diabetes	No effect	No effect	May worsen	May worsen (?)	Worsen
Hypokalemia	No effect	May correct	No effect	No effect	Worsen
Hyperuricemia	No effect	No effect	No effect	No effect	Worsen

Table 5–15   Drugs Causing Orthostatic Hypotension

Benzothiadiazides	Methotrimeprazine
Bretylium	Methyldopa
Captopril	Methysergide
Chlorisondamine	Minoxidil
Clonidine	Nifedipine
Cyclic antidepressants	Nitroglycerin
Furosemide	Pentolinium
Guanethidine	Phenothiazines
Guanidine	Phenoxybenzamine
Hexamethonium	Prazosin
Hydralazine	Procarbazine
Iopanoic acid	Reserpine
Levodopa	Thiothixene
Lidocaine	

produce proteinuria, reversible neutropenia, dermatitis, and angioedema. Enalapril (Vasotec) produces syncope in 1% of elderly patients who use the drug, as well as headache and dizziness. ACE inhibitors may cause hypotension in patients who are hypovolemic and taking diuretic therapy. Consequently, stopping diuretic therapy one week before beginning therapy with ACE inhibitors is generally recommended. The hypotensive effect of these drugs is also enhanced by the calcium channel blocker nifedipine — or significantly diminished by NSAIDs.

Over the past decade, the pharmacotherapeutic landscape for the treatment of hypertension has witnessed major tectonic shifts. Recently, physicians have been deluged by an avalanche of newly approved pharmaceuticals — from ACE inhibitors to long-acting, cardioselective beta-antagonists and combinations thereof — aimed at the primary treatment of hypertension.

Given the wide variety and proven efficacy of so many available agents, optimal antihypertensive therapy has become less a matter of selecting a drug that adequately controls diastolic and systolic blood pressure than of selecting an agent or regimen that is predictably associated with high patient compliance, a low incidence of adverse drug reactions, minimal interdrug toxicity, and preservation of quality of life, including cognitive and sexual function. As better-tolerated agents become available and long-term, large-scale studies on hypertension begin to yield statistically significant morbidity and mortality data, the focus has now shifted on the comparative ability of different antihypertensives to reduce total, cardiac, and stroke morbidity and mortality.

Left ventricular enlargement is a well-recognized marker of cardiac dysfunction of various causes and, in coronary artery disease, left ventricular volume is the best predictor of long-term survival. Dilatation of the left ventricle begins soon after an acute myocardial infarction and, in animal models, continues well after healing of the infarcted area has been documented histologically. This sustained enlargement of the left ventricle in animal models has been moderated by the long-term use of the ACE inhibitor captopril, with resultant improved survival.

One prospective, randomized, double-blind, placebo-controlled trial had three objectives: to determine whether left ventricular dilatation continues beyond the acute phase of myocardial infarction in humans; whether persistent ACE inhibition changes the long-term process; and whether captopril treatment improves exercise performance in patients with diminished left ventricular function without overt congestive heart failure.

Fifty-nine patients who had sustained a first myocardial infarction involving the anterior wall and with a radionuclide ejection fraction of 45% or less were randomized. Thirty patients received captopril in a blinded fashion beginning an average of 20 days after infarction and titrated to a target dose of 50 mg three times per day,

and 29 patients received placebo. The two groups were comparable in terms of coronary risk factors, peak creatine kinase concentration, pretreatment hemodynamics and functional status, and prior use of thrombolytic or angioplasty therapy. The study medication was added to optimal conventional therapy, including diuretics, digitalis, antiarrhythmics, and beta-blockade as deemed appropriate by the treating physician. Baseline catheterization was performed in all patients and repeated 1 year later, and exercise stress testing was performed quarterly.

At 1-year follow-up, left ventricular size as measured by end-diastolic volume increased significantly and left ventricular filling pressure remained elevated in the placebo group. In those treated with captopril, the increase in end-diastolic volume was not significant and filling pressure decreased. In a subset of patients with persistent occlusion of the left anterior descending artery and, therefore, at high risk for ventricular enlargement, captopril prevented further dilatation. The exercise duration in the captopril group consistently exceeded that in the placebo group at 3, 9, and 12 months.

The authors conclude that left ventricular enlargement following anterior myocardial infarction is a progressive process that may be moderated by treatment with captopril resulting in reduced filling pressures and improved exercise tolerance.

Salvage of ischemic myocardium in an effort to preserve left ventricular function in the setting of acute myocardial infarction has been a major focus of cardiologists in recent years. Primary care physicians, often entrusted with the long-term management of patients post-MI, have concentrated on risk factor modification and the use of antiplatelet or beta-blocker therapy to reduce the chances of recurrent infarction. This study provides preliminary evidence to suggest that it may become common to add ACE inhibitor therapy to the long-term outpatient treatment regimen of patients who have sustained a myocardial infarction.

Although the size of the study was small and restricted to those with anterior infarction and reduced ventricular function and the follow-up was only for 1 year, the salutary benefits of captopril therapy were significant. Coupled with results of other studies that have shown survival benefits in patients with congestive heart failure treated with ACE inhibition, it suggests that these agents interrupt a pathophysiologic sequence that promotes ventricular enlargement and dysfunction post-MI and in other situations causing heart failure.

It is interesting to speculate on the results of larger studies (currently ongoing) of longer term captopril therapy and whether any beneficial effects will be demonstrated with other ACE inhibitors. Most likely, evidence will continue to mount to support the use of ACE inhibitors as cornerstone therapy for heart failure precipitated by myocardial infarction and other causes.

Using data collected as part of the European MAPHY (Metoprolol Atherosclerosis Prevention in Hypertensives) Trial, a randomized, prospective study was designed to investigate whether metoprolol, a relatively beta-1-selective beta-blocker, given as initial antihypertensive treatment to white men aged 40 to 64 years, lowers cardiovascular complications of high blood pressure to a greater extent than thiazide diuretics. The investigators randomized 1,609 (8,110 patient years) patients to metoprolol and 1,625 (8,070 patient years) to a thiazide diuretic, with a mean follow-up time of 4.2 years. The mean dose of metoprolol was 174 mg/d and, of thiazide diuretics, 46 mg/d of hydrochlorothiazide. Both study groups achieved identical control of blood pressure using a fixed therapeutic schedule. The investigators randomized both previously treated patients and those with newly detected and untreated hypertension. The patients' diastolic blood pressure in the sitting position was 100 mm Hg or greater and less than 130 mm Hg at randomization. Since this was a study of primary prevention, previous myocardial infarction, angina pectoris, and stroke were exclusive criteria. Also excluded were patients with secondary hypertension, second- and third-degree atrioventricular block, cardiac failure, obstructive lung disease not well-controlled by beta-2 stimulants, and diabetes mellitus.

The investigators concluded that starting antihypertensive therapy in men with mild to moderate hypertension with the beta-1-selective beta-blocker — metoprolol — instead of a thiazide diuretic leads to a total mortality reduction of −68% to −17% (95% confidence limits). The lower total mortality can be ascribed to fewer deaths from coronary heart disease and stroke, a benefit that also extends to hypertensive smokers. Whether the improved mortality data are in any way specific to metoprolol or can be extended to other beta-blockers or nondiuretic antihypertensive drugs could not be answered by the present trial.

Several widely cited studies reported during the late 1970s and early 1980s proved conclusively that first-line treatment of hypertension with diuretics prevented or delayed several well-known complications of hypertension, including renal failure, heart failure, accelerated hypertension, and stroke. Despite these well-documented advantages, the effect of diuretics on reduction of deaths from coronary heart disease was not encouraging. This large, randomized study is significant, then, because it attempts to provide scientific proof that beta-blocker therapy used as initial therapy in mild to moderate hypertensives can lower total mortality from coronary heart disease better than thiazide diuretics.

Based on the findings from the MAPHY Trial, it is reasonable for physicians to use metoprolol as initial therapy for mild to moderate hypertension in white middle-aged men who have no previous history of heart dis-ease, stroke, or diabetes. Compared to thiazide diuretics, this agent can be expected to lower total mortality in both smokers and nonsmokers. The value of other beta-1-selective beta-blockers for primary prevention of death from coronary heart disease and stroke cannot be assessed from this study. (See Table 5–16.)

Table 5–16   Drug Interactions in Antihypertensive Therapy

Diuretics

Diuretics can raise lithium blood levels by enhancing proximal tubular reabsorption of lithium

NSAIDs, including aspirin, may antagonize antihypertensive and natriuretic effectiveness of diuretics

ACE inhibitors magnify potassium-sparing effects of triamterene, amiloride, or spironolactone

ACE inhibitors blunt hypokalemia induced by thiazide diuretics

Sympatholytic agents

Guanethidine monosulfate and guanadrel sulfate. Ephedrine and amphetamine displace guanethidine and guanadrel from storage vesicles. Tricyclic antidepressants inhibit uptake of guanethidine and guanadrel into these vesicles. Cocaine may inhibit neuronal pump that actively transports guanethidine and guanadrel into nerve endings. These actions may reduce antihypertensive effects of guanethidine and guanadrel

Hypertension can occur with concomitant therapy with phenothiazines or sympathomimetic amines

Monoamine oxidase inhibitors may prevent degradation and metabolism of released norepinephrine produced by tyramine-containing foods and may thereby cause hypertension

Tricyclic antidepressant drugs may reduce effects of clonidine and guanabenz

Beta-blockers

Cimetidine may reduce bioavailability of beta-blockers metabolized primarily by the liver by inducing hepatic oxidative enzymes. Hydralazine, by reducing hepatic blood flow, may increase plasma concentration of beta-blockers

Cholesterol-binding resins, i.e., cholestyramine and colestipol, may reduce plasma levels of propranolol hydrochloride

Beta-blockers may reduce plasma clearance of drugs metabolized by the liver (e.g., lidocaine, chlorpromazine, coumarin)

Combinations of calcium channel blockers and beta-blockers may promote negative inotropic effects on the failing myocardium

Combinations of beta-blockers and reserpine may cause marked bradycardia and syncope

ACE inhibitors. Nonsteroidal anti-inflammatory drugs, including aspirin, may magnify potassium-retaining effects of ACE inhibitors

Calcium antagonists

Combinations of calcium antagonists with quinidine may induce hypotension, particularly in patients with idiopathic hypertrophic subaortic stenosis

Calcium antagonists may induce increases in plasma digoxin levels

Cimetidine may increase blood levels of nifedipine

ANTIHYPERTENSIVE AGENTS: MANAGEMENT OVERVIEW

Since publication in 1984 of the last report of the Joint National Committee (JNC) on Detection, Evaluation, and Treatment of High Blood Pressure, there has been a significant decline in both national age-adjusted stroke mortality and in mortality associated with coronary artery disease. These impressive improvements have been accompanied by dramatic alterations in the pharmacologic and nonpharmacologic treatment of hypertension, the majority of which were addressed in the 1988 JNC report. Based on the latest scientific research, this comprehensive federal blueprint, produced under the auspices of a multimember committee chaired by Boston University's Aram V. Chobanian, represents state-of-the-art thinking regarding evaluation and management of high blood pressure.

Updating findings contained in previous reports, the 1988 JNC report is intended to serve as a guide for practicing physicians in their care of hypertensive patients and to guide health professionals participating in community-based high blood pressure programs. Directing its recommendations toward the treatment of 58 million Americans with high blood pressure, the 1988 white paper broadens the time-honored step-care approach to provide more flexibility for clinicians. Perhaps the most important change introduced by the JNC is the expansion of initial pharmacologic monotherapy to include both ACE inhibitors and calcium channel antagonists *in addition* to thiazide-type diuretics and beta-blockers recommended by the 1984 JNC report. Addressing special populations with management problems, the authors of the current report observe that, with respect to drug therapy, black patients usually do not respond as well to beta-blockers or ACE inhibitors as do whites and that diuretics are generally more effective monotherapy than either beta-blockers or ACE inhibitors. With respect to elderly hypertensives, the report notes the efficacy of calcium antagonists as monotherapy and recommends centrally and peripherally acting adrenergic inhibitors as step 2 drugs.

In addition to making specific pharmacologic recommendations, the step-care approach to antihypertensive therapy has been refined considerably. Its equation now includes implementation of one among three options in the event that, after a 1- to 3-month interval, the patient's response to the initial agent has been *inadequate* and is not experiencing significant side effects from the initial agent. In such cases, it is recommended that the physician 1) increase the dose of the initial drug if it was prescribed below the recommended maximum dose, 2) add an agent from another class, or 3) discontinue the initial choice and substitute a drug from another class. A step-down (i.e., drug withdrawal) option is also suggested for those patients with mild hypertension who have satisfactorily controlled their blood pressure through treatment for at least 1 year.

Comprehensive in its scope and presentation of adverse drug reactions and interactions, the 1988 JNC report makes a plea not only for a systematic, judicious approach to pharmacologic therapy of high blood pressure but for ongoing physician monitoring of the impact of such therapy on quality of life.

Although much of the 1988 JNC report confirms and highlights the significant improvements in stroke and cardiac morbidity that can be achieved with treatment of high blood pressure, there are some new wrinkles worthy of note in the pharmacologic treatment sphere, especially the addition — or, put another way, upgrading — of calcium blockers and ACE inhibitors to the revered step 1 class of monotherapy agents. For example, the inclusion of ACE inhibitors now provides a unique therapeutic option for those hypertensive patients who may also require treatment for chronic congestive heart failure, whereas hypertensive patients suffering from chronic stable angina are uniquely positioned to benefit from both the antianginal and blood pressure–lowering effects of a *single* agent (e.g., calcium blocker). Moreover, the elderly patient who requires treatment with a NSAID can, by using a calcium antagonist, be spared the potential potassium-retaining complications of combined NSAID-ACE inhibitor therapy. The addition of these two classes also provides salutary options for a number of patients — diabetics, asthmatics, and individuals with left ventricular dysfunction — who, under the 1984 JNC regimens, might have been adversely affected by the negative inotropic properties of beta-blockers or the alterations in plasma lipids and blood glucose associated with thiazide diuretics.

Recently, large clinical trials and meta-analytical studies have repeatedly demonstrated that antihypertensive therapy will reduce stroke morbidity and may reduce incidence and mortality of cardiovascular disease caused by hypertension. The elderly have been shown to be among the most compliant patients (HDFP trial) of any hypertensive age group. In spite of their fragility, careful antihypertensive therapy can be expected to prolong their useful lives.

Studies show that physicians are notably poor at judging the effect of hypertensive therapy on quality of life. Interestingly, patients were found to be only marginally better at assessing their general well-being in a British study of the effects of antihypertensive therapy. The *spouse or house mate* was the most sensitive indicator of adverse effect on well-being and, thus, is the individual to be queried by the physician to give the best assessment in this regard.

Failure of an antihypertensive regimen to lower blood pressure must not necessarily be assumed to be failure of the drug. Compliance must be verified before additional drugs are added to prevent hypotension.

Nonpharmacologic therapy must be tried first, but the clinician must be realistic about expectations for a change of long-established behaviors. Salt restriction, weight reduction, and avoidance of alcohol are all admirable goals if the patient can be persuaded.

In general, the elderly respond to all available antihypertensive agents. Some trials suggest they may respond to a calcium channel blocker better than to a beta-blocker or an ACE inhibitor, although any one of these classes may be used as monotherapy in the elderly.

Since concomitant diseases are prevalent in the elderly, tailoring therapy to these disorders and vigilant anticipation of side effects is the most important part of antihypertensive management. Hypertensives with angina may improve with a beta-blocker or a calcium channel blocker. Congestive heart failure is frequently accompanied by, and even caused by, hypertension. These patients benefit from diuretics and vasodilators of all types, especially ACE inhibitors.

NITRATE THERAPY

The sublingual (nitroglycerin) and oral (isosorbide dinitrate) nitrate preparations are the principal antianginal agents, and promote vasodilation of both venous and, to a lesser extent, arterial vascular beds. In the coronary beds, nitrates redistribute blood flow along collateral routes to the underperfused myocardium.[19]

Adverse drug reactions. Orthostatic hypotension occurs commonly in the elderly. Tolerance and cross-tolerance between nitrates develops with repeated usage. Headache occurs early in the use and with excessive doses. Angina may develop or worsen with sudden withdrawal of nitrates.

Adverse drug interactions. Orthostatic hypotension occurs with the antihypertensives, especially the calcium channel blockers, phenothiazines, and alcohol.

Management. Patients inexperienced with nitrates should lie down for the first few doses in case of hypotension. This is usually associated with dehydration.

The onset of action of nitroglycerin topical ointment is 20 to 60 minutes and transdermal patch is 40 to 60 minutes. These are adequate for prophylaxis but too slow to respond to the immediate need during angina. Only sublingual nitroglycerin or sublingual/chewable isosorbide with an onset of action of 1 to 3 minutes should be used for the acute anginal attack.

To avoid nitrate tolerance, a low-nitrate or nitrate-free period each 24 hours should be provided. Transdermal patch or ointment should be left on only for 14 to 16 hours and then removed. Oral nitrate such as isosorbide should be used three times per day with the last dose near the evening meal. Oral nitrate schedules that provide the last dose at bedtime are associated with tolerance. If angina persists, a beta-blocker or a calcium channel blocker should be added.

NONSTEROIDAL ANTI-INFLAMMATORY DRUGS (NSAIDs)

> **CURRENT NSAIDs**
> Aspirin
> Ibuprofen
> Indomethacin (Indocin)
> Diflunisal (Dolobid)
> Fenoprofen (Nalfon)
> Ketoprofen (Orudis)
> Meclofenamic acid (Ponstel)
> Naproxen (Naprosyn)
> Piroxicam (Feldene)
> Sulindac (Clinoril)
> Tolmetin (Tolectin)

Adverse drug reactions. After the psychotropic and cardiovascular drugs, the NSAIDs, including aspirin, are the most frequent causes of drug-related morbidity and mortality in the elderly. Important forms of toxicity include gastritis, peptic ulceration and blood loss, and renal insufficiency. All NSAIDs are associated with these adverse drug reactions although some studies have identified piroxicam (Feldene) and sulindac (Clinoril) as clinically safer with respect to renal toxicity. All NSAIDs, except aspirin, cause readily reversible inhibition of platelet function. Aspirin has an irreversible effect on platelet function that lasts for the life of the platelet, 4 to 7 days. All of the NSAIDs can cause allergic reactions ranging from rash to anaphylaxis in patients allergic to aspirin. Aspirin taken chronically even in recommended amounts by the elderly may lead to chronic salicylism, which is characterized by deafness, marked fatigue, confused and withdrawn behavior, metabolic acidosis, and noncardiogenic pulmonary edema. CNS effects include dizziness, anxiety, tinnitus, and confusion and may occur in up to 10 to 20% of the elderly on chronic salicylate therapy. Hepatic reactions are usually mild when they occur, but severe hepatitis has been reported. Aplastic anemia has also been reported with all of the available NSAIDs.

Women older than 65 seem to be at greatest risk of gastrointestinal bleeding and gastric perforation associated with NSAIDs. A history of gastrointestinal (GI) bleeding and concomitant diuretic therapy are the two risk factors identified in this group of patients that predict poor outcome. These patients are also frequently dehydrated. In one retrospective study, sulindac was a statistically significant more common cause of GI bleeding than ibuprofen. It is not clear whether this drug is more ulcerogenic than ibuprofen because of inadequate controls.

A review of Medicaid administrations for elderly patients from two states with diagnoses of nephritis, nephropathy, and hyperkalemia showed a strong correlation with NSAID use. Three distinct renal syndromes are now associated with NSAIDs:

1. Patients with dehydration, congestive heart failure, nephrosis, or pre-existing renal insufficiency develop acute renal failure within days of initiating NSAID therapy. The urine sediment is normal.
2. Acute interstitial nephritis may occur at any time but usually occurs after months of NSAID exposure. There is no eosinophilia or eosinophiluria or rash. Patients present with the nephrotic syndrome (usually edematous).
3. Chronic interstitial nephritis has been associated with high-dose NSAIDs and other analgesics for years. Papillary necrosis is frequently present.

Adverse drug interactions. NSAIDs increased the bleeding tendency of patients on *Coumadin anti-coagulants.* Mixing NSAIDs has no theoretical advantage and may delay excretion of one of the drugs. *Probenecid* reduces excretion of most NSAIDs. Ibuprofen, and probably all NSAIDs, blunt the antihypertensive effects of thiazides, beta-blockers, and ACE inhibitors. Diuretics, in general, have been associated with renal failure in some patients using NSAIDs. Specifically, triamterene and indomethacin, and HCTZ and ketoprofen, are interacting pairs reported to cause renal failure. *Lithium* levels may rise or fall and need to be monitored with concomitant NSAID therapy.[19]

Management. Elderly patients at risk of renal failure or GI bleeding need to be advised of these risks when taking OTC ibuprofen. If at all possible, NSAIDs should be reserved for acute inflammation associated with rheumatoid arthritis or osteoarthritis. GI blood loss is usually minimal even in predisposed patients during the first 7 to 10 days unless an active ulcer is present. After the acute flare, NSAIDs should be withdrawn in favor of acetaminophen for chronic pain control. Hypertensives should be warned that OTC ibuprofen and all NSAIDs may elevate blood pressure. Patients should be warned to stop NSAIDs if they become weak or dizzy or develop diarrhea, vomiting, or loss of appetite.

The NSAIDs piroxicam (Feldene) and sulindac (Clinoril) appear to have renal-sparing effects in the elderly population.

ORAL HYPOGLYCEMIC AGENTS

Management of non-insulin-dependent, type II diabetes mellitus usually relies on diet, weight control, exercise, and oral sulfonylurea agents (Table 5–17). Although newer oral sulfonylureas, such as glipizide (Glucotrol), appear to offer significant advantages in reducing adverse side effects, be aware of unusual manifestations of hypoglycemic syndromes in the geriatric population. Hypoglycemia, which can be precipitated by oral agents, is a frequently encountered metabolic derangement — especially in the frail elderly — and can present a broad range of neuropsychiatric syndromes and dysfunctions. Typically, CNS findings in the acutely hypoglycemic geriatric patient consist of confusion, mental impairment, delirium, focal deficits, or frank coma.

Physicians should maintain a high index of suspicion for hypoglycemic reactions in elderly patients with mild or progressive renal impairment (reflected in a decreased glomerular filtration rate) who are concomitantly taking an oral hypoglycemic agent. Because approximately two thirds of circulating insulin is metabolized in the renal parenchyma, patients with reduced renal mass who are taking insulin-releasing agents are especially prone to elevated circulating insulin levels and secondary hypoglycemia. Thus, in this clinical situation, oral sulfonylurea agents may precipitate hypoglycemia, even though the drug is being taken as prescribed and with adequate food intake. Initial treatment consists of IV glucose administration with $D_{50}W$ followed by patient education and readjustment of the sulfonylurea dose.

Large studies usually point to the first-generation sulfonylureas such as chlorpropamide (Diabinese) and tolbutamide (Orinase) as the agents most likely to cause hypoglycemia in the elderly population. Chlorpropamide has a long duration of effect (24 to 60 hours) and elimination half-life (35 hours) and should be used with caution in the elderly. Moreover, secondary drug interactions with phenylbutazone, sulfonamides, salicylates, and NSAIDs can precipitate an increased hypoglycemic effect among the first-generation oral agents.

A newer, more potent second-generation oral sulfonylurea agent, glipizide (Glucotrol), has a shorter half-life and more rapid onset of action, making it the current oral sulfonylurea of choice in the elderly population. Glyburide (Micronase, Diabeta) is another second-generation agent, but one study of its effects reported 57 cases of severe hypoglycemia, including 24 protracted cases and 10 fatalities. In contrast, glipizide caused neither long-lasting cases of hypoglycemia nor hypo-

Table 5–17 Pharmacologic and Pharmacokinetic Activity of Sulfonylurea Agents

Generic name	Brand	Daily dose range (mg)	Duration of effect (hr)	Elimination of half-life (hr)
Tolbutamide	Orinase	500–3,000	6–12	4–5
Tolazamide	Tolinase	100–750	10–16	7
Acetohexamide	Dymelor	500–1,500	12–24	5
Chlorpropamide	Diabinese	100–500	24–60	35
Glyburide	Micronase	2.5–20	24	10
Glipizide	Glucotrol	2.5–40	24	2–4

glycemia-induced fatalities in a 7-year study conducted by the Swedish Board of Health and Welfare's Adverse Drug Reaction Advisory Committee.[26,27]

Glyburide is also subject to erratic absorption and produces two active metabolites with 1/40 and 1/400 the potencies of the parent compound. The former metabolite is still five times more potent than the typical first-generation sulfonylurea and, therefore, can produce severe hypoglycemic reactions. In contrast, glipizide does not produce significantly active metabolic breakdown products.

Perhaps most importantly, among all oral sulfonylurea agents, glipizide has the unique capacity to induce a selective glucose (nutrient)-mediated insulin release that closely mimics in vivo insulin release patterns in response to postprandial nutrient loading. This selective release, which appears to be maintained as long as 48 months after glipizide therapy, offers special advantages and reduces adverse side effects in the elderly patient with type II diabetes. Finally, because glipizide, unlike the first-generation agents, is bound nonionically to serum proteins, it is less prone to producing hypoglycemia due to secondary drug interactions. Glipizide has a milligram-for-milligram potency equivalence with glyburide, and has been shown to reduce insulin requirements when used in type I diabetics.

Insulin versus oral agents for adult-onset diabetes. A major unresolved issue in management of non-insulin-dependent diabetes mellitus (NIDDM) is whether insulin or an oral agent is the treatment of choice for patients who fail dietary therapy. An intense debate among diabetologists has raged ever since the University Group Diabetes Program (UGDP) study cast some doubt on the safety of oral agent therapy. A small but statisically significant increase in cardiac deaths was found in patients treated with oral agents as compared to those treated with insulin. Proponents of oral agent therapy criticized the UGDP study design and argued that oral agents are ideally suited for NIDDM, since they act to lessen peripheral resistance to endogenous insulin, a major cause of NIDDM.

The issue of cardiovascular morbidity remains unresolved, although new data may be forthcoming. In the meantime, the advent of a more potent generation of oral agents raises the issue of how well these new preparations compare with insulin regarding control of hyperglycemia, risk of hypoglycemia, correction of hyperlipidemia, and other important risk/benefit parameters. A randomized, double-blind, placebo-controlled study of glyburide versus insulin for long-term metabolic control of NIDDM has just been reported, providing a prospective, controlled comparison of these two modes of therapy.

The study population consisted of 31 patients with NIDDM who failed to achieve normal glucose control on a program of diet alone. They were randomized to once-per-day insulin and glyburide placebo, or to glyburide and once-per-day placebo insulin injection. Active agent and placebo were adjusted according to fasting plasma glucose level to achieve a level of less than 115 mg/dL without hypoglycemia. Parameters monitored included weight, fasting serum glucose, hemoglobin A_{Ic}, triglyceride, cholesterol, high-density lipoprotein (HDL), and the ratio of HDL to cholesterol. Patients were observed for 9 months.

Both agents produced similar improvements in fasting blood sugar and hemoglobin A_{Ic} levels, similar degrees of weight gain, similar frequencies of mild symptomatic hypoglycemia, and significant reductions in serum lipid levels. Nearly normal degrees of blood glucose control were achieved. Patients in both treatment groups showed significant improvements in HDL levels and HDL: cholesterol, but those treated with insulin had a significantly greater improvement in these parameters than did those treated with glyburide.

The authors concluded that glyburide and once-per-day insulin therapy provide similar and very adequate degrees of glucose control in NIDDM patients who have failed on diet alone. Insulin appears to have the advantage of producing a more favorable lipid profile, although the long-term benefits of this effect are not known.

CHOLESTEROL-REDUCING AGENTS

According to the Framingham Heart Study, the prevalence of coronary artery disease in the diabetic patient is about twice that in the general population. Although the increased susceptibility to heart disease is almost certainly related in part to impaired glucose homeostasis, the patient with NIDDM is also susceptible to abnormalities in the lipoprotein metabolism that include increases in plasma VLDL triglycerides and VLDL and LDL cholesterol and decreases in HDL cholesterol. Based on epidemiologic studies in the general population, there is evidence to suggest that pharmacologic and/or dietary interventions that achieve beneficial effects on plasma lipid levels (i.e., reduction in serum LDL and VLDL cholesterol and elevation of HDL cholesterol) may decrease the risk of coronary heart disease in patients with NIDDM.

The investigators of this double-blind, randomized, placebo-controlled study employed lovastatin, a potent inhibitor of 3-hydroxy-3-methylglutaryl-coenzyme-A reductase, to determine whether significant reductions in plasma cholesterol levels could be achieved in 16 NIDDM patients on glyburide therapy with mild to moderate elevations of plasma lipids. Patients ranged in age from 41 to 70 years, with a mean age of 61 years. Based on plasma lipid levels determined at the beginning of the study and 28 days after therapy, the authors concluded that, when compared to placebo, lovastatin reduced total cholesterol by 26%, LDL by 28%, and LDL apolipoprotein B by 26%. In addition, lovastatin therapy reduced plasma triglycerides and VLDL cholesterol by 31% and 42%, respectively. Although there was no change in the plasma level of HDL cholesterol, the ratio of total cholesterol to HDL cholesterol fell by 29%. No side effects or abnormalities in the serum values of hepatic enzymes or creatine kinase were noted during short-term lovastatin therapy.

These investigators point out that, according to available data, an average reduction in total cholesterol levels of 26%, as observed with lovastatin therapy, should reduce the risk of coronary heart disease by about 50%. This reduction in risk, they conclude, should put patients with NIDDM at about the same baseline risk for heart disease as the general population.

The relative importance of multiple factors that place patients with NIDDM at increased risk for heart disease is not precisely known. Nevertheless, reduction of elevated plasma cholesterol and triglyceride levels with dietary or pharmacologic intervention is advisable in diabetic patients with risk factors for coronary artery disease. Although this study was conducted on a limited number of patients for a short period of time, it demonstrates the efficacy of lovastatin therapy in significantly reducing total cholesterol levels. Based on this data, lovastatin can be expected to improve the plasma lipid profile of patients with NIDDM at high risk for developing coronary heart disease.

ANXIOLYTIC AND SEDATIVE-HYPNOTIC DRUGS (Table 5–18)

Benzodiazepines. These agents are frequently used to relieve short-term anxiety in geriatric patients. Diazepam (Valium) has a longer half-life than most other benzodiazepines. Other such agents with long half-lives include chlordiazepoxide (Librium), flurazepam (Dalmane), clorazepate (Tranxene), and prazepam (Centrax). In general, these drugs should be avoided in the elderly population. Somnolence, confusion, and depression are the most common presenting symptoms of anxiolytic toxicity associated with long-acting benzodiazepines. Drugs with shorter half-lives, such as triazolam (Halcion), oxazepam (Serax), alprazolam (Xanax), and lorazepam (Ativan) are preferable anxiolytics for the

elderly. Benzodiazepines are also effective sedative hypnotics. Flurazepam is the most common, but, like diazepam, it has a long half-life. Thirty-nine percent of elderly patients receiving the usual 30 mg dose of flurazepam have significant CNS depression due to accumulation of the drug. A shorter-acting benzodiazepine, such as temazepam (Restoril) or alprazolam, may be an improvement, requiring only a dosage reduction.[4]

Midazolam (Versed) is a new ultra-short-acting parenteral benzodiazepine with excellent amnestic properties. It is particularly advantageous for inducing conscious sedation in elderly patients. An average dose not exceeding 1.0 to 1.5 mg of midazolam by slow IV infusion (0.018 mg/kg) is recommended. Versed has an average elimination half-life of about 2½ hours, and sedation usually occurs within 2 to 4 minutes. Because respiratory depression can occur, the use of midazolam should be restricted to settings where emergency intubation can be performed.

Cimetidine (Tagamet) and disulfiram (Antabuse) both inhibit metabolism of the long-acting benzodiazepines, diazepam and chlordiazepoxide. Oxazepam (Serax) is unaffected by these drugs. Alcohol potentiates the CNS depression of all benzodiazepines.

ANTIDEPRESSANTS

The elderly are particularly sensitive to the adverse effects of cyclic antidepressants (CAs). The most common presenting symptoms of CA toxicity include sedation, anticholinergic effects, adrenergic hyperactivity (tremulousness, sweating), and cardiovascular toxicity. Anticholinergic effects include dry mouth, constipation, blurred vision, urinary retention, decreased sweating, and hyperthermic reactions (Table 5–19).

Anticholinergic CNS effects — which may cause delirium, agitation, visual hallucinations, decreased thirst — precipitated by CAs are frequently underdiagnosed. Lack of sweating and decreased thirst can produce dehydration and electrolyte imbalances that can be fatal in the elderly population. Orthostatic hypotension due to anticholinergic toxicity can cause falls, myocardial infarction, and cerebrovascular events.

Cardiovascular effects due to antidepressant toxicity in the elderly include an anticholinergic effect which can

Table 5–18 Sedative-Hypnotic and Anxiolytic Drugs in the Elderly

Drug	FDA approved	Half-life (hr)	Usual initial dose for the elderly	Drug name
Flurazepam	Hypnotic	50–100 (major metabolite)	15 mg at bedtime	Dalmane
Temazepam	Hypnotic	5–15	15 mg at bedtime	Restoril
Oxazepam	Anxiolytic	5–20	10 mg three times a day	Serax
Diazepam	Anxiolytic	20–100 (major metabolite)	2 mg per day or twice a day	Valium
Lorazepam	Anxiolytic	10–20	0.5–2 mg/day	Ativan
Triazolam	Hypnotic	2.3	0.125 mg	Halcion
Alprazolam	Anxiolytic	12–15	0.25 mg–1.0 mg three times a day	Xanax

Table 5–19   Adverse Effects and Toxicity of Tricyclic and Tetracyclic Antidepressants

Structural class	Trade name	Young adult	Elderly	Sedative properties	Anticholinergic properties
Tricyclic					
Tertiary amine					
Amitriptyline	Elavil	100–300 mg	25–150 mg	+++	++++
Imipramine	Tofranil	100–300 mg	25–150 mg	++	+++
Doxepin	Sinequan	100–300 mg	25–150 mg	+++	++++
Trimipramine	Surmontil	100–300 mg	25–150 mg	+++	+++
Secondary amine					
Nortriptyline	Pamelor	50–100 mg	10–60 mg	+	+++
Desipramine	Norpramin	100–300 mg	25–150 mg	0	++
Protriptyline	Vivactil	20–60 mg	5–30 mg	0	+++
Dibenzoxazepine (amoxapine)	Asendin	150–300 mg	25–150 mg	++	+++
Triazolopyridine (trazodone)	Desyrel	150–400 mg	50–300 mg	+++	+
Tetracyclic maprotiline	Ludiomil	100–300 mg	25–150 mg	++	+++

increase the heart rate and a quinidine-like effect which may increase PR, QRS, and QTc intervals.

CA overdose has serious cardiotoxic effects that are *not* usually present at the therapeutic doses. Because of the cardiovascular effects associated with overdose, researchers anticipated an increased incidence of sudden death and arrhythmia among elderly patients using cyclic antidepressants. The Boston Collaborative Drug Surveillance Program, however, has demonstrated that neither occurs, even in the presence of organic heart disease, which is so common in the elderly.

Although pharmacologic treatment of depression is effective in the elderly, monoamine oxidase inhibitors should be avoided because of the risks of serious drug interactions and the frequency of orthostatic hypotension. Common practice dictates that agitated or anxious depressions should be treated with sedating drugs (amitriptyline or doxepin) and retarded depressions should be treated with less sedating agents (nortriptyline or desipramine). Orthostatic hypotension, which can cause falls, is probably the most dangerous side effect. Doxepin and nortriptyline cause fewer incidents of postural hypotension. Their major cardiac toxicity is interference with cardiac conduction. At high risk are patients with pre-existing bundle branch block or sinus node dysfunction.[28,29]

Doxepin has the fewest adverse effects on the heart. However, anticholinergic effects, such as dry mouth, urinary hesitance or retention, and constipation, are common. The most serious anticholinergic effect is confusion or delirium, for which the underlying cause frequently goes unrecognized in the emergency department setting. Amitriptyline and doxepin are the most potent anticholinergics, and desipramine is the least. Other miscellaneous side effects include increased appetite and weight gain, decreased seizure threshold, and increased anxiety.

ANTIPSYCHOTIC DRUGS

Several major psychiatric disorders in the elderly are treated with antipsychotic and neurologic agents. Com-

plications of this treatment include tardive dyskinesia (five times more common in the elderly), akathisias, dystonias, pseudoparkinsonism, and anticholinergic side effects similar to those discussed above (Table 5–20).

A major adverse reaction to neuroleptics is neuroleptic malignant syndrome (NMS), which is frequently unrecognized in the elderly. NMS consists of fever, rigidity, autonomic instability, and mental status changes.

With the widespread use of both cyclic antidepressants and antipsychotics, 12% of all elderly ambulatory patients and 25% of those hospitalized in nursing homes now receive two or more drugs with anticholinergic effects. In general, studies show that clinicians do not choose drugs within a given class to minimize anticholinergic effects. Consequently, suspect an anticholinergic reaction in elderly patients with symptoms of urinary retention, acute glaucoma, delirium, hallucinations, seizures, dysarthria, hyperthermia, tachycardia, and even heart block — especially if the patient has taken drugs in one or more of the anticholinergic classes.

ANTICOAGULANTS

Heparin and warfarin (Coumadin) cause complications in the elderly population. Oral anticoagulants are also associated with a high incidence of skin necrosis in obese, elderly women, especially in areas rich in fat (breast, buttock, and thighs).

Drugs can increase the anticoagulant effect in the elderly by the following mechanisms: inhibition of absorption, displacement of anticoagulant from binding sites, inhibition of hepatic microsomal enzymes, or other mechanisms not understood (Tables 5–21 through 5–23).

H₂ ANTAGONISTS

A commonly prescribed drug among the elderly population, cimetidine (Tagamet) can cause sedation and confu-

Table 5–20 Adverse Effects of Antipsychotic Medications in the Elderly

Drug and dose for elderly	Relative potency	Sedation	Extra-pyramidal	Anticholinergic	Orthostatic hypotension
Chlorpromazine (Thorazine) 10–25 mg b.i.d. t.i.d.	100	+++	++	+++	++
Thioridazine (Mellaril) 10–25 mg b.i.d. t.i.d.	95–100	+++	+	+++	++
Thiothixene (Navane) 2–3 mg	5	+	+++	+	+
Haloperidol (Haldol) 0.5–2 mg	2	+	+++	+	+
Fluphenazine (Prolixin) 0.5–2 mg	2	+	+++	+	+

Table 5–21 Possible Drug Interactions with Anticoagulants

Decrease vitamin K	Displace anticoagulant	Inhibit metabolism	Other
Antibiotics	Phenylbutazone	Chloramphenicol	Thyroid drugs
Cholestyramine	Salicylates	Allopurinol	Anabolic steroids
Mineral oil	Sulfonamides	Nortriptyline	Quinidine
	Sulfonylureas	Disulfiram	Glucagon
	Ethacrynic acid	Metronidazole	Cimetidine
	Mefenamic acid	Alcohol (acute ingestion)	
	Nalidixic acid	Phenylbutazone	
	Diazoxide		

Table 5–22 Drugs That Diminish Anticoagulant Drug Activity

Induction of enzymes	Increased procoagulant factors
Barbiturates	Estrogens
Glutethimide	Oral contraceptives
Ethchlorvynol	Vitamin K
Griseofulvin	
Phenytoin	
Carbamazepine	
Rifampin	
Chlorinated insecticides	

Table 5–23 Drugs Potentiating Anticoagulant Drug Effects

Inhibition of platelet aggregation	Inhibition of procoagulant factors	Ulcerogenic drugs
Salicylates	Quinidine	Phenylbutazone
Phenylbutazone	Antimetabolites	Oxyphenbutazone
Oxyphenbutazone	Alkylating agents	Sulfinpyrazone
Sulfinpyrazone	Salicylates	Salicylates
Indomethacin		Indomethacin
Dipyridamole		Adrenal corticosteroids

sion, especially in doses above 1,000 mg/day. Aside from this direct adverse reaction, side effects are very few (Table 5–24).

However, because cimetidine is a potent inhibitor of the P-450 hepatic microsomal oxidation enzymes, it blocks metabolism of many other drugs that may be taken concurrently, increasing their effect on plasma levels. This leads to a number of potentially dangerous drug interactions. In patients taking warfarin (Coumadin), the prothrombin time can rise 20 to 200%. Both diazepam (Valium) and chlordiazepoxide (Librium) can cause increased sedation. Theophylline levels can increase from the therapeutic to the toxic range in patients who are on cimetidine therapy. Toxic effects, such as bradycardia, hypotension, and arrhythmias, may appear with beta-blockers. Elevated levels of anticonvulsants, especially in the elderly, can be seen over a period of several days in patients taking carbamazepine (Tegretol) and phenytoin (Dilantin). With lidocaine, an increase in serum levels of 60 to 90% can occur with maintenance infusions in patients on cimetidine therapy.

The newer, selective H_2 antagonists, ranitidine (Zantac) and famotidine (Pepcid), produce very mild CNS depression and have the distinct advantage of not inhibiting the hepatic microsomal oxidation system. As a result, neither produces adverse secondary drug interactions such as those described with cimetidine.

BRONCHODILATORS

Aminophylline and theophylline represent the cornerstone of oral bronchodilator therapy for the elderly asthmatic, bronchitic, or cardiac patient. They are metabolized by the liver, and clearance is remarkably sensitive to hepatic dysfunction caused by disease (primary and hypoxia induced) or low-flow states (congestive heart failure and propranolol induced).

Complications of aminophylline include seizures, which may even occur at therapeutic levels, increased angina, palpitations, and arrhythmias. Nervousness and lack of sleep are also encountered in the geriatric population.

Table 5–24   Adverse Drug Interactions in Combination with Cimetidine (Tagamet)

- With warfarin, prothrombin time rises 20 to 200%.
- With diazepam (Valium) and chlordiazepoxide (Librium), increases sedation.
- With theophylline, increases in theophylline from therapeutic to toxic range (narrow therapeutic range).
- With beta-blockers, toxic effects may appear, such as bradycardia, hypotension, arrhythmias.
- With carbamazepine (Tegretol) and phenytoin (Dilantin), elevated levels of anticonvulsants, especially in the elderly, over several days.
- With lidocaine, 60 to 90% increase in serum levels occurred with maintenance infusion; study conducted in the elderly. Cimetidine therapy was new in these patients.

Aminophylline toxicity in the elderly may also mimic chronic organic brain syndrome, multi-infarct dementia, and psychosis. Draw blood levels on patients who have this constellation of symptoms and who are taking an aminophylline preparation.

Certain drug interactions may precipitate aminophylline toxicity. Cimetidine and other liver-metabolized antibiotics (erythromycin, clindamycin) decrease excretion of aminophylline. Ephedrine and other sympathomimetic agents in combination with aminophylline may cause excessive CNS stimulation, precipitating bizarre behavior and sleeplessness.

Epinephrine. Asthma is a reversible but serious respiratory condition that still claims more than 2,000 lives annually in the United States. For the past 80 years, the rapid reversal of acute bronchospasm and hypoxemia associated with asthma using subcutaneous epinephrine has been confirmed by numerous investigators. Despite its efficacy, many physicians are reluctant to administer subcutaneous epinephrine to acute asthmatics 40 years of age or older, especially those with concomitant heart disease or a history of hypertension, because of the potent cardiovascular effects of the drug. Cydulka and associates[29a] conducted a study to determine whether the administration of subcutaneous epinephrine (0.3 mL, 1:1,000) is associated with an increased risk of cardiovascular side effects — adverse hemodynamic consequences and arrhythmias — in patients more than 40 years of age as compared with patients younger than 40.

Conducting their prospective investigation in a large urban teaching hospital, these researchers administered three subcutaneous doses of 0.3 mL 1:1,000 epinephrine 20 minutes apart to 95 adult asthmatics 15 to 96 years of age during 108 asthma exacerbations. Thirty-nine of the 108 episodes occurred in patients over the age of 40, 48.7% of which were men. Patients were diagnosed as having an acute asthmatic attack if they had had an established history of reversible bronchospasm, dyspnea, or wheezing on presentation, and diminished peak expiratory flow rates. Individuals with a previous history of chronic obstructive lung disease, chronic bronchitis, or an acute myocardial infarction, as well as patients presenting with angina or those who had received epinephrine prior to admission, were considered ineligible. In addition, the use of aerosolized adrenergic agents was prohibited during the study period.

Heart rhythm and rate, blood pressure, respiratory rate, and clinical response were prospectively evaluated before, during, and after administration of epinephrine doses. The investigators found that initial systolic blood pressures were higher in the older than younger age group (146 ± 4.2 versus 130.6 ± 3.2 mm Hg), while the incidence of sinus tachycardia was not significantly different (49.3% older versus 59% younger) between the two groups. The only significant difference ($p < .0033$) between asthmatics in the two age groups occurred after the first dose of epinephrine when mean systolic blood pressure was observed to decrease by 9.5 ± 3.3 mm Hg in patients older than 40 years, while it increased 1.3 ± 1.9 mm Hg in the younger age group.

The authors noted there was no significant difference in the occurrence of ventricular arrhythmias between patients less than and older than 40 years of age, although isolated VPBs < 10/hr were observed after treatment in 11.6% of the younger patients and in 21.6% of those over 40 (p > .05). There were no adverse consequences from these ventricular irregularities. While atrial premature beats occurred significantly more often in the older than younger age group (32.4% versus 10.1%, p < .05), all atrial tachycardias resolved spontaneously without symptomatology or adverse cardiac consequences. Of special interest is the fact that mean systolic and diastolic blood pressures, heart rate, and respiratory rate decreased as bronchoconstriction was relieved and respiratory flow rates improved with epinephrine therapy in the older age group.

Clinical improvement was similar in each of the populations studied, with an average increase in peak flow rates of 47.1%, 24.5%, and 25.1% after the first, second, and third doses of subcutaneous epinephrine, respectively.

This study has important implications for the initial pharmacologic treatment of the adult asthmatic. A nonselective alpha- and beta-adrenergic agonist, epinephrine has long been considered standard therapy for acute asthma. It relaxes bronchial smooth muscle and constricts bronchial arterioles, reaching detectable serum levels within 5 to 10 minutes after subcutaneous injection, and attaining peak blood levels between 20 to 40 minutes. Because of its chronotropic effect on the sinoatrial node and positive inotropic effect on the myocardium, however, epinephrine can increase myocardial irritability and oxygen consumption, thereby precipitating cardiac arrhythmias in susceptible individuals.

While many practitioners routinely use epinephrine to relieve asthma in the young adult and pediatric patient, the proarrhythmogenic potential of epinephrine has deterred its use in older adults, especially those with preexisting cardiac disease or hypertension. This is unfortunate, since subcutaneous epinephrine is a relatively inexpensive, easily administered, and efficacious bronchodilator. In the older age group, many experts advocate aerosolized, inhaled selective sympathomimetic agents which, although just as efficacious as parenteral epinephrine, have been associated with fewer cardiovascular side effects. It should be noted, however, that the cost difference between injection and inhalation treatment is substantial. In most institutions, subcutaneous epinephrine 1:1,000 is approximately one third the cost of sympathomimetic inhalation therapy.

The results of this limited study suggest that use of subcutaneous epinephrine can probably be safely expanded to include selected asthmatic patients over 40 years of age, providing these individuals have not had a recent myocardial infarction and do not report anginal symptoms on presentation. The use of epinephrine in older patients with recent, silent myocardial infarction or severe coronary ischemia as determined by ECG findings was not specifically evaluated in this study and, therefore, the safety of its use in this population remains questionable.

Although the investigators report findings for 39 patients over the age of 40 years, they fail to indicate the mean age and specific breakdown of ages within the older population studied. Lacking such age-adjusted, fractionated data for the 40 years and older group, it is difficult to draw conclusions about the drug's overall safety in the "elderly" population, per se. In this regard, the authors conclude that a larger population must be studied before this modality can be recommended without reservation for all age groups. Moreover, in an age when selective, aerosolized bronchodilating agents are readily available — and have proven efficacy — the rationale for an expanded role for subcutaneous epinephrine therapy is debatable.

Optimal corticosteroid tapering schedule following exacerbation of asthma. Although corticosteroids have been known to be effective in the treatment of severe asthma for more than 30 years, no adequate data exist to help the physician determine how rapidly steroids can safely be withdrawn in patients who have experienced an acute exacerbation of their illness. Published recommendations run the gamut, from a few days to several months, but controversy persists, with some experts claiming that rapid tapering of corticosteroid therapy is associated with a higher exacerbation and hospital readmission rate, while other experts claim that long tapering schedules place patients at risk for complications of long-term corticosteroid therapy.

Given the clinical importance, economic implication, and widespread use of this outpatient prescribing practice, the investigators conducted a randomized, double-blind, placebo-controlled trial to determine whether a long corticosteroid tapering following an exacerbation of asthma reduced the likelihood of re-exacerbation and/or readmission to the hospital.

Non-steroid-dependent adult men (n = 43) hospitalized for asthma exacerbations and treated with steroids acutely during a 1-year period were randomly assigned to corticosteroid tapering regimens of 1 or 7 weeks, following an 8-day course of high-dose corticosteroid therapy. Specifically, the short taper consisted of 7 days using daily prednisone doses of 45, 30, 25, 20, 15, 10, and 5 mg; the long tapering consisted of each of the above doses for 7 days each for a total of 7 weeks.

With respect to clinical deterioration for each dosage schedule, this study found no significant difference between the long-taper and short-taper groups in the rate of re-exacerbation (41% versus 52%) or readmission (22% versus 21%) during the 12-week study period. Failure was defined as a re-exacerbation of asthma requiring additional high-dose corticosteroid therapy during the 12-week study period. Patients who did not have a re-exacerbation during the 12 weeks were evaluated with spirometry, with no significant differences occurring between the two groups. Those patients who required mechanical ventilation for their initial hospitalization (n = 7) or who reported more than 2 days of worse than usual dyspnea during the 12-week period (n = 20) had high rates of re-exacerbation (86% and 80%, respectively). And confirming the clinical impressions of some experts, the results of this trial also indicate that more patients in the long-term taper group reported corticosteroid side effects (41% versus 14%), including weight gain, edema, easy bruising, and acne. Based on rigorous statistical analysis (Cox's F test), the authors contend that their results provide reasonable certainty (90%) that a long taper does not result in a large reduction (50% or more) in re-exacerbations compared with a short taper. Moreover, they conclude that the relapse rate is high in this population regardless of the corticosteroid tapering regimen employed and that a long taper does not justify its routine use.

Corticosteroid therapy is pivotal to the management of exacerbations of asthma that fail to respond to conventional bronchodilator therapy. Curiously, despite the universal use of high-dose, short-course steroid therapy to treat this disorder, no previous studies have addressed the important question of how rapidly corticosteroid therapy should be withdrawn following an exacerbation. The value of conducting such a study is clear. If not associated with an increased readmission of treatment failure rates, the use of a short-term tapering schedule, because of its reduced likelihood of steroid-induced side effects, would have a significant clinical advantage over a long-term tapering regimen.

Based on this clinical trial, physicians can expect a short-term (7 days) tapering of prednisone therapy in adult men to be just as effective as a long-term (7 weeks) tapering regimen and to be associated with a significantly lower incidence of side effects. Although this recommendation will apply to large numbers of patients, three aspects of this study deserve comment.

First, the patients receiving systemic corticosteroids at the time of initial exacerbation were excluded from the study. Second, most of the patients in this study were older men (mean age, 63 years) with histories of heavy smoking and abnormal spirometry, whose clinical picture would be considered consistent with chronic obstructive pulmonary disease with a reversible component. This condition is frequently indistinguishable from asthma. And finally, those included in the study tended to have severe exacerbations as evidenced by the need for mechanical ventilation (16%) and high hospital readmission rates. These factors should be considered before extrapolating the results of this investigation to all outpatients with exacerbation of reversible airway disease.

SALICYLATES

More than 200 OTC preparations contain aspirin, which can adversely affect the elderly. Presenting symptoms can include gastritis with gastrointestinal blood loss leading to iron deficiency anemia and peptic ulcer with or without serious hemorrhagic manifestations. The elderly are particularly prone to chronic salicylate intoxication, which presents as tinnitus, confusion, respiratory alkalosis, and noncardiogenic pulmonary edema. Even patients taking therapeutic doses of salicylates are prone to chronic salicylism. Consequently, any elderly patient who presents with confusion, respiratory alkalosis, and pulmonary edema of unknown etiology should have a salicylate level drawn, even if the patient has taken salicylates as prescribed by a physician. The diagnosis depends on a thorough drug history and elevated blood salicylate level.

ANTIHISTAMINES

The early stages of diphenhydramine intoxication are characterized by acute psychosis, hallucinations, autism, loosened associations, affective blunting, and inappropriateness. As time passes, the symptom complex may become more similar to an acute brain syndrome with confusion, disorientation, inability to concentrate, and loss of short-term memory. These symptoms present an interesting differential diagnosis. However, based on the physical exam, drug overdose should always be suspected. Initial lab analysis should include serum electrolytes, prothrombin time, calcium, blood urea nitrogen (BUN), glucose, arterial gases, blood alcohol, and urine toxicologic screening. In addition, an ECG, chest and skull x-rays, and lumbar puncture may be necessary, depending on the clinical presentation.

A history of drug ingestion is frequently unreliable or unobtainable from the patient. Friends or relatives may be questioned concerning the availability of medications, prior history of drug use, and ingestion of hallucinogenic plants or seeds (jimsonweed, mushrooms). However, autonomic signs or symptoms may be the key to diagnosis. Anticholinergic poisoning is associated with tachycardia, mydriasis, flushing, hyperpyrexia, urinary retention, decreased intestinal motility, hypertension, dry skin, and decreased salivation. This clinical picture may be obscured by the frequency of hypertension, tachycardia, and mydriasis with many of the hallucinogens, including sympathetic stimulants (LSD, amphetamines) (Table 5–25).

A vast array of antihistamines, hypnotics, antidepressants, and tranquilizing agents pose significant anticholinergic activity. An increasing number of these

Table 5–25   Anticholinergic Agents

Antihistamines
Antiparkinsonian drugs
Antipsychotics (phenothiazines and butyrophenones)
Antispasmodics
Belladonna alkaloids
Ophthalmic products (mydriatics)
Plants (jimsonweed)
Thioxanthenes
Tricyclic antidepressants

drugs are now available in OTC preparation and may, in acute poisoning, produce a picture typical of central anticholinergic toxicity. This syndrome refers to an acute psychosis of delirium resulting from a primary blockade of cerebral cholinergic inhibitory pathways accompanied by signs of peripheral muscarinic blockage.

The presentation may vary from confusion, hallucinations, and convulsions to deepening coma and respiratory arrest. Toxic psychosis is a recognized complication of antihistamine poisoning. Ethanolamine derivatives, such as diphenhydramine, are distinct because of their proven safety and are noted for their sedative and anticholinergic properties (Table 5–26).

Clinical presentation of the diphenhydramine overdose patient depends on age. Adults commonly present with central nervous system depression, such as drowsiness, dizziness, and ataxia. Occasionally, there can be coma and cardiovascular collapse. Fever and flushing are not usually seen. Temporary ECG changes, such as prolonged QT interval, nonspecific ST-T changes, wandering pacemaker, and left bundle branch block, may be seen. A fatal dose in adults is approximately 20 to 40 mg/kg. In children, as little as 500 mg of diphenhydramine may be fatal. Children and young adults are remarkably susceptible to the anticholinergic action of this drug and commonly present with excitement, tremors, hyperactivity, hyperpyrexia, and tonic-clonic seizures.[30-32]

The central effects of antihistamines constitute their greatest danger in acute poisoning. The first report of toxic psychosis resulting from diphenhydramine was reported by Borman in 1947. Since then, there have been few reported cases. All the cases were characterized by amnesia for the entire toxic episode and returned to a

normal mental state within 48 hours. Possible predisposing factors to diphenhydramine-induced psychosis include parenteral administration, underlying psychosis, organic brain disease, combined use with other anticholinergic drugs, and reduced clearance of drug secondary to altered renal or hepatic function.

The treatment of a diphenhydramine overdose is generally supportive, particularly in regard to airway management and the maintenance of vital signs. The patient in a psychotic episode may require constant supervision for up to several days to guard against potentially serious complications, such as aspiration, accidental injury, hyperthermia, and seizures. Diphenhydramine is well absorbed following ingestion and is widely distributed throughout the body, including the CNS. The drug appears in plasma within 15 minutes and may reach peak concentrations within 1 hour. Gastric lavage or emesis should be initiated immediately on the patient's arrival at the emergency department. After emesis, administration of activated charcoal and a cathartic may help to minimize absorption. Forced diuresis, hemodialysis, and hemoperfusion are generally ineffective since little free drug remains in the plasma.

For a mild case of intoxication or in elderly, confused patients with uncertain cardiac status, one can manage the patient with conservative treatment and reassurance. Central nervous system depressants, which themselves have anticholinergic properties (phenothiazine), should be avoided. Convulsions may be treated with phenytoin at 10 to 15 mg/kg intravenously. Severe intoxications should be admitted to intensive care and monitored closely for cardiac arrhythmias, hypotension, and cardiovascular collapse.

The major controversy surrounding the treatment of any anticholinergic syndrome concerns the use of physostigmine (Antilirium). This drug is a reversible cholinesterase inhibitor capable of crossing the blood-brain barrier. Physostigmine (2 mg IV) has been shown to rapidly reverse coma, delirium, seizures, and other signs of the central anticholinergic syndrome. A patient may have dramatic symptomatic relief from low doses of intravenous physostigmine. However, the benefits of this therapy must be weighed against the major side effects, including seizures, cholinergic crises, bradyarrhythmias, and asystole. We feel that physostigmine should be reversed for use in patients with refractory tachyarrhythmias or convulsions.[33-35]

In summary, any patient with an acute onset of bizarre mental and neurologic symptoms should be suspected of poisoning by an anticholinergic drug, including antihistamines. A careful history, with specific attention to OTC drugs, is vital for confirming the diagnosis.

Table 5–26   Central Effects of Anticholinergic Toxicity

Anxiety	Hallucinations (visual/auditory)
Ataxia	Hyperactivity
Choreoathetoid movements	Lethargy
Coma	Loss of short-term memory
Delirium	Myoclonus
Disorientation	Paranoid ideation
Dizziness	Respiratory failure
Dysarthria	Seizures
Expressive aphasia	Tinnitus
Frank psychosis	Tremor

SUMMARY

Although the elderly constitute only 11% of the U.S. population, they consume approximately 20 to 30% of all

Table 5–27 Twenty Suggestions for Preventing Drug Toxicity in the Elderly

- Strive for a diagnosis prior to treating
- Take a careful drug history
- Know the pharmacokinetics of the drug(s)
- Adjust the dose
- Use smaller doses in the elderly
- Work to simplify the regimen
- Regularly review the regimen
- Avoid polypharmacy at all costs
- Use medication cards
- Keep a record of the Rx on the problem list
- Use medication diary (or containers, such as egg cartons, for daily doses)
- Have patient bring in all medicine bottles
- Check the labels
- Instruct family
- Destroy old medicines
- Use the services of visiting nurses
- Check serum drug levels when appropriate
- Support community education
- Consider overdose risk in elderly patients with clinically evident psychiatric conditions
- Be sure patients are aware that medicines can cause, as well as cure, illness

drugs (Table 5–27). Moreover, many of the elderly are simultaneously taking more than one prescription drug for more than one chronic condition, over variable periods of time; and they may supplement their prescription drugs with OTC medications and alcohol. For these reasons, this age group is at high risk for sustaining drug toxicity and adverse drug interactions.

One large study of hospitalized elderly patients with a mean age of 71 years found that each patient consumed an average of 3.1 prescription drugs and one OTC preparation. Initially, one sixth of the persons surveyed denied using OTC medications, but further questioning revealed that these patients did, in fact, take OTC drugs. Moreover, 50% of these elderly patients needed prompting to remember to take their medications, so noncompliance was a serious problem.

Among the implications of that study for the diagnosis and identification of adverse drug reactions in the emergency setting is the importance of focused assessment and interview techniques to examine drug behavior and compliance in the elderly, particularly for OTC drugs.

Finally, any elderly patient who presents to the emergency physician with nonspecific CNS, cardiac, or gastrointestinal signs and symptoms must have a careful drug history, including OTC medications, antiulcer agents, cardiac medications, and antihypertensives. Always consider adverse drug reactions, especially the anticholinergic syndrome, and secondary drug interactions, as a cause of illness.[1-8]

REFERENCES

1. Nolan L and O'Malley K: Prescribing for the elderly. I. Sensitivity of the elderly to adverse drug reactions, J Am Geriatr Soc 36:142–149, 1988.
2. Ouslander JG: Drug therapy in the elderly, Ann Intern Med 95:711–722, 1981.
3. Bliss MR: Prescribing for the elderly, Br Med J 282:203–206, 1981.
4. Larson EB et al: Adverse drug reactions associated with global cognitive impairment in elderly persons, Ann Intern Med 107:169–173, 1987.
5. Symposium: managing medication in an aging population: physician, pharmacist, and patient perspectives, J Am Geriatr Soc Suppl 30:11, 1985.
6. Cassel CK and Walsh JR, editors: Medical, psychiatric, and pharmacological topics, Geriatr Med 1:554, 1984.
7. Lamy PP: Geriatric pharmacology, Geriatrics 36(12):41, 1986.
8. Lamy PP: A "risk" approach to adverse drug reactions, J Am Geriatr Soc 36:79, 1988.
9. Shrimp LA et al: Potential medication-related problems in noninstitutionalized elderly, Drug Intell Clin Pharm 19:766, 1985.
10. Todd B: Drugs and the elderly: identifying drug toxicity, Geriatr Nurs 12:231, 1985.
11. American College of Physicians: Improving medical education in therapeutics, Ann Intern Med 108:145–147, 1988.
12. Leach S and Roy SS: Adverse drug reactions: an investigation on an acute geriatric ward, Age Ageing 15:241, 1986.
13. Knapp DA et al: Drug prescribing for ambulatory patients 85 years of age and older, J Am Geriatr Soc 32(2):138, 1984.
14. Report of the Royal College of General Physicians: Medication for the elderly, J R Coll Physicians Lond 18:7, 1984.
15. Albrich JM: Geriatric pharmacology. In Schwartz GR, Bosker G, and Grigsby JW, editors: Geriatric emergencies, Bowie, Md, 1984, Robert J Brady Co.
16. May FE, Stewart B, and Cluff LE: Drug interactions and multiple drug administrations, Clinical Pharmacol Ther 2:705, 1970.
17. Vestal RE: Drug use in the elderly: a review of problems and special considerations, Drugs 16:358, 1978.
18. Pickles H and Fuller S: Prescriptions, adverse reactions, and the elderly, Lancet 2 (8497):40, 1986.
19. Rizack MA and Hillman CDM: The Medical Letter handbook of adverse drug interactions, New Rochelle, NY, 1987, The Medical Letter.
20. Ray WA, Griffin MR, Schaffner W, et al: Psychotropic drug use and the risk of hip fracture, N Engl J Med 316:363, 1987.
21. Alegro S, Fenster PE, and Marcus FI: Digitalis therapy in the elderly, Geriatrics 38:93, 1983.
22. Lamy PP: Geriatric pharmacology, Geriatrics 36(12):41–49, 1986.
23. Williamson J and Chopin JM: Adverse reactions to prescribed drugs in the elderly: a multicenter investigation, Age Ageing 9:73, 1980.
24. Minardo JD et al: Clinical characteristics of patients with ventricular fibrillation during antiarrhythmic drug therapy, N Engl J Med 319:257, 1988.
25. Stults BM: Digoxin use in the elderly, J Am Geriatr Soc 30(3):158, 1985.
26. Leichter S: A prospective double-blind clinical trial of glipizide and glyburide in type II diabetes mellitus, Communication, 1986.
27. Melander A: Clinical pharmacology of sulfonylureas, Metabolism 36(2) (suppl 1), 1987.
28. Keller MB et al: Treatment received by depressed patients, JAMA 248(15):1848, 1982.
29. Litovitz T: Hallucinogens. In Hadden LM and Winchester JF, editors: Clinical management of poisoning and drug overdose, Philadelphia, 1983, WB Saunders Co.
29a. Cydulka R et al: The use of epinephrine in the treatment of older asthmatics, Ann Emerg Med 17:322–326, 1988.
30. Sachs BA: The toxicity of benadryl: report of a case and review of the literature, Ann Intern Med 29:135, 1948.
31. Loew ER, MacMillan R, and Katser ME: The antihistamine properties of benadryl, β-dimethylaminoethyl ether hydrochloride, J Pharmacol Exp Ther 86:229, 1946.
32. Kulig K and Rumack BH: Anticholinergic poisoning. In Haddad LM and Winchester JF, editors: Clinical management of poisoning and drug overdose, Philadelphia, 1983, WB Saunders Co.
33. Nigro SA: Toxic psychosis due to diphenhydramine hydrochloride, JAMA 203(4):139, 1968.
34. Nilsson E: Physostigmine treatment in various drug-induced intoxications, Ann Clin Res 14:165, 1982.
35. Rumack BH: Anticholinergic poisoning: treatment with physostigmine, Pediatrics 52:449, 1973.

SUGGESTED READINGS

American Society of Hospital Pharmacists: Antidiabetic agents-sulfonylureas, Drug Information TM '86 68:1579, 1986.

Amery A et al: Mortality and morbidity results from the European working party on high blood pressure in the elderly, Lancet 1:1349–1354, 1985.

Asplund K, Wilholm BE, and Lithner F: Glibenclamide-associated hypoglycemia: a report on 57 cases, Diabetologia 26:412, 1984.

Bauman JH and Kimelblatt BJ: Cimetidines as an inhibitor of drug metabolism: therapeutic implications and review of the literature, Drug Intell Clin Pharm 16:380, 1982.

Ben-Ishay D, Leibel B, and Stessman J: Calcium channel blockers in the management of hypertension in the elderly, Am J Med 81 Suppl 6a 81:30–34, 1986.

Blazer DG et al: The risk of anticholinergic toxicity in the elderly: a study of prescribing practices in two populations, J Gerontol 38(1):31, 1983.

Borland C et al: Biochemical and clinical correlates of diuretics therapy in the elderly, Age Ageing 15:357–363, 1986.

Christopher CD: The role of the pharmacist in a geriatric nursing home: a literature review, Drug Intell Clin Pharm 18:428–433, 1984.

Coope J and Warrender TS: Randomized trial of treatment of hypertension in elderly patients in primary care, Br Med J 293:1145, 1148, 1986.

Dall JLC: Maintenance digoxin in elderly patients, Br Med J 2:702, 1970.

Darnell JC et al: Medication used by ambulatory elderly: an inhome survey, J Am Geriatr Soc 34:1, 1986.

Douglas WW: Histamine and 5-hydroxytryptamine (serotonin) and their antagonists. In Goodman LS and Gilman A, editors: The pharmacological basis of therapeutics, ed 6, New York, 1979, Macmillan.

Downs GE, Linkewich JA, and DiPalma JR: Drug interactions in elderly diabetics, Geriatrics 36(7):45, 1986.

Duvoisin RC and Kat R: Reversal of central anticholinergic syndrome in man by physostigmine, JAMA 206(9):1963, 1968.

Egstrup K: Transient myocardial ischemia after abrupt withdrawal of antianginal therapy in chronic stable angina, Am J Cardiol 61:1219, 1988.

Emanueli A et al: Glipizede — new sulfonylurea in the treatment of diabetes mellitus: summary of clinical experiences in 1,064 cases, Arzneimittelforschung (Drug Res.) 22:1881, 1971.

Goldfrank LR and Melinek M: Locoweed and other anticholinergics (the telltale heart). In Goldfrank LR, editor: Toxicologic emergencies, New York, 1982, Prentice-Hall.

Granacher RP and Baldessarini RJ: Physostigmine: its use in acute anticholinergic syndrome with antidepressant and antiparkinson drugs, Arch Gen Psychiatry 32:375, 1975.

Granek E et al: Medications and diagnosis in relation to falls in a long-term care facility, J Am Geriatr Soc 35:505, 1987.

Greenblatt DJ and Shader RI: Anticholinergics, N Engl J Med 288(23):1215–1218, 1984.

Greenblatt DJ, Sellers EM, and Shader RI: Drug therapy: drug disposition in old age, N Engl J Med 306(18):1081, 1982.

Gryfe CI and Gryfe BM: Drug therapy for the aged: the problems of compliance and the roles of physicians and pharmacists, J Am Geriatr Soc 32(4):301, 1984.

Hall RCW et al: Anticholinergic delirium: etiology, presentation, diagnosis, and management. J Psychedel Drugs 10:237, 1978.

Hansten PD: Drug interactions, ed 5, Philadelphia, 1985, Lea & Febiger.

Heifetz S and Day D: Inadvertent chlorpropamide hypoglycemia — no longer once in a blue moon? N Engl J Med 316(4):223, 1987 (letter).

Hestand HE and Teske DW: Diphenhydramine hydrochloride intoxication, J Pediatr 90(6):1017, 1977.

Hoffman JR: Overdose with cardiotherapeutic agents, Geriatrics 38:51, 1983.

Hollifield JW and Slaton PE: Thiazide diuretics, hypokalemia, and cardiac arrhythmias, Acta Med Scand 647(suppl):67, 1981.

Hutchinson TA et al: Frequency, severity, and risk factors for adverse drug reactions in adult out-patients: prospective study, J Chronic Dis 39(7):533, 1986.

Iserson KV and Hackney KU: Antihistamines. In Haddad LM and Winchester JF: Clinical management of poisoning and drug overdose, Philadelphia, 1983, WB Saunders Co.

Jenike MA: Cimetidine in elderly patients: review of uses and risks, J Am Geriatr Soc 30(3):170, 1987.

Kramer MS et al: An algorithm for the operational assessment of adverse drug reactions. I. Background, description, and instructions for use. II. Demonstration of reproducibility and validity, JAMA 242(7):623–633, 1979.

Kranzelok EP, Anderson GM, and Mirik M: Massive diphenhydramine overdose resulting in death, Ann Emerg Med 11(4):212, 1982.

Lee JH, Turndorf H, and Poppers PJ: Physostigmine reversal of antihistamine-induced excitement and depression, Anesthesiology 43(6):683, 1975.

Leventhal JM, Hutchinson TA, Kramer MS, and Feinstein AR: An algorithm for the operational assessment of adverse drug reactions. III. Results of tests among clinicians, JAMA 242(18):1991, 1979.

Levy DW and Lye M: Diuretics and potassium in the elderly, J R Coll Physicians Lond 21(2):148, 1987.

McEvoy G, editor: American Hospital formulary service drug information 85, Bethesda, Md, 1985, American Society of Hospital Pharmacists, Inc., pp 12–13.

Monroe R, Jacobson G, and Ervin F: Activation of psychosis by combination of scopolamine and alpha-chloralose, Arch Neurol 76:536, 1957.

National Poison Center Network: Annual statistical report, Pittsburgh, 1979.

Plum F and Posner JB, editors: The diagnosis of stupor and coma, Philadelphia, 1982, FA Davis Co.

Podolsky S: Diabetes and aging: the type II patient. Abstract, 1986.

Spector R, editor: The scientific basis of clinical pharmacology: principles and examples, Boston, 1986, Little, Brown & Co.

Sternberg L: Unusual side reactions of hysteria from benadryl, J Allergy 18:417, 1947.

Thompson JF et al: Clinical pharmacists prescribing drug therapy in a geriatric setting: outcome of a trial, J Am Geriatr Soc 32(2):154, 1984.

Thompson TT, Moran MG, and Nies AS: Psychotropic drug use in the elderly, N Engl J Med 308(3):134, 1983.

Tilson HH: Social policy and drug safety, Clin Geriatr Med 2(1):165, 1987.

Tintinalli JE: Emergency psychiatric evaluation: medical history and physical exam. In Tintinalli JE, Rothstein RJ, and Krome RL, editors: Emergency medicine: a comprehensive study guide, New York, 1985, McGraw-Hill.

World Health Organization: Health care in the elderly: report of the technical group on the use of medications in the elderly, Drugs 22:279, 1981.

Wyngaarden JB and Severs MH: The toxic effects of antihistamine drugs, JAMA 145:277, 1951.

Poisoning

M. J. McMullen, M.D., F.A.C.E.P.

Toxicologic presentations in the elderly from both accidental therapeutic misadventures as well as deliberate ingestions and exposures are infrequently reported. However, with the increase in the aging population and aggressive therapeutic intervention for their medical problems, the potential for drug toxicity emergencies in this group is especially high. In addition, the older white man is vulnerable to the act of accomplished suicide, which he commits at a rate exceeding that for any other combination of age, sex, and race.[1] Of all fatalities from poisonings, there has been an increase in the percentage for the geriatric population from 8% in 1983 to 19% in 1986.[2] This increase was confirmed in 1987.[2b] This probably reflects greater recognition of the problem, as well as total increase in the number of poisonings.

This chapter will review the causes and clinical features of the three main types of poisoning in the elderly: iatrogenic, accidental, and deliberate self-poisoning. An understanding of the drug effects seen in the elderly due to changes in pharmacodynamics and pharmacokinetics will help in evaluating these patients and is included elsewhere in this text and in Greenblatt's review.[3] The management section is not intended to be a complete review of overdose treatment but rather will focus on the specific needs of the elderly. Preventative measures can hopefully slow the trend of increasing fatalities from poisonings and overdoses.

EPIDEMIOLOGY

Although the elderly constitute only 11% of the population of the United States, they use 25% of the nation's prescription drugs.[4] Chien and coworkers[5] reported that 83% of those people over 60 years of age were taking 2 to 6 drugs, and 14% were taking from 7 to 15 drugs routinely. Older persons often have multiple illnesses and may require multiple drugs for treatment. However, the large numbers of drugs used by the elderly contribute significantly to the chances of adverse reactions and misuse, either inadvertent or intentional.[6]

Iatrogenic Drug Poisoning

Adverse drug reactions in the elderly constitute a major clinical problem, accounting for 10 to 15% of hospital admissions.[7] A Federal Drug Administration (FDA) study of adverse drug reactions (ADRs) in the elderly, conducted from 1969 to 1983, listed 13 pharmacologic classes of drugs as being most commonly associated with reported problems (Table 6–1).[8] There were 200 specific drugs listed for which there had been over 50 reports of adverse reactions in geriatric patients. Diuretics, digoxin, oral hypoglycemics, histamine blockers, and nonsteroidal anti-inflammatory drugs (NSAIDs) were listed by Dr. Lamy of the University of Maryland as being the most common cause of ADRs in the elderly.[9]

Accidental Poisoning

It is well known that many elderly patients have difficulty taking medications as prescribed by their clinicians. Schwartz[10] found that 57% of a group of persons in the 60 to 75 age group made one or more medication errors, and 68% of persons over age 75 made one or more errors. The most frequent error was omission of medication, followed by lack of knowledge about medication, use of medications not prescribed by a clinician, and errors of dosage, sequence, and timing.

Table 6–1 Medications That Cause Adverse Drug Reactions in Geriatric Patients

The medications are numbered, beginning with the most frequently abused drug and ending with the least frequently abused one.

1. Antiparkinsonian
2. Antibiotics
3. Antiarthritics
4. Antiarrhythmics
5. Diuretics
6. Tranquilizers
7. Antihypertensives
8. Analgesics/antipyretics
9. Antidepressants
10. Radiographic
11. Adrenergic blocking agents
12. Anticonvulsants
13. Vasodilators

From FDA data base, 1969–1983.

Klein-Schwartz and associates[11] found that among patients referred to their center (Maryland Poison Center), the proportion of those older than 60 who had suffered accidental poisoning (83%) was much higher than the proportion of younger individuals in whom poisoning was accidental (55%). These accidental exposures have been classified as follows:

1. Confusional states. This category includes nursing home patients who, for no apparent reason, ate or drank substances stored within reach (e.g., cosmetics, flowers). In 13 instances, an inappropriate therapeutic dose was taken because of confusion, usually involving patients who had taken a second dose because they forgot they had taken the first.
2. Improper use of the product. These situations involved topical exposures or inhalation injuries that occurred while the product was being used for its intended purpose. In most of these cases, labels on the products containing directions were not followed. For example, mixing ammonia and bleach-containing products together released toxic chloramine gas.
3. Improper storage of an agent. The transfer from the original container to one that can be mistaken for a food or drink container is well documented.
4. Mistaken identities. Nonfood items were mistaken for food, and various substances (e.g., cleaning products) were mistaken for human therapeutic agents.

Of the 276 agents to which these older patients were exposed, drugs accounted for 148, household products for 42, personal care products for 34, plants for 7, and other miscellaneous agents for the remaining 57. The drugs most commonly involved were topical agents (e.g., pesticides), sedative hypnotics and minor tranquilizers, analgesics, cardiovascular drugs, antidepressants, and ethanol. The most common exposure site was in the patient's home (64%). Although only 27.4% of the study population received treatment in the emergency room, the probability of admission for the elderly person was significantly greater than that for younger adults and children.

Intentional Poisoning

The incidence of successful suicide is highest in the elderly; older persons taking an overdose are more likely to be making a real suicide attempt rather than a "gesture."[7] Physical and mental illnesses contribute to the problem of suicide among the aged, and some of the drugs prescribed for treatment are often accessible to the older person for misuse in suicide.[12] Digoxin, antianginals, oral hypoglycemics, and antihypertensives are commonly found in the homes of the elderly and are all potentially toxic.

A United Kingdom study by Edwards and Crome[13] showed a wide range of self-poisoning problems in those over the age of 65. Barbiturates were the most common cause of successful suicides.[5] The correlation between the increasing insomnia often associated with old age and the availability of barbiturates as a suicide means is still apparent. Benzodiazepines were the most common drug ingested, followed by tricyclic antidepressants and chlormethiazole (sedative-hypnotic). The elderly were more likely to use old-fashioned, and thus more toxic, household products, which may be taken accidentally or intentionally. Examples of such products include concentrated bleach, ethylene glycol, and hydrocarbon solvents.

The American Association of Poison Control Centers (AAPCC) began collecting uniform data from affiliated control centers in 1983. This National Data Collection System has compiled the largest poison exposure data base ever collected in the United States (Table 6–2). Because of the growth and development of this relatively new data collection project, extrapolations from the number of reported poisonings occurring annually in the United States cannot be made from these data alone. However, despite the limitations of the spontaneous reporting system, the absolute number of exposures still provides a general profile of the spectrum of poisoning cases detected, the population affected, and the severity.[2]

A review of the fatality data demonstrates that 71% were intentional ingestions or exposures; 14.5% were

Table 6–2 Human Poison Exposure Cases Reported to the American Association for Poison Control Centers

Year	Reported exposures	Total fatalities	Geriatric fatalities (%)
1983	251,012	95	8 (8.4)
1984	730,224	293	15 (5.1)
1985	900,513	328	48 (14.5)
1986	1,098,894	406	76 (18.7)
1987	1,166,940	397	76 (19.1)

listed as accidental.[2,14-16] Table 6–3 lists those categories most frequently implicated in poisoning fatalities among geriatric patients. Only fatalities deemed to be "probably" or "undoubtedly" related to the exposure are included. Analgesics, antidepressants, and cardiovascular and asthma drugs were implicated in the greatest number of deaths (Table 6–4). Interestingly, there were more fatalities from aspirin ingested alone than from acetaminophen. This may reflect greater aspirin utilization in the elderly or reflect only the influence of prior cardiovascular disease on aspirin survival.[2]

According to studies reported by Vestal in 1978, there is no evidence that the elderly are more sensitive to the therapeutic and toxic effects of digoxin than the general population.[4] The failure to treat early with digoxin-specific Fab fragments (secondary to limited availability) or the administration of grossly inadequate amounts occurred in 6 of the 11 fatalities (54.5%) in which digoxin was the primary agent.[2,16] However, with theophylline and the tricyclic antidepressants, the elderly do seem to be more sensitive to cardiac toxicity.[4] This, as well as availability, may be important factors in the trends noted above.

PATIENT PRESENTATION

The presentation of the poisoning victim may be simple and straightforward, as with many accidental ingestions or with suicide attempts who call for help or leave a note. More frequently, however, the initial presentation is obscure. It is not unusual for the diagnosis of poisoning to be made in the hospital when a drug screen test has been ordered as an afterthought, or after the patient has been admitted to a psychiatric ward, or even after death.

In healthy young adults, drug overdose is by far the most common cause of coma, whereas in the elderly the

Table 6–3   Profile of Geriatric Fatality Cases by Category of Substances and Products*

	Number of geriatric fatalities (%)
Analgesics	40 (19.4)
Cardiovascular drugs	32 (16.5)
Antidepressants	27 (13.9)
Asthma therapies	19 (9.8)
Cleaning substances	14 (7.2)
Gases and fumes	12 (6.2)
Alcohols/glycols	9 (4.6)
Sedative-hypnotics	9 (4.6)
Chemicals (cyanide, acid)	8 (4.1)
Insecticides/pesticides	4 (2.1)
Antipsychotics	3 (1.6)
Hydrocarbon solvents	3 (1.6)
Heavy metals (arsenic)	2 (1.0)
Miscellaneous	12 (6.2)

*Data from the American Association of Poison Control Centers (AAPCC), 1985–1987.

Table 6–4   Specific Drugs/Toxins Commonly Involved in Geriatric Fatalities in Order of Frequency*

1. Theophylline
2. Aspirin
3. Digoxin
4. Acetaminophen
5. Carbon monoxide
6. Amitriptyline
7. Alkaline cleaners
8. Ethylene glycol
9. Imipramine
10. Verapamil

*Data from the American Association of Poison Control Centers (AAPCC), 1985–1987.

causes of altered consciousness are numerous, e.g., stroke, infections, metabolic disturbances. Drug overdose should always be considered once other common causes have been ruled out.[13] Poisoning should also be suspected in the differential diagnosis of the following problems common in the elderly:

- Cardiac arrhythmias
- Pulmonary edema
- Parkinson's disease
- Cerebrovascular insufficiency
- Infection/sepsis
- Hypothermia
- Epilepsy
- Organic brain syndrome
- Major depression
- Acute psychosis
- Hepatic failure
- Uremia
- Head injury
- Glaucoma
- Metabolic disturbances
- Hypoglycemia

The diagnosis of poisoning in the elderly may be more difficult if there is a coexisting physical disease or if a drug with neurologic or cardiovascular effects has also been taken. For example, the psychiatric patient suffering from an overdose may also have concomitant head trauma, or the patient with a focal neurologic deficit may also be overdosing on a hypoglycemic agent.

Prior medical history, current medications, and allergies should all be determined from family and friends if the patient is unable to relate the information. Determine whether empty pill bottles were found nearby. Remember, ingestion of over-the-counter preparations can be toxic, particularly those containing aspirin, acetaminophen, and antihistamines. The patient should be asked whether any home remedies or self-treatments have been administered — the cure may have been worse than the disease.[17]

For the patient with obscure signs and symptoms or those that suggest exposure to toxins, a detailed occupational and vocational history should be obtained. The growth and diversification of hobbies have introduced a multitude of hazardous substances into the household. Elderly artists and craftsmen often face daily exposure to toxic substances, including solvents in paints, inks, and thinners; lead, cadmium, and other metals in pigments, pottery glazes, copper enamels, and silver solders; and dusts, such as silica and asbestos, in clays, talcs, and glazes. The basement studio may be poorly ventilated and messy, thus exposing the family as well as the hobbyist to toxic substances.[18]

Many elderly patients will deny completely that they have taken an overdose, and it may be equally difficult to elicit symptoms of an underlying psychiatric illness. In general, a patient with severe poisoning may present with coma, cardiac arrhythmias, metabolic acidosis, seizures, and gastrointestinal disturbances, either as symptom complexes or as isolated events. Hepatic, renal, respiratory, and bone marrow failures are delayed complications. When the patient's medications are known, a therapeutic drug level may be all that is needed to confirm your suspicions. In other cases, a toxicologic screen will be indicated.

CLINICAL EVALUATION

The physical examination can help to identify the agent and detect complications of the poisoning and underlying systemic disease.

Temperature. Pyrexia can occur with a great number of ingestions and a number of systemic disorders but is a hallmark of poisoning with anticholinergics, dinitrophenols, and salicylates. Hypothermia can develop because of exposure or hypoglycemia, or it can result from overdose with many agents (e.g., barbiturates, alcohol, and opiates).

Blood pressure. Hypertension is characteristic of sympathomimetic and anticholinergic agents. Almost all sedatives and hypnotics will cause hypotension if taken in large amounts.

Pupils. Mydriasis occurs with hypothermia caused by hypnotic drug poisoning and with the use of tricyclic antidepressants and phenothiazines. Miosis occurs with the use of opiates and organophosphate insecticides.

Breath. If the breath smells like silver polish, consider cyanide poisoning. A fruity odor may be detectable with diabetic ketoacidosis. Parathion smells like an insecticide. A cleaning fluid smell suggests carbon tetrachloride. The various hydrocarbons all have a characteristic odor.[17]

Skin. Diaphoresis points to hypoglycemia and myocardial infarction, but it is also seen in organophosphate or salicylate poisoning. Bullae occur in barbiturate, glutethimide, carbon monoxide, and tricyclic antidepressant poisoning. Anticholinergics, alcohol, and cyanide produce a pink, flushed skin. Carboxyhemoglobin may produce a cherry-red color, although this is not always obvious.[17]

Heart. Changes in heart rate or rhythm may be the presenting feature in many drug overdoses. Bradycardia is quite common with many drugs or disorders that cause central nervous system (CNS) depression, as well as

digoxin and beta-adrenergic blocking agents. Tachycardia, on the other hand, commonly results from stimulants, anticholinergic drugs, tricyclic antidepressants, and theophylline. Arrhythmias may be caused by all of these drugs and by all antiarrhythmic drugs, as well.[7]

Seizures. Common causes for seizures include cerebral hypoxia, hypoglycemia, direct toxic effect (i.e., tricyclic antidepressants), and loss of control of idiopathic epilepsy.

MANAGEMENT

The basic procedures of overdose and poison management in the elderly are identical to those followed for the general population. There are, however, age-specific considerations in both management techniques and potential complications from management.

All emergency treatment regimens, including toxicologic emergencies, begin with the "ABCs" — airway, breathing, circulation. In the elderly, the potential for airway compromise independent of the overdose must be kept in mind. A previous cerebrovascular accident, with residual difficulties with the gag relex or with swallowing, needs to be evaluated before ipecac is given or before lavage without endotracheal tube airway protection can be considered.

Loose-fitting dentures, the ability to sit up, and residual facial paralysis all must be taken into consideration in securing the airway of an elderly overdose victim. Decreased reserves in the respiratory and cardiovascular system are usual, and more careful assessment and monitoring are indicated in the geriatric population. Routine use of baseline arterial blood gases, oxygen saturation monitoring, and cardiac monitoring are indicated.

Naloxone should be given, 2 mg intravenously, in any suspected overdose victim who exhibits an altered level of consciousness. A blood sugar level, which can be checked at the bedside in less than 2 minutes, is preferred to the indiscriminate use of dextrose in elderly patients who present with an altered level of consciousness, where the exact etiology has not been determined. Request the following tests at the same time that decontamination procedures are initiated: laboratory samples for serum drug levels; toxicologic screening of serum, urine, and gastric aspirate; and baseline complete blood count, electrolytes, and renal and liver panels.

In the decontamination phase of care, unique characteristics of the elderly will modify treatment. The increasing likelihood of underlying chronic lung disease and predisposition to cardiac dysrhythmias must be taken into consideration when evaluating the need to administer high-flow oxygen to people who present with inhalation injuries. Oxygen should never be withheld if indicated, but close monitoring of the ventilatory status for loss of respiratory drive must be maintained.

Epinephrine is usually avoided for wheezing induced by respiratory irritants. Aminophylline bolus and maintenance doses are lowered by 25% from the standard adult dose for those over 65 years. The use of steroids, controversial in most inhalation injuries, is not contraindicated in the elderly, but their age-related pharmacokinetics have not been well defined.[4]

The decontamination of topical exposures will be the same in the elderly as in other patients. Friable skin, denuded surface areas, or chronic dermatologic disorders could theoretically enhance absorption of chemicals and toxins with a more serious intoxication than would have been otherwise expected. The increased susceptibility of the elderly to hypothermia must be kept in mind since there is a tendency to immediately undress and wash the entire body in a cold emergency department. Showers with controlled water temperature and higher flow of water are a better form of decontamination if the patient is able to stand and does not require electrical monitoring devices.

In gastrointestinal decontamination, ipecac or gastric lavage is indicated with appropriate attention to the airways as previously discussed. Activated charcoal should then follow, with some authors recommending using charcoal first, or instead of, ipecac or lavage.[19,20,30] In certain common overdoses such as theophylline, repetitive doses of activated charcoal have been shown to decrease the serum half-life of the drug.[19,21] However, concomitant use of cathartics, particularly magnesium citrate, has been associated with significant electrolyte imbalances. Very cautious use of cathartics and careful monitoring of serum electrolytes and fluid balance are essential in the elderly (Table 6–5).

Following the initial stabilization, ongoing supportive measures to evaluate and maintain stability of vital functions are required. Frequently, this is all that is needed to ensure a successful outcome. However, certain overdoses and poisonings, common in the elderly, have specific antidotes available that should be considered (Table 6–6). One needs to evaluate serum drug levels where available and the patient's overall clinical status to determine if these are indicated. The efficacy of N-acetylcysteine for acetaminophen intoxication is well established as are Fab fragments for digoxin toxicity.[22] The use of repetitive doses of activated charcoal for theophylline, tricyclic antidepressants, phenobarbital, cardiac glycosides, phenylbutazone, and carbamazepine was recently reviewed.[19] Hyperbaric oxygen for carbon monoxide is controversial but should be considered in the patient with moderate to high blood levels of carbon monoxide (> 40%) and/or cardiac or neuropsychiatric symptoms.[23,24] Chelating agents such as deferoxamine, dimercaprol (British anti-Lewisite [BAL]), calcium disodium edetate (EDTA), and penicillamine are indicated for symptomatic acute or chronic heavy metal intoxications. Recently ethylene glycol poisoning has been treated early (before renal failure) with the alcoholic dehydrogenase inhibitor 4-methylpyrazole.[29]

Table 6–5   Administration of Activated Charcoal

Initial dose: 1 gm/kg body weight
Repetitive doses: 0.5 gm/kg body weight q. 4 h

Procedure:

1. Suspend charcoal in water, 70% sorbitol, or saline cathartic until a soup-like consistency is obtained.
2. The slurry may be drunk or passed through a lavage tube.
3. If the patient vomits the dose, it may be repeated (protect airway).
4. Continue dosing every 4 hours until the patient is stable and serum concentrations are normal (alternate sorbitol and aqueous suspensions).
5. Concurrent therapy (i.e., diuresis, urine alkalinization, and dialysis) may be used as indicated.
6. During therapy, monitor fluid and electrolyte balance and gastrointestinal motility.

Contraindications:

1. Charcoal will not absorb caustic agents, some heavy metals, or aliphatic hydrocarbons.
2. Adynamic ileus or intestinal obstruction.
3. When specific antidotes (such as N-acetylcysteine or Mucomyst) are used concurrently with charcoal therapy, their dosage may need to be increased.

Modified from Flomenbaum NE, Goldfrank LR, Kulberg AG, et al: General management of the poisoned or overdosed patient. In Goldfrank LR, Flomenbaum NE, and Lewin NA, editors: Goldfrank's toxicologic emergencies, Norwalk, Conn, 1986, Appleton-Century-Crofts.

Hemoperfusion with charcoal or resin, and hemodialysis or peritoneal dialysis have the same indications as in any overdose. However, forced diuresis and urinary acidification/alkalinization must be performed with caution because of the potential for age-related renal insufficiency, fluid overload, congestive heart failure, and acid-base or electrolyte imbalance. Serum creatinine may not accurately reflect the renal function in a patient with a decrease in muscle mass due to normal aging.

Of those elderly patients treated in emergency departments for overdoses, 52% are admitted to the hospital, contrasting with 38% for the general adult population and 11% for children. Early management will frequently require intensive care unit admission to ensure careful monitoring of vital functions. All intentional overdose/poisoning patients should receive psychiatric

Table 6–6   Some Drugs with Specific Antidotes

Poison	Antidote
Acetaminophen	N-acetylcysteine (Mucomyst)
Anticholinergic agents	Physostigmine (Antilirium)
Carbon monoxide	100% oxygen
Cyanide	Sodium nitrate, sodium thiosulfate
Ferrous salts	Deferoxamine
Lead	EDTA*
Mercury (arsenic gold)	BAL*
Methanol (ethylene glycol)	Ethanol
Narcotics	Naloxone (Narcan)
Nitrites	Methylene blue
Organophosphates	Atropine, pralidoxime

*EDTA = calcium disodium edetate; BAL = British anti-Lewisite.

evaluation and treatment prior to discharge. In accidental poisoning situations, attention must be paid to the home or lifestyle factors that contributed to the problem. Preventive measures should be instituted before discharge.

PREVENTION

Efforts must be made by all those involved in the delivery of health care to the elderly, as well as the community as a whole, to prevent both accidental and intentional drug overdoses/poisonings in the aging population.

The level of seriousness of the attempted suicide and the incidence of successful suicide are highest in the elderly.[12,13,25] The drugs selected by the elderly are generally based on availability. As one can see from the AAPCC data, there were no deaths reported from stimulants or street drugs in the subset of patients over 65.[2,14-16] Instead, 77% of the elderly attempting suicide obtain the drugs from their physicians.[12] In attempting to identify the elderly who are at risk for suicide, several factors may be helpful. Sixty percent of the elderly who attempt suicide had a significant degree of physical disease; 80% suffered from depression, and only 13% indicated to someone else that they would try to kill themselves.[12] Social isolation, recent losses, lack of meaningful employment, poor economic situation, and poor self-image all contribute to an increased likelihood of suicide.[7,26] Signs and symptoms of depression should be aggressively sought by the physician, visiting nurse, and all who deal with the elderly. Specific questions about suicidal ideation need to be asked, and the answers need to be taken seriously. Old age and depression are not synonymous, and treatment of depression in the elderly is indicated.

The incidence of accidental ingestion and overdose, misuse of medications, and toxic chemical exposures may be decreased by several approaches (Table 6–7). The physician prescribing any medication should do so with the particular needs and circumstances of the elderly in mind. The first step is to determine if a drug is truly needed, and this will depend heavily on determining an accurate diagnosis rather than treating symptoms. One should always evaluate the possibility that the symptoms the patient is having may be due to a medication reaction. Decreasing or stopping a medication may be more appropriate than adding another one. If a medication is needed, the choice of which one to use should depend on known side effects, routes of metabolism, interactions with already prescribed drugs, and ease of scheduling doses. It is generally recommended that physicians start with lower doses in the elderly and check drug levels early and often, particularly for drugs with narrow therapeutic ranges.[4,7,11]

The physician should also discuss with the patient the correct method for taking the medication, the desired effect, and possible side effects. It is also important to provide clearly written instructions and a review of the information with those who will be assisting in the care of the patient. Limiting the total number of doses prescribed at one time, as well as the number of refills, is helpful. In one 1976 study of 130 elderly patients discharged from the hospital, 66 patients had deviated from their prescribed drug regimen within 10 days of discharge. Of those patients, 46 claimed they didn't understand their instructions, while the other 20 admitted to noncompliance.[27] Clear labeling, unit dose packaging, medication calendars or diaries, or weekly dose holders that can be filled by a friend or visiting health nurse may help prevent accidental misuse.[4,11,26,28]

In the area of nondrug toxic exposures, the importance of leaving products in their original container, reading all labels and warnings before using a product, and properly storing potentially dangerous substances are all appropriate preventive health measures to discuss with the elderly patient. A home evaluation by the public health department or visiting nurse service to review these areas could also prove beneficial.

Table 6–7   Preventing Drug Toxicity in the Elderly

- Strive for a diagnosis prior to treating.
- Take a careful drug history.
- Consider overdose risk in elderly patients with clinically evident psychiatric conditions.
- Know the pharmacokinetics of the drug(s).
- Use minimal drug doses.
- Simplify the treatment regimen — avoid polypharmacy.
- Destroy old medicines.
- Use medication cards, diary, or containers for daily doses.
- Make patient aware that medications can cause, as well as cure, illness.
- Instruct family members.
- Use visiting nurse services.
- Check serum drug levels when appropriate.
- Support community education.

SUMMARY

Elderly patients are at risk for both accidental and intentional overdose or poisoning from many of the drugs and products in their living environment. While management techniques are straightforward, the normal physiology of aging as well as concomitant chronic illnesses must be taken into consideration. Patient identification is frequently difficult. Therapeutic drug levels and toxicologic screening are often helpful. Preventive measures should be aggressively pursued by all members of the health care team.

REFERENCES

1. Rachlis D: Suicide and loss adjustment in the aging, Bull Suicidol (NIMH) 7:23–36, 1970.
2. Litovitz TL, Martin TG, and Schmitz B: 1986 annual report of the American Association of Poison Control Centers National Data Collection System, Am J Emerg Med 5:405–445, 1987.
2b. Litovitz TL, Schmitz BF, Matyunas N, et al: 1987 annual report of the American Association of Poison Control Centers National Data Collection System, Am J Emerg Med 6:479–512, 1988.
3. Greenblatt DJ, Sellers EM, and Shader RI: Drug disposition in old age, N Engl J Med 306:1081–1088, 1982.
4. Vestal RE: Drug use in the elderly: a review of problems and special considerations, Drugs 16:358–382, 1978.
5. Chien C, Townsend EJ, and Ross-Townsend A: Substance use and abuse among the community elderly: the medical aspect, Addict Dis 3:357–360, 1978.
6. Schernitski P, Bootman JL, Byers J, et al: Demographic characteristics of elderly drug overdose patients admitted to a hospital emergency department, J Am Geriatr Soc 28:544–546, 1980.
7. White A and Crome P: Common causes and clinical signs of poisoning in the geriatric patient, Geriatr Med Today 5:31–35, 1986.
8. Moore SR: Adverse drug reactions in geriatric patients in the United States, J R Soc Health 106:169–171, 1986.
9. Lamy PP: The elderly and drug interactions, J Am Geriatr Soc 34:586–592, 1986.
10. Schwartz D, Wang M, Zeitz L, et al: Medication errors made by elderly, chronically ill patients, Am J Public Health 52:2018–2021, 1962.
11. Klein-Schwartz W, Oderda GM, and Booze L: Poisoning in the elderly, J Am Geriatr Soc 31:195–199, 1983.
12. Benson RA and Brodie DC: Suicide by overdoses of medicines among the aged, J Am Geriatr Soc 23:304–308, 1975.
13. Edwards N and Crome P: The poison unit and the elderly, Geriatr Med 12:86–91, 1982.
14. Veltri JC and Litovitz TL: 1983 annual report of the American Association of Poison Control Centers National Data Collection System, Am J Emerg Med 2:420–443, 1984.
15. Litovitz TL and Veltri JC: 1984 annual report of the American Association of Poison Control Centers National Data Collection System, Am J Emerg Med 3:423–450, 1985.
16. Litovitz TL, Normann SA, and Veltri JC: 1985 annual report of the American Association of Poison Control Centers National Data Collection System, Am J Emerg Med 4:427–458, 1986.
17. Haddad L: General approach to poisoning. In Tintinalli JE, Rothstein RJ, and Krome RL, editors: Emergency medicine: a comprehensive study guide, New York, 1985, McGraw-Hill, pp 261–268.
18. Goldman RH and Peters JM: The occupational and environmental health history, JAMA 246:2831–2836, 1981.
19. Jones J, McMullen MJ, Dougherty J, et al: Repetitive doses of activated charcoal in the treatment of poisoning, Am J Emerg Med 5:305–311, 1987.
20. Curtis RA, Barone J, and Giacona N: Efficacy of ipecac and activated charcoal/cathartic, Arch Intern Med 144:48–52, 1984.
21. Lim DT, Singh P, Nourtsis S, and Dela Cruz R: Absorption inhibition and enhancement of elimination of sustained-release theophylline tablets by oral activated charcoal, Ann Emerg Med 15:1303–1307, 1986.
22. Rollins DE and Brizgys M: Immunological approach to poisoning, Ann Emerg Med 15:1046–1051, 1986.
23. Norkool DM and Kirkpatrick JN: Treatment of acute carbon monoxide poisoning with hyperbaric oxygen: a review of 115 cases, Ann Emerg Med 14:1168–1171, 1985.
24. Olsen KR: Carbon monoxide poisoning: mechanisms, presentation and controversies in management, J Emerg Med 1:233–243, 1984.
25. Proudfoot AT and Wright NS: The physical consequences of self-poisoning by the elderly, Gerontol Clin 14:25–31, 1972.
26. Tandberg D: How to treat and prevent drug toxicity. In Schwartz G, Bosker G, and Grigsby JW, editors: Geriatric emergencies: Brady's Series in Emergency Medicine. Bowie, Md, 1984, Robert J Brady Co., Prentice-Hall, pp 75–83.
27. Parkin DM, Henney CR, Quirk J, et al: Deviation from prescribed drug treatment after discharge from hospital, Br Med J 2:686–688, 1976.
28. Odera GM and Klein-Schwartz W: Poison prevention in the elderly, Drug Intell Clin Pharm 18:183–185, 1984.
29. Galliot M et al: Treatment of ethylene glycol poisoning with intravenous 4-methylpyrazole, N Engl J Med 319:97, 1988.
30. Dillion EC et al: Large surface area activated charcoal and the inhibition of aspirin absorption, Ann Emerg Med 18:547, 1989.

Neuropsychiatric Disorders

Evaluating the Elderly Patient with Neurologic Deterioration

Robert J. Grimm, M.D., F.A.C.P.

I am a very foolish fond man,
Fourscore and upward, not an
hour more or less,
And, to deal plainly,
I fear I am not in my perfect mind.

King Lear, Act IV, Scene vii

Aged nervous systems are heir to a number of catastrophes. As the neurologist Alex Comfort once remarked,[1] given the losses in speed, vision, and hearing associated with aging, the chances of being killed by bus number 10 increase. Inflexibility, loss of capacity, hesitancy, and a sensitivity to drugs are characteristic of the aged; an aged brain cannot take much abuse. Vulnerability rather than pathology is the marker. True, subdural hematomas, tumors, and dementias are common in the elderly. However, in the emergency department (ED), understanding and intervention are more serious tasks than mere labeling. Therefore in this chapter neurologic theory is presented first, followed by a discussion of clinical issues relevant to emergency evaluation of the aged.

THEORY

The Brain

The brain is an ensemble of parts and controlled physiologic variables including temperature, pH, glucose, PO_2, and osmolality that serve metabolic machinery supplied by autoregulated regional perfusion. If sufficiently altered, any one of these variables or combinations thereof can precipitate clinical deterioration. It is a matter of degree in the elderly; small changes are enough to cause major alterations in clinical function.

A 1,400-gram brain has an astronomical number of neurons and glia, with cyclic metabolic demands from a neuropil (gray matter) of extraordinary connectivity. The hallmark of the neuropil from crustacea to man is an inherent, stable rhythmicity. In addition to this first neurobiologic principle, there are others (Table 7–1).

Geriatric Neurology

Neurology is the study of derangements in this extraordinarily complex tissue called the brain. A variable or structure within the brain that is pushed beyond its limit may or may not be translated into a symptom. People differ in their ability to realize or express a symptom. It is symptoms, not signs, that provoke ED visits by the elderly.

Signs are another matter. They represent such observable losses as a flattened nasolabial furrow or Babinski's reflex — signs that may easily pass unnoticed. For example, after a 50% loss of dopaminergic neurons in the striatum (prior to the emergence of clinical signs such as the Parkinsonian gait or pill-rolling tremor) the ability to turn over in bed is lost. When would this be noticed and by whom?

Some signs are more easily heard than seen (e.g., dysarthria, a foot slap, or a palatal click). Other signs must be elicited to be seen, including the inability to converge the eyes, positional nystagmus, or loss of abdominal reflexes. An ED visit by an elderly patient means that something unpleasant has happened. It may not initially impress the emergency physician, but it did impress the oldster as unexpected or unwanted; or it may simply be an apprehension that is accompanied by no signs. Put another way, for older individuals who operate within a narrowed range and functional capacity, any loss is an issue. Aging is entropy, and small increments of disorder are enough to induce macro changes in the ability to cope with life.

The Aging Brain

Between the ages of 10 and 90, brain volume shrinks from 10 to 20%. At age 20, the brain/intracranial volume ratio = 0.92; at age 80, it falls to 0.83. This increases the bridging distance for veins (between dura and brain),

thus increasing the susceptibility to a subdural hematoma from trauma that, at the time, "seemed like only a bump."

There is a widely held belief that substantial numbers of neurons are lost during aging. There are approximately 46×10^6 cells per gram in the visual cortex of 20-year-olds; this number may drop to 24×10^6 by age 80, a 48% reduction. However, recent counts suggest a more optimistic view. Disappearance of large neurons from the frontal, temporal, and parietal cortexes in normal, aged brains are nearly matched by a corresponding increase in smaller neurons. For the most part, a reduction in cell volume, rather than in cell numbers, is observed. While awkward movement may be the legacy of such changes, barring vascular loss, degenerations, or bus number 10, *The New York Times* crossword puzzle may not be foreclosed by age.

But there *are* important physiologic changes that affect clinical events. For the first 50 years, the brain uses about 3.3 mL of blood/minute/100 grams or 2.7 liters per hour for a 1,400-gram brain. At age 75, with 10 to 15% less brain weight, the cerebral blood flow drops to 2.7 mL/minute/100 grams, a 25% reduction. There are also correlations between loss of brain weight and performance (Table 7–2).

After the age of 30, there is a gradual trade-off of speed for accuracy.[2] One may still be doing *The New York Times* crossword puzzle at age 75, but it will take 1.4 seconds more to copy a single letter than it did at age 20. This reflects more a matter of encoding delays and perceptual-motor responses than a matter of central processing. For those who keep themselves fit, there is hope. Payton Jordan qualified for the 1936 Olympic trials in the 200-meter dash with a time of 21.1 seconds. He ran the same distance in 25 seconds at age 61. The world's record at age 80 for the same distance was 41.2 seconds in 1979.

Neurologic Examination

Grandfather is spry and a raconteur at 80, but he's not the person he once was. Stooped and shortened, he totters and has lost his legendary strength. Muscle tone is increased, ankle jerks are gone, but his gag and cough reflexes remain. His voice has lost volume and is more hoarse; the speed of pupillary constriction to light, facial mobility, looking upward, and convergence are all diminished. There are losses in arm swing and grace on turns, and his joints are stiff. Gait is slower, and there is

Table 7–1   Neurobiologic Principles

- Gray matter has an inherent electrical rhythm; amplitude is inversely related to frequency.
- Loss of glucose, oxygen, or blood flow produces irreversible brain lesions.
- In general, central nervous system tissue is incapable of self-repair.
- Neural networks are discontinuous (synapses; neuropeptide "pulses").
- Brain is the principal integrator.
- The size principle: small motor neurons discharge before large neurons, thus smoothing performance.

Table 7–2   Brain Weight Lost with Age

Percentage	Function
5%	Decreased creativity; loss of "zing"
10%	Increased frustration; decreased judgment
15%	Deficits in memory and learning
20%	Dementia

less spring to his walk. He no longer can stand and put his pants on. Optic discs are a trifle indistinct; vision and hearing are less acute.

Slow to respond, his short-term memory is unreliable; he repeats himself; he ruminates. Known to Shakespeare and the ancients alike, such are the markers of age. The distance between normal performance and dysfunction shortens. Paresthesia, cognitive slips, trembling, timing errors, and disequilibrium emerge. Where recurrent, these little symptoms indicate a loss of redundancy, the signature of an aged brain.

Redundancy

Stanley Kubrick's film *2001: A Space Odyssey* contains a poignant scene that illustrates the loss of redundancy. At the movie's finale, the hero disables Hal, the demonic computer, by ripping memory circuit cards from the mainframe. Hal begins to sing the tune "Daisy," a self-check routine for system performance. Many cards (now chips) fall before you can detect any change in song quality. And so it is with the human brain: The earliest symptoms of dementia require a loss of, not just a few, but millions of neurons.

In discussing redundancy or the brain's capacity, we are really asking a question: "How much change can the brain withstand without a functional loss? At what point do symptoms or signs appear?" Such questions are tied to the principle of redundancy, the functional reserve of neurons in the elderly and the backup systems that ensure performance in the face of destabilizing influences.

Maximal redundancy is reflected in the neuropsychiatric makeup of normal, young adults (15 to 30 years of age) — a keen period in which age-specific mortality falls, learning is optimized, and endocrine and immune functions peak. Normal is as normal does, translating as a range of intellectual performance, gaits, gestures, ways of talking, and opinions. An epileptic fit, an old polio limb, paraparesis, blindness, or the blatherings of the demented represent a significant loss of redundancy. A similar point can be made with psychosis. Gericault's portrait of paranoia (Figure 7–1) would be recognizable in any culture. It was done in the early part of the nineteenth century for a textbook for the great Paris physician Philippe Pinel, who thought there was a facies of madness. Loss of redundancy for mind or body is the signature of aging.

Entropy

The work of the nervous system is information storage and its subsequent transfer from one neural station to another when needed for various programs or purposes. A faltering brain expresses itself by a loss of performance as denoted by the term entropy. Classically, entropy is a measure of the distribution of energy in a thermo-

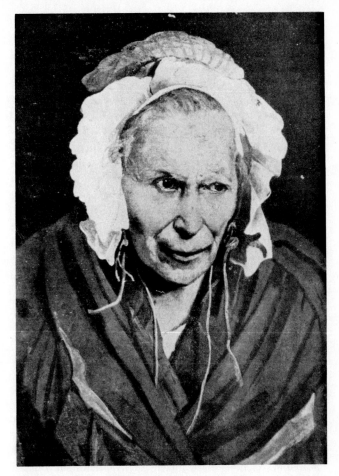

Figure 7–1 La vieille folle, Museum of Lyon, J. Gericault (1791–1824).

dynamic system unavailable for work or, to put it another way, a measure of disorder. As Gleick has remarked, the "inexorable tendency of the universe and any isolated system in it, to slide toward a state of increasing disorder."[3]

Culturally speaking, "order" is equated with social standards (e.g., "social order" versus "social disorder"). But for the brain and its maladies, such definitions are curiously backward. For the brain, too much order (literally speaking) spells trouble. For example, an awake, healthy brain is characterized by a low-voltage, fast (and mixed frequency) electroencephalogram (EEG) responding to an infinitude of sensory inputs in an active person; it is a busy, noisy brain with a central processor (neuropil) as stable as a Roman marketplace.

But if such activity is allowed to synchronize, the individual's mind is a blank (i.e., in an alpha wave pattern) or is in stage 4 slow wave. If the EEG pattern is one of hypersynchrony (high-amplitude, slow waves or frank spiking), the individual is either in a coma or having a seizure. Too much order can mean instability. Entropy represents the loss of functions associated with instabilities. In an older person, the order implicit in stereotyped performance, economy of expression (or its opposite), and limb stiffness (reduction in the degrees of freedom of movement at joints) may be the sign of entropy — the opposite face of redundancy.

Limit Cycles, Stability, and Catastrophes

Stability in any biologic system is the capacity to resist change. "Stable systems" are defined by limit cycles. If not pulled too far, a weight on a spring when released oscillates with a frequency, amplitude, and a die-away time course back to its original starting point.

However, if the pull exceeds the spring's elasticity, it suddenly gives way and irreversibly lengthens, its oscillations seeking a new, more stable cycle (higher amplitude, lower frequency). Such discontinuities or "jumps" have their counterparts in neurology in such phenomena as a convulsion, a dystonic reaction to a phenothiazine, or delirium.

Summary

For the neurologist, then, the concepts of redundancy, entropy, and catastrophe are exceedingly useful. Pathology is neither a focal nor a global lesion but rather a dysfunctional change somewhere in a system (e.g., ataxia can result from many lesion sites as can a faulty perception). When a system becomes unstable, a "catastrophe" (jump) occurs, entropy rises, and the transition is made to a more stable state, however transient or dysfunctional. For an aged brain at the "edge" of limit cycle stability for any particular biologic system you choose, a little fever or drop in cardiac output, a trivial level of drug toxicity, or a mild pneumonia is a potential trigger.

CLINICAL ISSUES

Confusion

Acute, rather than chronic, confusion brings the elderly person to the ED. Inattentiveness, irrelevancy, irritability, and restlessness are preliminary, early events in clinical deterioration. The process (e.g., a developing subdural hematoma) responsible for confusion may itself be chronic, and usually someone other than the patient notes an alarming change. The physician's first task is to identify or exclude end organ failure in the heart, lung, kidney, or liver. Are there focal neurologic signs — e.g., an exophoria (squint)? Has a Wernicke's encephalopathy emerged in a chronic (and concealed) alcoholic?

Brain tumors (metastatic, gliomas, and meningiomas) can also present with confusion precipitated by edema, hemorrhage, or a seizure. If located frontally, subdural hematomas, clots, and tumors may give no focal sign and, further, may not evoke nausea or vomiting in the elderly. The only history may be "My father seemed to have aged quickly in the last few months."

Confusion may also be hidden from view by retirement, depression, a long-forgotten consequence of gastrectomy (pernicious anemia), or intoxication. I once interviewed a healthy old woman in the ED who had been taken off a cross-country bus trip because of confusion. She had steadily downed bromides in anticipation of the family reunion. Any drug in the older brain can produce confusion. Ask the patient about neuroleptics, benzodiazepines, or any of the 600 over-the-counter anticholinergics. No drugs are entirely safe in the elderly, even those taken for routine ailments. Digoxin can cause petit mal status epilepticus, and the long-acting antihistamine meclizine given for dizziness is known to cause confusion.[4]

Suicide

Depression may be overshadowed by physical complaints or present as a pseudodementia featuring diminished concentration, sloppy hygiene, anorexia, or sleep disturbances. The elderly constitute 10% of the population but 25% of the suicides. (They are more successful suicides; the ratio of completed suicides to attempts in the elderly is 8:1.) A depressed elderly person may purposefully take an overdose, mix drugs, or fail to take a life-sustaining drug in a suicide attempt. With noncompliance rates of 25 to 90% in the elderly, a suicide attempt can be misconstrued as patient error.[5]

Weakness

Weakness is a companion to aging and, frequently, a symptom that is a prelude to disaster. Listen for the suggestion of uncertainty of performance — e.g., an "I used to, but now I can't" report. Somewhere in our brains a "decider" — should or shouldn't — exists. The brain reviews the readiness of motor programs and vetoes performances if conditions are unfavorable — stepping over a puddle, going up a ladder, taking the stairs, crossing an icy sidewalk, etc. It may be an atavism as revealed by visual cliff experiments in young animals who freeze when they come to a perceived cliff, prior to any experience with cliffs.

Single Limb Weakness

Limb weakness presenting in the elderly is a challenge; the problem is not a hemiparesis of sudden onset but a complaint of a single limb weakness. There are two causes of sudden single leg weakness. The first, an acute infarct of the femoral nerve in a diabetic (loss of the quadriceps), is diagnosed by history taking and treated with reassurance and disease control; it will improve with time and physical therapy. The other is an emergency: an acute retroperitoneal hemorrhage coupling psoas with quadriceps weakness. When this is recognized, immediate surgical consultation is required. If the clot is not evacuated, the nerve will be destroyed. Epidural bleeds produce unheralded, excruciating, and nonradiating back pain — a sign of aortic dissection or herniated disc. Weakness, reflex loss, and sensory changes follow.

Single arm weakness is rarely an ED issue in the acute setting except for cervical radiculopathy that occurs after an injury to the aged neck with foraminal spurs. This condition will be accompanied by an unbearable pain. A tardy ulnar paresis, when illuminated by some contemporary event, may present in the ED as acute weakness; pain is seldom an issue. Look for the telltale signs of muscle wasting in the hand, ulnar pattern sensory loss, and a positive Tinel's sign (tap-induced paresthesia) from the ipsilateral ulnar notch.

I once saw an elderly, insulin-diabetic woman with progressive hand weakness and numbness. She complained, "My legs feel weak." Her unusually brisk knee jerks (not accounted for by diabetes) came from a foramen magnum site meningioma pressing on the cord. The sensory changes in her hands were from cervical osteophytes, not diabetes.

Weakness in Both Legs

Bilateral leg weakness requires consideration of other etiologies. If proximal, it is characterized by a waddling gait as seen in temporal arteritis (polymyalgia rheumatica form). From any cause, the increased stretch reflexes of mild spasticity present as a sense of weakness. For leg weakness or aching associated with a sensory disturbance, one should consider the Guillain-Barré (GB) syndrome.[6] GB syndrome has a bimodal distribution with a first peak between ages 15 and 34 and a second greater peak between ages 50 and 74. Diagnosis in the elderly is overlooked because of its varied presentations, coexistence of other neurologic disease, and the belief that it only occurs in the young. Early recognition is vital if respiratory failure and cardiovascular collapse are to be avoided. GB syndrome may also present with leg aching and weakness elsewhere, e.g., the dribbling of saliva.

General Weakness

If not from thyroid or parathyroid dysfunction or as a mask for depression, weakness is often the initial presentation of a number of underlying neurologic and nonneurologic conditions. In the immunosuppressed patient, search for infection; if none is detected, suspect a central nervous system (CNS) lymphoma. A mild sensory neuropathy (absent stretch reflexes) and leg weakness can herald a remote effect of cancer, and if only one leg is involved, can suggest a retroperitoneal mass. Progressive weakness of amyotrophic lateral sclerosis (ALS) can present as weakness and weight loss. It may be detec-

table by letting the fingertips of the patient rest in your palm. Over a minute or so, note the fine "piano" twitches (fasciculations) of the fingers from dying motor neurons.

Late-Onset Myasthenia Gravis

Late-onset myasthenia gravis (MG) rarely presents as a primary event in the ED. Rather, myasthenics will come for other reasons such as aspiration or acute weakening secondary to fever (similar to the effect of heat on multiple sclerosis patients). Often, this is in combination with an erstwhile effort to keep up with their fever-driven weakness by taking more Mestinon (pyridostigmine, an anticholinesterase blocking agent). If the patients have also been on certain antibiotics (which potentiate their neuromuscular junction defect) or have been using any CNS depressant drug, there is more trouble. One elderly myasthenic came to the ED when she ran out of Mestinon. When I asked about symptoms (she looked perfectly well), she reported she used the drug to stop her chest pains. By slowing her heart rate (antiacetylcholinesterase effect of Mestinon), the drug reduced the body's cardiac work load, and angina ceased.

Ptosis and diplopia (as seen in younger myasthenics) may be absent in the elderly patient, but it is important to listen for a nasal voice, hoarseness, and difficulty in clearing secretions. MG is not the only condition that will give a nasal voice; another possibility is diphtheria, but botulism is more likely. Look for big pupils and a dry mouth in the context of a recent summer picnic or a sampling of home-canned vegetables.

Syncope

Fainting results from insufficient blood reaching the reticular core of the brainstem. Once the patient is down and gravity is out of the way, revival begins even after a Stokes-Adams attack. A few involuntary twitches are permissible; they do not mean epilepsy. Syncope is separable from cardiac arrest and coma on grounds of duration. Faints are reversible, without a prolonged confusion, and no appearance of dysarthria. Faints are distinguished from narcoleptic interludes, seizures, vertigo, fugues, and trances by other findings.

At midnight in the ED, I examined an elderly gentleman in a tuxedo who had passed out at dinner. He was awake and appeared perplexed; he was unable to speak or move the right body side of his body. His wife, who came to the ED with him, seemed nonplussed and assured me he would be all right. When I asked how she knew this she said, "Oh, this is the fourth time this has happened; he always recovers." In the morning, his neurologic deficits had vanished. Carotid ultrasound studies unmasked a subclavian steal syndrome and revealed a flow reversal from the left vertebral into the left subclavian artery that was stenosed at its origin.

In the elderly, chronic diseases frequently coexist, some or all of which can destabilize vascular control when standing (e.g., congestive heart failure, coronary artery disease, diabetes mellitus, and cerebrovascular disease). With aging, baroreceptor sensitivity falls with upright stance; both exercise and cough-induced Valsalva-like maneuvers can also drop perfusion pressure. Micturition syncope is rare in the elderly as are carcinoid tumors of the bladder wall (productive of facial flushes or episodes of wheezing with bladder emptying). Such regressions coupled with circuit-depressing drugs make syncope a classic example of control system failure; it doesn't take much to produce a 25-mm drop in systolic pressure and a fall.

Unsteadiness

Unsteadiness is the promise of an impending fall. It arises from deficits in the structure or metrics of gait or from problems with the body machinery per se (e.g., a painful knee or leg weakness). All movements have structure and metrics. Structure is the term given to the muscle composition or "scoring" of a movement. Metrics (measures) refer to a movement's energy, force, velocity, etc. Unsteadiness usually represents a problem in a central motor program, e.g., labyrinthine errors, loss of substantia nigra (Parkinsonism), hemiparesis, cerebellar disturbances, intoxication, or the first sign of a cervical myelopathy (median bar compression of the anterior spinal artery) unmasked by a fall. Unsteadiness means that a priority program (balance) is in trouble: it is safer to sit than walk. Brisk knee jerks (spasticity or labyrinthine disturbance) point to a program disorder; absent knee jerks suggest a neuropathy or the GB syndrome ("nonprogram" disorder).

Dizziness as Disequilibrium

There can be no precise meaning attached to the term dizziness. It must be individually defined in each patient. If not linked with syncope, vertigo, or "spaciness," let it stand for "disequilibrium," the inability to calibrate stance and motion — a worrisome symptom. Disequilibrium is the sine qua non for a critical loss of redundancy in a priority program in the brain. Equilibrium is an automatic brainstem program derived from a flexible mix of information supplied on-line by the eye, labyrinth, and proprioceptors. A sense of disequilibrium generates dread, uncertainty, and caution.

When elderly patients present with disequilibrium, the clinician should look for any recent change in vision (lens implant), spinal cord function, or sensory function in the feet. Determine whether or not the individual (with eyes open) can stand in a heel-toe position (modified Romberg test) without falling, probably the easiest way in the ED to assess whether or not vestibulospinal control has been lost (compensated for by vision). Acute disequilibrium in the elderly can result from a brainstem or cerebellar stroke, events usually accompanied by cranial nerve losses. A CT scan is mandatory since an acute cerebellar bleed or infarct can compress the brainstem within hours. A spinal tap is contraindicated if you suspect you are dealing with a posterior fossa mass, since it can result in herniation of the brain through the tentorium (especially in the presence of abscess). Cerebellar infarcts or bleeds provide the highest case-fatality rate for vascular insults. A neurosurgical consultation is mandatory as decompression may be lifesaving.

A discourse on dizziness, falling, and fainting in the elderly includes the following points: For postural hypotension from Valsalva maneuvers, consider a posterior fossa or foramen magnum meningioma, cough syncope, or a cerebellopontine angle (CPA) mass if accompanied by tinnitus, deafness, facial droop, and ataxia.

One afternoon I opened my waiting room door to call for a new patient. The woman turned her left ear toward me (contralateral to her sagging face) and staggered to the right as she stood up. Later, her friends told me that during meals food would drop unnoticed from her fork and while driving and talking, she would drift into the oncoming lane of traffic and have to be sharply alerted. During her professional work, there were also reports of inattentiveness and somnolence. A large right CPA meningioma was wrapped around cranial nerves VII and VIII and was also pressing on the superior colliculus, a structure that services an early step in subcortical attention and orientation. At surgery the third ventricle was enlarged indicative of intermittent hydrocephalus accounting for interludes of reduced consciousness.

There are other linkages between symptom and sign. These include:

- Dizziness and headache (posterior fossa mass)
- Dizziness with diplopia, dysarthria, and limb paresthesia (brainstem lesion)
- Dizziness with automatisms, amnesia, or hemisensory deficits (temporal lobe disturbance)
- Dizziness with palpitations and sweating (cancer)

Positional Vertigo and Traumatic Perilymph Fistulae

Positional disequilibrium (certain head movements or positions), after a seemingly trivial head blow or with the passage of time, raises false positional and acceleration signals in the labyrinth. As shown in Figure 7–2, otoconia from the macule of the utricle are sheared off by head trauma or degenerate with age. They float about and collect on the cupula of the posterior canal (cupulolithiasis), deflecting and destroying its normal zero buoyancy.

Such end-organ signal distortions provide the brainstem with erroneous information, which, in turn, pro-

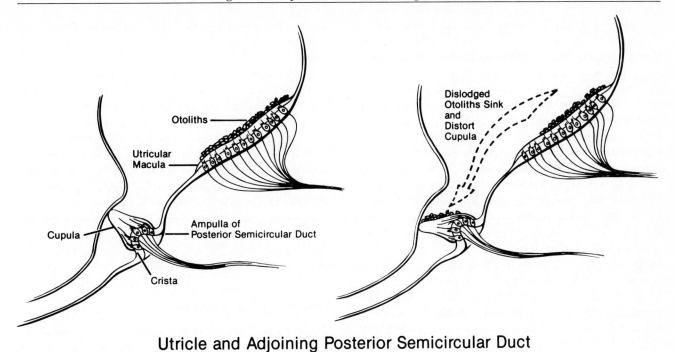

Otoliths

Utricular
Macula

Cupula

Ampulla of
Posterior Semicircular Duct

Crista

Dislodged
Otoliths Sink
and
Distort
Cupula

Utricle and Adjoining Posterior Semicircular Duct

Figure 7–2 Schematic diagram of mechanism of positional vertigo as produced by abnormal stimulation of cupula (cupulolithiasis).

vokes disequilibrium, mal d'embarquement phenomenon (hallucination of swaying after a ride on a boat, elevator, or escalator), or, even worse, a fall. There is also a curious interference with first-order cognition, which convinces the sufferer that he or she also has Alzheimer's disease.

Given the frequency of head injury, and the additional factor of age-based deterioration, the syndrome may be more common in the elderly than previously recognized. It can sometimes be brought out by Bárány's test, in which a backward head drop of 45 degrees (over the edge of an ED gurney) with the head turned to one side is followed by the onset at 2 to 20 seconds of nystagmus. Romberg's test (mentioned earlier) can also be modified and tried.

The elderly patient suffering from acute perilymph fistula caused by head or neck trauma (consciousness need not be lost) presents in the ED with acute dizziness and nausea, ataxia, tinnitus, and occasionally a sensorineural hearing loss. Otologic consultation is indicated.[7]

Strange Movements

Strange movements in the elderly are characteristically induced by neuroleptics. Huntington's chorea and Wilson's disease occur in younger age groups. Variants of parkinsonism with tremor, bradykinesia, and rigidity or progressive supranuclear palsy (PSP) patients, with their stiff necks and reptilian stare, seldom present initially in the ED. A Parkinsonian patient may have been on the floor 4 to 5 hours with an "off" response to long-time use

of antiparkinsonism drugs; in the PSP patient, the response is a backward fall or another pulmonary aspiration from an incompetent swallow.

The occasional hysteric with a bizarre gait disorder or the "shaking in boots syndrome" (orthostatic leg tremor) is occasionally found in the ED. Toxicity from neuroleptics must be considered for the older person with oral-facial dyskinesia (tongue thrusts) or akathisia (a ceaseless, rhythmical stepping in place). Such drugs are prescribed for the nonpsychotic elderly for aggressive behavior and confused states and for sedation. The greatest concern is the development of tardive dyskinesia (TD), a risk that approaches 40% chance in those over the age of 60. The brain is especially vulnerable, not only to TD but also to oversedation, postural hypotension, and the neuroleptic malignant syndrome (NMS); it is a fiction that NMS only occurs in the young. Hemiballismus from an infarct or cerebral hemorrhage in the deep brain near the region of the nucleus of Luys produces dramatic arm flings. The choreic movements of Creutzfeldt-Jakob disease (CJD) and chronic lithium intoxication are of smaller amplitude. Peculiar postures or fixed poses can be seen in schizophrenics. (In catatonia, an arm placed in a certain posture remains there.) The quality of "la belle indifference" (hysteric) can be measured against the disintegrated personality and lack of affect characteristic of psychosis.

Spells

A "spell" may be the only history a physician will get, but it speaks worlds. When a patient speaks of a spell, he/she has told you that it was a brief and novel event, that it passed without sequelae but raised enough alarm (usually from others) to trigger an ED visit. Spells can be divided into two groups: 1) those arising internally (in the brain per se) and 2) those initiated externally (by events outside the head). Seizures arising from an old cerebrovascular accident (CVA), a tumor, or anticonvulsant drug withdrawal are "spells" arising within the head. Orthostatic hypotension, cardiac arrhythmias, sick sinus syndrome, or "drop attacks" from basilar insufficiency (uncommon in the elderly) are events dictated by faults lying outside the head. An attack of Meniere's disease lies on the interface — arising inside the head but outside the brain. For Meniere's disease, knowing the patient's history is crucial.

The interesting thing about a first seizure in an elderly person is not the seizure itself but a question that arises from it. What intrinsic inhibitory mechanisms in the brain have fallen which prevent a seizure? For seizure occurrence, these mechanisms have been breached, the limit cycle stability has been exceeded, and the seizure begins. Tumors and late stroke sequelae (a CVA in the preceding two years) can do it. Such patients need to be hospitalized.

Dementia

Dementia alone rarely brings the elderly person to an ED. Strictly speaking, there are no acute dementias; there are acute psychoses and acute organic brain syndromes (e.g., delirium), but there is no acute Alzheimer's disease. But Alzheimer's or other dementias can worsen. In such cases, it is important to search for some other event that has altered the patient's social or motor behavior (i.e., unsteadiness, decreased awareness, a first seizure, no appetite). Never was the "it-doesn't-take-much" principle more apt. Dementia can be worsened by a mild urinary tract infection, a slight stroke, or an innocuous change in medicine, a subtle pneumonia, or a slowly expanding hematoma.

Senile dementia of the Alzheimer's type (SDAT) and multi-infarct dementia (MID) account for about 90% of ED dements. Pick's disease (knife edge zones of cortical atrophy usually in the temporal lobe) may be distinguishable from SDAT in the ED by elements of the Klüver-Bucy syndrome; the Pick's dementia patient wanders quietly about the ED bay examining everything by mouth.

Three uncommon dementias bear mentioning: progressive multifocal leukoencephalopathy (PML), Binswanger's disease, and CJD, the latter posing some risk for ED personnel.

PML is a multifocal demyelinating disease arising in the immunosuppressed person that is caused by the Creutzfeldt-Jakob virus (papova DNA virus) in 70% of patients. A person with this virus can present in the ED in a confused state — often someone previously treated for cancer or transplant survivors on immunosuppressive drugs.

Binswanger's disease is an atypical dementia characterized by confluent white and gray matter lacunas due to fibrinoid changes in long, penetrating white matter arteries. Hypertension is present in most cases. Binswanger noted that the disease begins slowly between 50 and 65 years of age with relentless mental deterioration and neurologic signs. Computerized tomography (CT) reveals symmetrical deep white matter lucencies. Between 1.6 and 5% of CT scans of adults show similar white matter changes. Consider Binswanger's disease when confronted by a history of a relentless neurologic decline, more neurologic signs than MID, and chronic hypertension with an unimpressive history of stroke.

Creutzfeldt-Jakob Disease

The demented patient with choreic jerks or generalized twitches may be chronically intoxicated with lithium or represent the end stage of Huntington's chorea, or have CJD. Caused by a prion (as opposed to virus), CJD is more infective than cholera stool.[8] It can be passed conjugally, by needle, and by corneal transplant. It is uniformly fatal, sharing this distinction with rabies and AIDS.

CJD involves all levels of gray matter including the spinal cord and has been clinically defined.[9] It is the most rapid moving of the dementias; it can destroy an individual within a year. Special precautions are to be taken (consult your lab) with procedures, blood drawings, or emergency surgery. In humans, CJD, kuru (New Guinea highlands), and Gerstmann-Strausser syndrome (two dementias often presenting first with cerebellar signs) have all been experimentally transmitted to animals. Scrapie of sheep and goats, mink encephalopathy, and chronic wasting disease of mule deer and elk are neurodegenerative diseases of similar design. Similarity of prions to genes regulatory for SDAT raises the question of the connection between aging, unrecognized prions, and gene regulation. Thus, the neurologic elderly in the ED remain a source of new biology and new questions.

ACKNOWLEDGMENTS

I wish to thank Dr. Nancy Grimm and Arnold Towe, Ph.D., for their review and critical comments.

REFERENCES

1. Comfort A: Confusion in the elderly: dementia, delirium, or pseudo-dementia. In Bosker G, editor: Updates in geriatric emergency medicine, Atlanta, 1988, American Health Consultants.
2. Strayer DL, Wickens CD, and Braune R: Adult age differences in the speed and capacity of information processing: 2 An electrophysiological approach, Psychol Aging 2:99–110, 1987.

3. Gleick J: Chaos: making a new science, New York, 1987, Viking Penguin Inc.
4. Molloy DW: Memory loss, confusion, and disorientation in an elderly woman taking meclizine, J Am Geriatric Soc 35:454–456, 1987.
5. Osgood NJ: Suicide in the elderly, Postgrad Med 72:123–130, 1982.
6. George J and Twowmey JA: The Guillain-Barré syndrome in the elderly: clinical and electrophysiological features of five cases, Age Ageing 14:215–219, 1985.
7. Grimm RJ et al: The perilymph fistula syndrome defined in mild head trauma, Acta Otolaryngol [Suppl 464] 1–40, 1989.
8. Prusiner SB: Prions and neurodegenerative diseases, N Engl J Med 25:1571–1579, 1987.
9. Brown P et al: Cruetzfeldt-Jakob disease: clinical analysis of a consecutive series of 230 neuropathologically verified cases, Ann Neurol 20: 597–602.

SUGGESTED READINGS

Blume HT: Immunological aspects of aging. In Terry RD and Gershon S, editors: Neurobiology of aging, New York, 1976, Raven Press.
Godfrey JB and Caird FI: Intracranial tumors in the elderly: diagnosis and treatment, Age Ageing 13:152–158, 1984.
Grimm RJ: Program disorders of movement. In Desmedt JE, editor: Motor control mechanisms in health and disease, New York, 1978, Raven.
Grimm RJ: Disorderly gaits, Neurologic Clinics 2:615–631, 1984.
Heilman KM: Orthostatic tremor, Arch Neurol 41:880–881, 1984.
Jagadha V et al: Atypical Wernicke's encephalopathy and dialysis, Ann Neurol 21:78–84, 1987.
Katzman R and Terry RD: The neurology of aging, Philadelphia, 1983, FA Davis Co.
Mahler M, Cummings JL, and Tomiyasa U: Atypical dementia syndrome in an elderly man, J Am Geriatr Soc 35:1118–1226, 1987.
Peabody CA and Warner D: Neuroleptics and the elderly, J Am Geriatr Soc 35:233–238, 1987.
Pereira M and Kaine JL: Polymyalgia rheumatica and temporal arteritis: managing older patients, Geriatrics 41:54–66, 1986.
Smith SJ and Kocen RS: Lithium associated with Creutzfeldt-Jakob-like syndrome, Neurosurg Psychiatry 31:120–123, 1988.
Strehler BL: Molecular and systemic aspects of brain aging: psychobiology of informational redundancy. In Terry RD and Gershon S, editors: Neurobiology of aging, vol. 3, New York, 1976, Raven Press.
Svenson J: Obtundation in the elderly patient, Am J Emerg Med 5:524–526, 1987.
Venna N: Dizziness, falling, and fainting: differential diagnosis in the aged, Geriatrics 41:30–40, 1986a.
Venna N: Dizziness, falling, and fainting: differential diagnosis in the aged, Geriatrics 41: 31–45, 1986b.

Focal Neurologic Lesions

Gideon Bosker, M.D., F.A.C.E.P.

The differential diagnosis and management of focal neurologic lesions represents one of the most important and challenging aspects of practicing emergency medicine. In a recent study, the emergency services of 3,152 elderly patients were evaluated; neurologic problems were reported by 400 men and 219 women. Neurologic problems were reported by 356 (58%) of those over 75. Of that number, 150 (24%) experienced cerebrovascular accidents; 204 (33%) were characterized by dizziness or syncope.[1-3]

The precise and accurate assessment of neurologic emergencies is complicated by the fact that loss of consciousness, altered mental status, confusion, and other nonspecific neurologic symptoms are frequently the initial complaints of such nonneurologic conditions (e.g., infection, metabolic derangements, collagen vascular disease, and toxicologic emergencies). Of all neurologic problems encountered by the emergency practitioner, focal neurologic lesions are especially common and problematic. In cases of craniocerebral trauma, for example, focal deficits or seizures are usually attributed to intracranial hemorrhage or acute contusional swelling. In those patients without a history of trauma, focal lesions are most often the result of cerebrooclusive disease, most notably thrombotic or embolic cerebral infarction.[4-6]

While many practitioners consider such "lumping" of causes convenient, many neurologic conditions will go undiagnosed and, consequently, untreated, unless a more systematic approach to focal neurologic emergencies is undertaken.[5-7] For example, focal manifestations of CNS derangements may be the first indication of transient ischemic attack (TIA), stroke, or intracranial malignancy, but they may also be the first indication of severe metabolic derangement, myocardial infarction, drug intoxication, dissecting aortic aneurysm, collagen vascular disease, or serious systemic or central nervous system (CNS) infections.[1,3,7] Consequently, the initiation of appropriate therapy in these patients depends upon the ability of the emergency physician to distinguish rapidly among various underlying etiologies and initiate appropriate therapy.

Part of this process requires a systematic diagnostic workup, recognizing the indications for emergency computerized tomography (CT) scanning. Specifically, the goal of the emergency physician is to detect focal brain injury that is amenable to surgical or pharmacologic intervention.[8,9] In the case of cranial trauma, recent studies[7,10,11] indicate that morbidity and mortality from epidural and subdural hematoma are increased when there is a delay between the injury and the operation. In one study, patients with acute subdural hematomas who underwent surgery within 4 hours of the time of injury had a 30% mortality rate, compared with a 90% mortality rate in those who had surgery more than 4 hours after the injury.[11-13]

The purpose of this chapter is to review those conditions that cause focal neurologic lesions and to outline methods of diagnosis, assessment, and management that can potentially reduce morbidity and mortality in this patient population.

GENERAL BACKGROUND

The most common cause of focal neurologic deficits is thrombotic cerebral infarction.[14-16] Since most thrombotic strokes cause abrupt neurologic deficit, this is an important differential point for establishing the diagnosis. Metabolic disorders, however, may also have an abrupt onset, so it is necessary, first, to distinguish stroke from other conditions (such as brain tumors and intracranial lesions) in which neurologic dysfunction usually progresses gradually, but in which the seizures or postictal focal paralysis may be the initial manifestations. Once conditions mimicking primary neurologic disorders have been eliminated, the emergency physician should attempt to identify which of the three categories of cerebroocclusive disease has occurred — thrombosis, embolism, or hemorrhage — since initial therapy will depend upon the underlying cause.

DIAGNOSTIC EVALUATION
Physical Examination

A rapid but comprehensive neurologic exam includes assessment of the following major neurologic functions:

- Mental status
- Station and gait
- Skull and spine
- Meninges
- Motor function
- Sensation
- Proprioception
- Cranial nerves
- Cerebellar function

Although nonspecific, initial vital signs may also give important information. For example, reflex sinus bradycardia and elevated systolic blood pressure are frequently encountered with catastrophic intracranial events such as subarachnoid intracerebral hemorrhage. The carotid pulses may reveal bruits, while the cardiac exam may suggest embolic causes for focal neurologic deficits: atrial fibrillation, paradoxical movement of the left ventricle (aneurysm with possibility of mural thrombus), and murmurs suggesting the presence of valvular disease associated with bacterial or marantic endocarditis.

Neurologic examination of the head-injured patient must be performed rapidly and precisely. The examination consists of noting the pupils' size, equality, and response to bright light; noting level of consciousness (Glasgow Coma Scale — best motor/verbal response, eye opening); and lateralizing extremity weakness. The standard definition of coma — the inability to open the eyes or to make any recognizable sound or follow commands — corresponds to a Glasgow Coma Scale (GCS) of eight or less. It should be noted that the GCS is not generally accurate if the patient is in shock or under the influence of alcohol or drugs but in other cases is generally a good predictor of clinical outcome.[12]

Although CT scans are performed on virtually all patients with severe head injury at the time of admission to the emergency department, the practitioner should be aware of those signs and symptoms that indicate tentorial herniation or upper brainstem dysfunction. These include pupillary dilatation with decreased or absent light reflex, stupor or coma and hemiparesis, flexor or extensor posturing, or bilateral flaccidity.[16]

The completion of a rapid neurologic exam must be accompanied by fluid resuscitation and other emergency measures as dictated by the presence of systemic injuries. A chest x-ray film and a lateral x-ray film of the cervical spine to rule out major neck injury should be obtained in all patients with multiple trauma and external evidence of head trauma. (See Table 8–1.)

Laboratory Examination

Because focal neurologic deficits are frequently the first manifestations of metabolic derangements,[17,18] the initial workup of such patients should include Dextrostix, which may reveal the presence of hypoglycemia or hyperglycemia. An elevated blood sugar level should alert the physician to the possibility of nonketotic hyperglycemic coma, which commonly presents with focal neurologic deficits.[18,19] Serum electrolytes may reveal the cause of a metabolic encephalopathy masquerading as a focal neurologic lesion. Look especially for hyponatremia or hypernatremia, hypomagnesemia, and hypophosphatemia (especially in alcoholic patients), hypokalemia (which can cause profound paralysis and weakness), hypocalcemia (which may be seen in patients with hypoparathyroidism and renal failure), and a large anion gap (which suggests metabolic acidosis).[1,5]

In those patients with a severely depressed mental status, arterial blood gases may reveal hypoxia or CO_2 narcosis. The presence of a quickly resolving lactic acidosis is strongly suggestive of antecedent seizure activity.

Table 8–1   Physical Examination of Patients with Tentorial Herniation

Finding	Number of patients (%) = 100
Cardiac arrest	7
Hypotension (systolic blood pressure less than 800 torr)	31
Major thoracic or abdominal injury	30
Lateralizing pupillary abnormalities	36
Single dilated pupil	63
Hemiparesis or hemiplegia	20
Asymmetric flexor or extensor posturing	11
Flaccidity	32

The electrocardiogram (ECG) may indicate the presence of a cardiac arrhythmia producing cerebral hypoperfusion and secondary focal neurologic deficits in the area of a previous cerebral thrombotic infarction.[20,21] Moreover, silent myocardial infarction may present as an embolic stroke secondary to a mural thrombus or a thrombotic stroke secondary to circulatory failure.[5,20,21] Consequently, all patients with focal neurologic deficits should be monitored with an ECG in the emergency department.

Electrocardiographic Evaluation

Rate and rhythm, most notably the presence of atrial fibrillation, may suggest a likely source of cerebral embolic infarction, while left ventricular hypertrophy (LVH) may suggest the possibility of long-standing hypertension and the presence of intracerebral hypertensive hemorrhage. A prolongation in the QT segment may be the first sign of hypocalcemia or hypomagnesemia, while peaked T waves may be due to hyperkalemia. The presence of U waves may suggest hypokalemia producing weakness, while ST elevation should alert the physician to the possibility of an acute myocardial infarction, with an associated stroke.[20] ST segment and T wave changes (in particular, symmetrical T wave inversion) are sometimes seen with an intracerebral catastrophe.

The incidence of ECG abnormalities in patients with spontaneous subarachnoid hemorrhage, cerebrovascular accident, head trauma, and various intracranial space-occupying lesions varies between 50 and 90%.[3,8,22] A primary, secondary, or coexistent relationship may occur between intracranial events and cardiac abnormalities. Primary cardiac disorders (for example, valvular heart disease, myocardial infarction, and atrial myxomas) may cause neurologic abnormalities by way of embolic phenomena and perfusion disturbances. On the other hand, common etiologic factors may result in coexisting atherosclerotic, cerebral, and coronary artery disease. Consequently, a thorough cardiac evaluation is mandatory in all patients who present with focal neurologic lesions.[20-22]

Computerized Tomography (CT) Scan

The CT scan is especially helpful in the diagnosis and assessment of patients with focal neurologic deficits and craniocerebral trauma.[11,14,23] It must be recognized, however, that temporal considerations exist that effect the false negativity of CT scanning in those patients with nontraumatic injuries. For example, in a bland (i.e., nonhemorrhagic) thrombotic or embolic stroke, only 25% of initial CT scans will be positive between 0 to 48 hours. Between 2 and 5 days, 60% will be positive, while more than 90% will indicate infarction at 7 days after the initial presentation.[3,13,14] This temporal profile reflects the fact that CT scanning diagnosis of cerebral infarction depends on the presence of cerebral edema, which is maximal at 48 to 96 hours following infarction.[1,3,13,14]

Intracerebral hemorrhage (greater than 1.5 cm in diameter) is detected with greater than 95% accuracy in patients with acute hemorrhage and focal neurologic deficits.[13,14] This is true for subdural hematoma, epidural hematoma, cerebellar hematoma, and subarachnoid hemorrhage (SAH) that extends into the ventricular system.[24] Chronic subdural hematoma may be difficult to detect when the hygroma is isodense with brain tissue.[25] Tumors, abscesses, and old areas of infarction are generally detected with high accuracy using the CT scan.

Indications for emergency CT scan of the head include head trauma, suspected subarachnoid hemorrhage, acute focal neurologic deficit plus a diminished level of consciousness, suspected cerebellar hemorrhage, status epilepticus, coma of unknown etiology, cardiovascular accident, or stroke-in-evolution if anticoagulation is being considered. Any patient in whom lumbar puncture is necessary, but who may have an intracranial mass or increased intracranial pressure, should have a CT scan prior to the procedure.[26]

A number of signs in both patients with head injuries and those with nontraumatic events should raise the index of suspicion for intracranial hematoma.

After the airway and circulation have been stabilized, immediate CT scanning should be performed on patients with the following symptoms:

1. Acute pupillary inequality of more than 1 mm (excluding local eye trauma, previous surgery, medication)
2. Persistent neurologic deficit (lateralized extremity weakness, confusion, aphasia)
3. Depressed skull fracture greater than 1 cm
4. Open cranial wounds with exposed brain or central spinal fluid (CSF) leakage
5. GCS of 8 or less
6. Deteriorating level of consciousness
7. Penetrating head injury[10]

Magnetic Resonance Imaging (MRI) Scan

In general, MRI is superior to the CT scan for demonstrating the presence of chronic subdural hematomas.[27] In those patients presenting with a focal neurologic deficit and a history of falls associated with an altered level of consciousness for more than 1 to 2 weeks, an MRI scan should be the initial procedure of choice to detect the possible presence of an isodense subdural hematoma.

Lumbar Puncture

Lumbar puncture is contraindicated in the presence of a focal neurologic deficit that is caused by craniocerebral trauma.[1,5,6] On rare occasions, it may be necessary, however, to employ this procedure in nontraumatic cases to distinguish between hemorrhagic and nonhemorrhagic infarction *when a CT scan is not available* and anticoagulation is contemplated. In the former, red blood cells may be seen with elevated protein, while bland infarction characteristically produces low-grade CSF pleocytosis, elevated protein, and minimally depressed glucose. Subarachnoid hemorrhage will present with grossly bloody CSF, and it is important to distinguish this finding from a traumatic tap. When available, CT scanning is always the preferred initial procedure of choice.

Arteriography

This procedure is reserved for the rapid diagnosis of subarachnoid hemorrhage, tumor, subdural or epidural hematoma, and ruptured aneurysm in those centers where CT scanning is not available. Arteriography should also be employed when carotid or aortic aneurysm with dissection is suspected.

CONDITIONS CAUSING FOCAL NEUROLOGIC LESIONS

Thrombotic Infarction

Cerebral occlusions result in well-described, sudden, focal neurologic deficits and occur without headache and vomiting, or with less severe headache and vomiting than intracerebral hemorrhages. Significant obtundation or depression of consciousness is unusual unless the occlusion involves a massive amount of brain, the brainstem, or a previously diseased brain. A full-blown deficit usually develops in seconds with emboli and from minutes to hours with cerebral thrombotic infarction. (See Table 8–2.)

Cerebral artery thrombosis usually develops at night during sleep, with symptoms perceived by the patient or by the family upon awakening in the morning.[28-30] As a rule, the patient falls asleep without a deficit and awakens with a hemiparesis or speech disturbance. By contrast, cerebral embolism is apt to occur at any time of the day or night and frequently occurs during periods of vigorous physical activity.[30] When evaluating the possibility of cerebral embolic infarction, it is essential to identify a source, if possible. Common sources include atrial thrombi (originating in elderly patients with long-standing chronic atrial or paroxysmal atrial fibrillation), valvular vegetations caused by bacterial endocarditis, thromboembolism in myocardial infarction, and, in patients with extracranial vascular disease, ulcerated plaques in the carotid system. It is, at present, a neurologic axiom that when atrial fibrillation and focal neurologic deficits coexist, cerebral embolization has occurred.[3,31]

As a rule, thrombotic cerebral infarction does not present with severe depression of consciousness unless the basilar artery system is involved or unless there has been massive internal carotid thromboembolism result-

Table 8–2　Stroke Syndromes

Stroke syndrome	Onset to maximal symptoms	Deficit duration
Occlusive		
Emboli	Seconds	> 3 weeks
Thrombi		
TIA*	Minutes	< 1 day
RIND*	Minutes–hours	> 1 day to < 3 weeks
Progressive	Hours–days	> 3 weeks
Completed	Minutes–hours	> 3 weeks
Lacunar	Minutes–hours	> 1 day
Hemorrhagic		
Subarachnoid	Seconds	> 1 day
Intracerebral	Seconds	> 1 day
Cerebellar	Seconds	> 1 day

*TIA = transient ischemic attack; RIND = reversible ischemic neurologic deficit.

ing in acute cerebral edema and secondary compression of brainstem structures.[4] Moreover, thrombotic infarction rarely causes seizures in the acute phase of the illness, although focal seizures do occur as a sequela in those regions that have been scarred as a result of the previous cerebral infarction. The diagnosis of thrombotic cerebral infarction should therefore be suspected in patients with hypercoagulable states due to malignancy, thrombocytosis secondary to collagen vascular disorders, hyperosmolar states, and hypernatremic dehydration, which can lead to venous thrombosis. (See Table 8–3.)

Embolic Infarction

Embolic infarction is the next most common cause of focal neurologic deficits.[3,5,16] As mentioned, embolic infarction usually occurs when the patient is awake and does not present with severely impaired mental status unless there has been a complete occlusion of the carotid artery leading to massive cerebral edema or unless the vascular insult involves the ascending reticular activating system (ARAS). The acute phase of embolic infarction may be accompanied by seizures, which can be either focal or diffuse, in up to 20% of the cases.[3] At present, it is recommended that patients who have had cerebral embolism due to an intracardiac thrombosis associated with atrial fibrillation be anticoagulated immediately with heparin therapy.[5,30] Anticoagulation should be preceded by CT scanning in order to exclude the possibility of hemorrhagic infarction. (See Table 8–4.)

Transient Ischemic Attack (TIA)

TIAs manifest as stereotyped, short-lived, focal neurologic deficits lasting, by definition, less than 24 hours. From the time of onset to the maximal deficit usually requires only a few minutes, and rarely lasts more than 8 hours. Most TIAs resolve within 15 to 60 minutes.[32] Although the definition of TIA is straightforward, management is complex and controversial. (See Table 8–5.)

In one study, 30% of the patients originally diagnosed as having TIAs were subsequently considered not to have had TIAs on review of their medical records by a stroke specialist.[31,33,35] Even neurologists perceive the management of TIAs as difficult, and physicians, in general, are frequently uncertain about how to best evaluate and manage such patients. From the point of view of emergency practice, the greatest clinical significance of TIAs is the fact that they are a harbinger of ischemic cerebral infarction, with its potentially devastating consequences. Estimates of the incidence of infarction following TIA vary, but in the absence of systematic treatment, approximately 5 to 10% of patients will have a stroke within a month and 12% will have one within a year. At the end of 2 years, a stroke will have occurred in an estimated 20 to 40% of TIA patients.[33,35] Therefore, the occurrence and the escalation of frequency of TIAs must be recognized and appropriate measures instituted so that the patient's risk of stroke will be reduced.

Transient focal deficits may be caused by neurologic disorders other than focal ischemia. Features in the history and physical examination may provide clues to these underlying disorders. For example, a throbbing unilateral headache (often occurring after disappearance or improvement of a focal deficit), scintillating scotomas, and accompanying nausea are suggestive of migraine, especially in younger patients. The presence of clonic motor activity and abrupt loss of consciousness followed by confusion or a history of epilepsy or traumatic brain injury is suggestive of a seizure disorder. A recent history of headache, a clouded sensorium, or a depressed level of consciousness with a focal neurologic deficit following a head injury may indicate a subdural hematoma. It is important to note that these may occur without any preceding head injury, especially in the elderly.

Table 8–3   Physical Findings Suggesting Specific Stroke Syndromes

Stroke syndrome	Findings
Emboli	Cholesterol plaques; atrial fibrillation; mitral stenosis murmur; recent myocardial infarction
Thrombi	Absent carotid pulse or (previously present) bruit; progression of findings over many hours
Lacunae	Hypertension; pure motor or sensory deficits; absence of "cortical" sensory findings and aphasias
Subarachnoid hemorrhage	Preretinal hemorrhage; nuchal rigidity; severe headache; nonfocal examination developing over seconds
Intracranial hemorrhage	Severe headache; focal examination developing over seconds; confusion
Cerebellar hemorrhage	Truncal and gait ataxia; nausea and vomiting; peripheral sixth or seventh cranial nerve palsies

Table 8–4   Diagnosis and Treatment of Stroke

Stroke syndrome	Diagnostics	Specific therapies to consider
Occlusive		
Emboli	CT*	Heparin anticoagulation
Progressive	CT and arteriogram	Anticoagulation or surgery
Completed	CT	—
Hemorrhagic		
Subarachnoid	CT ± LP*	Antifibrinolytics
Intracerebral	CT	—
Cerebellar	CT	Surgery

*CT = computerized axial tomography; LP = lumbar puncture.

Although systemic hypotension rarely produces focal symptoms, hemodynamic obstruction of a cerebral artery may produce a decrease in regional blood flow sufficient to cause dysfunction. In addition, cardiogenic emboli are well-known causes of TIA and stroke. Emboli arising from the heart may occur in association with valvular or nonvalvular atrial fibrillation, acute MI, adynamic wall segments following infarction, cardiomyopathy, mitral stenosis, or prosthetic heart valves. Mitral valve prolapse, especially in younger patients, may be associated with cerebral symptoms probably on an embolic basis. Occasionally, septic emboli will originate from a diseased endocardium. So-called paradoxic emboli originating in the lung or venous system and traveling through a patent foramen ovale may also occur. (See Figure 8–1.)

Acute therapy for TIAs includes antiplatelet agents (i.e., salicylates) and, when indicated, anticoagulants. Antiplatelet agents such as salicylates have been successful in reducing recurrences of TIAs, but have not as yet convincingly demonstrated a decrease in long-term stroke risk.[35,36] Except in atrial fibrillation, anticoagulation with Coumadin therapy does not appear to offer any advantage over aspirin (100 mg twice a day) in the treatment of TIAs, but does add significantly to an increased risk of hemorrhage. Thus, evidence at present supports the use of low-dose aspirin alone at the time of diagnosis.

Intracranial Hemorrhage

Hemorrhagic strokes, subarachnoid hemorrhage, and intracranial hemorrhage typically occur during stress or exertion. Precipitating events include sexual intercourse and Valsalva's maneuver. Recent evidence also suggests that alcohol consumption contributes to the incidence of hemorrhagic stroke, especially subarachnoid hemorrhage.[37,38] In most cases, focal deficits rapidly evolve, and many are associated with confusion, coma, or immediate death.

Excruciating headache is the cardinal symptom of intracranial hemorrhage, is classically described as "the worst in my life," and may be accompanied by nuchal rigidity on physical exam. Arteriovenous malformations (AVMs) may bleed into the subarachnoid space, but when they involve the cerebral parenchyma, lateralizing signs will be present. Lack of focal findings and age of presentation help to distinguish subarachnoid hemorrhage from intracerebral hemorrhage. Except for the occasional field cut, oculomotor palsy of aneurysmal compression, or focal seizure, lateralizing focal neurologic lesions are notably *absent* with subarachnoid hemorrhage. On the other hand, patients with intracranial hemorrhage are characterized by prominent focal findings because of the intraparenchymal location of the hemorrhage.

Intracranial hemorrhages are of two main types: intracerebral and extracerebral. In the elderly population,

Table 8–5   Differential Diagnosis of Transient Ischemic Attacks of the Brain

Brain tissue disorders	Blood vessel diseases	Blood elements
Brain tumors or expanding lesions: meningiomas and subdural hematomas	Atherosclerosis	Cardiogenic disorders (reduced cardiac output)
	Arteritides	Thrombocytosis
	• Cranial (temporal) arteritis	Polycythemia vera
	• Polyarteritis nodosa	Hyperviscosity syndrome
	• Systemic lupus erythematosus	Emboli: bacterial endocarditis
	• Rheumatoid arthritis	Prolapse of mitral valve
	Syphilis	Sinoatrial node disorders
	Drug abuse ("speed")	Oral contraceptives
	Migraine	Hypoglycemia
	Aneurysms	Electrolyte imbalance
	Arteriovenous malformations	Sickle cell anemia
	Homocystinuria	

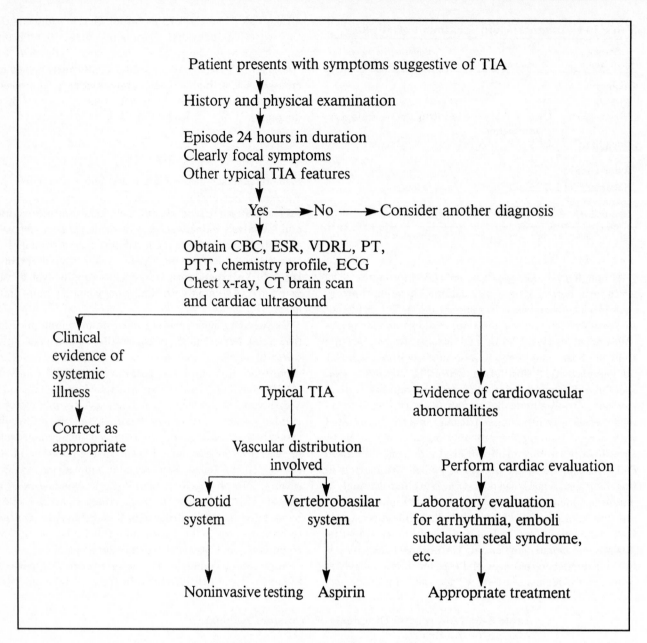

Figure 8–1　Emergency management of TIAs.

intracerebral hemorrhage is most often encountered as a complication of long-standing hypertension or anti-coagulation therapy. Hypertensive intracerebral hemorrhage has a predilection for certain sites and usually occurs, in order of frequency, in the thalamus, putamen, cerebellum, or brainstem. It most often develops when the patient is awake and active. It is especially important that the clinician be able to distinguish cerebellar hemor-

rhage or hematoma, since intracranial bleeding in this location is amenable to neurosurgical intervention.[39]

Spontaneous subarachnoid hemorrhage is usually the result of a ruptured intracranial aneurysm. Onset usually consists of a sudden severe headache during vigorous activity and, at times, is likened by patients to an abrupt blow on the head. Hemorrhagic infarction, which is the third most common cause of focal deficits in patients with cerebrovascular disease, should be considered in patients with hypertension and in those individuals taking anticoagulants, those who have had previous craniocerebral trauma, or those who have a history of unexplained headaches. Unlike thrombotic and embolic cerebral infarction, hemorrhagic infarction frequently presents with severe impairment of consciousness and/or seizure activity and may be accompanied by severe headache and nuchal rigidity.

Craniocerebral Trauma

Craniocerebral trauma can also produce focal neurologic deficits.[5,11,40] When traumatic lesions, including acute contusional swelling, subdural hematoma, epidural hematoma, intracerebral hemorrhage, and cerebral lacerations, cause focal deficits, impaired level of consciousness will usually be the dominant feature of clinical presentation. In a recent review of 85 patients diagnosed by CT scan as having subdural hematomas, it was found that 61 of the 85 patients (72%) were diagnosed within 24 hours of presentation. In addition, 45 of 57 (79%) with definite history or signs of cranial trauma were diagnosed within 24 hours, while only 16 of 28 (57%) without historical or physical evidence of trauma were diagnosed promptly. Focal neurologic signs were present in 32 of 57 (56%) with head trauma. In patients without head trauma who had subdural hematoma, 50% had focal neurologic signs.[1,7,10,40]

The study concluded that the presence of focal neurologic signs is a more sensitive indicator of the presence of subdural hematoma than is a positive skull series. Clinical suspicion of subdural hematoma is essential in any patient with or without a head injury, who has an unexplained depression of level of consciousness and/or focal neurologic signs. This suspicion should be entertained despite normal skull radiograms, and a CT scan should be obtained immediately after stabilization in the emergency department.

One investigation studied 128 patients who were admitted to a hospital trauma unit with acute subdural hematoma. It was concluded that those patients transferred from a lower level care facility, who suffered delays of several hours before receiving definitive surgical care, fared significantly worse than patients with equivalent trauma who were admitted directly to a trauma-I level hospital.[10,11] The mortality rate of transferred patients with acute subdural hematoma was 76% compared to 50% for patients who were directly admitted. The outcome was also worse for transfer patients who experienced a lucid interval, or those with alcoholic intoxication. The study concluded that delays associated with failure to admit patients with acute subdural hematoma directly to a head trauma center can cause an excessive mortality and morbidity — a situation that is potentially avoided by proper triage. In another study of

100 patients[16] presenting with tentorial herniation and history of head trauma, focal neurologic signs were seen in the majority of patients. Anisocoria was found in 63 patients. Hemiparesis or hemiplegia was detected in 20%, and unilateral or asymmetric flexor or extensor posturing in 11%. The worst motor response was opposite the dilated pupil in 22 patients and ipsilateral in 9 patients. Only 37% of this population presented with non-lateralizing neurologic findings.[16]

Spinal, Epidural, and Subdural Hematomas

The clinical symptoms and signs of subdural and epidural spinal hematomas consist of intensive pain localized in the neck or thoracic or lumbar spine.[41] In most cases, the pain comes suddenly, progresses rapidly, and quickly radiates segmentally to the arms, trunk, or legs, depending on the site of the hematoma. Within minutes, hours, or (seldom) days, progressive focal sensory and/or motor deficits develop corresponding to the level of the spinal cord compression. As a rule, these clinical signs and symptoms give no information about the cause of the bleeding (i.e., if it happened with or without anticoagulation or if it resulted from spinal trauma). In one study,[11] about 25% of all reported spinal hematomas occurred as a result of anticoagulation. With the general increase in the number of anticoagulated patients, this diagnosis should be maintained in all patients on Coumadin therapy.

Myelography using water-soluble, nonionic contrast agents is the most important examination for diagnosing a spinal, epidural, or subdural hematoma. After verification of the lesion by myelography, the spinal cord should be decompressed as quickly as possible, ideally by a laminectomy. In the event that the hematoma has resulted from overanticoagulation, coagulation factors, fresh frozen plasma, and vitamin K should be administered to patients taking anticoagulant drugs. Subsequent surgical decompression is then usually necessary.

Postictal State

That a focal neurologic deficit is the manifestation of a postictal phenomenon should always be considered in the evaluation of patients in the emergency department, since the presence of a seizure disorder may suggest a different diagnosis and treatment pathway. Nearly all types of focal neurologic deficits can be seen as a manifestation of a postictal event. Aphasia, hemiparesis, hemianopsia, hemianesthesia, and cortical blindness have all been reported following seizure activity. A number of other entities can also cause focal neurologic deficits, including migraine, collagen vascular syndromes, infection, tumor, hemodynamic instability, hypertensive encephalopathy, thrombotic thrombocytopenic purpura (TTP), cranial arteritis, and transient ischemic attacks.

NONCEREBROVASCULAR CAUSES OF FOCAL NEUROLOGIC DEFICITS

Metabolic Causes

Hyperosmolar states (hypernatremia, hyperglycemia), hypoxia, hypotension, carbon monoxide poisoning, hyponatremia, hypoglycemia, hypocalcemia, and hypophosphatemia can cause focal neurologic deficits.[1-5,42] CNS findings in patients with metabolic disorders may be diffuse or focal, with diffuse involvement producing alterations in consciousness that range from drowsiness to psychosis to coma. In general, these changes progress in severity as the metabolic derangement worsens, but they may, at times, develop rapidly.

Symptoms and signs of focal brain dysfunction resulting from metabolic derangement are especially common in the elderly. These abnormalities probably represent the unmasking of preexisting subclinical structural brain damage by profound metabolic changes within the brain that are induced by electrolyte or osmolar derangements.[43] The vast majority of diffuse and focal CNS abnormalities caused by metabolic derangements clear completely and promptly once the derangement is corrected.

The biochemical basis for focal neurologic deficits in metabolic disorders is unclear. However, alterations in brain cell volume seem to play a major role. Intracellular volume is determined by the effect of osmolarity and extracellular fluid. This relationship exists because cell membranes are freely permeable to water but impermeable to solute. Because tonicity between the two compartments must be equal in hypertonic states, intracellular dehydration results, which leads to CNS dysfunction.[2]

Hypoosmolar States

Hypoosmolarity is essentially synonymous with hyponatremia. A decrease in serum sodium concentration may be caused by sodium loss or by dilution of extracellular sodium by an increase in extracellular water absorption associated with syndrome of inappropriate ADH (SIADH). Clinical symptoms depend on both the actual level to which the serum sodium is depressed and the rapidity of the reduction in serum sodium. In general, nearly all patients with serum sodium levels less than 116 mEq/L will have neurologic findings.[44] These include nausea, vomiting, weakness, lethargy, confusion, or focal neurologic deficits. Myoclonus or asterixis may be noted as well as generalized grand mal or focal seizures. Prominent focal neurologic abnormalities may include aphasia or hemiplegia. Once the diagnosis is made, general therapeutic guidelines, including water deprivation and, when there is severe neurologic decompensation, administration of intravenous hypertonic saline, are recommended.

Hypernatremia

Hypernatremia elevates the serum osmolality and results in profound intracellular dehydration as water shifts into the extracellular space. Hypernatremia in the elderly is usually seen in the setting of neglect, which is usually accompanied by water deprivation. Cellular shrinking caused by hypernatremia may produce a number of vascular lesions including capillary congestion, subarachnoid and intracerebral hemorrhages, and cortical venous thrombosis with areas of venous infarction.

Neurologic manifestations occur in more than half of patients with serum sodium levels greater than 155 mEq/L,[45] and include altered sensorium, confusion, lethargy, stupor, and coma. Muscle weakness has also been reported, and while seizures are frequent, in contrast to hyponatremia, they most often occur during the period of rehydration and serum sodium correction.[45,46] Therapy for hypernatremia should be directed at the underlying cause; acute treatment consists of water replacement, usually in the form of 5% dextrose or D_5 ½ normal saline intravenously. Correction of hypernatremia must be undertaken slowly over a period of 48 to 72 hours to avoid rapid fluid shifts and precipitation of cerebral edema and seizures. (See Table 8–6.)

Hyperosmolar Nonketotic Hyperglycemia

Neurologic manifestations of diabetic ketoacidosis (DKA) are usually nonfocal and are characterized by progressive obtundation and coma. Most cases manifest drowsiness and weakness and severely affected patients will be comatose. Neurologic examination is usually unremarkable with normal pupillary light responses, intact extraocular movements, symmetrical reflexes, normal muscle tone, and the absence of focal findings.

The neurologic manifestations of DKA contrast markedly with those seen in hypoosmolar nonketotic hyperglycemia (HNKH). HNKH most commonly develops in previously undiagnosed, or untreated, adult onset diabetics and is especially common in women over the age of 65. Neurologic symptoms and signs may be present for days to weeks and usually progress from weakness, lethargy,

Table 8–6   Symptoms and Signs Suggesting Osmolar Disorders

Diffuse central nervous system abnormalities	Focal central nervous system abnormalities
Lethargy	Focal seizures
Confusion	Todd's (postictal) paralysis
Delirium and hallucinations	Hemianopsia
Stupor	Tonic eye deviation
Coma	Aphasia
Seizures	Nystagmus
	Hyperreflexia
	Sensory deficits

and fatigue until, finally, impairment of consciousness and even coma supervene. In the fully evolved clinical syndrome, the presenting features will typically include obtundation, dehydration, and marked hyperglycemia with ketosis and acidosis classically absent.[48,49]

Neurologic abnormalities in HNKH are distinct from those seen in DKA. Focal central nervous system signs are common in the former but rare in the latter. Focal deficits in HNKH include aphasia, homonymous hemianopsia, hemisensory deficits, hemiparesis, hemiballism, hyperreflexia, as well as simple and complex hallucinations. Brainstem dysfunction caused by cellular dehydration may be manifested by nystagmus and tonic eye deviation. Seizure activity, when present, is usually focal and may result in a Todd's postictal paralysis. In one study, focal nervous system abnormalities and/or seizures were seen in 40% of patients with HNKH.[18] (See Table 8–7.)

FOCAL SEIZURES

Seizures are rarely a manifestation of acute thrombotic cerebral infarction but do occur commonly as a long-term sequela of previous cerebral infarction. While the incidence of focal seizures is reported to be as high as 20% in acute cerebral embolic infarctions, they are more common as long-term sequelae of previous cerebrovascular accidents.[3,4] Focal seizures are seen in the elderly in the presence of focal slit hemorrhages and, especially, in ruptured saccular aneurysms, arteriovenous (AV) malformations, and ruptured mycotic aneurysms.

Patients with focal seizures accompanied by a severely depressed level of consciousness should be suspected of having an intracerebral hemorrhage, subarachnoid hemorrhage, or metabolic encephalopathy. Metabolic encephalopathies, especially those caused by hypo- and hyperglycemia, are also known to cause focal seizures with an altered level of consciousness. In the absence of craniocerebral trauma, and when cerebrovascular disease seems unlikely, an underlying metabolic etiology for focal seizures should be entertained and a thorough diagnostic evaluation initiated to rule out this possibility.

Epilepsy is the most common sequela of craniocerebral trauma and occurs in about 5% of all patients with closed head injuries and in as many as 50% of all patients with open wounds to the brain.[11,47] The interval between head injury and first seizure varies greatly. About 1% of head-injured individuals have one or more seizures (usually generalized) within moments of their injury, and somewhat larger numbers experience seizures within 24 to 48 hours after the incident.[1] Early seizures have a good prognosis as far as recurrence is concerned and are not ordinarily referred to as posttraumatic epilepsy. A number of other conditions commonly seen in the elderly — including hypertensive encephalopathy, hyperthermia, tumor, infection, and vasculitis — may also cause focal seizures.

SUMMARY

Focal neurologic lesions can result from a number of primary neurologic and nonneurologic disorders. In general, all patients who present to the emergency department with a focal neurologic deficit or seizure should have a thorough metabolic evaluation to rule out underlying electrolyte disorders. Once these are excluded, those patients who have an altered level of consciousness in combination with a focal deficit should have a CT scan to rule out a space-occupying lesion. Patients with cerebral occlusive disease, including TIAs, should be admitted to the hospital and appropriate anticoagulation therapy, when indicated, should be initiated. Those patients with craniocerebral trauma and focal neurologic deficits should have immediate neurosurgical consultation and CT scan to rule out the possibility of subdural or epidural hematoma.

Improvement in morbidity and mortality in patients with focal neurologic lesions can be improved by a systematic approach to evaluation and management of this challenging patient population.

CASE STUDIES

Case Study 1

A previously well 90-year-old white woman was brought to the emergency department by her 70-year-old daughter, who noticed that her mother had had a spell characterized by dizziness and confusion early that afternoon. During the spell, the patient nearly slipped to the floor but

Table 8–7 Hyperglycemic Disorders

	Diabetic ketoacidosis	Hyperosmolar nonketotic hyperglycemia
Serum glucose	Below 600 g/100 mL	Above 600 mg/100 mL
Serum ketones	4 +	0 to 2+ (at a 1:1 dilution)
Serum pH	Below 7.25	Normal (or above 7.25)
Serum osmolality	Below 350 mOsm/L	Above 350 mOsm/L
Seizures	Rare	Occur in 10–15% of patients; frequently focal
Focal abnormalities on neurologic exam	Absent	Frequent

managed to catch herself by holding onto a wall. This episode was followed by confusion and inappropriate behavior. The daughter stated that she had never seen this happen before and that her altered mental status was new. On physical exam, the patient was disoriented to time and place, moved all extremities, and had no focal neurologic findings. Babinski's reflexes were not present, there was no history of head trauma, and the patient was taking no medications. The patient admitted to having half a glass of wine that morning. Vital signs included a blood pressure of 170/90, heart rate of 86, respiratory rate of 24, and temperature of 37°C. The nurse who took the vital signs noted the possibility of "alcohol on the breath." The patient's private physician was called and recommended hospitalization.

Analysis

The nurse astutely noted the presence of alcohol on the patient's breath. A blood alcohol test was ordered and revealed a level of 167 mg%, which is legal intoxication. In a 90-year-old person, this level is high enough to cause serious alterations in mental status. The appropriate triage decision (discharge to home with recommendation for follow-up in a geriatric alcohol abuse therapy program) was made.

Alcoholism is much more common in the elderly than is generally recognized. It has been estimated that the incidence in the United States in those over 65 years of age is up to 9%. The majority of these patients are women, and about half the elderly alcoholics have always been heavy drinkers; in the remainder, the drinking habits start late in life, usually after bereavement or some other personal difficulty. Some of the elderly alcoholic patients are frankly depressed and, as with all alcoholics, may be extremely devious about their drinking habits and their means of obtaining alcohol.

The treatment of elderly alcoholics does not differ substantially from that in younger patients. The drug must be withdrawn and treatment given to prevent tremor, agitation, and delirium. If the problem is especially severe, or if the home circumstances are unsatisfactory, it may be necessary to admit the patient to a special alcohol rehabilitation unit. As with all alcoholics, the elderly require sympathy and support if the habit is to be cured.

Case Study 2

A 66-year-old white man with a history of mild hypertension and several recent bouts of a flu-like syndrome presented to the emergency department with fever and disorientation. According to his wife, the patient had suffered from coryza and muscle pains for three days and, on the day of admission, developed a mild cough and temperature of 102.2°F. At that time, profound disorientation and vomiting developed. Physical examina-

tion demonstrated a toxic-appearing white male with the following vital signs: temperature of 102°F, respirations of 26, heart rate of 100, and blood pressure of 150/100. Neurologic examination revealed that the patient was confused and disoriented to time and place. Cranial nerves demonstrated upward, downward, and lateral gaze nystagmus and mild impairment of upward gaze. Babinski's signs were not present. The remainder of the exam was essentially unremarkable, and the laboratory tests were not contributory. The patient was taking two to three aspirins per day for treatment of his flu-like symptoms and admitted to drinking five to six highballs per day.

Analysis

It was difficult for this patient, who appeared to have a life-threatening neurologic condition and who was disoriented, to give an accurate medical history. The patient's drinking history was obtained from the wife; this information, in combination with the neurologic findings, led to the suspicion that this patient may have acute Wernicke's encephalopathy. Because of the possibility of an intracerebral hemorrhage, subarachnoid hemorrhage, or other neurologic structural lesion, the patient was sent for a CT scan, after treatment with 220 mg of thiamine intramuscularly (IM). The CT scan and a lumbar puncture were both negative. By the time the patient returned from the CT scan, the upward and lateral gaze nystagmus had improved significantly and the patient's mental status was beginning to clear, which confirmed the diagnosis of acute Wernicke's encephalopathy.

In 1881, Carl Wernicke described Wernicke's encephalopathy — an illness characterized by paralysis of eye movement, ataxia of gait, and mental confusion. Russian psychiatrist S.S. Korsakoff described disturbance of memory related to alcoholism and to acute Wernicke's encephalopathy.

The diagnosis of acute Wernicke's encephalopathy is made on the basis of clinical features and the triad originally described by Wernicke — ocular palsy, ataxia, and mental confusion. The ocular signs are characterized by 1) nystagmus that is both horizontal and vertical; 2) paralysis or weakness of the external rectus muscle (cranial nerve [CN] VI); and 3) weakness or paralysis of conjugate gaze. While all three ocular manifestations usually occur together, they may occur in any combination.

Signs of alcohol withdrawal are shown by 15% of patients, and many show disturbances of consciousness and mentation. A global confusional state is the most common disorder of mentation.

The course of the illness is variable but is associated with substantial morbidity and mortality. There is a 17% mortality rate in the acute phase, with most deaths resulting from infection and decompensated liver disease due to cirrhosis. Those patients who do not recover respond to administration of thiamine in a fairly predictable manner. Ocular manifestations improve most dramatically with recovery beginning within minutes or hours and always within several days. While sixth cranial nerve palsies, ptosis, and vertical gaze palsies recover completely, usually within one to two weeks, vertical nystagmus may persist for several months. Horizontal gaze palsies usually recover completely, but in 60% of the cases, fine horizontal nystagmus persists. The global confusional state is almost always reversible with symptoms usually improving rapidly over minutes or hours. As the global symptoms recede, the defect in recent memory and learning (i.e., Korsakoff's psychosis) stands out more clearly. While about 85% of the patients follow this sequence of recovery, about 15% go on to manifest permanent Korsakoff's psychosis.

Korsakoff's psychosis is a sterotypical mental disorder consisting of two essential abnormalities of memory: 1) impaired ability to recall information heard before the illness (retrograde amnesia) and 2) impaired ability to acquire new information (anterograde amnesia).

Wernicke's encephalopathy is a medical emergency. Once the diagnosis is suspected, thiamine 200 mg intravenously or intramuscularly should be administered. This prevents the progression of the disease and reverses those lesions that have not yet progressed to the point of irreversible structural change.

Case Study 3

A 65-year-old white woman, previously in good health, was brought to the emergency department in an obtunded and confused state. According to her friends, she had been shopping on the day of her visit to the emergency department but "did not feel quite right" during the afternoon. During dinner, the patient experienced sudden onset of headache, dizziness, and persistent nausea and vomiting.

On physical examination, blood pressure was 180/100, pulse was 62, respiration was 24, and temperature was 97.4°F. On neurologic exam, the patient was able to follow very simple demands but was disoriented to time, place, and person. A peripheral right seventh CN and a right sixth CN palsy were present. The patient was able to move all extremities, and Babinski's reflexes were absent. The patient continued to have persistent vomiting, and a CT scan was performed.

Analysis

Neurosurgical emergencies in the elderly represent a difficult but important group of conditions with which the emergency physician should be familiar. Because of the difficulty in localizing and characterizing a clinical neurologic presentation, there is frequently a tendency to merely decide that "The patient needs to be admitted to the hospital" and to leave the responsibility of nitty gritty investigation to the attending physician. Unfortunately, there are several neurosurgical (nontraumatic) emergencies in the elderly for which the emergency department physician must have a high index of suspicion. Cerebellar hemorrhage is one of them.

It is important to diagnosis cerebellar hemorrhage on clinical grounds as early as possible. This particular lesion has been shown to be treatable surgically, in contradistinction to the majority of intracerebral hemorrhages, which are not especially benefited by clot evacuation. This elderly patient had a large cerebellar hemorrhage, a diagnosis that was suspected in the emergency department on the basis of sixth and seventh nerve palsies, persistent nausea and vomiting, dizziness, and the absence of hemiplegia. The clot was evacuated, and the patient recovered without any neurologic deficit.

The most common recorded complaints in patients with cerebellar infarction and hemorrhage are the sudden onset of nausea and vomiting, dizziness, and the inability to stand or walk or both. Headache is variable. On physical exam, prominent cerebellar signs include lateral appendicular ataxia, collateral gaze palsy (most commonly sixth CN), and peripheral facial palsy (seventh CN). At least two of the three signs were present in 73% of 26 patients in one large series in whom testing for all these signs was done.

According to one large study, the natural history of cerebellar hemorrhage and the poor results of patients subjected to prolonged observation should mandate prompt evacuation of the hematoma soon after onset in all cases in which the diagnosis has been confirmed. Although there is still some debate on whether to operate on comatose patients with brainstem signs secondary to cerebellar bleeding, results suggest that even these patients can have brainstem function restored following removal of the blood clot.

Case Study 4

A 70-year-old man was brought to the emergency department because of altered mental status. His wife, who slept in a separate bedroom, was awakened in the middle of the night by the husband's moaning and yelling. She found him on the floor, but he could not get up or be aroused.

The patient's physician called the emergency department and informed the staff that his patient, who had multiple intracerebral metastases, was coming to the hospital because of a sudden change in mental status. No other history was provided.

The patient was transported to the hospital by paramedics, who reported that the patient's mental status was severely depressed and who also noted that the patient had a left hemiparesis. On physical examination in the emergency department, the patient's vital signs were normal. The patient was a thin, elderly male who appeared weak. Neurologic exam revealed a patient who was virtually unresponsive except to deep pain, and who could not move his left arm and leg. Pupils were round, reactive, and equal to light, and no papilledema was detected.

The patient's wife informed the emergency department physician that her husband had recently been admitted to the hospital for chemotherapy for a tumor that had spread to his brain. "His brain has two or three spots . . . .The doctor thinks it's only a matter of time." The patient was observed in the emergency department for one-half hour without improvement. Laboratory tests were ordered including complete blood count (CBC), electrolytes, glucose, and blood urea nitrogen (BUN).

Analysis

A number of common diseases may be confused with one another in the elderly patient. Hypoglycemia is one of them, and this is precisely what this gentleman had. Laboratory tests revealed a glucose level of 31 mg/dL, and the patient's left hemiparesis and mental status resolved quickly after the administration of 50 mL $D_{50}W$. It took about one-half hour of talking with the patient's wife to determine that the patient was an insulin-dependent diabetic. She was so certain that her husband's condition was the result of the intracerebral metastases that she failed to provide the necessary historical information.

Despite the inadequate history, the prehospital and emergency department protocols for coma of unknown etiology apply to the elderly patient, as well as to the young. The patient was, after all, unresponsive, and proper protocol dictated that the patient should have received $D_{50}W$ on the basis of his coma alone, on the off-chance that hypoglycemia was a factor in his altered mental status. All comatose patients deserve a trial of $D_{50}W$ and thiamine 100 mg IM. Moreover, no alteration of neurologic function is inconsistent with hypoglycemia. Focal deficits, altered behavior, memory loss, and seizures have all been described as manifestations of profound hypoglycemia.

Case Study 5

A recently retired 67-year-old successful corporate executive was brought to the emergency department by his wife because of the acute onset of mental confusion. According to his wife, the patient had been swimming and exercising at the health club on a Saturday afternoon, as was his usual weekend routine. He was perfectly well when he left for the club, but upon returning for dinner she noted that he was acting "very strangely." The patient's wife noticed that her husband had forgotten to take off his swimming trunks and the water had soaked

through his pants. Additionally, the patient had forgotten his watch at the club, something he had never done before. The patient was unable to recall his visit to the health club in its entirety, and after noting that her husband was repeating the same questions over and over again, "Dear, how did my pants get wet? . . . Dear, how did my pants get wet? . . . ," she decided to bring him to the hospital.

On physical examination, the patient was a healthy appearing elderly gentleman, well dressed, ambulatory, and in no apparent distress. Vital signs were normal, and the patient had been well all his life and was not taking any medications. Except for the neurologic examination, his physical exam was totally unremarkable.

Neurologic exam revealed that the patient knew his name, phone number, place of birth, and wife's name but did not know who the president was, the date, or where he was. Although he was told on several occasions by the physician and nurse that he was at the hospital because of some "problems in the way he was thinking," the patient did not understand and he repeatedly looked around the examining room and every so often asked, "Where am I? . . . Why am I here? . . . What's wrong?" Moreover, each time the doctor and nurse entered his room, he asked, "Who are you? . . . Why am I here?" At times, his frustration at not knowing what was wrong and his perception that he was being deluged by a seemingly endless number of new doctors and nurses drove the patient to near-violence in the emergency department. The emergency physician had introduced himself to the patient at least seven times over a half-hour period.

The remainder of the neurologic exam was entirely normal. Electrolytes, CBC, and an alcohol level were unremarkable. The patient was admitted to the hospital.

Analysis

Many of those caring for this patient thought he was hysterical. Loss of memory for recent past events is a well-known sequel of certain clearly defined organic states including head injury, epilepsy, electroconvulsive (ECT) therapy, strokes, delirium, and acute hysteria. While sudden loss of memory without gross evidence of clouding of consciousness is often regarded as consciously motivated, these signs and symptoms are also consistent with a syndrome known as transient global amnesia (TGA), which most likely represents a thrombotic infarction of the vertebrobasilar system in the region of the hippocampus. Most patients report having developed TGA following some kind of stressful episode such as exertion. Many were known to have taken hot baths prior to the onset of symptoms, and there has been some speculation that vasodilation-induced local cerebral ischemia may play a role. This patient was admitted to the hospital, he had a normal CT scan, and his memory returned to normal over the next three to four days. The outlook for recovery in patients with TGA is excellent.

Case Study 6

A 70-year-old white man was found virtually unresponsive on the floor by his wife. According to her, he had collapsed suddenly with no mention of headache or chest pain. Upon arrival in the emergency department, the patient was semiconscious and able to follow simple commands but had an expressive aphasia. The patient had a history of hypertension but was otherwise well. Physical exam revealed a dense right-sided hemiparesis and hemianesthesia. The patient had paralysis of vertical gaze and nystagmus with left-sided gazing movements. Baseline chemistries, electrocardiogram (ECG), and CBC were normal.

Analysis

The presence of an upward gaze palsy in this patient is the key to the diagnosis. Paralysis or paresis of conjugate upward gaze, with or without pupillary abnormalities, is known as the Parinaud's syndrome and usually indicates a tumor or other structural lesion in the posterior third ventricle or pretectum. Parinaud's syndrome commonly can occur as a manifestation of hemorrhage, brainstem infarction, transtentorial herniation, obstructive hydrocephalus, and other lesions affecting the midbrain and pretectum.

A CT scan revealed a thalamic hemorrhage, which was treated conservatively. The patient's clinical status, including his ocular paresis, improved and the patient was discharged.

Case Study 7

A 72-year-old white man with a history of long-standing hypertension presented to the emergency department with aphasia. Over the past three days, the patient had noted mild headaches, and his wife noted that he had difficulty in choosing appropriate words. Physical examination revealed a pleasant white male with a blood pressure of 200/150, temperature of 98.6°F, respirations of 20, and heart rate of 96. Cardiac exam revealed normal S_1 and S_2, with an S_4 present. No friction rubs or S_3 were detected. The lungs were clear, and the abdomen was normal. The neck was supple and no bruits were heard. Neurologic examination revealed a Wernicke's aphasia with mild anomia. Babinski's signs were not present, and the remainder of the motor, sensory, and cerebellar exams were normal. The fundi revealed 4 + papilledema. There were no cholesterol retinal emboli or hypertensive hemorrhages.

Analysis

The differential diagnosis in this elderly patient includes transient ischemic attack (TIA), stroke in evolution, and a structural intracerebral lesion (tumor and hypertensive encephalopathy). Hypertensive emergencies may be categorized by any one or all of the following three: 1) hypertensive encephalopathy; 2) hypertensive pulmonary edema; and 3) dissecting thoracic aortic aneurysm. Hypertensive encephalopathy occurs when autoregulation of cerebral blood flow fails, leading to hypoperfusion of the brain and accompanying cerebral edema. Symptoms and signs in hypertensive encephalopathy include severe headache, altered mental status, irritability, lethargy, confusion, seizures, and a variety of focal neurologic signs and symptoms. Since hypertension may occur in intracerebral or subarachnoid hemorrhage, and in neurologic conditions, the diagnosis of hypertensive encephalopathy is, to some extent, a diagnosis of exclusion and should be made only after consideration has been given to the above-mentioned entities. In general, however, the sudden onset of neurologic signs and symptoms, combined with the absence of a prior history of hypertension or the absence of objective evidence for accelerated hypertension, diminishes the likelihood that hypertensive encephalopathy is the problem. Management of hypertensive crisis includes immediate lowering of the blood pressure with one of a number of agents including diazoxide and, preferably, nitroprusside when adequate hemodynamic monitoring is available. Hospitalization in an intensive care unit is recommended.

The aforementioned patient was treated with diazoxide 300 mg and 80 mg of furosemide intravenously; diastolic blood pressure was lowered to 190/100, and a nitroprusside drip was started. The Wernicke's aphasia resolved 8 hours after antihypertensive therapy.

Case Study 8

An 85-year-old white female with a history of insulin-dependent diabetes mellitus presented to the emergency department with left-sided hemiballism. She was recently discharged from the hospital with bilateral pneumococcal empyema. Physical examination demonstrated an elderly white female, conscious and alert with uncontrollable flailing movements of the left arm and leg. No intention ataxia or choreoathetoid movement was noted. Bilateral Babinski's signs were present. Cranial nerves II–XII were intact, the neck was supple, and the remainder of the physical exam was unremarkable except for decreased breath sounds in the left lung and the presence of a chest tube at the left midaxillary line. The patient was afebrile and normotensive. Initial laboratory studies were ordered and demonstrated a glucose of 1102 mg%, sodium of 149, and BUN 46; the remainder of the laboratory examination was unremarkable.

Analysis

The patient was treated with haloperidol with some improvement in the left-sided hemiballism. She was admitted to the intensive care unit where she was hydrated and treated with intravenous insulin. Hemiballism resolved completely after normalization of blood glucose. Her neurologic syndrome was felt to be a manifestation of her hyperosmolar state. Disorders of serum osmolality (hyponatremia, hypernatremia, and hyperglycemia) are quite common, especially in old people, and frequently produce nonspecific symptoms and signs. Diffuse weakness, malaise, anorexia, nausea or vomiting, and lethargy are common complaints. However, more than 50% of elderly patients with osmolar disorders present with signs of CNS dysfunction as the principal clinical manifestation. In a large series of patients with hyperglycemia of the nonketotic type (HNKH), the derangements in neurologic function were so pronounced that the majority of patients were diagnosed as having structural lesions, such as brain tumors or strokes.

CNS findings in patients with hyperglycemia and hyperosmolarity may be either diffuse or focal. Symptoms and signs of focal brain dysfunction frequently confuse the diagnosis, and these abnormalities may represent the "unmasking" of preexisting subclinical structure damage by profound metabolic changes within the brain that are induced by the osmolar derangement. Cerebral angiography and autopsy evaluation of patients who develop focal findings with osmolar derangement are usually normal.

The vast majority of both diffuse and focal CNS abnormalities will resolve completely and promptly when the metabolic disorders are corrected as in the case of the patient with hemiballism. In other cases, neurologic impairments may be permanent or death may result, especially if the diagnosis and treatment are delayed.

The syndrome of HNKH develops most commonly in previously undiagnosed or untreated adult-onset diabetes. Premonitory symptoms may be present for days and weeks, and include thirst, weakness, lethargy, and fatigue, until finally impairment of consciousness or other focal neurologic deficits supervene. In the fully developed syndrome, the presenting features typically include obtundation, dehydration, and marked hyperglycemia; ketosis and acidosis are classically absent, although modest acidemia and, occasionally, small quantities of plasma ketones may be detected.

The neurologic abnormalities in HNKH are distinct from those in diabetic ketoacidosis (DKA) in that focal central nervous system signs are frequently present and include focal and generalized seizures as well as deficits. The focal nervous abnormalities may reflect either cortical or subcortical damage. The former may include aphasia, homonymous hemianopsia, hemosensory deficits, hemiparesis, hyperreflexia with positive Babinski's signs, hemiballism, and simple or complex visual hallucinations. Subcortical dysfunction may include nystagmus and cranial nerve involvement, as well as autonomic nervous system disturbances producing hyperpnea or hypertension. Seizure activity is usually focal but may generalize. A focal Todd's (postictal) paralysis may be present. As a rule, focal deficits and seizure activity in HNKH are often notoriously resistant to drug therapy but usually resolve with corrections of the hyperosmolarity.

Case Study 9

An 81-year-old white woman with a history of congestive heart failure, chronic atrial fibrillation, hypertension, and left middle cerebral artery thrombotic infarction 15 years prior to admission was brought to the emergency department after having been found at home unconscious. Upon her arrival in the emergency department, the patient's vital signs included a heart rate of 84 (irregular), respirations of 24, blood pressure of 160/90, and temperature of 37.5°C. The patient was lethargic, confused, and disoriented and had a right-sided hemiparesis. ECG demonstrated peak T waves. Laboratory exam revealed a serum potassium of 6.7 and arterial blood gases consistent with metabolic acidosis: pH = 7.30, PCO_2 = 30, PO_2 = 117, and the lactic acid level was elevated.

Analysis

This case illustrates the diagnostic and therapeutic problems encountered in elderly patients with focal lesions who have several potential causes that may explain their clinical symptoms and signs. In this patient, the depressed level of consciousness and hemiparesis may have represented — especially because of chronic atrial fibrillation — an embolic cerebral infarction. However, relative preservation of consciousness in the presence of an extensive focal deficit is the rule in embolic thrombotic infarction, unless the upper part of the basilar arterial area is involved or unless massive brain swelling had occurred acutely, which, as a rule, usually evolves over 48 to 96 hours after the ischemic insult. Moreover, thrombotic or embolic infarction rarely causes severe depression of consciousness in the acute stage, unless a new infarction has occurred in the hemisphere opposite to that of an old infarction or unless there has been complete occlusion of a carotid artery, which may result in massive acute cerebral edema. The point to be stressed is that severe obtundation in combination with focal deficits should lead the physician to investigate other (i.e., noninfarction) causes such as intracerebral hemorrhage to explain the neurologic findings.

An obtunded state in combination with the right-sided hemiparesis in this patient could have been explained by a hypertensive intracerebral hemorrhage. Equally plausible, however, is the explanation that the patient's condition on arrival at the emergency department represented a postictal event, which was preceded by a focal seizure originating in the area of her old left middle cerebral artery infarction. It is apparently not well recognized that, while seizures are almost never the premonitory, first, or only manifestation of a thromboembolic infarction, they do commonly occur as sequelae of old infarctions.

Finally, it should be emphasized that metabolic derangements — most notably hyperosmolar states (hyperglycemia, hypernatremia), hyponatremia, hypocalcemia, hypomagnesemia, hypophosphatemia (diabetics, alcoholics), hypoglycemia, and hypokalemia — frequently cause focal neurologic deficits.

The patient's hyperkalemia was treated with 88 mEq of sodium bicarbonate, 25 g of 50% glucose intravenously, and 15 U of regular insulin intravenously. Within minutes, the patient became more arousable, and the hemiparesis improved dramatically. A repeat blood gas test demonstrated resolution of the lactic acidosis. What combination of factors was responsible for this patient's neurologic lesions? The most likely explanations are 1) that the patient had an undetected seizure (possibly precipitated by hyperkalemia or a cardiac arrhythmia) in the area of her old left hemisphere infarction and presented the emergency department with a postictal hemiparesis and confusional state or 2) that the entire clinical picture, including rapid resolution of focal neurologic deficits following sodium bicarbonate and insulin therapy, represented the natural history of a hyperkalemic metabolic encephalopathy.

It is interesting to note that this patient demonstrated enzymatic and electrocardiographic changes of a subendocardial infarction during her hospitalization, allowing speculation that an MI-induced arrhythmia may have given rise to an undetected seizure as suggested by the first alternative.

The patient had a CT scan two days after admission, which demonstrated only an old left hemisphere infarction without acute lesions. Her neurologic status had returned to normal within 24 hours after her admission.

Case Study 10

A 77-year-old white woman was brought to the emergency department with left-sided hemiparesis, fever, dehydration, and obtundation. The vital signs were blood pressure of 70/0, temperature of 38.9°C, respirations of 24, and pulse of 120. Urinalysis showed a full field of white blood cells and bacteria, and the arterial blood gases indicated severe metabolic acidosis. Volume repletion with D_5 normal saline and dopamine infusion were started; hemiparesis and mental status depression resolved in the emergency department after the blood pressure was raised to 120/70. Blood cultures performed in the emer-

gency department revealed gram-negative bacteremia. A lumbar puncture was normal, with no bacterial growth.

Analysis

This case illustrates that focal neurologic deficits can be induced by hypertensive, hypotensive, or hypoxic encephalopathies. Especially in old people, these abnormalities may represent the unmasking of preexisting subclinical structural damage by the profound hemodynamic or metabolic changes within the brain that are induced by hypotension or hypoxemia. It is speculated that many brain-affecting conditions — which are frequently divided into the categories of anoxic anoxia, anemic anoxia, and ischemic anoxia — can render previously infarcted areas of the brain and "border zones" of the cerebral cortex susceptible to activation (seizure) or dysfunction (deficit). In these patients, rapid institution of supportive therapy, which can include volume repletion, oxygen administration, correction of the anemia, or treatment of arrhythmias, may quickly correct the focal lesions as it did in this patient. Clearly an infectious process — meningitis or cerebral abscess — might have explained this patient's clinical presentation, but this diagnosis was not confirmed by subsequent studies performed during the hospitalization.

Case Study 11

A 70-year-old white female with a recent history of deep venous thrombosis presented at the emergency department with a chief complaint of fleeting numbness on the left side of her body and the inability to walk, because of falling to the left side. She had recently had an Austin-Moore prosthesis placed in the left hip and had been treated with an anticoagulant following a deep venous thrombosis during her hospitalization. The patient denied headache, neck pain, loss of consciousness, and seizures. Vital signs were normal except for a blood pressure of 150/108. The remainder of the physical was normal except for a well-healing scar on the left hip and for the neurologic exam, which revealed that the patient could not sit up without assistance and fell to the left side while attempting to walk. Mild left-sided weakness was also detected. Reflexes were noted to be symmetrical, and Babinski's reflexes were not present. In the emergency department, the patient's prothrombin time was noted to be 69.9 seconds (normal = 11 to 14 seconds). The patient was admitted to the hospital with a diagnosis of possible anxiety reaction.

Analysis

Over the next several hours, this patient developed obtundation, progressive left-sided hemiparesis, sustained clonus, and a Babinski's reflex on the left. A CT scan performed 12 hours after admission demonstrated a large intracerebral hematoma with intraventricular extension.

In this case, an intracerebral hematoma might have been suspected initially in light of the significantly prolonged prothrombin time in combination with a new neurologic deficit. While most intracerebral hemorrhages conform to the temporal profile of stroke, i.e., abrupt onset and rather rapid evolution of symptoms, intracerebral hemorrhage that results from an excess of anticoagulants may be remarkably slow in evolution. It should also be noted that, unlike thrombotic cerebral infarction, which usually has its onset during sleep, hemorrhages usually have their onset while the patient is active and awake. Though headache is generally considered to be an accompaniment of intracerebral hemorrhage, it is absent or insignificant in almost 50%. Similarly, nuchal rigidity is frequently found, but is so often absent that failure to find it should not detract from this possibility. Both nuchal rigidity and headache are more likely to occur when an intracerebral hemorrhage extends into the ventricular system, causing subarachnoid irritation. Focal and generalized seizures are more frequently encountered in cerebral hemorrhage than in either thrombotic or embolic infarction.

Following thrombotic and embolic cerebral infarction, hemorrhage is the third most common cause of "stroke." In order of frequency, the most common sites of hypertensive hemorrhage are: 1) putamen and internal capsule; 2) cerebral white matter; 3) thalamus; 4) cerebellar hemisphere; and 5) pons. Because these sites are in close proximity to the deep gray matter and/or brainstem, intracerebral hemorrhage is frequently accompanied by impaired consciousness, which is a differential point in distinguishing it from thrombotic or embolic infarction without hemorrhage. This neurologic finding may be accompanied by focal deficits or seizures; when accompanied by impaired consciousness, it favors the diagnosis of hemorrhage over thrombotic or embolic infarction.

Intracranial bleeding as a complication of anticoagulant therapy may occur in sites of predilection for hypertensive hemorrhage or elsewhere. When precipitated by heparin therapy, early treatment with fresh frozen plasma and vitamin K is indicated. When hemorrhage is associated with aspirin or antiplatelet agents, fresh platelet infusions in massive amounts may be required.

Case Study 12

A 66-year-old blind female with chronic renal failure and non-insulin-dependent diabetes was brought to the emergency department with a markedly depressed mental status accompanied by right arm and leg hemiparesis. Physical exam revealed the following vital signs: temperature of 36°C, respirations of 24, pulse of 110 and regular, blood pressure of 212/118. Neurologic exam demonstrated profound right-sided hemiparesis, a severe expressive aphasia, and a Babinski's reflex on the right. Cardiac and pulmonary exam were normal. Blood samples for CBC and electrolytes were drawn, and an ECG revealed left axis deviation and left ventricular hypertrophy with strain.

Analysis

This elderly patient with a markedly depressed mental status and hemiparesis was suspected of having an intracerebral hypertensive hemorrhage. While waiting for the laboratory exam, the patient was scheduled to have a CT scan. Prior to transfer to the radiology department, the serum glucose obtained in the emergency department was found to be 26 mg/dL. The patient's neurologic deficit resolved with the administration of 50 ml $D_{50}W$.

Hypoglycemia is a common metabolic derangement, and it may precipitate many focal neurologic lesions, including deficits and seizures. Other neurologic findings may include confusional states, delirium, and coma. Hypoglycemia may be suspected as the initial diagnosis in a patient with renal failure who is taking oral hypoglycemic therapy, because insulin is metabolized by the kidney; therefore, patients with reduced renal mass who are taking insulin-releasing hypoglycemic agents are prone to hyperinsulinemia and hypoglycemia. This is one clinical setting in which oral hypoglycemic agents may precipitate hypoglycemia, even though the oral agent may be taken in normal amounts and in the presence of adequate food intake. In most other cases of hypoglycemia induced by oral agents, there has been excessive ingestion of these agents in a suicide attempt or markedly reduced food intake. This case illustrates an emergency in which hypoglycemia was not considered as the initial diagnosis but should have been in view of the history. Other diseases in which hypoglycemia should be considered are severe liver disease, insulin-dependent diabetes, Addisonian crisis, and beta-cell tumor of the pancreas.

REFERENCES

1. Bosker G: Manuscript in preparation, 1990.
2. Lowenstein SR et al: Care of the elderly in the emergency department, Ann Emerg Med 15:5, 1986.
3. Ernest MP: Emergency diagnosis and management of brain infarctions and hemorrhages. In Ernest MP, editor: Neurologic emergencies, New York, 1983, Churchill Livingstone.
4. Toole JF: Vascular diseases — etiology and pathogenesis. In Rowland LP, editor: Merritt's textbook of neurology, Philadelphia, 1984, Lea & Febiger.
5. Rosen P et al: Emergency medicine, ed 2, St. Louis, 1987, CV Mosby Co.
6. Schwartz G et al: Principles and practice of emergency medicine, Philadelphia, 1988, WB Saunders.
7. Bowers SA et al: Outcome in 200 consecutive cases of severe head injury treated in San Diego County: a prospective analysis, Neurosurgery 6:237–241, 1980.
8. Adams HP et al: Pitfalls in the recognition of subarachnoid hemorrhage, JAMA 244:794–796, 1980.

9. Ramirrez-Lassepas M et al: Value of computerized tomography scan in the evaluation of adult patients after their first seizure, Ann Neurol 15:536–543, 1984.

10. Gennarelli TA: Emergency department management of head injuries, Emerg Med Clin North Am 2:749–760, 1984.

11. Stone JL et al: Acute subdural hematoma: direct admission to a trauma center yields improved results, J Trauma 26:445–558, 1986.

12. Hockberger RS et al: Blunt head injury: a spectrum of disease, Ann Emerg Med 15:2, 1986.

13. McMicken DB: Emergency CT head scans in traumatic and atraumatic conditions, Ann Emerg Med 15:3, 1986.

14. Calandre L et al: Clinical-CT correlations in TIA, RIND, and strokes with minimum residuum, Stroke 15:663–666, 1984.

15. Khaw KT et al: Prediction of stroke-associated mortality in the elderly, Stroke 15:244–248, 1984.

16. Andrews BT et al: Is computed tomographic scanning necessary in patients with tentorial herniation? Results of immediate surgical exploration without computed tomography in 100 patients, Neurosurgery 19(3):409, 1986.

17. Auer RV: Progress review: hypoglycemic brain damage, Stroke 17:699, 1986.

18. Arieff AJ et al: Nonketotic hyperosmolar coma with hyperglycemia, Medicine 51:73–74, 1972.

19. Khardori R et al: HNKH, Am J Med 77:899–904, 1984.

20. Komrad MS et al: Myocardial infarctions and stroke, Neurology 34:1403–1409, 1984.

21. Tobias SL et al: Myocardial damage and electrocardiographic changes in acute cerebrovascular hemorrhage: a report of three cases and reviews, Heart Lung 16:521–525, 1987.

22. Kelley RE et al: Cerebral ischemia and atrial fibrillation: prospective study, Neurology 34:1285–1291, 1984.

23. Gurusinghe NT et al: The value of computerized tomography in aneurysmal subarachnoid hemorrhage, J Neurosurg 60:763–770, 1984.

24. Hosoda K et al: Magnetic resonance images of chronic subdural hematomas, J Neurosurg 67, 1987.

25. Duffy GP: Lumbar puncture in subarachnoid hemorrhage, Lancet 2:1103–1104, 1982.

26. Olendorf WH: Magnetic resonance imaging versus computerized tomography, West J Med 142:54–62, 1985.

27. Adams JP et al: CT and clinical correlations in recent aneurysmal subarachnoid hemorrhage: a preliminary report of the Cooperative Aneurysm Study, Neurology 33(8): 981, 1983.

28. Schmidley JW et al: Agitated confusional states in patients with right hemispheric infarctions, Stroke 15:883–885, 1984.

29. Lehman LB: Coma in the elderly: evaluation and treatment, Hosp Pract, June 15, 1987.

30. Harrison MJG and Marshall J: Atrial fibrillations, TIA's and completed strokes, Stroke 15:441–442, 1984.

31. Bucknall CA et al: Physicians' attitudes to four common problems: hypertension, atrial fibrillation, transient ischemic attacks, and angina pectoris, Br Med J 293:20, 1986.

32. Furlan AJ: Transient ischemic attacks: strategies for minimizing stroke risk, Postgrad Med 75:183–189, 1984.

33. Neugebauer R et al: Seizures in public places in New York City, Am J Public Health 76(9):1115, 1986.

34. Morris PJ et al: Transient ischemic attacks, New York, 1982, Marcel Dekker.

35. Wolf PA et al: Epidemiologic assessment of chronic atrial fibrillation and risk of stroke: the Framingham study, Neurology 28:973–977, 1978.

36. Gill JS et al: Stroke and alcohol consumption, N Engl J Med 315:1041–1046, 1986.

37. Donahue R et al: Alcohol and hemorrhagic stroke, JAMA 255:2311–2314, 1986.

38. Melamed N et al: Cerebral hemorrhage: a review and reappraisal of benigh cases, Arch Neurol 41:425–428, 1984.

39. Vicaro S et al: Emergency presentation of subdural hematoma: a review of 85 cases diagnosed by computerized tomography, Ann Emerg Med 11(9):475–478, 1982.

40. Mattle H et al: Nontraumatic spinal epidural and subdural hematomas, Neurology 37:1351–1356, 1987.

41. Tuhrim S et al: Management of transient ischemic attacks, Am Fam Physician 34(4):162, 1986.

42. Bindu T et al: Seizures in relation to head injury, Ann Emerg Med April 4, 1987.

43. Braaten JT: Hyperosmolar nonketotic diabetic coma: diagnosis and management, Geriatrics 42:83–92, 1987.

44. Miller M: Fluid and electrolyte balance in the elderly, Geriatrics 42:65–76, 1987.

45. Ashouri OS: Severe diuretic-induced hyponatremia in the elderly, Arch Intern Med 146:1355, 1986.

46. Mahler ME: Seizures: common causes and treatment in the elderly, Geriatrics 42:73–78, 1987.

47. Snyder ND et al: Hypernatremia in the elderly patient, Ann Intern Med 107:309–319, 1987.

48. Sterns RH: Severe symptomatic hyponatremia: treatment and outcome, Ann Intern Med 107:656–664, 1987.

49. Wachtel TJ: Predisposing factors for the diabetic hyperosmolar state, Arch Intern Med 147: 1987.

Dementia, Confusion, and Altered Mental Status

Robert Rafal, M.D.

Review of chronic dementias

Definitions and classifications of neuropsychologic
 disorders

Diagnosis of reversible causes of dementia

Alzheimer's disease and other degenerative disorders
 producing progressive dementia

Acute mental deterioration

 Presenting symptoms and signs of dementia

 Acute worsening of dementia

Evaluation of the acutely confused patient

 Diffuse encephalopathies: metabolic, toxic, anoxic,
  traumatic, epileptic, and infectious (meningitis,
  encephalitis)

 Structural lesions in the brain causing altered
  mental status

This chapter will discuss the evaluation of the patient who is brought for emergency care because
of "confusion." The diagnosis of an altered mental
state is more difficult in the elderly because the causative
condition may present with more subtle symptoms and
signs and because there is a problem of sorting out
relevant acute factors from chronic factors. Because
dementia is so common in the elderly, it is a special challenge to the emergency department physician who must
determine 1) if the patient's condition represents a substantial change from previous level of function, and, if so,
2) if the acute mental disturbance indicates the presence
of an acute neurologic disorder, or, 3) if it is based on an
exacerbation or decompensation of a chronic dementia
due to nonneurologic causes (e.g., psychosocial factors or
covert, intercurrent systemic illnesses).

To approach this problem rationally and systematically, physicians must be familiar with those medical and
neurologic disorders that can cause acute confusional
states. In addition, they must also have an appreciation
for the types of dementia, their component mental symptoms, and their pathophysiology. This review, therefore,
will be divided into two parts: 1) an overview of the
chronic dementias and 2) acute mental deterioration.

REVIEW OF CHRONIC DEMENTIAS

As people grow older, it is normal for mental processes to
undergo change. By the end of adolescence, memory
capacity is already beginning to decline slowly, and it becomes increasingly difficult to learn new things. After the
age of 65, reaction time also tends to slow down, but this
is because we tend to be more cautious, not necessarily
because we are becoming less intelligent. Brain scans
using computerized tomography (CT) have shown that it
is common for the size of our brains to begin to shrink.
For these reasons, there is a historical tendency for
people, including physicians, to believe that "senility" in
the elderly is a normal process.

It is now known that such an assumption is not medically valid and that it may unnecessarily prejudice the
care and quality of life of senior citizens. Many people in
their seventies, eighties, and nineties continue to be
productive and independent and to enjoy the use of their
intellect, even though their memories may not serve
them as well as they once did. Severe mental impairment, producing a loss of independence, is never normal
at any age and indicates the presence of disease requiring medical evaluation.

The evaluation of a demented person includes:

1. Functional analysis and characterization of the component mental symptoms and signs (This analysis is
 based upon both history and mental status examination as well as psychometric testing when appropriate.)

2. Identification of the associated abnormalities on neurologic examination (e.g., localizing signs, Parkinsonian features, gait disorders)
3. Consideration of coexisting (and potentially causative or contributing) systemic illness
4. Integration of data from neurodiagnostic studies and other laboratory tests

The purpose of a comprehensive evaluation of the demented patient is first, of course, to exclude a potentially curable or reversible cause, but, and of equal importance for the patient whose disease cannot be cured, the goal is to define the individual's prognosis, limitations, and retained capacities so that an appropriate private management program may be formulated. The first step in the evaluation process listed above (i.e., the functional analysis of the character and severity of the component mental symptoms and signs) is important both for guiding the physician toward a correct etiologic diagnosis and in guiding psychosocial managment of the patient with a progressive dementia. For this reason, this chapter will first review some concepts and neuropsychologic definitions that are necessary to proceed with a systematic analysis of the patient's mental condition.

DEFINITIONS AND CLASSIFICATIONS OF NEUROPSYCHOLOGIC DISORDERS

The first distinction to be made in assessing mental function is between disorders in the *level* of consciousness and disorders of the *content* of consciousness. The level of consciousness refers to how alert and/or how arousable the individual is. Conditions that produce somnolence or stupor will inevitably result in impaired cognitive abilities, and the differential diagnosis is similar to that applied to the problem of stupor or coma. On the one hand, the diagnostic approach is rather different in the patient who is alert but whose content of consciousness is disrupted by disorders of memory, attention, language, etc.

Disorders in the content of consciousness may be either *global* or *selective* — that is, an individual may be impaired due to a selective loss of memory, the ability to read, write, speak, recognize objects, or do arithmetic, while other mental functions remain intact. Disease processes that affect localized brain regions, such as stroke or tumor, are likely to produce such selective deficits. Diffuse neurologic diseases will produce a global deficiency in mental function. While loss of memory is almost universal in these conditions, there are always other associated mental defects such as loss of language, reasoning, judgment, the ability to calculate, spatial orientation, or the ability to move about safely. A diffuse neurologic disease that produces chronic global impairment (either progressive or irreversible) is called a *dementia*. An acute global mental impairment of sudden onset and self-limited duration is called a *delirium*.

It is useful to approach the problem of evaluating the patient with an organic mental disorder by analyzing the condition in terms of three different components: cognitive, affective, and conative.

Cognitive deficits. Refers to disturbances of specific mental functions such as language (aphasia), writing (agraphia), reading (alexia), memory (amnesia), and recognition of objects (agnosia). A mental status examination that systematically examines such functions will provide valuable clues as to whether the individual has a selective cognitive disorder or more global dysfunction, which suggests the presence of dementia.

Affective disorders. Refers to mood disturbances such as depression or euphoria. A characteristic of organic mental disorders is emotional lability — that is, mood changes that are inappropriate and unpredictable and for which the patient does not seem to have any control of expression.

Conative disorders. Refers to an inability to plan and initiate goal-directed behavior. The term is used to indicate the presence of a defect in motivation that is organically based. Conative disorders are characteristic of frontal lobe lesions and diffuse cortical diseases. When conative dysfunction is the salient or presenting feature or an organic mental syndrome, it is often misinterpreted as a psychiatric problem. Patients may insidiously become apathetic and disinterested. They may stop pursuing past hobbies and interests, sit for long periods of time without moving, become disinclined to see old friends, and lose interest in family. Initially, family and friends may interpret these changes as laziness or perhaps depression.

It is not until this disturbance of motivation and goal-directed behavior causes patients to begin neglecting their own personal hygiene that families and friends may become suspicious of something wrong with brain function. For this reason, it is not unusual for patients with slowly progressive dementias (especially those involving chiefly frontal lobes) to show symptoms that are not recognized as being due to early dementia. They may be diagnosed as having psychiatric problems and receive inappropriate treatment based on this supposition. They may be unable to work but, lacking a medical diagnosis, are denied disability benefits. For years these patients and their families may be left hanging, with the disease going unrecognized until the nature of the condition is recognized.

DIAGNOSIS OF REVERSIBLE CAUSES OF DEMENTIA

Once the physician has diagnosed the mental disorder as being an organic and diffuse dementia, the next thing is to determine the exact cause and, specifically, to rule out conditions that may be cured or arrested. Reversible causes of dementia may be related either to general systemic illnesses or to specific neurologic diseases.

Among the most common general medical illnesses causing dementia are metabolic disorders and nutritional deficiencies.[1] Hypothyroidism can result in mental abnormalities that may be completely reversed with replacement therapy. Occasionally, significant mental impairment may be the presenting symptom with the other stigmata of the disease being less conspicuous. Pernicious anemia resulting from B_{12} deficiency may cause a mental deterioration even before anemia develops.[2] Almost always, however, there are other neurologic symptoms and signs. The early occurrence of very distressing paresthesias and dysesthesias in the lower extremities is quite characteristic.

Pernicious anemia is one of those neurologic dementia-producing illnesses often dominated by psychiatric symptoms such as paranoia, dramatic personality change, or even overt psychosis. Thiamine deficiency, as typified by the malnourished alcoholic, classically results in Korsakoff's syndrome in which severe memory impairment is the main finding. Multiple vitamin deficiencies, including thiamine and folic acid, commonly coexist with other neurologic degenerative diseases such as Alzheimer's disease. When elderly individuals, especially those living alone, begin to fail intellectually, they become less able to provide for their own needs and to maintain adequate diets. The results are nutritional deficiencies, including vitamin inadequacy, which accelerate the dementing process.

Cardiopulmonary diseases may also cause, or contribute to, dementia. These diseases may produce diffuse cerebral hypoxia and/or ischemia leading to an acute organic mental syndrome. However, ischemia may also result in a more insidious, slowly progressive decline in mental function. Patients with aortic stenosis may have periods of bradycardia (or other arrhythmias) that are covert and occur chiefly during sleep. Similarly, patients with chronic obstructive pulmonary disease may have borderline oxygen saturation that is considered to be "adequate" when tested during the day. However, they may also have superimposed periods of sleep apnea causing significant oxygen desaturation which, over a period of time, will produce a progressive decline in mental abilities. Therefore, patients with valvular disease, chronic congestive heart failure, cardiac arrhythmias, or pulmonary disease who begin to decline mentally require very careful reevaluation with special attention directed towards monitoring cardiopulmonary function during sleep.

Tumors may produce insidious and slowly progressive dementia in the elderly. This is especially true of slow-growing, extraaxial (that is, outside the substance of the brain) masses such as chronic subdural hematomas or meningiomas. Subdural hematomas can occur in the elderly after a relatively minor injury not documented at the time of presentation. Mental status changes may dominate the clinical picture without localizing findings, headache, or depressed level of consciousness. CT scanning is adequate for ruling out most intracranial lesions. However, one warning is necessary with regard to chronic subdural hematomas; if they are bilateral, they may be isodense with the brain and, hence, not visualized on the CT scan. When such isodense subdural hematomas are bilateral, they may produce no shift of midline structures. In this case, the only clue is that the ventricles look inappropriately small, and the sulci are not seen. This so-called "hypernormal" pattern on CT scanning should raise the index of suspicion of possible bilateral subdural hematoma; isotope brain scanning may be used to make the diagnosis in these cases, or, occasionally, it may be necessary to perform angiography.

Another common cause of dementia is cerebral vascular disease. One stroke, even a fairly large one, may be devastating to the individual in terms of producing specific functional deficits but may not produce a global dementia. However, an elderly individual who has had numerous small strokes scattered throughout the brain can, over time, become demented. This is particularly true in hypertensive patients. This entity is called multi-infarct dementia. In a patient with multiinfarct dementia who acutely becomes more confused, it may be difficult to determine whether the individual has had another small stroke or whether there has been some other factor causing the acute decompensation. The advent of MRI scanning demonstrates more precisely the nature of the insult, including the white matter changes.[3]

Another uncommon, treatable cause of dementia is communicating hydrocephalus. Communicating hydrocephalus implies that the ventricles empty normally, but the cerebrospinal fluid (CSF) is not properly absorbed over the surface of the brain. Communicating hydrocephalus is common following hemorrhage, trauma, or meningitis. When it occurs without any obvious cause in a middle-aged or elderly person, it may produce an insidiously progressive dementia without marked elevation of cerebrospinal fluid pressure. This form of communicating hydrocephalus is what is referred to as "normal pressure hydrocephalus syndrome."

Most physicians are aware of this and are familiar with the fact that it consists, clinically, of a triad of symptoms — dementia, gait disorder, and incontinence. However, *any* dementia may, terminally, produce these three symptoms. The point being emphasized is that these individual component symptoms have a very specific character in the normal pressure hydrocephalus syndrome. The dementia is characterized by pronounced psychomotor retardation, with markedly prolonged latencies. A careful examiner may, after doing a detailed mental status evaluation, determine that the patient's mental faculties, individually, are not as severely impaired as they may appear on casual inspection and that the marked slowness of responses gives the patient the appearance of being more demented than he or she really is. The gait disorder in normal pressure hydrocephalus is that of a gait apraxia. Postural righting reflexes are impaired; but, in addition, the gait has a stuck-to-the-floor character such that patients seem to have difficulty in shifting their weight from one foot to the other and seem to be held to the floor by magnets. Finally, although incontinence is common in severely demented patients, it is unusual for it to be an early or marked feature in the patients who are mildly demented. In summary, the diagnosis of normal pressure hydrocephalus should be suspected in patients who have an emerging dementia characterized by marked slowness of response and psychomotor retardation, gait difficulties, and the early onset of incontinence. A CT scan, in a typical case, shows markedly enlarged ventricles but with relative sparing of the cortex such that cortical atrophy is not conspicuous. The diagnosis must be confirmed by radioisotope cisternography.

There are two abnormal findings on cisternography that are important. First, the isotope is seen, within 6 to 12 hours after injection into the lumbar space, entering the ventricular system. Ventricular reflex is abnormal. However, ventricular reflex occurs in Alzheimer's disease and other neurologic conditions in which ventricles are dilated. Therefore, ventricular penetration of the isotope itself does not confirm the diagnosis of communicating hydrocephalus. In order to make the diagnosis of hydrocephalus, the most important radioisotope finding is *persistence* of ventricular penetration. That is, if the isotope remains in the ventricular system and does not diffuse over the surface of the brain for 48 hours, the study can be interpreted as confirming the clinical diagnosis of communicating hydrocephalus.

A ventriculoperitoneal shunt may be quite dramatic in reversing the dementia and other symptoms of normal pressure hydrocephalus. A beneficial result is most likely to occur in patients in whom all three clinical components of the triad are present, in whom the cisternogram is unambiguously confirmatory, and in whom the CT scan shows little or no cortical atrophy. However, even in such carefully selected cases, only about half of the patients who are operated upon will improve.

Lumbar puncture has a continuing place in the evaluation of dementia to rule out chronic infections. The diagnosis of tertiary central nervous system syphilis in a demented patient with positive blood serology can be confirmed by a spinal fluid examination revealing elevated protein and positive CSF serology. Chronic basilar meningitis due to the fungus *Cryptococcus neoformans* can produce a slowly progressive dementia. Previously, the diagnosis was based upon the findings of spores on India ink preparations of the spinal fluid or growth of the fungus on culture. Currently, the most direct and sensitive way of making the diagnosis is to study the spinal fluid for cryptococcal antigen. In addition, always be aware of AIDS as a possible cause of dementia, as well as opportunistic infections resulting from impaired immunity resulting from AIDS.

ALZHEIMER'S DISEASE AND OTHER DEGENERATIVE DISORDERS PRODUCING PROGRESSIVE DEMENTIA

The most common cause of dementia in the elderly is Alzheimer's disease. This is a degenerative disorder of unknown cause in which nerve cells of the cerebral cortex die, and the cortex becomes atrophic. The disorder is named after the German neuropathologist who first described the histopathologic abnormalities that consist of nerve cell degeneration and reactive gliosis (scarring). Specific changes found in degenerating nerve cells include neurofibrillary tangles (that stain with silver stain) and senile plaques.

Only recently has the prevalence of Alzheimer's disease really been appreciated and the malignant nature of the process fully recognized. Although the deterioration in mental function does not directly cause death, patients ultimately stop eating and become malnourished and immobilized so that they are prone to intercurrent infections. Alzheimer's disease does shorten the life span, and it has been estimated that it is the fifth or sixth largest killer in the United States. There is a progressive increase in the incidence of the disease with increasing age. When the onset begins before the age of 65, the current convention is to refer to that entity as "presenile dementia of the Alzheimer type"; in patients afflicted after the age of 65, "senile dementia of the Alzheimer type." Approximately 5% of the population over age 65 are suffering from a severe dementia and, if mild cases are included, this percentage may be as high as 10%. Of all the elderly patients with chronic dementias, approximately two thirds will be victims of Alzheimer's disease.

Two areas of the brain seem to be most prone to early involvement by Alzheimer's disease: the frontal lobe and the hippocampus. The hippocampus, located within each temporal lobe, is critical to new learning and storing new memories. It is for this reason that forgetfulness and memory problems are the commonest early manifestations of Alzheimer's disease. Disease affecting the frontal lobe results in personality changes. Although such personality changes may be quite dramatic with the emergence of paranoia, delusions, irritability, and depression, it is also not uncommon for the consequences of frontal lobe dysfunction to emerge more insidiously in the form of a conative disorder as discussed earlier. Although memory disorders, personality changes, and conative dysfunction are the most common presenting symptoms of Alzheimer's disease, the illness can affect more posterior areas of the brain first to produce atypical presentations. Alzheimer's disease patients can present with aphasias (typically anomia or word-finding difficulties) or apraxias (for example, patients who wake up one morning and find that they are unable to dress themselves).

The diagnosis of Alzheimer's disease is made chiefly on clinical grounds by documenting a history of slowly *progressive* and *global* impairment of mental function, and the systemic exclusion of treatable/reversible causes of dementia as discussed above. Radiographic procedures such as a CT scan are used to confirm the clinical diagnosis.

In a typical CT scan from a patient with advanced Alzheimer's disease, the cerebral gray matter is completely destroyed. There is a marked enlargement of the cortical sulci with secondary dilatation of the ventricles. This ventricular enlargement, in which the CSF filled spaces expanded to replace the shrunken brain, is referred to as "hydrocephalus ex vacuo." There is dilatation of the temporal horns of the lateral ventricle. The hippocampus of the temporal lobe sits in the floor of the temporal horn. Therefore, since degeneration of the hippocampus is one of the early pathologic features of Alzheimer's disease, dilatation of the temporal horn of the lateral ventricles is very often the earliest radiographic abnormality seen in this disease.

CT scanning in a dementia workup should include careful attention to the region of the temporal lobe. In some patients with dementia who have a variant of the so-called lobar atrophies, the degenerative process may selectively involve a local area of the cerebral cortex and remain relatively confined until the course is quite advanced. An example is Pick's disease, which characteristically involves the frontal poles and the very anterior part of the temporal lobes. In these patients there is asymmetric atrophy of the temporal horn.

In the patient who has a typical clinical history of Alzheimer's disease and has dramatic CT scan changes of cortical atrophy, the diagnosis generally poses no problem. However, the limitations of diagnosing Alzheimer's disease radiographically must be fully appreciated. Generally, there is relatively poor correlation between the clinical severity of the dementia and the appearance of the atrophy as estimated on CT scan. Moreover, it has been clearly established that cortical atrophy occurs with advancing age even in neurologically normal individuals. Therefore, the presence of moderate cortical atrophy in the 55-year-old patient who is becoming demented would be highly significant and confirmatory of the diagnosis of Alzheimer's disease; in a 75-year-old patient a similar degree of cortical atrophy may not necessarily be pathologic. On the other hand, in a 66-year-old individual with early Alzheimer's disease, the CT scan may appear normal (especially if there has not been careful radiographic attention to the region of the temporal lobes). The point being emphasized is that the CT scan, whether normal or abnormal, must be interpreted with caution and correlated carefully with the clinical history and examination findings. The only definitive way to diagnose the disease during life is through cortical biopsy, looking for the characteristic histologic changes of Alzheimer's disease. Only rarely, however, is it

necessary to resort to such an invasive diagnostic approach. In most cases, the diagnosis should be established on the basis of history of progression and global deterioration of mental function, a comprehensive medical and neurologic evaluation to exclude other, treatable causes of dementia, and radiographic studies to confirm the diagnosis.

The cause of Alzheimer's disease is not known. It was once attributed to "hardening of the arteries" or poor circulation to the brain and has been related to arteriosclerosis. However, it is now known that Alzheimer's disease is not secondary to arteriosclerosis. The primary disorder is in the nerve cells, not in the blood vessels. The cause of this neuronal degeneration remains unknown, but there are some clues.

Recently, it was found that nerve cells from Alzheimer's disease patients have increased amounts of aluminum. The reason for this chemical change, or its significance in terms of a causal relationship to the disease, is unknown. There are also unexplained but marked abnormalities in glutamate metabolism. Research has also suggested that there may be a genetic predisposition towards Alzheimer's disease. However, only in very rare families will the disease be clearly genetic in any predictable sense. If, in a given family, there is a strong history that many members have become demented early in life, then other family members are probably at significantly greater risk of an early dementia. Some studies have suggested that the presence of dementia in parents puts an offspring at double the risk of developing the disease later in life (i.e., the risk goes from 4% to 8%). However, even if this suggestion is confirmed by future genetic studies, the odds will still favor the child of an Alzheimer's disease patient; the presence of Alzheimer's disease in only one elderly parent does not mean that the children will inevitably meet a similar fate. There are certain rare degenerative, dementia-producing illnesses that have been proven to be caused by small infectious agents similar to viruses (slow virus infections). However, there is no compelling evidence that this is true for Alzheimer's disease; the disease has not been transmissible to primates through inoculation of human brain tissue. Some preliminary research suggests that certain immunologic factors contribute to the development of the disease, but this hypothesis requires a great deal more research. In patients with Alzheimer's disease, a decrease in the receptor enzyme for the neurotransmitter, acetylcholine, is found. Acetylcholine is produced in the nerve cells of the cerebral cortex and is the means by which the cells "talk to each other." Since the cells of the cerebral cortex are degenerating and dying in Alzheimer's disease, it is not surprising that the chemicals in them would also decrease. There is no direct evidence that this chemical defect is in any way a cause of the disease. However, this biochemical finding has given rise to some strategies for drug therapy. Efforts have been made to improve mental function in Alzheimer's disease patients by giving agonists that increase acetylcholine activity. However, to date, therapeutic trials of such agents as lecithin, choline, and physostigmine have been disappointing.

ACUTE MENTAL DETERIORATION

Acute deterioration in mental function can be subdivided into three broad categories: 1) chronic dementias presenting initially as acute mental deterioration; 2) chronic dementias with acute worsening of mental symptoms; and 3) confusion in a nondemented individual with an acute neurologic illness.

Presenting Symptoms and Signs of Dementia

Anxiety and depression are common early manifestations of dementia, which may have somatic manifestations leading the patient to seek medical care. It is important to differentiate a serious depression with signs of dementia (so-called pseudodementia) from other forms of dementia because of the treatment potentials in the former condition.[4] The patient may come to the emergency department with vague complaints such as headache, indigestion, discomfort, weakness, or fatigue that the patient cannot clearly define and to which the doctor cannot ascribe a cause. Hysteria and hypochondriasis do not usually begin late in life, and in the elderly, "functional" disorders usually indicate a more serious underlying systemic, neurologic, or psychiatric illness. Therefore, when a previously healthy and stable individual begins frequenting the emergency department with apparent functional complaints, the physician should suspect an emerging depression, a dementia, or both.

Dementia may be heralded by an acute, florid psychosis, including hallucinations, paranoid delusions, and even catatonia. When a psychotic disturbance occurs with no previous history of psychiatric symptoms, an underlying dementia should be strongly suspected.

Dementing illnesses may progress insidiously without being recognized for long periods of time as long as the individual maintains normal routines and is not stressed. As is the case with chronic illnesses affecting other organ systems, mental function in a slowly developing dementia may remain "compensated" and asymptomatic as long as the reserve capacities of the individual's mental capabilities are not overtaxed. In this situation, however, even a minor physical, social, or emotional stress may cause the individual to *decompensate*. This may occur with a minor head injury, emotional stress such as the death of a loved one, a move to a new location, or an intercurrent medical illness such as the flu or pneumonia. When this occurs, an elderly individual who has been living independently and "getting by" may be brought to the emergency department acutely confused and dis-

oriented. When this kind of decompensation occurs, there may be no obvious precipitating factor.

Acute Worsening of Dementia

Just as dementia can present acutely, as discussed above, it may also deteriorate acutely. Therefore, whenever a patient with a "mild" dementia becomes acutely confused, the challenge will be to determine whether the individual's mental reserve is "decompensating" as part of the progression of the dementia or whether there is an acute insult to the brain superimposed upon a chronic dementia. The second diagnosis is, of course, one of exclusion and is one that is never easy to make with confidence.

Perhaps the most common and frustrating example of this kind of problem is represented by the "found-on-the-floor syndrome." Every emergency department physician is familiar with this problem. An elderly individual who has been, perhaps, a bit forgetful but living independently is found on the floor of his apartment in a confused and disoriented state. The presence of pressure sores and dehydration indicates that the individual probably was on the floor for several days. Other than lethargy and confusion, there are no neurologic findings. There are a number of possibilities that may explain the situation. One is that the individual simply lost his balance and fell to the floor. Being too frail to get back on his feet, he lay there for days. The resulting social isolation and the effects of dehydration and hyponatremia combined to result in an acute confusion. Another possibility is that the individual may have had a "small stroke," possibly involving the vertebrobasilar arterial distribution and resulting in confusion and poor balance but without other clear localizing findings. Alternatively, the individual may have lost his balance and fallen, struck his head, and had a mild concussion resulting in confusion. The individual may have a small metastatic brain tumor that caused a convulsion and resulted in a fall to the floor and confusion. Or a cardiac arrhythmia with syncope may have caused the patient to fall. Also, an anoxic period resulting in encephalopathy may have produced the confusion.

Obviously, the five possibilities listed above are just part of the list of causes. They are intended only to highlight the protean possibilities and the diagnostic difficulties that this situation poses to the emergency department physician. It emphasizes the importance of considering acute neurologic illnesses even in patients with known chronic dementias. Some of these may leave no objective sequelae that can be confirmed with neurodiagnostic studies; for example, a minor concussion, a small stroke, or a brief period of anoxia may leave no findings that can be detected using the electroencephalogram (EEG), CT scan, or spinal fluid analysis when the patient is brought to the emergency department 2 days later. On the other hand, the presence of a cardiac arrhythmia in a patient brought to the emergency department in a confused state should at least raise the suspicion of a possible cerebral anoxic episode. A CT scan can be obtained to rule out a chronic subdural hematoma; an EEG may give some evidence for an active epileptic disturbance in a patient who had a seizure 2 days before. For these reasons, a patient who is "found-on-the-floor" should be carefully evaluated, and consideraton should be given to the various diagnostic possibilities so that treatable or curable conditions may be detected.

EVALUATION OF THE ACUTELY CONFUSED PATIENT

The approach to the patient who has been mentally normal previously, and becomes acutely confused, does not differ greatly from the approach to the younger patient with confusion. However, although the diagnostic process and differential diagnosis are similar, the statistical probabilities of certain entities are different. For example, encephalitis, Korsakoff's syndrome, and psychomotor status epilepticus are much more common causes of confusion in younger people; in the elderly, these disorders are relatively rare, and vertebrobasilar insufficiency is a common cause of confusion.

The differential diagnosis of an altered mental state parallels that of depressed levels of consciousness in stupor or coma. The following discussion, therefore, will proceed by separating disorders causing acute mental changes into two broad categories, diffuse encephalopathies and structural lesions on the brain.

Diffuse Encephalopathies: Metabolic, Toxic, Anoxic, Traumatic, Epileptic, and Infectious (Meningitis, Encephalitis)

Electrolyte imbalance and prerenal azotemia from dehydration may precipitate or contribute to confusion as in the "found-on-the-floor syndrome" discussed above. Patients should be admitted for gradual rehydration and nutritional support, while their neurologic status is carefully monitored. Until the mental state starts improving, suspicion must be maintained that some other, covert process may be involved in the encephalopathy.

Cerebral and/or myocardial anoxia, due to hypotension or cardiac arrhythmia, should be suspected in any confused patient who is found to be hypotensive or who has cardiac arrhythmias, aortic stenosis, or carotid bruits. An acute myocardial infarction (MI) should be ruled out, and electrocardiogram (EKG) monitoring should be considered during the first day or two in the hospital.

Blood gas determination is a frequently neglected but an important part of the evaluation of any elderly, confused patient. Therapeutically, it is important to identify and correct even mild hypoxia in order to optimize cerebral function. Blood gas determinations are also useful diagnostically in identifying metabolic or toxic encephalopathies. Respiratory alkalosis may provide a clue to the presence of salicylate intoxication or pulmonary embolus. Respiratory alkalosis is common in encephalopathy accompanying sepsis and may be an important clue to the presence of sepsis in the absence of other symptoms and signs.

Search for a covert infection is important in the evaluation of any confused geriatric patient; the elderly can become very sick with systemic infections without developing fever, leukocytosis, or (with meningitis) nuchal rigidity. Whenever sepsis is suspected as the underlying cause of confusion in an elderly patient, every effort should be made to identify the source of infection in the emergency department with appropriate studies (chest or sinus x-rays, urinalysis, lumbar puncture). (See Chapter 22.)

The elderly may be very sensitive to sedative, narcotic, or hypnotic medications. Intoxication with these agents is a common cause of stupor and confusion and should be considered in any geriatric patient with a depressed level of consciousness. Anticholinergic medications have been implicated, and delirium has been reported from diuretics, digoxin, cimetidine, antihypertensives, antiarrhythmic drugs, and even nonsteroidal antiinflammatory medications.[5] Respiratory acidosis from hypoventilation should increase the physician's suspicion of narcotic/hypnotic medication intoxication. Other drugs, for example those used in treating Parkinson's disease, don't depress the level of consciousness, but do produce an agitated delirium. Vivid visual hallucinations, which the patient knows are not real, are quite characteristic of toxic delirium from psychoactive medication. The tendency to hyperventilate in a patient with an agitated delirium will usually produce a mild respiratory alkalosis.

It is unusual for epileptic disorders to present, for the first time, as confusional states in the elderly, but it does occur. One example was of a patient who came to see me because she felt "confused." She was playing a game with her young grandchildren and could not remember the rules. When I examined her, there were no localizing findings. She seemed alert, composed, and lucid. The only abnormal observation on mental status examination was that she had difficulty with word finding and naming objects. The EEG showed a generalized spike and wave abnormality. Treatment with anticonvulsants resulted in her mental state and EEG returning to normal. The diagnosis of epileptic twilight state should be suspected whenever there are dramatic fluctuations in mental state from one minute to the next. In general, it is helpful to remember that there are two types of disorders that can result in rapid and fluctuating changes in mental states, namely, epileptic disorders and vascular insufficiency. An EEG is indicated, as an emergency procedure, in any patient with a confusional state of uncertain cause and in whom there are marked or rapid fluctuations in the level of consciousness or the mental state.

The CT scan is overutilized in evaluating patients in the emergency department while the EEG is underutilized. As discussed below, a CT is an appropriate emergency procedure in any patient with a depressed level of consciousness to rule out an intracranial lesion. In the patient who is confused, but without a depressed level of consciousness, a CT scan can be done electively after admission to the hospital. If the patient has a subdural hematoma or a brain tumor, it will not disappear in an hour or two. On the other hand, if the patient has an epileptic encephalopathy, the chance of making the diagnosis will be lost if an EEG is delayed until the next day, when the patient's mental state has returned to normal.

In the case of the patient whose situation is discussed above, the cause of her seizure disorder was never determined. A diagnosis of idiopathic epilepsy was made. Usually when seizures occur for the first time in an elderly individual, there is some underlying neurologic disease. The two most common causes are cerebral vascular disease and brain tumors. Seizures related to cerebral vascular disease may be either a later complication of a stroke or its presenting symptom. Seizures following a stroke can begin a month or even years after a stroke. While seizures resulting from stroke are usually associated with large strokes that produce at least some degree of permanent, residual deficit, at times the individual may have made a complete functional recovery by the time the first seizure occurs. Focal seizures may herald a cerebral infarction. Strokes due to cardiac embolus are generally considered to have a higher incidence of acute seizures.

Structural Lesions in the Brain Causing Altered Mental Status

Lesions can be divided into two broad groups: 1) extra-axial masses such as subdural hematomas that press on the brain but do not destroy it and 2) intra-axial (parenchymatous) lesions in the substance of the brain. Subdural hematomas produce their effect on mental status through increased intracranial pressure. Therefore, subdural hematomas almost always produce altered mental states in which there is a depressed level of consciousness and in which psychomotor retardation is a conspicuous symptom. Localizing neurologic findings may be absent. Intraaxial lesions, on the other hand, usually will produce some localizing findings on careful examination such as mild hemiparesis, aphasia, or visual field defect. However, tumors involving some relatively "silent" areas of the brain can grow to be quite large and produce quite pronounced and global changes in mental function without localizing findings. Tumors involving the frontal lobes are notorious for mimicking degenerative disease. Or multiple small tumors scattered throughout the brain

may produce mental deterioration without any localizing findings until later in the course of the disease.

Cerebral vascular insufficiency is probably the most common cause of acute changes in mental states in the elderly but can be the most difficult to diagnose. When a hemiparesis or hemiplegia accompanies the change in mental state, the diagnosis is seldom missed. However, there are certain specific syndromes of vascular insufficiency that can produce confusion without localizing findings. Emergency department physicians should be familiar with these syndromes, since the diagnosis must be made, or at least suspected, on clinical grounds alone. Changes in the CT scan due to stroke seldom occur within the first 48 hours (even with large strokes); therefore, the correct and early diagnosis must be based on clinical skill.

The anterior and middle cerebral arteries are branches of the internal carotid artery. Together they constitute the "anterior circulation" and they are lateralized; the right carotid artery supplies the right cerebral hemisphere and the left carotid artery supplies the left hemisphere.

The anterior cerebral artery supplies the frontal pole of the hemisphere, as well as the medial aspect of the cortex. The hemiparesis, resulting from anterior cerebral artery ischemia, is generally greater in the leg than in the upper extremities or face and may not be appreciated unless the function of the lower extremities is specifically examined.

The posterior cerebral arteries are both branches of a single blood vessel, the basilar artery. Vertebrobasilar insufficiency may therefore produce bilateral cerebral ischemia, which results in confusion, without hemiplegia or other obvious localizing signs. The incidence of posterior circulation ischemia disease increases in older people in relation to anterior circulation strokes. Posterior circulation ischemia may be the most common cause of acute confusion in the elderly; it is certainly the most commonly undiagnosed cause.

Emergency department physicians should be aware of the protean neuropsychologic manifestations of posterior cerebral artery ischemia. These episodes are often transitory, and the emergency department physician may be the only person in the position to make the diagnosis. The symptoms of vertebrobasilar insufficiency may be divided into two classes: 1) symptoms due to infratentorial ischemia affecting the brainstem and cerebellum and 2) supratentorial ischemia compromising the cerebral cortex of the occipital and temporal lobes. Ischemia to the brainstem frequently produces an impaired level of consciousness. Midbrain ischemia especially will produce somnolence often associated with relatively subtle localizing findings such as unequal and irregular pupils. Infratentorial ischemia also will frequently produce more obvious symptoms of dysarthria, vertigo, nystagmus, ataxia, and dysphagia. For these reasons, vertebrobasilar insufficiency, which produces brainstem ischemia, is usually not difficult to diagnose.

When the posterior circulation ischemia is restricted to the posterior cerebral artery distribution, sparing the brainstem, the diagnosis of cerebral ischemia may not be so obvious. Ischemia in the distribution of one, or both, posterior cerebral arteries will often result in a generalized, global confusional state; visual impairment and memory loss are the dominant symptoms. The posterior cerebral arteries supply the occipital lobes, and ischemia unilaterally produces a visual field loss. Bilateral occipital ischemia may produce agnosia for faces or objects or, if sufficiently severe, may result in cortical blindness. The posterior cerebral arteries also supply the basal and mesial temporal lobes bilaterally. This distribution includes the hippocampus of the temporal lobes, which is critical for memory function. Ischemia restricted to the temporal lobes bilaterally results in severe memory impairment and, if the brainstem and occipital lobes are not affected, there may be no visual impairment or other cognitive deficits besides memory. The prototype of this syndrome is transient global amnesia. The patient may be completely alert and lucid but will ask the same questions over and over again, being unable to remember any new information presented to him.

When posterior cerebral artery ischemia is relatively selective, involving either the temporal or occipital lobes, it can be easy to identify distinct conditions such as amnesia and agnosia as discussed above. However, it is more common for the ischemia to be more diffuse, affecting the occipital and temporal lobes of both hemispheres, and the result is that of a global confusional state. Patients may be somnolent or manifest an agitated delirium. In such patients, it can be difficult to formally evaluate visual or memory function and, if vertebrobasilar insufficiency is not considered in the differential, the diagnosis is frequently missed. Special attention should, therefore, be directed to evaluating vision in any confused, elderly patients, since visual abnormalities are often the key to the diagnosis. Even when patients are too confused to cooperate during examination, there are certain observations that can be made. Does the patient turn toward the examiner? Does he or she establish eye contact or track the examiner with the eyes? Blink to a visual threat? If turning to look at the examiner, will he or she do so from both sides or tend to neglect one area?

SUMMARY

This chapter reviews the problem of acute confusion in the elderly. In approaching this problem in the emergency department, the physician must determine if the patient's condition represents a substantial change from the previous level of function. If so, is the acute change in mental function based upon an exacerbation or decompensation of a chronic dementia that is not due to a new neurologic problem (e.g., psychosocial factors, intercurrent systemic illness)? Or, rather, does it signify the presence of an acute neurologic illness? To approach this problem systematically, the emergency department physician must appreciate the multiple symptomatology of dementia.

This chapter first reviews chronic dementing illness. It distinguishes those medical and neurologic causes of dementia that can be cured or arrested from irreversible degenerative disorders. Alzheimer's disease and related disorders are discussed in some detail, including prevalence, morbid anatomy, symptoms and signs, radiographic features and diagnostic criteria, current concepts of etiology, and neurochemical pathophysiology.

The second section of this chapter deals with acute mental deterioration in the elderly. Dementia may present acutely and bring the patient to the emergency department with psychoneurotic complaints, psychotic episodes, or acute delirium. The differential diagnosis of acute confusion is divided into two broad catagories — diffuse encephalopathies (including metabolic, toxic, anoxic, traumatic, epileptic, infectious) and structural lesions (including tumors, hematomas, and infarction). The appropriate applications of chemistry studies, CT scanning, and EEG are discussed. Special attention is directed to posterior circulation ischemia and infarction as a common, but frequently unrecognized, cause of acute confusion in the geriatric population.

REFERENCES

1. Blass JP and Plum F: Metabolic encephalopathies in older adults. In Katzman R and Terry RD, editors: The neurology of aging, Philadelphia, 1983, FA Davis Co.
2. Lindenbaum J et al: Neuropsychiatric disorders caused by cobalamin deficiency in the absence of anemia or macrocytosis, N Engl J Med 318:720, 1988.
3. Gamache FW: Update in cerebrovascular disease, Med Times 117:21, 1980.
4. Blazer D: Depression in the elderly, N Engl J Med 320:164, 1989.
5. Lipowski ZJ: Delirium in the elderly patient, N Engl J Med 320:578, 1989.

SUGGESTED READINGS

Gershon S and Radkin A, editors: Aging. Vol 2. Genesis and treatment of psychologic disorders in the elderly, New York, 1975, Raven Press.
Joynt FJ and Shoulson I: Dementia. In Heilman K and Valenstein E, editors: Clinical neuropsychology, New York, 1979, Oxford University Press.
Katzman R and Terry RD: The neurology of aging, Philadelphia, 1981, FA Davis Co.
Strub RL and Black RW: Organic brain syndrome, Philadelphia, 1981, FA Davis Co.
Wells CE: Dementia, ed 2, Philadelphia, 1977, FA Davis Co.

Emergency Geropsychiatry

Richard C. U'Ren, M.D.

GUIDELINES

All clinicians working in an emergency department are faced with older patients whose symptoms are not easily placed in the usual psychiatric versus medical categories. The reason for this is simple: the rate of both medical and psychiatric disorders, particularly senile dementia, increases in frequency with age. As a result, there is not only an overlap between medical and psychiatric symptoms, but also a greater likelihood that medical problems will be accompanied by psychiatric symptoms and vice versa. This represents both the challenge and frustration of geriatric practice.

Many clinicians working in an emergency department have a greater familiarity with medical and surgical problems than they do with psychiatric disorders. Accordingly, some guidelines for the evaluation of the older patient in the emergency room from a psychiatric perspective are in order.

Collect essential information about the patient from as many sources as possible.

From the psychiatric standpoint, essential information consists of the following:

- A description and brief history of the main complaint for which the patient was brought to the emergency room. This should include specific details about the presenting problem, usually defined by such terms as "confusion," "depression," "agitation," or "paranoia." How did the patient specifically *show* agitation or confusion? Under what circumstances did it appear? Suddenly or slowly? How long ago did it start? What have

the consequences been for the patient or the family (or other caregivers) since the onset of the problem? Why did the problem warrant a trip to the emergency room?
- An elicitation of other psychiatric signs and symptoms antecedent to or accompanying the main complaint. The three psychiatric conditions that account for the majority of morbidity in older patients are delirium, dementia, and depression. All three disorders can coexist in the same patient, and all three disorders may be caused or exacerbated by medical illnesses and pharmacologic agents.
- Delirium, which is also called "an acute confusional state," can be recognized by a sudden change in mental status characterized by disorientation to time and place, difficulty focusing and maintaining attention, easy distractibility, and lethargy or hyperalertness. Other signs are a fluctuation in the level of the patient's consciousness so that disorientation is more evident at one time of the day than another; insomnia; extreme difficulty with recent memory; depression; and paranoid thoughts.
- Dementia, or chronic confusion, is usually characterized by a memory loss that has been slowly progressive for several years. Intellectual deterioration (manifested by an inability to balance a checkbook, play cards, read a map, or deal with household problems) and personality changes (withdrawal, irritability, apathy, belligerence, or aggression) are also common. Since dementia predisposes individuals to delirium, disentangling the two conditions clinically in a particular case can be difficult. Without a clear history of dementia, it is best to diagnose only delirium in a confused older person when the clinician suspects the two conditions of coexisting. Only when the delirium has cleared can a proper assessment of basic intellectual abilities be carried out.
- Depression may present in the emergency department as severe agitation, profound apathy and withdrawal, or suicidal thoughts, feelings, or attempts. A substantial number of patients brought to the emergency room with depression have suffered previous episodes of affective disorders earlier in their lives, so questions

about past personal history of psychiatric disorders are critical for clues to diagnosis. Low mood, lack of energy, joylessness, fatigue, poor appetite, trouble sleeping, weight loss, difficulty with memory and concentration, crying spells, and, occasionally, delusions of poverty or of somatic functioning (perineal pain, a delusion that one's bowels are clogged, a sensation that one's brain has disappeared, etc.) constitute a picture of what psychiatrists call a "major depressive disorder." Depressive symptoms are common in delirium and dementia. However, it is almost axiomatic that the more a patient complains of memory loss, the more likely he or she is to be depressed, not delirious or demented. In patients with dementia, it is family members or other care providers who notice (and complain about) the patient's memory loss.

- An inventory of past and present medical conditions. This is crucial for the simple reason that so many medical disorders may cause delirium, worsen dementia, or trigger depression.[1] Medical disorders prominent in the genesis of delirium in the elderly include cardiac failure, pulmonary and genitourinary infections, chronic respiratory disease, dehydration, and electrolyte disturbance. Medical disorders can cause the dementia syndrome also. Alzheimer's disease and multi-infarct dementia (or a combination of the two) are the two disorders responsible for most cases of dementia in the aged; however, medical conditions such as hypothyroidism, normal pressure hydrocephalus, diabetes, brain tumors, syphilis, cyanocobalamin (B_{12}) deficiency, and — more recently — the acquired immune deficiency syndrome (AIDS)[2] can be identified in some patients. Even more important than identification of possible arrestable or reversible causes of dementia is the identification of medical conditions, often unrecognized, that cause "excess disability" — disability in excess of what the underlying dementing process causes. Hearing and visual problems, cardiac conditions, and infections are all responsible for excess disability.[3]

It is apparent, from the literature in the field, that virtually any medical condition, particularly if it is chronic or disabling, can be associated with some degree of depression. Various cancers, endocrine abnormalities (especially hypothyroidism and diabetes), and congestive heart failure are among the more prominent.[4]

- A survey of pharmacologic agents that the patient is currently using, including over-the-counter (OTC) drugs. Pharmacologic agents, like medical disorders, can be responsible for the entire gamut of psychiatric disorders in the aged. Delirium can be precipitated by any drug with a strong anticholinergic effect, which includes tricyclic antidepressants, antipsychotics, and anti-Parkinson agents; by benzodiazepines; by cardiac medications (most prominently digoxin and prop-

ranolol); and any analgesics, antihypertensives, and corticosteroids. Dementia-like syndromes can be seen with benzodiazepines, antihypertensives, bromides, barbiturates, and corticosteroids. Depression is a well-known complication of reserpine and corticosteroid preparations, but digoxin, antihypertensives, opioid analgesics, stimulants, and benzodiazepines have also been responsible for individual cases of depression. In all three of the major psychiatric disorders in the aged, also, alcohol as a cause or a contributor to a particular clinical syndrome should never be overlooked.

- A mental status examination. The more subjective part of this examination rests on a clinician's impressions of the patient: level of alertness, ability to maintain attention, appearance and behavior, attitude toward the examiner, speech pattern, and form and content of thought. The more objective part of the exam, based on the patient's answers to specific questions, is still inadequately carried out in most emergency departments. Questions about gross orientation — the most common mental status questions that emergency physicians ask about — have a high degree of specificity for the presence of cognitive impairment but possess only a low degree of sensitivity. This means that intellectual impairment is often undetected in older patients brought to emergency departments.[5]

At the very least, all patients should be tested on three items that comprise the Composite Decision Rule (CDR). First, the patient should be asked about the date: the day, the month, the year. Second, the patient should be asked to memorize three unrelated words — "honesty," "brown," and "tulip" are common examples. The patient is then asked to repeat the words immediately upon hearing them and again after 5 minutes. Third, the patient should be asked to count backwards from 100 by sevens. This is known as the Serial Sevens test. The first five digits are counted. It is preferable to lead up to this question by asking the patient first to count backwards from 10 by ones. If successful, ask the patient to count backwards from 20 by threes. If that task has failed, there is no reason to go on to the Serial Sevens question. The patient who does not want to do numbers at all should be asked to spell "world" forward, then backwards. The ability to spell "world" backward is considered comparable to performing the Serial Sevens test successfully.

The first question in the Composite Decision Rule is directed toward orientation. As an item to detect cognitive impairment it possesses low sensitivity and high specificity, which means that a substantial number of cognitively impaired individuals will answer the question correctly, though few unimpaired individuals will miss it. The second and third questions possess high sensitivity but low specificity, which means that few cognitively impaired patients will get them right but that a proportion of normal people will also miss them. Combining these items, however, makes for a screening instrument with a very acceptable sensitivity and specificity for the detection of cognitive impairment in the elderly.

The only other instrument that can be recommended for an emergency screening on a routine basis is the Short Portable Mental Status Questionnaire (SPMSQ).[6] This is primarily a memory-orientation test. The questions can be memorized easily by clinicians working in the emergency room, and the scoring is standardized. The usefulness and sensitivity of the test can be increased by asking the patient to recall three words 5 minutes after presentation, but this question should not be counted as one of the items in the scoring of the SPMSQ.

The ten questions in the SPMSQ are:

1. What is the date today? _____
    Month   Day   Year
2. What day of the week is it? _____
3. What is the name of this place? _____
4. What is your telephone number? _____
4A. What is your street address? _____
    (Ask only if patient does not have a telephone)
5. How old are you? _____
6. When were you born? _____
7. Who is the President of the U.S. now? _____
8. Who was President just before him? _____
9. What was your mother's maiden name? _____
10. Subtract 3 from 20 and keep subtracting 3 from each new number, all the way down.*

The scoring is done in the following manner:

0–2 Errors   Intact intellectual functioning
3–4 Errors   Mild intellectual impairment
5–7 Errors   Moderate intellectual impairment
8–10 Errors Severe intellectual impairment

Allow one more error if the patient has had only a grade school education.

Allow one less error if the patient has had education beyond high school.

Allow one more error for black patients, using identical educational criteria.*

More comprehensive mental status screening examinations include the Cognitive Capacity Screening Examination (CCSE) and the Mini-Mental State Examination (MMSE).[7,8] These instruments, which contain more items and therefore test a wider range of cognitive functions than the Composite Decision Rule or the SPMSQ, take longer to administer and usually require a written form while interviewing the patient. For these reasons they cannot be recommended for routine screening in the emergency department.

Assume that every patient brought to the emergency room has an undetected medical condition that may be responsible for the psychiatric presentation.

Studies in the community and in the clinic uniformly document a high rate of previously undetected medical problems among older patients.[9-15] There is no reason to think that the rate is any lower among patients brought to an emergency room. Because of the close relationship between medical illnesses and psychiatric symptoms, a complete medical review, a physical examination, and routine laboratory studies should be carried out on all elderly patients seen in the emergency room. Common medical conditions that cause delirium, dementia, or depression were mentioned on page 108.

Assume that all older patients brought to an emergency department have been prescribed — or are taking on their own — medications or drugs that might explain their psychiatric symptoms.

Pharmacologic agents, alone or in combination, are among the commonest causes of delirious states. They can also aggravate dementia and cause depression. Levodopa, digoxin, and corticosteroids are all triple-threat players in the genesis of these psychiatric disorders, as is alcohol. Common nonspecific presentations that indicate chronic alcohol abuse include deteriorating self-care, impaired cognitive function, incontinence, falls, and hip fractures. Overmedication with antipsychotic or benzodiazepines may result in sedation and apathy that can mimic (or worsen) dementia. OTC medications such as Sominex, Sleep-Eze, and Compoz contain atropine-like agents that can be responsible for delirium, while Nervine contains bromide, which can cause delirium or dementia. With prolonged use, amphetamines and methylphenidate can cause paranoid or schizophrenic-like syndromes and, if withdrawn, can be responsible for severe depression and suicidal thoughts.

Be cognizant of safety issues.

The majority of older patients evaluated in an emergency department will not be violent. But a few will. Patients with delirium and dementia represent the bulk of emergency room admissions for assaultiveness, but older patients with paranoid schizophrenia may also be brought, or sent, for evaluation. Such patients can be dangerous.

Control of behavior takes precedence over everything else in patients who are agitated and assaultive when they arrive in the emergency department. The patient should be taken to a secure, private room and approached by the physician in a confident, direct, nonthreatening manner. The patient should not be crowded. If the patient does not calm down and violence seems possible, a show of force by at least five people — one for each limb and one to administer medication or to apply restraints — is necessary.

Leather restraints are preferable to cloth restraints, which may impede circulation and cause neurological problems if tied improperly. If a chemical restraint is necessary, droperidol (Inapsine) can be administered intramuscularly (IM) at a dose of 2.5 mg (1 ml) and be repeated within 20 minutes. Alternatively, haloperidol, 2 to 5 mg IM, can be given if droperidol, which is quicker acting, is not available.[16]

During these procedures, the physician should try to explain to the patient what is being done, why, and what the results will be in an attempt to make the experience less terrifying. In the majority of instances, excluding only a few patients with acute alcoholic intoxication, further psychiatric evaluation in the hospital will be necessary for patients who are agitated enough to require the procedures just described. Civil commitment procedures — a "doctor's hold" — will also have to be initiated in the majority of these cases.

Document what you find and what you do.

The initial presentation of the patient — what the leading complaint was and how the patient looked and behaved in the emergency department — is a critical part of the diagnostic process, and the initial findings must be recorded. Careful documentation is also imperative when treatment is administered in the emergency room, particularly when it must be done either against the patient's wishes or carried out because the patient is judged incompetent to make his or her own decisions. Notes pertaining to the patient's understanding, judgment, and ability to give consent are mandatory, as are remarks relevant to the patient's medical and psychiatric status. Any procedures carried out should be documented, as should the rationale that prompted them.

COMMON PRESENTATIONS

Psychiatrically, the majority of older patients who are brought to an emergency room fall into one of four categories:

- Those with a sudden change of mental status manifested by confusion, disorientation, paranoid thoughts, incoherence, and unusual or atypical behavior. This picture spells delirium, often superimposed on a dementing process. Undetected medical illness or use of pharmacologic agents should be prime etiologic suspects in this group.
- Those with a history of a gradual deterioration of memory and intellectual capacities whose behavior has become unacceptable or unmanageable. Aggressiveness, belligerence, uncooperativeness, wandering, paranoia, sundowning, and shouting are some common ex-

amples. This picture spells dementia, often exacerbated by undetected medical disorders, pharmacologic agents, or changes in the patient's environment.

- Those with somatic symptoms, particularly pain, who also admit to insomnia, low mood, sleep disturbance, fatigue, lack of energy, trouble thinking, poor memory, and suicidal thoughts. This group represents patients with depression, with and without significant medical disorders.
- Those with a variety of psychiatric symptoms or problems. Included here are chronic mental patients, usually those with paranoid schizophrenia, who have aged; chronic alcoholics; patients with grief reactions; individuals with situational problems manifested by anxiety or milder degrees of depression; patients brought to the emergency department, usually by the police, with paranoid delusions that have developed for the first time in old age; and the occasional elderly manic patient. Of this miscellaneous group, paranoid schizophrenics are probably the most poorly served in emergency departments because they are categorized immediately as "mental patients" and significant medical problems or untoward pharmacologic effects are overlooked.

In terms of the major psychiatric diagnostic categories, delirium is the condition that every physician should know backward and forward, because it represents a true medical and psychiatric emergency. The cause is often an acute medical condition that, if left unrecognized or untreated, may be fatal to the patient. Patients with dementia are brought to the emergency department either when delirium is superimposed on dementia or when agitation, aggressiveness, or assaultiveness gives concern to relatives or caregivers. The major risk of depression is suicide. Accordingly, the psychiatric emergencies to be considered in greater detail in this chapter are delirium, aggressive behavior, depression, and suicide.

Delirium

Delirium, which is also referred to as an acute confusional state, is characterized by an impairment of higher mental function in a patient who shows a clouding of consciousness. The clinical picture of delirium reflects a widespread dysfunction of brain tissue. It is frequently due to disease processes outside the central nervous system (CNS), is not associated with neuropathologic changes in such cases, and is often reversible once its causes are identified and corrected.

The hallmark of delirium is a clouding of consciousness, a condition that often fluctuates in intensity during the day or from day to day. Clouding of consciousness, a cumbersome phrase, refers to changes in the level of alertness and to disturbances of awareness. It varies from the mildest impairment of thinking, attending, perceiving, and remembering to the extreme of coma. Four states of consciousness are usually distinguished: full alertness, lethargy, semicoma, and coma. Some patients with delirium, however, will show hyperalertness though some degree of memory or impairment and disorientation will always be present. The state of a patient's consciousness can be determined by observing the intensity of stimulation needed to arouse the patient, the patient's response, and the patient's behavior after the stimulation has ceased. Estimates of the incidence of delirium in older patients differ so widely — up to 100-fold — that it is impossible to cite an accurate figure. Delirium is, however, probably the most common organic mental disorder that physicians will confront in their work with older patients.

Whatever its incidence, delirium is a serious condition in the elderly. For the first month of illness, mortality rates range from 17 to 25%. Mortality may be as high as 30% within 3 months of the initial episode.[17] Medically ill patients diagnosed as delirious during their first admission have significantly higher mortality rates than patients who are demented, depressed, or cognitively intact. Rabins and Folstein[18] found that 23% of delirious patients died during admission. Recovery from a delirious episode is inversely related to both age and to duration of the episode.

In one study, 75% of patients whose delirium had lasted less than 7 days had recovered by the time of discharge, whereas only 12% of patients whose delirium had lasted over 7 days were recovered by time of discharge. The presence of delirium in the course of a medical illness should alert the clinician to a patient who has a higher risk of dying.

Clinical Features

The onset of delirium is rapid and can progress from normality to gross disturbance in a matter of hours to days.[19] Early symptoms and signs are nonspecific and may include anxiety, depression, irritability, insomnia, or sometimes vivid nightmares. Patients may seem absent-minded and complain of difficulty in concentrating. As the condition of delirium develops, patients may lose the thread of their conversations or be unduly distracted by noises outside the room.

Disorientation to place and especially to time, as well as loss of recent memory, are constant features and vary in degree from mild to severe. Perceptual disturbances such as misinterpretations, illusions, delusions, hallucinations, and paranoid thoughts and feelings are common. Speech may be rambling or incoherent at times. Restlessness and agitation or lethargy may be present. A fluctuating course, in which the patient appears relatively normal at one time of the day and extremely confused at another, is another common feature. Insight may

vary with the fluctuating level of consciousness, and a wide range of emotional reactions — anxiety, depression, fear, irritability, or panic — can be seen, though apathy is probably the most common.

Delirium is always worse at night. The elderly patient who suddenly becomes anxious, restless, and disoriented during the night should always be suspected of having early delirium. In fact, the sudden onset of strange behavior at night (wandering, disorientation) combined with periods of memory loss and confusion, personality change, and a recent physical illness (e.g., a cold that has turned into a pneumonia) is one of the most common presentations of delirium in an emergency department. Unfortunately, these patients are often triaged to psychiatry, not medicine, because of their behavioral changes.

There are noisy and quiet forms of delirium. The noisy form, marked by restlessness, agitation, fear, anxiety, illusions, and hallucinations, is usually associated with alcohol or drug intoxication or withdrawal, but it may occur with almost any medical illness. The quiet form of delirium is more common among the elderly patients and presents as drowsiness or lethargy, poor concentration, and distractibility. The form of delirium may also alternate between the noisy and quiet varieties in any one patient.

Subacute delirious states come on more gradually and follow a more leisurely and protracted course. Often associated with medical conditions such as anoxia, uremia, hepatic failure, subdural hematoma, and hypothyroidism, they possess clinical features of both delirium and dementia and may be hard to distinguish clearly from other conditions.

Etiology

In most cases of delirium, one should look for multiple causes rather than a single cause. Conditions that predispose to the development of delirium in older patients are an unfamiliar environment, inadequate sensory input, lack of reassurance, hearing and visual defects, sleep disturbances, previous brain damage, drug addiction or a history of such, and dementia. In a number of cases, the first symptom of an undetected dementia is delirium precipitated by a seemingly trivial event. It may be, however, that even in the absence of dementia, the aging brain is particularly vulnerable to the development of delirium. The precipitating causes of delirium are listed in Table 10–1.

As the table shows, an enormous variety of physical illnesses can cause delirium. Cardiovascular conditions, infections, and drugs are responsible for the majority of delirious states in the elderly. Congestive heart failure, myocardial infarction, various arrhythmias, pneumonia, chronic respiratory disease, and urinary infections as well as major strokes or transient ischemic episodes are

Table 10–1   Causes of Delirium

Cardiovascular
  Congestive heart failure
  Myocardial infarction
  Transient ischemic episodes and major strokes
  Arrhythmias
    Atrial fibrillation
    Heart block
  Pulmonary embolism
  Hypertensive crises
  Aortic stenosis
  Subdural hematoma
  Temporal arteritis

Fluid, Electrolyte, and Metabolic Disturbances
  Dehydration
  Hypoglycemia and hyperglycemia
  Kidney disease (in women)
  Liver disease
  Chronic diarrhea

Drugs
  Digitalis
  Sedatives (i.e., benzodiazepines)
  Antidepressants
  Steroids
  Alcohol
  Barbiturates
  Anticonvulsants
  Neuroleptics
  Antihistamines
  Diuretics
  Anti-Parkinson agents
    (propranolol, methyldopa, guanethidine, clonidine)
  Antihypertensive agents
    (propranolol, methyldopa, guanethidine, clonidine, hydralazine)

Infections
  Pneumonia
  Urinary tract infections, especially pyelonephritis
  Pelvic sepsis (secondary to diverticulitis)
  Cellulitis
  Cholangitis, cholecystitis
  Neurosyphilis
  Tuberculosis
  Cerebral abscess

Endocrinopathies, Underactivity, or Overactivity
  Thyroid
  Beta cells of pancreas
  Parathyroid glands
  Adrenal glands
  Hypopituitarism

Other
  Neoplasm, primary and metastatic, particularly from lung, breast, or bowel
  Respiratory insufficiency (e.g., COPD,* asthma)
  Fractures (fat embolism)
  Surgery (e.g., black patch delirium, complications of anesthesia)
  Hypothermia
  Severe pain (e.g., herpes zoster, glaucoma)
  Epilepsy
  Vitamin deficiency: thiamine, nicotinic acid, folic acid, B_{12}
  Functional psychiatric conditions: depression, mania, and paranoid states

*COPD = chronic obstructive pulmonary disease.

among the many causes. Digitalis, steroids, levodopa, antihypertensive agents, and oral antidiabetic agents as well as the tricyclics and benzodiazepines may all produce delirious states. Also, dehydration and electrolyte disturbances, hypothermia, carcinomatosis, and severe pain caused by herpes zoster, glaucoma, a toothache, or fecal impaction may cause confusional states, particularly if dementia is already present.

Delirium tremens, perhaps the commonest form of delirium in younger individuals, is not nearly as common among the elderly. But there are, of course, exceptions. Patients taking benzodiazepines often show a withdrawal syndrome when their medication is discontinued abruptly.[20] Insomnia, agitation, tremulousness, hypotension, hyperthermia, hallucinations, disorientation, and even seizures may be seen. In most cases, withdrawal occurs after a patient has been taking one of the benzodiazepines for a substantial period of time: months to years. It is becoming increasingly apparent, however, that withdrawal symptoms can occur with the use of ordinary doses for prolonged periods; for example, some patients experienced withdrawal symptoms after the dis-

continuation of alprazolam (Xanax), in some cases on as low a dose as 1.5 mg a day for as short a period of time as 8 weeks.[21] When withdrawal symptoms occur, the offending drug should be readministered and then tapered much more slowly.

Evaluation

The evaluation of delirium occupies a central place in acute geriatric medicine. Its importance can hardly be overemphasized since delirium is a more common early symptom of physical illness in older patients than fever, pain, or tachycardia.[22] If unrecognized or untreated, many of the diseases causing the delirium may lead to permanent cognitive impairment in normal older persons, hasten intellectual decline in those with dementia, or cause death.

Therefore, underlying physical causes should always be searched for. Whenever an older patient develops psychiatric symptoms in a short period of time — hours to days — delirium is the prime diagnostic consideration. An older person with serious physical problems who is taking several medications is at risk to develop delirium. It is more fruitful to look for several contributing causes of delirium rather than just one cause. Minor degrees of renal impairment and/or anemia often contribute to, though they may not cause, delirium.

Careful physical and neurologic examination is, of course, mandatory as is a mental status examination. Physically, the patient is almost always ill, seriously so in many acute delirious states. Asterixis and multifocal myoclonus are two neurologic signs that strongly suggest delirium, but they are often absent in older patients. Abnormalities on the mental status examination that should alert the clinician to the presence of delirium include lethargy or unusual hyperalertness, diminished awareness, distractibility, disorientation, an inability to remember recent events, and a fluctuating clinical picture, in which the patient is almost normal at certain times and quite confused at others. On the SPMSQ, the patient may show an inability to subtract serial threes from 20, to remember the date or the day of the week, or to recall three words after a distraction. Necessary laboratory examinations include a complete blood count (CBC) and erythrocyte sedimentation rate, urinalysis and culture, chest x-ray, arterial blood gases, an electrocardiogram (ECG), a chemistry panel, a qualitative Venereal Disease Research Laboratory (VDRL) test, thyroid-stimulating hormone (TSH) and free T_4, cyanocobalamin and folic acid levels, and a test for occult blood in the stool. Drug screening, an electroencephalogram (EEG), and a lumbar puncture may be necessary in selected cases. CT scan and MRI scanning may be used to evaluate the possibility of a stroke or other lesion.[23] If abnormalities are detected on the physical examination or through laboratory or ancillary investigations, the patient should be admitted to a medical ward for observation and treatment. If no medical abnormalities are detected, the older patient presenting with an abrupt change of mental status should be admitted to the psychiatric ward for further observation and evaluation. Beware, however, of early manifestations of meningoencephalitis, which has confusion as a symptom in greater than 90% of cases.[24] These patients require urgent treatment.

Differential Diagnosis

The most important disorder from which delirium needs to be distinguished is dementia. The alteration in level of consciousness is the main distinguishing feature. Delirium is marked by a change in the *level* of consciousness whereas dementia is characterized by a change in the *content* of consciousness. Fluctuations in level of awareness and alertness, insomnia, illusions, visual hallucinations, and vivid subjective experiences always favor the diagnosis of delirium. The onset and length of illness are also distinguishing points between the two conditions. If signs and symptoms have developed rather suddenly within hours or days, the diagnosis has to be delirium: dementia invariably has a longer history. When delirium is superimposed on a previously undiagnosed dementia, it may be hard to tell the two conditions apart on clinical grounds alone, but careful questioning will usually elicit a story of increasing forgetfulness, minor episodes of disorientation, or personality changes that point toward an underlying dementia.

Both manic and depressive episodes can initially present as delirium. After a few days, however, the delirious features usually subside and the more typical picture of mania or depression becomes apparent. A past history of mania or depression should raise the possibility of these psychiatric diagnoses. To complicate matters further, serious medical illnesses can precipitate mania (as well as depression) in predisposed patients.

Clinical Features

Tricyclic antidepressants may cause not only an acute delirium episode with peripheral autonomic signs but also a more subtle subacute delirium marked by various degrees of disorientation, forgetfulness, a protracted course, and even intermittent episodes of urinary or bowel incontinence. Acute confusional episodes should not be too quickly attributed to transient ischemic episodes if the patient does not have neurologic symptoms and signs, though the occurrence of confusion without paresis following infarction in the area supplied by the right middle cerebral artery is not uncommon.[25] Mild episodes of acute confusion *may* occur in the course of senile dementia but other causes of delirium should be conscientiously sought before dementia is accepted as the explanation. If a delirious state persists after a stroke, an EEG should be requested in order to rule out an epileptic confusional state caused by underlying brain damage.

Course and Prognosis

Once the responsible medical conditions are identified and corrected, delirium usually subsides within several weeks. Great variation in the clinical course can be seen, however. Some patients recover very quickly while others take a protracted, fluctuating course, especially after a stroke, that may last weeks to months and end in recovery or leave the patient with residual brain damage. Delirium due to drugs may last weeks to years, and the delirium that comes on as a symptom of drug withdrawal may appear within a week after the drug (e.g., benzodiazepines) is stopped. When delirium is superimposed on a dementia, the dementia often becomes permanently worse. Following recovery from a delirium, patients may pass through a transitional period lasting a week or two in which they show abnormalities of thought (e.g., paranoid thoughts), of mood (e.g., depression or anxiety), of behavior (e.g., restlessness or lethargy), or of memory (e.g., amnesia) without clouding of consciousness.

Management

Emergency physicians have two responsibilities when managing the delirious patient. One is to make the diagnosis and try to identify the etiology, and the other is to ensure the safety of the patient and others. The diagnostic process was discussed above.

It is best to avoid restraints and medication with the delirious patient if possible, but some patients who are thrashing about and who are in danger of hurting themselves (or others) will obviously require restraints, medications, or both. For the patient who is very combative and highly confused, restraints should be applied first and then medication administered. The restraints can then be removed, cautiously, as the medication takes effect. Sedatives should be used, also, when the patient is excessively restless, agitated, fearful, or in danger of exhaustion. The benzodiazepines, especially chlordiazepoxide and diazepam, are often the drugs of choice in the treatment of delirium in younger and middle-aged patients, but they should *not* be the drugs of choice in the treatment of older patients because of their long elimination half-lives, their subsequent tendency to accumulate in the body, and their propensity to increase the patient's confusion. Haloperidol is the drug of choice instead and can be given by mouth (0.5 to 5 mg every 1 to 2 hours until restlessness subsides) or by IM injection (2 mg repeated every hour as needed). Haloperidol produces sedation without excessive drowsiness and has fewer hypotensive and anticholinergic effects than phenothiazines such as chlorpromazine or thioridazine. The most common side effects are a drug-induced Parkinson's syndrome or a subjective feeling of restlessness called akathisia.

Aggressive or Assaultive Behavior

Aggressive or assaultive acts among the elderly are committed usually by individuals with dementia, some of whom are suffering from a superimposed delirium, most of whom are not.[26] Since most demented patients in the United States live at home or with relatives (only 5% of individuals over the age of 65 live in nursing homes), most complaints about aggressiveness come from family members, though complaints from nursing home staff are also common. Aggressiveness, defined as either a threat of violence or an actual act of physical violence without a weapon, can assume a variety of forms. Hitting, pushing, scratching, and biting are the most frequent. Aggressiveness often occurs in the context in which the demented individual is asked or forced to do something he/she is not inclined to do at the moment, such as bathing, eating,

returning after wandering away, or going back to bed. In many instances, the troublesome behavior has become repetitive (and wearing to caregivers) by the time the family or the nursing home calls or brings the individual in to the emergency room.

If either a family member or a nursing home staff member calls the emergency department about an elderly individual who is being aggressive or assaultive at the moment, the police, who can authorize ambulance service, should be notified. If the patient is still aggressive on arrival, he or she should be taken into a secure, quiet room and managed in the way described earlier in the chapter. The physician or triage nurse should then seek to understand the situation as comprehensively as possible by taking a history in a calm, unhurried manner from the patient and anyone who knows the patient and the situation. Phone calls to relatives and nursing home staff should be made in order to elicit all relevant information. Special attention should be paid to the parts of the medical and psychiatric examination that were mentioned in the introduction to this chapter: medical status, medication history, psychiatric history, psychiatric symptoms, recent upheavals, and the mental status examination. The point of this effort is to make a diagnosis, which should guide treatment.

Details of the context in which the aggressive behavior occurred should be elicited carefully since they will allow the clinician to decide how seriously to take the aggressive act. An assaultive act that is premeditated, based on a self-perceived threat to the patient and involving the use of a weapon, is a quite different act than a reflexive striking out by a confused and disoriented nursing home resident. When and where the assaultive act occurs, what the provocation was, what was said by the patient, what the nature of the violent act was, who was hurt, and any other observations surrounding the aggressive behavior should be determined if possible. The observation that one person hit another with his cane does not constitute a complete history. One always needs to learn about the circumstances.

A complete physical and neurologic examination should be carried out since so many medical conditions may cause the acute or chronic confusional states that may lie behind aggressive behavior. Silent myocardial infarctions, strokes, infections, and drug intoxication should always be kept in mind in acute conditions.

The decision to seek psychiatric consultation or to recommend hospitalization depends on the circumstances. As a rule, physicians should not hesitate to seek psychiatric consultation (if it is available) if they are uncertain about their ability to evaluate the patient's condition, particularly the psychiatric aspects of it. In general, however, there are several reasons why all patients who are brought to the emergency department because of aggressive or assaultive behavior should be considered seriously for admission to the hospital. First, many individuals who are demented and living at home or in a nursing home have not yet been evaluated adequately. Second, caregivers are usually desperate for help by the time they send an individual to the emergency room and may need a respite from care themselves. Third, a careful evaluation of the problem behavior as well as attempts to manage the problem — through either social measure or psychopharmacologic agents — can often be done more effectively on a psychiatric ward than in a private home or in a nursing home, where access to psychiatric expertise is often unavailable. Fourth, most patients with dementia have more than one behavioral problem. These may need to be observed and evaluated also. Fifth, a stay in the hospital offers the opportunity to evaluate the suitability of the patient's present living situation.

Older patients who actually commit a violent act — one characterized by a threat to use, or actual use of, a weapon — constitute an entirely different group than demented or delirious aggressive patients. They are much more likely to have a diagnosis of late-onset schizophrenia, a condition coming on in late middle age or after that is associated with paranoid delusions with or without hallucinations. Almost none of this group live in nursing homes, and they do not show significant cognitive impairment. Most importantly, their threats pose a significant danger to other people. They are paranoid, and their violence is aimed at their alleged persecutors. Admission to a psychiatric unit is mandatory for such patients.

Paranoid symptoms are a common feature of several psychiatric disorders in old age. They are most common, of course, in association with dementia. Patients with a dementing illness usually believe someone is stealing their jewelry, money, or clothes, when, in fact, they have hidden or misplaced those articles themselves. Paranoid symptoms are a common feature of delirium, and they may also occur in mania and severe cases of depression. However, it is only when those symptoms constitute the leading feature of the psychiatric disorder — as they do in late-onset schizophrenia — and are associated with violence that the most serious concern of the clinician is necessary.

Depression

Depressive symptoms are common in the elderly. More then 10% of older people experience significant symptoms of depression at any given time.[27] Depressive symptoms exist on various spectra, ranging from mild to severe, few to many, and mildly bothersome to totally incapacitating.[28] Because of the wide range of symptoms and severity, estimates range from 10% to over 40%.[29]

The current classification of depressive disorders is more sophisticated than the old reactive versus endogenous or neurotic versus psychotic categories.[30]

In the elderly, the four most common types of depression are:

- Major affective disorders
- Dysthymic disorders
- Organic affective disorders
- Adjustment disorders with depression

A fifth category should also be added. This category would be composed of older patients whose depressive symptoms are not numerous, intense, and incapacitating enough to qualify them for a major affective disorder but also whose symptoms lasted so long — 2 years — that they would qualify for the diagnosis of a dysthymic disorder. These individuals should simply be referred to as patients with depressive symptoms.

Of the various kinds of depression, the most important for the emergency physician to recognize is the depressive phase of a major affective disorder. The criteria for this diagnosis are quite explicit. They include:

1. A dysthymic (or depressed) mood *or* loss of interest or pleasure in all or almost all activities and pastimes.
2. At least four of the following symptoms, which must be present virtually every day for at least 2 weeks:
   - Insomnia or hypersomnia
   - Poor appetite or significant weight loss *or* increased appetite and significant weight gain
   - Psychomotor agitation or retardation
   - Loss of pleasure in usual activities or decrease in sexual desire
   - Loss of energy, fatigue
   - Feelings of worthlessness, self-reproach, or excessive or inappropriate guilt
   - Difficulty thinking or concentrating (which includes indecisiveness or slowed thinking)
   - Recurrent thoughts of death, suicidal ideation, wishes to be dead, or a suicide attempt

Major affective disorders themselves are of two varieties: the more common is called "major depression," the less common is referred to as a "bipolar disorder." There is only one feature that distinguishes them: a person who has a history of a manic episode at any time in his or her life will by convention fall into the bipolar category.

An individual is said to be suffering from an organic affective syndrome if there is a disturbance in mood — occasionally mania but in most cases depression — and, in addition, at least two of the symptoms listed above as criteria for a major depression. There must also be evidence from the history, physical examination, or laboratory tests that a specific organic factor, either a medical disorder or a pharmacologic agent, is etiologically related to the disturbance.

Dysthymic disorder refers to a state of chronic depression, present most of the time during a 2-year period, that is marked by at least three of the depressive symptoms listed under 1 and 2 (above). The symptoms of this disorder are not, however, of sufficient number or intensity to meet the criteria for a major depressive episode. The essential feature of an adjustment disorder with depression is the onset of depressive symptoms within 3 months of an identifiable psychologic stressor.

Causes

Genetic factors are extremely important in the genesis of the two types of major affective disorder.[31] A history of affective disorder in at least one close family member will be present in 90% of bipolar patients and 50% of patients with major depression. Various losses occur more frequently as individuals age. These losses — financial security, health, a spouse — are often associated with depressive symptoms. Numerous physical illnesses may cause depression.[32] Any medical condition associated with systemic involvement and metabolic disturbance can have profound effects on mental functioning and affect in the elderly. The most common are fever, dehydration, reduced cardiac output, electrolyte disturbances, hypoxia, and hyponatremia. Cancer, particularly of the pancreas, lung, and bowel, is often associated with depression, as are endocrine disorders, particularly hypothyroidism and hyperparathyroidism. Congestive heart failure, myocardial infarction, and strokes, as well as Alzheimer's and Parkinson's diseases, are also common causes. There is, in fact, no chronic disorder that cannot be associated with depressive symptoms.

Pharmacologic agents also cause depressive symptoms in a great many instances. Antihypertensives, narcotic analgesics, digitalis, corticosteroids, estrogens, and benzodiazepines are among the common offenders.

Differential Diagnosis

Depressive symptoms are common in many psychiatric and medical illnesses. The presence of depression in viral illnesses, hepatitis, and pancreatic cancer is well known, but the high rate of depressive symptoms in strokes, Parkinson's disease, and Alzheimer's disease is less well appreciated.[33-35]

In some elderly patients, it can be difficult to distinguish between Alzheimer's disease — or for that matter any dementing illness — and depression. Apathy, loss of motivation, lack of energy, social withdrawal, difficulties with memory, and psychomotor slowing are common features of both conditions. When depression alone produces this picture, the condition is called "pseudodementia."[36,37]

Two caveats are in order, however. First, it is often impossible to separate dementia and depression in some patients because depressive symptoms themselves are very common in Alzheimer's disease, especially in the early stages. Second, depression *can* cause severe cognitive impairment that can mimic severe dementia exactly. Whenever depression is part of a patient's history, whenever depressive symptoms coexist with cognitive impairment, and whenever the clinical picture is atypical for dementia (e.g., recent onset of impairment, depressive complaints), the patient should be considered to have depression that is either associated with the dementia or is, in the rare instance, the cause of dementia itself.[38] Depression associated with Alzheimer's disease responds well to antidepressant therapy.

Suicide

Individuals over 65 account for 12% of the population but 25% of suicides. Each year, 5,000 to 8,000 Americans kill themselves, but the real figure may be at least twice that because of underreporting.

Suicide rates increase steadily in men after age 40. The suicide rate for white males over 85 — 50/100,000 of the population — is higher than that for any other age group. This is not true for women, who show the higher suicide rates between the ages of 50 to 54 and whose rates of suicide decline to a low of 4/100,000 in the age group over 85.[39,40]

The reasons for this marked difference between men and women are conjectural. It may be that women are better prepared to cope with the practical tasks of everyday living, which makes it easier for them to live alone once they are widowed. It may be that many women are better at forming intimate bonds with friends outside marriage and have more to fall back on once their husbands die. And it may be that men have more of their self-esteem tied up in work, status, and control, so that retirement brings a greater feeling of uselessness than it does for women.

Older people make relatively few suicide gestures. They are more successful at killing themselves than younger people. Men are more likely to kill themselves violently, with guns or by hanging, whereas women take drug overdoses, especially barbiturates.

Older people rarely kill themselves for just one reason. Suicide results when unhappy circumstances and events accumulate. Losses of various kinds are common in old age and sap a person's morale and will to live. The closer in time the losses occur, and the more unexpected they are, the greater their inimical effect can be.

Management

As in the case of delirium, the emergency room physician's first task with depression is to recognize it. All older patients should be asked about their mood and their level of interest and pleasure in usual activities and pastimes, as well as their sleeping pattern, their appetite, and whether they have gained or lost weight recently. Other prominent symptoms of depression are a sense of hopelessness or despair about the future, crying spells, an inability to make decisions, difficulty in concentrating, regret or guilt about past events, a feeling that one's mind and body are slowed down, and thoughts of suicide. Somatic symptoms of all kinds are very common in depression and are frequently the presenting complaints of depressed patients.[41]

Although suicidal risk is increased in virtually all psychiatric patients, those with depression and alcoholism run the highest lifetime risk of committing suicide: 15%.[42] If either of those conditions is identified, the emergency physician's second task is to assess the suicidal potential of the patient. An awareness of risk factors is of help. These are listed in Table 10–2.

While most depressions that result in suicide are severe, not all are, and individuals with milder depressions are also at risk. Severe insomnia, even in the absence of depression, increases suicidal risk. Homosexuals, especially those who are aging, depressed, or alcoholics, present a higher suicidal risk than heterosexuals.

There is no evidence that questions about suicidal thoughts and feelings increase the risk of suicide. On the contrary, many patients feel relief when they are asked about their feelings. Physicians should explicitly ask about suicidal intent since they are often the last professionals to see a suicidal individual alive. About 75% of the people who kill themselves consult a physician shortly before they do so. One study revealed that 90% of elderly suicides had seen a physician within 3 months of their deaths. Within a week of suicide, 47% had visited a physician.

To evaluate a patient's state of mind about suicide, the following sequence of questions can be useful:

How does the future look to you?

Does life ever seem hopeless?

Do you ever wish it would end?

Have you thought about ending it?

Have you ever thought about how you'd do it?

How close have you come?

Do you have a gun (or drugs) at home?

Relatives should also be asked about symptoms and signs of depression in the patient and expressions of hopelessness or suicidal intent. The more specific the patient's plan for suicide, the greater the risk of its actually occurring.[43] Unfortunately, though, many older suicidal patients do not talk about their intentions. Indirect clues may be helpful in assessing suicidal intent in such cases. An attitude of hopeless resignation, absence of any plans for the future, a wish to rejoin a recently deceased spouse, euphoria following a depression, bad dreams (e.g., of falling into a void), self-deprecating remarks ("People would be better off if I weren't around."), and behavioral clues — giving away one's pos-

Table 10–2   Risk Factors for Suicide[42-45]

- Age over 55
- Male
- Presence of a painful or disabling physical illness, especially in a man who was robust and energetic
- Lives alone
- History of prior suicide attempts
- Family history of suicide
- History of drug or alcohol abuse
- Depression, especially associated with agitation, hypochondriasis, excessive guilt or self-reproach, delusions, insomnia, and a sense of hopelessness
- Decreased income or debt; unemployment
- Bereavement
- Suicidal preoccupation and talk
- Is near the end of a depressive illness, when energy returns but low mood persists
- Well-defined plans for suicide

sessions, for instance — are all indicators of high suicide potential.[44] More direct comments, such as "I won't be here tomorrow," are also indicators.

As a general rule, any older man who is brought to the emergency department having attempted suicide should be hospitalized immediately, preferably after psychiatric consultation.[45] If the attempt is judged serious and the patient, male or female, is alcoholic, depressed, suffering from a serious medical illness, or experiencing a recent bereavement, the need for hospitalization is particularly urgent. A person who sincerely wants to take his life should not be considered adequately protected unless he or she is hospitalized. If the patient refuses hospitalization and the suicide risk is judged to be great, involuntary admission will be necessary. Once admission is arranged, the physician should see to it that suicidal precautions for the patient have been written in the patient's chart and that the rationale for admission has been documented there also.

In some cases, the physician may be uncertain about the risk of suicidal potential even after evaluation of the patient. Psychiatric consultation is encouraged, but if this is not immediately available and the physician decides to send the patient home, he or she should see to it that the patient will not be alone, that all pills and firearms are removed from the house, that a return appointment is set up for the next day, and that the patient — or relatives — can contact the physician at any time. This kind of a plan is usually more practicable with younger patients, who make many more suicidal gestures and kill themselves at a much lower rate than older individuals, but it may have applicability to occasional older patients as well.

For patients who are suffering from a major depressive disorder but who are not at risk for suicide, psychiatric hospitalization should be considered when 1) their suffering is intense; 2) their ability to care for themselves at home is impaired; and/or 3) their personal support network is wearing thin: individuals with depression are often difficult to be around because of their complaints, their irritability, and their indecisiveness.

Those who do not require hospitalization — or refuse it — should be referred for outpatient treatment. Initiating treatment of major depression in an emergency room with tricyclic antidepressants is not recommended for several reasons. First, since the onset of the effect of the tricyclic antidepressant is delayed (often 2 to 3 weeks), there is no advantage of starting them in the emergency room. Second, patients need a thorough medical workup including laboratory studies and ECG before starting medication. Third, tricyclic antidepressants can be associated with adverse effects — hypotension and heart block are among the most worrisome examples — that require ongoing monitoring. Fourth, most clinicians are more comfortable prescribing some medications than others. If the patient is given one pharmacologic agent in the emergency room and the clinician prefers to prescribe another instead, no time has been saved. Treatment of depression is best given in the context of an ongoing relationship where both effects and side effects can be monitored carefully and regularly.

REFERENCES

1. Small GW and Jarvik LF: The dementia syndrome, Lancet 2:1443–1446, 1982.
2. Naria BA, Jordan BO, and Price RW: The AIDS dementia complex: I. Clinical features, Ann Neurol 19:517–524, 1986.
3. Larson EB et al: Caring for elderly patients with dementia, Arch Intern Med 146:1909–1910, 1986.
4. Ouslander JG: Physical illness and depression in the elderly, J Am Geriatr Soc 30:593–599, 1982.
5. Klein LE, et al: Diagnosing dementia: univariate and multivariate analyses of the mental status examination, J Am Geriatr Soc 33:483–488, 1985.
6. Pfeiffer E: A short portable mental status questionnaire for the assessment of organic brain deficit in elderly patients, J Am Geriatr Soc 23:433–441, 1975.
7. Jacob JX, et al: Screening for organic mental syndromes in the medically ill, Ann Intern Med 86:40–46, 1977.
8. Folstein MF, Folstein SE, and McHugh PR: "Mini-mental state": a practical method of grading the cognitive state of patients for the clinician, J Psychiatr Res 12:189–198, 1975.
9. Williamson J et al: Old people at home: their unreported needs, Lancet 1:1117–1120, 1964.
10. Wells CE: Geriatric organic psychoses, Psychiatr Ann 8:57–73, 1978.
11. Liston EH: Delirium in the aged. In Jarvik L and Small G, editors: Psychiatr Clin North Am 5:49–66, 1982.
12. Epstein LJ and Simon A: Organic brain syndrome in the elderly, Geriatrics 22:145–150, 1967.
13. Hodkinson HM: Mental impairment in the elderly, J R Coll Physicians Lond 7:305–317, 1973.
14. Simon A and Cahan RB: The acute brain syndrome in geriatric patients. In Mendel WM and Epstein LJ, editors: Acute psychotic reaction. Psychiatric Research Reports of the American Psychiatric Association 16:8–21, 1963.
15. Kovar MG: Health of the elderly and use of health services, Public Health Rep 92:9, 1977.
16. Steinhart MJ: The use of haloperidol in geriatric patients with organic mental disorder, Curr Ther Res 33:132, 1983.
17. Weddington WW: The mortality of delerium, Psychosomatics 23:1232, 1982.
18. Rabins PU and Folstein MF: Delerium and dementia, Br J Psychiatry 140:149, 1982.
19. Varsamis J: Clinical management of delirium. In Hendrie HC, editor: Psychiatr Clin North Am 1:71–80, 1978.
20. Ayd F: Benzodiazepine withdrawal phenomena — new insights, Psychiatr Ann 14:133–134, 1984.
21. Browne JL and Hauge KL: A review of alprazolam withdrawal, Drug Intell Clin Pharmacol 20:837–841, 1986.
22. Hodkinson HM: Common symptoms of disease in the elderly, Oxford, 1976, Blackwell.
23. Gamache FW: Update in cerebrovascular disease, Med Times 117:21, 1989.
24. Schwartz GR: Herpetic meningoencephalitis. In Schwartz GR et al: Emergency medicine: the essential update, Philadelphia, 1989, WB Saunders Co.
25. Mesulam MM et al: Acute confusional states with right middle cerebral artery infarctions, Neurol Neurosurg Psychiatry 39:84–89, 1976.
26. Petrie WM, Lawson EC, and Hollander MH: Violence in geriatric patients, JAMA 248:443–444, 1982.
27. Blazer D: Depression in the elderly, N Engl J Med 320:164, 1989.
28. Blazer D and Williams CD: Epidemiology of dysphoria and depressions in an elderly population, Am J Psychiatry 137:439–444, 1980.
29. Cohen D and Eisdorfer C: Depression. In Calkins F, editor: The practice of geriatrics, Philadelphia, 1986, WB Saunders Co.
30. Diagnostic and statistical manual of mental disorders, third edition, revised, Washington DC, 1987, American Psychiatric Association, pp 222–224.
31. Schlesser MA and Altshuler KZ: The genetics of affective disorder: data, theory, and clinical applications, Hosp Community Psychiatry 34:415–422, 1983.
32. Rodin G and Voshart K: Depression in the medically ill: an overview, Am J Psychiatry 143:696–705, 1986.
33. Robinson RG and Price TR: Post-stroke depressive disorders: a follow-up study of 103 patients, Stroke 13:635–641, 1982.
34. Mayeux R et al: Depression and Parkinson's disease. In Hassler RG and Christ JF, editors: Advances in neurology, vol 40, New York, 1984, Raven, pp 241–250.
35. Reifler BV et al: Dementia of the Alzheimer's type and depression, J Am Geriatr Soc 34:855–859, 1986.
36. Kiloh LG: Pseudo-dementia, Acta Psychiatr Scand 37:336–351, 1961.
37. Wells CE: Pseudodementia, Am J Psychiatry 136:895–900, 1979.
38. Reifler BV, Larson E, and Hanley R: Coexistence of cognitive impairment and depression in geriatric outpatients, Am J Psychiatry 139:623–629, 1982.
39. McIntosh JL: Suicide among the elderly: levels and trends, Am J Orthopsychiatry 55:288–293, 1985.
40. Blazer D, Bachar JR, and Manton KG: Suicide in late life: review and commentary, J Am Geriatr Soc 34:519–526, 1986.
41. Guze SB and Robins E: Suicide among primary affective disorders, Br J Psychiatry 117:437–438, 1979.
42. Miles CP: Conditions predisposing to suicide: a review, J Nervous Ment Dis 164:231–246, 1977.
43. Hawton K: Assessment of suicide risk, Br J Psychiatry 150:145–153, 1987.
44. Barraclough B: Suicide in the elderly, Br J Psychiatry (special publication 6) 87–97, 1972.
45. Fuchs R: Presentation of depression in an emergency setting. In Bassuk EL and Birk AW, editors: Emergency psychiatry, New York, 1984, Plenum, pp 219–232.

Coma and Cerebrovascular Syndromes

Mohamud Daya, M.D., F.A.C.E.P., and Gary Young, M.D., F.A.C.E.P.

Coma
Mohamud Daya

Pathophysiology

Initial management

Approach to the comatose patient

General examination

Neurologic examination

Diagnostic techniques

Differential diagnosis

Hyperosmolar hyperglycemic nonketotic coma

Head injury

Myxedema coma

Drug overdose

Hypoglycemia

Coma and altered states of consciousness are frequently encountered in elderly patients. Coma, which can be defined as a pathologic state of total unresponsiveness to all external stimuli, is a medical emergency. Coma in the elderly is of particular challenge since reduced cerebral reserves and underlying medical illnesses markedly limit the amount of additional neurologic injury that can be tolerated. A rapid and organized approach to the elderly patient with coma is thus essential to optimize recovery. In this regard, the three most important aspects of management include the following:

1. Maintenance of life by preserving respiration and circulation
2. Preservation of existing neural tissue
3. Prevention of additional injury
4. Arriving at a diagnosis and initiating definitive management

PATHOPHYSIOLOGY

Conscious behavior consists of two components, awareness and arousal. The cerebral hemispheres are responsible for awareness while the brainstem maintains arousal. A central core neuronal network in the brainstem — the reticular activating system (RAS) — is responsible for arousal. The RAS is linked to the cerebral hemispheres via the diencephalon. To produce coma, a pathologic process must either affect both cerebral hemispheres (bihemispheric) or the RAS (brainstem). Conditions producing these effects can be divided into three clinical processes (Table 11–1):

1. *Supratentorial masses* that compress or displace the brainstem downward
2. *Subtentorial lesions* that directly displace or destroy the brainstem
3. *Metabolic derangements* that cause diffuse bihemispheric brain dysfunction

Supratentorial and subtentorial processes can be grouped together as structural causes of coma, which represent one third of all cases. The remaining two thirds

119

Table 11–1   Common Causes of Coma

Supratentorial mass lesions — secondarily encroach upon deep diencephalic structures so as to compress or damage physiologic ascending RAS*

    Epidural hematoma
    Subdural hematoma
    Intracerebral hematoma
    Cerebral infarct with edema
    Brain tumor
    Brain abscess

Subtentorial lesions — directly damage the brainstem central core

    Brainstem infarct
    Brainstem tumor
    Brainstem hemorrhage
    Cerebellar hemorrhage
    Cerebellar abscess

Metabolic and diffuse cerebral disorders — widely depress or interrupt brain function owing to reduction in cerebral metabolism or blood flow

    Anoxia or ischemia
    Concussion and postictal states
    Infection (meningitis and encephalitis)
    Subarachnoid hemorrhage
    Exogenous toxins
    Endogenous toxins and deficiencies
    Major organ failure

*RAS = reticular activating system.

are due to metabolic or toxicologic causes. The pathogenesis of metabolic coma most likely involves multiple effects such as impaired energy supplies, membrane-potential changes, neurotransmitter abnormalities, and, possibly, ultrastructural changes. Separation of coma into metabolic and structural causes is useful in that structural coma usually requires computerized tomography (CT) scanning and neurosurgical consultation.

INITIAL MANAGEMENT

The emergency management of coma, which begins in the prehospital setting and is continued in the emergency department, is the same regardless of etiology. Initial intervention includes the following steps.

Ensure Oxygenation

Brain function is critically dependent on oxygen; therefore, the presence of a patent airway and adequate ventilation are paramount. Unconscious patients frequently experience tongue prolapse with resultant airway obstruction. This can be corrected with the chin-lift maneuver along with using an oral or nasopharyngeal airway. The elderly are particularly prone to tongue prolapse as a result of hypotonic facial musculature. Patients with absent gag reflexes should be intubated to reduce the risk of aspiration. With suspected trauma, the

usual principles regarding cervical spine precautions must be adhered to during airway management. Next, the adequacy of respirations must be assessed. Clinical evaluation should include measurement of arterial blood gases. One should aim for a PaO_2 of 100 mm Hg and $PaCO_2$ of 30 to 35 mm Hg. Those with shallow respirations and rates less than 8/minute will usually require ventilatory assistance.

Ensure Adequate Circulation

Cerebral blood flow (CBF) must also be maintained to ensure adequate nutrient supply. Usually, a systolic blood pressure (SBP) of 100 mm Hg is acceptable. In the elderly, preexisting hypertension and altered cerebral autoregulation may require a higher SBP to maintain CBF. Fluids should be administered cautiously to avoid precipitating pulmonary edema.

Draw Blood

All patients should have an intravenous (IV) line established and blood drawn for the following analysis: complete blood count (CBC) with differential, electrolytes, glucose, blood urea nitrogen (BUN), creatinine, Ca^{+2}, PO_4, and liver function tests. Additional tubes should be obtained in case further metabolic and/or toxicologic studies are required.

Administer Glucose

The brain is completely dependent on glucose as its energy source. Protracted hypoglycemia results in irreversible brain injury. Treatment consists of 25 g (50 mL of 50% solution) of glucose administered to all comatose patients. A Dextrostix can be a useful guide to glucose administration.

Administer Thiamine

Glucose administration in the face of malnourishment or alcoholism can precipitate Wernicke's encephalopathy. Therefore, all patients should receive 1 to 2 mg/kg thiamine IV concurrent with glucose administration.

Administer Antidote

Administer 2 mg of naloxone intravenously in all cases to reverse possible narcotic depression. This dose may be repeated as needed. Propoxyphene, codeine, and "designer" opioid drugs may require large doses of naloxone (10 to 14 mg) for reversal.[1]

APPROACH TO THE COMATOSE PATIENT

After initiating the aforementioned therapy, the clinician should embark on a search for the underlying etiology. A detailed history and physical exam with an emphasis on the neurologic system will usually allow categorization of the cause into metabolic or structural etiologies. This approach is not infallible, however, since focal neurologic deficits, which are the hallmark of structural coma, can occasionally be seen with metabolic lesions. During the early phase of evaluation, the clinician must be able to detect herniation syndromes, which result from the pressure effect of mass lesions. Early recognition and prompt neurosurgical intervention can be lifesaving in these patients.

Although obtaining a history directly from the patient is impossible, friends and relatives can relay valuable information. The physician should inquire whether the onset of coma was abrupt or gradual, and note any antecedent neurologic symptoms such as ataxia, vertigo, headache, vomiting, or fever. Current medications, as well as any history of drug and alcohol abuse, should also be recorded. Search for any history of trauma either prior to or following the onset of coma. Document the presence of any underlying hepatic, renal, cardiac, or neoplastic disease, as well as any psychiatric illnesses. The presence of any confusion or delirium preceding the coma should be recorded.

GENERAL EXAMINATION

Although the neurologic exam is vital in determining the etiology of coma, the general exam can contribute significant clues. A thorough step-by-step assessment of the following areas can be most rewarding.

Vital Signs

1. Temperature alterations, although nonspecific, can reflect a number of disease processes. Hyperpyrexia can be associated with infection, pontine hemorrhage, heat stroke, hyperthyroidism, subarachnoid hemorrhage, and poisoning with anticholinergics, amphetamines, or cocaine. Hypothermia suggests underlying hypothyroidism, hypoglycemia, cold exposure, hypothalamic injury, or intoxication with barbiturates or alcohol.

2. Respiratory patterns can sometimes be used to specify the level of dysfunction. Normal respiration implies an intact brainstem. Cheyne-Stokes respiration is typical of bihemispheric disease. Apneustic breathing (prolonged respiration followed by an expiration pause) suggests a pontine lesion while ataxic (irregular) respiration suggests medullary dysfunction. Hyperventilation is usually compensatory for underlying metabolic acidosis. Central neurogenic hyperventilation (deep, rapid breathing) resulting in respiratory alkalosis is seen with both metabolic and structural coma.

3. Cushing's triad, characterized by hypertension, bradypnea, and bradycardia, indicates raised intracranial pressure with the presence of a herniation syndrome. Hypertension alone may be a manifestation of hypertensive encephalopathy.

Skin. Useful clues are the presence of needle track marks in the intravenous narcotic addict and blisters in barbiturate or carbon monoxide poisoning. Icterus occurs in hepatic failure, and a petechial rash is characteristic of meningococcemia.

Head. Examine specifically for signs of trauma such as scalp laceration, hematoma, or depression. Raccoon eyes and Battle's sign suggest basilar skull fracture. Search for the presence of hemotympanum, cerebrospinal fluid otorrhea, and rhinorrhea.[2]

Neck. Palpate for deformity, soft tissue swelling, and nuchal rigidity. With suspected head trauma, any movement of the neck should be preceded by radiographic clearance of the cervical spine. Meningismus, when present, suggests meningitis or subarachnoid hemorrhage. Look for scars suggestive of previous thyroidectomy.

Chest. Cardiac murmurs or dysrhythmias, such as atrial fibrillation, may be complicated by cerebral embolism.

Abdomen. Ascites, caput medusae, and hepatomegaly reflect hepatic failure. Multiple masses raise the possibility of neoplastic disease.

Breath. Specific breath odors associated with alcohol, acetone (DKA), musk (hepatic failure), and uremia (renal failure) are valuable clinical clues.

NEUROLOGIC EXAMINATION

A detailed neurologic examination with specific emphasis on the following will usually allow categorization of the coma as either metabolic or structural and permit localization of the lesion.

Level of Consciousness (LOC)

This should be assessed and recorded in the form of a narrative description of the patient's response to stimuli. Alternatively, the Glasgow Coma Scale (GCS) (Table 11–2) can be used to record the level of consciousness. The LOC cannot separate metabolic from structural coma; however, rapid deterioration from the baseline strongly suggests a structural process accompanied by herniation.

Eyes

1. *Funduscopic* examination allows direct visualization of precipitating events. These include subarachnoid

Table 11–2   Glasgow Coma Scale

		Score
E — Eye Opening	Spontaneous	4
	To command	3
	To pain	2
	None	1
V — Verbal Response	Oriented	5
	Confused but appropriate	4
	Inappropriate	3
	Incomprehensible	2
	None	1
M — Motor Response	Follows command	6
	Localizes pain	5
	Withdraws (flexes)	4
	Flexor posturing	3
	Extensor posturing	2
	None	1
	$E_4 + V_5 + M_6$ =	15
	$E + V + M < 7$ =	COMA

hemorrhage (subhyaloid hemorrhages), diabetes (microaneurysm, dot-blot hemorrhages), hypertension (flame hemorrhages), and raised intracranial pressure (papilledema). Venous pulsations, when present, indicate the absence of raised intracranial pressure.

2. *Pupils* should be examined for size, shape, and reaction to light, both direct and consensual. The third nerve nucleus (CN III) is relatively resistant to metabolic disturbances, and, therefore, pupillary abnormalities suggest structural coma. An exception occurs with the ingestion of drugs that affect the autonomic nervous system. Atropine is associated with fixed dilated pupils and glutethimide with midposition, unreactive pupils. Examples of structural lesions leading to abnormalities include pinpoint and reactive pupils of pontine hemorrhage resulting from bilateral interruption of the sympathodilator fibers. A unilateral dilated pupil can occur from uncal herniation secondary to a supratentorial lesion or from a unilateral midbrain process. In the elderly, the presence of cataracts and glaucoma along with prescribed eye medications makes the interpretation of pupillary findings difficult.

3. Accurate assessment of *eye movement* is the most important step in determining the etiology of coma. Evaluation of ocular movements reflects the function of cranial nerves III, IV, VI, and VII as well as the medial longitudinal fasciculus (MLF), which links the ipsilateral VI nerve nucleus with the contralateral III nerve nucleus. The intimate association of these structures with the brainstem RAS makes it highly unlikely that a structural process exists in the face of intact oculomotor responses.

At rest, the patient should be examined for the presence of spontaneous conjugate roving eye movements. When present, these indicate an intact function-

ing brainstem. In the absence of spontaneous movement, the oculocephalic and oculovestibular reflexes are used to evaluate ocular motor function.

The oculocephalic (doll's eye) reflex is present only with coma and provides data on brainstem function. It requires movement of the head and is contraindicated with suspected neck injury. Movement of the head in one direction normally results in the eyes moving conjugately in the opposite direction. A normal oculocephalic response suggests an intact brainstem, making structural coma less likely.

The oculovestibular (caloric) reflex tests both the brainstem and the supratentorial control of conjugate eye movements. The head should be elevated 30 degrees and the ears examined to ensure that the tympanic membranes are intact. After 50 ml of cold water is injected into the ear, the patient is observed for the following responses:

a. Conjugate deviation of the eyes toward the cold ear with a fast bilateral nystagmus away from the ear. This indicates intactness of both the brainstem and cerebral hemispheres, implying a functional comatose state (pseudocoma).

b. Bilateral conjugate deviation toward the cold ear without any nystagmus. This indicates an intact brainstem and, in the presence of normal pupillary response, suggests metabolic coma.

c. No ocular response is an ominous sign reflective of severe brainstem dysfunction. The etiology can be structural or metabolic. Barbiturate and ethchlorynol intoxication are examples of reversible metabolic causes.

d. Unilateral tonic deviation toward the cold ear suggests a brainstem lesion affecting the MLF, resulting in intranuclear ophthalmoplegia.

4. The corneal reflex, which interconnects cranial nerves V and VII, is also useful in assessment of brainstem function in coma. A normal response consists of brisk bilateral lid closure when the cornea is touched with a wisp of cotton. Evaluation of the remaining cranial nerves adds little additional information of use in determining the etiology of coma.

5. Motor system evaluation includes an assessment of tone, movement, and reflexes. Lower brainstem damage can result in generalized flaccidity while generalized hypertonia frequently accompanies metabolic coma. The presence and symmetry of movement, either spontaneous or in response to stimuli, is very informative. Appropriate response signifies an intact motor system from cerebral cortex to limb. Reflex decorticate or decerebrate posturing indicate hemispheric or upper brainstem dysfunction, respectively. Focal motor deficits usually indicate structural coma but can also be seen with metabolic coma. In the elderly, the absence of focal motor deficits is a more useful finding because of the frequent presence of preexisting neurologic deficits. Tendon and plantar

reflexes are also useful in evaluating the corticospinal tract. Focal abnormalities suggest structural damage whereas symmetric brisk reflexes often accompany metabolic coma.

DIAGNOSTIC TECHNIQUES

Diagnostic testing in coma serves primarily to confirm the clinical diagnosis. With suspected metabolic coma, blood analysis should include glucose, calcium, electrolytes, liver, and renal function tests. Arterial blood gases should be obtained to exclude hypoxia, hypercarbia, and acidosis. A CBC with differential is useful in suspected sepsis or meningitis. In the elderly, however, the CBC can be normal in the face of overwhelming infection.

Toxicology screening is also an important part of the metabolic coma workup. Initially, a qualitative urine screen for alcohol, barbiturates, benzodiazepines, opioids, tricyclic antidepressants, and other sedative-hypnotics is valuable. Positive urine screens, where appropriate, may be followed by quantitative serum testing.

With suspected structural coma, a CT scan of the head should be obtained promptly. Although usually diagnostic, a normal CT scan does not always exclude structural coma. The CT scan may appear normal with early cerebral infarction, small brainstem lesions, and isodense subdural hematomas.

The lumbar puncture (LP) is useful in suspected cases of meningitis or subarachnoid hemorrhage. In the patient with suspected meningitis who has no features of structural coma, an LP should be done immediately and antibiotics started empirically. Cerebrospinal fluid analysis should include protein, glucose, cell count with differential, Gram stain, and culture. The initial workup for suspected subarachnoid hemorrhage is the CT scan. However, up to 10% of cases may have a normal CT scan necessitating an LP to establish the diagnosis. Although not as readily available, magnetic resonance imaging (MRI) is superior to CT in certain areas such as the brainstem.

DIFFERENTIAL DIAGNOSIS

Having performed a thorough neurologic and general examination, the clinician should attempt to categorize coma into metabolic, supratentorial, structural, or infratentorial structural etiologies (Figure 11–1). It is important to recognize, however, that all unresponsive patients are not necessarily in coma. Organic and psychogenic processes that produce comalike states must first be excluded.

Organic causes include the abulic state (akinetic mutism) and the locked-in syndrome. The abulic state is characterized by awakeness with very slow response to verbal commands. It is a result of bilateral frontal lobe depression leading up to huge delays in information processing. Destruction of the corticospinal and corti-

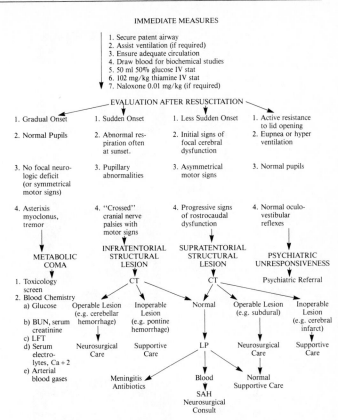

Figure 11–1 Management algorithm for comatose patients.

cobulbar tracts in the cerebral pons results in the locked-in syndrome. These patients appear awake but are paralyzed and speechless. Since vertical eye movements are preserved, the patients can communicate by looking up or down.

Catatonia and hysterical coma are examples of psychogenic unresponsiveness. These patients usually demonstrate marked resistance to eye opening with rapid closure upon release. Catatonia is also characterized by increased motor tone and sustained limb posture. The neurologic exam is usually normal, and oculovestibular testing demonstrates conjugate deviation with rapid nystagmus. An interview using amobarbital can be helpful in releasing patients from functional coma.

Having ruled out comalike states, one can proceed with coma categorization. Patients with supratentorial structural coma may present with either bilateral (uncal) or central herniation (Figure 11–2). Both are characterized by an orderly progression and accelerated loss of neurologic function in a rostrocaudal fashion. Recent head trauma, headache, or focal symptoms may antedate coma. The presence of asymmetric motor deficits is a cardinal feature. Early lateral herniation is characterized by ipsilateral pupillary constriction secondary to oculomotor nerve compression. Increasing herniation results in ipsilateral and then bilateral dilated pupils. This is followed by marked neurologic deterioration with deepening coma, abnormal respiratory patterns, and flexor and then ex-

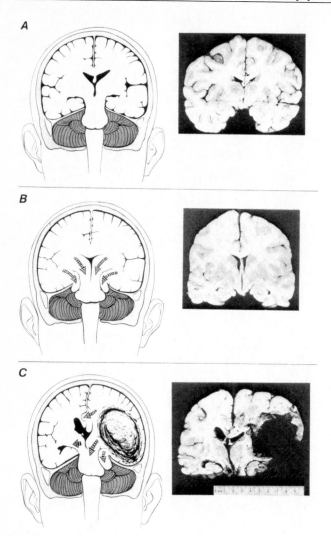

Figure 11-2 Intracranial shifts from supratentorial lesions. (From Plum F and Posner JB: The diagnosis of stupor and coma, ed 3, Philadelphia, 1980, FA Davis Co.)

tensor posturing. In contrast, central herniation begins with worsening coma as a result of diencephalic compression. The pupils are initially normal but dilate with increasing compression. The same progressive abnormalities in respiration and posture seen with lateral herniation quickly follow. Suspected supratentorial lesions require early CT scanning and neurosurgical consultation.

Infratentorial structural coma is characteristically sudden in onset and associated with pupillary response abnormalities as well as signs of brainstem dysfunction. These include miosis, dysconjugate gaze, ocular deviation, internuclear ophthalmoplegia, and cranial nerve palsies along with the absence of oculocephalic and oculovestibular reflexes. Occipital headache, vomiting, vertigo, ataxia, diplopia, and nystagmus may precede coma. Disturbances in respiratory pattern such as Cheyne-Stokes respiration and ataxic and apneustic breathing are also prominent. A CT scan should be ob-

tained early since certain infratentorial mass lesions (e.g., cerebellar hemorrhages) are amenable to neurosurgical decompression.

Metabolic coma is characterized by a gradual onset and the absence of definitive neurologic signs. Confusion and disorientation frequently precede the onset of coma. Motor abnormalities, when present, are usually symmetric. Although lateralizing findings are rare, they may occasionally be seen with hypoglycemic coma or hyperosmolar nonketotic coma. Additional features include the presence of asterixis, tremor, and myoclonus. Pupillary reaction to light is usually preserved as are the oculocephalic and oculovestibular reflexes. Exceptions to this include drug intoxications involving the opiates, anticholinergics, barbiturates, and glutethimides. A distinct feature is the absence of rostrocaudal deterioration in neurologic function. The diagnosis of metabolic coma is established conclusively by blood chemical and toxicologic analysis.

Structural coma, when associated with rapid clinical deterioration, suggests the presence of intracranial hypertension. Measures to reduce the intracranial pressure (ICP) should be instituted promptly to reduce the risk of herniation. Patients should be intubated and hyperventilated to a $Paco_2$ of 25 mm Hg. Administration of 2 g/kg of a 20% mannitol solution also helps reduce the ICP. Diuretics and steroids may be of value in certain cases. Once again a stat CT scan and urgent neurosurgical consultation should be obtained.

HEAD INJURY

Head trauma occurs frequently in the geriatric population. In one study, patients over 65 accounted for 14% of admissions to a head and spinal cord unit.[2] Whereas motor vehicle accidents are the primary cause of head injury in the young, falls account for the majority of the injuries in the elderly.[3] Additional epidemiologic differences include a 1:1 male/female ratio and the frequent presence of underlying medical illnesses. Although trauma may be the primary process underlying the coma state, the possibility of a toxic-metabolic process and secondary head trauma should not be overlooked. Cervical spine immobilization should be employed in all patients with head trauma and altered levels of consciousness.

Cerebral atrophy accompanies aging and predisposes the patient to developing an intracranial hemorrhage following trauma. The subdural hematoma is the most common kind and can present in an acute or delayed fashion. The enlarged subdural space allows for more tolerance of mass effect and hence a late presentation.[4] Classically, the chronic subdural hematoma is characterized by a head injury followed by progressive deterioration with coma as a terminal event. Recent studies suggest that chronic subdural hematomas enlarge as a result of recurrent hemorrhage and not osmotic changes as previously thought.

Following initial stabilization, the association of head trauma and an altered level of consciousness mandates emergent CT scanning along with neurosurgical consultation. Extracranial problems should also be sought and corrected. A rapid and aggressive approach can do much to improve the outcome in these patients. Unfortunately, preexisting reduced cerebral reserve allows for poor tolerance of further insult, and many are unable to return to their previous level of functioning.

HYPEROSMOLAR HYPERGLYCEMIC NONKETOTIC COMA

Hyperosmolar hyperglycemic nonketotic coma (HHNK) is a common metabolic derangement seen in elderly diabetics and characterized by severe hyperglycemia, hyperosmolality, glycosuria, dehydration, and the absence of ketoacidosis.[5]

HHNK is most common in the older population with a mean age of 60 and occurs more often in women than men. At the time of presentation, one third of the patients are known diabetics, usually controlled by diet or oral hypoglycemic agents. In two thirds of the cases, HHNK is the initial presentation of the diabetic state. HHNK has been associated with a number of precipitating factors, including infection, myocardial infarction, abdominal emergencies, recent surgeries, and prescribed medications (in particular, the thiazide diuretics).

The basic defect is a relative deficiency of insulin that results in decreased peripheral utilization of glucose and the breakdown of lipids as an alternate source of energy. Unlike diabetic ketoacidosis, it appears that sufficient insulin exists in HHNK to prevent the intrahepatic oxidation of free fatty acids to ketoacids.

The resulting hyperglycemia leads to intracellular dehydration as a result of fluid shift along the osmotic gradient. Concurrent osmotic diuresis results in significant extracellular fluid and electrolyte losses, leading to a state of extreme dehydration (intracellular and extracellular).

The clinical picture is usually that of an institutionalized patient brought to attention following a subacute decline in the level of consciousness. There may be a history of recent polyuria, polydipsia, and polyphagia. The patient is usually dehydrated with dry mucous membranes, sunken eyeballs, and decreased skin turgor. Mental status abnormalities range from mild drowsiness to coma. Neurologic signs and symptoms are prominent with 15% of the patients exhibiting focal seizure activity. Focal neurologic deficits, such as hemiparesis and hemisensory loss, are also common. As a result, a cerebrovascular accident is often misdiagnosed. Severe dehydration may present with shock and cardiovascular collapse.

The diagnosis is confirmed by documenting hyperglycemia and the absence of ketoacidosis. The latter may be performed at the bedside utilizing the nitroprusside serum test for ketones. Acetone breath and Kussmaul respirations are notably absent. Useful laboratory tests include glucose, electrolytes, BUN, creatinine, osmolality, and arterial blood gases. Typically, the glucose is greater than 800 mg/dL, and the osmolality is greater than 350 mOsm/kg. The alterations in mental status correlate directly with the serum osmolality. Extracellular dehydration results in hypernatremia and an elevated BUN. The total body sodium and potassium are usually depleted as a result of osmotic diuresis. A mild lactic acidosis is also characteristic. Precipitating factors should be searched for in all cases.

Treatment includes replacement of fluid and electrolyte losses, restoration of glucose homeostasis, and the correction of possible precipitating factors. Debate continues over the ideal replacement fluid. In general, patients with cardiovascular collapse require normal saline. Stable patients, especially those with hypernatremia greater than 150 mEq/L, should receive one-half normal saline. Potassium can be added once it is established that the patient is producing urine. Insulin is administered to all patients initially as a bolus of 0.1 unit/kg. Glucose should be administered once the blood glucose drops to 250 mg/dL to avoid precipitation of cerebral edema. Lastly, all patients should be observed for the development of arterial and venous thrombosis, which frequently accompany HHNK.

MYXEDEMA COMA

Hypothyroidism is a chronic illness with generalized body slowing secondary to decreased thyroid hormone. Myxedema coma is a rare life-threatening manifestation of hypothyroidism. It has an incidence of 0.1% and is most common in the winter months. There is a 3.5:1 female/male ratio and one half of the patients are between 60 and 70 years old. Usually the underlying hypothyroidism is known but occasionally it is undiagnosed and presents a formidable clinical challenge. Most cases are associated with a precipitating factor, usually a respiratory infection. Other intercurrent processes that may precipitate myxedema coma include congestive heart failure, anemia, cerebrovascular accident, noncompliance with replacement therapy, trauma, and drugs — especially the beta blockers. These stresses worsen the hypothyroid state, which, if uncorrected, can progress to coma. Despite early diagnosis and treatment, the mortality rate for myxedema is 40 to 50%.[6,7]

Hypothyroidism can result from primary, secondary, or tertiary causes (Table 11–3). The most common causes are autoimmune destruction (Hashimoto's disease) and surgical or radioiodide therapy for Graves' disease. Symptoms of hypothyroidism include weight gain, fatigue, cold intolerance, constipation, and hoarseness. Physical findings include facial edema, macroglossia, dry yellow skin, sinus bradycardia, and delayed reflexes. Myxedema

Table 11–3   Etiology of Hypothyroidism

Thyroid insufficiency (primary)	Pituitary or hypothalamic insufficiency (secondary or tertiary)
Idiopathic	Tumors
Autoimmune (Hashimoto's thyroiditis)	Infiltrative disease (sarcoidosis)
Radioactive iodine therapy of Graves' disease	
Surgical therapy of Graves' disease	
Congenital enzymatic defect in thyroid hormone biosynthesis	

Table 11–4   Treatment of Complicating Illness of Myxedema Coma

Intercurrent Illness
1. Search vigorously for a clinically suppressed infection while realizing that a normal temperature in myxedema coma is inappropriately high.
2. Carefully search for other intercurrent illness associated with myxedema coma.

Hypothermia
1. Avoid external heat sources.
2. Cover with blankets.

Respiratory Acidosis
1. Monitor arterial blood gases.
2. Use respiratory support system if necessary.

Hyponatremia
1. Free water restriction is usually sufficient.
2. If clinically needed, use saline with the administration of furosemide.

Hypoglycemia
1. Use glucose in parenterally administered solutions.
2. Administer hydrocortisone sodium succinate (Solu-Cortef) 300 mg/daily.

Hypotension
1. Usually responds to thyroid hormone replacement.
2. If needed, use vasopressor agents. Monitor cardiovascular system closely.

Thyroid Hormone Replacement
1. Administer L-thyroxine (T_4) 400 μg intravenously or 100 to 200 μg orally each day.
2. Administer triiodothyronine 12.5 μg by nasogastric tube every 8 hours.

coma is the most extreme presentation of hypothyroidism. The coma is related directly to a deficiency in the thyroid hormone level. In myxedema, hypoventilation with resistant hypercarbia and hypoxia is common. Hypothermia, hypotension, and bradycardia are also characteristic features. Common diagnostic test abnormalities include hyponatremia, hypochloremia, hypoglycemia, low-voltage electrocardiogram (ECG), and an enlarged heart on chest x-ray. Serum thyroxine, triiodothyronine, thyroid-stimulating hormone (TSH), and triiodothyronine resin uptake should be measured. The results, although not available emergently, are useful to support the clinical impression.

Myxedema coma is a medical emergency and must be treated rapidly. Therapy must be initiated on the basis of clinical judgment. Definitive therapy requires thyroid hormone replacement in the form of IV L-thyroxine or enteral triiodothyronine. In addition, all patients require supportive therapy along with a search for intercurrent illness (Table 11–4). Intravenous steroids should be administered to all patients to cover for possible associated adrenal unsufficiency (secondary or tertiary cases).

DRUG OVERDOSE

Depression and suicide are common, often unrecognized problems in the older population. The elderly are subject to many losses, in particular self-esteem, financial, health, and companionship. Furthermore, they have access to a large variety of prescription and nonprescription medications. Common intentional ingestions include the benzodiazepines, tricyclic antidepressants, barbiturates, cardiovascular agents, and narcotic analgesics, especially propoxyphene (Darvon). In addition, physical changes associated with aging often result in accidental ingestion of various medications. *Thus, drug overdose should be suspected in all elderly patients who present with an altered level of consciousness.*

Propoxyphene is prescribed commonly in this age group, primarily because of reduced side effects. However, its toxicity in overdoses is high, particularly in the elderly. In one series reporting propoxyphene deaths,[1] 35% of cases were over 65. There is a short delay between ingestion and the onset of serious symptoms. Respiratory depression and seizures are the primary features, followed by cardiac failure and eventually cardiac arrest. Naloxone can reverse propoxyphene toxicity and should be administered to all obtunded patients. Large doses may be required in suspected propoxyphene poisoning.

The management of suspected overdoses should include stabilization of cardiovascular function followed by methods to decrease absorption and increase elimination. Ipecac is usually contraindicated in obtunded patients. Most require gastric lavage following protection of the airway. Lavage effluent can be sent for toxicologic analysis. Following lavage, the patient should receive 1 g/kg of activated charcoal and a cathartic. Blood and urine toxicologic screens are useful in identifying the ingested toxin. Methods to increase elimination — such as multiple-dose activated charcoal, alkaline diuresis, dialysis, or hemoperfusion — should be used when indicated. Similarly, antidotes when available should be used in the appropriate setting.

HYPOGLYCEMIA

The human brain is totally dependent upon glucose as its source of energy. Hypoglycemia — a fall in glucose concentration that results in central nervous system dysfunction — is a common medical emergency. Hypoglycemia has protean manifestations with considerable individual variation, and delay in diagnosis may result in irreversible neuronal damage. Although there is poor correlation between the blood glucose level and symptom onset, adult hypoglycemia generally exists when the blood glucose falls below 50 mg/dL.[8]

The presence of hypoglycemia signifies a disturbance in glucose homeostasis normally achieved by a complex interaction between insulin and the counterregulatory hormones (epinephrine, corticosteroids, glucagon, and growth hormone). Sudden hypoglycemia usually presents with manifestations of acute hyperepinephrinemia such as diaphoresis, tachycardia, palpitations, tremor, and nervousness. Slower developing hypoglycemia is characterized by neuroglycopenic features such as headache, focal neurologic deficits, memory loss, coma, and seizures (Table 11–5).

The most common physiologic approach is to characterize the hypoglycemia as either fasting, postprandial, or exogenous. Fasting hypoglycemia usually occurs 5 to 6 hours after a meal. Causes include insulinoma, extrapancreatic tumors that produce insulin-like substances, deficiency of counterregulatory hormones, and severe hepatic disease. Postprandial hypoglycemia is manifest 2 to 4 hours after a meal and is secondary to excess insulin release. Common causes include early diabetes mellitus and alimentary tract dysfunction following gastrectomy.

Exogenous (toxic) hypoglycemia is very common; most cases involve insulin, alcohol, or oral hypoglycemic agents. Insulin coma may be precipitated by many factors — in particular, dietary changes and improper insulin dosage (either accidental, intentional, or iatrogenic). Alcohol metabolism interferes with hepatic gluconeogenesis. Thus, when combined with poor glycogen stores secondary

Table 11–5 Signs and Symptoms of Hypoglycemia

Adrenergic activation	Disturbed cortical function
Beta stimulation	Weakness
Tremulousness	Headache
Tachycardia	Blurred or double vision
Palpitations	Disturbed intellectual function
Diaphoresis	Amnesia
Faintness	Incoordination or paralysis
Anxiety	Seizures
Hunger	Coma
Gastric hypermotility	Brainstem dysfunction
Nausea	

to inadequate carbohydrate intake, this results in alcoholic hypoglycemia. Oral hypoglycemic agents (sulfonylureas) are common causes of hypoglycemia in the elderly. Glucopenic reactions to these agents are usually more profound because of the long duration of their presence and physiologic effect. Drug-drug interactions may potentiate the hypoglycemic effect of these agents and should be considered in all cases of sulfonylurea hypoglycemia.

Suspected hypoglycemia should be treated promptly with intravenous or oral glucose solutions. All patients with hypoglycemia-induced altered mental status or coma should receive 50 ml of 50% glucose by IV bolus followed by a continuous infusion of glucose until the patient is able to eat. Patients with primarily adrenergic manifestations, who have an intact swallowing mechanism, are candidates for oral glucose replacement therapy. In the prehospital setting, glucagon 1 mg intramuscular (IM)/subcutaneous (SC) may be used in the presence of adequate glycogen stores to reverse hypoglycemia. Sulfonylurea hypoglycemia can persist for days requiring prolonged therapy with intravenous glucose infusions.

Cerebrovascular Disease
Gary Young

Cerebral blood flow and metabolism

Causes of cerebral ischemia and infarction

Transient ischemic attacks

Cerebral infarction

Large cerebral artery thrombotic occlusion

Anterior cerebral ischemia

Vertebrobasilar insufficiency

Small vessel or lacunar infarcts

Cerebral embolism

Intracerebral hemorrhage

Subarachnoid hemorrhage

Computerized tomography scanning, magnetic resonance imaging, and lumbar puncture

Evaluation and management of patients with cerebrovascular syndromes

Workup and management of selected complications

Specific therapies

Prophylactic antiplatelet therapy

Prophylactic and therapeutic anticoagulant therapy

Thrombolytic therapy

Biorheologic therapy

Approximately 600,000 new strokes occur in elderly patients annually in the United States. These account for about 250,000 deaths, third only to heart disease and cancer. The morbidity of strokes among elderly survivors remains high; the Framingham stroke study found that 16% of survivors are institutionalized, 31% required assistance in self-care, and 71% had decreased vocational function.[9] Despite these alarming statistics, the incidence of new strokes has decreased by almost one half during the past 30 years, probably due to recognition and treatment of risk factors. Hypertension is the major risk factor for stroke in the elderly and the only risk factor for which treatment has been shown to decrease complications.[10] Heart disease is another important risk factor; cerebral embolism may result from atrial thrombi associated with atrial fibrillation (AF) and mural thrombi after myocardial infarction (MI). The finding of a carotid artery (CA) bruit suggests CA stenosis; this is also a sign of a patient at risk for a coronary ischemic event.[11] The finding of cholesterol emboli (Hollenhorst plaques) on funduscopic examination of the retina represents showering of emboli from an ipsilateral CA ulcerative plaque, which is the cause of approximately half of all transient ischemic attacks (TIAs).[12] Other risk factors for stroke are similar to those for atherosclerotic vascular disease in general (see Table 11–6). The most common site for atheroma formation involving the cerebral circulation is the CA bifurcation, followed by the basilar artery (BA) and vertebral artery (VA).

CEREBRAL BLOOD FLOW AND METABOLISM

The brain weighs approximately 2% of the total body weight, but it receives 15% of the cardiac output and re-

Table 11–6   Risk Factors for Cerebrovascular Disease

Hypertension
Transient ischemic attack
Asymptomatic carotid bruit
Cholesterol retinal emboli
Male sex
Age
Cigarette smoking
Hypercholesterolemia
Diabetes mellitus
Polycythemia
Hyperuricemia
Oral contraceptive pills
Cardiac disease
  Atrial fibrillation
  Mitral valve disease
  Mural thrombus
  Left-sided chamber enlargement
  Left ventricular aneurysm
  Congestive heart failure
  Large myocardial infarction
  Coronary artery disease

quires 25% of the extractable oxygen.[13] The brain contains no stores of glycogen, and it requires 70% of the circulation glucose, which is its sole metabolic substrate.[13] The direct relationship between the rate of local brain metabolism and the rate of local cerebral blood flow (CBF) is governed by a mechanism known as *autoregulation*. Autoregulation of CBF is controlled by small arterioles in the brain over a range of mean systemic BP from 50 to 150 mm Hg.[14] CBF is normally approximately 50 ml/100 g/min; the brain can survive on about half this much perfusion. But the average CBF to the area surrounding an acute cerebral infarction is less than one quarter of normal perfusion.[14]

Interventions meant to ameliorate cerebral ischemia must be introduced promptly because complete neuronal recovery probably cannot occur after more than 2 hours of cerebral arterial occlusion.[15] This is certainly true for the infarcted brain tissue itself, but in clinical terms it is particularly important for the potential salvation of the areas of brain bordering the actual infarct, known as the "ischemic penumbra."[16] Improvement in local cerebral perfusion may prevent the loss of more cerebral cells from this ischemic penumbra.

Autoregulation is usually dysfunctional during an acute cerebrovascular insult. Interventions designed to increase brain perfusion to the brain may even prove counterproductive. Because cerebral vessels supplying the ischemic region are already maximally dilated, consequently use of vasodilators to dilate all cerebral vasculature may result in an "inverse steal" syndrome.[14] In this case, any "discretionary" CBF may be shunted to areas of normal brain where cerebral blood vessels not injured by the ischemic process will be more likely to relax with vasodilator therapy. On the other hand, the involved cerebral vessels may be so damaged by the ischemic process that they cannot respond to endogenous or exogenous vasodilatory stimuli. The use of vasopressors to enhance systemic perfusion of the diseased cerebral vessels may further worsen already elevated intracranial pressure.

CAUSES OF CEREBRAL ISCHEMIA AND INFARCTION

Acute cerebral infarction usually occurs secondary to the occlusion of cerebral arteries by thrombi or emboli; angiography has revealed corresponding arterial occlusion in over 90% of patients.[17] The major causes of cerebral ischemia in the elderly are stenosis, thrombotic occlusion of carotid or cerebral arteries , and emboli from the proximal carotid artery or cardiac sources. Occlusion of cerebral arteries probably results in incomplete ischemia because of collateral blood flow.[15,16] Not all focal neurologic deficits secondary to lack of CBF are caused by cerebrovascular thromboembolism; there are many other etiologies, especially in the older patient, including tumor, vasculitis, and hypoperfusion syndromes (see Table 11–7).

Table 11-7 Less Common Causes of TIA-Stroke Syndromes

Brain tumors: primary or metastatic

Cardiac "masses": mural thrombi due to MI or AF; atrial myxoma

Valvular disease: left-sided mitral or aortic stenosis or regurgitation, infectious endocarditis, artificial prosthetic valves

Arteritis: temporal arteritis, systemic lupus erythematosus, periarteritis nodosa

Hypercoagulable state: thrombocytosis, polycythemia, anticoagulation therapy, leukemias, sickle cell anemia

Hypocoagulable state: thrombocytopenia, bleeding diatheses, coagulopathies, leukemias

Infectious: meningoencephalitis with arteritis; viral, fungal, bacterial, tuberculosis, syphilis, and mycotic aneurysm

Parasitic: malaria, schistosomiasis, trichinosis

Cerebral thrombophlebitis: postpartum, postoperative, infectious, dehydration

Metabolic: hypoglycemia, hyperglycemia

Vascular: dissecting aortic aneurysm, complications of arteriography, aneurysms, arteriovenous malformations

Trauma: carotid or vertebral arteries and brain trauma

Vasospasm: classic migraine headache with persistent deficit, subarachnoid hemorrhage

Systemic hypotension: hypovolemia, arrhythmias, shock, antihypertensive therapy

Toxicologic: cocaine, amphetamine, OTC sympathomimetics

Other important causes include inflammation of cerebral vessels due to infection (e.g., syphilis or tuberculosis), temporal arteritis, and collagen vascular diseases.[10] Because of the gratifying response of these latter etologic conditions to available therapies (i.e., antibiotics or immunosuppressive agents), exhaustive workups (e.g., cultures and serologies) and invasive tests (e.g., angiograms and septomeningeal biopsies) may be justified. Focal cerebral ischemia can also occur during hypoperfusion of brain tissue due to any cause of hypotension or shock, including overly aggressive antihypertensive therapy, especially in elderly patients with underlying focal atherosclerotic cerebrovascular disease.[10] Other causes for acute neurologic deficits also include direct trauma to the carotid or cerebral arteries, subarachnoid, intracerebral hemorrhages and mass lesions such as subdural or epidural hematoma.

The differential diagnosis of an acute CVA includes cranial and peripheral nerve disorders (e.g., Bell's palsy and nerve root compressions), demyelination disorders (e.g., multiple sclerosis), focal or generalized seizures (i.e., Todd's paralysis), classic migraine headaches (elderly patients may present with unusual forms of migraine equivalents),[19] and metabolic disorders (e.g., hypoglycemia or hyperglycemia, which are usually reversible).

TRANSIENT ISCHEMIC ATTACKS

Transient ischemic attacks (TIAs) put patients at high risk for a subsequent cerebral infarction, although only about 15% of strokes are preceded by TIAs.[20] TIAs of the anterior circulation were first described by Fisher as "prodromal fleeting attacks of paralysis, numbness, tingling, speechlessness, [and] unilateral blindness."[21] The Advisory Committee for the Classification of Cerebrovascular Disease defines TIAs as temporary and focal neurologic deficits due to presumed cerebral ischemia from which complete recovery occurs within 24 hours.[22] Most TIAs are, in fact, fleeting, usually lasting only from 2 to 3 minutes up to 10 to 15 minutes; 88% of TIAs resolve within 1 hour. Most patients with neurologic deficits lasting more than 1 hour have had a completed stroke.[23] The entity called RIND (resolving ischemic neurologic deficit) is defined as a focal neurologic finding that lasts more than 24 hours. Most often, it results from hemispheric cerebral infarction, which gradually improves within 3 weeks.[4]

The neurologic deficit due to a TIA usually corresponds to an anatomic distribution consistent with an ischemic syndrome. Ischemic syndromes can be divided into those involving the anterior cerebral circulation (i.e., the distribution of the middle cerebral arteries [MCAs] or anterior cerebral arteries [ACA]) and the posterior cerebral circulation (i.e., the distribution of the posterior cerebral artery [PCA] and vertebrobasilar [VB] artery system). The diagnosis of TIAs or infarctions in the distribution of the anterior cerebral circulation is usually straightforward (i.e., *unilateral* facial or extremity weakness or numbness, aphasia, and monocular blindness). The same cannot be said with respect to the posterior circulation (see later discussion). Characteristically, vertebrobasilar insufficiency causes *bilateral* neurologic symptoms or signs involving both cranial nerves and extremities.

Diagnosis of a TIA is usually based on the history. Data from many studies suggest that the diagnosis of TIA is either incorrect in about 30%[24] of patients or in disagreement in 35%[25] of patients.[25] Infarcts, hemorrhages, and mass lesions can all present like TIAs. In one study[26] 7 of 22 patients diagnosed with TIAs demonstrated infarcts on CT and 17 had infarcts detectable on MRI. In another study[27] 8 of 21 patients diagnosed with TIAs had positive CTs and 16 had positive MRIs. In a third study[28] 13 of 60 TIA patients had focal CT abnormalities, whereas 42 had abnormal MRIs. Amaurosis fugax, temporary partial or complete monocular blindness, is a classic symptom of an anterior circulation TIA, but in the elderly it can be mimicked by glaucoma, vitreous hemorrhage, retinal detachment, papilledema, migrainous aura, and even ectopic "floaters."[12]

Because of time delays before presentation, by the time the emergency physician examines the patient with a history consistent with a TIA, the neurologic examination is frequently normal. If a patient in the emergency department has a neurologic deficit that apparently clears or improves (i.e., a scenario consistent with the diagnosis of TIA), the patient may still have had a minor cerebral infarction. If such a patient is discharged, it is common for the patient to return within the next day or days with a more severe, fixed stroke deficit.

Therefore, when an elderly patient presents with a history consistent with TIA, this should be considered a sign of unstable cerebral ischemia. There are patients with "crescendo" TIAs, which occur many times over a few hours or days; these patients are at very high risk of cerebral infarction.[20,29] The risk of a stroke is highest in the days and weeks following a TIA. One study of 49 patients who had a stroke following a single TIA found that half of these patients had their strokes within 24 hours of the TIA; and in another study of 51 patients who had strokes preceded by multiple TIAs, the stroke occurred within 10 days of the first TIA in half of the cases.[30]

The long-term prognosis of a patient with a TIA follows the "rule of threes": in the absence of therapeutic intervention, one third of patients with TIAs go on to have CVAs, one fourth of these within 1 month; one third of patients will have at least one more TIA; and the last one third will have no further ischemic events.[20,31] It is not possible to predict which patients will go on to have a cerebral infarction without first delineating the cause and the anatomy of the TIA. Most, if not all, elderly patients presenting with a history of a TIA should be admitted for observation for a possible stroke and for an expeditious workup to rule out remediable etiologies and to start treating risk factors (see Tables 11–6 and 11–7).

CEREBRAL INFARCTION (Table 11–13)

The major neuropathologic mechanisms causing cerebral ischemia or infarction are thrombosis, embolism, and hemorrhage. Clinically, one cannot reliably predict whether embolic or thrombotic mechanisms underlie a given patient's neurologic syndrome or whether the stroke has been the result of or is complicated by hemorrhage. Clinically, small cerebral hemorrhages in strategic locations may mimic TIAs or nonhemorrhagic infarction. The major types of cerebral ischemic stroke syndromes include the following:

1. Large cerebral artery thrombotic occlusion
2. Small vessel (lacunar) infarcts
3. Carotid artery emboli
4. Cardiac emboli
5. Intracerebral hemorrhage (ICH)
6. Subarachnoid hemorrhage (SAH).

Although figures vary from study to study, it is fairly consistent among reported series of patients that each of the stroke syndromes listed above comprises from 10 to 30% of all cases. Cerebral ischemia can also result from cerebral hypoperfusion secondary to any form of shock or in association with cardiac events, especially in elderly patients with atherosclerotic cerebral vessels. Areas of the brain most vulnerable to these episodes of hypoperfu-

Table 11–8   Common Causes of Seizures in Elderly Patients Presenting to an Emergency Department

1. Idiopathic
2. Alcohol or drug withdrawal
3. Reduction of or abrupt withdrawal of anticonvulsant drugs
4. Head trauma
5. Cerebral anoxia
6. Intracranial infection
   a. Abscess
   b. Subdural empyema
7. Intracerebral hemorrhage
8. Toxic-metabolic
   a. Hypoglycemia
   b. Hypocalcemia
9. Brain tumor
10. Subdural hematoma
11. Cortical vein thrombosis

sion are known as "watershed" zones where the major cerebral arteries anastomose.[10,16] Any of the aforementioned etiologies may produce a seizure, but this complication is most commonly seen with cerebral embolism and intracranial hemorrhage (Table 11–8). Urgent therapy is indicated for this complication (Tables 11–9 and 11–10).

The course of a completed stroke may worsen within the first 72 hours because of extension of the thrombosis or hemorrhage, further embolic events, or edema formation. The prognosis of completed strokes is that one fourth of patients die as a result of, or from a complication related to, their CVA; about half of those stroke patients over 70 years of age die; 10% of CVAs in older patients occur in association with an acute MI.[31] About 50% of deaths that occur in patients with acute cerebral infarction are due to myocardial ischemia or cardiac arrhythmias; another 5% are related to herniation secondary to

Table 11–9   Commonly Used Anticonvulsant Drugs and Routes of Administration

Name	Loading dose	Maintenance dose
Phenytoin (Dilantin)	15–18 mg/kg IV, PO	5 mg/kg/day in one or two divided doses PO, IV
Phenobarbital	15–20 mg/kg IV, IM, PO	1–2 mg/kg IV, IM, PO
Carbamazepine (Tegretol)	Not clinically useful	400–12,000 mg/day or more in three or four divided doses with monitoring of blood levels, PO
Valproic acid (Depakene, Depakote)	1,000 mg per rectum in selected cases	15–60 mg/kg/day in three divided doses, PO
Ethosuximide (Zarontin)	Not clinically useful	250–750 mg/day, PO
Primidone (Mysoline)	Not clinically useful	300–750 mg/kg/day in three divided doses, PO
Diazepam (Valium)	5–10 IV slow push	Not recommended for maintenance

Table 11–10 Therapeutic Levels of Commonly Used Anticonvulsants

Drug	Therapeutic level
Phenytoin (Dilantin)	10–20 µg/ml
Phenobarbital3	20–45 µg/ml
Primidone (Mysoline)	7–15 µg/ml primidone (active metabolite is phenobarbital found at levels of 10–40 µ/ml
Valproic acid (Depakene, Depakote)	50–100 µg/ml
Carbamazepine (Tegretol)	4–12 µg/ml
Ethosuximide (Zarontin)	40–100 µg/ml

increased ICP; and most of the remainder are a consequence of pulmonary complications, such as aspiration pneumonia or pulmonary embolism.[31] Thus, it is imperative that patients with stroke syndromes be admitted to the hospital for monitoring, evaluation of any accompanying illnesses, and prevention of complications.

LARGE CEREBRAL ARTERY THROMBOTIC OCCLUSION

Cerebral artery occlusions (Tables 11–11 to 11–13) account for one fourth to one third of all stroke syndromes. The most likely locations for atherosclerotic lesions are the ICA, MCA, VA, and BA. Infarcts at these sites are caused by reduced perfusion through a narrowed lesion, a thrombotic occlusion, or an intraarterial embolus from a proximal occlusive arterial lesion. Hypertension, hypercholesterolemia, and smoking are the major risk factors. These patients are very likely to have concomitant coronary and peripheral vascular disease with a high incidence of angina, myocardial infarct, and cardiac death.

Large vessel thrombosis usually presents with a fluctuating and gradual but, ultimately, progressive course. On the other hand, quite often the elderly patient will

Table 11–11 Common Symptoms of Transient Ischemic Attacks

Carotid TIA
  Hemiparesis or monoparesis
  Hemiparesthesia or monohypesthesia
  Hemihypesthesia or monohypesthesia
  Aphasia
  Monocular visual loss (amaurosis fugax)
  Homonymous hemianopia
  Combination of the above

Vertebrobasilar TIA
  Monoparesis, hemiparesis, or quadriparesis
  Paresthesia, hypesthesia, in various combinations over one or both sides of the body or face
  Loss of vision, bilateral or unilateral homonymous hemianopsia
  Ataxia
  Hearing loss, unilateral or bilateral
  Combination of the above

Table 11–12 Differential Diagnosis of Transient Ischemic Attacks

Atheromatous embolus
Hypoglycemia
Lacunar strokes
Cerebral embolism of cardiac origin
Hypoperfusion syndromes
Seizures
Migraine
Hypertensive encephalopathy
Multiple sclerosis
Nonatherosclerotic arteriopathies
Hematologic disorders

awaken in the morning with a completed stroke. The patient may have a headache. There is often a history of TIAs. The neurologic deficits are variable, depending on which cerebral vessel is occluded, including brainstem syndromes. The location of the thromboembolic event for a specific deficit can also be variable. Although unilateral weakness and numbness with aphasia is the classic presentation for an MCA hemispheric stroke, a clinically indistinguishable presentation can be precipitated by an acute vascular event involving either the basal ganglia, internal capsule, or pons. At the time of presentation to the ED, the CT scan may or may not reveal a decreased density in the location of the infarct, especially with brainstem infarcts. MRI scans are more sensitive, detecting abnormalities earlier and more often, including after brainstem infarcts.[26-28] The CSF should be clear, unless hemorrhagic transformation occurs within the first 2 or 3 days as a result of bleeding from weakened blood vessels. Delayed hemorrhage or edema with herniation can occur at 48 to 72 hours. The prognosis is fair and is related to the amount and location of the infarcted brain tissue.

Anterior Cerebral Ischemia

The blood supply to the anterior cerebral circulation is derived from the internal carotid arteries (ICAs), which

Table 11–13 Classification of Cerebrovascular Infarction

I. Arterial disease
  A. Occlusion of the lumen with distal infarction
    1. Thrombosis
    2. Embolus
    3. Arteriopathies (infective and noninfective)
    4. Trauma and mechanical compression
    5. Dissecting aneurysm
    6. Spasm (migraine, angiography)
  B. Hypoperfusion with infarction in border zone territories
    1. Hypotension
    2. Arrhythmia
    3. Valvular lesion
II. Venous disease
  A. Aseptic thrombotic occlusion
  B. Septic thrombotic occlusion

enter the circle of Willis to anastomose with the posterior cerebral circulation. Each ICA gives off an ophthalmic artery before bifurcation into the middle cerebral artery and the anterior cerebral artery; the two anterior cerebral arteries are connected by the anterior communicating artery. Transient or permanent ipsilateral visual deficits result from emboli entering an ophthalmic artery and its branch, the central retinal artery. Thus, amaurosis fugax, or monocular blindness, is a hallmark of disease in the carotid artery. From a hemodynamic standpoint, the MCA is the continuation of the ICA while the ACA takes off at a right angle from the bifurcation; thus, emboli in the ICAs usually involve the MCA territory. Typical anterior cerebral circulation ischemic syndromes result from obstruction of one of the following arteries:

1. The *ICA syndrome* causes symptoms and signs of a hemispheric cerebral infarction comparable to the MCA syndrome. Contralateral findings of hemiplegia, homonymous field defect, hemianesthesia, and gaze palsy are associated with aphasia (with dominant, usually left hemisphere involvement) or hemineglect (with nondominant hemisphere involvement). With a hemispheric infarction of ICA origin, massive edema can cause acute increases in ICP, resulting in obtundation and even coma with death due to unilateral cerebral herniation through the tentorium.

2. The MCA is the most frequent site of intracranial cerebral artery thrombosis. The *MCA syndrome* results in neurologic findings similar to those seen in the ICA syndrome. The potential exists for massive swelling and herniation. When branches off the MCA are involved, the neurologic deficit will be greater in the face and arm than in the leg. If a lower extremity is involved in an MCA infarction, it is not due to cortical ischemia but rather to internal capsule involvement.

3. The *ACA syndrome* produces more findings involving the contralateral leg than the face and arm. Urinary incontinence is often present. If both ACAs arise from a single trunk, then occlusion of the lone trunk may cause bilateral parasagittal infarction and a state of anarthria with paraplegia.

Vertebrobasilar Insufficiency

The vertebral arteries (VAs) come off the aorta and flow cephalad to form the basilar artery (BA), which then bifurcates to form the posterior cerebral arteries (PCAs). The PCAs communicate with the anterior cerebral circulation through the posterior communicating arteries. Vertebrobasilar insufficiency (VBI) is common, accounting for almost half of all TIAs.[32] For VBI to be properly diagnosed, the symptoms must localize to the distribution of a major artery in the VB system or a major branch (e.g., the PCAs or the posterior or anterior inferior cerebellar arteries) that supplies the brainstem, cerebel-

lum, and occipital lobe. The symptoms must be sterotypical and recurrent. The following symptoms alone are insufficient to diagnose VBI[23,32]: isolated memory loss, confusion, dysarthria, diplopia, dizziness, syncope, ataxia, and vertigo. VBI syndromes may produce these symptoms but usually only in association with other neurologic symptoms or signs consistent with brainstem ischemia. For example, true syncope is not a "drop attack," in which the patient often drops to his knees or falls to the ground because of sudden and transient loss of postural tone in the legs without loss of consciousness; on the other hand, a "drop attack" should not be labeled as a TIA in the absence of other neurologic symptoms associated with VBI.[12] The differential diagnosis of VBI in the elderly includes some of the entities noted in previous sections as well as such disorders as acoustic neuroma and vestibular disease (Tables 11–14 and 11–15). As opposed to anterior circulation stroke syndromes, in which hemiparesis and hemianesthesia involve contralateral extremities, VBI results in alternating ischemic syndromes, which produce ipsilateral CN palsies, contralateral hemiplegia, and ipsilateral cerebellar signs. VBI is usually due to the obstruction of one of the following arteries:

1. The *paramedian arteries* supply midline structures in the brainstem; ischemia causes deficits of cranial nerves III, IV, VI, and XII, the pyramidal motor tract, and proprioception. At the level of the midbrain, partial ophthalmoplegia is associated with contralateral hemiparesis. At the level of the pons, paralysis of conjugate gaze (internuclear ophthalmoplegia) and contralateral hemiparesis are associated with loss of position and vibratory sense. At the level of the medulla, hemiparalysis of the tongue occurs with contralateral hemiparesis.

2. The *circumferential arteries* are divided into short arteries (supplying the brainstem) and long arteries (brainstem and cerebellar hemispheres). Associated neurologic deficits involve cranial nerves V, VII, VIII, IX, and X, the spinothalamic sensory tract, the cerebellar peduncles, and the central fibers of the sympathetic nervous system. A classic presentation is that of Wallenberg's lateral medullary syndrome due to occlusion of a VA or the posterior inferior cerebellar artery, which causes ipsilateral facial numbness, palate and vocal cord paresis, nystagmus, and Horner's

Table 11–14   Common Causes of Acute Vertigo

Labyrinthine	Central
Acute labyrinthitis	Vascular
Positional	Vertebrobasilar insufficiency
Ménièr's disease	Posterior fossa stroke or
Middle ear infection	hemorrhage
Drug induced or toxic	Infections
	Vestibular nerve inflammation
	Secondary to herpes zoster
	Multiple sclerosis

Table 11–15 Commonly Used Vestibular Sedatives

Generic name	Trade name	Usual adult dose	Route of administration
Meclizine	Antivert	12.5–25 mg q6h	PO
Promethazine	Phenergan	25 mg	PO, IM, IV
Dimenhydrinate	Dramamine	25–50 mg q6h	PO, IM, IV
Diphenhydramine	Benadryl	25–50 mg q6h	PO, IM, IV
Scopolamine	Trans-dermScop	0.5 mg	Cutaneous patch
Prochlorperazine	Compazine	10.0 mg q4–6h	IM, PO
Diazepam	Valium	5.0 mg tid	PO
Clonazepam	Klonopin	0.5 mg bid or tid	PO

syndrome associated with contralateral pain and temperature loss and ataxia.

3. The *internal auditory artery* off the BA or off the anterior inferior cerebellar artery; ischemia causes sudden ipsilateral deafness, vertigo, unsteadiness, and vomiting and presents like Ménière's disease, but the deafness is permanent.

4. *BA occlusion* (BAO) can progress quickly after the patient presents with most of the VBI-associated symptoms noted above, plus numbness around the lips or face associated with hemiparesis and hemisensory loss on contralateral limbs. Further progression can result in bilateral infarction of the pons, manifested by quadriplegia with bilateral lower CN paralysis (the "locked-in" syndrome), and death due to medullary infarction. Acute BAO is a life-threatening emergency requiring rapid diagnosis by angiography and definitive treatment with anticoagulation, thrombolysis, or vascular surgery.

5. *PCA syndromes* are variable because the PCA supplies blood to the upper brainstem (via the interpeduncular branches), the thalamus (thalamoperforating branches), and the occipital cortex. Resultant neurologic findings include the following:

   a. Thalamic syndrome of Déjérine (contralateral sensory loss, both deep and cutaneous; minimal, transitory hemiparesis; homonymous hemianopsia; and hyperpathic "thalamic" pain)

   b. Central midbrain (oculomotor palsy, contralateral hemiplegia, paralysis of upward gaze, and intention tremor)

   c. Subthalamic infarction (hemiballismus, hemiathetosis, and hemiataxia)

   d. Unilateral cortical infarction (homonymous hemianopsia or quandrantanopsia and alexia without agraphia in the dominant hemisphere)

   e. Bilateral cortical infarction, which can arise from a single occlusion at the bifurcation of the BA into both PCAs or from bilateral embolization. The result is cortical blindness, in which case the patient may be unaware of the blindness (denial) and confabulate when asked to identify objects (Anton's syndrome).

VBI can be associated with a relatively nondiseased VB arterial system because of shunting of blood away from the posterior circulation to supply either the anterior circulation (i.e., to compensate for carotid artery disease) or the ipsilateral upper extremity (i.e., the subclavian artery steal syndrome). In these two situations, angiography is indicated because they represent syndromes in which vascular surgery may benefit posterior circulation ischemic syndromes.

SMALL VESSEL OR LACUNAR INFARCTS

Small vessel thrombosis or lacunar infarcts are associated with chronic hypertension.[33] These syndromes result from occlusion or hemorrhage involving the penetrating branches off any of the major cerebral arteries, usually the MCA or PCA. The MCA gives off the lenticulostriate arteries, which supply the basal ganglia and the internal capsule. The PCA gives off thalamoperforating branches, which supply the posterior thalamus, and interpeduncular branches, which supply the upper brainstem and cerebellum. These straight perforating branches are small terminal arteries, which develop either atherosclerotic occlusion or aneurysmal dilation secondary to hypertension. Rupture of microaneurysms in these arteries produces hypertensive ICH syndromes involving deep structures. Occlusion of small perforating arteries produces small infarcts known as lacunes. There are five relatively distinct lacunar infarct syndromes[33]:

1. Pure motor hemiplegia may result from infarction of the corona radiata, internal capsule, pons, or medullary pyramid, causing weakness of the face, arm, and leg on one side of the body without sensory, visual, aphasic, or cognitive abnormalities

2. Pure sensory stroke involving the thalamus or internal capsule, causing numbness or paresthesias in the face, arm, and leg on one side of the body without motor, visual, or cognitive abnormalities

3. The dysarthria–clumsy hand syndrome consisting of facial weakness, ataxia of the hand, dysarthria, dysphagia, and some hemiparesis due to infarct of the internal capsule or the pons

4. Homolateral ataxia with hemiparesis consisting of weakness and ataxia of the arm and/or leg on the same side of the lesion in the pons, internal capsule, or corona radiata

5. Multiinfarct dementia

Although combined sensory and motor deficits without cognitive abnormalities can be caused by lacunar infarcts, they are more often caused by large artery disease or intracerebral hemorrhage. The onset of a lacunar infarct is usually gradual, but it may be sudden. The patient usually does not complain of headache nor should the consciousness be altered. There may be a history of stereotypical TIAs. The CT scan is classically normal, but it can reveal a relatively small hypodense lesion or even a loculated hemorrhage. MRI is again more sensitive. The CSF should be clear. The treatment is generally supportive with long-term control of hypertension.

CEREBRAL EMBOLISM

Cerebral emboli arise from CA or cardiac sources; the embolic material consists of small platelet aggregates or large mural clots, respectively.[34] Cerebral emboli can also consist of valvular vegetations, metastatic tumor, or air or nitrogen bubbles. Embolic infarction usually has a sudden, often apoplectic onset associated with a rapid loss of consciousness from the awake state, followed by the maximum deficit at the outset in 80% of cases.[34] A small percentage of patients have a stepwise or progressive course during the first 24 to 48 hours caused by distal migration of the embolus. There may be unilateral headache, opposite the side of the neurologic findings. The patient or family may give a history of similar prior episodes, especially in the setting of cardiogenic emboli. Within one to two days, the CT scan will reveal a decreased density in the peripheral cerebral cortex; there may be many such defects on CT, involving the vascular supply of more than one cerebral artery. This finding is consistent with multiple embolic events, many of which may have been clinically silent.[26] The CSF is usually clear. An ECG may reveal a recent MI; most mural thrombi that embolize do so in the first month after an acute MI.[34] In patients with cardiogenic emboli, the risk of another embolus is approximately 15% over the first 2 weeks. Anticoagulation is recommended in nonhemorrhagic embolic infarction. The patient's rhythm should be monitored for abnormal rhythms, especially atrial fibrillation. The prognosis following an embolic stroke is fair to poor, worse in patients with cardiogenic emboli because of the underlying cardiac disorder and because the neurologic deficit is usually more severe owing to the larger size of the embolic material or to the occurrence of multiple embolic events.

INTRACEREBRAL HEMORRHAGE

There are two broad categories of intracerebral hemorrhage (Table 11–16). ICH is most often caused by rupture of a penetrating cerebral artery which has undergone aneurysmal dilation secondary to chronic hypertension.[35] Hypertensive intracerebral hemorrhage is most common in deep structures, especially the putamen but also in the subcortical white matter, thalamus, pons, and cerebellum. Less common is the more superficial, so-called lobar ICH associated with arterial rupture at the site of vascular degeneration (e.g., secondary to hypertension or vasculopathies) or of vascular anomalies (e.g., aneurysms and arteriovenous malformation).[35] In these patients, ICH can be caused by an abrupt increase in BP, caused by excessive use of sympathomimetic agents, especially

Table 11–16   Classification of Intracranial Hemorrhage

Intracerebral	Extracerebral
Hypertensive	Subarachnoid
Hemorrhagic infarction	Subdural
Arteriovenous malformation	Traumatic
Clotting disorder	Spontaneous clotting
Liver disease	disorder
Leukemia	Epidural
Thrombotic	
thrombocytopenic purpura	
Anticoagulant therapy	
Hemorrhage into tumor	

over-the-counter (OTC) medications with phenylpropanolamine. Both types of ICH syndromes usually present very abruptly over minutes, but the leakage of blood from ruptured cerebral arteries can be gradual over hours.

The first symptoms result from ischemic effects at the site of hemorrhage. Progressive focal neurologic deficits result, but because there are no sensory nerves within the cerebral parenchyma, headache is absent or minor if the hematoma is small or if blood has not been released into the subarachnoid space. Enlarging hematomas increase ICP and cause headaches, vomiting, and deterioration in mental status. By the time the emergency physician evaluates the patient with an ICH, the systemic BP is usually very elevated. This is an autoregulatory mechanism whereby the systemic hypertension is an attempt to perfuse the brain despite a very elevated ICP. One should avoid the urge to lower the BP until the extent of the ICH can be visualized on CT scan[38] (Figure 11–3).

ICH that occurs in patients receiving anticoagulant agents develops more slowly. These hemorrhages often involve the cerebellum, the site of approximately 10% of such cases.[39] It is important to recognize the early, so-called toxic signs of a posterior fossa mass effect secondary to a cerebellar hemorrhage (or infarction with edema formation), because surgical evacuation of the posterior fossa can be lifesaving and patients tolerate the removal of a cerebellar mass surprisingly well. Signs include severe headache, nausea and vomiting, nystagmus and ophthalmoplegia, severe ataxia, or inability to stand. Hemiparesis occurs very late after an acute cerebellar event, and by the time that coma supervenes from acute herniation, the mortality rate is high. ICH is also very common after head trauma, especially in patients with poor liver function or who are taking anticoagulants.[36]

The CT scan is excellent at detecting hematomas due to ICH as hyperdense, well-circumscribed lesions. The location, size, and spread of the hematomas are well-defined, as are surrounding edema and pressure on adjacent structures. MRI also readily detects ICH and can better estimate the age of the bleeding. Lumbar puncture is rarely necessary nor indicated in these patients. The exception would be the patient with such a small ICH

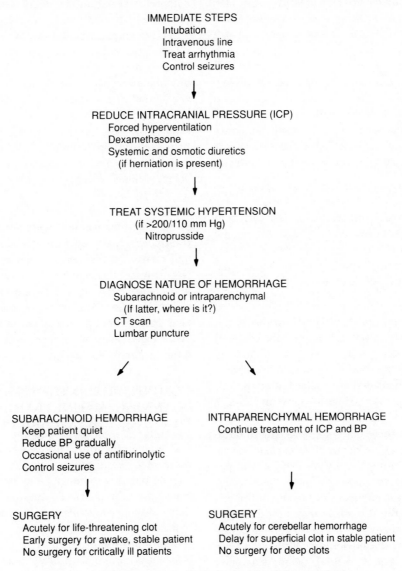

Figure 11–3 Management scheme for intracranial hemorrhage.

(less than 10 ml) that it is not visualized on the CT scan, in which case SAH would be included in the differential diagnosis and an LP would be appropriate. The LP will detect blood in the CSF in about 80 to 90% of hemorrhages that rupture into the ventricles or subarachnoid space.[37]

SUBARACHNOID HEMORRHAGE

Although the incidence of other CVAs has declined over the past two decades, SAH has not.[40] SAHs account for about 10% of CVAs, including about half of CVAs in patients below the age of 45 years, with a peak age range between 35 and 65 years. The majority of SAHs are due to rupture of an aneurysm, usually a Berry aneurysm in the anterior portion of the circle of Willis at the base of the brain. Unruptured aneurysms are found in about 3% of patients at autopsy; they are rare before the age of 20

years. In up to 50% of cases, an alert patient with an aneurysm may have a small, sentinel SAH or other warning symptoms caused by aneurysm expansion. It is extremely important to make the diagnosis at this point because the prognosis of a patient with a SAH is directly related to the state of consciousness at the time of intervention. About one third of patients with SAH die with the initial hemorrhage, one third subsequently suffer significant morbidity and mortality, and one third recover relatively or completely intact. Other causes of SAH include trauma, infection, vasculitis, bleeding diathesis, tumor hemorrhage, hypertensive crises, and iatrogenic interventions.

The patient with an SAH classically complains of the "worst headache of my life"; this headache is caused by meningeal irritation from the blood and by an increase in ICP. Also characteristic is the sudden onset of the headache, often during exertion, associated with the instant release of blood under arterial pressure. A sudden increase in ICP can cause vomiting and even syncope, followed later by decreased alertness, restlessness, and stiff neck with meningismus and photophobia. Funduscopic examination may show preretinal bleeding in up to 20% of patients with SAH. Paralysis and other focal neurologic signs are usually absent because bleeding is around and not into the brain, but local collections of blood or edema can cause compression and vasospasm can cause infarction of adjacent structures. These focal signs are characteristic for the location of the following aneurysms:

1. ICA-posterior communicating artery aneurysms are associated with ipsilateral third cranial nerve.
2. MCA bifurcation aneurysms are associated with contralateral facial weakness and aphasia or visual neglect.
3. Anterior communicating artery aneurysms are associated with bilateral leg weakness or numbness and positive Babinski signs.

The most common and significant complications in patients who survive the initial SAH are rebleeds and vasospasm. Rebleeds occur in 30 to 40% of patients by the end of the first month and have a fatal outcome in about 80%. The peak incidence of a rebleed after the initial "sentinel" bleed from an SAH occurs between 2 and 7 days. Vasospasm is an even more common cause of morbidity and mortality in these patients, occurring in 60 to 80% of patients. The peak incidence of vasospasm occurs between days 4 and 12 after the initial SAH; 30% of patients with vasospasm develop neurologic deficits secondary to ischemia. Vasospasm occurs at the site of the initial bleed where the cerebral vesssels were first damaged by the original hemorrhage, then made irritable and susceptible to vasospasm by the surrounding blood.

Other complications related to SAH include extension into the brain, ventricles, and even the subdural space requiring evacuation; cardiac arrhythmias necessitating early ECG monitoring of these often young patients; electrolyte abnormalities associated with diabetes insipidus or the syndrome of inappropriate secretion of antidiuretic hormone; and communication hydrocephalus. Cardiac arrhythmias are most likely during the initial hours or days after the SAH; they occur secondary to catecholamine release, which affects repolarization as suggested by ECG changes involving ST segment and T wave changes and prolonged QT intervals. The communicating hydrocephalus may be acute and severe secondary to the rapid pooling of blood in the basal cisterns. This results in a worsening headache and decreasing mental status because of increased ICP. Acute hydrocephalus may require immediate ventricular drainage. Most often, communication hydrocephalus develops gradually secondary to a blockage of CSF reabsorption at the base of the brain. This subacute hydrocephalus may necessitate placement of a ventri-

culoperitoneal shunt for increased ICP. Chronic normal pressure hydrocephalus may subsequently develop.

A CT scan performed soon after an SAH usually shows blood in the subarachnoid space and basal cisterns. The CT scan may be normal in up to 10% of SAHs on the first day (usually with small bleeds), in about 75% of cases by the second day, and about half of cases by the third day after the SAH.[33] Lumbar puncture will detect red blood cells in the CSF in virtually all cases of SAH from 1 to 2 hours until 48 to 72 hours after the bleed. The CSF may reveal xanthochromia, which requires 2 to 4 hours to develop, becomes maximal at 36 hours, and may be present for 7 to 10 days.[42]

The prognosis of patients with SAH is directly related to delay in management and severity (Table 11–17). The treatment of patients with SAH depends upon neurologic and mental status presentation at the time of diagnosis (see below). Because of the poor prognosis associated with delay in the diagnosis and management of the initial SAH, it is of utmost importance for the physician to keep SAH in mind in any patient coming to the emergency department with new onset of a sudden, severe or different type of headache.

COMPUTERIZED TOMOGRAPHY SCANNING, MAGNETIC RESONANCE IMAGING, AND LUMBAR PUNCTURE

A CT scan of the brain reveals a hypodense defect in most cases of cerebral infarction due to thrombosis or embolism, but these changes may only be evident 24 to 48 hours after the onset of symptoms.[26,41] CT is even more likely to be normal with small lacunar infarcts, although hypodense abnormalities may also be apparent on presentation and are usually seen within 1 or 2 days. CT is usually normal with brainstem infarction, whereas a brainstem hemorrhage may be visible on CT. Many patients with a clinical diagnosis of thrombosis are found to have an ICH on CT scan. Any hemorrhagic infarct produces an area of increased density that is readily visible on CT. CT reveals blood in the subarachnoid spaces (i.e., within the sulci and ventricles and at the basal cistern) within the first hours after the onset of symptoms in almost all cases of SAH. The yield of CT in patients with SAH diminishes over time to below 50% after 2 to 3 days. The addition of a contrast CT study to a non-

Table 11–17 Hunt-Hess Scale

Grade	Clinical description
0	Asymptomatic
I	Mild headache
II	Moderate to severe headache, nuchal rigidity, can have oculomotor palsy
III	Confusion, drowsiness, or mild focal signs
IV	Stupor or hemiparesis
V	Coma, moribund, and/or extensor posturing

contrast study is not necessary for the emergency department patient appearing with an acute stroke syndrome. With contrast enhancement, infarcts may mimic tumors, but this is generally not associated with the significant mass effect that occurs with tumors. However, in some instances of large MCA infarcts, a mass effect caused by edema may be present, but serial CT scans can help clarify the diagnosis. Contrast can also cause artifacts due to enhancement, which suggest the presence of an SAH.

Although many neurologists are correct in recommending that CT scanning be delayed for 1 to 2 days to allow higher yield in visualizing the nonhemorrhagic infarct, the emergency physician may wish to obtain an early CT scan in patients with suspected TIAs or CVAs to rule out an ICH or to increase the yield of picking up a SAH. Although less common, CT scan is very good at detecting or ruling out potentially treatable lesions that may appear like a TIA or CVA (i.e., subdural hematomas, brain tumor, or metastatic disease), in which case contrast is usually helpful. Although MRI scans are more sensitive than are CT scans, clinically CT is still more useful than MRI because of its greater availability and its ability to rule out most of the important differential diagnostic considerations.

MRI scanning has enhanced our diagnostic capabilities in patients with TIAs and stroke.[26-28] MRI is more sensitive than CT in documenting cerebral infarcts, and it will reveal abnormalities consistent with infarcts earlier (see previous section on TIA). Thus, there are some situations where MRI is likely to detect an abnormality but CT may not document the process. This is clearly the case in patients with posterior fossa lesions, especially brainstem infarcts. MRI is also more likely than CT to detect cerebrovascular lesions (e.g., aneurysms, vascular malformations, and sagittal sinus thrombosis). MRI may be best reserved for patients in whom the CT scan does not reveal an abnormality in a patient with a clinical picture consistent with a CVA. On the other hand, MRI may miss some early hemorrhages and later reflect degenerative changes over an area larger than the documented stroke on CT scan. MRIs are less readily available, more expensive, and require more patient cooperation than CT; the added sensitivity in picking up ischemic lesions does not often lead to any significant change in management. In summary, because MRI is more sensitive but less specific than CT, MRI scans should probably be obtained only after neurologic or neurosurgical consultation because MRI only infrequently offers a clinically relevant advantage over CT scan.

Lumbar puncture has largely been replaced by CT and MRI in the workup of patients with TIAs and CVAs. But if anticoagulation therapy is contemplated, some authors recommend that a lumbar puncture be done, whereas other authors find that the CT is sensitive enough in ruling out ICH.[38,42] If lumbar puncture is performed, no cells are expected in the CSF with large or small vessel thrombosis. If the CSF is clear, then 6 to 24 hours should elapse after the lumbar puncture before anticoagulation is begun to decrease the risk of a lumbar epidural hematoma. Although the CSF is clear in the majority of cases of emboli, CSF with only 50 to 500 red blood cells mm^3 is suggestive of an embolus with some associated hemorrhage. A large number of red blood cells (>1000/mm^3) in association with an elevated pressure (>200 mm Hg) suggests hemorrhage somewhere within the CNS that has ruptured into the CSF. About 10% of ICHs show no cells in the CSF and do not have an elevated pressure because the rupture was only into the cerebral tissue without communication with the CSF. Virtually all SAHs show bloody CSF, if not immediately, then within 2 to 4 hours, which persists for at least 48 to 72 hours. SAHs will begin to show xanthochromic CSF within 2 to 4 hours; the xanthochromia persists for 7 to 10 days. White blood cells may sometimes be seen after thrombosis or an embolus, but the possibility of inflammation (vasculitis or cerebritis) or infection (encephalitis or meningitis) should be considered.

EVALUATION AND MANAGEMENT OF PATIENTS WITH CEREBROVASCULAR SYNDROMES

The primary goal in the management of patients with cerebrovascular disease is prevention by treating hypertension and other risk factors (e.g., cerebral, cardiac, and systemic), in part because the therapies for cerebrovascular disease after the event are not particularly efficacious. Any patient presenting with a TIA(s) or stroke should be expeditiously evaluated to determine the pathophysiology (i.e., thrombosis, embolism, or hemorrhage), underlying etiology (e.g., cerebral, carotid, cardiac, or systemic), and whether the anterior or posterior circulation is at risk.

A patient initially having a TIA-like picture should be admitted to the hospital, for many reasons: (1) the patient may have actually had a CVA that may worsen with progressive ischemia, edema, or bleeding over the next few days; (2) the patient may develop a stroke, because the patient is at greatest risk of having a stroke soon after a TIA; (3) medical problems must be actively sought as the cause of the presumed TIA because medical problems are usually more treatable and potentially more reversible; and (4) if a patient's medical problems are not stabilized, cerebral hypoperfusion may result in progressive neurologic morbidity or the patient's survival may be at risk.

The workup of a patient with a TIA should include a CT scan without contrast dye to rule out an acute bleed and a CT scan with contrast to evaluate any mass lesion. Lumbar puncture may be necessary to definitively rule out an SAH. Holter monitoring and echocardiography are considered sufficient screening tests to rule out cardiac embolic sources in most patients.[35] Further CA workup (i.e., noninvasive studies or angiography) depends on the TIA involving the anterior circulation and the patient being a potential surgical candidate (i.e., carotid endarterectomy). The patient with TIAs involving the posterior circulation rarely benefits from a noninvasive assessment of the carotid arteries. Further cardiac workup (i.e., catheterization) depends on the TIA being caused by a cardiogenic embolus and the patient being a candidate for either long-term anticoagulation or cardiac surgery.

The elderly patient presenting with a stroke syndrome should be admitted to the hospital for these reasons: (1) medically, because an acute cardiac event or other medical problem may be the underlying cause and because completed strokes often result in the death of the patient; (2) neurologically, because the stroke can progress in 15 to 25% of patients as progressive ischemia, bleeding, or edema develops; and (3) socially, because the patient and family require assistance with rehabilitation and time to assimilate the severe disturbance to their home and work environment caused by the event.

The management of a patient with an acute cerebrovascular syndrome is all too often expectant, even with the introduction of neurologic ICUs for observation and monitoring. At this time of dynamic change in the cerebrovascular status of the patient, in consideration of the selective vulnerability of the ischemic penumbra, it is important to do no harm. Reports of adverse neurologic outcome with the use of CNS depressant drugs, such as diazepam and haloperidol and some antihypertensive agents,[43,44] and a report of improved motor performance with the one-time administration of oral d-amphetamine compared with placebo[45] suggest that the emergency physician must choose pharmaceutical interventions carefully. Another seemingly simple decision, whether or not to administer intravenous fluids, has become clearer with the empiric observation that most CVA patients are dehydrated and that the administration of saline will decrease serum viscosity and improve cerebral perfusion.[46,47] This does not apply to patients having dense hemiplegia from a large MCA infarct; fluid in these patients should be relatively restricted because they are prone to develop cerebral edema on the second or third day. The use of dextrose in water is to be discouraged because it will not improve cerebral perfusion as much as saline. Furthermore, the administration of dextrose will increase the serum glucose concentration and hyperglycemia is associated with larger strokes.[48]

Many therapeutic interventions have been studied, but the treatment of such a complex multifactorial process will require multimodal therapy, as most of the unifactorial therapies used to date have proven relatively unsuccessful in improving neurologic outcome and survival.[47] Another reason for the apparent lack of benefit from most of the therapies studied is that early intervention has not been emphasized, because too often the patient delays seeking medical care and the practitioner delays working up the patient and administering treatment.[15] For example, a randomized controlled prospective study of modified hypervolemic hemodilution with phlebotomy to a goal hematocrit of 35% has shown that mortality was reduced and functional activity improved in stroke patients.[50] However, when the treatment was reproduced in a community hospital setting, there was no benefit,[41] probably because patients were entered into the study up to 48 hours after the CVA and there was another 48-hour delay in reaching the goal Hct. The lack of blood supply to the ischemic penumbra remains a primary problem, and efforts to minimize the degree of injury by optimizing perfusion to the injured brain (e.g., vasopressors and vasodilators, antiplatelet and anticoagulant therapies, thrombolytic and biorheologic agents, and others; see below) have had at best mixed results.[46,47] Therapies that enhance resistance to ischemia by decreasing brain metabolism to better match the decreased perfusion of substrates (e.g., hypothermia, general anesthesia, free radical scavengers, lactate mobilization, neurotransmitter inhibition, and others) have demonstrated even less potential, because these interventions have not been shown to be practical or of much benefit (see Table 11–18).

WORKUP AND MANAGEMENT OF SELECTED COMPLICATIONS

Subarachnoid hemorrhage (SAH). Bed rest should be prescribed for patients with SAH who are stable and who are not going to early surgery; the heads of their beds should be elevated as their BP is gradually lowered to a low normal range. Some or all of the following medi-

Table 11–18   Investigated Therapies for Acute Cerebrovascular Disease

Ancrod
Aspirin
Barbiturates
Calcium channel blockers
Carotid endarterectomy
Corticosteroids
Dextran
Dipyridamole
Extracranial-intracranial bypass
Hemodilution
Heparin
Naloxone
Pentoxiphylline
Prostacyclin
Stimulants
Sulfinpyrazone
Thrombolytics
Ticlopidine
Warfarin

cations should be administered: sedatives, stool softeners, antitussives, antiemetics, anticonvulsants, antispasmodics (e.g., nimodipine), and perhaps antifibrinolytic agents and steroids. Nimodipine (Nimotop), a calcium channel blocker, crosses the blood-brain barrier. One study has demonstrated that nimodipine prevented some of the neurologic complications of delayed ischemia secondary to vasospasm that occur following SAH.[51] Another controlled trial found benefit in CVA patients when nimodipine therapy was begun within 12 hours.[52]

Concern about vasospasm often dictates the timing of neurovascular surgery in patients with SAH due to aneurysms.[41] If the initial "warning bleed" is properly diagnosed, the patient may undergo clipping of the aneurysm within 1 to 2 days, before the peak risk of vasospasm begins at 3 to 4 days. Otherwise, neurovascular surgery is usually delayed until the second week after the initial SAH when the blood vessels are more stable and the patient is at less risk from vasospasm and rebleeding. However, early surgery is often preferred to eliminate the risk of rebleeding by clipping the aneurysm accompanied by irrigation of the blood at the site of the SAH, which theoretically decreases the risk of vasospasm. Early surgery also allows pharmacologic therapy to be oriented toward the prevention of vasospasm without fear of inducing rebleeding; this phase of therapy includes the administration of IV fluids to increase the perfusion pressure. Studies show that delayed surgery at 10 to 14 days may be of equal benefit with respect to overall patient outcome, assuming the patient has not had a rebleed in the interim. One can be more certain of the diagnosis by this stage, and the neurosurgeon's dissection will be easier because there is less brain edema. The routine use of antifibrinolytic agents (such as epsilon aminocaproic acid or tranexamic acid) is no longer recommended because of ischemic complications. The routine use of steroids has also come under question and should be left up to the admitting physicians.

Hypertension is usually the primary risk factor for, but not necessarily a complication of, ischemic cerebrovascular events. An elevated BP in the setting of acute cerebral ischemia does not necessarily mandate treatment.[37] In fact, overly aggressive antihypertensive therapy can cause or worsen acute cerebral ischemia. Hypertension in this setting is usually secondary to an autoregulatory, compensatory mechanism attempting to increase cerebral blood flow to the ischemic region of brain against a gradient caused by an acute increase in ICP. Overly aggressive antihypertensive therapy will cause further ischemia to the border zone by causing relative hypotension for the collateral circulation to the ischemic penumbra. Most authorities now favor observing the patient's BP for at least the first few hours of a CVA. If bedrest, oxygen, and IV hydration do not result in a lowering of the initially high BP to below 200/120, then the CT scan usually reveals an ICH. A minority of neurologists theorize that

lowering the BP to approximately 10 mm Hg above the patient's baseline level of hypertension may stabilize the amount of ICH. Rarely, a patient may present with hypertensive encephalopathy looking just like an acute CVA.

Increased intracranial pressure (ICP) complicates the condition of about 10 to 15% of patients with acute CVAs, both early and late secondary to extension of the infarct, hemorrhage, or edema. Also, an obtunded stroke patient can hypoventilate and become hypercarbic, resulting in an increase in ICP secondary to vasodilatation from the elevated partial pressure of carbon dioxide (PCO_2). When coupled with concomitant hypoxia, the increased ICP can be associated with futher neurologic determination. An increase in ICP can result acutely from the mass effect associated with bleeding (e.g., from an ICH or an SAH) and subacutely from hydrocephalus (e.g., SAH) or edema formation (e.g., large MCA infarct). A large ICH will result in a hematoma mass and an abrupt increase in ICP, resulting in a rapid deterioration in mental status associated with focal neurologic deficits. A retrospective study showed that nonsurgical management of large clots (those found to be greater than 50 ml) was associated with a 90% mortality rate. Whereas nonsurgical management of smaller clots (less than 50 ml) were associated with only a 10% mortality rate.[53] Later, the edema associated with an ICH of any size or associated with a large MCA thrombosis will result in a gradual increase in ICP over the next 2 to 3 days associated with a gradual decrease in the patient's mental status with or without further progression in the neurologic deficit.

Increased ICP (above 15 mm Hg or 20 cm H_2O) is associated with decreased cerebral perfusion pressure (CPP = mean arterial pressure [MAP] minus ICP), which should be maintained above 50 mm Hg. Patients at risk for increased ICP (i.e., large ICH or MCA infarcts) and patients displaying signs of increased ICP (e.g., SAH with obtundation) may best be monitored with a ventriculostomy catheter (to drain off CSF during acute ICP spikes) or at least a subarachnoid bolt. The emergency physician must be cognizant of the fact that any stimulation of the patient can result in increased ICP (e.g., any induction of coughing or straining on the part of the patient, especially during nasogastric or endotracheal intubation). It has been taught that the head of the bed should be elevated to 30 degrees, but recent studies comparing invasive measurements of ICP with MAP monitoring via arterial lines have found that some patients' brains actually perfuse better while they are lying flat.[46] This is especially likely in the dehydrated patient whose systemic BP drops in the upright position. In patients with increased ICP, it is important to avoid a precipitous drop in BP and not to administer hypotonic IV fluids. Sudden increases of ICP are best treated with hyperventilation of the PCO_2 down to 25 to 30 mm Hg in the emergency department and, in the ICU or OR, drainage of CSF. The osmotic agent mannitol is helpful to temporarily ameliorate early herniation by drawing free water out from the brain; it is also a free radical scavenger.[46,47] Furosemide is also helpful, especially in combination with mannitol, because of its diuretic activity.[38,39] However, mannitol and furosemide take longer to work and are often less dramatic in their effects on ICP, so they are often used only in the patient en route to the operating room for definitive management of an underlying mass lesion that is responsible for an abrupt increase in ICP.

Neurosurgery may be necessary to manage the patient deteriorating from an acute mass effect.[46] The best responses to surgical evacuation of an ICH are seen in patients with increased ICP secondary to relatively superficial "lobar" hematomas. A large hemispheric ICH may necessitate late surgical decompression when cerebral edema supervenes and incipient herniation occurs. Although patient outcomes in these late cases are generally poor, surgical decompression is the only potentially effective therapy. Surgical decompression may be especially helpful in relieving brainstem compression caused by a cerebellar hematoma or a cerebellar infarct with edema formation. The best timing and response to cerebellar evacuation occur when the patient is displaying so-called toxic signs of a posterior fossa mass effect. By the time hemiparesis and coma supervene, neurosurgery probably will not be beneficial. A recent report of a series of patients with cerebellar hemorrhages and infarcts found that the presence of hydrocephalus was the most important factor in the survival of these patients.[55] The authors concluded that an indication for surgery in patients with cerebellar strokes is the presence of hydrocephalus, in which case ventricular drainage may be effective and evacuation of the cerebellar clot or the cerebellum itself not necessasry.

Cerebral edema is a common complication of a CVA, and it is difficult to treat. Cerebral edema occurs when reperfusion to the infarcted brain occurs during the time that a temporary blood-brain barrier defect exists.[46] This occurs after the first 24 hours and peaks at 48 to 96 hours. For this reason, patients with dense hemiplegia should have fluids relatively restricted (as opposed to the therapy of patients with mild to moderate strokes who are usually dehydrated and should be rehydrated with saline; see earlier discussion). Patients with large MCA hemispheric infarcts are especially prone to develop extracellular edema, which raises the ICP and results in obtundation. The patient may require airway management with intubation to prevent aspiration and to induce hyperventilation in an attempt to decrease the ICP. The use of mannitol is only temporary and may lead to a rebound hyperosmolar state, which may worsen the cerebral edema. Furosemide may be helpful in association with relative dehydration; it also decreases CSF formation. Steroids are not helpful in either preventing or treating the edema associated with CVAs because the extracellular edema is secondary to a cytotoxic mechanism, as opposed to the vasogenic edema associated with brain tumors where steroids are helpful. The risks associated with the use of steroids further complicate their use in the unstable CVA patient; for example, the propensity to increase BP or cause hyperglycemia. Of course, a brain tumor with edema or hemorrhage may appear like a TIA or cause a CVA.

Bleeding may be the cause of or may be associated with the initial event or delayed as a nonhemorrhagic infarct deteriorates into an hemorrhagic stroke after 24 to 48 hours.[46] This results from rupture of cerebral arteries that were damaged by the original ischemic event. The vessels become further damaged by the extracellular edema that occurs after 24 to 48 hours. The combination of hemorrhage and edema formation results in increased ICP and a deterioration of the patient's mental and neurologic status. This is a not uncommon reason for patients initially diagnosed as having a TIA to return to the emergency department after 1 to 2 days, at which time their initially subtle neurologic deficit becomes more obvious and fixed, or for the hospitalized patient to deteriorate while under observation. Another example of delayed deterioration would be in the patient with an embolic stroke, which can be associated with acute bleeding. When combined with subacute edema, the bleeding can be the cause of increased ICP. Of course, the initial SAH is often followed by a secondary rebleed, which is usually much more devastating and which makes obvious any initial misdiagnosis of the "sentinel" SAH.

SPECIFIC THERAPIES
Prophylactic Antiplatelet Therapy

The great majority of patients with TIAs or small CVAs receive daily acetylsalicylic acid (aspirin, ASA) as antiplatelet therapy. The use of ASA therapy in the prophylaxis of patients at risk for CVAs is not controversial, except for the proper dosage and duration of therapy. ASA therapy decreases the risk of CVA by 50 to 75% by blocking platelet aggregation via irreversible inhibition of prostaglandin pathway enzyme reactions for the life of the platelet. ASA may be more helpful in males (per a Canadian study[56]), but it has been shown to prevent strokes in females (per a later French study[57]). Published studies have used ASA for 6 to 12 months after TIA or chronically at doses ranging from 300 mg every other day to 1200 mg daily. A meta-analysis of studies involving approximately 29,000 patients showed that vascular mortality is decreased 15% and nonfatal CVAs or MIs are decreased 30% by ASA.[58] The issue with dosing concerns the fact that lower doses of ASA may preferentially block the enzyme cyclooxygenase and the production of thromboxane (the "antiplatelet" or antithrombotic effect). But too much ASA also blocks the next step in the prostaglandin pathway, the endothelium's production of prostacyclin (an inhibitor of platelet aggregation and a vasodilator). ASA therapy is not recommended by some authors for primary prevention in low-risk patients, because it may be associated with an increased risk of hemorrhagic strokes.

Ticlopidine (Ticlid) also inhibits platelet aggregation for the remainder of the platelet life span; it interferes with a different pathway than ASA. A recent randomized trial compared ticlopidine at a dose of 500 mg daily with ASA 1300 mg daily.[51] Ticlopidine was found to be somewhat more effective than ASA in preventing strokes. However, the side effects in the ticlopidine group consisted of severe but reversible neutropenia and increased total cholesterol levels. Dipyridamole and sulfinpyrazone have not shown consistent benefit in the prevention of strokes, with or without concomitant ASA therapy.

Prophylactic and Therapeutic Anticoagulant Therapy

Heparin has many complex and contradictory effects on thromboembolic mechanisms.[60,61] It activates antithrombin III immediately, but antithrombin III levels subsequently decrease. Heparin enhances platelet aggregability, but it can cause thrombocytopenia. The use of chronic anticoagulant therapy with warfarin is associated with significant risk of minor and major, life-threatening bleeding episodes. No patient with a TIA or CVA should receive anticoagulant medication at any time unless the cost-benefit ratio is decidedly positive. Administration of prophylactic heparin followed by warfarin in patients who have had a large MI with a mural thrombus can decrease the risk of embolic CVA by more than 50%. These patients have not had a CVA, so their cerebrovascular risk with anticoagulation is very small. On the other hand, the value of the use of anticoagulant agents in preventing CVAs in patients following TIAs remains largely unproven. Their use in selected patients can decrease the incidence of stroke, but the risk of hemorrhage often offsets anticipated benefits. One study found that 16% of patients receiving heparin continued to have TIAs, 7% had a stroke, and 12% had bleeding complications.[62] Prophylactic heparin therapy has also been recommended for patients with TIAs in the hope of preventing a stroke during the high-risk period within the next few days or weeks. Short-term heparinization for this indication is best justified in certain high-risk subgroups, especially patients with cardiogenic emboli. However, the patient with an embolus to the brain secondary to infectious endocarditis should never receive anticoagulant agents because of significant risk of hemorrhagic transformation. At best, there is a suggestion that anticoagulation after a TIA is slightly beneficial in preventing CVAs during the first few months following the TIA, but this may be no more efficacious than antiplatelet therapy.

There are anecdotal reports of benefit from acute heparinization in patients with progressing strokes, especially if the neurologic deficit is initially mild to moderate. But one problem is clinical: the recognition of CVA progression is difficult. Most progressing CVAs occur in the setting of an acute occlusion of an ICA, which places the patient at risk of retrograde thrombosis of the MCA and a large hemispheric infarct, or of the BA, which places the patient at risk of a brainstem infarct. Acute BA occlusion is the only absolute indication for early heparinization in a patient with either TIA or CVA.[46,47] The second problem is that in controlled clinical trials, heparin has not been shown to benefit the larger, unselected group of patients with a progressing "stroke-in-evolution."[46] Nevertheless, some authors continue to argue for early heparinization in a patient with progressing stroke.

The value of anticoagulation in preventing another stroke in a patient after a first stroke is also uncertain. A recent study did not find benefit from the use of heparin in an attempt in improve the neurologic deficit of patients with stable stroke.[63] The risk of transforming a nonhemorrhagic stroke into a hemorrhagic stroke is highest during the first week or two after the initial insult. Waiting at least 1 week before initiating anticoagulation will significantly decrease the risk of CNS hemorrhagic complications. Patients with stroke secondary to cardiogenic emboli that places the other hemisphere at risk should generally receive anticoagulant agents.[34] This assumes that the initial CT scan and a follow-up CT scan after at least 2 to 4 days rule out delayed hemorrhage or excessive edema formation and that the BP is controlled. Anticoagulation should not be excessive so a low-dose heparin infusion without an initial bolus or full-dose warfarin without initial heparinization is recommended starting 7 to 10 days after the stroke.[46]

Risk factor intervention, especially control of hypertension, is essential in the management of patients with TIAs or cerebral infarction. If a patient has a TIA or a small stroke while compliant with either ASA or coumadin, then either another diagnostic workup is indicated (i.e., is the correct underlying cause being treated?) or the patient's therapy may need to be advanced (i.e., from ASA to systemic anticoagulation or from warfarin to carotid endarterectomy) because the patient is at risk of developing a permanent deficit.

THROMBOLYTIC THERAPY

Thrombolytic therapy is also being actively investigated, despite the fact that pilot studies with streptokinase revealed an unacceptably high incidence of cerebral hemorrhage and currently a recent CVA is a contraindication to coronary thrombolytic therapy.[64,65] There are anecdotal reports of patency in an arteriographically proven occlusion with the use of intraarterial tissue plasminogen activator (tPA) within 2 hours of the event[66] and of success with the use of intraarterial tPA in patients with acute MCA and VBA occlusions.[67] There is hope that the newer clot-specific agents, such as tPA, will be less likely to transform a bland infarct into a hemorrhagic event. However, the relatively high dose of tPA necessary for IV administration in MI patients has led to as many hemorrhagic CVAs as has streptokinase.[65] Thus, thrombolytic therapy remains investigational for CVA patients.

The risk of bleeding associated with the use of thrombolytic therapy is probably increased with the coadministration of antiplatelet or anticoagulant therapy. The spontaneous hemorrhagic conversion rate in cerebral infarction has been reported between 0 and 43%.[56,57] The administration of thrombolytic agents for coronary thrombolysis has been associated with a less than 2% risk of intracerebral hemorrhage in patients without clinically manifest prior cerebrovascular disease.[64,65] To date clinical trials of late IV infusion of streptokinase or urokinase in patients with completed strokes have supported a general contraindication to their use in CVA patients because of inconsistent benefit associated with bleeding rates from 0 to nearly 50%.[68,69] Del Zoppo[65] listed concerns regarding the use of thrombolytic agents in the treatment of acute stroke, including the necessary dose rate, the true potential benefits versus the true risk of ICH, and the clinical parameters to success (i.e., functional outcome versus documented recanalization). Successes have been reported even with the delayed administration of thrombolytic agents in patients with central retinal vein thrombosis[70] but not with central retinal artery occlusion. Intraarterial internal carotid artery administration of urokinase has benefited comatose patients with documented sagittal sinus thrombosis with lateral sinus extension.[71] However, cerebral hemorrhage frequently accompanies sinus thrombosis.

BIORHEOLOGIC THERAPY

The viscosity of blood is determined by the hematocrit (patients with Hct's above 40% have larger infarcts), platelet and erythrocyte aggregability, erythrocyte flexibility, fibrinogen levels, and the blood flow rate.[49,50] CBF varies inversely with blood viscosity, which is increased in dehydrated patients. The majority of patients with CVAs are either clinically dehydrated or at risk of not taking in enough fluids orally. CBF is increased by intravenous hemodilution therapy, which decreases viscosity. As noted previously,[46,47,49] hemodilution with crystalloid (i.e., saline, not dextrose) or colloid solutions to an Hct goal of less than 35% within 24 hours of presentation has been shown to be of benefit experimentally in the treatment of patients with CVAs. Saline is preferred over dextrose in free water because free water increases the risk of cerebral edema and because a serum glucose above 140 mg/dl is associated with a larger stroke. Numerous authors have written about the adverse outcome in stroke patients with hyperglycemia.[48] Therefore, saline appears to be the best choice as an IV solution early in the management of these patients.

Recently investigated pharmacologic interventions to decrease serum viscosity have also shown promise. *Pentoxyphylline* (Trental), a methylxanthine derivative, is approved for the treatment of intermittent claudication because it has been shown to lower the blood viscosity by improving red blood cell deformability. Pentoxyphylline has been shown to benefit a subgroup of CVA patients, those with lacunar infarcts in progression, during the first 24 to 48 hours.[72] However, it did not alter mortality and there was no difference in outcome after 1 month; there were no significant side effects. *Ancrod* is a defibrinating enzyme extracted from the Malayan pit viper; it induces hypofibrinogenemia.[73] Ancrod decreases the viscosity of blood to improve flow properties; it does not affect coagulation profiles or platelet activity. It is still too early to determine if this agent will demonstrate clinical benefit in patients with acute CVAs. Colloid solutions (e.g., low molecular weight dextran), crystalloid substitutes (e.g., hydroxyethyl starch), and oxygen-carrying agents (e.g., Fluosol-DA) are also being actively studied for their beneficial effects on blood viscosity in patients with CVAs.[46,47]

Finally, *prostacyclin* (epoprostenol, prostaglandin I2) is a potent vasodilator produced by the endothelium in response to ischemia; it also has beneficial effects against platelet aggregation in the microcirculation. Atherosclerotic vessels have a decreased ability to synthesize prostacyclin, but exogenous administration can partially overcome this defect. Prostacyclin also potentiates the anticoagulation effects of heparin. However, three trials have shown inconsistent administration of prostacyclin.[74,75]

REFERENCES

1. Madsen PS et al: Acute propoxyphene self-poisoning in 222 consecutive patients, Acta Anaesthesiol Scand 28:661–665, 1984.
2. Galbraith S: Head injuries in the elderly, Br Med J 294:325, 1987.
3. Tinetti ME and Speechly M: Prevention of falls among the elderly, N Engl J Med 320:1055, 1989.
4. Pathy MS: Subdural hematoma. In Pathy MS, editor: Principles and practices of geriatric medicine, New York, 1985, John Wiley & Sons.
5. Ragland G: Nonketotic hypersomolar coma. In Tintinalli JE, Rothstein RJ, and Krome RI, editors: A study guide in emergency medicine, New York, 1985, McGraw-Hill.
6. Ragland A: Myxedema coma. In Tintinalli JE, Rothstein RJ, and Krome RL, editors: A study guide in emergency medicine, New York, 1985, McGraw-Hill.
7. Hamberger S and Collier RE: Myxedoma coma, Ann Emerg Med 11:156–159, 1982.
8. Malouf R and Burst JC: Hypoglycemia: causes, neurological manifestations and outcome, Ann Neurol 17:421–430, 1985.
9. Gresham GE et al: Residual disability in survivors of stroke — the Framingham study, N Engl J Med 293:954–959, 1975.
10. Dyken MR et al: Risk factors in stroke, Stroke 15:11–15, 1984.
11. DiPasquale G et al: Cerebral ischemia and asymptomatic coronary artery disease: a prospective study of 83 patients, Stroke 17:1098–1101, 1986.
12. Pellegrino TR: Vascular syndromes, Emerg Med Clin North Am 5:751–764, 1987.

13. Siesjo BK: Cerebral circulation and metabolism, J Neurosurg 60:883–889, 1984.

14. Strandgaard S and Paulson OB: Cerebral autoregulation, Stroke 15:413–419, 1984.

15. Barsan WG et al: Early treatment for acute ischemic stroke, Ann Intern Med 111:449–450, 1989.

16. Astrup J, Siesjo BK, and Symon L: Thresholds in cerebral ischemia — the ischemic penumbra, Stroke 12:723–725, 1981.

17. Solis OJ et al: Cerebral angiography in acute cerebral infarction, Rev Interv Radiol 2:19–25, 1977.

18. Lacy JR et al: Brain infarction and hemorrhage in young and middle-aged adults, West J Med 141:329–335, 1984.

19. Fisher CM: Late-life migraine accompaniments, Stroke 17:1033–1042, 1986.

20. Marshall J: The natural history of transient ischemic cerebrovascular attacks, J Med 131:309–324, 1964.

21. Fisher CM: Occlusion of the internal carotid artery, Arch Neurol Psychiatry 65:346–377, 1951.

22. Committee on Cerebrovascular Diseases: Classification and outline of cerebrovascular diseases. II, Stroke 6:564–616, 1975.

23. Caplan LR: TIAs: we need to return to the question, "What is wrong with Mr. Jones?" Neurology 38:791–793, (editorial) 1988.

24. Dykey ML et al: Cooperative study of hospital frequency and character of transient ischemic attacks, JAMA 237:882–887, 1977.

25. Kraaijeveld CL et al: Interobserver agreement for the diagnosis of transient ischemic attacks, Stroke 15:723–725, 1984.

26. Awad I et al: Focal parenchymal lesions in transient ischemic attacks: correlation of computed tomography and magnetic resonance imaging, Stroke 17:399–402, 1986.

27. Salgado E et al: Proton magnetic resonance imaging in ischemic cerebral vascular disease, Ann Neurol 20:502–507, 1986.

28. Kinkle P: Nuclear magnetic resonance imaging. In Baker AB and Joynt RJ, editors: Clinical neurology, vol 1, Philadelphia, 1987, Harper & Row.

29. Muuronen A and Kaste M: Outcome of 314 patients with transient ischemic attacks, Stroke 13:24–31, 1982.

30. Gautier JC, Julliard JBE, and Loron PHL: Time interval between transient ischemic attacks and cerebral infarction, Stroke 18:298, 1987.

31. Bounds JV et al: Mechanism and timing of deaths from cerebral infarction, Stroke 12:474–477, 1981.

32. Pessin MS, Caplan LR, and Hedges TR: Posterior cerebral artery territory stroke, Stroke 21:15–19, 1986.

33. Fisher CM: Lacunes: small, deep cerebral infarcts, Neurol 15:774–779, 1965.

34. Cerebral Embolism Task Force: Cardiogenic brain embolism, Arch Neurol 43:71–84, 1966.

35. Horning CR, Dorndorf W, and Agnolj AL: Hemorrhagic cerebral infarction: a prospective study, Stroke 17:179–185, 1986.

36. Levine S and Welch KMA: Cocaine and stroke, Stroke 22:25–30, 1987.

37. Lavin P: Management of hypertension in patients with acute stroke, Arch Intern Med 146:66–68, 1986.

38. Caplan LR et al: Lumbar puncture and stroke, Stroke 18:544A–546A, 1987.

39. Heros RC: Cerebellar hemorrhage and infarction, Stroke 13:106–109, 1982.

40. Biller J, Godersky J, and Adams H: Management of aneurysmal subarachnoid hemorrhage, Stroke 23:13–17, 1988.

41. Davis JM et al: Cranial computed tomography in subarachnoid hemorrhage: relationship between blood detected by CT and lumbar puncture, J Comput Assist Tomogr 4:794–796, 1980.

42. Marton KI and Gean AD: The diagnostic spinal tap, Ann Intern Med 104:880–885, 1986.

43. Porch B, Wyckes J, and Freeney DM: Haloperidol, thiazides and some antihypertensives slow recovery from aphasia, Soc Neurosci Abstr 11(part I):52, 1985.

44. Schallert T, Hernandez TD, and Barth TM: Recovery of function after brain damage: severe and chronic disruption by diazepam, Brain Res 379:104–111, 1986.

45. Davis JN et al: Amphetamine and physical therapy facilitate recovery of function from stroke: correlative animal and human studies. In Raichle M and Powers W, editors: Cerebrovascular diseases: fifteenth research (Princeton) conference, New York, 1987, Raven Press.

46. Grotta, J: Current medical and surgical therapy for cerebrovascular disease, N Engl J Med 317:1505–1516, 1987.

47. Sila CA and Furlan AJ: Drug treatment of stroke: current status and future prospects, Drugs 35:468-476, 1988.

48. Helgason CM: Blood glucose and stroke, Stroke 23:1-6, 1988.

49. Aberg A et al: Multicenter trial of hemodilution in acute ischemic stroke. 1. Results in the total population, Stroke 18:691–699, 1987.

50. Strand T et al: A randomized controlled trial of hemodilution therapy in acute ischemic stroke, Stoke 15:980–989, 1984.

51. Allen GS et al: Cerebral arterial spasm — a controlled trial of nimodipine in patients with subarachnoid hemorrhage, N Engl J Med 308:619–624, 1983.

52. Gelmers HJ et al: A controlled trial of nimodipine in acute ischemic stroke, N Engl J Med 318:203-207, 1988.

53. Helweg-Larsen S et al: Prognosis for patients treated conservatively for spontaneous intracerebral hematomas, Stroke 15:1045–1048, 1984.

54. Rosner MJ and Coley IB: Cerebral pressure, intracranial pressure, and head elevation, J Neurosurg 65:636–641, 1986.

55. Shenkin HA and Zavala M: Cerebellar strokes: mortality, surgical indications, and results of ventricular drainage, Lancet 2:429–432, 1982.

56. The Canadian Cooperative Study Group: A randomized trail of aspirin and sulfinpyrazone in threatened stroke, N Engl J Med 299:53–59, 1978.

57. Bousser MG et al: "AICLA" controlled trial of aspirin and dipyridamole in the secondary prevention of athero-thrombotic cerebral ischemia, Stroke 14:5–14, 1983.

58. Antiplatelet Trialist's Collaboration: Secondary prevention of vascular disease by prolonged antiplatelet treatment, Br Med J 296:320–331, 1988.

59. Hass WK et al: A randomized trial comparing ticlopidine hydrochloride with aspirin for the prevention of stroke in high-risk patients, N Engl J Med 321:501–507, 1989.

60. Miller VT and Hart RG: Heparin anticoagulation in acute brain ischemia, Stroke 22:7–11, 1987.

61. Sherman DG et al: Antithrombotic therapy for cerebrovascular disorders, Chest 59:241–246, 1986.

62. Putman SF and Adams HP Jr.: Usefulness of heparin in initial management of patients with recent transient ischemic attacks, Arch Neurol 42:960–962, 1985.

63. Duke RJ et al: Intravenous heparin for the prevention of stroke progression in acute partial stable stroke: a randomized controlled trial, Ann Intern Med 105:825–828, 1986.

64. Sloan MA: Thrombolysis and stroke — past and future, Arch Neurol 44:748–764, 1987.

65. Del Zoppo GJ: Thrombolytic therapy in cerebrovascular disease, Stroke 23:7–11, 1988.

66. Brott TG et al: Very early therapy for cerebral infarction with tissue plasminogen activator (tPA), Stroke 19:133, (abstract) 1988.

67. Nenci GG et al: Thrombolytic therapy for thromboembolism of vertebrobasilar artery, Angiology 34:561–571, 1983.

68. Fletcher AP et al: A pilot study of urokinase therapy in cerebral infarction, Stroke 7:135–142, 1976.

69. Aldrich MS, Sherman SA, and Greenberg HS: Cerebrovascular complications of streptokinase infusion, JAMA 253:1777–1779, 1985.

70. Kwaan HC, Dobbie JG, and Fethenhour CL: The use of anticoagulants and thrombolytic agents in occlusive retinal vascular disease. In Paoletti R and Sherry S editors: Thrombosis and urokinase, London, 1977, Academic Press.

71. Zeyner GL: Survey of progress: vascular recanalizing techniques in interventional neuroradiology, J Neurol 231:287–294, 1985.

72. Pentoxifylline Study Group: Pentoxifylline in acute ischemic stroke, Stroke 18:298, 1987.

73. Hossman V et al: Controlled trial of ancrod in ischemic stroke, Arch Neurol 40:803–808, 1983.

74. Huzzynski J et al: Double-blind controlled trial of the therapeutic effects of prostacyclin in patients with completed ischemic stroke, Stroke 16:810–814, 1985.

75. Hsu CY et al: Intravenous prostacyclin trial, Stroke 18:352–358, 1987.

SUGGESTED READINGS

Easton JD: Disorders of consciousness. In Stein JH, editor: Internal medicine, ed 1, Boston, 1983, Little, Brown & Co.

Emeads J: An approach to the comatose patient, Med Clin North Am 1:3076–3083.

Hamburger S, Rush DR, and Bosker G: Endocrine and metabolic emergencies, Bowie, Md, 1984, Robert J Brady Co.

Henry GL and Little N: Neurologic emergencies: a symptom orientated approach, New York, 1985, McGraw-Hill.

Hoffer ED: Coma and altered mental status. In Hoffer ED, editor: Emergency problems in the elderly, Oradell, NJ, 1985, Medical Economics Co, Inc.

Moy MM and Shaffer MA: Neurologic emergencies. In Judd RL, Warner CG, and Shaffer MA, editors: Geriatric emergencies, Rockville, Md, 1986, Aspen.

Needham CW: Neurosurgical signs, Springfield, Ill, 1986, Charles C Thomas Publisher.

Plum F and Posner J: Diagnosis of stupor and coma, ed 3, Philadelphia, 1980, FA Davis Co.

Ragland A: Hypoglycemia. In Tintinalli JE, Rothstein RJ, and Krome RL, editors: A study guide in emergency medicine, New York, 1985, McGraw-Hill.

Ragland A: Myxedema coma. In Tintinalli JE, Rothstein RJ, and Krome RL, editors: A study guide in emergency medicine, New York, 1985, McGraw-Hill.

Roy CW, Pentland B, and Miller JD: The causes and consequences of minor head injury in the elderly, Injury 17:220–223, 1986.

Svenson J: Obtundation in the elderly patient: presentation of a drug overdose, Am J Emerg Med 5:524–526, 1987.

SECTION
V

Cardiovascular Disease

Generalized Chest Pain

Dennis P. Price, M.D., F.A.C.E.P.

The elderly patient with chest pain may represent one of the more challenging diagnostic problems. Some basic assumptions regarding such pain should be made.

First, until an initial, even brief, evaluation of the patient is made by a physician, assume the worst possible cause for the pain. Knowing the severity, duration, and location are only a small part of the evaluation. Some seemingly minor pains have dangerous causes. Consequently, the patient should be seen immediately. This necessity for speed has been accentuated within the past 5 years because of the widespread use of thrombolytic agents and reperfusion strategies.[1] There is a compelling need for early therapy when indicated.

Second, after your initial evaluation, even if you feel there is no life-threatening cause for the patient's pain, assume that the potential exists and still maintain a high index of suspicion for the possibility of myocardial infarction.

Third, all complaints in some way represent a change in the pattern of the elderly patient's health, regardless of how chronic they may sound initially. For instance, the patient may have been having exertional pain for years, and initially you may see no change in its pattern. You then find that the patient has been more short of breath lately, experiences more dyspnea with exertion, and is unable to perform daily activities due to fatigue. The patient's pain pattern hasn't changed, but superimposed upon it is an angina equivalent. Understanding your elderly patient and the disease process, and assuming that a change has occurred in the patient's health pattern, will help you make the diagnosis.

DISEASE CLASSIFICATION — SPECIFICITY VERSUS URGENCY

The number of diseases associated with chest pain is great. Emergency evaluation is largely clinical; laboratory and other tests, however, may be helpful. We sometimes treat before obtaining a complete history or physical examination (i.e., impending cardiac or respiratory arrest, life-threatening arrhythmias, tension pneumothorax).

It follows then that a more useful method of classification would be based on urgency (see Table 12–1). For instance, those conditions that should be diagnosed immediately (i.e., within minutes) are myocardial infarction, acute aortic dissection, transection of the aorta (usually a history of severe injury), and tension pneumothorax. Others can be diagnosed within minutes to a few hours: pericarditis, nontension pneumothorax, pneumonia, and pulmonary embolism. Finally, there are those conditions that need no specific diagnosis urgently, such as myofascial pain, rib fracture, esophagitis, and so forth.

Reevaluation and Reassignment of Risk

The patient often requires more than just a history and physical examination to determine the risk associated with his pain. After an initial evaluation and assignment of risk, early, aggressive eliciting of other important facts must occur if the patient is to receive effective and efficient care.

Old charts, emergency department records, x-rays, and electrocardiograms (ECGs) are helpful, as well as clinical information accompanying such materials, such as previous complaints, blood pressures, and medicines.

The Patient's Family

A candid talk with the family may not only further define the patient's symptoms but may also shed light on nonmedical factors. The patient may have recently lost a spouse or may be worried about or seeking separation

Table 12–1   Degree of Urgency in Treating Chest Pain

Most urgent	Urgent	Nonurgent
Acute myocardial infarction	Pneumothorax (nontension)	Musculoskeletal pain
Aortic dissection	Pneumonia	Herpes zoster
Aortic transection	Pleurisy	Esophagitis
Tension pneumothorax	Pericarditis	
	Pulmonary embolism	

from the family because he or she feels like a burden to them. On the other hand, the family may have fears about the older patient's failing health.

The Physical Examination

The physical examination must focus on the following key points.

Vital signs. If there is any question of irregularity, the pulse should be taken apically. Premature beats, both atrial and potentially troublesome ventricular premature beats, may be missed if only the radial pulse is palpated. This is because the ejection fraction of the premature beat is usually small. This is particularly true of atrial fibrillation. It is not uncommon to have a radial pulse of 80 or 90 recorded and then to find, when you examine the patient, that the apical rate is between 130 and 150.

Blood pressure should be recorded in both upper extremities; marked differences may be your first clue to serious central pain syndromes. Differences may be your earliest clue to an aortic dissection.

The respiratory rate and pattern are likewise helpful. Inspiration is usually longer than expiration, and the rate is somewhere between 12 and 14. Tachypnea is commonly seen in moderately advanced states of shock, early in myocardial infarction, and often in vasovagal states with severe pain. This sign is a highly sensitive indicator of severe abnormalities, although unfortunately not specific.

The patient's temperature should be obtained per rectum. It is not uncommon to find a 2° to 3°C difference between oral and rectal temperatures. Smoking, techniques in taking the temperature, tachypnea, and states of hydration may all lead to errors in taking oral temperatures.

The physical exam should also make note of sweating (anticholinergic activity), color (oxygenation and hematocrit), and temperature of the skin (perfusion). Abnormalities of any of the above usually indicate serious disease and the need for measures such as placing the patient on a cardiac monitor, doing an ECG, and measuring arterial blood gases. In the elderly patient, try to perform these studies quickly and calmly so as not to add to the patient's general anxiety.

The rest of the exam starts from the neck down and includes five key points.

1. *Neck.* Examine the neck for jugular venous distension. The internal jugular venous system is probably the most reliable evidence of abnormality but the most difficult to read. However, if one is attempting to read elevated right ventricular filling pressures, it is acceptable to read the external jugular system. Carotid pulses should be palpated bilaterally for equality, upstroke (ejection fraction), and strength (core perfusion) and auscultated for murmurs. Be careful not to massage the carotid excessively, as this may inadvertently cause bradycardia.

2. *Lungs.* The lungs should be auscultated for rales and wheezes, which, if present, must be interpreted in relation to the cardiac exam. If rales and wheezes are associated with an S_3 gallop, they usually indicate elevated left ventricular pressure and primary cardiac disease. If no S_3 gallop is heard, rales and wheezes usually indicate intrinsic lung disease or congestive heart failure. One must also evaluate for signs of consolidation and effusion.

3. *Heart.* Probably the most important part of the cardiac exam is feeling for the apex beat. Lateral displacement indicates an enlarged or a displaced heart. You should also listen for adventitious sounds such as rubs. Murmurs should be noted as well, both their presence and absence.

4. *Abdomen.* The abdominal exam must be thorough. Note areas of tenderness, bowel sounds, size of the liver (tenderness of the liver may indicate congestive heart failure), abnormal masses and pulsations, and, most importantly, femoral pulses.

5. *Neurologic exam.* The neurologic findings associated with serious cardiovascular disease are usually not subtle. One should pay particular attention to mental status, the content of consciousness, the strength in the extremities, and the deep tendon reflexes. Usually, changes in these result from the effects of serious cardiovascular disease and sometimes from thyroid disease, which is mentioned elsewhere as a sometimes unsuspected cause of geriatric emergencies.

MYOCARDIAL ISCHEMIC SYNDROMES

Myocardial infarction. The pain of myocardial ischemia represents the most urgent pain to which a physician must respond (Table 12–2). The onset of infarction may be associated with bradyarrhythmias and tachyarrhythmias with secondary hypotension and its complications. These rhythms may also deteriorate to complete heart block or ventricular fibrillation. The first few hours after the infarction are the most dangerous in terms of arrhythmias and sudden death, and the most fertile for reperfusion therapies.[2,3]

The pain of myocardial infarction is usually localized in the center of the chest anteriorly and is described as squeezing, pressure-like, or choking. The classic patient may even give Levine's sign, which is a clenching of the

Table 12–2   Differential Diagnosis of Chest Pain

Disease	Characteristics	Physical findings	Laboratory evaluation
Myocardial ischemia	Pressure-like pain; risk factors may be present	Nonspecific	ECG* normal or ST-T wave changes
Aortic dissection Aortic transection Tension pneumothorax	Sudden onset of ripping pain; hypertensive history; no good response to morphine	Pulse defects common in proximal dissection; aortic regurgitation if valve ring deformed; look for signs of pericardial tamponade	Normal ECG Widened mediastinum on chest x-ray; aortic arteriography confirms diagnosis
Pericardial or pleural diseases	Stabbing-like chest pain; circumstances surrounding case aid in specific diagnosis	Pleural rub; pericardial three-component friction rub	Chest x-ray may show effusion, infiltrate, enlarged cardiac silhouette; ECG may show ST-T wave elevations diffusely
Pneumonia	Teeth-chattering chill; productive cough	Fever; signs of consolidation	Chest x-ray with suggestive infiltrate
Pulmonary embolism with hemorrhage	Sudden onset of dyspnea; correct clinical setting and predisposing factors	Tachypnea Right ventricular heave or S_3 gallop	Low PO_2; ECG with right ventricular strain pattern; chest x-ray may show infiltrate if hemorrhage is present
Pneumothorax	Sudden onset of pain and dyspnea	Decreased breath sounds over involved lung	Chest x-ray shows collapsed lung especially in expiratory film
Gastrointestinal	Past history usually suggestive; relationship to eating usually elicited	Exam may be normal; may show signs of peritoneal irritation or volume instability	Stool guaiac may be positive; oral cholecystogram, upper gastrointestinal series, endoscopy may be indicated to aid in diagnosis
Musculoskeletal	Pain diffused or localized; may be related to activity level	Areas of tenderness often found	X-ray may disclose abnormal calcifications, unsuspected fracture, and osteoporosis

*ECG = electrocardiogram.

fist in front of the sternum (though this is rare — less than 1%).

The elderly patient may not present such a classic picture. Previous somatic diseases, such as cervical arthritis, shoulder bursitis, and dental disease, may cause a referral of cardiac pain to different areas.[4] This is thought to occur through a mechanism of facilitation, whereby pain impulses follow previous pathways established by somatic pain stimulations. Previous somatic pain thus alters the pattern of visceral (cardiac) pain.

Atypical symptoms may also cause myocardial infarction to go unrecognized in the elderly. In a retrospective study, Uretsky and colleagues studied patients with documented myocardial infarctions admitted to the Boston City Hospital and found that 26 of the 102 patients did not present with symptoms of chest pain. The mean age of these patients was 69.1 years as compared to 58.7 years for the more typical group. The most frequent complaints were dyspnea — seen in 14 patients, abdominal or upper gastric distress — seen in 5 patients, and fatigue — seen in 4 patients. This group had a significantly greater median delay between the onset of symptoms and 1) arrival at the hospital, 2) examination by a physician in the emergency department, 3) diagnosis of possible myocardial infarction, and 4) transfer from the emergency department

to the intensive care unit. Mortality in this atypical myocardial infarction group was 50%, compared with 18% in the group with chest pain.[5]

The history of the patient just prior to the onset of symptoms is also helpful. Had he become increasingly tired? Had she been having more shortness of breath? Had paroxysmal nocturnal dyspnea increased? All of these changes may be indicative of ischemic disease.

One should also look for associated symptoms of infarction such as nausea, vomiting, sweating, light-headedness, eructation, and syncope. Of course, as with patients of all ages, the traditional coronary disease risk factors such as hypertension, abnormal lipid profile, and positive family history of coronary disease should be determined.

On physical exam, one must pay careful attention to the blood pressure. Frequently, it is elevated during the early stages of myocardial infarction; however, it may also be low. If the patient is driven by a predominantly catecholamine response, the pulse will be elevated. If the patient is exhibiting a vasovagal reaction to myocardial ischemia, the blood pressure and pulse may be low. Make note of jugular venous distension, the pulses in both carotids and the patient's extremities, murmurs, and the presence of an S_3 or S_4 gallop.

If you think a patient has sustained a myocardial infarction, the first laboratory study to do is an ECG. In many cases of myocardial infarction, abnormalities on an ECG may only develop during the course of the patient's hospital stay. If the patient is a candidate for thrombolytic therapy, a complete laboratory examination, including tests of clotting ability and liver function, is needed. See Chapter 14 for details of administration.

Pain can be treated with intravenous morphine sulfate if there are no contraindications. Enough morphine should be administered to reduce the individual's pain by 80% or 90%. Allow the patient to titrate his or her own morphine dose; that is, it should be reduced to the level where the patient's anxiety is decreased. This allows for easier evaluation and is easily reversed with naloxone hydrochloride (Narcan).

Administer intravenous lidocaine (Xylocaine) even in the absence of signs of ventricular irritability, since the drug is safe and effective in reducing the incidence of ventricular fibrillation.[6,7] This is particularly important because classic warning arrhythmias may not occur before all episodes of ventricular fibrillation, or they may occur almost concurrently with the onset of ventricular fibrillation.[8]

The loading dose of lidocaine should be adjusted so that the patient receives 200 mg in 20 minutes: 100 mg immediately and then, 20 minutes later, another 100 mg if there were no complications from the initial dose. Also start a continuous drip with the first dose of lidocaine at 2 to 3 mg per minute. In cases of congestive heart failure, shock, and liver disease and in patients over 70 years of age, the loading dose should be reduced by 50%, and infusion rates should be between 1 and 2 mg per minute.

Unstable angina. The elderly patient with angina who presents with chest pain must be evaluated carefully. Any change in the pattern of the patient's angina must be sought. This includes both frequency and duration of the attacks, the level of activity bringing on the attacks, dyspnea associated with the angina, and increasing fatigue.

Other precipitating causes of ischemic pain must be sought, such as low-output states as seen with arrhythmias, hypovolemia from various causes, uncontrolled hypertension with concomitant increase in the afterload to the left ventricle, and worsening congestive heart failure.

Aortic dissection. Chronic stress placed on the aortic wall, perhaps from long-standing hypertension and age, causes changes in the aorta wall. These changes consist of deterioration of the collagen and elastic tissue with cystic changes. These changes are seen in some degree in all people as they age but are usually marked in people with aortic dissection.

An aortic dissection begins with a tear of the intimal lining of the aorta and subsequent bleeding into the medial layer or sometimes just from a spontaneous bleed into the media.

The patient commonly presents with pain that is immediately severe, in contrast to an acute myocardial infarction, which has a slightly longer initial course. The patient may describe the pain as tearing or ripping. He may have nausea, vomiting, sweating, and a syncopal episode. If the dissection is proximal, just distal to the aortic valve, most of the pain will be anterior. If distal dissection occurs, the pain may be felt in the upper back. Characteristically, the pain is not relieved with the usual doses of morphine.

The physical exam will usually disclose hypertension and tachycardia. Hypotension with this disease usually indicates pericardial tamponade or rupture through the adventitial layer of the aorta with subsequent hypovolemia. With proximal dissection, pulse losses may occur as the hematoma dissects along through the aorta. Careful palpation of carotid, brachial, radial, and femoral pulses should be done repeatedly and recorded. This is most accurately done by taking the blood pressure in the extremity. Special attention should be paid to murmurs, especially aortic regurgitation secondary to deformation of the valve ring by the hematoma. A friction rub may be caused by blood leaking into the pericardial sac.

The ECG may show signs of hypertension such as left ventricular hypertrophy. Classically, there will be no signs of acute infarction unless the coronary os has become obliterated by dissection. The chest x-ray may show a widened mediastinum and abnormalities of the aortic silhouette, and a left pleural effusion may be found, indicating blood in the left pleural space. The diagnosis is confirmed by aortic arteriography.

Pericarditis. The causes of pericarditis are numerous: viral, bacterial, fungal, parasitic, neoplastic, and uremic. It may be secondary to drug use, trauma, connective tissue disease, or irradiation of the chest for tumors. In addition, it may be due to hemorrhage resulting from anticoagulant therapy and is often seen 2 to 4 weeks after an acute myocardial infarction (Dressler's syndrome).

The pain may be pleuritic — stabbing in nature and varying with respiration — or similar to that of myocardial infarction. It may be intermittent and often is accentuated or alleviated by positional changes. Classically, it is improved by leaning forward.

Hypotension may indicate decreased filling of the cardiac chambers secondary to cardiac tamponade. The physician should be on the alert for signs of pulsus paradoxus. This is easily determined by having the patient breathe normally and listening for the Korotkoff sounds. In the normal individual, they initially will be interrupted during inspiration for about 5 mm Hg before being heard continuously during inspiration and expiration. The difference between the discontinuous and continuous Korotkoff sounds is the pulsus paradoxus. A difference of more than 10 mm Hg is considered abnormal. Abnormalities may be seen with cardiac tamponade, asthma, and congestive heart failure. Pericarditis that produces a large amount of fluid in a short time is more likely to cause problems with tamponade than an effusion that develops slowly; the latter gives the pericardium time to compensate and stretch. Jugular venous distension may be noted if an effusion is interfering with cardiac filling.

A three-component friction rub is often heard when the patient sits forward during either forced inspiration or expiration, and the stethoscope is pressed firmly on the chest. When there is only one component to the rub, it may indicate a short systolic murmur and not a rub at all. The rub may be transient, which is quite characteristic of the disease.

The ECG shows diffuse ST-T wave elevation in a nonfocal distribution. The chest x-ray may show pleural effusions or infiltrates if the pleura is involved as well. The cardiac silhouette may be enlarged if an effusion is present.

Pleuritic pain. The causes of pleuritic pain are similar to those of pericardial pain. There are, however, two — namely, pneumonia and pulmonary embolism — that deserve particular attention in the elderly.

Most pleuritic pain is sharp, stabbing, and surprisingly localized. The patient may describe shortness of breath rather than pain; however, careful questioning may reveal that pain is causing her to avoid taking a deep breath. True dyspnea suggests involvement of the pulmonary parenchyma or impingement on the parenchyma such as from an effusion. Chills and productive cough suggest an infection. Sudden onset of dyspnea suggests pulmonary embolism.

Pulmonary embolism with hemorrhage (hence the pleuritic pain) is usually seen in individuals who have been on bed rest, have incompetent valves in the venous system of their legs, are postoperative, have hemiplegia, have sustained local trauma, or have heart failure.

The physical examination may reveal a temperature elevation suggesting a viral or bacterial pneumonia. The lung exam may disclose signs of consolidation such as increased breath sounds; localized, wet rales; and dullness to percussion over the involved area. You may also find signs of pleural effusion, namely, decreased breath sounds at the bases, e to a changes above the effusion, as well as dullness over the effusion.

Laboratory tests are essential in working through the differential diagnosis of pleuritic chest pain. The chest x-ray should be obtained in both the posterior-anterior and lateral projections; if an effusion is present or suspected, decubitus films are needed. Arterial blood gases may not only aid in the differential diagnosis but indicate the need for oxygen therapy; thus, tests should be obtained early in the course of the patient's evaluation. If the patient is coughing up sputum, a Gram stain may reveal a predominant organism that would dictate antibiotic therapy. A ventilation/perfusion scan is indicated if a pulmonary embolism is suspected.

Pneumothorax. Normally, a negative atmospheric pressure in the intrapleural space holds the lung adjacent to the parietal pleura. When air enters the pleural space, secondary to rupture of an emphysematous bleb, or trauma, the lung tends to collapse. The amount of collapse correlates with the amount of air that has entered the space.

The symptoms generally are dyspnea and pleuritic pain over the involved lung field. However, in the elderly, pneumothorax may present as an acute respiratory decompensation. Blood pressure and pulse are generally normal. The diagnosis is confirmed by chest x-ray done in both a posterior-anterior and lateral projection. The posterior-anterior film must be done in both inspiration and expiration. The latter is important so that a subtle pneumothorax is not missed. An expiration film makes the pneumothorax easier to see because the vasculature is more prominent in a less expanded lung. Also, there is less negative intrapleural pressure at the end of expiration.

Esophagitis. Esophagitis presents as retrosternal pain described as burning and may be associated with a sour taste in the mouth. The pain may radiate, starting in the epigastric area and moving upwards. The condition is usually made worse by bending over or lying down and may be more common after a heavy meal.

The physical exam is generally unrewarding. Characteristically, pain is immediately relieved with antacids. Using a mixture of antacids and 2 to 3 ml 2% viscous lidocaine has been successful. Of course, a history must be highly suggestive of esophagitis before relying on the information obtained from an antacid challenge because of the possibility of the placebo effect.

Peptic ulcer. Gastric ulcers increase in incidence in the older population, reaching a peak about the sixth decade. The symptoms are less well defined than with duodenal ulcer. Duodenal ulcer symptoms typically improve after eating and with antacids. Gastric ulcers, on the other hand, may actually be worsened with eating. The pain is usually in the epigastric region and described as burning and gnawing.

In uncomplicated disease, the physical exam generally reveals normal vital signs and, at times, some mild epigastric tenderness. The rectal exam, which should be done in all cases where peptic ulcer is suspected, will sometimes reveal heme-positive stool and, in severe cases, melena.

Tachycardia or orthostatic blood pressure changes with assuming the upright position — that is, a pulse rise of 30 or greater or systolic blood pressure drop of 20 to 30 mm Hg after 1 minute of standing — suggest volume depletion and serious bleeding.[9]

Gallbladder disease. The incidence of gallstones increases with age and must be considered as a cause of chest pain in the elderly patient. The pain of gallbladder disease is due to obstruction of either the cystic or the common duct. The pain is sudden in onset, reaches its maximum intensity quickly, and is often associated with nausea and vomiting. If the stone passes or falls back into the gallbladder, the pain subsides. The physical exam at that time may reveal only mild or no right upper quadrant tenderness. If the stone stays impacted in the cystic duct or the common bile duct, the pain will continue. On exam you may be able to feel tenderness or a mass in the right upper quadrant.

Musculoskeletal pain. Various musculoskeletal conditions are associated with chest pain, such as bursitis and arthritis of the shoulders. Fractures resulting from osteoporosis are another source of pain. If the pain is caused by a fracture, the onset is abrupt; arthritis and bursitis are more vague in onset.

The physical exam may disclose tenderness in an area. Of course, finding such an area does not rule out cardiac disease, so if the history is suggestive of other causes, further evaluation is warranted.

Skin. The incidence of herpes zoster, another disease commonly seen in the elderly, increases with age. The pain is burning or aching and usually is in a dermatome distribution. The rash may occur along with the symptoms or as late as 4 to 5 days after the onset of the symptoms. The pain, which may be extremely severe, may occur days, weeks, or months after the rash (postherpetic neuralgia).

REFERENCES

1. Grines CL and O'Neill WW: Emergency treatment and triage strategies for acute myocardial infarction in the reperfusion era. In Schwartz GR, editor: Emergency medicine: the essential update, Philadelphia, 1989, WB Saunders Co, p 17.
2. Simons ML et al: Improved survival after early thrombolysis in acute myocardial infarction, Lancet 2:578, 1985.
3. Gruppo Italiano per lo Studio della Streptochinasi nell Infarcto Miocardico (GISSI): Effectiveness of intravenous thrombolytic treatment in acute myocardial infarction, Lancet 1:397, 1986.
4. Henry JA: Cardiac pain referred to site of previously experienced somatic pain, Br Med J 2:1605–1606, 1978.
5. Uretsky BF et al: Symptomatic myocardial infarction without chest pain: prevalence and clinical course, Am J Cardiol 40:498–503, 1977.
6. Lie KL, Wellens HJ, and Durrer D: Lidocaine in the prevention of primary ventricular fibrillation: a double-blind randomized study of 212 consecutive patients, N Engl J Med 291:1324, 1974.
7. Harrison DC: Should lidocaine be administered routinely to all patients after acute myocardial infarction? Circulation 58:581–584, 1978.
8. Lie KL, Wellens HJ, and Durrer D: Characteristics and predictability of primary ventricular fibrillation, Eur J Cardiol 1:379, 1974.
9. Knopp R, Claypool R, and Leonardi D: Use of the tilt test in measuring acute blood loss, Ann Emerg Med 9:72–75, 1980.

SUGGESTED READINGS

Alonzo AA, Simon AB, and Feinleib M: Prodromata of myocardial infarction and sudden death, Circulation 52:1056–1062, 1969.
Baughman DJ: Pain of myocardial infarction reproduced by precordial palpation, JAMA 241:1328, 1979.
Dallen JE et al: Pulmonary embolism, pulmonary hemorrhage and pulmonary infarction, N Engl J Med 296:1431–1435, 1977.
Darsee JR: Eructonesius without inferior myocardial infarction, N Engl J Med 298:221–222, 1978.
Solomon HA, Edwards AL, and Killip T: Prodromata in acute myocardial infarction, Circulation 52:463–471, 1969.
Stowers M and Short D: Warning symptoms before major myocardial infarction, Br Heart J 32:833–838, 1970.

Assessment and Detection of Acute Coronary Ischemia

Gideon Bosker, M.D., F.A.C.E.P., **Jeffrey S. Jones**, M.D.,
Steven Romisher, M.D., **and Dennis P. Price**, M.D., F.A.C.E.P.

Assessment of myocardial infarction

History and physical examination

   Warning symptoms

   Silent myocardial infarction

The electrocardiogram in the geriatric patient

   Background

   Electrocardiogram

Cardiac syncope

Cardiac enzymes

Differential diagnosis

Disposition and triage

The elderly patient with acute coronary ischemia represents one of the most challenging diagnostic problems in emergency medicine. In the previous chapter the importance of rapid diagnosis of myocardial infarction was emphasized because of the possibilities of reperfusion therapies. The goal of the emergency department evaluation is to determine which of three triage options — a coronary care unit, an intermediate care unit, or discharge — is most appropriate when there is a possibility that a patient is having an acute myocardial infarction.[1] Until an initial, even brief, evaluation of the patient is made by a physician, the clinician must assume the worst possible cause for the chest pain. Knowing the severity, duration, and location of the pain syndrome is only a small part of the entire evaluation. Since some seemingly minor pains have dangerous etiologies, the elderly patient with chest pain should be seen immediately.

When a patient presents to the emergency department with acute chest pain or other manifestations of acute coronary ischemia, the physician is faced with two related but separate issues. First, the diagnosis must be determined as accurately as possible. Second, a quick decision must be made about whether to admit the patient to the hospital.[2] Since the diagnosis of myocardial ischemia may remain uncertain even after the history, physical examination, and emergency laboratory tests have been evaluated, the disposition is often aided by the knowledge of differential diagnostic possibilities, prognostic implications of electrocardiogram (ECG) findings, and available triage options.

The variable presentation of acute myocardial infarction (MI) in the elderly is generally well recognized, with the absence of chest pain and increased incidence of pulmonary symptoms reported to be characteristic.[3-5] As a rule, however, all chest complaints in the elderly should be considered to represent a change in the pattern of the patient's health, regardless of how chronic these complaints may seem initially. For instance, an elderly patient may have been experiencing exertional pain for years, and, initially, the clinician may detect no change in its pattern. Later, however, the emergency physician may discover that the patient has been more short of breath lately, has experienced more dyspnea on exertion (DOE), and is unable to perform daily duties due to fatigue. In such cases, the patient's pain pattern has not changed, but superimposed on it may be the anginal equivalent. In addition, the elderly are prone to silent MI and have altered presentations and well-described prodromal symptoms that can be recognized by the astute clinician. This chapter focuses on assessing the elderly patient with chest pain, sifting out the disease processes that produce this symptom, and reviewing the assessment and triage of acute coronary ischemia in the elderly. Table 12–2 offers useful information to assist a differential diagnosis.

ASSESSMENT OF MYOCARDIAL INFARCTION

One of the most important considerations in assessing coronary ischemia in the elderly is whether the patient has a previous history of MI or angina pectoris.[6] If such a history can be elicited, the clinician should direct his or her questioning to determine how the patient's current pain level compares with those of previous episodes. For example, is the pain the same as that of a previous MI? Is the pain similar to the patient's chronic anginal pattern but worse in intensity, duration, or frequency, or does it fail to respond to the usual treatment? Is there new onset of shortness of breath or DOE? If the answer to one of these questions is yes, then there is little doubt that the patient has worsening ischemic heart disease and that a new myocardial infarction is a compelling possibility.

In those elderly patients presenting with chest discomfort, the pain of myocardial infarction is usually localized in the center of the chest anteriorly and is described as squeezing, pressure-like, or choking.[7] The classic patient may even produce Levine's sign, which is a clenching of the fist in front of the sternum. This finding occurs in less than 1% of patients.[2] A significant percentage of elderly patients, however, may not present with such a classic picture (Figure 13–1).

Atypical symptoms may also cause myocardial infarction to go unrecognized in the elderly. In a retrospective study, researchers documented people with myocardial infarctions who were admitted to Boston City Hospital and found that 25%[8-10] of those patients did not present with symptoms of chest pain as their initial chief complaint. The mean age of patients presenting without chest pain was 69 years old, compared to 58 years for the more typical group. The most frequent complaints for the atypical group were dyspnea, abdominal or epigastric distress, and fatigue. In addition, the elderly group had a significantly greater median delay between the onset of symptoms and 1) arrival at the hospital; 2) examination by a physician in the emergency department; 3) diagnosis of possible MI; and 4) transfer from the emergency department to the intensive care unit. Mortality in this atypical MI group was 50% compared with 18% in the group with chest pain.[9,10]

A comprehensive study[6] of 777 elderly hospitalized patients suggests that the spectrum of presentation changes significantly with increasing age. Based on those findings, the clinician should be aware that chest pain and discomfort are less frequently reported, although present in the majority of patients up to the age of 85 years. In those over 85, shortness of breath is more common than chest pain. Syncope, stroke, and acute confusion become more common in patients over 75 and are often the *sole* presenting symptom in patients over the age of 85. Shortness of breath, although the most frequently reported symptom in patients over the age of 85, is equally common at all ages and occurs in about 30 to 34% of all elderly patients studied.[5] Thus, in patients aged 85 years or over, an atypical presentation of myo-

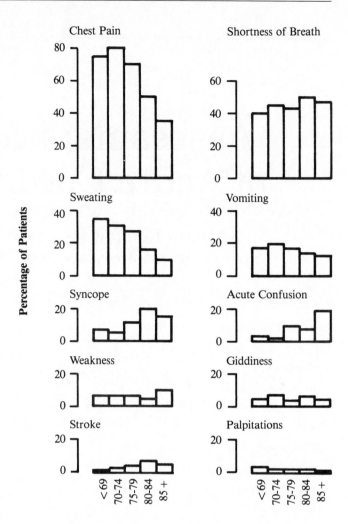

Figure 13–1 Presenting symptoms of acute myocardial infarction in elderly patients. (Reprinted with permission from Bayer J et al: J Am Geriatr Soc 34:263–266, 1986.)

cardial infarction is the rule. Consequently, in the "elder" elderly, the emergency department physician should screen for myocardial ischemia in virtually all acutely ill patients with pulmonary, cardiac, or neurologic abnormalities.

Silent myocardial ischemia is increasingly being recognized in even the younger patient with coronary artery disease. With recent advances in frequency-modulated and amplitude-modulated ambulatory ECG monitoring (which measure myocardial ischemia through detection of ST-segment depression with a 98% specificity), we have become aware that over 75% of all ischemic episodes in all patients with coronary artery disease are asymptomatic.[2] This has led to a new realization that angina pectoris is just *one component* of what is now called the *total ischemic burden* of the heart. There is strong evidence to suggest that the total ischemic burden, especially in the elderly, is the best predictor of patient outcome in myocardial ischemia.

Part of the explanation for silent myocardial ischemia relates to another newly described concept called the *ischemic cascade*. Studies in human patients undergoing percutaneous transluminal angioplasty (PTCA) show a predictable sequence of events in the ischemic myocardium. There is initially a supply-demand imbalance, followed by ventricular diastolic dysfunction with increased wall stiffness and elevated end-diastolic pressures (leading to the symptom of dyspnea). This is predictably followed by ventricular systolic dysfunction with hypokinesis on the ventriculogram. The latter is followed by the development of ST-segment abnormalities. It is only after the development of the ST-segment abnormalities that angina (chest pain) develops and, at that, not in all patients.

Therefore, we now know that pain is a late and insensitive feature of myocardial ischemia, and the pathophysiologic events preceding it occur much more frequently and in equal severity with or without pain.

If we correlate these findings with the knowledge that the aging heart "normally" exhibits a progressive impairment to diastolic filling (due to increasing wall stiffness), we can begin to understand the much higher incidence of symptoms such as dyspnea, fatigue, and syncope in the elderly patient. This patient cannot tolerate moving down the ischemic cascade and develops symptoms so powerful that the variable chest pain that might otherwise be noticed by a younger counterpart is either not noticed or is obscured and not reported.

The altered presentation of MI is summarized in Table 13-1. Chest pain was the most frequently reported symptom and was present in the majority of patients in all age groups. There was, however, a fall in the frequency of reports of classical chest pain as the patients became older.[5,11] In the oldest age group, this symptom was replaced by shortness of breath. Sweating and vomiting were uncommon in the absence of chest pain, and both were less frequently reported with increasing age. Syncope, acute confusion, or stroke became increasingly common in those over the age of 70 and were encountered in 14.9 to 21% of elderly patients in this age group.[5]

Many theories have been advanced to explain the absence of pain in MI and the increasing frequency of shortness of breath in the elderly.[12] It is hypothesized that a failure in the perception of pain in the elderly may be due to a higher pain threshold, autonomic dysfunction, damage to sensory autonomic fibers from previous myocardial ischemia, or cortical failure secondary to cerebrovascular or other neurologic disease. The decreasing incidence of sweating with increasing age and its usual association with chest pain suggests that autonomic function may indeed have a significant influence on the symptomatology of these elderly patients. Alternatively, the presence of chest pain may be overshadowed by the overwhelming intensity of other symptoms, such as severe shortness of breath, or the problem may simply be a failure of expression due to stroke, poor memory, or confusion.[13]

Table 13–1   Presentation of Myocardial Infarction in the Elderly

Symptom	< 70 (N = 125) No.	%	70–74 (N = 243) No.	%	75–79 (N = 181) No.	%	80–84 (N = 140) No.	%	85+ (N = 88) No.	%	Total (N = 777) No.	%	Statistical significance*
Chest pain	95	(76.0)	193	(79.4)	123	(67.9)	71	(50.7)	33	(37.5)	515	(66.3)	< .0001
Shortness of breath	47	(37.6)	104	(42.8)	74	(40.9)	66	(47.1)	38	(43.2)	329	(42.4)	NS†
	13	(10.5)	27		24		31		23		118		
Syncope	11	(8.8)	20	(8.2)	27	(14.9)	30	(21.4)	16	(18.0)	104	(13.4)	< .005
	5		10		20		21		16		72		
Stroke	2	(1.6)	5	(2.1)	9	(5.0)	12	(8.6)	6	(6.8)	34	(4.4)	< .02
	2		5		7		12		6		32		
Acute confusion	4	(3.2)	6	(2.5)	15	(8.3)	11	(7.9)	17	(19.3)	53	(6.8)	< .0001
	3		4		13		11		15		46		
Weakness	9	(7.2)	17	(7.0)	14	(7.7)	8	(5.7)	9	(10.2)	57	(7.3)	NS
	7		7		9		7		6		36		
Giddiness	7	(5.6)	16	(6.6)	7	(3.9)	7	(5.0)	4	(4.5)	41	(5.3)	NS
	4		3		2		5		4		18		
Palpitations	5	(4.0)	4	(1.6)	3	(1.7)	2	(1.4)	1	(1.1)	15	(1.9)	NS
	0		1		1		1		1		4		
Vomiting	23	(18.4)	51	(21.0)	33	(18.2)	24	(17.1)	14	(15.9)	145	(18.7)	NS
	0		6		7		8		7		28		
Sweating	45	(36.0)	79	(32.5)	49	(27.1)	24	(17.1)	12	(13.6)	209	(26.9)	< .0001
	3		5		6		2		2		18		
Arterial embolus	1	(0.8)	2	(0.8)	0		0		0		3	(0.4)	NS
	1		2		0		0		0		3		
Silent	2	(1.6)	5	(2.1)	3	(1.8)	4	(2.8)	3	(3.3)	17	(2.2)	NS

From Bayer AJ: Changing presentation of myocardial infarction with increasing old age, J Am Geriatr Soc 34:263–266, 1986.

*P value reflects change in symptoms as a function of age.

†NS = not significant.

HISTORY AND PHYSICAL EXAMINATION

The history of the elderly patient just prior to the onset of symptoms is especially helpful in elucidating coronary ischemia. A number of key historical points will set the stage for subsequent evaluation. Has the patient become increasingly tired? Has there been more shortness of breath? Has paroxysmal nocturnal dyspnea or dyspnea on exertion increased? Since these alterations in clinical status may represent anginal equivalents in the elderly, all of these changes may be indicative of coronary ischemia. In addition, you should ask about recent changes in medications — including withdrawal of beta-blockers or calcium channel blockers — that might precipitate cardiac failure and secondary myocardial ischemia.[14]

The clinician should also look for associated symptoms of infarction such as vomiting, lightheadedness, and syncope. On physical examination, you should pay careful attention to the blood pressure. Frequently, it is elevated during the early stages of infarction; however, it may also be low. If the patient is driven by a predominantly catecholamine response, the pulse will be elevated. If the patient is exhibiting a vasovagal reaction to inferior myocardial infarction, the blood pressure may be inordinately low. Make note also of jugular venous distension and pulses in both carotids and in the extremities. The presence of murmurs, especially mitral insufficiency associated with papillary muscle dysfunction — which carries an ominous prognosis — and the presence of an S_3 or S_4 gallop should be noted. In addition to obtaining a detailed history of signs and symptoms, the emergency evaluation of elderly patients also includes ECG, chest x-ray, creatine kinase (CK), electrolytes, and complete blood count (CBC).

Warning Symptoms

It is well known that up to 55%[16] of elderly patients who develop documented MI experienced specific symptoms days or weeks before the actual event. Given the high incidence of prodromal complaints, it is important that the clinician be aware of the specific nature of warning symptoms in elderly patients prior to documented MI. Maintaining a high index of suspicion for prodromal symptoms associated with myocardial ischemia gives ground for the hope that MI might be averted in many instances and that inappropriate discharges from the emergency department can be minimized.

To achieve this, the clinician should recognize the early symptoms of coronary heart disease. In one large study,[16] 180 patients in the hospital with proven MI were questioned during their recovery about unusual symptoms they experienced during the 2 months prior to the diagnosis of infarction. Approximately 70%[16] of these patients admitted to such symptoms, and more than half said they had experienced either the onset or an inten-

sification of attacks of chest pain. Other symptoms were described by 13% of the patients, particularly tiredness and breathlessness. Of the original group, 37% of the patients received only reassurance.[16] (See Figure 13–2.)

About half of these patients described pain extending across the chest. This usually occurred at the midsternal level, but sometimes it occurred above and, occasionally, below. Almost one third of this group described the prodromal pain as being localized in the midline. In nearly half of the patients, the prodromal pain occurred only on effort and was relieved by rest. In 30%, it had a crescendo course, becoming progressively more easily induced, more frequent, more severe, and more widespread until it culminated in the episode that finally necessitated admission to the emergency department. This was especially true of those patients who had suffered from long-standing angina. In most patients, the pain occurred mainly on effort, though sometimes at rest, and in 20% of the entire group, the attacks occurred mainly at rest; sometimes these attacks were brief but in nearly half the cases they lasted for over 30 minutes. The incidence of prodromal symptoms was approximately the same in those patients with previous infarction and those without and occurred in equal frequency in those with and without a history of chronic angina pectoris.

More than 33% of the patients with prodromal cardiac pain consulted their physicians about their symptoms in the month preceding admission.[16] Most were advised to rest and did so. Although MI is widely believed to strike without warning, this study[16] suggests that the clinician should be aware that the majority of patients admitted to the hospital through the emergency department for MI are able to recall premonitory symptoms extending for days and often weeks before admission. The fact that over one third of patients with prodromal cardiac pain

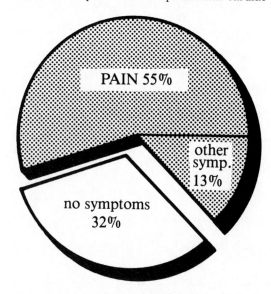

Figure 13–2 Percentage of elderly patients with symptoms of prodromal pain prior to diagnosis of myocardial infarction. (Reprinted with permission from Br Heart J 32:833–838, 1970.)

who consulted with physicians received only reassurance, reflects the difficulty of diagnosing coronary artery disease even when an ECG is freely available.

Silent Myocardial Infarction

As discussed earlier, the diagnosis of MI in the elderly is easily missed.[17] Of patients admitted to the hospital, almost 30% have atypical presenting features and in some patients the event is completely silent.[9,18,19] In the Framingham study,[10] more than 25% of MIs in all age groups were discovered only through the appearance of new diagnostic ECG evidence during routine biennial ECG examinations. Of these unrecognized infarctions, almost half were "silent," while the remainder were associated with atypical symptoms. The proportion of all infarcts that were unrecognized was higher in older women and men. Interestingly, unrecognized — or "silent" — infarctions were just as likely as recognized ones to cause death, heart failure, or stroke, which has important prognostic and triage implications for the emergency physician. Recurrent infarctions were more likely to be recognized than were first infarctions.

Among patients 75 years or older, 39% had infarctions that were unrecognized.[9] Thus, all chest discomfort syndromes, however undramatic, should be viewed as possibly cardiac in origin, and this message needs to be transmitted to the population at large in terms that do not cause undue alarm. The incidence of mortality from MI in the elderly increases with age; recognition of an MI, however, becomes more difficult. Since accurate diagnosis must precede appropriate treatment, it is clear that the emergency physician must be careful not to miss atypical presentations.

THE ELECTROCARDIOGRAM IN THE GERIATRIC PATIENT

Background

Despite the decline in cardiovascular mortality during the past decade, acute MI still claims over 600,000 lives annually; at least half of these deaths occur in individuals aged 65 years or older.[20] Published data indicate that over 30% of elderly subjects with ECG evidence of MI failed to manifest clinically[21] and less than 20% of elderly patients with acute infarction present with classic symptoms. Most symptoms, thus, were secondary to impaired cardiovascular function, resulting in low cardiac output or congestive heart failure.[17]

Electrocardiogram

Electrocardiographic diagnosis of acute infarction may be complicated by preexisting left bundle branch block (LBBB), prior infarctions, cardiac amyloidosis, emphysema, or chest deformities.[22-24] Septal infarction is par-

ticularly difficult to diagnose due to the usual reduction of the first vector of heart activation, resulting from senile infraseptal fibrosis. This is manifested by the disappearance of the R wave in V_1 and V_2 and the Q wave in aVL, V_5, and V_6. Finally, the ST segment and T-wave abnormalities may be the only ECG signs of nontransmural infarction; however, their presence should be interpreted with caution in elderly subjects, since they may be associated with left ventricular hypertrophy, paced rhythm, and other nonacute conditions.[23,24]

There are a number of characteristics in electrocardiograms of the aging of which the clinician must be aware when assessing patients with acute chest pain and electrocardiographic abnormalities. Although the resting heart rate falls little with age, there is a general decrease in the heart rate response to exercise.[23] Most elderly people experience a decline in the number of pacemaker cells in the SA node[25]; this change can be as dramatic as an 80% loss of nodal cells between the ages of 60 and 75 years.[25] Although pronounced changes in the atrioventricular (AV) node have not been described, there are several age-related changes seen in the bundle of His. These include a loss of specialized muscle cells and an increase in fibrous and adipose tissue depositions, as well as amyloid infiltration.[20]

In view of the degenerative changes that occur in the cardiac conduction system with aging, it is not surprising that several features of the ECG are altered in the elderly, many of which have important clinical implications. These changes involve the duration of the PR-QT intervals, orientation of the electrical axis, duration and morphology of the atrial and ventricular complexes, and characteristics of the ventricular repolarization. (See Table 13–2.) To accurately interpret any ECG in an elderly patient with chest pain, it is important to establish a reasonable baseline.

Table 13–2 Characteristics of Electrocardiograms in the Aging

1. The incidence of abnormal ECG increases with age and heart disease.
2. Probable insignificant electrocardiographic (ECG) findings in the elderly include left axis deviation without evidence of left anterior hemiblock, lower wave amplitudes, longer intervals, and isolated premature contractions.
3. T-wave inversions and ST segment depression have too many noncardiac causes to be specific.
4. Bradycardias (sinus bradycardia, sinus arrest, exit block, and second- or third-degree atrioventricular block) are rare in normal subjects.
5. The specific ECG abnormalities that correlate strongly with heart disease are atrial fibrillation, left bundle branch block, and nonspecific intraventricular conduction delay.
6. Myocardial infarction patterns, left anterior hemiblock, and right bundle branch block do not correlate with the presence of clinical disease but may reflect anatomic disease.
7. With the exception of left ventricular hypertrophy, prognosis for a specific ECG abnormality remains that of the underlying disease.

P Wave

P-wave notching, slurring, and loss of amplitude are so common in the aged that they lose diagnostic significance when interpreting ECGs in elderly patients being evaluated for MI. In addition, the percentage of missing P waves increases with age.

First-Degree Atrioventricular Block

All available data indicate that the prevalence of first-degree AV block, defined as a PR interval greater than 0.21 second, increases with age.[26] In a broad range of geriatric patients, the prevalence is approximately 10%, but in nonagenarians, the prevalence rises to 35%.[23-26] A prolonged PR interval in these patients is usually not associated with clinical heart disease, and when first-degree AV block is an isolated finding, it should not affect disposition of patients with chest pain.

QRS Complex

The duration of the QRS interval tends to be greater in the aged, owing to slight slowing of the conduction system, but it is never prolonged to 0.12 second or longer in the absence of a bundle branch block.

Ventricular Hypertrophy

Left ventricular hypertrophy (LVH) is one of the most common ECG abnormalities in the elderly. The actual prevalence ranges from 1% to 40% depending on the criteria used in diagnosis. The Framingham study indicated that electrocardiographic evidence of LVH increased in frequency with age and paralleled the distribution of systemic hypertension. The data also suggested that LVH is a poor prognostic sign, even in the absence of clinical evidence of heart disease.

Bundle Branch Block

The overall prevalence of bundle branch block in young military populations is considerably less than 1%, while in the elderly the prevalence is as high as 42%.[29] In almost all series of elderly patients, right bundle branch block (RBBB) occurs slightly more often than LBBB. In a collected series of aged persons, researchers have found left anterior hemiblock (LAH) in 36%, RBBB in 6%, and LBBB in 3% of all subjects studied.[24-26]

The prognosis of bundle branch block depends on its etiology. In the elderly, bundle branch block is usually due to fibrocalcific changes in the conduction system rather than to ischemic heart disease. Persons with isolated LBBB have been shown to have a slightly higher incidence of heart disease and subsequent mortality than age-matched controls. Generally, RBBB is considered a benign condition and only when associated with left anterior hemiblock is it accompanied by an increased incidence of heart disease.

Arrhythmias

The prevalence and complexity of most arrhythmias are increased in older populations. Routine ECG recordings performed in the nonhospitalized elderly reveal an incidence of 10% in both atrial and ventricular premature beats.[24] Ambulatory ECG recordings revealed that in patients studied for a 24-hour period, the elderly show a substantial prevalence of isolated supraventricular (88%) and ventricular (80%) ectopic beats.[22-26] Supraventricular tachyarrhythmias were found in 30% of the elders, with 26% displaying more than 100 atrial ectopic beats over the 24-hour monitoring period.[4,12,22-25] There was also a high incidence of complex arrhythmias including ventricular couplets and short runs of ventricular tachycardia. Thus, when evaluating patients with acute chest pain, the clinician should be aware that the mere presence of premature systoles in older patients does not necessarily imply the presence of acute ischemia, nor is it an indication for antiarrhythmic treatment. (See Table 13–3.)

Atrial Fibrillation

Atrial fibrillation occurs in 2 to 8% of all elderly subjects.[22] A higher frequency is reported in hospitalized geriatric patients and in the very old (i.e., octagenarians). It is universally considered an abnormal ECG finding, and the vast majority of subjects with atrial fibrillation have demonstrable heart disease. The hemodynamic consequences of atrial fibrillation are related to the rapidity of ventricular response. If the ventricular rate is 60 to 90 beats per minute, which allows adequate ventricular filling, then the rhythm is usually well tolerated, even in the aged.[27]

The emergency management of new onset atrial fibrillation varies between institutions and individual physicians. Because atrial fibrillation often occurs in elderly

Table 13–3 Prevalence of Electrocardiogram Abnormalities in Subjects 65 Years or Older

Entity	Percent
Abnormal electrocardiogram	54
One-degree atrioventricular block	9
Left axis deviation (> − 30°)	36
Right axis deviation (≥ + 120°)	2
ST-T wave changes	17
Left bundle branch block	3
Right bundle branch block	6
Interventricular conduction delay	2
Premature atrial systole	10
Premature ventricular systole	9
Atrial fibrillation	7

patients and is associated with coronary artery disease, patients presenting for the first time are often selected for admission to the coronary care unit to exclude the possibility of acute MI. In one study[1,28] reviewing 245 patients with atrial fibrillation admitted to an intensive care unit, evaluation of a number of clinical variables during the initial assessment indicated that elderly patients with MI could be distinguished from others by the presence of left ventricular hypertrophy, electrocardiographic evidence of old MI, typical cardiac chest pain, and duration of cardiac symptoms less than 4 hours. The presence of two or more of these features identified all patients with acute MI and seven others at high risk for serious cardiac complications.[28] These findings suggested that new onset atrial fibrillation, in the absence of clinical predictors suggesting MI, does not warrant routine admission to the coronary care unit.

Sinus Bradycardia

It is significant that bradycardias (sinus bradycardia, sinus arrest, sinoatrial exit block, and second-degree or third-degree AV block) are rare in normal elderly subjects.[29,30] As a result, these findings in symptomatic patients presenting to an emergency department indicate the need for corrective therapy and hospitalization.

ST-T Wave

The most commonly observed age-related ECG changes involve ventricular repolarization. The ST segment flattens and the T-wave amplitude diminishes. ST depression is usually found in the left precordial leads, especially in V_4 and V_5. The amplitude of the T wave decreases slightly with advancing years, and low or notched T waves are not uncommon. Inverted T waves in leads I and II and precordial leads V_4 to V_6 indicate myocardial damage or ischemia.[22-26]

Several studies[23-27] indicate that the incidence of nonspecific ST-T wave changes is nearly 17% in subjects over the age of 70. In the elderly, the multiple noncardiac causes of T-wave inversions and ST segment depressions — obesity, hypoglycemia, metabolic factors, drugs, and aging changes in the chest — result in a loss of specificity and diagnostic value. If noncardiac causes can be excluded, the ST-T wave changes in the resting ECG have the same prognostic implications in the elderly as in the middle-aged population.

CARDIAC SYNCOPE

Cardiac syncope, the presenting symptom in 9 to 21% of elderly patients with acute MI,[31] results from transient reduction in cerebral perfusion precipitated by a primary decrease in cardiac output. Unlike vasovagal syncope, cardiac syncope may occur in the recumbent or supine position. Consequently, loss of consciousness in an elderly

patient should always suggest cardiac syncope until proven otherwise. The cardinal manifestation of cardiac syncope is loss of consciousness, which can occur in any position, unlike vasovagal syncope that classically occurs in the upright position. The patient may experience a brief premonitory weakness, palpitations, or chest pain, depending on the cause of cardiac syncope. It is estimated that 4 to 7 seconds[31] of asystole are required for the patient to lose consciousness in the upright position, and as long as 20 to 30 seconds if the patient is recumbent; therefore, a brief premonition in the supine position is not inconsistent with cardiac syncope. There are multiple types of cardiac syncope, including bradyarrhythmias, tachyarrhythmias, and mechanical obstruction to cardiac output.

Cardiac syncope resulting from atrioventricular block[32] is perhaps the most common type of bradyarrhythmic cardiac syncope. A syncopal episode associated with this arrhythmia is known as Stokes-Adams-Morgagni syndrome.[31] When patients develop heart block, there is sudden interruption of intraventricular conduction, and asystole will exist for 10 to 90 seconds before any ventricular rhythm begins. During this period of asystole, a dizzy spell or frank syncopal episode may be experienced by the patient. Often, the clinical picture is one of an elderly individual who complains of brief episodes of dizziness or presyncope that occurs without warning, often two to three times per day. These episodes frequently occur over a period of several weeks. If the diagnosis is not made and a pacemaker is not implanted, 50% of these patients will be dead within one year.

Supraventricular tachyarrhythmias are the most common cause of cardiac-induced syncopal episodes in the elderly. One study[33] reported 46 patients with dysrhythmias that correlated with symptoms of dizziness or loss of consciousness. In this series, 18 patients had supraventricular tachycardias, 10 had ventricular tachycardias, and the remaining 18 had other types, including conduction disturbances.[33]

Usually, ventricular rates not exceeding 180 beats per minute do not reduce cerebral blood flow. However, elderly patients have a much lower tolerance to tachycardias because of combined cardiac and cerebrovascular disease. Therefore, tachycardias with rates as low as 140 may reduce cerebral blood flow sufficiently to produce syncope.

CARDIAC ENZYMES

There has been much controversy about the use of cardiac enzymes for identifying patients with acute MI in the emergency department. A number of studies[34,35] have suggested that cardiac enzymes are only of limited value for identifying patients with acute MI in the emergency department. More recent studies,[36] however, suggest that the cardiac enzyme (CK) value has significant sensitivity and positive predictive value for patients with MI. In one study[36] of 252 patients presenting to an emergency department with chest pain, the ECG correctly identified 66% of patients with acute MI who were evaluated within 4 hours of onset of symptoms. In this group of "early presenters," the CK values were elevated in only 9% of the patients. However, among elderly patients evaluated 4 hours *after* the onset of their symptoms, the ECG was helpful in diagnosing acute MI in only 36% of the patients, while the CK levels were high in 63%, adding significantly to the accuracy of diagnosis of MI in patients already evaluated with ECG. The study suggests that the determination of serum CK levels in the emergency department is of value in the evaluation of elderly patients complaining of chest pain for 4 or more hours after the onset of symptoms.[36]

Elderly patients with an ECG pattern of old MI present special difficulties in diagnosis. A high rate of error in analyzing the infarct's age (i.e., recent or new) has been reported.[22-25] In one study, an old MI pattern was recorded in the emergency department ECG tracings of 12 patients who had no previous ECG available for comparison. Half of these patients, all with high CK levels, ultimately proved to have acute MI.[36] Therefore, the determination of serum CK levels can be helpful in distinguishing new MI from old MI in elderly patients in the emergency department.

The overall results of these studies[34-36] suggest that in the elderly population the CK test does not increase the diagnostic sensitivity of the ECG in patients evaluated less than 4 hours from the onset of their symptoms. However, in patients evaluated later than 4 hours from the onset of pain, the diagnostic sensitivity of the ECG is lower than in patients seen shortly after the onset of pain, and the CK becomes the most sensitive single test at this time. As many as 34% of the patients with acute MI arriving later than 4 hours from the onset of symptoms would have been missed had a CK been omitted from the initial diagnostic battery.[36] Since the majority of elderly patients with acute MI arrive at the emergency department more than 4 hours after the onset of symptoms, the CK test plays a very important role in the evaluation of this subgroup of patients.

DIFFERENTIAL DIAGNOSIS

A pseudoinfarction pattern on ECG has been associated with a number of noncardiac diseases, including acute pancreatitis, perforated gastric and duodenal ulcers, gallbladder disease, acute appendicitis, pneumoperitoneum, rapid blood loss, and some acute abdominal conditions associated with shock and severe metabolic stress.[37] In addition to the intraabdominal catastrophes, various central nervous system and pulmonary diseases are also known to mimic electrocardiographic changes of acute MI in the elderly. Therefore, the aforementioned conditions should be considered in the differential diagnosis of all elderly patients presenting with new, unexplained ECG abnormalities.

Frequently, the history, ECG, CK, and physical examination cannot definitely establish that an acute MI is occurring in an elderly patient. One of the first priorities, then, is to exclude the possibility that a local musculoskeletal abnormality is causing chest discomfort. For example, costochondral or chondrosternal disorders can cause localized chest pain that is reproduced by palpation. The pain of an intercostal muscle cramp, which is commonly noticed at rest, may also be exacerbated by local pressure or inspiration. Similarly, inflammation of the subacromial bursa, the supraspinatus tendon, or the deltoid tendon can cause pain in the clavicular or shoulder area that may radiate to the anterior chest or down the arm. The gastrointestinal discomfort of a duodenal ulcer or cholecystitis may include an epigastric or substernal component. The discomfort of acid-peptic disease may be provoked by aspirin, alcohol, or certain foods and is usually relieved by ingestion of bland foods or antacids. Discomfort related to a hiatal hernia is commonly at its worst when the patient is supine. It may present as a classic substernal burning relating to esophageal reflux and acid irritation, or the reflux may precipitate esophageal spasm, which produces pain that may be indistinguishable from that of myocardial ischemia.[38] (See Figure 13-3.)

Some cardiac disorders other than acute coronary ischemia can also present with chest discomfort. For example, myocardial ischemia caused by valvular aortic stenosis or asymmetric septal hypertrophy is indistinguishable from the angina caused by coronary artery disease. Pericarditis (which is commonly associated with coronary artery disease) can be caused by viral infections, bacterial infections, uremia, and other inflammatory processes and can manifest two distinct pain syndromes. As a rule, the pain is intensified by inspiration and by being in the supine position. The hallmark of pericarditis is a pericardial friction rub, which should always be sought as part of the physical examination of elderly patients with acute chest pain. (See Figure 13-4.)

DISPOSITION AND TRIAGE

Although an ECG is a mandatory part of the emergency evaluation of any elderly patient with possible ischemic heart disease, the definitive disposition of such patients depends upon the interpretation of a number of clinical, historical, and laboratory parameters and tests. A completely normal ECG makes the diagnosis of acute MI very unlikely. Only 1% of patients above the age of 30 who present to emergency departments with acute chest pain and normal ECGs will have acute MI, while only another 4% will eventually be diagnosed as having unstable angina.[22-26] In the elderly, about 50% of all patients with acute MI will have new findings of ST elevation of Q waves in two or more leads upon presentation.[24] Approximately another 25% will have new ECG findings of ischemia or strain without ST elevation.[23,24] Thus, only about 15% of all acute MIs will present to the clinician

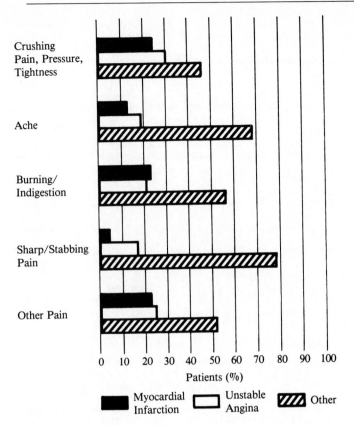

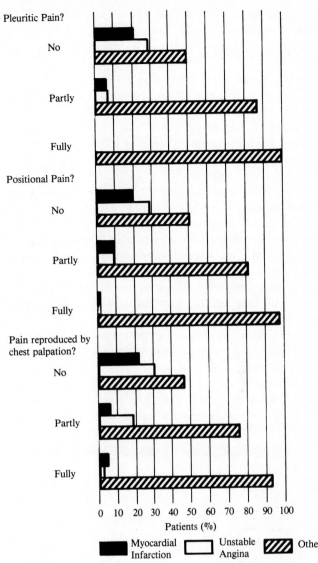

Figure 13–3 Types of chest pain syndromes in patients with myocardial infarction, unstable angina, and other types of chest pain. (Reprinted with permission from Goldman L: Hosp Pract, July 15, 1986; drawn by Albert Miller.)

with ECGs that do not show any new changes of ischemia, strain, or infarction.[24-26]

Unfortunately, reliance only on the elderly person's ECG would miss about 15 to 29% of all MIs.[3,9] As a result, a clinical history is the most important determinant of triage and disposition in this group.

In one study,[39] the first ECG obtained on presentation for suspected MI was examined for its usefulness in predicting clinical course and triage. High-risk patients were identified if ECG diagnoses included MI, ischemia, left ventricular hypertrophy, left bundle branch block, or paced rhythm. These patients constituted approximately one third of the total group study and manifested a significantly greater incidence of serious events, the need for invasive diagnostic procedures, and death than the lower risk patients whose initial electrocardiograms did not manifest the above ECG findings. Thus, elderly patients with low-risk ECGs can safely be treated in an intermediate care unit, thereby reducing costly coronary care unit admissions.[39]

SUMMARY

The diagnosis of acute coronary ischemia and MI in the elderly is easily missed. Atypical presentations, silent MI warning prodromes, and syncope are common. Moreover, chest pain in the elderly may be a manifestation of a

Figure 13–4 Pain precipitants in myocardial infarction, unstable angina, and nonischemic conditions. (Reprinted with permission from Goldman L: Hosp Pract, July 15, 1986.)

number of other disease processes.[40] Because cardiac pain tends to be less intense in the elderly, the classic description of crushing retrosternal chest pain radiating to the jaw and left arm is frequently absent in the geriatric patient. Instead, this subgroup presents with "anginal equivalent" syndromes such as aching shoulders, complaints of indigestion, and interscapular ache, or complaints of extreme weakness, fatigue, shortness of breath, confusion, or focal neurologic deficits. Typical signs and symptoms of congestive heart failure may also be absent or obscured by the coexistence of other pathologic processes such as pulmonary edema, chronic obstructive lung disease, anemia, or obesity.

The differential diagnoses of chest pain are long. The most common disorders include myocardial ischemia and infarction, pulmonary embolism, aortic dissection, tension pneumothorax, simple pneumothorax, pneumonia, pericarditis, pleurisy, rib fracture, costochondritis, esphagitis, and herpes zoster in the thoracic distribution. Physical examination should focus attention on the ABCs (airway, breathing, circulation) first. Are the respirations labored or not? The presence of rate, rhythm, and character of pulse should be noted. The blood pressure should be measured in both arms if aortic dissection is a possibility. The level of consciousness, color of the skin, presence of diaphoresis, and anxiety should all be noted. Abdominal examination is important to rule out gallbladder disease, pancreatitis, esophagitis, and peptic ulcer disease.

The electrocardiographic interpretation of the elderly patient with chest pain should be made with the full understanding of common preexisting ECG abnormalities in this patient population.[22-26] And, finally, the CK level may be of value in patients who present to the emergency department with onset of symptoms that are 4 or more hours in duration.

With an awareness of common prodromal symptoms, atypical presentations, and difficulties in interpretation of laboratory and electrocardiographic tests, it may be possible to improve accuracy of triage and disposition and to avoid the medicolegal risks of discharging elderly patients from the emergency department who have acute coronary ischemia.[41-44]

On the other hand, we can also assist in speeding the treatment with thrombolytic agents or reperfusion strategies, which might include coronary bypass or transluminal angioplasty.[45]

REFERENCES

1. Friedman HZ et al: Cardiac care unit admission criteria for suspected acute myocardial infarction in new-onset atrial fibrillation, Am J Cardiol 59(8):866–869, 1987.
2. Goldman L: Acute chest pain: emergency room evaluation, Hosp Pract, July 15, 1987.
3. Presentation of myocardial infarction in the elderly, Lancet 2:1077–1078, 1986 (editorial).
4. Unrecognized myocardial infarction, Lancet 2:1379, 1984 (editorial).
5. Bayer AJ et al: Changing presentation of myocardial infarction with increasing old age, J Am Geriatr Soc 34:263–266, 1986.
6. Pathy MS: Clinical presentation of myocardial infarction in the elderly, Br Heart J 29:190–199, 1967.
7. Pacy H et al: Chest pain as an emergency in general practice, Aust Fam Physician 11(11):861–865, 1982.
8. Urestsky BF et al: Symptomatic myocardial infarction without chest pain: prevalence and clinical course, Am J Cardiol 40:498–503, 1977.
9. Cohn PF et al: Frequent episodes of silent myocardial ischemia after apparently uncomplicated myocardial infarction, J Am Coll Cardiol 8(4):982–985, 1986.
10. Kannel WB and Abbott RD: Incidence and prognosis of unrecognized myocardial infarction: an update on the Framingham study, N Engl J Med 311:1144–1147, 1984.
11. Moss AJ: Cardiac disease in the elderly, Prac Geriatr, vol 29, 1986.
12. Katz P, Dube D, and Calkins E: Aging and disease, Prac Geriatr, vol 29, 1986.
13. Gerstenblith G et al: Disorders of the heart. In Gerstenblith G et al: Principles and practice of geriatric medicine, Philadelphia, 1985, WB Saunders Co.
14. Harris R: Clinical geriatric cardiology, Philadelphia, 1986, JB Lippincott.
15. Maisel AS et al: The murmur of papillary muscle dysfunction in acute

16. Stowers M and Short D: Warning symptoms before major myocardial infarction, Br Heart J 32(6):833–838, 1970.
17. Webb CR: Myocardial infarction, Geriatrics 41(2):89–90, 95–97, 100, 1986.
18. Alonzo AA, Simon AB, and Feinleib M: Prodromata of myocardial infarction and sudden death, Circulation 52:1056–1062, 1969.
19. Blodstein M: The characteristics of non-fatal myocardial infarctions in the aged, Arch Intern Med 98:84–90, 1956.
20. Pomerance A: Cardiac pathology in the elderly. In Noble RJ and Rothbaum DA editors: Geriatric cardiology, Philadelphia, 1981, FA Davis Co.
21. Podell RN: Delay on hospitalization for myocardial infarction, J Med Soc NJ 77(12):813–816, 1980.
22. Willius EA: The heart in old age: a study of 700 patients seventy-five years of age and older, Am J Med Sci 182:1–12, 1981.
23. Olbrich O and Woodford-Williams E: The normal precordial electrocardiogram in the aged, J Gerontol, pp 510–522, 1985.
24. Rodstein M: The ECG in old age: implications for diagnosis, therapy, and prognosis, Geriatrics 32:76–79, 1977.
25. Bachman S, Sparrow D, and Smith LK: Effect of aging on the electrocardiogram, Am J Cardiol 48:513–516, 1981.
26. Camm AJ and Ward DE: Clinical electrocardiography. In Martin A and Camm AJ, editors: Heart disease in the elderly, Chichester, England, 1984, John Wiley & Sons, Ltd.
27. Simonson E: The effect of age on the electrocardiogram, Am J Cardiol 29:64–73, 1972.
28. Stark ME and Vacek JL: The initial electrocardiogram during admission for myocardial infarction: use as a predictor of clinical course and facility utilization, Arch Intern Med 147(5):843–846, 1987.
29. Fleg JL: Cardiovascular emergencies. In Wilson LB, Stimson SP, and Baxter CR, editors: Handbook of geriatric emergency care, 1984, University Park Press.
30. Mather HG: Cardiac emergencies, Practitioner 225(1358):1093–1096, 1981.
31. Sequeira M: Evaluation of syncope and dizziness in the elderly patient, Geriatric Emergencies 3:19–39, 1984.
32. Rodstein M, Brown M, and Wolloch L: First-degree atrioventricular heart block in the aged, Geriatrics 23:159–163, 1968.
33. Van Durne JP: Tachyarrhythmias and transient ischemic attacks, Am Heart J 89:538, 1975.
34. Hedges JR et al: Use of cardiac enzymes identifies patients with acute myocardial infarction otherwise unrecognized in the emergency department, Ann Emerg 16(3):248–252, March 1987.
35. Lee TH et al: Evaluation of creatine kinase and creatine kinase-MB for diagnosis of myocardial infarction: clinical impact in the emergency room, Arch Intern Med 147(1):115–121, 1987.
36. Viskin S et al: The importance of creatine kinase determination in identifying acute myocardial infarction among patients complaining of chest pain in an emergency room, Cardiology 74(2):100–110, 1987.
37. Thomas I et al: Electrocardiographic changes in catastrophic abdominal illness mimicking acute myocardial infarction, Am J Cardiol 59(12):1224–1225, 1987.
38. Konu V: Myocardial infarction in the elderly, Acta Med Scand Suppl 604:1–68, 1977.
39. Schor S et al: Disposition of presumed coronary patients from an emergency room: a follow-up study, JAMA 236(8):941–943, 1976.
40. Grant AP and Dowey KE: The associations of acute stroke and myocardial infarction in elderly medical emergencies, Ir J Med Sci 149(1):15–18, 1980.
41. Bloom BS and Peterson OL: End results, cost and productivity of coronary care units, N Engl J Med 288:72–78, 1973.
42. Detsky AS et al: Prognosis, survival and the expenditure of hospital resources for patients in an intensive care unit, N Engl J Med 305:667–672, 1981.
43. Hofvendahl S: Influence of treatment in a CCU on prognosis in acute myocardial infarction, Acta Med Scand Suppl 189:285–291, 1971.
44. Hill JD, Holdstock G, and Hampton JR: Comparison of mortality of patients with heart attacks admitted to a coronary care unit and an ordinary medical ward, Br Med J 2:81–83, 1977.
45. Detre K et al: Percutaneous transluminal coronary angioplasty in 1985 and 1977–81, N Engl J Med 318:265, 1988.

myocardial infarction: clinical features and prognostic implications, Am Heart J 112(4):705–711, 1986.

Intervention in Acute Myocardial Infarction

Michael Sequeira, M.D., F.A.C.E.P., and Louis A. Cannon, M.D.

Because of the high prevalence of myocardial infarction (MI) and its atypical presentation in the elderly, coronary heart disease requires the practitioner to maintain a high index of suspicion when caring for the geriatric population. Despite reductions in cardiovascular morbidity and mortality, cardiac disease is still the leading cause of death among people over the age of 65. Of all deaths in this age group, 40% are caused by cardiac disease; ischemic heart disease accounts for 80 to 90% of total mortality. Random studies of otherwise normal elderly patients living at home demonstrate that over 40% have clinical evidence of coronary heart disease, with over 50% of those over the age of 75 manifesting clinical evidence of cardiac disease.[1]

With recent studies suggesting that such valuable infarct-limiting measures as coronary thrombolysis, percutaneous transluminal angioplasty (PCTA), and beta blockade are time-dependent in their efficacy, it is now particularly important to recognize MI in the elderly as early in the course of its evolution as possible. A frustrating, occasionally troublesome aspect of this necessity is that elderly patients with MI present with such strikingly different patterns, making timely diagnosis that much more difficult. These facts underscore the need for clinicians to become aware of the various modes of presentation of MI in the elderly if they are to have any impact in stemming its morbidity and mortality in this age group.[2-4]

The purpose of this chapter is to outline the unique and polymorphous presentations and management strategies of MI in the elderly. Atherosclerotic risk factors and their impact in the elderly, changes in the aging cardiovascular system, diagnostic tools for MI, the pathophysiology of coronary heart disease, treatment of MI and its complications, and postmyocardial infarction management in the elderly patient will also be discussed in detail.

PHYSIOLOGIC CHANGES OF THE CARDIOVASCULAR SYSTEM IN THE ELDERLY

Among the myriad changes in the cardiovascular system that predictably occur with aging is the change in the *intrinsic heart rate,* which after pharmacologic denervation with simultaneous cholinergic and adrenergic blockade, declines with age. In addition, cardiac output steadily declines with age at an approximate rate of 1% per year. This is corroborated by studies measuring maximal oxygen consumption ($\dot{V}O_2$ max). There is a progressive and gradual decline in total blood volume with an increase in circulation time. Therefore, the decrease in cardiac output represents a decrease in stroke volume with only minimal decrease in heart rate. Since the duration of mechanical systole is unaltered, systolic ejection rate is reduced and systemic peripheral vascular resistance is increased.[5,6]

In the elderly, minimal changes in cardiac output are generally observed at rest. However, with exercise, there is a smaller increase in cardiac output accompanied by disproportionate rise in left-sided filling pressures (wedge pressure), indicating an impairment to left ventricular filling. This impaired diastolic filling may explain why older individuals are more likely than younger ones to develop breathlessness and other symptoms of left ventricular failure during ischemia/infarction and during tachycardia.

PATHOLOGIC CHANGES IN THE AGING CARDIOVASCULAR SYSTEM

Coronary Artery Disease

The most important cause of heart disease in the elderly is coronary artery disease, but not all elderly patients have coronary artery disease. In those patients with congestive heart failure, only 50% have ischemic disease associated with transmural MI. In out-of-hospital sudden death, ischemic heart disease is found in over 62% of patients over 65 years of age. As many as 20% of elderly patients have clinically unsuspected ischemic pathology at autopsy.[7,8]

Risk Factors in the Elderly[9]

Age itself is a risk for the development of atherosclerotic disease. Patients who are otherwise at low risk for atherosclerotic disease develop atherosclerotic disease with advancing age. Atherosclerotic risk increases from approximately 1% at 40 years of age to 10% at 70 years of age in males with no other risk factors for coronary heart disease. In contrast, high-risk males have a 60% probability of having atherosclerotic disease at age 40 and by age 70 there is an 80% risk.[3-5] Derived from the Framingham Heart study, these data suggest that although age is an independent risk factor, other risk factors such as systolic hypertension (elevated blood pressure), elevated serum cholesterol, diabetes, and cigarette smoking remain additional risk factors for cardiovascular disease.

The major risk factor in elderly patients is an elevated blood pressure. It has been estimated that 50% of the cardiovascular sequelae of untreated hypertension in males and 40% in females appear before such evidence can be detected by routine examination. Thus, hypertension is the most common and treatable contributing risk factor for cardiovascular disease in the elderly. Physical inactivity is arguably a risk factor in elderly patients. However, while regular physical activity certainly seems to be desirable, there is no clear indication that associates it with reduced cardiac morbidity and mortality.[3]

Although cigarette smokers still have a slightly higher coronary mortality at 75, the relative risk for acquiring atherosclerotic heart disease from cigarette smoking diminishes with advancing age. The benefit of smoking cessation has been demonstrated in patients over 65 years of age. It has also been convincingly shown that younger persons reduce their risk significantly. The *overall* death rate is much lower in persons who give up smoking despite the lack of change in the rate of new coronary attacks. Therefore, there is adequate reason to advise elderly persons to give up smoking cigarettes.

In a similar vein, hypercholesterolemia is also a weak predictor of cardiovascular risk in elderly persons, and there is no convincing evidence that lowering the cholesterol decreases the risk. Patients with diabetes mellitus have an increased risk of cardiac failure that is secondary to abnormal myocardial function. There is little evidence that control of hyperglycemia improves cardiovascular mortality.

Neither coffee nor moderate use of alcohol seems to be associated with an increased cardiovascular risk. The currently available evidence shows no clear-cut proven benefit to be produced by the prophylactic use of aspirin or beta-blocking agents or by reduction of emotional stress in asymptomatic elderly patients, although a number of studies in these areas are currently underway. The role of emotional stress is particularly controversial, and there is no way to make quantitative measurements. On the other hand, life-style improvements and stress reduction are almost universally recommended for older patients, regardless of conclusive evidence on their merit.

Myocardial Hypertrophy

This is the second most common pathologic finding in the elderly. Multiple factors may contribute to this. Of course, the most important factor is hypertension, although other factors such as aortic valvular or ischemic heart disease do play a part.

Amyloidosis

Senile cardiac amyloidosis is a specific type of amyloid disease that has distinctive age and pathologic characteristics. It seems to be immunologically distinct from the other types of amyloidosis. Generally, 50% of the patients older than 70 develop amyloidosis. The functional significance of this phenomenon is debatable. The conducting system is rarely affected. Severe cardiac involvement, however, can lead to progressive and refractory heart failure.[10]

Valvular Heart Disease[11,12]

Degenerative valvular disease has two forms: calcification and mucoid degeneration. Calcific degeneration is one of the most common findings of cardiac pathology in elderly patients. It occurs in up to one third of patients over 75 years of age. The calcification appears initially at the base of the aortic cusp, probably related to repeated mechanical stress during normal valve action. With progression, calcification can extend toward the rest of the cusp, but it rarely involves the cusp's free edges.

Mitral annular calcification is found in over 10% of patients who are older than 50 years at autopsy. Women apear to be affected four times more often than men. This is usually an incidental finding but may be associated with some mitral regurgitation, conduction abnormalities, or endocarditis. Mucoid degeneration of the mitral valve can also occur. This leads to redundancy and eventual prolapse but is not usually associated with significant valvular insufficiency. The main concern here is the development of spontaneous chordal rupture.

Changes in the Conducting System[3]

The number of pacemaking cells in the sinoatrial node decreases with age so that by the age of 75 only 10% of the intrinsic pacemaker cells remain. There is also concomitant atrial fibrosis and degeneration. There appear to be no age-related changes in the atrioventricular (AV) node; however, there seems to be a progressive loss of bundle of His fibers with age.

Lev's disease is manifested by chronic AV block due to the loss of conducting fibers in the proximal left bundle and occasionally the bifurcating bundle. Lenegre's disease is a diffuse disease involving the middle and distal portions of the conducting system. Together, these two diseases account for a significant proportion of second- and third-degree block in the elderly.

THE PATHOPHYSIOLOGY OF MI

The majority of elderly patients with acute MI have atherosclerotic occlusive lesions in multiple coronary arteries. There is no uniform mechanism that leads to total occlusion and subsequent myocardial necrosis in all patients. Some of the mechanisms at work include superficial damage in areas of atherosclerotic plaques involving the endothelium and subendothelium, leading to platelet aggregation, adhesion, and thrombin generation. Thrombin production promotes more platelet aggregation and subsequent fibrin polymerization with formation of thrombus.

Another potential mechanism is plaque damage with ulceration, tearing, exposure of collagen, and subsequent formation of thrombus in situ. Hemorrhage can also occur in the plaque, due to damage of the supportive perivascular tissue. This leads to luminal occlusion per se or, through the formation of thrombi, to exposure of collagen to blood flow. Lastly, coronary spasm in the vicinity of an atherosclerotic plaque may induce marked diminution of blood flow with subsequent stasis and thrombosis with platelet aggregates. These may, in turn, perpetuate vasospasm mediated by the release of thromboxane A_2 from aggregated platelets.

During the early hours of acute transmural (Q wave) MI, one or more of the aforementioned mechanisms is usually present, precipitating thrombosis of the involved coronary artery. Coronary arteriograms performed within 4 hours of the onset of symptoms of infarction show that 80% of patients have total coronary occlusion. Complete occlusion, however, can be demonstrated angiographically in only 65% of patients studied 12 to 24 hours after symptoms. Angiographic studies performed prior to coronary thrombolysis show that a thrombotic coronary artery occlusion is present in about 80 to 90% of MIs.[13]

Thus, it is generally accepted that complete thrombotic occlusion of a coronary artery is the principal cause of acute MI. Other evidence indicates, however, that a thrombus is not always present in the initial hours of infarction. This suggests that some other event, or a combination of events, may initiate infarction and precede thrombus formation. Thus, it may be that coronary spasm and/or recanalization of the thrombus may play important roles in the pathogenesis of acute myocardial necrosis.

Transmural Versus Nontransmural MI

It appears that spontaneous lysis of the occluding thrombus is a frequent phenomenon and may have profound implications for the pathogenesis of transmural versus nontransmural infarction. Eighty percent of patients with transmural (Q wave) infarction will have complete occlusion of the thrombosed artery 1 to 5 weeks after infarction, while only 19% of patients with nontransmural (non-Q wave) infarction demonstrate complete occlusion at this time point. It is possible that complete occlusion occurs transiently in nontransmural infarction and that early reperfusion spares a portion of the myocardium at risk. In addition, the infarct size of nontransmural infarction is smaller than in transmural infarction, although the incidence of infarct extension is higher in nontransmural infarction. The extent of obstructive coronary disease seems to be similar in both transmural and nontransmural infarction. The in-hospital mortality is lower in nontransmural infarction, but late (1-year) mortality rates are similar in patients with both types of infarct patterns. Thus, it appears that transient complete occlusion of the coronary artery is the pathogenic mechanism of nontransmural infarction.

Perfusion Changes After Coronary Occlusion

After coronary occlusion, the progression and severity of myocardial changes will vary. Ischemic changes initially occur in the subendocardium, with temporal extension toward the epicardium. The infarcted myocardium becomes dysfunctional, contributes little to ventricular ejection, and is detectable on ventriculogram as a hypokinetic or asynergic segment.

As expected, these changes initiate a vicious cycle of myocardial ischemia. Initially, as left ventricular filling pressure increases from the normal 5 to 10 mm Hg to 15 to 30 mm Hg, hypoperfusion of both the endocardium and myocardium occurs because of increased wall tension. Next, myocardial ischemia causes a generalized vasodilatation of the coronary resistance vessels. This favors blood flow away from the subendocardium toward the epicardium. As systemic vascular resistance increases in response to the resultant lower cardiac output, cardiac output decreases further while myocardial oxygen demand increases. Finally, myocardial ischemia predisposes to ventricular and supraventricular arrhythmias. This cascade results in a marked decrease in the threshold for ventricular fibrillation.

ESTABLISHING A DEFINITIVE DIAGNOSIS

In general, the practitioner will make a clinical diagnosis of acute MI based on three factors: 1) a history compatible with myocardial ischemia; 2) ECG changes on the electrocardiogram; and 3) cardiac enzyme changes. Usually, a patient needs at least two of these factors for the diagnosis of MI to be definitive. However, the elderly patient can present both with understated or atypical complaints and peculiarities in cardiac enzyme levels. The only factor that doesn't exhibit an age-related peculiarity is the electrocardiogram.

SYMPTOMS OF MI IN THE ELDERLY[14-16]

The classic presentation of crushing substernal chest pain, which radiates into either arm or to the jaw and is associated with shortness of breath, nausea, and diaphoresis, is in fact extremely rare in elderly patients over 75 years of age. Various clinical retrospective and prospective studies have shown that chest pain may be ab-

sent in up to 65% of elderly patients with MI. Dyspnea is the most common symptom of acute MI in patients over 85, occurring in about 35 to 45% of patients. MI may also present as a syncopal attack, confusion, or cerebral infarction.

Other symptoms encountered in the elderly include generalized sudden onset of weakness; isolated, unexplained nausea or vomiting; unexplained fall of blood pressure; abdominal pain; sudden onset of confusion; or even a cerebral infarction. Elderly diabetic patients may present with the sudden and unexplained onset of ketoacidosis.

Those patients who present with chest pain may have their symptoms altered by chronic disease involving structures, referred to as thoracic dermatomes, which may lower pain threshold and cause the pain of infarction to be isolated in the jaw, neck, shoulder, or arms. When these factors are combined with poor memory, altered pain perceptions, less active life-styles, and diminished expectations of elderly patients, one can see how difficult it may be to confirm the diagnosis of MI. It is important to have an extremely high index of suspicion for MI in any patient who suddenly presents with syncope, breathlessness, fatigue, abdominal pain, or any of the other manifestations cited above.

SIGNS OF MI IN THE ELDERLY

The first signs of MI may be severe if the patient has had a ventricular dysrhythmia, marked bradycardia with poor output, or abrupt left ventricular failure that has not subsided as compensatory reflex mechanisms came into play.

In mild cases, the patient may appear well, with dry skin and normal pulse and blood pressure, and complain only of prolonged substernal discomfort. If the patient did not present with chest pain, he or she may only be slightly short of breath and may actually be feeling quite normal after an initial syncopal episode. In more severe cases, the patient may appear acutely ill and may have marked hypotension with low cardiac output, tachycardia, diaphoresis, and a gray, ashen appearance due to peripheral cyanosis. If cerebral perfusion is impaired, the patient may be acutely confused and may have either a tachycardia or bradycardia.

At the onset of acute MI, the temperature is usually normal. The fever, which occasionally occurs with younger patients at 24 to 72 hours due to myocardial necrosis, may not, and usually does not, develop in the elderly patient.

Finally, the patient with severe circulatory impairment may present in clinical shock with hypotension, poor peripheral perfusion with cool extremities, confusion, and cyanosis. The patient may be in cardiogenic shock with evidence of acute pulmonary edema, with respiratory crackles, jugulovenous distention, hepatic venous congestion, and an S_3 on examination.

ELECTROCARDIOGRAPHIC FINDINGS AND MI

The appearance of new diagnostic Q waves (0.04 second or greater in duration and 1 mm in depth) accompanied by evolving repolarization abnormalities characterize transmural infarction. Because of the imprecise ECG morphologic correlations, the current designation of "Q wave" and "non-Q wave" infarction is the preferable terminology at this time. Q waves reflect an absence of electrical activity from an area of necrotic myocardium and appear in the leads specific for the area of infarction. Therefore, an inferior infarction will show Q waves in leads 2, 3, and F; an anteroseptal infarction has Q waves in leads V_1, V_2, and V_3; anterolateral infarction shows Q waves in leads V_1, AVL, and V_4 through V_6; anterior infarction demonstrates Q waves in leads V_1 through V_4; and a high anterolateral infarction shows Q waves in only lead V_1 and AVL.

Tall, peaked T waves nearest the injured area are the earliest electrocardiographic change of acute transmural infarction. These are soon followed by the development of a ST elevation with a classic coved configuration. Other changes suggesting transmural infarction include the development of a tall initial R wave in lead V_1 (true posterior infarction), a loss of initial R wave forces in leads V_1 through V_4 (anteroseptal infarction), and a general loss of voltage in the extremity leads (lateral infarction).

A non-Q wave infarction, however, is diagnosed by the development of at least 1 mm of a horizontal downsloping ST segment depression or recent T-wave inversion in two or more leads. Either of these changes must persist at least 24 hours to confirm a non-Q wave infarction as the diagnosis.

It should be emphasized that a single, normal, unchanged ECG does not exclude the diagnosis of acute MI. This is especially important considering the abnormal presentation of the elderly patient. If the clinical suspicion is high enough, then management must proceed as if the patient has had an infarction, since the early period of the infarction is characterized by the highest incidence of life-threatening dysrhythmias. It should be pointed out that the absence of normal Q waves does not necessarily rule out the diagnosis of an acute transmural infarction in the initial hours after coronary occlusion, since there may be a lag before the ECG evidence of myocardial necrosis develops.

CARDIAC ENZYME DETERMINATION OF MI

In the absence of specific changes on the ECG of characteristic ST segment elevations, serum enzyme levels provide reliable evidence of myocardial necrosis. When ischemia disrupts the integrity of the myocardial solid membrane, intracellular enzymes are released into the circulation. It should be remembered that a small area of myocardium may infarct and may do so without generating a diagnostic elevation of cardiac serum enzymes. Three enzymes commonly considered for serial measurements for diagnosing acute MI include creatine kinase (CK), lactic dehydrogenase (LDH), and serum glutamic oxaloacetic transaminase (SGOT).

The time course and pattern of enzyme elevations may be helpful. Serum CK rises within 4 to 6 hours following an acute MI, peaks at 12 to 18 hours, and usually returns to normal in 2 days. CK-MB isoenzyme levels are important to determine regardless of the level of the CK. However, CK-MB levels will frequently peak earlier than the total CK levels and at 6 to 8 hours may actually be normal at the time the total CK peaks.

The range of CK concentrations in the serum of elderly subjects is relatively low compared with expected values established in younger patients. This may be due to age-related declines in skeletal muscle mass or CK activity in striated muscle. Elderly patients with suspected MI are more likely than younger patients to have elevated CK-MB fractions in association with normal CK levels. Several studies have shown that these patients are at high risk of subsequent cardiac mortality. Therefore, it is recommended that all elderly patients have a routine CK isoenzyme determination, regardless of the total level of the CK.

LDH levels may be helpful in diagnosing MI, primarily because the levels peak late and stay elevated for prolonged periods. This is important because the frequently overlooked symptoms of MI in the elderly combine with other factors, such as altered mental status and poor social support, to delay the arrival of the patient. LDH levels begin to rise about 12 hours following an acute MI and peak at approximately 48 to 72 hours. The levels do not return to normal for up to 7 to 10 days. Since LDH may be found in many different organs and elevation is found in many disease processes, specific measurement of LDH isoenzymes is also helpful here as it is with CK. Specifically, it is the LDH-1 isoenzyme that, when greater than LDH-2, indicates the presence of myocardial necrosis since in the normal patient, LDH-2 exceeds the level of LDH-1.

The third cardiac enzyme, the SGOT, is usually not necessary to draw except for corroboration. This enzyme rises within 8 to 12 hours following an acute MI, peaks at 24 to 48 hours, and returns to normal in 4 to 5 days. Practically, the SGOT is unnecessary and shouldn't be drawn on a routine basis. If the CK levels with the CK-MB fraction are elevated, this, in conjunction with either the patient's history or characteristic ECG changes, confirms the diagnosis of MI. It is, therefore, not necessary to draw the SGOT or the LDH. If, however, there is concern that the patient had a MI more than 2 days prior, but less than 14 days prior, to the time of evaluation then the LDH enzyme assay with isoenzyme fractionation will be valuable. Other methods of determining acute MI will be discussed in a later section.

Nuclear Medicine Testing[17]

The indications and the proper deployment of nuclear testing for suspected MI are useful to know because of the frequently questionable and ambiguous histories and potentially undiagnostic myocardial enzyme studies that may occur in elderly patients presenting with potential MI. In addition, elderly patients may present late in the course of the infarction, and it is important to know — for their postinfarction and prospective management — whether or not the patient has had an MI. The radioisotope studies currently in use are the thallium 201 scan and the technetium 99 pyrophosphate scan.

Thallium 201

Coronary perfusion studies using thallium 201 in patients with previous MI have shown that the myocardium supplied by the artery may have normal coronary blood flow at rest, but hypoperfusion and altered distribution flow during the stress of exercise. Quantitative thallium 201 scans have been used to determine the location, extent, and persistence of myocardial ischemia at the time of the acute infarction and later before hospital discharge. Transient ischemia can be observed by comparing rest and exercise abnormalities. Perfusion defects in areas distant from that of the acute infarction indicate additional areas of ischemia. Multiple thallium 201 defects usually predict multivessel and more extensive disease with a greater likelihood of left ventricular dysfunction.

In addition, right ventricular infarction can be diagnosed by radioisotope studies and abnormal radionuclide uptake can be localized to the right ventricle, or localized hypokinesis of the right ventricle may be evident on gated blood pool angiography. Technetium scans have also shown that up to 30% of inferior infarctions have associated right ventricular infarction.[17]

On the thallium scan, the isotope goes where blood flow goes, such that areas that receive no blood flow do not image. Therefore, the thallium scan is what is known as a "cold spot" scan. The disadvantage of this, of course, is that areas of old infarction, new infarction, and ischemia all may show up as potential defects in the thallium scans. In addition, the thallium isotope scans do not show small perfusion defects and reproducibility is variable unless maximal exercise is performed.

Technetium Pyrophosphate

In contrast, intravenous technetium pyrophosphate has the advantage of being actively taken up by acutely infarcted myocardial cells, producing discrete well-localized "hot spots" in transmural acute infarction. Technetium pyrophosphate has limitations in nontransmural, non-Q wave infarction, because diffuse uptake can be seen. Such uptake may also occur in the absence of infarction, and it will cause false-positive interpretations. In general, the technetium scan has about a 93 to 95% sensitivity with about an 83 to 86% specificity. Thus, the imaging is relatively sensitive but is somewhat less specific. Patients with unstable angina have been shown to have false-positive results; however, these patients generally manifested a diffuse pattern. Pyrophosphate imaging should be performed roughly 48 to 72 hours after the onset of infarction. This is the time of greatest likelihood of achieving a positive result. The infarct images generally become negative approximately 7 to 10 days after the infarction. However, positive scans have been noted to remain positive even weeks after the scan. Thus, it is an ideal test for a patient who presents with an equivocal picture of MI who may be anywhere from 3 to 7 days postinfarction.[17]

Radioisotope Ventriculogram

Radioisotope techniques can also be used to evaluate wall motion abnormalities in left ventricular function. There are two of these methods. The first is by the recording of images during both systole and diastole after a bolus injection of technetium-labeled albumin "gated" (synchronized) to the ECG. In these gated pool studies, disturbances in wall motion can be recognized and localized areas of hypokinesia or dyskinesia can be noted. Ejection fraction can be determined from the difference between the systolic and diastolic isotope image. The second method is by the so-called single pass nucleotide angiogram in which technetium 99 pertechnetate is given intravenously, and a computerized summated series of cardiac cycles is obtained. These cycles resemble a dye dilution curve. Localized abnormalities of wall motion and ejection fraction can be noted. Both methods correlate reasonably well. Radioisotope special techniques such as radionuclide angiography to determine wall motion abnormalities are still research procedures, involving expensive equipment and highly technically trained physicians, and are not essential in most patients with acute MI.

Echocardiography

An easier and more useful method for determining left ventricular function and wall motion abnormalities is two-dimensional echocardiograms. Localizing a global ejection fraction and regional wall motion by two-dimensional echocardiograms may be the earliest finding in acute coronary occlusion. The presence of extensive wall abnormalities outside the immediate acute infarcted area is associated with more severe disease and a worse prognosis for survival.

EFFECTS OF CORONARY ARTERIES ON COMPLICATIONS OF ACUTE MI

The coronary circulation is usually regarded as a three-vessel system. The right coronary artery arises from the right sinus of Valsalva and follows the anterior AV groove around the acute margin to the crux of the heart. There it gives rise to the posterior descending branch or branches supplying the inferior and posterior surface of the left ventricle, as well as the posterior aspect of the interventricular septum. It also provides the main blood supply of the right ventricle.

In approximately 60 to 70% of the patients seen, the right coronary artery supplies the sinus node; in 90%, it supplies the AV node. Obstruction of the right coronary artery, which can occur anywhere in its course, typically results in an inferior infarction. Conduction disturbances in the AV node are a relatively common association although isolated infarction of the right ventricle is rare and usually occurs only when severe right ventricular hypertrophy is present. Some involvement of the right ventricle in patients with inferior wall infarction is common and occurs in up to 30 to 40% of the patients. Occasionally (in about 10% of the cases) the right coronary artery is nondominant and does not reach the crux of the heart, nor does it supply a significant portion of the left ventricle. In these individuals, the posterior descending branch is supplied by the circumflex artery. Because the sinus node is usually supplied by the right coronary artery, it is, therefore, not infrequent to find significant bradydysrhythmias associated with inferior wall infarctions in up to 40% of the individuals in the first 2 hours after infarction.

The left coronary artery arises from the left coronary sinus of Valsalva. The main stem of the artery quickly divides into two branches — the left anterior descending artery (LAD) and the circumflex vessels. The LAD usually provides the major supply of blood to the left ventricle. This artery runs down the anterior interventricular groove to the apex of the heart, where it turns and runs up the posterior intraventricular sulcus for a variable length.

During its course, the LAD gives off branches that penetrate the anterior two thirds of the septum and anastomose with septal branches of the posterior descending artery. All these branches supply the anterolateral aspect of the left ventricle via its diagonal branches. Atherosclerotic lesions of the LAD commonly occur at its origin and shortly after the origin of the first septal and diagonal branches. Occlusion of the LAD proximal to the origin of its largest branches may result in infarction involving the interior, lateral, apical, and septal surfaces of the left ventricle. Right bundle branch conduction disturbances are common. Occlusion of the artery after the origin of the diagonal and septal branches results in a smaller infarction of the anterior wall.

The circumflex artery, the most variable of the three vessels, runs posteriorly in the AV groove towards the crux of the heart. Its major branches are obtuse marginal branches that supply the posterolateral surface. Often, the circumflex artery becomes a small vessel after the origin of these main marginal branches. When occlusive lesions occur, they result in infarction of the true posterior wall and the posterolateral aspect of the left ventricle. In about 10% of the cases, the circumflex artery is dominant, supplying the AV node as well as the posterior descending artery.

MANAGEMENT OF ACUTE MI AND ITS COMPLICATIONS

For many years, the treatment of acute MI consisted simply of palliative measures such as bed rest, oxygen, maintenance of blood pressure and urine output, the prevention of pulmonary and systemic embolization, and measures that had one primary goal: to allow the infarct to heal. With the introduction of careful cardiac monitoring in the early 1960s and the development of coronary care units (CCUs), a progressive decrease in in-hospital deaths by prompt and effective treatment of ventricular arrhythmias and conduction disturbances occurred.

In the last decade, with increasing evidence that infarct size is the primary determinant of in-hospital and long-term mortality and morbidity and with better understanding of acute MI as a dynamic process, the focus of therapeutic efforts has shifted toward the limitation of infarct size. The initial efforts toward this goal involved measures to decrease the myocardial oxygen demand. Although some of these efforts were successful, they do not match the more recent efforts in acutely increasing myocardial or coronary blood supply. These efforts will be discussed in a later section.

General Measures
Coronary Care Unit (CCU)[16,18-22]

Elderly patients with a diagnosis of acute MI or suspected MI should be admitted to the CCU. That the CCU can make a significant difference in morbidity and mortality in the elderly has been reconfirmed in a prospective study by Sagie and colleagues. Their study[20] showed a difference in mortality of 24% versus 46% in those elderly patients admitted to the CCU as compared with those patients admitted to a routine hospital ward. This confirms previous studies that showed a CCU mortality of 16 to 40% compared with a ward mortality of 43 to 95%.[19-22,23]

In the CCU, the patient should, like younger patients with acute MI, have an intravenous line placed. Oxygen should be placed at moderate flow rates and should be dictated by any potential degree of arterial hypoxemia that may have resulted from acute pulmonary congestion. Of course, patients with a previous history of chronic obstructive pulmonary disease should have low-flow oxygen placed by nasal cannula.

Control of Chest Pain

The patient's chest pain should be treated on admission to the emergency department. Sublingual or buccal nitroglycerin should be given to the patient as long as the systolic blood pressure remains above 100 mm Hg. Patients who have blood pressures between 90 and 100 mm Hg should be given low-dose nitroglycerin. The advantage of buccal nitroglycerin is that if the patient were to develop hypotension after the administration of the nitroglycerin, the undissolved portion of the nitroglycerin tablet can be removed. The same advantage exists with cutaneous administration of nitroglycerin. The other advantage of either buccal or cutaneous nitroglycerin is that they have more prolonged duration of action, lasting up to 4 to 6 hours. Studies have shown that repeated nitroglycerin in a stepped, graded fashion can relieve chest pain as quickly as the administration of intravenous narcotic agents.

If chest pain has lasted more than 30 minutes and remains unrelieved by nitrates, then small incremental dosages of morphine sulfate should be given at intervals of 5 to 10 minutes. Morphine sulfate will be effective in treating the patient's reaction to the pain and provide the hemodynamic benefits of venodilatation. Slight arterial dilatation will decrease preload and afterload, left ventricular and diastolic pressure, and myocardial oxygen demand. Myocardial oxygen demand is also decreased by the attendant decrease in the anxiety of the patient and his or her pain response.

Prevention of Primary Ventricular Fibrillation

Lidocaine prophylaxis to prevent ventricular fibrillation still remains a controversial issue. The prevailing opinion, however — based on the fact that patients can develop life-threatening ventricular arrhythmias without prior ventricular ectopy — is to administer routine intravenous lidocaine in the initial hours after an acute MI to prevent ventricular fibrillation. The proper dosage for lidocaine in the elderly, especially those over 70 years old, is to halve the initial loading bolus, the infusion rate, as well as the total loading dose given. Therefore, patients should receive 0.5 to 1 mg/kg of lidocaine as an initial bolus, followed by a 0.25 mg/kg load up to a total loading dose of 1.5 mg/kg. Infusion rates should begin at 1 mg/minute and increase to a total of 2 mg/minute. Even at these lower doses, signs and symptoms of lidocaine toxicity — such as altered mental status and seizures — should be carefully watched for. After the first 12 hours, lidocaine prophylaxis should be used only in the presence of persistent ventricular ectopy; the benefit of lidocaine's prophylactic use diminishes after

that time interval, and its toxicity increases with the duration of its usage.[24]

Thrombolytic Therapy in Acute MI

It is now widely accepted that the administration of thrombolytic drugs, given within the first few hours of acute MI, not only effects a significant reduction in mortality of the patients but also effects a significant reduction in infarct size in subsequent congestive heart failure.[25-29] Data are rapidly accumulating that support the belief that generalized intravenous administration of a thrombolytic agent, if given in the first 4 hours after the onset of symptoms, will have such benefit. In general, studies such as the GISSI and ISIS-2 study have shown that intravenous streptokinase produces at least a 20% reduction in mortality. The thrombolysis in MI (TIMI) trials has shown significant improved effectiveness of the thrombolytic agent, tissue-type plasminogen activator. It proved to be even more effective than streptokinase, producing reperfusion of affected myocardium in 66% of the patients, compared with 36% of patients treated with intravenous streptokinase.

In general, studies with thrombolytic agents have shown that anterior wall infarctions or multiple location infarctions seem to respond better than inferior or lateral wall infarctions. In addition, patients in cardiogenic shock are more likely to benefit from the thrombolysis treatment. Treatment is least likely to demonstrate obvious benefit for patients with stable inferior wall infarcts, non-Q wave infarcts, or ST segment depression infarcts.

The best reperfusion results are seen in patients treated within 2 hours of symptom onset, although considerable benefits are seen in patients treated within 4 hours and sometimes even within 6 hours of symptom onset. Studies in which streptokinase and prehospital care have been given have shown that treatment given in less than 2 hours saved approximately one half of the involved myocardium while treatment begun after 2 hours spared one fifth of the myocardial tissue at risk.

The general complications of thrombolysis revolve around bleeding complications. So far it does not seem that tissue plasminogen activator (TPA) has a lower incidence of subsequent bleeding complications. It is unclear whether the bleeding complications associated with TPA or streptokinase are solely the result of the thrombolytic agent or the anticoagulation that is administered to the patient after thrombolysis.

Contraindications to thrombolytic therapy basically revolve around those patients who either are actively bleeding or have a high risk of bleeding. These include patients with documented active internal bleeding, history of cerebrovascular accident (CVA), recent (within 2 months) intracranial or intraspinal surgery or trauma, intracranial neoplasm, arteriovenous malformation or aneurysm, known bleeding diathesis, or severe uncontrolled hypertension. Other relative risk factors listed include patients with recent cardiopulmonary resuscitation (CPR) and who are older than 75 years of age.

Thrombolysis in the Elderly

Most of the studies involving thrombolysis and acute MI do not address the specific efficacy and side effects of thrombolytic therapy in the elderly patient. Only two studies — the GISSI and ISIS-2 — have examined the effect of thrombolysis in the elderly. The GISSI study showed that advanced age is not an absolute contraindication to thrombolytic therapy and that the subsequent complication rate was no higher in the elderly than in younger patients. The study did show, however, that patients younger than 65 years seemed to show a greater benefit from thrombolytic therapy than older patients did. The ISIS-2 study demonstrated that elderly patients had outcomes as successful as those in the 65 and under age group. This GISSI study did not correlate the time from presentation with age, which may be a significant factor in the elderly patient. Most of the other studies on thrombolysis — including streptokinase given intravenously, intracoronary, and TPA — empirically exclude patients over the age of 75. This is done because studies with anticoagulation show that the incidence of significant intracranial hemorrhage and life-threatening hemorrhage in other regions of the body increases significantly in patients in this age group. There is no convincing evidence, however, that shows that elderly patients without a history of CVA or uncontrolled hypertension should automatically be excluded from the benefits of thrombolytic therapy. Further investigations are obviously needed on the specific efficacy of thrombolytic therapy in patients over 65 years old.

Because of the urgency required for institution of thrombolytic therapy and knowledge of the significance of diagnostic time delays in the elderly patient with acute MI, the practitioner should be prepared to make the diagnosis as quickly as possible. Predesigned protocols that would automatically include and exclude pertinent patients should be developed. These include drawing the appropriate laboratory tests, performing an ECG, preparing and administering the thrombolytic agent, notifying the appropriate consultation, and administering antidysrhythmic prophylaxis.

Percutaneous Transluminal Coronary Angioplasty

There is increasing evidence that emergency percutaneous transluminal and coronary angioplasty (PTCA), when combined with thrombolytic therapy, can produce even higher rates of coronary recanalization.[30] PTCA appears to be a logical choice in acute MI and avoids the hemostatic problems of thrombolysis and the resulting less severe coronary stenosis, as it provides a more effective preservation of ventricular function. Initial reports demonstrate that this technique can be used safely with a high incidence of recanalization and good clinical results. Emergency PTCA in acute MI without thrombolytic therapy may have a particularly useful role as an alternative to treatment in patients with contraindications to thrombolysis, who failed to achieve "effective reperfusion" after thrombolysis.

Coronary Artery Bypass Grafting (CABG)

CABG is another well-established and safe method to restore myocardial perfusion. This approach to myocardial reperfusion is clearly not applicable at present to the majority of patients with acute MI, and its attractiveness has decreased with the recent availability of intravenous thrombolysis and PTCA. There are, however, some groups of patients with acute MI who could benefit from this approach:

1. Patients with multivessel coronary disease or left main coronary artery stenosis
2. Patients in whom thrombolysis or PTCA has achieved no effective reperfusion and their myocardial ischemia persists
3. Patients with associated mechanical complications of acute MI, such as acute mitral regurgitation

Agents That Decrease Myocardial Oxygen Demand

The majority of patients with acute MI, especially elderly patients with confusing presentations, present beyond the theoretical cutoff time for immediate myocardial reperfusion and seek medical attention because of persistent or recurrent chest pain. The therapeutic effect in this phase (after 6 hours from the onset of pain) is to limit the infarct size by decreasing the myocardial oxygen demand and by treating any subsequent complications of MI, since thrombolytic therapy will usually not be efficacious.

Beta-Adrenergic Blocking Agents

The use of beta-blockers has become one of the most attractive pharmacologic interventions for limiting infarct size.[31] These agents reduce myocardial oxygen consumption by reducing heart rate, blood pressure, and cardiac inotropy. They also redistribute blood flow to ischemic areas and augment collateral blood flow. Beta-blockers have also been shown to alter myocardial substrate use toward glucose, shift the oxyhemoglobin dissociation curve to the right, and inhibit platelet aggregation. Objective evidence of infarct size limitation by the use of beta-blockers when given early in acute MI has been reported in several studies. There is no evidence at the current time that beta-blockers significantly decrease in-hospital mortality. Beta-blockers should be given intravenously to achieve the immediate effects, and, preferably, short-acting preparations should be used.

Patients who will be good candidates for the use of beta-blockers include those with persistent chest pain or evidence of ischemia and those with hyperkinetic circulatory response (hypertension and tachycardia) who have no evidence of left ventricular failure or conduction disturbances. Propranolol and metoprolol both have been shown to be effective in these situations. These agents should be carefully administered. Therapy should be discontinued as soon as the heart rate is reduced to less than 50 beats/minute, or the blood pressure is reduced to less than 100 mm Hg; if therapy is not discontinued at these times, other known complications of beta-blockade, including exacerbation of congestive failure and bronchospasm with decreased peripheral perfusion, may ensue. A promising new agent in this regard is the ultrashort-acting intravenous agent esmolol. The effective half-life of this drug in the circulation is less than 5 minutes, since it is destroyed by the red blood cells. Esmolol is a combined beta-1 and beta-2 agent and its use in infarct limitation remains to be studied.

Calcium Channel-Blocking Agents

The previously optimistic expectation that calcium channel-blocking agents would reduce the infarct size and improve mortality from MI has not been fulfilled. Nifedipine, for example, not only did not decrease the infarct size but in one subgroup, patient infarct size was actually increased — possibly from reflex tachycardia induced by the hypotension from nifedipine. Studies with diltiazem in patients with Q-wave infarction, diminished ejection fraction, and congestive heart failure have also produced disappointing results. It is only in recurrent or persistent ischemia after MI that the calcium antagonist may play a role when the suspected pathogenetic mechanism of coronary occlusion is coronary vasospasm or when the use of beta-blocking agents and nitrates is not well tolerated or contraindicated.

Nitroglycerin and Other Nitrates

There are several animal and clinical studies that demonstrate the effectiveness of nitrate preparations, especially intravenous nitroglycerin, in decreasing infarct size and controlling persistent and recurrent ischemia. The advantage of intravenous nitroglycerin is that its use and effects are easily controlled. Intravenous nitroglycerin is especially indicated in the subset of normotensive patients with evidence of left ventricular failure (pulmonary capillary wedge pressure more than 18 mm Hg and a cardiac index of less than 2.5 liters/minute/m^2).

Nitroglycerin should be started at 10 µg/minute with the dose being increased by 10 µg every 5 to 10 minutes until angina is controlled or tachycardia and hypotension occur. If the patient's condition stabilizes for an interval of 48 hours and no reinfarction has occurred, intravenous nitroglycerin should be withdrawn slowly and oral nitrates started. The recurrence of angina is a clear indication for early coronary arteriography and potential revascularization procedures.

Intra-Aortic Balloon Counterpulsation

Intra-aortic balloon counterpulsation (IABC) is a well-established method for the circulatory support of patients with cardiogenic shock resulting from a variety of causes and has been used in acute myocardial ischemia because it not only decreased myocardial oxygen demand but also increased coronary blood supply. The disadvantage of IABC is the significant rate of complications and the logistic difficulties associated with its use. It can be used effectively, however, in those patients with severe angina that persists after appropriate use of other interventions previously described.

COMPLICATIONS OF ACUTE MI

Ventricular rhythm disturbances remain the most common cause of mortality in nonhospitalized as well as hospitalized patients. The incidence does not seem to be any different than in the younger patient, nor are any of the other tachydysrhythmias. The incidence of complete AV block does not appear to be any different from the general MI population as well.

At the present time, premature ventricular contractions (PVCs) occur in over 80% of CCU patients with acute MI. As stated previously, patients with only occasional PVCs after the initial hours probably do not warrant antidysrhythmic prophylaxis. Suppressive therapy is recommended, however, for patients with more malignant and complex ventricular ectopy, including frequent premature beats (more than 5/minute), multifocal premature contractions, runs or salvos of premature beats, or frequent combinations of premature beats such as bigeminy or trigemini. In these cases, the initial bolus dose of lidocaine for the elderly patient is 0.5 mg/kg, repeated every 2 to 5 minutes to a total of 1.5 mg/kg. An additional sustaining infusion should be begun at 1 mg/minute and increased after each bolus to a maximum of 1.5 mg/kg. Again, it should be noted that the incidence of lidocaine toxicity increases with the time of administration.

Ventricular tachycardia occurs in about 10 to 20% of elderly patients in the CCU with acute MI. It frequently terminates spontaneously but has devastating consequences if it progresses to ventricular fibrillation. If the patient is stable (does not have continuing chest pain, shortness of breath, evidence of pulmonary edema, hypotension, or abnormal mental status), then acute suppressive therapy with lidocaine, procainamide, or bretylium tosylate is indicated. If the patient with ventricular tachycardia is unstable (has chest pain, shortness of breath, pulmonary edema, hypotension, or abnormal mental status), then the patient should be defibrillated with an initial energy level of 50-watt seconds, increasing wattage to 100, 200, and 360 until the patient is converted after sedation, as dictated by the individual's condition. Ventricular fibrillation occurs in about 10 to 15% of patients during the initial hours after infarction. Of course, the patient with ventricular fibrillation should be defibrillated with initial levels being approximately 200-watt seconds. The recommendations of the American Heart Association for subsequent defibrillation follow. After the initial defibrillation, the patient should have two more successive defibrillations, at 200- to 300-watt seconds and then at 360-watt seconds with as little delay as possible, after ensuring that the patient has remained in ventricular fibrillation.

After the initial three shocks, the patient should then be given epinephrine (5 to 10 ml of the 1:10,000 concentration) and intubated. If the patient remains in ventricular fibrillation and still has no pulse, then the patient should be defibrillated again at 360-watt seconds. If this, in turn, is not successful, then acute suppressive therapy with lidocaine (beginning at 1 mg/kg) should be begun, followed by another defibrillation: subsequent alternating defibrillations with doses of lidocaine at 0.25 mg/kg for the elderly should be instituted. After the initial 1 mg/kg bolus of lidocaine, bretylium can be used instead in alternation with the defibrillations. The bretylium should be given initially at 5 mg/kg, followed by 10 mg/kg to a maximum of 30 mg/kg.

Finally, accelerated idioventricular rhythm (slow ventricular tachycardia) occurs in up to 30% of elderly patients in the early hours to days after infarction. This rhythm results from progressive slowing of the sinus pacemaker with subsequent ventricular escape. This rhythm consists of wide uniform QRS complexes with a rate of 80 to 100 beats/minute. It is vital to distinguish this rhythm from the more rapid ventricular tachycardia that poses a much more ominous prognosis. An accelerated idioventricular rhythm does not need to be suppressed since it represents the residual lower functioning pacemaker driving the heart. The rhythm rarely causes symptoms or hemodynamic consequences, although digitalis toxicity should be excluded as the cause in this situation.

Bradydysrhythmias

Sinus bradycardia is a common transient arrhythmia that occurs in approximately 20% of patients with inferior infarction, especially within the initial 2 to 4 hours

after the onset of infarction. It occurs so frequently, primarily because of the fact that the sinoatrial node is supplied by the right coronary artery as mentioned previously. Significant evidence has accumulated to support the theory that the sinus bradycardia is a protective reflex and decreases myocardial oxygen demand. As such, it should not be treated with atropine, unless it produces hemodynamic consequences or is associated with underlying premature ventricular contractions.

The treatment of the various AV blocks differs according to the degree of block and the location of the infarction. First-degree AV block and Mobitz I (Wenckebach) second-degree AV block generally require only observation. However, some authorities advocate standby pacemaker placement for the Mobitz I (Wenckebach) second-degree AV block. Certainly, the recent acceptance and proven efficacy of external pacemakers has allowed more frequent prophylactic placement of its paddles without invading the patient. Complete AV (third-degree) block in patients with inferior MI demands a pacemaker only if it produces hemodynamic sequelae.

In contrast, patients with anterior infarction (and either a Mobitz II second-degree AV block or a complete heart block) should have temporary electrical pacing. These patients have been shown to have over 80% in-hospital or early posthospitalization mortality. The reason for the disparity in mortality between inferior and anterior MI with a Mobitz II second-degree heart block and complete heart block can be explained by the anatomic concepts for inferior MI mentioned above; both heart blocks frequently occur from temporary ischemia of the AV node. Unless there is a specific, extremely rare, infarction of the AV node, these blocks tend to be temporary. In anterior infarction, however, heart block develops from massive destruction of the myocardial electrical pathways that extend along the ventricular septum. Complete heart block due to AV node ischemia in patients with inferior infarction usually resolves in 7 to 10 days. It occurs two to three times more commonly in patients with inferior infarction.

Temporary transvenous pacemaking is also recommended in new onset right bundle branch block and left anterior hemiblock, especially when these are associated with first-degree AV block. The association of a left anterior or posterior hemiblock with a right bundle branch block in patients with anterior MI is an ominous sign most likely leading to sudden complete heart block. This certainly necessitates the placement of a temporary transvenous pacemaker.

Elderly patients with MI do, however, have a higher incidence of pulmonary edema and cardiogenic shock. This suggests and correlates with a higher incidence of pre-existing heart disease and/or generalized decline in myocardial reserve. Approximately 60 to 80% of in-hospital mortality from MI in the elderly occurs from cardiogenic shock and another 15% from acute pulmonary edema.

The classification of Killip and Kimball,[32] in which patients with postinfarction congestive heart failure are classified according to the severity of the failure shows the direct correlation between the degree of heart failure and mortality in MI. The Killip classification is a little bit more useful in that it does not require invasive hemodynamic monitoring. In brief, the Killip classification divides patients into four classes. Class I patients have uncomplicated MI with no evidence of heart failure. Class II patients have mild to moderate congestive heart failure with an S_3 and pulmonary inspiratory crackles less than or equal to halfway up the lungs. Class III patients have severe congestive cardiac failure with inspiratory crackles over one half of the lung fields, and class IV patients are in cardiogenic shock.

The treatment of post-MI left ventricular failure involves a stepped-up approach. Intravenous diuretics such as furosemide are used for all degrees of heart failure. Caution should be exercised in those patients who have never taken furosemide before since its venodilatory effect may cause an abrupt drop in blood pressure. Therefore, small doses such as 20 mg should be used initially until the patient's response can be judged. For moderate and severe heart failure, intravenous vasodilator therapy is indicated; in the presence of MI, intravenous nitroglycerin is the drug of choice and should be started at a dose of 5 to 10 μg/minute. For severe heart failure, dobutamine should be added to the intravenous nitroglycerin to maintain pulmonary capillary wedge pressure in the range of 18.

For those patients who present with hypotension in the postinfarction period, a trial of volume replacement is indicated in all cases in which the pulmonary capillary wedge pressure is less than 18 and in all cases of right ventricular infarction. However, if the pulmonary capillary wedge pressure is greater than 18 or if the patient is in cardiogenic shock, then progressive use of dopamine and/or dobutamine is advised.

The incidence of CVA from MI is also higher than in the general population with acute MI. Reports have shown incidences of 2 to 4% in elderly patients with acute MI.[33]

Of the other infrequent but predictable potential complications of acute MI, cardiac rupture is found most frequently in elderly patients.[34,35] It usually occurs 3 to 12 days following an infarction and is often heralded by the reappearance of chest pain, which is associated with a normal sinus rhythm at the onset of the hypotension (electromechanical dissociation). The other complications of acute MI do not seem to have a higher incidence in the elderly. Acute mitral regurgitation is usually seen complicating posterior MI, and ventricular septal rupture frequently complicates anterior and anteroseptal infarctions — both occur during the first week after infarction.

Right ventricular infarction, which as previously stated occurs in about one third of the cases of inferior infarction, is heralded by the onset of hypotension, distended neck veins, hepatic congestion, clear lung fields, and chest pain. In this situation, right precordial ECG leads will show the characteristic ST elevation of infarction. There seems to be a slightly higher incidence of right ventricular infarction in the elderly patient than in the younger population.

MYOCARDIAL SALVAGE

Without prompt intervention, the reversibly ischemic myocardium will proceed rapidly to irreversible cell necrosis, with loss of ventricular function and the subsequent risk of malignant arrhythmia, loss of mechanical function, and death. The emergency physician has many therapeutic options, but all require rapid data acquisition, assessment of possible contraindications, and timely institution of therapy. Interventions for myocardial salvage may be divided into two general categories: those that promote clot lysis with reperfusion of nutrients and oxygen, and those that influence myocardial oxygen consumption by improving flow to ischemic areas and reducing the oxygen requirements of compromised tissue. These agents have several goals: to decrease the risk of reexpansion and reinfarction, to preserve left ventricular function, to decrease the incidence of serious arrhythmias, to decrease the risk of sudden and infarct-related death, and to preserve the quality of life by preserving left ventricular ejection fraction.

The last decade has left us with a plethora of literature on the thrombolytic treatments; however, nonthrombolytic therapy is an important primary treatment of myocardial infarction or adjunct in patients where lytic therapy is either contraindicated or efficacy reduced because of delayed presentation. Thrombolytic agents, beta-blockers, and intravenous nitrates have documented efficacy, while some calcium channel blockers have been beneficial only in well-defined subgroups and have increased mortality in others. All therapies entail risk and may precipitate hemorrhage, congestive heart failure, or serious arrhythmias, or worsen ischemia or cause hypotension. Physicians must be cognizant of the benefits and contraindications, routes and dosages for administration, and the indications for the variety of available therapeutic options.

Thrombolytic Myocardial Salvage

The pathophysiology of myocardial infarction is thought to involve fissuring or rupturing of an atherosclerotic plaque precipitating platelet activation and intracoronary thrombus formation. In the early hours of acute MI, mortality may be reduced up to 50% by thrombolytic therapy. The most dramatic benefits have been reported when treatment is given within 6 hours of the onset of chest pain, but some centers have reported beneficial effects on mortality up to 24 hours after the onset of symptoms.[36] Three thrombolytic agents are generally available: streptokinase, tissue plasminogen activator, and urokinase. The advantages and disadvantages of the agents are outlined in Table 14–1. Another agent, anisoylated plasminogen activator complex (APSAC), may soon be available.

Indications

The decision to use thrombolytic therapy must be made with caution but without delay. The sooner therapy is implemented the greater the likelihood for coronary patency and myocardial salvage. Any patient coming to the emergency care unit with chest pain lasting more than 30 minutes and less than 6 hours, associated with 1 mm or more of ST segment elevation in two or more contiguous leads (inferior, anterior, lateral, posterior, or septal distributions) should be evaluated for thrombolytic therapy.

These indications, however, are not absolute; strict application of these recommendations may exclude patients likely to benefit from lytic therapy. Patients may have stuttering symptoms for hours from intermittent or partial coronary artery occlusion before complete occlusion takes place; a strict 4- or 6-hour restriction for thrombolytic therapy would not work to the patient's benefit in this situation.

The use of lytic therapy in uncomplicated inferior wall MI is also debatable. "Uncomplicated inferior infarctions" have a tendency to turn complicated rapidly with right ventricular involvement, arrhythmia, and heart block. Right coronary artery occlusion, while less often associated with death or cardiogenic shock, is highly detrimental in the event of occlusion of the left anterior descending system because it would preclude the development of right-to-left collateral flow. Therefore, the decision

to implement thrombolytic therapy must take into account the individual presentation, the underlying pathophysiology and coronary anatomy, and the risks to that patient.

Contraindications

A rapid assessment of patient contraindications must be made before implementing lytic therapy (Table 14–2). A list of contraindications to thrombolytic therapy should be posted in rooms where cardiac patients are treated. This will facilitate assessment and help to ensure that contraindications are not forgotten in the haste to implement therapy. However, therapy should be administered by weighing any potential risk against the known benefits of early therapy. For instance, a patient with a history of right main and circumflex coronary artery occlusions resuscitated from ventricular tachycardia in the field with a chest thump and half a dozen chest compressions, who presents with anterior ST segment elevation and pain, would probably greatly benefit from keeping his only viable coronary artery open regardless of the relative contraindications from cardiopulmonary resuscitation. Common pitfalls for inappropriate thrombolytic therapy should also be considered before initiating therapy (Table 14–3).

Therapy

Once the decison to implement thrombolytic therapy has been made, preparation and implementation must pro-

Table 14–1 Advantages and Disadvantages of Selected Thrombolytic Therapies

Agent	Advantages	Disadvantages
Streptokinase (Kabikinase, Streptase)	Least expensive Long half-life Low rate of reocclusion Easy to administer Most cost-effective With MI < 3 hr old	Potentially antigenic Systemic lytic state Depletes plasminogen May precipitate hypotension
Urokinase (Abbokinase)	No antigenicity Less plasminogen depletion Relatively clot-selective	More expensive Limited clinical experience
Tissue plasminogen activator (Activase)	Clot specific Most effective with clots > 3 hr old	Most expensive High rate of reocclusion

Table 14–2 Contraindications to Thrombolytic Therapy[63]

Absolute contraindications
  Active internal or major external hemorrhage
  Cerebrovascular accident within 6 months

Relative contraindications

Major risk factors
  Major trauma
  Prolonged cardiopulmonary resuscitation
  Associated uncontrolled hypertensive emergency
  Major surgery within 10 days
  Ongoing severe gastrointestinal hemorrhage
  Previous cerebrovascular accident

Minor risk factors
  Pregnancy
  Age >75 years
  Minor trauma
  Thrombus or endocarditis of left side of heart
  Diabetic retinopathy
  Inflammatory bowel disease
  Endotracheal intubation
  Catheter or needle in internal jugular or subclavian vein
  Current anticoagulation or hemostatic disorder
  Cavitary lung, hepatic, or renal disease

From Thrombolytic therapy in thrombosis. A National Institutes of Health Consensus Development Conference (symposium), Ann Intern Med 93:141–144, 1980.

Table 14–3   Common Pitfalls of Thrombolytic Therapy

Pericarditis
Early repolarization variant
Left ventricular hypertrophy pattern
Remote ventricular aneurysm
Ascending aortic dissection with coronary artery involvement
Remote myocardial infarction with incomplete ST resolution

ceed rapidly, because delays threaten the potential for optimal myocardial salvage. Two peripheral intravenous lines should be placed, one for the thrombolytic agent and the second for other drugs such as lidocaine or nitroglycerin. An attempt should be made to keep blood sampling, especially arterial punctures, to a minimum after initiation of thrombolytic therapy. A third heparin-locked line is often useful for blood draws or inadvertent complications.

A baseline laboratory evaluation (complete blood count, clotting parameters with PT, PTT, and fibrinogen, renal and cardiac profile) should be performed, but in the absence of known or suspected abnormalities, therapy should not be delayed while waiting for the results. Lines should be carefully secured, especially in patients who will be transported by helicopter or who may need ground transport to a tertiary care facility for urgent catheterization, angioplasty, or intra-aortic balloon pumping. Once patient preparation is complete, the risks and benefits of therapy explained, and patient identification rechecked, thrombolytic therapy should be started.

Streptokinase. Streptokinase is usually administered by IV infusion of 1.5 million units over 30 minutes to 1 hour. Either 100 mg IV push of hydrocortisone (or comparably dosed steroid) as well as 50 mg IV push of diphenhydramine can be administered before or during the infusion of streptokinase to keep allergic reactions to a minimum. Therapy should be initiated at 400 to 500 units/kg/min and reduced to 200 to 250 units/kg/min if blood pressure declines. Streptokinase produces a disseminated lytic state for up to 48 hours. Although heparin therapy is not necessary, most studies have used heparin without a bolus after streptokinase administration. If heparin is used, it should be started after the streptokinase infusion is complete and should be adjusted to maintain the activated partial thromboplastin time in the range of 60 to 90 seconds.

One hour after administering streptokinase, an increase in fibrin degradation products should be noted to ensure that a systemic lytic state has been initiated. Large amounts of antistreptolysin antibodies may negate the effects of streptokinase. Therefore, if fibrin degradation products are not elevated or if fibrinogen is not depressed, the presence of antistreptolysin antibodies should be presumed and either another lytic agent used or the dosage of streptokinase increased. Another reason for lack of sustained efficacy may be depletion of plasminogen, a substrate needed for thrombolytic effect. In such patients the administration of fresh frozen plasma may restore plasminogen levels to that needed for efficacy. Therapy should also include aspirin (160 to 325 mg/day) to impede platelet aggregation on existing thrombus, although this may increase the risk of bleeding complications.

ECGs should be obtained at least every hour for the first 4 hours and cardiac creatine kinase enzymes followed up closely. Clinical parameters of reperfusion are not always reliable but include the development of reperfusion arrhythmias (usually accelerated idioventricular rhythm), relief of pain, resolution of ST segment elevation, and early peaking of CK enzymes. The efficacy of peripheral intravenous streptokinase averages approximately 50% by angiography and 84% when noninvasive parameters of recanalization are studied.[28,37]

Complications are mainly related to bleeding and include a relatively rare incidence of intracranial hemorrhage (0.9% compared with 0.6% in controls).[38] Fever, urticaria, and flushing occur as well as nausea, vomiting, and headaches. Gastrointestinal bleeding is seen in approximately 5 to 10% of patients, and hypotension may occur if the medication is administered too rapidly.[39] Since streptokinase is antigenic, a repeat administration at a later time may precipitate an allergic reaction. Therefore, streptokinase should only be administered during one infarction period and not repeated at a later date.

Tissue Plasminogen Activator (TPA). In a study comparing the efficacy of two regimens for TPA, a weight-adjusted dosing regimen appeared to be the most efficacious with the least number of side effects.[40] We have found a modified weight-adjusted dosage regimen, shown in Table 14–4, to be easily and safely administered. The total dose given is equal to the patient's weight (kg) plus 30 mg not to exceed 120 mg in total. Care should be taken not to shake the preparation because active drug may be lost in the foam created. Tubing should be flushed with D5W before administering the TPA bolus. In addition, the same tubing used for the bolus should also be used for the maintenance drip since some active drug may bind to the tubing, creating an additional loss for each tubing set used. The first dose is a 10 mg bolus given intravenously. An infusion rate is then immediately started so that the first hour of infusion equals the patient's weight (kg) minus 10 ml/hr (not to exceed 80 ml/hr). Maintenance therapy should continue for 3 hours at a rate of 10 ml/hr.

Patients should also be given 106 to 325 mg of aspirin at the start of therapy. Heparin should be started 60 to 90 minutes after the TPA is administered by giving a 5,000 to 10,000 unit bolus followed by maintenance therapy with 1,000 units per hour. Delaying the initiation of heparin therapy decreases the risk of bleeding complications while maintaining efficacy.[41]

Table 14–4   Weight-Adjusted TPA Protocol

Preparation	Administration
Two peripheral IVs	TPA dose
1. Nitroglycerin or	Total: Wt (kg) + 30 mg
lidocaine line	Mix 50-mg vial with
2. TPA line	50 ml sterile water
	Do not shake tube
Third Line	10 mg bolus IV push
3. Heparin lock (16 or 18 g)	Place remainder in sterile
for labs	bag and infuse:
	Hour 1 (max 80 ml/hr)
Labs	Wt (kg) – 10 ml/hr
CK, SGOT, LDH	Hours 2, 3, 4
Renal profile	10 ml/hr
CBC	Do not interrupt infusion
PT, PTT, fibrinogen	Heparin
	60–90 minutes after TPA
	infusion give:
	5–10,000 units bolus
	Maintenance:
	1,000 units/hr
	Aspirin
	160–325 mg immediately

Adapted from Dean E et al: University Hospital Department of Cardiology: acute interventional cardiology program protocol, 1988–1989.

ECGs and laboratory evaluation should follow the same protocol as for streptokinase. Since TPA is a naturally occurring human protein, allergic reactions and antibodies do not pose a problem. As with streptokinase, clinical indexes of reperfusion may also be unreliable.

Despite TPA's relative clot specific nature, the incidence of bleeding is directly related to the cumulative dose given. The incidence of intracranial hemorrhage rises fourfold when the dose of TPA is 150 mg rather than 100 mg.[39] Other complications include gastrointestinal bleeding, hematoma formation at the site of catheters, and continual oozing at the site of venipuncture.

TPA versus streptokinase. In the current era of cost containment and fixed DRG reimbursement for thrombolytic therapy and MI, it is imperative to examine the costs of agents that are similar in beneficial and adverse effects. Both streptokinase and TPA are highly effective agents in the early hours of infarction, and coronary artery patency rates have been roughly equal in studies examining the effectiveness of both these therapies early in the course of infarction. Until recently, however, head-to-head trials have been lacking. In a timely study comparing the efficacy of streptokinase versus intravenous TPA in acute MI less than 3 hours old, there was no difference in angiographic patency between the two therapies administered early in the course of MI.[42] This study and others comparing the complication rate of the two agents show some advantage for TPA. However, they also indicate an increased prevalence of reocclusion and recurrent ischemia with TPA, which may counterbalance the benefits of a lower side effect profile.

In an analysis of the incremental cost-effectiveness of alternative strategies for the treatment of acute MI, Steinberg found the additional cost per presumed life saved to be $64,571 greater for those patients treated with TPA instead of streptokinase for acute MI (using data from previous studies that assumed a mortality rate of 11.3% for conventional treatment, 10.0% for streptokinase, and 9.3% for TPA).[43] Since both agents are extremely effective in fresh clots less than 3 hours old, the potential cost savings to the medical system for equal efficacy by using streptokinase in the early hours of infarction would be even more impressive — without loss of effective treatment for our patients.

Since the difference in cost between TPA and streptokinase is significant, streptokinase appears to be the more cost-effective agent in the early hours of coronary artery occlusion. TPA is the more efficacious agent when administered between 3 and 6 hours of chest pain and is probably the preferred agent in that time period regardless of cost. Since a systemic lytic state is not created with TPA and since reocclusion may be a problem, aspirin and heparin therapy in these patients is of prime importance.

Urokinase. Urokinase is a nonallergenic plasminogen activator that is relatively clot-selective. It is more expensive but less allergenic than streptokinase. Urokinase is administered intravenously over 60 minutes, starting with a 40 mg dose. An additional 20 to 40 mg may be given if signs of reperfusion are lacking. The published clinical experience with this agent is limited to less than 100 patients and further studies are needed.[44]

APSAC. The search for a more ideal thrombolytic agent that can be given quickly, with a high rate of coronary recanalization and a low rate of reocclusion has led to the development of anisoylated plasminogen streptokinase activator complex (APSAC). Current studies utilize a 30-unit dose administered over 5 minutes. Heparin is not needed until 4 hours after administration and coronary patency approaches 70% with a 24-hour reocclusion rate of only 5%.[45] Further studies are in progress and early results are promising.

Nonthrombolytic Myocardial Salvage

So much attention has been given to thrombolytic myocardial salvage that nonthrombolytic therapies are frequently considered secondary forms of therapy. There is no reason to allow an infarct to expand while the patient progresses into florid congestive heart failure because he or she did not meet the strictest criteria for thrombolytic therapy. Nonthrombolytic therapies are powerful agents used alone or as adjuncts to thrombolytic therapy. A substantial amount of data has been collected regarding the beta-blockers, nitrates, and calcium channel blockers, as well as other therapeutic agents.

Beta-Blockers

Beta-blockers decrease myocardial oxygen consumption by lowering blood pressure and heart rate and decreasing contractility. They also counter the adverse effects of excessive catecholamines and decrease arrhythmogenesis in the periinfarct period. Their beneficial effect on mortality stems largely from an observed decrease in sudden death, predominantly in the early days after infarction. Their main action is thought to be prevention of ventricular septal rupture and malignant ventricular arrhythmias.[46] Beta-blockers can be used intravenously or orally at the onset of MI or be initiated several days later. Pooled data indicate that the best results come from starting intravenous beta-blocker therapy early and continuing the therapy orally for 1 to 2 years. The pharmacologic properties of commonly used beta-blockers are shown in Table 14–5. The initial intravenous management will be reviewed here because this is most pertinent to the emergency physician. The two most widely studied intravenous beta-blockers, atenolol and metoprolol, and a newer fast-acting, short half-life, intravenous beta-blocker, esmolol, will be discussed.

Indications. The indications for beta-blocker therapy in acute MI are the same as those for the thrombolytic agents except for the lack of stringent time constraints for administering therapy. Therefore, they become of prime importance for the patient with stuttering symptoms or without clear-cut onset of pain. They are also ideal agents in patients with absolute contraindications to lytic therapy or in those with relative or minor contraindications from whom the physician chooses to withhold lytic treatment. They are powerful primary agents or adjuncts to thrombolysis and are particularly effective in patients with hypertension, tachycardia, ventricular or atrial ectopic rhythm, tachyarrhythmias, or those with a hyperadrenergic state.

Contraindications. The contraindications to beta-blocker use in MI are reviewed in Table 14–6. Paradoxically, the patients most likely to benefit from beta-blocker therapy are those whom physicians are often least likely to treat, that is, patients with a history of heart failure, low ejection fraction, or history of previous MI. This is an unfortunate paradox because a patient with a borderline ejection fraction or history of heart failure who is actively infarcting the remainder of the myocardium may not receive beta-blocker therapy and yet may be the patient most likely to benefit — especially in the absence of thrombolytic therapy. Therefore, the risks of beta-blocker therapy must be compared to the benefits; if trepidation exists, a fast-acting beta-blocker with a short half-life such as esmolol may be a useful alternative.

Therapy. Continuous rhythm and intermittent blood pressure monitoring should be performed. More invasive hemodynamic monitoring measures are often difficult and unnecessary in the hemodynamically stable patient in the emergency department. Two large-bore intravenous lines should be placed and atropine kept at the bedside for possible hemodynamically significant bradycardia. In the event of bradycardia unresponsive to atropine, isoproterenol should be avoided since use of the selective beta-one receptor (cardiac) blockers may cause preferential agonist effects on peripheral beta-two receptors, contributing further to hypotension. If atropine is ineffective, patients will usually respond to time and fluids; however, glucagon may be used to increase heart rate by a non-beta receptor mechanism and appears to be the drug of choice in massive beta-blocker overdose or unresponsive beta-blocker toxicity. This degree of refractory bradycardia would certainly be unusual in the routine treatment of MI and rapid acceleration of the heart rate would be deleterious to myocardial oxygen consumption. Therefore, glucagon should be withheld unless serious refractory bradycardia with hypotension is present, and therapy usually starts with 1 mg of glucagon administered intravenously over 10 minutes.[47]

1. Atenolol. Therapy should start with an immediate IV of 5 mg, given over 5 minutes. If complications develop, the injection should be stopped and may cautiously

Table 14–5 Pharmacologic Properties of the Beta-Blockers

Generic name	Trade name	Half-life (hours)	Elimination (hepatic/renal)	Dosages
Nonselective				
Propranolol	(Inderal)	3–6	Hepatic	10–20 mg qid
Timolol	(Blocadren)	3–4	80%/20%	1--20 mg bid
*Pindolol	(Visken)	3–4	60%/40%	15–30 mg qd
Nadolol	(Corgard)	14–24	Renal	40–80 mg qd
Selective				
*Acebutolol	(Sectral)	3–4†	60%/40%	200–600 mg bid
‡Metoprolol	(Lopressor)	3–4	Hepatic	100–200 mg bid
‡Atenolol	(Tenormin)	6–9	Renal	50–100 mg qd
‡Esmolol	(Brevibloc)	9 min	RBC esterase	50–200 µg/kg/m

*Intrinsic sympathomimetic activity.
†Diacetolol, active metabolite present for 8–13 hours.
‡May be used intravenously in AMI.

Table 14–6 Contraindications to Beta-Blockers in Acute Myocardial Infarction

Major contraindications
  Heart rate persistently <50
  Systolic blood pressure persistently <100 mm Hg
  Second- or third-degree heart block
  Severe heart failure
  Severe bronchospasm

Relative contraindications
  Poor peripheral circulation
  Implanted pacemaker
  Impaired AV conduction (PR >0.24 ms)
  Status post-resuscitation
  Ongoing inotropic (catecholamine) administration

be restarted when the patient is hemodynamically stable. If after 10 minutes the initial heart rate has not dropped to 60 to 70 beats/minute, up to 5 mg is given again intravenously. Ten minutes after the IV doses are complete, 50 mg of atenolol is given orally followed by another 50 mg 12 hours later. Therapy should continue at 50 or 100 mg twice daily.[46]

2. Metoprolol. Intravenous injection of 15 mg of metoprolol (5 mg at a time with 2-minute intervals between injections) is administered and heart rate and blood pressure are closely monitored. If heart rate and blood pressure have not been lowered sufficiently, it should be repeated using 5 mg at a time to maintain adequate pulse and pressure effect. If after 15 minutes the heart rate and blood pressure have been lowered sufficiently with adequate drug effect, 100 mg of metoprolol is given orally. Maintenance therapy of 100 to 200 mg orally every 12 hours is then administered.[48,49]

3. Esmolol. Esmolol is a recently released ultra–short-acting (t1/2 of 9 minutes) cardioselective beta-blocker. Its short half-life allows for rapid reversal of drug effect and rapid titration to a desired hemodynamic target. Clinical studies have shown esmolol to be an effective and safe method to lower blood pressure and heart rate in patients with MI or unstable angina — even in patients where beta-blockers might routinely be withheld because of contraindications such as elevated pulmonary capillary wedge pressure. The drug is usually administered from a 10 mg/ml solution given in infusion periods of 250 to 500 µg/kg/min for 1 to 2 minutes followed by 4- to 5-minute infusions of 25-300 µg/kg/min. The condition of most patients will stabilize between 50 and 150 µg/kg/min, and hemodynamic effects usually completely reverse within 30 minutes of drug termination.[50]

Nitrates

Intravenous nitrate therapy used during the course of acute MI has the potential to limit infarct size and expansion, as well as lower the incidence of infarct-related complications and mortality.[51,52] Therapy must be expedient and judicious because the greatest benefits occur with early therapy and harmful effects may be produced if the mean blood pressure drops too low. Nitrates act to alter the balance of oxygen supply and demand by increasing the flow to ischemic areas. They dilate fixed stenotic segments and also increase the blood supply by relieving any associated coronary artery spasm. Decreases in elevated left ventricular diastolic pressure (preload) and afterload all favorably decrease myocardial oxygen demand. These potential benefits must be carefully titrated against the potential to worsen ischemia through a reflex increase in heart rate (which increases myocardial oxygen consumption) or lower blood pressure, further decreasing coronary artery perfusion pressure. Coronary perfusion pressure roughly equals the intraaortic diastolic pressure minus the left ventricular end-diastolic pressure. Therefore, diastolic hypotension is tolerated poorly by patients with high wedge pressures or elevated left ventricular end-diastolic pressures. Further decreases in coronary perfusion may additionally increase infarct size.

Several studies have demonstrated a statistically significant reduction in mortality and myocardial enzyme release in groups of patients treated with either nitroprusside or nitroglycerin during acute MI.[54] Nitroprusside has proven to be an effective agent, particularly in those patients with hypertension; however, the potential for a paradoxical decrease in flow to poorly perfused areas, the "coronary steal phenomenon," has limited its widespread acceptance.

Therapy. Many effective nitrates are available for the treatment of acute MI (Table 14–7) with several forms capable of delivering some form of nitrate therapy during episodes of acute ischemia. Generally, therapy should start with sublingual NTG while another form of therapy that delivers more continuous blood levels is prepared.

Intravenous nitroglycerin is the therapy of choice in acute ischemic syndromes as it allows for pain control with ease of blood pressure titration. Endpoints used in studies for nitroglycerin therapy have been inconsistent, although there is agreement that rapid or overaggressive blood pressure lowering is deleterious. Examples of useful endpoints include: 1) not more than a 10% decrease in mean blood pressure (but never below a mean of 80 mm Hg), 2) a 10% decrease in systolic blood pressure (but never below a systolic blood pressure of 90 mm Hg), and 3) a maximum dose of 200 µg/min. Hemodynamic endpoints are perhaps more applicable than absolute dose limitations, since patients on high doses of nitrates at home may exhibit tolerance to the usual doses of nitroglycerin and will require larger doses for the desired effects.

Indications and contraindications. All patients with acute ischemic syndromes are candidates for nitrate therapy unless they are hypotensive. Therapy in hypoten-

Table 14–7   Nitrates Commonly Used as Adjuncts in Treatment of Acute Myocardial Infarction

Medication	Dosage	Onset	Side effects
Intravenous NTG	Variable	1–2 min	Headaches, flushing, hypotension
Sublingual NTG	0.3–0.6 mg	2–5 min	Headaches, flushing, hypotension
Aerosol NTG	0.4 mg	2–5 min	Headaches, flushing, hypotension
Oral ISDN	5–30	15–30 min	Headaches, flushing, hypotension
2% Ointment	½–2 in	20–60 min	Skin reaction
Transdermal	5–10 mg	30–60 min	Skin reaction

sive patients should only be performed in those patients with pulmonary artery catheters to allow for continuous monitoring of ventricular filling pressures, cardiac outputs, and vascular resistance. Therefore, use of intravenous nitrates in this setting generally should not be attempted in the emergency care unit. Those patients who are preload dependent for adequate output such as those with right ventricular infarction are particularly prone to develop hypotension during the course of therapy.

Patients requiring short-term helicopter transport without invasive monitoring in place may benefit from application of nitropaste to allow for ease of application and a short half-life if the paste is wiped off. It is not necessary to place an arterial line in patients receiving intravenous nitroglycerin; however, vigilant blood pressure monitoring or intermittent timed monitoring is advisable, especially in the initial phase of therapy titration.

Intravenous nitroglycerin. Nitroglycerin is now usually issued to pharmacies in a stable powder that is mixed with ethyl alcohol and sterile water to place in solution. Once in solution the preparation must be refrigerated, kept sterile, and protected from light. Solutions should generally be used within 4 weeks and are then diluted in 5% dextrose in water to approximately 60 µg/ml. Infusions should be made through a standard to infusion pump starting at 5 µg/min and increased by 5 to 20 µg/min every 3 to 5 minutes. The average infusion rate required to lower mean blood pressure is highly variable with a dose of 45 ± 34 µg/min in normal patients and 54 ± 39 µg/min in hypertensive patients.[53,54] It is imperative that therapy be started as early as possible and should continue for 36 to 48 hours even if pain has subsided completely.

Other Therapies

Aspirin and other antiplatelet agents. Platelet activation and aggregation at the site of atherosclerotic plaque rupture or fissuring is thought to be one of the underlying mechanisms for coronary thrombosis and MI. Several trials have evaluated the effects of aspirin given on the day of MI and continued for at least 4 to 5 weeks. The largest of these was the ISIS-2 trial, which found significant reductions in nonfatal reinfarction (44%) and in mortality (21%).[36] Although there may be a higher incidence of complications in patients given both a throm-

bolytic agent and aspirin, especially in patients undergoing catheterization, most studies still utilize both therapies concurrently. Therefore, aspirin should be given in doses of 160 to 325 mg/24 to 48 hours. If lytic therapy is administered, the decision to initiate aspirin concurrently should be individualized based on the potential for bleeding if urgent catheterization, angioplasty, or invasive monitoring is indicated.

Calcium channel blockers. Calcium channel blockers have the theoretic potential to limit infarct size by reducing blood pressure, heart rate, and contractility. Therefore, it may seem surprising that the calcium channel blockers, so routinely used in stable angina, are under the heading of "other therapies." However, at least two trials involving verapamil, four involving nifedipine, and one involving diltiazem, have failed to show a substantial reduction in mortality, morbidity, or enzyme release.[54-56]

In only one study that specifically dealt with non–Q wave MI diltiazem was shown to reduce early recurrent infarction. However, a small nonsignificant excess of deaths and a substantial number of side effects were noted.[57] The potential benefit of these compounds is probably limited at the current time by their negative inotropy, chronotropy, and risk of side effects. In certain instances, however, where beta-blockers and lytic therapy are contraindicated or pose substantial risks to the patient,[58,59] the calcium channel blockers may be used as adjunctive therapy with other agents. Currently, the available data do not support the use of calcium channel blockers in the face of acute transmural MI.

Hyaluronidase. Hyaluronidase is a naturally occurring enzyme usually extracted from bovine testes, thought to increase the diffusion of nutrients to ischemic zones by depolymerizing surrounding mucopolysaccharides. There are no serious side effects of hyaluronidase, but studies have shown variable degrees of efficacy in terms of mortality and infarct size. Although the side effect profile is minor, further studies are needed to assess the efficacy of this agent.[60]

Free radical injury: superoxide dismutase and catalase. Activated oxygen species containing one unpaired electron (superoxide anion and hydroxyl radical) may react with critical cell components such as sulfhydryl-containing amino acids and unsaturated fatty acids to increase the myocardial injury of reperfused ischemic myocardium. Thus, treatment with a free radical scavenger such as catalase or superoxide dismutase (SOD) may reduce infarct size, improve myocardial salvage, and promote left ventricular recovery. One purpose of the thrombolysis and angioplasty in acute MI (TAMI) trials is to examine the efficacy of a 10 mg/kg bolus followed by an infusion of 0.2 mg/kg/hr infusion of SOD to prevent segmental wall motion abnormalities and prevent impairment of ejection fraction. Although this is an exciting and promising area of interest, studies have been largely confined to animals and have had mixed results.[61,62]

Angioplasty in acute myocardial infarction. Since a significant residual coronary artery stenosis remains in approximately 70% of patients after thrombolysis, it seemed reasonable to perform immediate catheterization and angioplasty in patients given thrombolytic therapy for acute MI.[58] Supporting this approach was the potential for an immediate diagnosis of high-risk coronary anatomy and immediate therapeutic intervention through angioplasty. On the negative side was the difficulty of obtaining 24-hour catheterization facilities, the cost to implement them, and the potential for hemorrhagic complications. Several studies have now concluded that immediate catheterization and angioplasty are associated with no differences in long-term outcome (ejection fraction or death). A higher incidence of reocclusion, bleeding, and the need for emergency bypass surgery has also been shown, further solidifying the case for a conservative approach.[57,58] One subgroup at particular risk, who should be catheterized immediately, are those patients with unrelieved pain and ST segment elevation. With this exception, immediate angioplasty offers no clear advantage to delayed elective catheterization and angioplasty in those patients thought to have reperfused on clinical grounds and is potentially dangerous.

Conclusion

The progression from a quiescent atherosclerotic plaque to an area of exposed endothelium with active thrombus formation and total coronary artery occlusion is swift.[63,64] Delays in therapy decrease the chance of myocardial salvage and increase the risk of cell death and myocardial necrosis. Thrombolytic therapy should be initiated with either streptokinase or with TPA if the patient presents within the first 3 hours of onset of pain or with TPA if presentation is delayed beyond 3 hours. Sublingual nitroglycerin or another fast-acting nitrate should be administered until an intravenous nitroglycerin drip is prepared, and nitrates should be titrated to relieve pain without adverse hemodynamic effects. Beta-blockers may be used as effective primary agents if thrombolytic therapy is contraindicated or as adjunctive therapy. Aspirin should be administered as soon as possible to patients not receiving streptokinase, and heparin sould be started 60 to 90 minutes after TPA administration. Treatment

with calcium channel blockers cannot be justified at the present time unless they are specifically indicated for persistent pain or arrhythmias and contraindications exist to other forms of therapy. Several agents such as APSAC, hyaluronidase, catalase, and superoxide dismutase are not yet ready for routine clinical use. Immediate catheterization and angioplasty should be reserved for those patients with continued pain and ST elevation refractory to standard therapy.[57-64] Table 14–8 gives an algorithm for acute myocardial infarction. A complete and comprehensive scheme for myocardial salvage in selected elderly patients (75 years old or younger) is presented in the Appendix to this chapter.

LOGISTIC PROBLEMS OF THE ELDERLY IN THE POSTINFARCTION PERIOD

Although the patient psychosis prevalent in early years of CCU management has virtually disappeared today, a prolonged CCU stay, with its associated isolation and disruption of normal eating and sleeping habits, still frequently causes confusion in the elderly patient. During this confusion, intravenous lines and other life support devices may be disconnected. Patients who are confused

Table 14–8 Algorithm for Treatment of Acute Myocardial Infarction

Acute Myocardial Infarction

↓

Check pitfalls
Assess contraindications

↓

If blood pressure >100
Intravenous Nitroglycerin
and

Beta-blockers contraindicated or <3 hours old	or 3–6 hours old	Thrombolytics contraindicated or >6 hours old
Streptokinase (or TPA)	TPA Aspirin Heparin in 60–90 minutes	Beta-blockers Atenolol Metoprolol Esmolol and Aspirin

Consider: 1. All patients monitored with oxygen and IV
2. Beta-blockers as adjuncts or primary treatment in all patients unless contraindicated
3. Calcium channel blockers only if beta-blockade is contraindicated
4. If pain and ST segment elevation persist, urgent catheterization and/or angioplasty

may actually get out of bed and fall, suffering significant complications. Attendant cerebral hypoxia or the characteristically excessive reaction of the elderly toward sedatives and other medications, particularly lidocaine, may exacerbate the psychosis and the confusion. Prolonged bed rest may result in pulmonary atelectasis or deep venous thrombosis with or without subsequent pulmonary embolism. Bed rest also can cause profound weakness and deconditioning (elderly patients who are submitted to bed rest lose over 40% of their strength after just 4 days) and increase the risk of pneumonia. Furthermore, anticoagulation has been shown to have increased risk of cerebral, gastrointestinal, and pericardial bleeding in elderly patients.

SUMMARY

New advances in emergency coronary revascularization with thrombolytic agents and balloon angioplasty dictate the diagnosis of MI in as timely a manner as possible. However, the variable presentation of the pathogenesis and pathophysiology of MI in the elderly along with other psychosocial factors make this early arrival of the patient less likely. The symptoms of MI have been reviewed with the emphasis that chest pain is a relatively infrequent presenting symptom. Other peculiarities of MI in the elderly include the fact that CK levels are frequently normal in the elderly, necessitating isoenzyme determination in all cases for the diagnosis of MI.

Much work needs to be done with regard to further delineating the differences in presentation and management of MI in the elderly if we are to continue in our progress of limiting its extremely high morbidity and mortality.

REFERENCES

1. Applegate WB and Graves MHS: Acute myocardial infarction in elderly patients, South Med J 77:1127–1132, 1978.
2. Konu B: Myocardial infarction in the elderly, Acta Med Scand Suppl 604:9–68, 1977.
3. Pomerance A: Cardiac pathology in the elderly. In Noble RJ and Rothbaum DA, editors: Geriatric cardiology, Philadelphia, 1981, FA Davis Co.
4. Wroblewski M, Mikulowski T, and Steen B: Symptoms of myocardial infarction in old age: clinical case, retrospective and prospective studies, Age Ageing 15:99–104, 1986.
5. Gerstenblith G, Lakatta EG, and Weisfeldt ML: Age changes in myocardial function and exercise response, Prog Cardiovasc Disease 19:1–21, 1976.
6. Kostis JB et al: The effect of age on heart rate in subjects free of heart disease, J Circulation 65:141–145, 1982.
7. Kennedy RD, Andrews GR, and Caird RI: Ischemic heart disease in the elderly, Br Heart J 39:1121–1125, 1977.
8. Rothbaum DA: Coronary artery disease. In Noble FJ and Rothbaum DA, editors: Geratric cardiology, Philadelphia, 1981, FA Davis Co.
9. Keannell WB and Gordon T: Evaluation of cardiovascular risk in the elderly: the Framingham study, Bull NY Acad Med 54:571–573, 1978.
10. Cornwell GG and Westermark R: Senile amyloidosis: a protein manifestation of the aging process, J Clin Pathol 33:1146–1152, 1980.
11. Fulkerson PK et al: Calcification of the mitral annulus, Am J Med 66:967–977, 1979.
12. Pomerance A: Aging changes in the human heart valve, B Heart J 29:222–230, 1967.
13. American Heart Association: Text book for advanced cardiac life support, Dallas, Texas, 1986.
14. Pathy MS: Clinical presentation of myocardial infarction in the elderly, Br Heart J 29:190–199, 1967.
15. Beahrmann JH, Hipp HR, and Heyer HE: Pain patterns in acute myocardial infarction, Am J Med 9:156–163, 1950.
16. Berman ND: The elderly patient in the coronary care unit. I. Acute myocardial infarction, J Am Geriatr Soc 27:145–149, 1979.
17. Berger HR and Zaret EL: Nuclear cardiology, N Engl J Med 305:799–808, 1981.
18. Condini MA: Management of acute myocardial infarction, Med Clin N Am 70:769–791, 1986.
19. Marshall RM, Blount SG, and Brenton E: Acute myocardial infarction: influence of the coronary care unit, Arch Intern Med 122:472–480, 1968.
20. Sagie A et al: Acute transmural myocardial infarction in elderly patients hospitalized in the coronary care unit versus the general medical ward, J Am Geriatr Soc 35:915–919, 1987.
21. Thanavaro S et al: In-hospital prognosis of patients with first nontransmural and transmural infarctions, Circulation 61:29–33, 1980.
22. Wenger NK: Management of acute myocardial infarction patients. Special report: acute myocardial infarction, Atlanta, 1987, American Health Consultants Inc.
23. Williams BO et al: The elderly patient in a coronary care unit, Br Med J 2:451–455, 1976.
24. DeSilva RA et al: Lidocaine prophylaxis in acute myocardial infarction: an evaluation of randomized trials, Lancet II:855–858, 1981.
25. European Cooperative Study Group: Streptokinase treatment in acute myocardial infarction, N Engl J Med 301:797–802, 1979.
26. Kennedy JW et al: Western Washington randomized trial of intracoronary streptokinase in acute myocardial infarction, N Engl J Med 309:1477–1482, 1983.
27. Rentrop KP: Thrombolytic therapy in patients with acute myocardial infarction, Circulation 71:627–631, 1985.
28. TIMI Study Group: The thrombolysis in myocardial infarction (TIMI) trial, N Engl J Med 312:932–936, 1985.
29. White HD et al: Effect of intravenous streptokinase as compared with that of tissue plasminogen activator on left ventricular function after first myocardial infarction, N Engl J Med 320:817, 1989.
30. Hartzler GO et al: Percutaneous transluminal coronary angioplasty with and without thrombolytic therapy for treatment of acute myocardial infarction, Am Heart J 106:965–973, 1983.
31. Braunwald E et al: Role of beta-adrenergic blockade in the therapy of patients with myocardial infarction, Am J Med 74:113–123, 1983.
32. Killip T and Kimball JT: Treatment of myocardial infarction in a coronary care unit: a two-year experience with 250 patients, Am J Cardiol 20:457–464, 1967.
33. Thompson PL and Robinson JS: Stroke after acute myocardial infarction: relation to infarct size, Br Med J 2:457–459, 1978.
34. McDonald JP: Presentation of acute myocardial infarction on cardiac rupture, Br Heart J 13:37–42, 1951.
35. Patch IL: Aging of cardiac infarcts and its influence on cardiac rupture, Br Heart J 13:37–42, 1951.
36. ISIS-2 (Second International Study of Infarct Survival) Collaborative Group: Randomized trial of intravenous streptokinase, oral aspirin, both or neither among 17,187 cases of suspected acute myocardial infarction, Lancet 2:349–360, 1988.
37. Rentrop KP: Thrombolytic therapy in patients with acute myocardial infarction, Circulation 71:627–631, 1985.
38. Yusuf S et al: Intravenous and intracoronary fibrinolytic therapy in acute myocardial infarction: overview of results on mortality, reinfarction and side-effects from 33 randomized trials, Eur Heart J 6:556–585, 1985.
39. Faxon DP: The risk of reperfusion strategies in the treatment of patients with acute myocardial infarction, J Am Coll Cardiol 12:52A–57A, 1988.
40. Topol EJ et al: Comparison of two dose regimens of intravenous tissue plasminogen activator for acute myocardial infarction, Am J Cardiol 61:723–728, 1988.
41. Topol EJ et al: A randomized controled trial of intravenous tissue plasminogen activator and early intravenous heparin in acute myocardial infarction, Circulation 79:281–286, 1989.
42. Magnani BV and PAIMS Investigators: Plasminogen Activator Italian Multicenter Study (PAIMS): comparison of intravenous recombinant

single-chain human tissue-type plasminogen activator (rtpa) with intravenous streptokinase in acute myocardial infarction, J Am Coll Cardiol 13:19–26, 1989.

43. Steinberg EP et al: Cost and procedure implications of thrombolytic therapy for acute myocardial infarction, J Am Coll Cardiol 12:58A–68A, 1988.

44. Van De Werf F, Nobuhara M, and Collen D: Coronary thrombolysis with human single-chain urokinase-type plasminogen activator (pro-urokinase) in patients with acute myocardial infarction, Ann Intern Med 104:345–348, 1986.

45. Bonnier HJ et al: Comparison of intravenous anisoylated plasminogen streptokinase activator complex and intracoronary streptokinase in acute myocardial infarction, Am J Cardiol 62:25–30, 1988.

46. ISIS-1 Collaborative Group: Mechanisms for the early mortality reduction produced by beta-blockade started early in acute myocardial infarction, Lancet 1:921–923, 1988.

47. Agura ED, Wexler LF, and Witzburg RA: Massive propranolol overdose: successful treatment with high-dose isoproterenol and glucagon, Am J Med 80:755–757, 1986.

48. Ryden L et al: A double-blind trial of metoprolol in acute myocardial infarction: effects on ventricular arrhythmias, N Engl J Med 308:614–618, 1983.

49. MIAMI Trial Research Group: Metoprolol in Acute Myocardial Infarction (MIAMI). A randomized placebo-controlled international trial, Eur Heart J 6:199–226, 1985.

50. Kirshenbaum JM et al: Use of an ultrashort-acting beta-receptor blocker (esmolol) in patients with acute myocardial ischemia and relative contraindications to beta-blockade therapy, J Am Coll Cardiol 12:773–780, 1988.

51. Jugdutt BI: Intravenous nitroglycerin infusion in acute myocardial infarction: myocardial salvage, Cardiovasc Rev Rep 5:1145–1163, 1984.

52. Michorowski BL, Senaratne MPJ, and Jugdutt BI: Myocardial infarct expansion, Cardiovasc Rev Rep 8:42–47, 1987.

53. Jugdutt BI and Warnica JW: Intravenous nitroglycerin therapy to limit myocardial infarct size, expansion, and complications. Effect of timing, dosage, and infarct location, Circulation 78:906–919, 1988.

54. Wilcox RG et al: Trial of early nifedipine in treatment in patients with suspected myocardial infarction, Br Heart J 55:506, 1986 (abstract).

55. Multicenter Diltiazem Post-infarction Research Group: The effect of diltiazem on mortality and reinfarction after acute myocardial infarction, N Engl J Med 319:385–392, 1988.

56. Gibson RS et al: Diltiazem and reinfarction in patients with non-Q wave myocardial infarction, N Engl J Med 315:423–429, 1986.

57. TIMI Research Group: Immediate versus delayed catheterization and angioplasty following thrombolytic therapy for acute myocardial infarction: TIMI IIA results, JAMA 260:2849–2858, 1988.

58. Topol EJ et al: A randomized trial of immediate versus delayed elective angioplasty after intravenous tissue plasminogen activator in acute myocardial infarction, N Engl J Med 317:581–588, 1987.

59. De Bono DP (European Cooperative Study Group): The European Cooperative Study Group Trial of intravenous recombinant tissue-type plasminogen activator (rtpa) and conservative therapy versus rtpa and immediate coronary angioplasty, J Am Coll Cardiol 12:20A–23A, 1988.

60. MILIS Study Group: Hyaluronidase therapy for acute myocardial infarction: Results of a randomized, blinded, multicenter trial, Am J Cardiol 57:1236–1242, 1986.

61. Gallagher KP et al: Failure of superoxide dismutase and catalase to alter size of infarction in conscious dogs after three hours of occlusion followed by reperfusion, Circulation 73:1065–1076, 1986.

62. Ambrosio G et al: Reduction in experimental infarct size by recombinant human superoxide dismutase: insights into the pathophysiology of reperfusion injury, Circulation 74:1424–1433, 1986.

63. Thrombolytic therapy in thrombosis. A National Institutes of Health Consensus Development Conference (symposium), Ann Intern Med 93:141–144, 1980.

64. Dean E et al: University Hospital Department of Cardiology: acute interventional cardiology program protocol, 1988–1989 (adapted with permission).

SUGGESTED READINGS

Alderman EL et al: Randomized comparison of intravenous versus intracoronary streptokinase for myocardial infarction, Am J Cardiol 54:14–19, 1984.

Brand Von Brener M, Landowne M, and Shock NW: Changes in cardiac output with age, Circulation 12:557–566, 1955.

Chatterjee K and Pommerly WW: Vasodilator therapy for acute myocardial infarction and chronic congestive heart failure, J Am Coll Cardiol 1:133–153, 1983.

Coon WW and Willis PW: Hemorrhagic complications of anticoagulant therapy, Arch Intern Med 133:386–392, 1974.

Gerstenblith G et al: Echocardiographic assessment of a normal adult aging population, Circulation 56:273–278, 1977.

Hotvendahl S: Influence of treatment in coronary care unit on prognosis of acute myocardial infarction, Acta Med Scand 519[suppl]:1–78, 1971.

Port S et al: Effect of age on response of left ventricular ejection fraction to exercise, N Engl J Med 303:1133–1137, 1980.

Thrombolytic Therapy for Acute Myocardial Infarction

Goal: *To initiate thrombolytic therapy within 20 minutes of the patient's arrival to the emergency department.*

PATIENT SELECTION

Candidates

1. Patients presenting with continuing symptoms and ECG abnormalities consistent with acute myocardial infarction (MI), both of which persist after nitroglycerin therapy.
2. Patients with duration of symptoms less than 6 hours.

Absolute Contraindications

1. Previous history of any CVA or CNS tumor.
2. Surgery, any hemorrhagic event, or major trauma within 2 weeks.
3. Pregnancy.
4. Suspected aortic dissection.
5. Blood pressure >200 systolic or >110 diastolic after initial sedation.

Relative Contraindications

1. Active bacterial endocarditis.
2. Known left heart thrombus.
3. CPR with rib fractures.
4. Known bleeding tendency.
5. For streptokinase or APSAC:
   a. Previous streptokinase or APSAC administration.
   b. Blood pressure <90 mm Hg.
6. Age ± 75.

EMERGENCY DEPARTMENT PROCEDURE

Triage Personnel

- Immediately escort any patient with chest discomfort to a monitored bay by stretcher or wheelchair.
- Immediately notify the physician-nurse team that you have brought in a patient with chest pain.
- Remain at the patient's bedside and initiate the protocol for cardiac chest pain until the physician-nurse team arrives.

ECG Technician

- Respond and have the ECG done within 10 minutes of initial *stat* page.

From Thrombolysis Review Committee, Good Samaritan Hospital, Portland. Prepared by Michael Sequeira, M.D., F.A.C.E.P. Committee members: Alan Ames, M.D., F.A.C.C., Suzanne Hall, M.D., F.A.C.C., Ronald Shutz, M.D., F.A.C.C., David Schuetze, R.Ph.

Emergency Department Nurse

- Order a *stat* ECG.
- *Notify* the emergency physician of the patient.
- Initiate *oxygen* therapy.
- Attach *ECG monitor*.
- Assess *vital signs*.
- Establish a large-bore IV lifeline.
  - NOTE: If thrombolytic therapy is indicated, *two additional* IV lines (or one additional *double lumen* catheter) will need to be established with minidrip tubing.
  - Avoid any unneccessary arterial or venous punctures. Attempt to draw venous samples from indwelling catheters either during insertion or after. Avoid any IM injections.
- Administer *nitroglycerin* 0.4 mg SL unless systolic BP$_{syst}$ <90 mm Hg.
- Draw baseline *laboratory* data[†]:
  - CK with isoenzymes
  - CBC (including platelet count)
  - Multichem battery
  - PT, PTT, fibrinogen
  - Open heart screen
  - Urinalysis (should not delay protocol)
  - Research protocol labs (if a likely candidate) — draw 20 ml extra for special coagulation tubes
- *Repeat nitroglycerin* in 5 minutes if chest pain persists.
- Repeat vital signs at least every 10 minutes.
- Record *ECG rhythm strip* every 15 minutes. Use the lead that shows the maximum ST segment elevation.
- Show the ECG to the emergency physician *immediately* upon completion if the ED physician is not already at the bedside.
- Have the Unit Coordinator *notify the Pharmacy Department* that there is a potential thrombolysis candidate *and give the weight of the patient.*
- Call the OHI research nurse if the possibility for thrombolysis is good.

Emergency Department Physician

- *Evaluate patient and ECG* for the diagnosis of acute MI as soon as possible. If he/she is with another patient, evaluate the ECG brought to him/her by the nurse. A rectal exam with a stool guaiac should be included in the patient's evaluation.

- *Review Patient Selection Criteria* and assess suitability of the patient for thrombolytic *and* beta-blocker therapy.
- Consider the patient for any current AMI research protocol. Consult list of inclusion and exclusion criteria.
- *Order thrombolytic therapy* if all criteria are met and patient possesses no contraindications. *Concurrently* (while thrombolytic agent is being prepared):
  - Administer *metoprolol* 5 mg IV push, q 5 min × 3 (NOTE: reassess patient after each dose).
  Do *not* give if patient has:
    - History of asthma, chronic obstructive pulmonary disease, congestive heart failure
    - Wheezing or signs of CHF on initial examination
    - Blood pressure <90 mm Hg
    - Heart rate <60 bpm
    - Atrioventricular block
- Place *nitroglycerin ointment*: 1 inch on upper chest.
- Administer *aspirin*: 160 mg (2 baby aspirin) chew.
- *Order nitroglycerin infusion*, to begin at 5 µg/min (nitroglycerin ointment should be wiped off whenever the nitroglycerin infusion is begun). The nitroglycerin infusion can be increased by 5 µg/min every 3–5 min according to patient tolerance and therapeutic response.
- Immediately place a call to the patient's primary care physician and cardiologist if he/she has one. If patient does not already have a primary care physician, call a cardiologist.
- If patient does not clearly meet inclusion criteria, or if any questions arise with regard to the suitability of the patient for thrombolysis, then discuss this with the patient's primary care physician and/or a cardiologist before initiating any thombolytic therapy.
  - In this case, if the patient's primary care physician or his/her designated call physician does not respond within 20 minutes, then the ED physician should then contact a cardiologist.
- Institute *prophylactic lidocaine* (1.5 mg/kg initial IV bolus with an initial 2 mg/min IV infusion followed 2–5 minutes later with another 0.5 mg/kg IV bolus).
NOTE: All doses of lidocaine should be reduced under the following circumstances: age ≥70 years, CHF, BP <90 mm Hg, hepatic insufficiency, concomitant cimetidine therapy.
- Transfer patient to CCU as condition allows.

PHARMACY/IV PROCEDURE

- Have thrombolytic agent prepared and delivered to the ED for infusion 5 minutes after it is ordered.
- The *priorities* for the pharmacist on duty will be the following (in order of importance):

1. Thrombolytic agent preparation and delivery
2. Nitroglycerin infusion preparation and delivery
3. Heparin infusion
- If current AMI research protocol patient, follow the designated protocol.

[†]Tubes to be drawn: one lavender, one green, one mottled red, one large red, one blue.

THROMBOLYTIC AGENTS
(to be prepared by the Pharmacy/IV Department)

Streptokinase

1. *Preparation and dosage*: 1.5 million units added to 50 ml of normal saline for a final volume (including overfill) of 60 ml.
2. *Administration* should be given over a separate, dedicated IV line): by IV infusion pump over 60 minutes (set at 60 ml/hr).
   NOTE: When the infusion bag is empty, spike a new bag of 50 ml normal saline and run at the same rate until empty. This will complete the infusion of the remaining drug from the tubing.

TPA (alteplase)

1. *Preparation*: 100 mg reconstituted in 100 ml of sterile water to give a concentration of 1 mg/ml.
2. *Dosage and administration* (should be given over a separate, dedicated IV line):
   A. If patient weight is ≥65 kg (143 pounds): *100 mg total dose*, divided as follows:
      i. *First hour* dose: 60 mg, given as:
         a. Loading dose: 10 mg IV over 2 minutes (may set pump at 300 ml/hr for 2 minutes)
         b. First hour infusion: 50 mg over 60 minutes.
      ii. *Second hour* dose: 20 mg IV, infused over 60 minutes.*
      iii. *Third hour* dose: 20 mg IV, infused over 60 minutes.*
   B. If patient weight is <70 kg: *1.25 mg/kg total dose*, divided according to the attached chart.

TPA (Alteplase) Dosing Chart

Weight (kg)	Total dose	Loading dose (over 2 min)	Infusion rate: Dose (mg)= Rate (ml/hr) First 1hr	Second 1hr*	Third 1hr*
>65	100 mg	10 mg (10 ml)	50 ml/hr	20 ml/hr	20 ml/hr
60–64	77 mg	8 mg (10 ml)	39 ml/hr	15 ml/hr	15 ml/hr
55–59	71 mg	7 mg (10 ml)	36 ml/hr	14 ml/hr	14 ml/hr
50–54	65 mg	7 mg (10 ml)	32 ml/hr	13 ml/hr	13 ml/hr
45–49	59 mg	6 mg (10 ml)	29 ml/hr	12 ml/hr	12 ml/hr
40–44	53 mg	5 mg (10 ml)	26 ml/hr	11 ml/hr	11 ml/hr

*The infusion bottle will run dry before the end of the infusion time. When the infusion bottle is empty, spike a bag of normal saline (5 ml) and run at the rate stated above. This will ensure that the patient receives the entire dose remaining in the tubing.

CORONARY CARE UNIT PROCEDURE

- General treatment for myocardial infarction, and continue therapy begun in the emergency department.
- If this is a research patient, follow the designated protocol. Preprinted orders are available.
- Begin *heparin* 4–8 hours after the initiation of streptokinase or 2 hours after the initiation of TPA. Give 100 units/kg IV bolus followed by 900–1,000 units/hour IV infusion and titrate to keep the PTT between two and three times the control.
- Avoid any unnecessary arterial or venous punctures. Attempt to draw venous samples from indwelling catheters. Avoid any IM injections.
- Record *ECG rhythm strips* every 15 minutes for 3 hours after the initiation of thrombolytic therapy, then hourly for the next 4 hours. Use the lead that shows the maximum ST elevation.
- Order *12 lead ECG* after thrombolytic therapy completed, then q 8 hours × 2, q AM × 2, and as necessary for any recurrence of chest pain or suspected ischemia.
- *Laboratory* to be ordered:
  - CK with MB: 10, 14, 18, and 22 hours after the onset of the chest pain/MI symptoms.
  - CK with MB: daily for the next 12 days.
  - Fibrinogen 1–4 hours after the onset of thrombolytic therapy and in the morning.
  - CBC and electrolytes in the morning following thrombolytic therapy.
  - PTT as needed to keep between two and three times the control.
- Continue *aspirin* every morning.
- If previous IV *metoprolol* was tolerated, continue metoprolol: 25–50 mg PO every 6 hours for 48 hours, starting 15 minutes after the last IV bolus or as soon as the clinical condition allows. Continue as indicated.

Clinical Parameters to Monitor

- **Indicators of occult or gross hemorrhage:** NOTE
  — If any of these occur, the nurse should discontinue the heparin and thrombolytic agent infusion(s), draw a PTT and fibrinogen level, and contact the doctor immediately.
  —*melena*: Hemetest all stools and record this on the bedside chart
  —*hematemeses*
  —*hemoptysis*
  —*unusual leg or back pain* (this may herald the onset of retroperitoneal hemorrhage)
  —*change in CNS status*

- **Reocclusion or reinfarction**
  —The majority of reocclusions occur within the first few days while the patient is in the CCU. A strong correlation between inadequate anticoagulation and reinfarction exists. Therefore, it is important for the patient to take adequate anticoagulant medication.

CHECKLIST FOR THROMBOLYSIS CANDIDATES

Thrombolytic agent _____

Patient weight _____

Approx. time of onset of symptoms _____

Time of arrival in ED _____

Time thrombolysis begun _____

ECG called _____

ECG response _____

Check the Appropriate Categories and Include This in the Patient's Chart

_____ 1. Continuing symptoms and ECG abnormalities (ST segment elevation of ≥ 1 mm at 0.02 sec after the end of the QRS in at least 2 of 2,3, avF or of V_{1-6}) consistent with acute myocardial infarction, both of which persist after nitroglycerin therapy.

_____ 2. Duration of symptoms less than 6 hours.

Absolute Contraindications

_____ 1. Previous history of any CVA or CNS tumor.

_____ 2. Surgery, hemorrhagic event, or major trauma within 2 weeks.

_____ 3. Pregnancy.

_____ 4. Suspected aortic dissection.

_____ 5. BP >200 systolic or >110 diastolic after initial sedation.

Relative Contraindications

_____ 1. Active bacterial endocarditis.

_____ 2. Known left heart thrombus.

_____ 3. CPR with rib fractures.

_____ 4. Known bleeding tendency.

_____ 5. For streptokinase or APSAC: a) previous streptokinase or APSAC administration; b) BP <90 mm Hg.

_____ 6. Age ≥ 75 years.

Contraindications for *Metoprolol*

_____ 1. History of asthma, COPD, or CHF.

_____ 2. Wheezes or CHF on initial examination.

_____ 3. BP must be >90 mm Hg.

_____ 4. Heart rate must be >60 beats/minute.

_____ 5. Atrioventricular block.

R.N. _____

M.D. _____

Valvular Cardiac Emergencies

Louis A. Cannon, M.D.

Significant valvular heart disease usually arises in youth or middle age; however, because of the long natural history of these lesions and the development of valvular abnormalities with aging, the physician frequently encounters valvular disease in the elderly. The gradual decline of left ventricular reserve may make previously well-tolerated lesions clinically significant. A valve that is the site of an anatomic lesion is subject to abnormal mechanical stress and premature degenerative changes. Such changes as sclerosis, fibrosis, and calcification influence the progress of valvular lesions and may result in new hemodynamically significant disease.

The aging process itself, which is accompanied by a decrease in vascular elasticity, may alter symptoms and physical findings in the elderly. Consequently, evaluation of the severity and clinical significance of many lesions may be made more difficult. For example, a systolic murmur occurs in approximately 50% of the elderly population and may represent a benign process such as aortic sclerosis or be the harbinger of hypertrophic obstructive cardiomyopathy.[1] In the following chapter, we will discuss the evaluation of valvular disease in the aged with specific emphasis on the presenting signs and symptoms and on the potential benefit of medical and surgical intervention.

AORTIC STENOSIS

Aortic stenosis (AS) is present in approximately 4% of the elderly.[2] There are several etiologies of AS that can largely be classified by the age in which the symptoms appear. In patients less than 60 years of age, rheumatic heart disease is the most common etiology. Rheumatic AS is always accompanied by mitral stenosis or regurgitation. Between 60 and 75 years of age, calcification of a congenitally bicuspid valve is more common. Bicuspid aortic valves become stenotic in two thirds to three fourths of individuals with this abnormality. AS in the very elderly (over 75 years old) is usually due to simple degeneration or "wear and tear" of a previously normal tricuspid valve.

Aortic valve calcification (aortic sclerosis) is a common entity — present in more than 55% of patients over 90 years old. Only 5% of these patients have enough calcification to produce obstruction.[3] The natural history of the progression from aortic sclerosis to AS is unknown. However, greater than 60% of symptomatic patients with AS have been aware of the presence of a systolic murmur for over 10 years.[4] Characteristically, these are early systolic ejection murmurs with minimal transmission to the carotid arteries, grade 1 or 2 over 6 in intensity, and a well-preserved A_2 with normal splitting of S_2. The benign nature of these heart sounds is confirmed by documenting a normal carotid pulse, absence of left ventricular hypertrophy by physical examination, electrocardiogram (ECG), and a normal or mildly reduced aortic valve orifice as disclosed by echocardiography. The aging process is certainly not a static one. The diagnosis of aortic sclerosis on the patient's records should arouse suspicion of a developing obstruction in the newly symptomatic patient.

History and Symptoms

Patients with aortic valve stenosis may be asymptomatic until late in the course of the illness. Symptoms in the elderly are similar to those experienced by the younger patient and include angina pectoris, dizziness, syncope, and left heart failure (Table 15–1). Once the elderly patient becomes symptomatic, he or she is at increased risk of sudden death. The median survival without definite surgical intervention is 2 to 5 years. It is therefore important for clinicians to recognize AS in symptomatic patients and initiate appropriate diagnostic and therapeutic measures.

The symptoms of severe AS are often attributed to other disease entities in the elderly. Since arteriosclerosis is so prevalent in the age group, angina pectoris may be mistakenly attributed to coronary artery disease. Likewise, dizziness and syncope are often considered to have a vascular or neurologic origin.[5] Syncope in AS can be caused by atrial or ventricular arrhythmias, or it can be related to an inability of the cardiac output to meet the body's demands during exercise. Left ventricular failure in AS comes from left ventricular hypertrophy, fibrosis, and ischemia.[6] Patients complain of exercise intolerance and fatigue. About half of elderly patients with AS will have congestive heart failure, often precipitated by the occurrence of atrial fibrillation.[7] Dyspnea is often a late symptom of AS and may be incorrectly diagnosed as a pulmonary disorder. It may present as orthopnea, paroxysmal nocturnal dyspnea, or frank pulmonary edema. Although sudden death has classically been associated with AS, it is rarely the presenting manifestation.

Clinical Findings

Many of the classic findings of aortic stenosis (Table 15–1) may be absent or attenuated in the elderly. Initially, blood pressure is normal, but as the disease progresses, systolic blood pressure falls and pulse pressure narrows. Older patients, however, have a loss in aortic compliance secondary to atherosclerosis and senescent changes. Systolic blood pressure may be normal or even slightly elevated with maintenance of a normal pulse pressure. The classic — slowly rising, delayed — carotid pulse (parvus et tardus) may be difficult to appreciate as well.

The most reliable physical sign associated with critical AS is the crescendo-decrescendo quality of the ejection murmur, which peaks in mid to late systole, and a decreased or absent second heart sound. The systolic murmur may be unimpressive and unusually low in pitch because of the depressed cardiac output or an increased chest anteroposterior diameter. Often murmur and associated thrill can be best appreciated at the base of the neck, where the senile uncoiled aortic arch may be palpated. As the stenosis increases in severity, the splitting of S_2 becomes narrowed and occasionally reversed (paradoxical splitting). Aortic valve leaflets that are still mobile may have an early systolic ejection click, but increasing age, fibrosis, and calcification usually reduce this finding.[8]

The ECG usually shows left ventricular hypertrophy and secondary repolarization changes ("strain pattern"). In the aged with emphysematous changes and an increased chest diameter, the ECG voltage may not be impressive, and an interventricular conduction delay often will be present that masks hypertrophy. Radiologic

Table 15–1   Symptoms and Signs of AS

Symptoms
  Angina pectoris
  Dizziness and/or exertional syncope
  Dyspnea on exertion
  Left ventricular failure (paroxysmal nocturnal dyspnea, fatigue, orthopnea, exercise intolerance)

Physical Findings
  Narrow pulse pressure (< 20 mm Hg)
  Systolic hypotension (90–114 mm Hg)
  Pulsus parvus and tardus
  Enlarged, sustained left ventricular impulse
  Early systolic ejection click
  Decreased or absent aortic component of S_2
  Harsh, crescendo-decrescendo (ejection) systolic murmur along the right sternal border, radiating into the carotid arteries decreased intensity with Valsalva's maneuver
  S_4 common; S_3 when left ventricular (LV) failure present

Electrocardiogram
  LV hypertrophy with strain
  Left atrial enlargement

Chest X-ray
  LV enlargement
  Prominent ascending aorta
  Aortic valve calcification

evaluation often discloses a normal to slightly enlarged cardiac silhouette but is usually not sensitive enough to pick up valvular calcification on a routine basis.

Echocardiography is one of the most useful tools for the diagnosis of valvular heart disease. Demonstration of good aortic leaflet mobility and systolic separation in an adult is quite sufficient to exclude significant AS.[9] Conversely, however, failure to visualize systolic leaflet separation does not establish the diagnosis of AS but, rather, suggests the need for further evaluation.[10] Recently, pulsed Doppler examination has been successful in quantifying the severity of stenotic and regurgitant lesions; its use with M-mode and two-dimensional echocardiography makes these the noninvasive diagnostic procedures of choice.[11]

Many clinicians, however, still prefer the definitive data provided by cardiac catheterization. Heart rate, cardiac output, and valvular gradients are determined and used to calculate effective aortic valve orifice size. Angiography also documents the state of left ventricular contraction, concomitant valvular regurgitation, and the condition of the coronary arteries. Approximately half of patients with severe AS also have coronary artery disease.[6]

Treatment

Physical exertion should be limited in elderly people with moderate to severe AS. Isometric forms of exercise are contraindicated, although routine, light exertion such as walking is permitted. Appropriate prophylaxis for bacterial endocarditis should be administered (see Table 15–2). Patients who present with signs and symptoms of congestive heart failure can be treated with salt restriction and diuretics. However, these patients depend on adequate preload (ventricular filling) to maintain cardiac output, and overdiuresis may be life threatening. Nitrates may be cautiously tried for treatment of chest pain, although they may exacerbate syncope and orthostatic hypotension.[12]

Patients with AS who develop atrial fibrillation may suffer marked hemodynamic deterioration due to loss of atrial kick. The treatment of choice for hemodynamically significant atrial arrhythmias is electrical cardioversion. In the event that a significant bradycardia unresponsive to medical therapy is present, pacemaker therapy may be indicated.

While medical therapy is sufficient for asymptomatic patients with valvular AS, symptomatic patients with severe stenosis require surgical intervention. Advanced age is no longer a contraindication to cardiac valve replacement. Improved patient care and operative techniques have reduced mortality of elective single valve replacement to 3% and to 5 to 10% for combined cardiac revascularization and valve replacement. This compares quite favorably with the 80 to 90% 2-year mortality of pa-

Table 15–2 Antibiotic Prophylaxis Against Bacterial Endocarditis

Dental and Respiratory Tract Procedures	
Oral	Pen-Vee-K 2 g 1 hour before procedure and 1 g 6 hours later
	or
	Erythromycin 1 g 1 hour before procedure and 500 mg 6 hours later
Parenteral	Ampicillin 1–2 g plus gentamicin 1.5 mg/kg IM or IV 30 minutes before procedure, repeated 8 hours later
	Vancomycin 1 g 1 hour before procedure given slowly IV; repeat dose not needed
Genitourinary and Gastrointestinal Procedures	
Oral	Amoxicillin 3 g 1 hour before procedure and 1.5 g 6 hours later
Parenteral	Ampicillin 2 g plus gentamicin 1.5 mg/kg IM or IV 30 minutes before procedure, repeated 8 hours later
	or
	Vancomycin 1 g given slowly IV, plus gentamicin 1.5 mg/kg IM or IV both given 1 hour before procedure, and may repeat above 8–12 hours later

tients with unoperated, symptomatic AS.[13] One alternative to surgery is through the use of balloon valvuloplasty. A catheter with a balloon tip is placed in the aortic orifice and inflated in order to open the stenotic valve. This procedure has recently been shown to be effective even in calcific disease.[14] Improvement in lifestyle is usually dramatic following aortic valve replacement or valvuloplasty.

HYPERTROPHIC CARDIOMYOPATHY

The first significant description of hypertrophic cardiomyopathy was in 1958. Since that time multiple synonyms have been used for the condition, including idiopathic hypertrophic subaortic stenosis (IHSS), asymmetric septal hypertrophy (ASH), and muscular subaortic stenosis. Anatomically, there is unexplained myocardial hypertrophy, especially involving the interventricular septum, which contributes to an outflow tract pressure gradient possibly also related to abnormal mitral valve motion. This disorder merits consideration in the present discussion because it has elements of both congenital and valvular heart disease and is often considered an example of both.

Hypertrophic obstructive cardiomyopathy (HOCM) is currently understood to be a familial illness, genetically transmitted as an autosomal dominant trait with high penetrance. Although it is generally regarded as a disease of young or middle-aged people, several studies report that the elderly constitute one fourth to one third of patients with HOCM.[15-17] It is not known whether these older patients represent a group with late-onset HOCM or have a slowly progressive form of cardiomyopathy compatible with decades of asymptomatic disease. There are twice as many women as men in this group, although men are more likely to become symptomatic when older.[16]

There is a common tendency to overlook this disease in the elderly since signs and symptoms of HOCM are often attributed to coronary or valvular disease. In many instances, the correct diagnosis of HOCM is made only at the time of cardiac catheterization performed in pursuit of another diagnosis or at autopsy.[15]

History and Symptoms

Elderly patients may become symptomatic for the first time in the seventh or eighth decade. The chief symptoms are similar to those of younger patients with dyspnea, angina, fatigue, and impaired level of consciousness. The clinical presentation is often difficult to distinguish from valvular AS and Table 15–3 identifies helpful clinical findings useful in this differentiation.

Dyspnea is the most common symptom of HOCM. It is caused by increased left atrial and pulmonary venous pressure that is a direct result of decreased compliance of the left ventricle.[18] Angina pectoris is also a common symptom, present in approximately 35 to 50% of elderly patients.[16] Although the chest pain often has atypical features (prolonged duration, occurrence at rest or with no relation to exertion, and often not relieved by nitrates), evidence demonstrates that ischemia does occur in the hypertrophied myocardium even in the absence of significant coronary artery disease.[19] The neurologic symptoms associated with HOCM may be due to the reduced cardiac output or may accompany generalized cerebrovascular disease. These symptoms include transient ischemic attack, stroke, dizziness, and syncope.

Table 15–3   Distinguishing AS and HOCM

	Valvular AS	HOCM
Carotid upstroke	Delayed	Rapid, bisferious
Aortic valve closure (A$_2$)	Decreased	Normal
Ejection click	Common	Uncommon
Location of murmur	Aortic area or apex	Left lower sternal border (LSB)
Radiation	Carotids	LSB, axillae, midsternum
Effect of maneuvers:		
Valsalva's	Decreased	Increased
Standing	Decreased	Increased
Hypovolemia	Decreased	Increased
Squatting	No change	Decreased

Other nonspecific symptoms of HOCM are fatigue, palpitations, and pulmonary edema.

Hypovolemia (e.g., dehydration, gastrointestinal bleeding) may exacerbate symptoms of HOCM in three ways.[20] First, diminished venous return leads to decreased ventricular filling upon which a hypertrophic ventricle is particularly dependent for adequate stroke volume. Second, decreased ventricular filling promotes obstruction of the left ventricular (LV) outflow tract by facilitating the apposition of the anterior mitral leaflet and septum. Third, a reflex sympathetic response enhances contractility, increasing the bulging of the septum, and accelerates the heart rate, thus reducing the ventricular filling period.

Clinical Findings

The auscultatory hallmark of HOCM is a midsystolic crescendo-decrescendo murmur at the apex or left sternal border. The murmur is rarely transmitted to the carotid arteries and tends to increase in length toward the lower left sternal border and apex where it is often pansystolic because of associated mitral incompetence. The gradient and the murmur will increase with provocative maneuvers that increase contractility, decrease preload, or decrease afterload such as Valsalva's strain, standing, amyl nitrite, and exercise. In contrast, maneuvers that increase preload or afterload such as squatting and isometric handgrip will decrease the gradient and the murmur. There typically is a loud fourth heart sound. The second heart sound in severe outflow obstruction is paradoxically split for the same reasons as in valvular AS. However, if either an ejection click or an aortic diastolic murmur is heard, the presence of HOCM is unlikely.

The carotid pulse rises rapidly in HOCM since there is no obstruction in early systole. As obstruction develops, the pulse declines in midsystole and then has a secondary rise. This bisferious pulse is seen in 94% of younger patients and in 40 to 70% of the elderly. When present, the brisk carotid upstroke is a key clinical sign in differentiating HOCM from valvular AS. The apical precordial impulse is often displaced laterally, is abnormally forceful, and is enlarged. It may have a bifid character that is related to the early rapid and the late ventricular ejection phase or may be "triple" when the presystolic distention of the noncompliant ventricle becomes palpable.[21] A systolic thrill is common at the apex or left sternal border.

Chest x-ray findings are variable and include left ventricular hypertrophy and a widened cardiothoracic ratio greater than 50%. Calcification of the mitral annulus has been noted in a number of patients with HOCM but is rarely visible on routine radiography. Electrocardiographic findings in these patients include left ventricular hypertrophy, left atrial enlargement, and various conduction disturbances such as left bundle branch block and accessory pathways. Occasionally, deep Q waves or QS patterns, simulating myocardial infarction, occur in anterolateral or inferior leads. In more advanced forms of the disease, atrial and ventricular arrhythmias may be found.

Echocardiography is the most helpful technique for the recognition of HOCM. M-mode or two-dimensional studies reveal left ventricular hypertrophy, usually involving the interventricular septum, narrowing and obstruction of the left ventricular outflow tract, and a systolic anterior motion of the mitral valve. The anterior motion of the mitral leaflet appears to be due to a systolic "sucking" of the mitral apparatus into the left ventricular outflow tract. Cardiac catheterization usually reveals a pressure gradient within the chamber of the left ventricle that is separated from a subaortic chamber by the apposition of the mitral valve and the thickened septum.

Treatment

Emergency management of HOCM necessitates aggressive hydration and withdrawal of potentially deleterious medications, such as digitalis, nitrites, and beta-adrenergic agents. Since the mid-1960s, propranolol has been the mainstay of therapy in symptomatic patients. By decreasing heart rate and the force of contraction, it increases cardiac filling, increases heart size, and subsequently decreases the gradient across the obstructed ventricle. Patients note a decrease in all the principal cardiac symptoms with routine doses of propranolol (160 to 320 mg/day).[22] Unfortunately, beta blockade has not been shown to decrease the frequency of serious arrhythmias.

Verapamil also appears to decrease the patient's symptoms, reduce outflow obstruction, and improve exercise capacity. Average doses approximate 360 mg/day of verapamil; however, only limited data are currently available regarding other calcium channel blockers.[22] When initiating therapy with verapamil, caution must be exercised in patients with preexisting conduction disease to avoid the potential for complete heart block. Recently, treatment with disopyramide[23] or amiodarone[24] has appeared very promising.

Atrial fibrillation is seen in approximately 10% of all patients with HOCM.[22] It may lead to rapid hemodynamic compromise, and immediate cardioversion may be lifesaving. The risk of systemic embolization with cardioversion is equivalent to that seen in patients with mitral valve disease, and anticoagulation should be considered. Surgical intervention is an option for the suitable patient with HOCM who does not respond to medical management. Operative therapy usually consists of septal myectomy via a transaortic approach. Successful operation often produces lasting clinical and hemodynamic improvement and may prevent secondary left ventricular hypertrophy.

AORTIC REGURGITATION

The clinical course of aortic regurgitation (AR) depends largely on the chronicity of the lesion. Chronic AR in the elderly develops as a result of atherosclerosis, hypertension, valvular deformity (e.g., congenital, sclerotic, rheumatic, or postendocarditic), or aortic root dilatation (e.g., aortitis, atherosclerosis, or myxomatous degeneration). The regurgitant lesion can be very well-tolerated and is often asymptomatic for 10 to 15 years.

In acute AR, no time has been allowed for compensatory left ventricular hypertrophy or dilatation to develop, so that cardiac failure may occur following the abrupt increase in volume overload. Common etiologies of acute AR are shown in Table 15–4. Damage to a native or prosthetic aortic valve by bacteria or fungi is the most common cause. Dissection of the ascending aorta can result in acute AR in approximately 65% of patients.[25] This may be due to intimal dissection of the hematoma or from disruption of the valve leaflets themselves. Blunt chest trauma may bring about AR by causing aortic dissection, leaflet tears, or avulsion of commissural attachments. Spontaneous rupture or prolapse has been associated with fenestrated and myxomatous degeneration of the aortic leaflets.[25]

History and Symptoms

Patients with chronic AR usually remain asymptomatic for a longer period of time than patients with isolated AS. Awareness of an abnormal pulsation in the neck or precordium, especially in the recumbent position, may be the first symptom to appear. Palpitations, pounding

Table 15–4   Common Etiologies of Acute Aortic Insufficiency

Infectious endocarditis
  Gram-positive organisms
    Staphylococcus aureus
    Streptococcus pneumoniae
  Gram-negative organisms
    Neisseria meningitidis
    Haemophilus influenzae
  Fungi

Aortic dissection
  Traumatic
  Hypertensive
  Connective tissue disorders

Spontaneous leaflet rupture
  Myxomatous degeneration
  Fenestrated cusp rupture
  Trauma

Prosthetic valve dysfunction

Postoperative
  Faulty incision of
    stenotic aortic valve

head, and fatigue are other subjective manifestations experienced by these patients. These complaints may be present for years before symptoms of congestive heart failure develop. Syncope is rare, and angina pectoris is less frequent than in patients with AS; however, nocturnal angina associated with sweating and palpitations may be a disturbing and prominent symptom in some patients.[26] Some individuals may remain asymptomatic despite dilated, poorly functioning left ventricles.

In acute AR, the manifestations of the underlying disease, commonly bacterial endocarditis or acute aortic dissection, usually predominate. The majority of patients are men who present with symptoms suggestive of severe heart failure with peripheral hypoperfusion. Because of the marked increase in myocardial oxygen consumption, myocardial ischemia is common in acute AR, even in the absence of coronary artery disease.

Clinical Findings

The physical signs and laboratory findings in chronic and acute AR also differ (Table 15–5). The classic signs of chronic AR include a hyperdynamic precordium, soft S_1, bisferious pulse, and accompanying loud systolic ejection murmur. The typical diastolic murmur of chronic AR is a high-frequency holosystolic decrescendo murmur after the aortic component of S_2. The duration of the murmur reflects the severity of disease more reliably than its

Table 15–5 Differential Features of Severe AR

	Acute	Chronic
Etiology	Endocarditis	Rheumatic heart disease
	Aortic dissection	Dilatation of the aortic root
Heart Failure	Early, sudden	Late, insidious
Physical Examination		
Systolic pressure	Normal or decreased	Increased
Pulse pressure	Narrow	Widened
Arterial pulse	Single contour, decreased	Bisferious, hyperdynamic
Peripheral arterial signs	Absent	Present
Left ventricular (LV) impulse	Normal	Displaced, hyperdynamic
Aortic regurgitant murmur	Medium pitched, short	High pitched, extended
Aortic systolic murmur	Grade 3 or less	Grade 3 or more
Third heart sound	Common	Uncommon
Fourth heart sound	Consistently absent	Usually absent
Electrocardiogram	Sinus tachycardia	LV hypertrophy and strain
Chest X-ray	Pulmonary venous congestion; normal cardiac silhouette	LV enlargement; aortic valve calcifications; poststenotic dilatation

intensity. The murmur is loudest along the left sternal border in AR secondary to organic valvular disease and loudest along the right sternal border when regurgitation is secondary to aortic root dilatation. A low, middiastolic apical rumble (Austin Flint murmur) is also likely to be heard accompanying pure AR. Pistol shot femoral artery pulsations, bounding carotid pulses, and capillary pulsations are commonly observed with chronic AR and relate to the hyperdynamic peripheral circulation. With significant chronic AR, the chest x-ray demonstrates progressive cardiac enlargement and prominence of the ascending aorta. As the severity of aortic incompetence increases, the ECG discloses the pattern of left ventricular hypertrophy and strain, although in the early phases it may show a volume overload pattern characterized by prominent Q waves and large symmetric upright T waves in the left precordial leads.

The clinical features of acute AR depend on the magnitude of the regurgitant flow and the suddenness of its onset. When aortic valve incompetence is severe, it leads to elevated left ventricular end-diastolic and pulmonary venous pressures due to the abrupt regurgitation of a large volume of blood into a noncompliant left ventricle. Patients are almost uniformly acutely and seriously ill with congestive heart failure. Low cardiac output and systemic vasconstriction may result in pale, cool distal extremities sometimes with peripheral cyanosis. Tachycardia is so consistent that its absence cautions against the diagnosis of acute AR. With advanced left ventricular failure, the pulse pressure narrows considerably. This not only tends to minimize the peripheral signs of aortic incompetence but may make the diastolic component inaudible and, hence, obscure the diagnosis.[21] The chest x-ray will not show the dilated ventricle of chronic insufficiency but will exhibit the lung findings of pulmonary congestion or edema. Radiographic evidence of aortic dissection (i.e., widened mediastinum and abnormal aortic knob) may be appreciated. The ECG may be normal or show ST and T wave changes suggestive of myocardial ischemia.

Two-dimensional and Doppler echocardiography are the procedures of choice for diagnosing, detecting the etiology, and grading the severity of acute and chronic AR. Although useful in detecting regurgitation, radionucleotide angiography (RNA) is most helpful in acute AR for quantifying the percentage of regurgitant flow. Cardiac catheterization provides the definitive diagnosis of acute AR but is much less practical in the acute setting and is most often used in the preoperative evaluation of aortic valve replacement.

Treatment

Patients with chronic AR who manifest left ventricular failure should be treated with digoxin and diuretics. Oral afterload reducers, such as hydralazine or prazosin, may be added if necessary. Patients with acute AR may derive benefit from prompt treatment with nitroprusside or a combination of nitroprusside and dopamine. The purpose of vasodilator therapy is the reduction of impedance to forward flow as well as the reduction of regurgitation, while improving peripheral tissue perfusion. Because of its predictable response, ease of titration, and short half-life, sodium nitroprusside is the drug of choice in this setting. It can be initiated at 0.25 µg/kg/minute and increased by 5 µg/minute every 5 to 10 minutes until the desired effect is reached. A useful goal in vasodilator therapy is cautious reduction in the diastolic blood pressure of no lower than 50 to 60 mm Hg or to a mean arterial pressure of 15 to 20 mm Hg from baseline.[24] However, this should be viewed as a temporary measure to stabilize the patient prior to definitive surgical therapy. Aortic balloon counterpulsation is contraindicated in aortic valve insufficiency.

Because infective endocarditis is the most common cause of acute AR, the empiric use of antibiotics is indicated after appropriate blood cultures have been obtained. However, most cases of acute AR will require emergency or urgent surgical intervention. An emergency valve replacement carries less risk than delay and further hemodynamic compromise, even for the patient with infective endocarditis.[28]

The surgical management of elderly patients with chronic AR remains controversial. In general, individuals who are severely symptomatic (New York Heart Association Functional Class III or IV) should undergo aortic valve replacement in order to ameliorate symptoms and extend longevity.

Symptomatic patients with normal left ventricular function and only a mild increase in left ventricular volume will do better postoperatively than will those with enlarged, poorly contractile left ventricles. Compromised ventricular function preoperatively, however, does not preclude the operation in symptomatic patients because most of these patients' symptoms will alleviate even if ventricular function does not normalize.[29] In asymptomatic or minimally symptomatic patients, close continued serial follow-up is necessary in order to detect the onset of the resting left ventricular dysfunction and to recommend the optimal timing for surgical intervention.

MITRAL STENOSIS

In elderly patients, mitral valvular stenosis usually results from rheumatic heart disease (Figure 15–1). This condition is almost always acquired before the age of 20 years but may not manifest clinically until several decades later. The typical patient with mitral stenosis (MS) has relatively mild valvular obstruction and becomes symptomatic either because of the development of other cardiac abnormalities or through arterial embolism. Various autopsy series have reported an incidence of 2.5 to 5% of rheumatic mitral valve disease in older patients. Only 40 to 65% of the elderly were able to provide a history of rheumatic fever or chorea.[30]

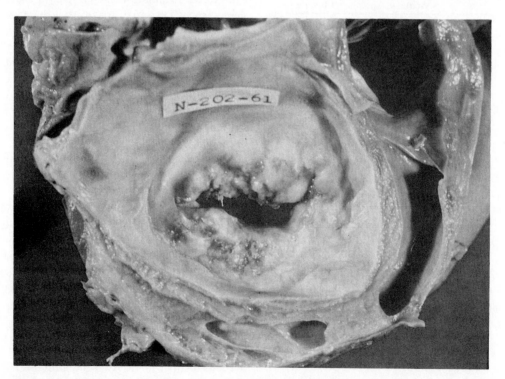

Figure 15–1 Longitudinal section of the heart showing mitral valvular stenosis secondary to rheumatic heart disease.

In addition to rheumatic fever, calcification of the mitral annulus can also cause narrowing of the mitral orifice severe enough to produce obstruction. The incidence of mitral annular calcification (MAC) is 8.5 to 10% at autopsy in patients beyond the age of 50. Not only the absolute incidence of MAC but also its predilection for women increases with progressive aging.[31] This condition is thought to be a normal degenerative process of the cardiac fibrous skeleton that begins at birth and progresses to old age. It appears that increased valve stress may accelerate the annular calcification. MAC is frequently associated with AS, HOCM, mitral valve prolapse, and arterial hypertension. Formerly regarded as a benign marker of the elderly heart, MAC is now known to predispose affected patients to atrial fibrillation, subacute bacterial endocarditis, arterial emboli, and high-grade atrioventricular block.[32]

History and Symptoms

The natural history of mitral stenosis is related to several factors: the severity of stenosis and its stable or progressive nature, the presence of atrial arrhythmias, the degree of pulmonary hypertension, and occurrence of complications such as systemic embolism. Patients with stable mitral stenosis often show moderate reduction of effort tolerance but adapt themselves well to the disability.[33] Acute decompensation may be precipitated by upper respiratory infection, sepsis, myocardial infarction, pulmonary emboli, anemia, noncompliance with medications, or arrhythmias.

The most common presenting symptom (80%) in patients with mitral stenosis is shortness of breath on exertion. The dyspnea is due to pulmonary congestion and may be accompanied by hemoptysis. Other clinical manifestations are outlined in Table 15–6, including chronic cough, chest pain, and hoarseness from laryngeal nerve damage with progressive left atrial enlargement. In the later stages of mitral stenosis, pulmonary arterial vasoconstriction develops as a response to the chronic pulmonary venous hypertension. This may ameliorate the symptoms of dyspnea but leads to right ventricular failure with fatigue, hepatic congestion, ascites, and peripheral edema. Presenting symptoms due to systemic embolism are infrequent in patients with mitral stenosis. Embolism is more common after onset of atrial fibrillation and tends to occur later in the disease.

Clinical Findings

The physical signs in patients with mitral stenosis vary with the severity of the valvular lesion and also with the amount of increase in pulmonary vascular resistance. The patient with mitral stenosis may exhibit the characteristic "mitral facies" appearance with a malar flush and ruddy complexion. The blood pressure is usually low

Table 15–6 Symptoms and Signs of Mitral Stenosis

Symptoms
  Dyspnea on exertion
  Hemoptysis
  Pulmonary edema (orthopnea, paroxysmal nocturnal dyspnea)
  Chest pressure
  Right ventricular failure (ankle edema, fatigue, anorexia, abdominal swelling)

Physical Findings
  Mitral facies
  Prominent jugular "a" wave
  Peripheral hypoperfusion
  Pulmonary congestion
  Parasternal right ventricular impulse
  Loud first heart sound
  Opening snap
  Diastolic murmur with presystolic accentuation
  Right ventricular failure (jugular venous distention, hepatomegaly, peripheral edema, Graham Steell's murmur)
  Tricuspid regurgitation murmur

Electrocardiogram
  Atrial fibrillation
  P mitrale
  Right axis deviation
  Right ventricular hypertrophy

Chest X-ray
  Left atrial enlargement
  Right ventricular hypertrophy
  Mitral valve calcification
  Enlarged pulmonary artery
  Pulmonary venous congestion

normal, and the pulse may be irregularly irregular secondary to atrial fibrillation. The carotid pulse upstroke and amplitude are unremarkable. The left ventricular impulse is small or absent; a parasternal right ventricular impulse may be palpable.

The cardinal auscultatory features of mitral stenosis are an accentuated first heart sound, an early diastolic opening snap, and an early to middiastolic rumble with presystolic accentuation. The murmur is often heard best with the patient in the left lateral position, using the bell of the stethoscope and the apex of the heart. Patients with more severe degrees of mitral stenosis have a holodiastolic murmur and a short interval between S_2 and the opening snap. In patients with pulmonary hypertension, the pulmonic component of the second heart sound is loud, and mild functional pulmonary incompetence may ensue with the early diastolic blowing murmur of Graham Steell. Finally, because of the common association of mild mitral regurgitation, aortic valve disease, or tricuspid disease, their corresponding murmurs may be present.

There is a certain number of patients in whom the mitral diastolic murmur is difficult to elicit or may actually be absent. It is important to have a high index of suspicion regarding "silent" mitral stenosis in patients whose clinical features suggest heart disease. Radiographic findings include left atrial enlargement and pulmonary vascular redistribution secondary to pulmonary venous hypertension; right ventricular enlargement and dilatation of the pulmonary artery may also be present. Calcification of the mitral annulus is recognized by echocardiography or by the "inverted C" pattern of calcification seen on the chest x-ray. The ECG is often the most important initial clue in the diagnosis of mitral stenosis. The P wave may be broad and/or notched (P mitrale). Individuals with pulmonary hypertension and right ventricular hypertrophy (RVH) frequently demonstrate right axis deviation.

The echocardiogram has become the most important noninvasive diagnostic tool. M-mode echocardiography shows thickened mitral valve leaflets with reduced mobility; two-dimensional echo allows accurate calculation of valve orifice size and left ventricular function. Catheterization is not required to make the diagnosis of mitral stenosis but may be indicated to aid in planning mitral valvular surgery.

Treatment

The treatment of mitral stenosis as it relates to the emergency physician depends primarily on the recognition and initial management of acute complications. Congestive heart failure should be treated with oxygen, upright posturing, diuretics, and preload reduction. Sustained tachycardias are poorly tolerated by patients with mitral stenosis; atrial fibrillation with a rapid ventricular response is most common in this situation. Ventricular rate should be controlled at 70 to 90 beats/minute with digoxin and, if needed, propranolol. Propranolol will be much more effective than digoxin in patients with normal sinus rhythm to keep the heart rate from increasing with exercise. In the elderly patient, the difficulty of restoring sinus rhythm, or of maintaining it, is so great that it is usually not worth more than a single attempted cardioversion, and this only if the appearance of atrial fibrillation is recent.[33]

It has been estimated that at least 20% of all patients with mitral stenosis have at least one arterial embolus in a lifetime. In some cases, the embolus may be the first sign of cardiac disease. Cerebral emboli are most common, with renal, splenic, and other systemic sites also frequently involved. In an elderly person with atrial fibrillation and acute neurologic deficits, one must always look carefully for the auscultatory signs of mitral stenosis. Further emboli can often be prevented with the use of long-term oral anticoagulant therapy.

Mild hemoptysis may occur secondary to a temporary rise in pulmonary venous pressure (e.g., exercise). Rarely, life-threatening hemoptysis may require airway protection and emergency bronchoscopy. Any bleeding diathesis should be corrected immediately. Another important aspect of emergency care for the patient with mitral stenosis is to prevent seeding of the affected valve. Bac-

terial endocarditis prophylaxis is mandatory whenever an invasive procedure is initiated in the emergency care unit.[34]

Mitral valve surgery is recommended for the NYHA Functional Class II or III patient whose calculated mitral valve area is less than 1 cm^2. Commissurotomy may be possible if the valve is not calcified and subvalvular disease is not extensive. This procedure usually provides relief of mitral stenosis for at least 10 years.

MITRAL REGURGITATION

The mitral valve may be incompetent from disease affecting any part of the functional mitral valve apparatus: left ventricular wall, papillary muscles, chordae tendineae, mitral valve leaflets, mitral annulus, or left atrial wall. In the elderly, the more common etiologies of mitral regurgitation (MR) include mitral valve prolapse, coronary artery disease and its complications, and degenerative changes (Table 15–7). Rheumatic mitral valve disease is seen in 2 to 3% of the geriatric population; MR is the dominant lesion in two thirds.

Although mitral valve prolapse (MVP) usually becomes symptomatic in the third through fifth decades, attention has recently focused on MVP as a cause of significant morbidity in the aged.[35] This syndrome is due to a mismatch between the size of the mitral valve apparatus and the left ventricular cavity. The "redundant" mitral valve prolapses into the left atrium as the left ventricle shrinks past a critical volume during systole. The natural history of MVP remains unclear; it is not known if the condition occurs abruptly or represents a disease process that has progressed to the point at which it has become clinically recognizable. MVP is characterized by a midsystolic click and late systolic apical murmur. Approximately 4% of the elderly develop significant MR (holosystolic murmur) associated with disabling chest pain and arrhythmias.[36] Prophylaxis for bacterial endocarditis is needed with the possible exception of some patients who have a click without an associated murmur.

Postinfarction mitral incompetence due to papillary muscle and/or ventricular wall dysfunction occurs commonly in the aged and usually does not require aggressive

Table 15–7   Etiologies of MR in the Elderly

Rheumatic heart disease
Mitral valve prolapse
Ischemic heart disease
   Papillary muscle dysfunction
   Acute myocardial infarction
Degenerative changes
   Mitral annular calcification
   Myxomatous leaflet degeneration
Spontaneous idiopathic chordal rupture
Bacterial endocarditis
Trauma, blunt and penetrating
Left ventricular dilatation

therapy. Because of marginal blood supply, the papillary muscles are very sensitive to coronary artery disease. Rupture of a papillary muscle typically occurs 12 to 48 hours after myocardial infarction and is most commonly associated with inferior wall necrosis. Complete transection of the papillary muscle is usually fatal and, fortunately, occurs in only 2 to 5% of acute myocardial infarctions. More commonly, acute MR is the result of transient papillary muscle dysfunction or ruptured chordae tendineae.

Degenerative changes in the mitral valve are a common cause of MR in the elderly, and the effects of abnormal wear and tear on a slightly abnormal valve may be important in the development of mitral incompetence. Atrophy of valve tissue, stretching or tearing of the chordae tendineae, and myxomatous degeneration are frequently found during operations in both acute and chronic cases.[37] Functional MR may also follow left ventricular dilatation from cardiomyopathy, because the dilated, poorly contractile mitral annulus does not allow adequate coaptation of the mitral valve leaflets in systole.

History and Symptoms

The symptoms manifested by a patient with MR depend on the degree of regurgitation, its rate of progression, pulmonary artery pressure, and the presence of associated heart disease.[38] Patients with chronic MR may remain asymptomatic for decades. The left atrium bears the brunt of the load and in chronic cases dilates and becomes extremely compliant.[37] The left atrial pressure is usually less than 20 mm Hg so that dyspnea is not a prominent complaint.[37] Left atrial dilatation eventually leads to atrial fibrillation, but since there is no obstruction to mitral diastolic flow, patients with MR withstand this arrhythmia better than do patients with any degree of mitral stenosis. Eventually, however, left ventricular failure develops in severe MR, and patients note exercise intolerance, fatigue, and weakness. Palpitations occur frequently, especially with the onset of atrial dysrhythmias.

In contrast, acute MR frequently presents as a catastrophic event, the natural history of which depends upon etiology. In general, as blood attempts to regurgitate into the noncompliant left atrium, pressure rises to very high levels and acute pulmonary edema quickly develops. Dyspnea is the principal presenting symptom. As long as the left ventricular function remains competent, cardiac output is maintained in the face of pulmonary edema. However, if the condition is not recognized and corrected, reflex pulmonary vasoconstriction and symptoms of right-sided failure may result. Once the left ventricle fails (hours to days), cardiac output is severely compromised and hemodynamic collapse occurs with shock.[38]

It is important that the diagnosis of acute MR be considered in every patient presenting with sudden onset of pulmonary edema, with or without a new systolic murmur. Keep in mind that acute MR does not necessarily imply severe MR; if the rupture of a few chordae occurs, left ventricular failure will not ensue, even though pulmonary edema may be a presenting feature.[38]

Clinical Findings

Elderly patients with chronic MR of a moderate or severe degree present with typical clinical findings (Table 15–8). The systolic escape of blood into the left atrium with its subsequent diastolic return results in a large total ventricular systolic stroke volume. Both events explain a hyperdynamic left ventricular impulse displaced to the left (left ventricular enlargement), a systolic thrill at the apex, the ausculatory features of a diastolic filling sound (S_3), and an apical holosystolic murmur that radiates to the left axilla.[21] There is no strict correlation between the murmur's intensity and the severity of mitral incompetence; however, if the murmur is confined to late systole instead of beginning with S_1, the MR usually is due to papillary muscle dysfunction or mitral valve prolapse and is not severe.[38] Chest x-rays and electrocardiography show left ventricular and atrial enlargement; in addition, the chest films usually show signs of pulmonary venous congestion.

Patients with severe acute MR generally are seriously ill with left ventricular congestive heart failure. The api-

Table 15–8 Differential Features of Severe MR

	Acute	Chronic
Initial symptoms	Dyspnea, tachypnea, pulmonary congestion	Exertional dyspnea, fatigue, palpitations
Physical Findings		
Left ventricular (LV) impulse	Normal	Displaced
Right ventricular (RV) impulse	Increased	Normal
Precordial thrill	Frequent	Uncommon
Jugular vein pulsation	Increased "a" wave	Normal
Carotid pulse	Rapid upstroke and falloff	Normal or collapsing
Mitral regurgitant murmur	Loud, harsh decrescendo in late systole	Holosystolic
Murmur radiation	Base of heart	To axillae
Electrocardiogram	Sinus tachycardia	Atrial fibrillation; P mitrale; LV hypertrophy with strain
Chest X-ray	Pulmonary edema; normal cardiac silhouette	Left atrial and ventricular enlargement

cal impulse is usually active, with prominent thrusts and a systolic thrill. Acute right ventricular pressure overload may cause jugular venous distention, with a prominent "a" wave and a left parasternal lift. Sinus tachycardia is common and distinguishes the acute syndrome from chronic MR, in which atrial fibrillation is the rule. Auscultatory signs may be obscured by the pulmonary congestion. The harsh apical regurgitant murmur starts with S_1 and may end before S_2 because left ventricular and atrial pressures equalize before the end of systole.[39] This early systolic murmur may be extremely difficult to distinguish from AS, acute ventricular septal defect, and HOCM. A prominent S_4 gallop points toward acute MR as the small left atrium tries to discharge the acute volume overload.[24] The chest x-ray will show evidence of congestive heart failure with a normal cardiac silhouette. The ECG is generally nondiagnostic, although sinus tachycardia, evidence of acute myocardial infarction, or large, negative terminal P forces in lead V_1 (suggestive of atrial volume overload) may be present.

Doppler echocardiography can accurately detect and grade the severity of the MR, while two-dimensional studies are useful in determining the cause of the regurgitation. Radionucleotide angiography and cardiac catheterization are used in a similar manner to the workup of AR.

Treatment

The therapeutic principles of acute MR are very similar to those of acute AR — ensuring adequate oxygenation and ventilation, loop diuretics, morphine, nitrites, and afterload reduction. Nitroprusside increases forward output in MR by decreasing afterload and may lead to improved mitral valve function by decreasing left ventricular volume. In cases of extreme hypotension, concurrent amrinone or dobutamine infusion may be attempted, although the resultant vasoconstriction may exacerbate myocardial ischemia and regurgitation. In contrast to acute AR, the use of intra-aortic balloon pumping (IABP) is indicated in severe cases that are unresponsive to pharmacologic measures. The optimum regimen is often a combination of IABP counterpulsation and nitroprusside infusion. The majority of patients can be stabilized with medical management, but most require surgical mitral valve replacement within 1 year of presentation.[11]

ACUTE RHEUMATIC FEVER

Acute rheumatic fever (ARF) is characteristically a disease of childhood and young adult life; however, about 10% of the cases occur in patients over 60.[40] Despite this prevalence, ARF is often misdiagnosed in older patients. Most clinically recognized cases present with nonspecific symptoms such as fatigability, malaise, fever, and arthralgia. Evidence of antecedent streptococcal infection

is usually absent, and only one third of the patients will have a prior history of rheumatic fever or rheumatic heart disease.

Acute polyarthritis and carditis (e.g., changing murmurs and transient prolongation of the PR interval) are the most common signs of ARF in the elderly. The other major Jones criteria are often absent. The course of ARF in the elderly is usually protracted, with chronic recurrences and a low incidence of permanent cardiac damage.[41] Sclerotic lesions of the mitral, aortic, and tricuspid valves may occur with repeated episodes. Chronic joint immobility and pain may cause permanent disability, but successful medical and surgical interventions now allow the elderly patient with rheumatic heart disease to attain a long and high-quality life.[42]

INFECTIOUS ENDOCARDITIS

In the 1960s it was realized that the pattern of infectious endocarditis had changed and that increasingly it was becoming a disease of elderly patients, often with no antecedent valve disease. Recent studies from large community hospitals have noted more than 50% of their cases of endocarditis to be in patients over age 60.[43,44] The changing pattern is due in part to the introduction of antibiotics, decline in rheumatic fever, use of prosthetic valves, and increasing survival to ages where degenerative valve diseases become common, as do symptoms requiring diagnostic and surgical procedures likely to produce bacteremia.

As with many diseases in this age group, the clinical presentation may be atypical and many of the classic findings may not be found. In a recent study by Terpenning and colleagues, endocarditis was misdiagnosed in 68% of patients beyond age 60.[43] Symptoms may be very vague, consisting only of generalized weakness or malaise. Arthralgias, myalgias, or headache may be noted. Fever, although present in 82% in one geriatric series,[45] is usually low grade, and new or changing murmurs are heard infrequently. Older patients are less often tachycardic and may be hypotensive on admission to the hospital. About one third of all elderly patients present with neurologic signs, most commonly confusion, seizures, and focal deficits. The "classic" skin lesions of endocarditis (petechiae, Osler's nodes, Janeway's lesions, and splinter hemorrhages) are usually not part of the presenting symptom complex but should be sought on history and physical exam.

The most common sources of infection in the aged are invasive vascular procedures, dental work, skin lesions, and bowel or anorectal sources. However, more than 40% of these patients have no identifiable source of infection.[43] *Staphylococcus aureus* and *Streptococcus viridans* are the organisms isolated most frequently in all age groups. Enterococci, *Streptococcus bovis,* and coagulase-negative staphylococci are more common in the elderly.

The definitive diagnosis is made in suspected cases by finding positive blood cultures; however, these are not available at initial presentation.

Laboratory abnormalities in endocarditis are nonspecific. Anemia is common, usually normochromic and normocytic. The white blood cell count may be elevated, normal, or depressed. Microscopic hematuria, often present, suggests microemboli to the kidneys. The erythrocyte sedimentation rate is usually elevated.[27] Echocardiography may show the valvular vegetations in up to 50% of cases; lesions must be at least 2 mm in diameter for adequate visualization (Figure 15–2).

Treatment of endocarditis should be based on the results of blood cultures and sensitivities with at least 4 weeks of intravenous antibiotic therapy. Life-threatening complications of acute infectious endocarditis are still a problem despite the availability of effective antimicrobial agents. Problems include cardiac failure, destructive intracardiac lesions and abscesses, pericarditis, myocarditis, and heart block in addition to central nervous system (CNS) and systemic embolization.[46]

Prevention of acute endocarditis involves prevention of all causes of bacteremia that may subsequently affect the cardiac valves. Prophylactic antibiotics are administered to patients with established valvular disease who undergo invasive dental procedures, manipulation of infected foci, urethral catheterization of an infected bladder, and sigmoidoscopy. Antibiotic prophylaxis is currently recommended for those patients with prosthetic valves, rheumatic or other acquired valvular heart disease, hypertrophic cardiomyopathy, mitral valve prolapse with systolic murmur, history of bacterial endocarditis, most congenital malformations, and patients who have had corrected systemic-pulmonary shunts. Prophylaxis is not recommended for those elderly patients who have undergone coronary artery bypass surgery or have a known or corrected secundum atrial septal defect if the correction was more than 6 months previous. Table 15–2 lists the regimens for antibiotic prophylaxis preceding dental and surgical procedures.

PROSTHETIC VALVE COMPLICATIONS

Open heart surgery has been established long enough for its late sequelae to be appearing in geriatric age groups, and valve replacement in patients over 65 years of age is now a common procedure. Despite refinements in design, no valve, currently, is free of potential serious complications, which may occur early after surgery or be delayed for years after implantation.

Prosthetic heart valves may be classified into two basic types: tissue (bioprosthetic) valves and mechanical prostheses. The tissue valves most commonly used are stent-mounted porcine aortic valves or bovine pericardial valves. Their advantages are low thrombogenicity and minimal hemolysis. Durability is the major drawback, with a valve failure rate of approximately 5% after 4 to 5 years.[48] Mechanical valves are much more durable but, in contrast, are highly thrombogenic and are more likely to cause significant hemolysis. The three mechanical prostheses currently implanted most often are the caged ball, tilting disk, and, more recently, the bileaflet designs.[47] If

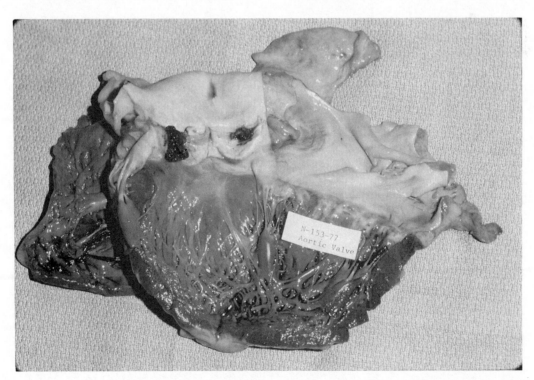

Figure 15–2 Valvular vegetations on the aortic valve from infectious endocarditis.

the patient cannot provide information about the valve implanted, the valve type and location usually can be determined radiographically. A detailed guide to the radiographic identification of prosthetic heart valves is given by Morse and colleagues[49] and Mehlman and Resnekov.[50]

Thromboembolic phenomena are the most frequent life-threatening complications of artificial valves and may present as myocardial infarction, sudden stroke, or peripheral arterial occlusion. Ball or disk movement may be impeded by a thrombus on the cage, and, occasionally, the valve orifice becomes occluded by a pannus or thrombus (Figure 15–3). Although less of a problem, thrombosis may also occur on bioprosthetic valves, especially in the mitral position. Presentation may be as acute as cardiogenic shock or as subtle as shortness of breath, low perfusion syndrome, or transient ischemia. To prevent thrombosis, patients are often put on warfarin, which in turn can lead to bleeding complications, which must be identified and treated immediately, particularly in postoperative patients.

The turbulence and gradients produced by the lateral flow characteristics of ball valve prostheses may cause considerable hemolysis of red cells. Most people are able to compensate for the hemolysis and only 10 to 15% of patients with the older design mechanical valves will develop anemia.[51] Prosthetic valve dysfunction results from wear on the ball or disk, which may then become acutely fixed in either the open or closed position. They may fragment, rupture, or shrink, producing catastrophic stenosis or incompetence. Symptoms suggestive

of mechanical dysfunction are increased angina, heart failure, and syncope. Chest radiographs should be done to confirm the correct position of the prosthesis. Doppler echocardiography, cinefluoroscopy, or angiography may be necessary for definitive diagnosis.

Prosthetic valve endocarditis (PVE) develops in 2 to 3% of patients per year and may present as a febrile illness, systemic embolization, a new murmur of valvular regurgitation or stenosis, or hemodynamic deterioration.[52] PVE that develops within 2 months of surgery has a 72% mortality and is commonly caused by staphylococci or gram-negative rods. Late-onset PVE occurs more than 60 days after valve replacement, has a 45% mortality, and is most often due to *Streptococcus viridans* or *Staphylococcus epidermidis*. Because the infection is at the site of a foreign body, the prognosis for recovery with antibiotic therapy is worse than in native valve endocarditis. Recurrent infection after one trial of medical therapy is generally an indication for replacement of the valve.[53] Other indications for surgical valve replacement include 1) persistent sepsis from an infected prosthesis[54]; 2) recurrent emboli; 3) obstruction and persistent leakage; and 4) heart failure secondary to valve dysfunction. The operative mortality remains very high.

One of the reasons for difficulty with antibiotic therapy has been the recent emergence of methicillin-resistant strains of *Staphylococcus aureus*.[55] These strains are also resistant to other antibiotics such as the aminoglycosides. Infection with these organisms becomes more difficult to treat although there has been some success with combination therapies.

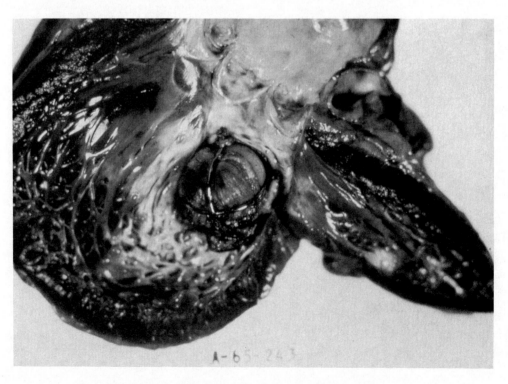

Figure 15–3   Prosthetic ball valve occluded by a thrombus.

REFERENCES

1. Duthie EH, Gambert SR, and Tresch D: Evaluation of the systolic murmur in the elderly, J Am Geriatr Soc 29:498–502, 1981.
2. Pomerance A: Pathogenesis of aortic stenosis and its relation to age, Br Heart J 34:569–574, 1972.
3. Waller BF and Morgan R: The very elderly heart: valvular heart disease. In Waller BF, editor: Contemporary issues in cardiovascular pathology: cardiovascular clinics, Philadelphia, 1988, pp 361–408, FA Davis Co.
4. Lombard JT and Selzer A: Valvular aortic stenosis: clinical and hemodynamic profile of patients, Ann Intern Med 106:292–298, 1987.
5. Tresch DD: Atypical presentation of cardiovascular disorders in the elderly, Geriatrics 42:31–46, 1987.
6. Richards AM et al: Syncope in aortic valvular stenosis, Lancet 2:1113–1116, 1984.
7. Selzer A: Medical progress: changing aspects of the natural history of valvular aortic stenosis, N Engl J Med 317:91–98, 1986.
8. Roberts WC, Perloff JK, and Constantino T: Severe valvular aortic stenosis in patients over 65 years of age, Am J Cardiol 27:497–506, 1971.
9. Stapczynski JS: Valvular heart disease. In Tintinalli JE, Rothstein RJ, and Krome RL, editors: Emergency medicine: a comprehensive study guide, New York, 1985, pp 170–177, McGraw-Hill Book Co.
10. Fulkerson PK and Foreman DW: Calcific aortic stenosis: a condition of increasing importance for the geriatric patients, Geriatr Med Today 4:67–70, 1985.
11. Janz TG: Valvular heart disease: clinical approach to acute decompensation of left-sided lesions, Ann Emerg Med 17:201–208, 1988.
12. Simpson PC and Bristow JD: Recognition and management of emergencies in valvular heart disease, Med Clin North Am 63:155–172, 1988.
13. Kay HR, Goel IP, and Mundth ED: Valve replacement in the elderly: special considerations and results, Geriatrics 37:109–114, 1982.
14. Isner JM et al: Treatment of calcific aortic stenosis by balloon valvuloplasty, Am J Cardiol 59:313–317, 1987.
15. Shenoy MM et al: Hypertrophic cardiomyopathy in the elderly: a frequently misdiagnosed disease, Arch Intern Med 146:658–661, 1986.
16. Krasnow N and Stein RA: Hypertrophic cardiomyopathy in the aged, Am Heart J 96:326–336, 1978.
17. Whiting RB et al: Idiopathic hypertrophic subaortic stenosis in the elderly, N Engl J Med 285:196–200, 1971.
18. Frank S and Braunwald E: Idiopathic hypertrophic subaortic stenosis: clinical analysis of 162 patients with emphasis on the natural history, Circulation 37:759–763, 1968.
19. Maron BJ et al: Medical progress: Hypertrophic cardiomyopathy; interrelations of clinical manifestations, pathophysiology and therapy, (first of two parts), N Engl J Med 316:780–789, 1987.
20. Miller KP et al: Hypotension and a transient murmur in an elderly woman, Hosp Physician 32:45–51, 1986.
21. Brandenburg RO, editor: Office cardiology. Philadelphia, 1980, FA Davis Co.
22. Maron BJ et al: Medical progress: Hypertrophic cardiomyopathy; interrelations of clinical manifestations, pathophysiology and therapy (second of two parts) N Engl J Med 316:844–849, 1987.
23. Pollick C: Muscular subaortic stenosis: hemodynamic and clinical improvement after diisopyramide, N Engl J Med 307:997–999, 1982.
24. Paulus WJ et al: Effects of long term treatment with amiodarone on exercise hemodynamics and left ventricular relaxation in patients with hypertrophic cardiomyopathy, Circulation 74:544–554, 1986.
25. Morganroth J et al: Acute severe aortic regurgitation: pathophysiology, clinical recognition and management, Ann Intern Med 87:223–232, 1977.
26. Panidis IP and Segal BL: Aortic valve disease in the elderly. In Frankl WS and Brest AN, editors: Valvular heart disease: comprehensive evaluation and management, Philadelphia, 1986, pp 289–311, FA Davis Co.
27. Rippe JM and Csete ME, editors: Manual of intensive care medicine, Boston, 1983, Little, Brown & Co.
28. Symbas PN et al: Surgical treatment of aortic regurgitation and aortico-left ventricular discontinuity, J Thorac Cardiovasc Surg 84:291–296, 1982.
29. Nishimura RA et al: Chronic aortic regurgitation: indications for operation–1988, Mayo Clin Proc 63:270–280, 1988.
30. Bell MH and Mints GS: Mitral valve disease in the elderly. In Frankl WS and Brest AN, editors: Valvular heart disease: comprehensive evaluation and management, Philadelphia, 1986, pp 313–324, FA Davis Co.
31. Fulkerson PK et al: Calcification of the mitral annulus: etiology, clinical associations, complications and therapy, Am J Med 66:967–977, 1979.
32. Savage DD et al: Prevalence of submitral (annular) calcium and its correlates in a general population-based sample (the Framingham study), Am J Cardiol 51:1375–1378, 1983.
33. Rothbaum DA, editor: Geriatric cardiology, Philadelphia, 1981, FA Davis Co.
34. Limas CJ: Mitral stenosis in the elderly, Geriatrics 26:75–79, 1971.
35. Kolibash AJ et al: Mitral valve prolapse syndrome: analysis of 62 patients aged 60 years and older, Am J Cardiol 52:534–539, 1983.
36. Naggar CZ, Pearson WN, and Seljan MP: Frequency of complications of mitral valve prolapse in subjects aged 60 years and older, Am J Cardiol 37:1209–1212, 1986.
37. Sokolow M and McIlroy MB: Clinical cardiology, Los Altos, Calif, 1986, Lange Medical Publications.
38. Kusiak V and Brest AN: Acute mitral regurgitation: pathophysiology and management. In Frankl WS and Brest AN, editors: Valvular heart disease: comprehensive evaluation and management, Philadelphia, 1986, pp 257–280, FA Davis Co.
39. DePace NL, Nestico PF, and Morganroth J: Acute severe mitral regurgitation: pathophysiology, clinical recognition, and management, Am J Med 78:293–306, 1985.
40. Caird FI and Dall JLC: The cardiovascular system. In Brocklehurst JC, editor: Textbook of geriatric medicine and gerontology, New York, 1985, pp 257–258, Churchill Livingstone.
41. Kjorstad H: Rheumatic fever in the aged: report on a hospital series from Oslo, Acta Med Scand 158:337–344, 1957.
42. Harris R, editor: Rheumatic fever and rheumatic heart disease. In Clinical geriatric cardiology: management of the elderly patient, Philadelphia, 1986, pp 270–291, JB Lippincott Co.
43. Terpenning MS, Buggy BP, and Kauffman CA: Infective endocarditis: clinical features in young and elderly patients, Am J Med 83:626–634, 1987.
44. Vanezio FR et al: Infective endocarditis in a community hospital, Arch Intern Med 142:789–792, 1982.
45. Applefield MM and Hornick RB: Infective endocarditis in patients over age 60, Am Heart J 88:90–94, 1974.
46. Weinstein L: Life-threatening complications of infective endocarditis and their management, Arch Intern Med 146:953–957, 1986.
47. Harrison EC et al: An emergency physician's guide to prosthetic heart valves: identification and hemodynamic function, Ann Emerg Med 17:194–200, 1988.
48. Lipson LC et al: Long term hemodynamic assessment of the porcine heterograft in the mitral position: late development of valvular stenosis, Circulation 64:397–402, 1981.
49. Morse D, Steiner RM, and Fernandez J: Guide to prosthetic cardiac valves, New York, 1985, Springer-Verlag.
50. Mehlman DJ and Resnekov L: A guide to the radiographic identification of prosthetic heart valves, Circulation 57:613–623, 1978.
51. Wilson WR et al: Prosthetic valve endocarditis, Mayo Clin Proc 57:155–161, 1982.
52. Watanakunakorn C: Prosthetic valve endocarditis, Prog Cardiovasc Dis 22:181–187, 1979.
53. Bell BB, Shapiro EP, and Zieve PD: Common cardiac disorders revealed by auscultation of the heart. In Barker LR, Burton JR, and Zieve PD, editors: Principles of ambulatory medicine, Baltimore, 1986, pp 765–767, Williams & Wilkins.
54. Shulman ST et al: Special report. Prevention of bacterial endocarditis: a statement for health professionals by the Committee on Rheumatic Fever and Infective Endocarditis of the Council on Cardiovascular Disease in the Young, Circulation 70:1123A–1127A, 1984.
55. Brumfitt W and Hamilton-Miller J: Methicillin-resistant Staphylococcus aureus, N Engl J Med 320:1188, 1989.

Syncope and Dizziness

Michael Sequeira, M.D., F.A.C.E.P.

Syncope and dizziness in the elderly patient represent a challenge to the clinician and require an appreciation of the complex changes that can occur in multiple organ systems in this age group. Vari- ous series have shown that of the visits by the elderly to ambulatory care facilities, up to 30% are for some complaint of syncope and/or dizziness. Between 3 and 5% of medical admissions to a community hospital are for the evaluation of syncope and up to 85% of these patients are over 65 years of age. There is a yearly incidence of syncope of 6% in elderly institutionalized patients with a recurrence rate of up to 30%.[1-5]

Not only are syncope and dizziness common in the elderly patient, but they also carry significant prognostic import. In one study of patients over 60 years old who presented with syncope, there was a 21% incidence of major morbidity or death in the 6 months after presentation.[6] This compares with a 6% incidence of major morbidity or death in a corresponding 6-month follow-up in patients less than 60 years old. Silverstein and associates have shown that of those syncopal patients over the age of 60 who are admitted to medical intensive care units, there is a 1-year mortality of 6% in those patients with noncardiovascular diagnoses and 19% in patients with cardiovascular causes.[7] In addition, their study shows that patients with unexplained syncope had a 1-year mortality rate — 1.5 times that of the age-standardized American white population. Elderly patients who have the simple diagnosis of vasodepressor syncope had a 16% major morbidity over the ensuing 6-month follow-up.[1] The reasons for this disturbing figure are multiple, for the elderly are particularly susceptible to the consequences of falls that can result from syncope.[8] Fractures, subdural hematomas, aspiration pneumonia, soft tissue injuries, loss of independent function, and toxic effects of treatment are potential life-threatening consequences of syncope in elderly patients. Of the patients who sustain a hip fracture, up to 20% will not survive 1 year; of those patients who do survive, one fifth of them will never walk again.

Syncope presents a diagnostic challenge to the clinician for other reasons as well. As with many other symptoms of geriatric medicine, syncope may be the atypical manifestation of very important diseases that are usually not expected to produce it. In elderly patients, several age-

and disease-related impairments may critically reduce cerebral blood flow to the threshold of the maintenance of consciousness. Any acute process that further affects cerebral blood flow or oxygen delivery can then present as syncope. Therefore, diseases such as pneumonia, bronchitis, or myocardial infarction or everyday stresses such as hyperventilation, postural change, cough, or Valsalva's maneuver may present atypically as syncope in the elderly. For instance, syncope has been reported to be the presenting manifestation of myocardial infarction in 10 to 20% of elderly patients. In addition, hyperventilation can critically reduce cerebral blood flow by up to 40% in the elderly patient, thereby causing enough of a decrease in cerebral blood flow to cause syncope when it otherwise would not.

Thus, the reason for the high incidence of syncope in the elderly population is that a combination of many processes reduces cerebral blood flow, including normal degenerative processes and coexisting disease processes. Various disease processes that may coexist, including atherosclerosis and its many complications — such as coronary insufficiency and carotid disease, degenerative processes of the autonomic and central nervous system, chronic obstructive pulmonary disease, and hypertension — can combine with the various other "normal" physiologic changes that occur with aging to produce the ideal changes that can result in the frequent recurrence of syncope in the elderly patient.

The purpose of this chapter is to examine the problem of syncope and dizziness; to review the various age-related physiologic changes that occur in the elderly patient with regard to the problem of syncope and dizziness; to define the symptom categories of syncope, dizziness, lightheadedness, and vertigo; to review the multiple causes of these symptom categories as well as their pathophysiology; to present a diagnostic approach to elderly patients presenting with such symptoms; and to review pertinent therapeutic maneuvers that may potentially save a geriatric patient's life.

SYMPTOM CATEGORIES

The physician must be able to carefully identify and help the patient identify the significant differences between syncope, faintness or presyncope, lightheadedness, vertigo, and seizure disorders. *Syncope* primarily comprises a generalized weakness of muscles and inability to stand and is associated with a transient loss of consciousness. *Presyncope* or *faintness* contrasts with syncope in that there is no loss of consciousness, but there is a sense of giddiness and lack of strength with a sensation of impending loss of consciousness.

Patients who have syncope usually experience it in an upright position, either sitting or standing, and have ample warning of the impending faint through a sense of "not feeling good." A sense of giddiness is accompanied by

the sensation of swaying of surrounding objects. Patients yawn or gape, see spots before their eyes, and hear ringing in their ears. Nausea may accompany these symptoms, sometimes with vomiting. There is a notable pallor or ashen-gray complexion to the skin. The patient is usually profusely diaphoretic. The deliberate onset frequently allows patients to protect themselves from injury, and a hurtful fall from syncope is rare. Loss of consciousness may occasionally be averted if the patient assumes a recumbent position before he or she passes out. Patients usually remain unconscious for a period of seconds to minutes but may be unconscious for as long as 20 to 30 minutes. They usually lie motionless, but a few clonic jerks of the limbs and face may occur. Generalized tonic-clonic movements do not occur although occasional urinary incontinence (but not fecal incontinence) may be noted. Once patients awaken, their color returns. They may experience sensations of being weak and may actually lose consciousness again if arising too quickly. Headache, drowsiness, and mental confusion are unusual after a syncopal episode; if these occur, they usually imply the presence of a convulsion.

It is important for the physician to help patients specify whether the complaint of dizziness represents lightheadedness or vertigo. *Lightheadedness* usually refers to a sensation of giddiness or faintness while vertigo refers to a feeling of whirling rotation. Patients with vertigo have no alteration of consciousness or no sensation of an impending faint. The key symptom of *vertigo* is the sensation of motion, which the patient may perceive as veering, staggering, imbalance, or momentary disequilibrium, although many with vertigo may describe the classic sensation of spinning or rotation. The patient may often describe the sensation of being pulled to one side or to the ground as if drawn by a magnet — the phenomenon of impulsion. The feeling of impulsion is particularly characteristic of vertigo. All but the mildest forms of vertigo are accompanied by diaphoresis, pallor, nausea, and vomiting. As a rule, the patient can walk only with difficulty or not at all if the vertigo is intense. Most patients have previously experienced a sensation of vertigo after normal activities such as riding a merry-go-round. When queried specifically, they often readily recognize the similarity between their symptoms and those previous experiences. If they cannot be specific in distinguishing their "dizziness," provocative maneuvers, which will be described later, may be indicated to attempt to reproduce symptoms they have experienced.

PATHOPHYSIOLOGY

Syncope, essentially, is a result of a temporary hypoperfusion of the brain, which causes generalized cerebral ischemia and a sudden cessation of cerebral metabolism (Table 16–1). The human body has several mechanisms that can operate to ensure brain perfusion while in the

Table 16–1   Causes of Syncope and Dizziness

1. Vasodepressor syncope
2. Seizure
3. Orthostatic syncope
   a. Hypovolemia or adrenal insufficiency
   b. Prolonged recumbency
   c. Physical deconditioning
   d. Venous insufficiency
   e. Peripheral neuropathies or drugs
   f. Autonomic insufficiency
   g. Micturition syncope
4. Cardiac syncope
   a. Morgagni-Adams-Stokes syndrome
   b. Bradyarrhythmias
   c. Tachyarrhythmias
   d. Sick sinus syndrome
   e. Aortic stenosis
   f. Idiopathic hypertrophic subaortic stenosis
   g. Massive myocardial infarction
   h. Pulmonary embolism
   i. Atrial myxoma
   j. Carotid sinus syncope
5. Cerebrovascular causes
   a. Drop attacks and akinetic fainting spells
   b. Atherosclerosis
6. Hypoglycemia
7. Narcolepsy
8. Hyperventilation
9. Vertigo

upright posture. Approximately 75% of the total blood volume is contained in the venous bed and any interference with venous return may lead to a reduction in cardiac output. Perfusion of the head may still be maintained as long as systemic arterial vasoconstriction occurs. But if this adjustment fails, serious hypotension may occur. A decrease in cerebral perfusion to less than half of the normal rate will result in syncope. The pooling of blood in the extremities is usually prevented by a combination of pressor reflexes, which induce arteriolar and venular constriction; reflex tachycardia by means of aortic and carotid reflexes; and improvement of venous return through muscular activity of the limbs and increased respiratory rate.

Age-Related Physiologic Changes Predisposing to Syncope

Multiple age-related and degenerative processes alter these compensatory mechanisms and make the elderly patient vulnerable to syncope. The accumulation of these age- and disease-related conditions — conditions that threaten cerebral blood flow or reduce oxygen content in the blood — may bring cerebral oxygen delivery dangerously close to the threshold needed to maintain consciousness. Any additional stress that further reduces cerebral blood flow or blood oxygen content may precipitate syncope. Diabetes impairs the normal compensatory increase in cerebral blood flow that occurs in response to hypocardia, and hypertension resets the min-

imum blood pressure required to maintain cerebral autoregulation and, therefore, presents symptoms of cerebral hypoxia. Normal aging is associated with progressive irreversible changes in many of the physiologic mechanisms maintaining vascular homeostasis. These include alterations in the baroreflexes, heart rate, and the extracellular volume regulation.

Baroreflexes

Baroreflex sensitivity decreases with age. In older people, the compensatory bradycardic response to acute increases in blood pressure induced by phenylephrine has been shown to be blunted. Additionally, the compensatory tachycardia that results from acute decreases in blood pressure induced by nitroprusside has also been shown to be blunted in elderly patients. The natural evolution of these two facts is that elderly patients are, therefore, more sensitive to vasodilators unless able to compensate for sudden drops in blood pressure from such entities as acute hemorrhage. Intravascular volume shifts can occur from coughing, Valsalva's maneuver, or the abrupt assumption of the upright posture. In addition, the age-related stiffening of the carotid arteries and aortic arch may reset baroreflex sensitivity by producing less tonic input to the vasomotor center for any given level of blood pressure. This may possibly explain an increase in basal systemic blood pressure with age.

Heart Rate

In the elderly, the compensatory tachycardic response to such diverse stimuli as hypoxia, hypercarbia, isometric hand grip, exercise, cough, and isoproterenol is blunted.[5] Despite this effect, there is a more sustained plasma norepinephrine response to the upright posture in normal elderly men. This implies that a diminished heart rate response to upright posture results from a decrease in sensitivity to adrenergic stimulation of the aged heart. This corresponds to studies that show a progressive decrease in beta receptors of the heart with age. Therefore, another compensatory reflex to blood pressure changes — heart rate — is impaired as a normal concomitant of aging.

Extracellular Volume Regulation

Basal plasma renin and aldosterone concentrations are diminished by 30 to 50% in elderly patients. Because of this, the aged kidney takes longer to conserve sodium when salt intake is restricted. The patient cannot, therefore, tolerate relatively minor intravascular volume losses and poor oral intake, for instance, because of this progressive inefficiency and sodium conservation.

Virtually all of the homeostatic mechanisms that normally maintain intravascular volume and blood pressure within narrow limits become variably impaired with age, making the older patient especially vulnerable to syncope and dizziness. When the effects of various disease processes and drugs, which may affect vascular homeostasis, are added to these derangements, the reason for the high incidence of syncope and dizziness in the elderly patient is evident.

TYPES OF SYNCOPE

Vasodepressor Syncope

Vasodepressor or vasovagal syncope is perhaps the most frequently encountered type of syncope, accounting for approximately 40% of syncopal episodes. Vasodepressor syncope carries a worse prognosis in the elderly than with younger patients. Approximately 16% of the elderly patients experiencing vasodepressor syncope have major morbidity or mortality in the intervening 6 months, whereas less than 1% of patients under 30 who present with this type of syncope are at such risk.

This is the common faint experienced by most normal people. Regardless of the precise mechanism, all of these patients experience hypotension accompanied by an inappropriate slowing of the heart rate. The setting is very important in the diagnosis of vasovagal syncope. Typically, these spells occur after an emotional upset, in crowded warm rooms, or during prolonged standing, as seen in children during school assemblies or in soldiers during parades or inspections. They also occur after injurious shocking events, or prolonged bed rest, and during pain and fasting. Mild blood loss, poor physical condition, anemia, fever, and organic heart disease also will predispose a person to vasovagal syncope. Such fainting spells occur in approximately 5% of normal blood donors (Table 16–2). Full meals and warm baths, which cause diversion of blood away from the brain to the viscera and extremities, also predispose people to these spells.

Patients are always standing or sitting in the premonitory phase before these spells. Very characteristically, there is a spectrum of premonitory symptoms that lasts for at least a few seconds and usually for a few minutes or longer. Symptoms consist of weakness, nausea or diaphoresis, a sensation of impending loss of consciousness, diminished hearing, graying of vision, nausea, and epigastric distress. Patients feel weak and confused and are pale and sweaty. Physiologically, there is first a marked fall in arterial pressure and systemic

Table 16–2   Scenario for Vasodepressor Syncope

1. Emotional distress
2. Prolonged standing in warm, crowded rooms
3. During pain
4. After prolonged bed rest or fasting
5. Mild blood loss
6. Anemia
7. Fever

vascular resistance that is most notable in the skeletal muscular beds. Cardiac output may be within normal limits, but it fails to exhibit the expected increase that normally occurs with hypotension. Cardiac output then declines when vagal activity leads to marked bradycardia replacing tachycardia, which results in a further lowering of arterial pressure and a reduction of cerebral perfusion. Recovery comes after the patient assumes the recumbent position, although pallor and weakness often persist. Episodes may recur within a half hour if the patient attempts to stand again. Usually no specific therapy is needed, although pretreatment with atropine in predisposed individuals can reduce this type of syncope. In the emergency department, an IV infusion of dextrose and normal saline is usually all that is required, along with monitoring. Adrenergic agents are rarely necessary.

Orthostatic Syncope

This type of syncope affects elderly patients who have a disproportion between blood volume and vascular capacitance or a chronic defect or instability of vasomotor reflexes. The character of the syncopal attack is similar to that of the vasovagal or vasodepressor type of syncope. However, the effect of posture is the cardinal feature here. Sudden rising from the recumbent or sitting position is the circumstance in which it is most likely to happen. Elderly patients are particularly predisposed to this type of syncope. They frequently lack physical conditioning and undergo prolonged illness and recumbency. Their flabby muscles allow more pooling of blood in their legs, and they frequently have venous insufficiency, which increases the capacity for the pooling of blood in the legs. Furthermore, elderly patients are subject to neuropathies, which are more frequent in their age group. The elderly diabetic patient who gets diabetic neuropathy, which may affect the autonomic nervous system, is particularly at risk. Diabetic neuropathy is very rare in juvenile diabetics. In addition, there is a higher incidence of the chronic complications of alcoholism (including peripheral neuropathy and other degenerative neuronal processes) that occur in geriatric patients (Table 16–3).

Table 16–3   Causes of Orthostatic Hypotension

1. Disproportion between circulating blood volume and vascular capacity
   a. Venous varicosities
   b. Hypovolemia (due to bleeding, dehydration, etc.)
2. Autonomic dysfunction
   a. Postsympathectomy
   b. Pharmacologic sympathectomy
   c. Autonomic neuropathy
      • Chronic postganglionic
      • Chronic preganglionic
      • Part of diffuse neuropathies
3. Drug induced (See Table 16–4)
4. Micturition syncope

Furthermore, there are more geriatric patients receiving antihypertensive, vasodilator, and antiparkinsonism drugs — all of which may predispose them to orthostatic hypotension (Table 16–4).

Loss of vasoconstrictor reflexes in the resistance and capacitance vessels of the lower extremities, as mentioned above, leads to orthostatic hypotension and syncope. Elderly patients are particularly predisposed to specific abnormalities known as primary autonomic insufficiency or dysautonomias. These defects may occur either in peripheral (postganglionic) or central (preganglionic) neurons.

Chronic Postganglionic Autonomic Insufficiency

Chronic postganglionic autonomic insufficiency is a disease of middle-aged and elderly individuals who gradually become troubled by a chronic orthostatic hypotension occasionally in conjunction with sphincter disturbances, impotence, and anhidrosis. Approximately 5 to 10 minutes after these patients arise, their blood pressure drops at least 35 torr, and the pulse pressure narrows. These occurrences are not associated with pallor, nausea, or an increase in pulse rate. The characteristic lack of pulse increase with a pressure drop marks orthostatic hypotension due to autonomic insufficiency from any cause. In this particular syndrome, men are affected more than women. The condition is relatively benign but seemingly irreversible. In this type of autonomic insufficiency, the neurons of the sympathetic ganglia degenerate. The resting serum levels of norepinephrine are subnormal because of the failure of its release from postganglionic endings, and there is a characteristic denervation hypersensitivity to exogenously administered norepinephrine. Upon standing, unlike the normal individual, there is little if any rise in norepinephrine levels. In this type, as well as in chronic preganglionic autonomic insufficiency, levels of plasma dopamine beta-hydroxylase are subnormal. The most effective treatment for this type of orthostatic hypotension is fluorohydrocortisone (oral dose 0.5 to 2.0 mg/day) and salt loading to increase blood volume, supplemented by mechanical devices to prevent blood pooling, such as Jobst or Sigvaris stockings.

Table 16–4 Drugs Causing Orthostatic Hypotension

Benzothiadiazines	Minoxidil
Bretylium	Methotrimeprazine
Chlorisondamine	Methyldopa
Clonidine	Methysergide
Furosemide	Nitroglycerin
Guanacline	Pentolinium
Guanethidine	Phenoxybenzamine
Hexamethonium	Phenothiazines
Hydralazine	Procarbazine
Iopanoic acid	Reserpine
Levodopa	Thiothixene
Lidocaine	Tricyclic antidepressants

Chronic Preganglionic Autonomic Insufficiency

In this type of primary orthostatic hypotension, variable impotence, sphincter disturbances, and anhidrosis may be combined with any one of three or more disorders of the *central* nervous system. These include 1) tremor, extrapyramidal rigidity, and akinesia (Shy-Drager syndrome), 2) progressive cerebellar degeneration, and 3) a variable extrapyramidal and cerebellar disorder (striatonigral degeneration). These syndromes frequently lead to disability and often death within a few years. In this central type of primary autonomic insufficiency, the lateral horn cells of the spinal cord degenerate. In addition, the resting levels of norepinephrine are normal, and there is no hypersensitivity to injected norepinephrine. Further, there has been greater success with the use of sympathomimetic amines such as tyramine (which releases norepinephrine from postganglionic endings) supplemented by a monoamine oxidase (MAO) inhibitor (to prevent destruction of the amine). Propranolol has also been indicated to be effective.

Micturition syncope is considered another variant of orthostatic syncope. This type of syncope usually occurs in males presumably because of the upright posture for micturition. It has been variably attributed either to an unconscious Valsalva's maneuver or to vagal impulses. It is probably more frequent in the elderly male because of increased incidence of bladder outlet obstruction due to prostatic hypertrophy and/or carcinoma that is seen in these patients.

Cardiac Syncope

Approximately 30 to 35% of syncopal episodes in the elderly patient result from some type of cardiac dysfunction. The morbidity and mortality of cardiac syncope is significantly higher than with other types of syncope, with a mortality rate of 19% in patients admitted to a medical intensive care unit.[6]

Cardiac syncope results from transient reduction in cerebral perfusion from a primary decrease in cardiac output. It is the one specific cause of syncope that may occur while the patient is in the recumbent or supine position. Loss of consciousness in an elderly patient, especially when sitting or supine, must *always* suggest cardiac syncope until proven otherwise. The cardinal manifestation of cardiac syncope is loss of consciousness, which can occur in any position. The patient may experience a brief premonitory weakness, palpitations, or chest pain, depending on the cause of the cardiac syncope. It is estimated that 4 to 7 seconds of asystole are required for the patient to lose consciousness in the upright position and as long as 20 to 30 seconds if the patient is recumbent so that such brief premonition is not inconsistent with cardiac syncope. There are multiple types of cardiac syncope, including bradyarrhythmias, tachyarrhythmias, and mechanical obstruction to cardiac output.

Cardiac syncope, resulting from atrioventricular block, is perhaps the most common type of bradyarrhythmic syncope; syncopal episodes associated with this arrhythmia are known as the Morgagni-Adams-Stokes syndrome.[9] When patients develop heart block, there is a sudden interruption of intraventricular conduction, and asystole will exist (the warm-up period) for 10 to 90 seconds before any ventricular rhythm begins. During this period of asystole, a dizzy spell or syncope may be experienced by the patient. Often the clinical picture is that of an elderly individual who complains of brief episodes of dizziness and presyncope that occur without warning, often two to three times per day. These episodes frequently occur over a period of several weeks. If the diagnosis is not made and a pacemaker not implanted, 50% of these patients will be dead within 1 year.

Patients who develop complete heart block usually have prior evidence of conduction disease if, in fact, previous electrocardiograms (ECGs) are available. Perhaps the most frequent cause of conduction disturbance in the elderly patient is an age-related fibrodegenerative disease initially described by Lev in which a fibrotic disruptive process typically involves the proximal fascicles high in the muscular septum. Another idiopathic degenerative process, which involves fibrocalcific degeneration of the conducting pathways, was first elucidated by Lenegre. There are, of course, other causes of chronic progressive heart block. Calcific encroachment into the atrioventricular (AV) node and His-Purkinje system, usually in association with aortic valve calcification, is also a relatively frequent cause. Iatrogenic heart block may result from cardiac surgery or valve replacement. In addition, syphilis, Chagas' disease, amyloid disease, and other cardiomyopathic syndromes must be considered in the etiology as well as ischemic heart disease. Other more exotic causes of complete heart block include such infectious diseases as acute rheumatic fever, diphtheria, and toxoplasmosis; degenerative diseases — such as Friedreich's ataxia and muscular dystrophy — and carcinomatous diseases involving the heart (including rhabdomyosarcoma, lymphoma, metastatic carcinoma, and hemochromatosis) also contribute. Trauma and drugs (including digitalis, quinidine, procainamide, lidocaine, and phenytoin) are also causes.

Previous ECGs, as intimated above, may help one suspect the occurrence of complete heart block. Variable patterns that may have been present in these patients include right bundle branch block and left anterior hemiblock — perhaps the most frequent pattern in patients subsequently developing complete heart block, right bundle branch alone, left anterior hemiblock alone, or left bundle branch block alone. A chief problem is the prediction of or the likelihood of progression to complete heart block in patients with bundle branch block on a baseline ECG. Prospective follow-up studies with previously asymptomatic patients suggest that documented or suspected heart block develops in only 4 to 6% of cases observed for 3½ years. However, patients with chronic bifascicular and trifascicular conduction abnormalities show a higher incidence of subsequent heart block when they have histories of syncope (17%) than when they do not (2%).[10] There is no difference in sudden or nonsudden death, however.

Approximately 2% of all patients presenting with complete heart block will have reversible conduction failures from acute myocardial infarctions, digitalis intoxication, or hyperkalemia. Life expectancy in most of the patients who present with complete heart block is normalized after the insertion of a permanent transvenous pacemaker.

Tachyarrhythmias

Supraventricular tachycardias are the most commonly occurring cause of cardiac syncopal episodes. Van Durme reported a series of 46 patients with dysrhythmias that correlated with symptoms of dizziness or loss of consciousness. In his series, 18 patients had supraventricular tachycardia, 10 had ventricular tachycardia, and the remaining 18 had a number of other types, including conduction disturbances.[11]

Usually, ventricular rates not exceeding 180 beats per minute do not reduce cerebral blood flow. However, elderly patients have a much lower tolerance due to combined cardiac and cerebral vascular disease. Therefore, tachycardias with rates as low as 140 may reduce cerebral blood flow to the point of causing syncope.

It is often difficult to establish whether or not dysrhythmias are the cause of symptoms. For example, among many of the patients in this series complaining of dizziness, a full week of continual monitoring disclosed complex dysrhythmias that were not correlated with symptoms while a large number of patients (42%) had only frequent premature atrial or ventricular contractions without symptoms. Thus, monitoring does not establish unequivocally whether the previous symptoms in these two groups of patients have been caused by high-grade or more prolonged dysrhythmias.

Unless monitoring reveals an arrhythmia that is correlated with symptomatology, this type of study may be inconclusive. Arrhythmias may occur in the absence of symptoms and, therefore, be given uncertain importance. Conversely, often several or more monitoring periods are necessary to establish the diagnosis in patients with symptoms that are ultimately shown to correlate with arrhythmias. A study by Clark and Glassar has shown, during monitoring, the frequent occurrence of atrial or ventricular premature beats and/or couplets that have no correlation with symptoms.[12] Other studies have shown so-called dangerous warning arrhythmias in up to 15% of elderly asymptomatic normal patients.[13]

Sick Sinus Syndrome

Sick sinus syndrome is frequently associated with syncope in elderly patients. Two thirds of the patients with this syndrome are over 70 years old. The sinus node is the normal determinant of cardiac rhythm. With advancing age, sinus impulse formation is typically slow. Symptoms can arise from extreme slowing, from pauses caused by failure of impulse formation (sinus arrest), or from failure of the impulse to exit the sinus and excite the atria. Symptomatic sinus node failure often occurs in the absence of underlying myocardial or coronary disease and involves lower pacemakers that would otherwise provide a reasonably fast escape rhythm and prevent symptoms.

Concomitant atrial degeneration can result in paroxysms of atrial tachycardia, flutter, or fibrillation when these alternate with episodic sinus failure. This is called "bradycardia-tachycardia syndrome." Episodes of tachyarrhythmia further suppress sinus node impulse formation, and the asystole that follows spontaneous termination of tachyarrhythmia is usually the source of symptoms. Further degeneration eventually leads to permanent atrial fibrillation, eliminating the possibility of symptomatic asystole. Embolization is also an important cause of morbidity in sick sinus syndrome. Paroxysms of atrial fibrillation as well as asystolic periods can result in atrial thrombi that dislodge upon the return to sinus rhythm.

Most cases in which the diagnosis is based on sinus bradycardia in sick sinus syndrome are characterized by episodic dizziness when the sinus rate falls intermittently below 45 beats per minute. In patients with sinus bradycardia or slow atrial fibrillation, the heart rate characteristically fails to increase by more than 25% after intravenous administration of 1 mg of atropine. This relative tolerance to atropine is one of the presumptive diagnostic criteria for sick sinus syndrome. Others include sinus pauses greater than 2 seconds, prolonged sinus node recovery time after abrupt termination of rapid atrial pacemaking (greater than 1,250 msec), symptomatic sinus bradycardia, inappropriate sinus bradycardia, or the bradycardia-tachycardia syndrome. None of these criteria stands alone in clinching the diagnosis, however.

The prognosis for untreated sick sinus syndrome is not as threatening as other conduction problems. In sick sinus syndrome, supraventricular escape rhythms generally alleviate the symptoms before morbidity or death occurs. As noted above, supratachyarrhythmias in sick sinus syndrome arise in the setting of bradycardia. The equivalent tachyarrhythmias in trifascicular block are ventricular tachycardia or fibrillation. As sick sinus syndrome worsens, the permanent atrial fibrillation actually ameliorates the symptoms. Therefore, pacemakers are indicated for repeated or disabling symptoms after inciting drugs (propranolol, digitalis, and many antihypertensives) have been excluded, if recording implicated these bradyarrhythmias causing the symptoms. In the event of a recorded bradyarrhythmia during symptomatic epi-

sodes, the best predictor of pacemaker efficacy is probably sinus node recovery time.

Cardiac Syncope Due to Mechanical Obstruction to Blood Flow

Syncope may also arise due to a number of factors that may suddenly inhibit blood flow from the heart, including valvular aortic stenosis (AS). Severe critical AS occurs in elderly patients who have bicuspid aortic valves, which usually become symptomatic in the sixties. Patients with tricuspid aortic valves, which subsequently undergo aortic sclerosis with calcification and severe stenosis, become symptomatic usually in their late sixties or seventies.

In valvular AS, the main characteristic of syncope is its appearance during exercise. The mechanism of syncope in this condition has not been definitively worked out, but the two best explanations include 1) sudden failure of the heart, induced when the level of exercise exceeds the functional ability of the left ventricular, and 2) initiation of ventricular tachycardia or fibrillation probably related to relative myocardial ischemia. Valvular AS seldom presents as syncope at rest unless the patient has an unusually far-advanced disease with a coexistent severe congestive heart failure. Many elderly patients have mild AS, and syncope, when present, is best explained by some other mechanism.

Hence, before an episode of syncope is considered to be caused by the valvular obstruction, proof that the stenosis is severe becomes essential. Clinical evidence of severity includes a small, slowly rising arterial pulse (not always present in older individuals with inelastic arteries); left ventricular heave; fourth sound; absence of aortic closure sound; prolonged, late-peaking, harsh systolic murmur; and fluoroscopic evidence of valve calcification. Cardiac catheterization with direct pressure measurements across the valve is required to prove the severity of stenosis and, if all factors point to this, to prove that it is the cause of syncope. Valve replacement is recommended in most circumstances, especially if more than one episode of syncope has previously taken place.

Idiopathic hypertrophic subaortic stenosis (IHSS) may also produce a variant of exertional syncope. About one third of patients with this syndrome are older than 60. Like AS, IHSS may present with angina in 20 to 35% of patients, dyspnea in 25 to 40% of patients, or syncope in 25 to 30% of patients. The degree of outflow obstruction in IHSS is, by nature of the obstruction, dynamic and varies markedly from moment to moment. Typical settings for syncope in IHSS are immediately after exercise and during paroxysmal tachycardia. In the postexertional type, the patient, after he or she ceases exercising and rests for a minute, subsequently slumps into unconsciousness. Possibly, the mechanisms for this outflow obstruction include catecholamine release and tachycardia, which are associated with the peripheral pooling that occurs secondary to vasodilation in the exercise and sudden lack of the muscular pumping that augments venous return. All these combine to increase the subvalvular obstruction by decreasing the cardiac chamber size or increasing the cardiac inotropy.

In addition, supraventricular tachycardias are fairly common in IHSS and, when present, may provoke a marked augmentation in the degree of stenosis and, therefore, syncope. Hallmarks in the diagnosis of IHSS include the quickly rising arterial pulse, left ventricular heave, lower left sternal border ejection-type systolic murmur and fourth sound, augmentation of the systolic murmur with measures that decrease venous return (such as Valsalva's maneuver or amyl nitrite), and the appearance of a pseudoinfarct pattern on the ECG, simulating an anterior or anteroseptal myocardial infarction (MI). Most patients with IHSS can usually be treated with beta blockade and concomitant discontinuation of digitalis and nitrate therapy. Surgical correction is rarely needed but is reserved for particularly refractory cases.

Pulmonary embolism can also cause loss of consciousness. In this situation, the embolism is usually massive. Syncope is the presenting symptom in approximately 9% of all patients with pulmonary emboli. Thames and colleagues have shown, in a retrospective study, that syncope usually occurs only in those patients with a massive embolism who present with syncope.[13] Usually, there is associated acute cor pulmonale and/or complete right bundle branch block indicating acute right heart strain.

There are other more rare causes for cardiac syncope due to mechanical obstruction. Included among them is atrial myxoma, which may present with intermittent variable syncope that may perhaps relate to a particular position that may correlate with "plopping" of the tumor into the mitral orifice. Other uncommon causes of mechanical obstruction include acute pulmonary hypertension and prosthetic valve malfunction.

Carotid Sinus Hypersensitivity

Carotid sinus hypersensitivity or syncope is a relatively rare but important cause of syncope in the elderly patient due to its potentially reversible outcome. The carotid sinus is normally sensitive to stretch and gives rise to sensory impulses carried by the nerve of Hering, a branch of the glossopharyngeal nerve to the medulla oblongata. Massaging one or both of the carotid sinuses, particularly in elderly patients, may produce one or more of the following responses: 1) a reflex bradycardia — the so-called vagal type of response; 2) a reflex drop in arterial pressure without bradycardia — the so-called depressor type of response; or 3) a mechanical interference with circulation to the ipsilateral cerebral hemisphere with occlusion of the contralateral carotid artery — the so-called central type of response. Atropine will block the cardioinhibitor component of this response but not the vasodepressor component. In the 1930s, Sigler studied the response to carotid sinus massage in over 700 people and found that the frequency and magnitude of cardioinhibitory and vasodepressor responses increased with age. Persons with arteriosclerosis, hypertension, diabetes mellitus, and other pathologic changes such as scars, tumors, and lymph nodes overlying the carotid body have a higher incidence and degree of this response.

The stimulus for carotid sinus syncope may be the turning of the head to one side or the wearing of a tight collar; in a few reported cases, shaving over the involved carotid sinus was the stimulus.[14] As might be imagined, this was a common problem in the era of high-starched collars. This is now infrequently encountered and, when encountered, it is usually in elderly patients who have diabetes or severe atherosclerosis. Drugs that enhance cardiac vagal tone, such as digitalis or propranolol, may also augment or produce carotid sinus hypersensitivity.

The provocative test for this syndrome is a very *brief, light* massage over the carotid artery. During this procedure, an intravenous line should be in place with the patient placed supine; ECG monitoring must be done, and atropine should be at the bedside prior to testing. It should be assured that the patient does not have digitalis toxicity, and that there are no carotid bruits. A positive test consists of 3 or more seconds of asystole, dizziness associated with lesser slowing of the pulse, or blood pressure decline greater than 30 mm Hg or a 33 mm Hg or more fall in diastolic and systolic blood pressure. The value of the test in clinical practice is limited by the occurrence of false positive findings of up to 20% in patients over 60 years old as well as many false negative tests in patients subsequently documented to have this type of syncope. The test may be hazardous. It was reported that 5 out of 19 patients with carotid sinus syncope had to be resuscitated after the performance of the provocative maneuver. This maneuver should not be repeated once it has been found to be positive. Therapy for those patients with recurrent syncope caused by this type of vagally induced asystole is the placement of a permanent transvenous pacemaker. Atropine (0.5 mg orally 4 times a day) may be tried out but is frequently ineffective in alleviating symptoms.

Certain other vagally mediated syndromes should be identified here. Vagal or glossopharyngeal neuralgia is one of these types of reflex fainting. The sequence of events in glossopharyngeal neuralgia is always pain, then syncope; in this instance, the pain is localized at the base of the tongue, the pharynx, the tonsillar area, and the ear, and may be triggered by pressure at these sites. Sectioning the appropriate branches of the ninth or tenth cranial nerves may relieve the condition. The cardiovascular effects are attributable to reflex excitation of the dorsal motor nucleus of the vagus nerve via collateral fibers from the nucleus of the tractus solitarius.

When recurrent syncope and carotid sinus sensitivity are caused wholly by the depressor type of response with hypotension, a pacemaker cannot prevent syncopal attacks. Medical management with ephedrine (25 to 50 mg 3 times daily) may benefit some of these patients. Refractory cases with hypotension (in which persistent, severe, recurrent syncope is unresponsive to medical management) may be alleviated by surgical denervation via stripping the internal, external, and common carotid sheaths below the bifurcation. However, there have been a few fatalities from transient hypertension in the week following surgery, and overall risk of stroke or death following this procedure is 1 to 2%. So this is, perforce, a rather drastic measure indicated only for those patients with truly intractable symptoms that are not compatible with a normal life.

Tussive and Defecation Syncope

Defecation syncope, too, probably arises from diminished cardiac output from an impeded venous return induced by Valsalva's maneuver during defecation. Nine cases of defecation syncope have been described in elderly patients who lost consciousness after arising from bed at night and defecating or after manual disimpaction. It has been postulated that a reflex hypotension may result from sudden decompression of the rectum. However, investigators have been unable to show any significant blood pressure changes on rapid deflation of an intrarectal balloon. The exact mechanism of defecation syncope, therefore, remains unknown. This is a relatively rare condition that may result from sudden paroxysms of coughing, usually presenting in elderly men who have chronic bronchitic pulmonary emphysema. The diagnosis is usually made when taking a history where it will be disclosed that the patient suddenly becomes weak and loses consciousness after a paroxysm of hard and persistent coughing. It is postulated that the high intrathoracic pressure created by coughing is, in essence, a very severe Valsalva's maneuver, which effectively impedes venous return through the heart and causes a subsequent sudden and marked decrease in cardiac output. Again, this syndrome usually occurs in the elderly patient who has resting compromise in cardiac output and cerebral perfusion.

Syncope Due to Cerebrovascular Disease

Syncope in the elderly patient is frequently attributed to transient ischemic attacks (TIAs). However, most often follow-up studies have shown that this diagnosis is frequently mistaken, especially in patients presenting only with syncope without other associated symptoms. Loss of consciousness must, perforce, involve nonperfusion of the reticular activating system, and as such, TIAs in the carotid distribution usually do not involve loss of consciousness. Vertebrobasilar system TIAs, however, may involve loss of consciousness; however, as mentioned above, syncope alone is the exception rather then the rule. Other symptoms associated with vertebrobasilar insufficiency (including diplopia, dysarthria, bilateral weakness, bilateral visual loss, and vertigo) usually accompany loss of consciousness. One specific manifestation of vertebrobasilar TIA that both signals its origin and is relatively pathognomonic of vertebrobasilar insufficiency is the so-called "drop" attack or akinetic collapse. In this type of episode, patients usually do not lose consciousness but experience sudden inescapable paralysis of their extremities, especially the legs, falling to the floor helplessly. This usually signifies TIA of the brainstem, and these attacks are characterized by "tunnel vision," speechlessness, or ptosis.

It must be noted that although the possibility of transient cerebral ischemic attacks must always be considered in older patients who complain of spells of dizziness, virtually all symptoms commonly associated with the usual TIAs are focal in nature, whereas patients with a complete loss of consciousness generally fall into a different diagnostic category. Thus, if a careful description of the patient's symptoms indicates that the event was focal in nature, cerebrovascular disease should be the primary consideration. It should be noted, however, that a combination of extracranial occlusive disease and hypotension from another cause, even if only moderate in severity, may lead to syncope in the geriatric patient. Noble[15] reported eight patients who had carotid artery stenosis associated with carotid sinus sensitivity. Recurrent syncope in these patients occurred during hypotensive episodes that were only mild or transient. As previously noted, syncope in elderly patients also occurs during relatively brief runs of supraventricular tachycardia. Bilateral tight carotid stenosis or unilateral stenosis with occlusion of the contralateral carotid is particularly likely to predispose such patients to syncope.

SEIZURES AND SYNCOPE

Seizure disorders must be in the differential diagnosis of transient loss of consciousness in the elderly patient. Seizures are usually marked by an abrupt loss of consciousness. Unlike syncope, seizures usually occur without warning in more than 50% of cases. As with Stokes-Adams attacks, an abrupt loss of consciousness may occur in the supine position, independent of the patient's activity level or posture and without warning (Table 16–5). A careful interview of the patient and witnesses may help distinguish the occurrence of the seizure from syncope. Although 50% of seizures occur without warning, the remainder present with a brief momentary premonitory syndrome or aura. This aura usually does not include weakness, dizziness, or graying of vision but,

Table 16–5 Differentiation Among Syncope, Stokes-Adams Syndrome, and Seizures

History	Syncope	Stokes-Adams syndrome	Seizure
Position	Usually upright	Upright/supine	Upright/supine
Skin color	Pale	Pallor/cyanosis	No change
Injury	Rare	Frequent	Frequent
Episode length	Short	Variable	Long
Tonic/clonic jerks	Few	Few	Frequent
Tongue biting	Rare	Rare	Frequent
Incontinence	Rarely urinary	Rarely urinary	Frequent urinary or fecal
Postictal	Promptly lucid	Promptly lucid	Return to consciousness slow; headache; confusion; weakness prolonged

rather, does include discrete neurologic symptoms such as an auditory phenomenon, a queasy stomach, complex visual experiences, or unpleasant olfactory sensations. The seizure can occur even during sleep and may be induced by monotonous music or loud noise. It may begin with a cry as the air is emitted and forced through the closed glottis. Characteristically, the eyes turn either to one side or upward although this sign is of little value in localizing the side of the neurologic deficit. There is usually stertorous breathing and cyanosis rather than pallor. Frequently, tachycardia rather than a slow thready pulse is present.

Perhaps the most characteristic and distinguishing feature between seizures and syncope is the postictal phenomenon. Frequently, patients have been injured during their seizure episode — an occurrence most unlikely in syncope where patients have premonitory warnings to allow them to protect themselves. The period of unconsciousness does tend to be longer in epilepsy than in syncope; urinary and fecal incontinence are frequent in epilepsy and rare in syncope. The return of consciousness, as mentioned, is prompt in syncope and slow in epilepsy. Mental confusion, headache, and drowsiness are common sequelae in epilepsy while these are rare in the postsyncopal period. Physical weakness with clear sensorium usually characterizes the postsyncopal sensorium. Of course, the occurrence of frequent tonic-clonic movements is much more characteristic of a seizure disorder.

The occurrence of a seizure with sudden loss of consciousness without an aura is to be emphasized, however. In a recent study, 52% of patients known to be epileptic

had experienced such episodes prior to seizures; at other times, they were isolated events. The majority of these episodes were less than 3 minutes in duration. Thus, sudden, unexplained loss of consciousness can be an ictal event even when brief in duration.[16]

The electroencephalogram (EEG) is not a definitive diagnostic test. In some studies, up to 20% of patients with documented epilepsy had a consistently normal EEG taken during seizures, whereas 50% were normal on first tracings. Specific seizure activity — spikes and short waves — was present in only about half the patients with abnormal EEGs, depending on the number of EEGs and whether they were obtained after sleep deprivation. The remaining patients had only nonspecific EEG findings.[17]

OTHER CONDITIONS CAUSING EPISODIC WEAKNESS AND FAINTNESS BUT NOT SYNCOPE

Anxiety in the hyperventilation syndrome must be considered in patients presenting in this manner. A careful history will frequently reveal the characteristic scenario associated with these attacks. The giddiness of anxiety is frequently interpreted as a feeling of faintness without actual loss of consciousness. Such symptoms are usually not accompanied by facial pallor and not relieved by recumbency. Diagnosis is usually made on the basis of associated symptoms and part of the attack may be reproduced by hyperventilation for 2 to 3 minutes.

Two of the mechanisms known to be involved in these attacks are reduction in carbon dioxide as a result of hyperventilation and the release of epinephrine. Hyperventilation results in hypocapnia, alkalosis, and cerebrovascular spasm, which may in its most severe form actually cause an occasional loss of consciousness. Usually, the associated symptoms of perioral or extremity tingling, lightheadedness, and association with known stressful situations will, along with lack of other known serious causes of syncope, cause the practitioner to make this diagnosis. It should be mentioned that this type of syncope, although more frequently occurring in the younger patient, may occur in the elderly patient, but it should be a diagnosis of exclusion.

Hypoglycemia may cause occasional episodes of faintness, weakness, and even loss of consciousness. The clinical picture is usually one of confusion or, in the severe form, loss of consciousness. In patients with hypoglycemia, there is generally some relationship between spells and meals. In the reactive type, symptoms develop several hours after carbohydrate intake. Fasting hypoglycemia may be due to hepatic insufficiency, insulinoma, or some other organic cause. Patients with reactive hypoglycemia experience the *gradual* onset of sweating, palpitations, and hunger, which can progress to confusion but rarely to syncope. Overt loss of consciousness or seizures related to hypoglycemia suggest that the etiology is organic or that the patient has taken insulin. In contrast to the period of unconsciousness in syncope that lasts from seconds to minutes, the duration of altered consciousness is more prolonged in patients who are severely hypoglycemic and usually falls into the category of confusion or coma.

Narcolepsy is another syndrome that may present with recurrent episodes of akinesis or sudden weakness or paralysis of the musculature. However, narcolepsy, per se, is usually associated with more specific symptom complexes:

1. Irreversible somnolence when the patient is relaxed
2. Cataplexy — the sudden loss of muscle tone — usually occurs after stimuli such as coughing, laughing, or being startled
3. Sleep paralyses, which are brief periods of immobility on awakening or on falling asleep
4. Hypnagogic hallucinations (vivid dreams)

Any combination of these factors may be noted. The occurrence of any of these symptoms in association with the cataplexic episodes will aid in the diagnosis. This usually is a diagnosis in young patients, but the disease may occasionally remain undiagnosed and present in an older age group. Another type of periodic weakness or paralysis, which causes episodic akinetic attacks without true loss of consciousness, is found in patients who develop sudden periodic paralysis. True periodic paralysis is a syndrome usually diagnosed in younger patients. However, the akinetic episodes associated with this may be associated with primary hyperaldosteronism (Conn's syndrome) or other causes of severe hypokalemia (including diuretic abuse or use).

VERTIGO, DIZZINESS, AND FEELINGS OF DISEQUILIBRIUM

The symptoms of vertigo were described in a previous section in this chapter. There are four basic systems involved that orient the body to its environment:

1. Visual orientation, which requires accurate reception of visual impulses and oculomotor coordination to supply information about the body and its surroundings
2. Labyrinthine function, which primarily assesses changes in body position and in the direction of motion
3. Proprioceptors (located in the joints and muscles), which are important to all reflex, postural, and volitional movements
4. Cerebellar, brainstem, and basal ganglia, which integrate all the information from the above receptors and allow for postural adjustments

Dysfunction of any of the components listed above will cause a relative disorientation of the body to its environment and cause subjective "dizziness."

Visual malfunction may give a sensation of intermittent "dizziness" or giddiness, especially when the patient changes position in space. Visual clues used by the patient to descend stairs or maneuver about are no longer properly received. An example of this occurs in elderly patients who must suddenly wear bifocal lenses. They will feel dizzy or giddy until they adjust to their new perceptions.

Peripheral sensory neuropathy may also cause intermittent dizziness or disorientation of the body to its environment. With decreased sensation and/or proprioception, the patient progressively loses the awareness of his limb position when walking. The results are imbalance and dizziness, which are caused by the walker's over-reliance on visual and labyrinthine responses to achieve a sense of stability. This disability is often alleviated by use of an aluminum walker, which will allow the patient to achieve more awareness of spatial orientation through the trunk and upper extremities of the body.

In practice, it is not difficult to distinguish true vertigo from other causes of dizziness. The feelings of rotation and impulsion earmark vertigo, as well as its important ancillary symptoms of nausea, vomiting, tinnitus, deafness, nystagmus, and staggering. Oculomotor dysfunction can cause spatial disorientation, especially when the patient looks in the direction of the involved muscle.

In approaching the vertiginous patient, the practitioner should attempt to distinguish the source of the dysfunction causing the symptoms.

Peripheral Versus Central Vertigo

It is helpful to divide true vertigo into peripheral and central causes (Table 16–6). In general, vertigo due to peripheral and end-organ dysfunction is more severe. This kind of vertigo is markedly enhanced by, and adjusts to, posture change and has much more prominent ancillary symptomatology. Furthermore, vertigo of peripheral origin tends to parallel the nystagmus present. In central lesions, there is often marked nystagmus with little or no vertigo. The nystagmus is most prominent on looking toward the side of the lesion, and the fast component of

Table 16–6 Distinguishing Peripheral and Central Causes of Vertigo

Peripheral dizziness	Central dizziness
Prominent	Usually mild
Markedly postural	Minimal change with posture
Symptoms abate with postural adjustment	Symptoms persist despite postural change
Ancillary symptoms (nausea, vomiting, diaphoresis) prominent	Ancillary symptoms mild, if present at all
Symptoms characterized by exacerbation and remissions	Associated neurologic signs (facial paresis, weakness, dysphagia)

the nystagmus usually changes with looking in different directions in central causes of vertigo. In acute labyrinthine and vestibular nerve disorders, the nystagmus is usually more prominent on looking toward the good ear. In peripheral vestibulopathy, the patient falls *toward* the side of the lesion and *away* from the fast component of the nystagmus. In central lesions, such as cerebellar infarction, the patient falls *toward* the side of the lesion and *toward* the fast component of nystagmus.

Common examples of peripheral causes of vertigo include otitis media, Ménière's disease, acute labyrinthitis, vestibular neuronitis, and posttraumatic vertigo. Ménière's disease is the classic example of a peripheral cause of vertigo. Ménière's disease consists of a characteristic triad of vertigo, tinnitus, and deafness. The underlying mechanism probably relates to swelling of the endolymphatic space. Attacks in this disease are severe and abrupt, last from minutes to hours, and are associated with tinnitus, a feeling of fullness in the ear, high-tone deafness with auditory recruitment, and other ancillary symptoms of severe vertigo. The vertigo lasts 1 to 2 hours, not seconds or days. Treatment includes sedatives, fluids, antihistamines, and antiemetics during the attack. Prophylactically, some patients use diuretics and sodium restriction. Surgical therapy is recommended in some cases.

Vestibular neuronitis refers to severe vertigo, often lasting several days without deafness or tinnitus. Caloric testing shows hypofunction of the affected side, which serves to distinguish it from labyrinthitis. Treatment is symptomatic.

Patients with Bárány's benign positional vertigo experience paroxysms of vertigo lasting for only a few seconds after lying down, sitting up, or suddenly changing their head position. There is no hearing loss, calorics are normal, and the disorder is self-limited. Treatment with meclizine is usually beneficial.

Central Causes of Vertigo

Temporal lobe epilepsy (complex partial seizures) should be considered. The symptom of vertigo is a rare component of the aura of such seizures, and the vertigo is usually a prelude to a more complex seizure process in which the patient will exhibit repetitive movements, automatisms, and altered consciousness.

Among central etiologies of vertigo, the early recognition of acoustic neuroma is important. Acoustic neuroma begins from sheath cells of the vestibular portion of the eighth cranial nerve in the internal auditory canal; thus, tinnitus, decreased hearing, and dizziness or disequilibrium are early complaints. As the tumor grows into the cerebellopontine angle, cranial nerve dysfunction (loss of corneal reflex, facial weakness) and cerebellar signs become prominent. Diagnosis is not difficult once there is obvious central nervous system involvement. Early recognition depends on ordering brainstem auditory evoked responses and x-rays of the internal auditory canal in patients with dizziness, unsteadiness, and/or symptoms referable to the eighth cranial nerve (tinnitus and decreased hearing). Sizable lesions of the acoustic nerve are detected by computerized axial tomography scan. Small lesions are detectable by posterior fossa myelography.

Posterior fossa tumors may cause a vertigo or dizziness. These would be associated with cerebellar and other brainstem signs. Vascular disease (vertebrobasilar insufficiency) may also cause vertigo. These, as noted before, however, are usually associated with other brainstem symptoms, including diplopia, slurred speech, numbness, trouble swallowing, or signs such as cranial nerve dysfunction, motor, or sensory loss. Dizziness or vertigo will only be the *first* sign of vertebrobasilar insufficiency, but most patients have accompanying signs or symptoms of brainstem dysfunction within months of the onset of vertigo.

Cerebellar hemorrhage or infarction may begin with the acute onset of dizziness, vomiting, inability to walk or stand, and severe headache. As pointed out elsewhere in the book, cerebellar hemorrhage is very important to diagnose as it can lead to rapid death via brainstem compression; treatment is surgical evacuation of the clot. Strength and sensation are usually normal unless brainstem compression occurs. The patient may also have trouble looking to the side of the lesion (gaze paresis).

Basilar migraine may be associated with vertigo and is characterized by symptoms in the basilar artery territory. There may be associated visual disturbances (including scotomata), tinnitus, blackouts, and associated complaints of throbbing occipital headache when the symptoms subside.

Vertigo of brainstem origin spares auditory function. The nystagmus here is coarse, protracted, and variable; it is more severe on lateral gaze. Vertigo here again does not occur alone and will accompany symptoms arising from other brainstem dysfunctions.

THE DIAGNOSTIC APPROACH TO THE PATIENT WITH SYNCOPE AND DIZZINESS

Elderly patients admitted to the emergency department or into practitioners' offices who have had transient unconsciousness or presyncopal episodes should be treated as presenting with a major symptom with potentially serious sequelae. They should not be kept waiting in the waiting room and should immediately be admitted into the department and onto a bed. A cardiac monitor should be placed, an intravenous line started, and, in the absence of other contraindications, at least low-flow oxygen administered. A history should then be taken from the patient with the intention of interviewing appropriate witnesses, especially if the patient does not have knowledge of the events surrounding his or her loss of consciousness. A careful history and physical examination will reveal the cause of the syncope or dizziness in up to 70% of cases.

In the history, careful differentiation of the several conditions causing diminished cerebral blood flow must be made. When faintness is related to primary cardiac pathology, there is usually a combination of dermal pallor and cyanosis. On the other hand, when peripheral circulation is at fault, pallor is usually a striking manifestation and is not accompanied by cyanosis or respiratory disturbances. When the primary disturbance is in the cerebral circulation, the face is likely to be florid and the breathing to be slow and stertorous.

During the attack, a heart rate faster than 150 beats per minute indicates an ectopic cardiac rhythm, while a striking bradycardia at less than 40 beats per minute suggests complete heart block. In a patient experiencing faintness or syncope attended by bradycardia, one must distinguish between a reflex vasovagal attack and cardiogenic or a Stokes-Adams type of bradycardia. Of course, the ECG is decisive and must be taken in any elderly patient who presents with syncope. Approximately 4% of the patients have no historical indication of cardiac syncope in which an ECG will reveal the subsequent cause.

Careful delineation of symptoms before the patient's loss of consciousness (premonitory symptoms), during the event, and after the event will allow the practitioner to place the patient in diagnostic categories that will aid in the diagnosis.

With regard to premonitory symptoms, attention must be placed on the period of time during which the attack develops. If the attack begins over a period of seconds, carotid sinus syncope, postural hypotension, sudden AV block, ventricular standstill, or fibrillation is likely. When the symptoms develop gradually during a period of several minutes, hyperventilation or hypoglycemia should be considered. The occurrence of syncope during or after exertion would, of course, suggest aortic outflow obstruction.

The position of the patient at the onset of the attack is important. Epilepsy and syncopal attacks due to hypoglycemia, hyperventilation, or heart block are likely to be independent of posture. Faintness associated with a decline in blood pressure and with tachycardia usually occurs only in the sitting position, whereas faintness associated with orthostatic hypotension is likely to occur shortly after the change from the recumbent to the standing position.

Associated symptoms must also be noted. These include palpitations and numbness and tingling of the hands and face, which are frequent accompaniments of hyperventilation. Genuine convulsions during the attack will also prove diagnostic.

Careful query should be made about the duration of the attack. When the duration is brief (i.e., a few seconds to a few minutes), carotid sinus syncope or one of the syncopal forms of postural hypotension is most likely. A duration of a few minutes but less than an hour suggests hypoglycemia or hyperventilation.

In the physical examination, certain procedures should always be carried out in the patient with syncope. Orthostatic blood pressures with the patient lying, sitting with legs dangling, and standing should be performed, taking careful note of *both* blood pressure *and* pulse. A drop in blood pressure without a pulse rise, as indicated before, should indicate a primary autonomic disturbance causing the orthostatic hypotension. As with any patient, note carefully any abnormal vital signs. The thrust of the physical examination should be towards the detection of localizing neurologic signs, a careful cardiopulmonary examination with specific attention towards suspicious murmurs, abnormal pulse or pulse formation, and bruits.

PUTTING IT ALL TOGETHER — THE RED FLAGS AND THE ESP MNEMONIC

Bosker and Sequeira have encapsulated all of the dangerous aspects of syncope into an appropriate mnemonic device.[18] They term this the ESP approach to syncope. This approach divides the diagnostic assessment of syncope into three distinct phases, the *E*arly premonitory phase, the *S*yncopal phase, and the *P*ostsyncopal phase. Each of these phases has a mnemonic to signify the respective red flags or situations in which syncope could be potentially dangerous.

In the early premonitory phase, the appropriate mnemonic for the dangerous situations is summarized by **SCENT**:

Supine posture when syncope occurs.

Cardiac symptoms occur just before the syncope (chest pain, shortness of breath, palpitations).

Elderly patients should always be considered to have a serious cause of their syncope.

No warning to the syncope should always imply cardiac or neurologic cause.

Trauma associated with the syncope is important because the patient with benign syncope usually can protect himself or herself from the fall.

The syncopal phase: Red flags can be organized under the mnemonic **TIPS**.

Tongue biting

Incontinence of urine but especially of stool

Prolonged duration of loss of consciousness

Seizure activity

The postsyncopal red flags are organized under the mnemonic **CHAN**.

Confusion

Headaches

Abnormal vital signs

Neurologic dysfunction (especially focal dysfunction)

Provocative Maneuvers

When indicated, certain maneuvers, such as the Hallpike test, may help the practitioner to elucidate the cause of the syncope. This test involves placing the patient in a sitting position and explaining that the examiner will quickly push the patient's head to the pillow on the examining table. The physician holds the head firmly, instructs the patient to keep his eyes wide open, and throws the head back directly looking for nystagmus. The maneuver is repeated with the head turned to the right and left sides to test all six labyrinths. Again, the patient should report any feelings similar to those of his symptoms and any nystagmus should be noted.

In addition, the patient's head can be hyperextended for a period of up to 2 minutes to see if the components of the symptomatology are reproduced. This maneuver will, on occasion, further decrease borderline vertebrobasilar circulation and reproduce symptoms of vertebrobasilar TIAs.

When hyperventilation is accompanied by faintness, the pattern of symptoms may be reproduced by having the patient breath rapidly and deeply for 2 to 3 minutes. An easy way to do this is to hold a paper towel approximately 2 feet away from the patient and to have him or her blow at it for the desired time. This test is frequently of therapeutic value as well because the underlying anxiety tends to be alleviated when the patient learns that the symptoms can be produced simply by controlling breathing.

Other maneuvers may be undertaken, as specified in the previous section, including controlled carotid massage and induction of the Valsalva's maneuver in investigating possible tussive syncope. In relevance to provocative testing, it should be emphasized that the crucial point is not the symptoms produced; the provocative maneuvers frequently will induce those symptoms in healthy, normal people. But, rather, the crucial point is whether the *exact* pattern of symptoms that occur spontaneously can be reproduced artificially. Laboratory exams — such as an ECG and tests for serum electrolytes and glucose — can look for specific electrolyte abnormality such as hypokalemia. This abnormality may either cause arrhythmias or be associated with episodic weakness or may indicate other metabolic problems. In addition, as circumstances may dictate, appropriate radiographic examination should be made on parts of the body possibly injured during or after the syncopal episode. We have discussed the potential value and the drawbacks of continuous Holter monitoring of the patient's cardiac rhythm and also discussed the value and drawbacks of EEG testing.

After the history/physical examination and appropriate laboratory testing, there still remains an approximate 10% of patients who have syncope without an identifiable cause. Work on this subsegment of patients has been variably rewarding. Recent studies by DiMarco and colleagues have shown that intracardiac electrophysiologic tests may reveal a potential dysrhythmic cause of the patient's syncope in up to 60% of patients with previously unidentified causes for their syncope.[19] Since this is an invasive test, it probably should be reserved for those patients with intractable symptoms.

SUMMARY

In summary, the complaint of loss of consciousness, faintness, or dizziness in the elderly patient is a very serious complaint and should be honored as one would honor the complaint of chest pain. A careful systematic history and physical examination of the patient will frequently reveal the cause of the patient's symptoms. Multiple studies have shown that there is a higher incidence of both cardiac and cerebral causes for transient loss of consciousness in the geriatric patient. In turn, loss of consciousness due to cardiac causes has been shown to carry a significant morbidity and mortality in the subsequent follow-up period. A careful consideration of all the potential causes of syncope, carotid sinus syncope, cerebral vascular disease, and seizures should always be undertaken. With a carefully developed systematic approach to this problem, we should be able to minimize the potential morbidity to these high-risk patients.

REFERENCES

1. Besu CT: Syncope in the elderly, J Am Geriatr Soc 24:126, 1976.
2. Branch WT: Syncope and dizziness. In Branch WT, editor: Office practice of medicine, ed 2, Philadelphia, 1987, WB Saunders Co.
3. Lipsitz LA: Syncope in the elderly institutionalized population: prevalence, incidence, and associated risk, Q J Med 55:45, 1985.
4. Lipsitz LA: Syncope in the elderly, Ann Intern Med 99:92–105, 1983.
5. Kapoor W et al: Syncope in the elderly, Am J Med 80:419, 1986.
6. Day SC et al: Evaluation and outcome of emergency patients with transient loss of consciousness, Am J Med 73:15, 1982.
7. Silverstein MD et al: Patients with syncope admitted to medical intensive care units, JAMA 248:1185, 1982.
8. Tinetti ME and Speechley M: Prevention of falls among the elderly, N Engl J Med 320:1955, 1989.
9. Pomerantz B and O'Rourke RA: The Stokes-Adams syndrome, Am J Med 46:941–946, 1969.
10. Surawicz B: Prognosis of patients with chronic bifascicular block, Circulation 60:40, 1979 (editorial).
11. Van Durme JP: Tachyarrhythmias and transient cerebral ischemic attacks, Am Heart J 89:538–540, 1975.
12. Clark PI et al: Arrhythmias detected by ambulatory monitoring: lack of correlations with symptoms of dizziness and syncope, Chest 77:722, 1980.
13. McAnulty JH et al: A prospective study of sudden death in high-risk bundle-branch block, N Engl J Med 299:209, 1978.
14. Cohn FL: Carotid sinus syndrome, J Neurosurg 45:78, 1976.
15. Noble RJ: The patient with syncope, JAMA 237:1272, 1977.
16. Ercaw BL: When loss of consciousness is not caused by epilepsy, Geriatrics 38:431, 1977.
17. Hughes JR and Drachman DA: Dizziness, epilepsy and EEG, Disease Nerv Sys 38:431, 1977.
18. Bosker G and Sequeira M: The sixty-second syncope assessment. In The 60-second EMT: rapid BLS/ALS assessment, diagnosis, and triage, St Louis, 1988, The CV Mosby Co.
19. DiMarco JP et al: Intracardiac electrophysiologic techniques in recurrent syncope of unknown cause, Ann Intern Med 95(5):542, 1981.

Sudden Death and Cerebral Resuscitation

Michael Sequeira, M.D., F.A.C.E.P.

Sudden death and cerebral resuscitation are particularly relevant and controversial subjects in the elderly population. Most victims of sudden death are over 60 years old, and cardiac arrest is one of the biggest killers of the elderly. Since 1960, when Kouwenhoven[1] reported the capacity to generate cardiac output with external cardiac massage, our knowledge of and experience with resuscitation have blossomed. A new discipline — resuscitology — has emerged, which in turn has even created a new disease — the postresuscitation disease or syndrome.

Along with this scientific progress, philosophical and ethical problems have naturally developed: the right to die and living wills, do not resuscitate (DNR) orders, and questions grappling with the risks and benefits of resuscitation on different patient subsets. It soon became apparent that our new efforts in resuscitation were creating a legion of brain-damaged, dysfunctional patients that were further burgeoning an already medically burgeoned society. The elderly are often among the patient subsets in which sudden death and resuscitation are frequently discussed. Daily decisions are made on elderly patients about whether or not to resuscitate them or continue life-sustaining measures, and, not infrequently, these decisions are based on little more than the patients' advanced age. Ironically, however, there is very little age-specific evidence about sudden death, hypoxic encephalopathy, the postresuscitation syndrome, or cardiopulmonary-cerebral resuscitation.

Today the clinician must know the essential facts about sudden death and cardiopulmonary-cerebral resuscitation. The purpose of this chapter will be to review pertinent epidemiologic aspects of sudden death as it occurs in the aged patient, its causes, prodromal symptoms, and current knowledge about its prediction. Postcardiac arrest, global cerebral ischemia, anoxia, the mechanisms of cerebral cellular injury, and the current status of prevention and minimization of damage and preservation of available brain tissue and function will then be reviewed.

It is hoped that by this review clinicians will approach the problems associated with sudden death, resuscitation, and postresuscitation with a better understanding and will base their literal life-and-death decisions on a foundation of scientific fact rather than supposition.

SUDDEN DEATH IN THE ELDERLY

Sudden death accounts for about 15% of all deaths in the elderly and about 60% of all deaths from coronary artery disease in the elderly. In the United States, 72% of the deaths from cardiovascular disease occur in patients over the age of 65. Of all patients dying suddenly, the majority — 65 to 80% — will be over 60 years of age. In fact, the average age of the patient who dies suddenly is 60 years of age. Therefore, sudden death is an important problem in the elderly patient.[2-4]

There is little disagreement in the literature that the incidence of sudden death increases with age up to the age of 60. However, there is conflicting data about the relative incidence of sudden death after the age of 60. The Framingham study found that the incidence of sudden death actually decreases with age after 60 while other studies failed to show this correlation. The probable reason for a tailing off of sudden death in the elderly is the increasing incidence of other disease processes and the eventual mortality associated with their progression.

The general risk of major complications after a coronary event also increases with age. The relationship is not linear but, rather, exponential with a rapidly increasing complication rate beginning at about the age of 55 years. Since age is not amenable to intervention, some authors consider age a risk marker rather than a risk factor. Because of the powerful effect of increasing age on posthospitalization complication rates, most studies either restrict the age range of the population being studied or else use any of a variety of age-correcting or age-grouping techniques.

In patients observed for up to 15 years after a myocardial infarction, the sudden death rate for this postinfarction group was very high and increased for each decade from 30 to 79 years.[5] However, as the Framingham study also found, the sudden death rates did not increase as rapidly with age in this group as the rates of the population at large in the same area. That is, the risk of sudden death was far greater for each decade in men who had recovered from an infarction than in the general population, but this differential diminished with increasing age. Thus, this showed a greater relative risk of sudden death in the younger age group.

Studies of postmyocardial infarction patients have shown that increasing age is a consistent, very heavy risk factor for sudden death. Age was weighted equally with a previous history of exertional dyspnea and with Q waves on the initial electrocardiogram (ECG) in the Peel prognostic index. Norris[6] found that age was of about equal relevance to long-term survival as to short-term survival. Moss,[7] using a stepwise discriminant analysis technique for predicting survival in the posthospital phase of myocardial infarction, observed that age was one of the most important factors in identifying patients with increased mortality risk.

Most sudden deaths are not totally unexplained; often, the patient has had coronary or hypertensive heart disease or has recently sought medical care for symptoms that were disregarded or misinterpreted. One study showed that about one third of the patients had seen a physician within 2 weeks before death complaining of various prodromal symptoms. This is a particular problem with the elderly, due to the increasing problems of symptom obscuration, competing medical problems, mental deterioration, and overpowering and distracting symptoms. A frequent complaint seen in these prodromal visits is the progression of increasing fatigue (38%). Other nonspecific complaints such as difficulty sleeping (13%), combined with the cardiopulmonary complaints such as chest pain (13%), shortness of breath (18%), coughing (12%), syncope (2%), dizziness (9%), and palpitations (4%), accounted for the major proportion of these visits. *This simply reinforces two general occurrences in geriatric patients: the importance of general, seemingly unimportant symptoms and the variable presentation of common medical problems.*

CAUSES OF SUDDEN DEATH AMONG GERIATRIC PATIENTS

Studies examining the causes of sudden death have been hampered by the variable definitions used. The World Health Organization has defined sudden cardiac death as death occurring within 24 hours of the onset of illness or injury. Using this classification, cardiovascular disease caused sudden death in about 60% of cases. Respiratory disease accounted for about 15%, central nervous system disease for about 15%, digestive and urogenital disease about 7%, and miscellaneous causes were cited in approximately 4% of all cases.

Spain[8] separated cases of sudden death occurring within 1 hour of symptom onset from those occurring within 24 hours of symptoms onset. He found that deaths occurring within 1 hour of symptom onset were due to coronary heart disease in 91% of male patients and 51% of female patients. Of deaths occurring up to 24 hours after onset of symptoms, 55% were due to coronary heart disease.

Hinkle and Thaler[9] have proposed a classification to determine the cause of cardiac death. Their classification has been validated by a multicenter prospective evaluation of mortality after acute myocardial infarction. This study showed clearly that death within 1 hour of the onset of symptoms was specific for arrhythmic death.

Neither 1- nor 24-hour periods were useful in identifying the mechanism of death.

Despite the high (90%) incidence of advanced coronary artery disease in elderly patients with sudden cardiac death, the majority of them have not died as a direct result of an acute myocardial infarction. Pathologic evidence of acute myocardial infarction is found in less than 50% of victims of sudden cardiac death. In addition to severe diffuse coronary atherosclerosis, old myocardial infarcts are also often found. All of this strongly suggests that sudden cardiac death results from arrhythmias, and, of these, ventricular fibrillation is by far the most common.

In addition, the recurrence rate of ventricular fibrillation in victims of sudden cardiac death is high: about 30% in the first year and 50% by 3 years. Subsequent studies with coronary arteriography of survivors of out-of-hospital ventricular fibrillation demonstrate a high prevalence of advanced atherosclerosis in one or more major coronary arteries. Three fourths of these patients had abnormalities of left ventricular wall motion, an indication of the likelihood of previous myocardial infarctions. Of the patients who were resuscitated but died in subsequent months, at least two thirds had recurrent sudden death. The latter suggests that the final event was similar to the initial event, usually ventricular fibrillation.

Sudden death occurring after 2 hours of symptoms is less often secondary to ventricular arrhythmias, although coronary heart disease still accounts for at least half of these cases. Other frequent causes of sudden death in the elderly are overwhelming sepsis and other cardiac disorders such as myocarditis, cardiomyopathy, aortic stenosis or aortic dissection, cerebral hemorrhage, shock due to multiple causes, or bowel obstruction. Even the so-called cafe coronary, often mistaken for sudden cardiac death, is found more frequently in the elderly patient because of the higher incidence of dysphagia and esophageal obstruction due to stricture formation and carcinomatous involvement.

PREVENTION OF SUDDEN DEATH

Sudden death can be prevented by identifying the high-risk patient and utilizing long-term approaches designed to prevent cardiac arrest and by efficient management of cardiac arrest or acute myocardial ischemia with a special eye toward brain preservation and resuscitation. The latter will be discussed in the section on cerebral resuscitation. Since most deaths due to coronary heart disease occur suddenly, usually owing to ventricular fibrillation, successful resuscitation depends upon how quickly trained bystanders and medical personnel can reach the patient and institute appropriate measures to sustain the patient until defibrillation can be accomplished. There is no doubt that lives have been saved in communities where specially equipped, trained paramedics are available and can reach the patient within 2 to 3 minutes, recognize arrhythmias, administer atropine or lidocaine, and accomplish defibrillation.

As was previously mentioned, about two thirds of the patients who are resuscitated had premonitory symptoms in the preceding 1 to 2 weeks, and one fourth of them saw a physician in the preceding 1 to 2 days, not necessarily for a recognizable cardiac complaint. Because so many sudden deaths are unwitnessed or occur so soon after the development of acute symptoms that the mobile coronary care team cannot arrive in time, it can be fairly stated that most patients with ventricular fibrillation do not survive — even those resuscitated during the acute phase. Thus, primary prevention of sudden death — identifying the high-risk patient and attempting to modify those risks — is by far the most desirable and cost-effective approach for the patient.

Identifying the Elderly Patient at Risk for Sudden Cardiac Death

As previously mentioned, age is an independent, very heavy risk factor for sudden death. As a result, clinicians caring for the aging patient must be even more meticulous in detecting and treating other risk factors that patients may have. In general, the risk factors for sudden arrhythmic death are the same risk factors as for coronary artery disease: male, diabetes mellitus, cigarette smoking, very low-density lipoproteinemia, and a family history of premature atherosclerosis. Several other studies have shown that psychologic and social factors such as a low level of education or a relatively high alcohol consumption appear also to be risk factors. Although regular strenuous physical activity reduces the possibility of sudden death, patients at risk for sudden arrhythmic death are more likely to collapse during or just following exercise than during sedentary activities. In addition, the high incidence of both coronary disease and coronary deaths in the lumberjacks of northeastern Finland indicates that strenuous physical activity does not effectively protect against coronary disease or sudden death.

More and more proof is emerging that validates efforts in risk factor modification regarding improvement in the morbidity and mortality of coronary heart disease. There is ample evidence that stopping smoking allows patients to very rapidly return to the risk level of nonsmokers. Cigarette smoking has been shown to lower the ventricular fibrillation threshold through catecholamine release. Filter cigarette smoking has not been shown to decrease mortality rates.

Since hypertension has been shown to be a major risk factor not only for coronary heart disease but also for left ventricular hypertrophy, which is thought to be an independent cause of arrhythmia and sudden death, its control is especially important in the elderly patient. We now know that even diastolic pressures of 90 mm Hg and systolic pressures of 160 mm Hg increase the risk of coronary artery disease (CAD) and stroke several fold and must be meticulously monitored and controlled.

It has finally been shown that the reduction of serum cholesterol will reduce the incidence of all cardiovascular events. This proof was recently provided by the Lipid Research Clinics' Coronary Primary Prevention Trial.

Hypokalemia, hypomagnesemia, and prolongation of the QT interval also increase the risk of an arrhythmic death. Elderly patients are prone especially to the development of hypokalemia and hypomagnesemia from their frequent use of diuretics and from the unrecognized presence of malnutrition, both of which can severely deplete total body potassium and magnesium stores. Multivariate analyses of various risk factors list age, left ventricular ejection fraction, and the presence of complex ventricular ectopy (greater than or equal to 10 PVCs/hour or three or more repetitive ectopic beats) as independent predictors for a subsequent episode of cardiac arrest.

A significant advance in the management and detection of sudden death and coronary events in general has already been mentioned in the previous chapter on coronary ischemia — i.e., the detection and treatment of silent myocardial ischemia, the total ischemic burden. Since sudden cardiac death has been overwhelmingly linked to the presence of advanced coronary artery disease and since arrhythmias frequently occur secondary to myocardial ischemia, it makes powerful empiric sense that the control of previously unrecognized and untreated silent myocardial ischemia would make a significant impact upon the incidence of sudden death and coronary morbidity and mortality in general.

There is now strong evidence to suggest that the total ischemic burden, which consists mostly of silent ischemic episodes, does relate to the incidence of sudden coronary events such as sudden death. Using amplitude-modulating Holter monitoring for 48-hour periods, many investigators have shown that patients in whom silent episodes totaled $\geq$ 60 minutes/24 hours had a much poorer prognosis than those with fewer episodes. Moreover, treatment of these episodes, which are most likely due to coronary spasm, with nitrates, beta-blockers, and calcium channel blockers has a significant impact on the incidence of sudden death and subsequent coronary events.

With the use of intracardiac electrophysiologic studies, there has been increasing progress in identification and treatment of the high-risk arrhythmia patient with recurrent ventricular tachycardia and/or ventricular fibrillation. Using these techniques, electrophysiologists have been able to tailor specific antiarrhythmic agents for each specific patient. Yet the 1-year mortality for these patients is still high (about 16%).

The advent and use of a new device, the automatic implantable cardioverter/defibrillator (AICD), has been shown to significantly improve mortality and incidence of sudden cardiac death in these high-risk patients. This device monitors cardiac rhythm continuously and is designed to detect ventricular fibrillation or ventricular tachycardia and deliver automatically a discharge of 25 joules within 20 seconds. Initial trials with AICDs have been extremely promising, even though the devices were placed in patients with extremely high-risk profiles. Data from several centers implanting the AICD demonstrate that overall 1-year mortality and sudden cardiac death are significantly reduced in selected patients. For instance, Mirowski[10,11] showed a decrease in sudden death from 16.6 to 2%; Echt and colleagues[12] showed a corresponding decrease from 10.1 to 1.8%; Luceri[13] and colleagues from 9.5 to 0%; and Marchlinski and colleagues[14] from 12.9 to 0%.

These data with the AICD are even more dramatic when compared with mortality statistics for similar but nonmatched patients who were treated with antiarrhythmic drugs. In a large series, Echt and colleagues[12] demonstrated that the 1-year mortality rate for patients treated with antiarrhythmic agents guided by electrophysiologic study was 16% in those patients who responded to the drug and 40% in nonresponders. The sudden cardiac death rate was 10% for responders and 26% in nonresponders.

SURVIVAL AFTER CARDIAC ARREST IN THE ELDERLY

Many studies on survival after cardiac arrest exclude age in their data for the reasons mentioned above. Those studies that do examine the relationship of age to the outcome of resuscitation are conflicting in their results, which relates to the different conditions of each study. Linn and Yurt[4] have done the only specific study of cardiac arrest in geriatric patients. They found that the survival data for those over 60 was 23% (those discharged from the hospital), a survival rate equivalent for that seen in the group under the age of 60. Eisenberg's data,[15] however, showed that being over 60 years old was associated with worse survival in a study of out-of-hospital deaths. These data revealed that the elderly had about a 15 to 20% greater chance of dying from out-of-hospital cardiac arrest. An important difference in these two studies is the fact that Linn's patients were already in the hospital. A study by Tresch[15a] showed that although elderly patients had a higher mortality rate from cardiac arrest (28% survival vs 47% in those less than 70 years of age), the duration of the hospital stay for elderly survivors was not longer, the elderly did not have more residual neurologic impairments, and their survival following hospital discharge was similar to that in younger patients. A recent study by Murphy[15b] reported a 22%

initial survival and only 3.8% survival to discharge of elderly patients, with the poorest outcome occurring in those patients with out-of-hospital unwitnessed arrest, CPR lasting more than 15 minutes, and with asystole and electromechanical dissociation. The neurologic outcome of these patients was poor, with only 1.6% discharged back to their homes, and most of the survivors having some degree of neurologic or physical deficit. This study was retrospective, with no younger control group and no correlation with down times, so that definitive conclusions cannot be drawn from these data. There is no other evidence that shows that the elderly patient does any worse than the younger patient when there is correction for other conditions.

Despite all of the progress in the identification and primary and secondary prevention in patients at high risk for sudden death, we still cannot identify all of these patients, particularly since sudden death is the initial manifestation of coronary heart disease in about one fourth of the patients. Also, as we have already seen, preventative measures will not and cannot always be successful. Therefore, we must continue to advance our knowledge and skills in the treatment of cardiac arrest and in the preservation of that critical organ of human existence — the brain. This will be the subject of the rest of this chapter.

CEREBRAL RESUSCITATION

It has become clear that our current methods of resuscitation are just not doing the job when it comes to leaving a patient with an intact brain and a functional existence. In fact, as we will later discuss, our current resuscitative practices may actually make things worse with regard to maintaining cerebral function and integrity during and after the resuscitation.

The bulk of past resuscitative efforts have concentrated on *cardiac* resuscitation, and it was only after significant progress was made in this field that we found that the brain did not fare well in the process. We now have enough survival data to establish that 20 to 40% of *survivors* of cardiac arrest and resuscitation have permanent neurologic damage of variable severity. With optimal conditions of implementation of basic life support within 4 minutes and advanced life support within 8 minutes of arrest, we can resuscitate about 50% of out-of-hospital cardiac-induced ventricular fibrillation patients and bring them to the hospital alive. Of these surviving patients, half (50%) will survive to be discharged from the hospital alive. Of these patients (25% of the total), up to 50% will have permanent neurologic damage. Thus, *under optimal conditions of resuscitation,* only about 10% of patients who have out-of-hospital ventricular fibrillation will be resuscitated and remain neurologically intact.

Despite all of our advances, the old concept of the "4-minute barrier" of certain anoxic neuronal deaths still by and large holds true. Furthermore, studies on resus-citated patients have shown that if advanced life support and definitive resuscitation is not achieved within 15 to 20 minutes after arrest, then neurologic prognosis remains poor, regardless of the duration of initial anoxia and arrest.

What makes this all the more frustrating is that we have known since 1963 that cerebral neurons have the capacity to survive and recover both structurally and functionally after up to 60 minutes of total anoxia. Therefore, ischemic anoxic brain death may be the result of other mechanisms that occur after the insult and the resuscitation.

The conclusion from all of this data is that our current resuscitation techniques, primarily centered upon heart resuscitation, are not adequately resuscitating the brain. Out of this has come the necessary and total revamping of our approach to cardiopulmonary resuscitation (CPR). CPR has now become CPCR — cardiopulmonary *cerebral* resuscitation.[16,17] Every aspect of current resuscitation methods is being examined from the standpoint of increasing survival of the brain. New drugs, methodologies, and instruments are developing; in some cases, old techniques (open chest cardiac massage) are enjoying renewed emphasis — all in the interest of brain resuscitation.

The purpose of this section will be to review our current methods of brain resuscitation and to review the complex events that occur during the total anoxia of circulatory arrest, the ischemia of resuscitation, and the postresuscitation period — events that can contribute to permanent brain damage. We will also review the current efforts in cerebral resuscitation and indicate future avenues of study to prepare readers to better assimilate the inevitable growth of knowledge in this field in the near future and prepare them to *wisely* incorporate these into their practices.

BASIC PATHOPHYSIOLOGY

Although it is only 2% of the total body weight, the brain receives about 16% of the body's total cardiac output and utilizes 20% of the body's total oxygen consumption. This attests to the brain's high metabolic activity in activities such as cell organelle synthesis, neurotransmitter substance synthesis, axoplasmic transport, and the maintenance of transmembrane potentials through ionic pumps.

Because of this high metabolic rate, it is easy to understand that the brain is the most sensitive organ in the body to ischemia. Other organs have the capacity to survive for hours after an ischemic insult, but the brain uses up over 90% of its adenosine triphosphate (ATP) stores within 1 minute of total ischemia. Certain portions of the brain are more sensitive than others to ischemia and, therefore, have the lowest threshold for injury in this circumstance. In general, the higher up the neuraxis and the more complex its function (and, therefore, the higher the energy requirements), the more ischemically vulnerable is the part of the brain. This is consistent with the neurologic deficits most frequently and typically seen after resuscitation from cardiac arrest (i.e., in low-level neurologic impairment). Typically, the cerebral cortex and especially the hippocampus (responsible for memory), the cerebellum (coordination), the basal ganglia (consciousness), and the cerebral cortex (intellect and motor function) are the most sensitive to neurologic sequelae following cardiac arrest.

The brain has certain minimum blood flow requirements to maintain its function and cellular integrity. Progressive functional and metabolic disturbances are manifested by increasing the severity and duration of the ischemia. At flow rates above 35% of normal, the neurons can maintain normal ATP content by stimulation of anaerobic glycolysis despite compromised oxygen delivery. Restoring normal oxygen and substrate delivery results in rapid cell recovery. When cerebral blood flow falls to about 35% of normal, the electroencephalogram (EEG) becomes silent, but the neurons can continue to pump ions across cell membranes and thus maintain a normal intracellular milieu. At the range of 15 to 30% of normal flow, glucose availability becomes rate limiting and cellular ATP content declines. Lactic acidemia depresses anaerobic ATP production by inhibition of phosphofructokinase (PFK), the rate-limiting enzyme in glycolysis. Lactic acid accumulation increases cellular osmolality and contributes to intracellular edema. At this level of blood flow, the brain lacks the energy required to maintain the transmembrane ionic relationships. At this stage, progression to irreversible injury may occur even after reperfusion.

However, it is believed that as long as cerebral flow is maintained above 20% of the normal rate, cellular viability is maintained. Fall of cerebral blood flow below this critical threshold of 20% of normal is believed to compromise neuronal viability. Flow rates to the brain that are less than 10% of the normal rate result in rapid depletion of ATP, and all anabolic and catabolic metabolism breaks down. This event has been termed "the ischemic freeze" by Jennings. Severe cellular acidosis can develop and leads to protein and membrane degeneration. Release of lysosomal enzymes may follow. Lactate accumulation has been correlated with irreversible ischemic cellular injury.

Thus, we see that consciousness requires at least 50% of normal cerebral blood flow. Neuronal function requires at least 35% of normal blood flow. Neuronal cell viability requires at least 30 to 35% of normal blood flow, and the maintenance of membrane integrity and cell viability requires at least 20% of normal cerebral blood flow.

CPR AND CEREBRAL BLOOD FLOW

Standard external (closed chest) CPR (SECPR) provides borderline cerebral blood flow under the best of conditions. SECPR has been shown to generate forward cardiac output primarily by the generation of intrathoracic

pressure fluctuations that, in conjunction with one-way valving in the extrathoracic vasculature, produce forward blood flow and, secondarily, by compression of the heart between the sternum and vertebral column. Sternal compressions can produce systolic pressure peaks of 100 mm Hg and more, but the diastolic pressure produced may be as low as 10 mm Hg. Epinephrine raises the diastolic pressure to a small degree — about 5 to 10 mm Hg. However, the systolic central venous, right atrial, jugular venous, and intracranial pressures are increased almost as much as arterial pressure, and this leads to minimal perfusion pressures. Coronary and cerebral arteriovenous perfusion pressures of at least 30 to 40 mm Hg are required to maintain cerebral blood flows of 30 to 35% of normal. These low perfusion pressures limit SECPR to maximum cerebral blood flows of 30% of normal flow and often less than 10% of normal.

As we have seen, ideally SECPR should be capable of uniformly reperfusing the heart and brain with oxygenated blood with at least 20% of their normal blood flow for up to 20 minutes of normothermic circulatory arrest without advanced life support measures and perhaps up to 30 minutes to cover transportation in out-of-hospital arrest. It has been shown that the ability of SECPR to produce cerebral perfusion pressures adequate for cerebral blood flows (CBF) of at least 20% of normal depends in large degree upon the arrest time without CPR (down time). In a laboratory demonstration, it was shown that CPR can generate cerebral blood flows of up to 50% of normal only when it was started within 2 minutes of the arrest. CPR started even 5 minutes after the onset of arrest generated CBFs of only about 20 to 25% of normal. CPR started more than 10 minutes after the onset of arrest produced minimal to no cerebral blood flow.

The important concept here is not so much the actual times but the negative correlation of CBF with "down time." This is substantiated by case reports suggesting that SECPR started immediately upon collapse has occasionally continued for hours and been followed by complete cerebral recovery after restoration of spontaneous circulation. On the other hand, several minutes of arrest with CPR, when followed by SECPR longer than 15 minutes, was rarely followed by complete cerebral recovery. The superior resuscitation rates achieved by cities with massive bystander participation, such as Seattle, Washington; Lincoln, Nebraska; and Oslo, Norway, are also at least partially explained by this phenomenon (along with more increased awareness of the lay public and more rapid access of the emergency medical services [EMS] system, leading to the quicker delivery of definitive, advanced cardiac life support [ACLS] treatment).

CPR AND "TRICKLE PERFUSION"

More and more, some resuscitologists are not only questioning the efficacy of SECPR, but they are also implicating the potential deleterious effects induced by CPR that is begun too late or continued for too long. Providing only about 20 to 30% of normal cerebral blood flow, SECPR may actually provide only a trickle of perfusion — enough to feed the damaging enzymatic reactions to be described but not enough to enable neurons to maintain their viability. In fact, there is evidence that *no flow* to the brain may perhaps cause less damage than the 10 to 20% of normal cerebral blood flow that most CPR attempts produce.

The reason for this relates to the fact that anaerobic metabolism and lactate production cease after about 5 minutes of circulatory arrest but can continue if a trickle of blood flow is provided. Continued substrate delivery also results in increased accumulation of lactic acid in the brain and other tissues. As we have seen, this produces progressive biochemical abnormalities, retards recovery of electrical activity, and produces irreversible tissue damage. Some studies have shown that there is worse functional recovery following 30 minutes of 10% cerebral blood flow than after 30 minutes of no flow, with severe mitochondrial injury from a massive increase in neuronal lactate.

Current data indicate that CPR markedly loses its effectiveness with time. Survival is only about 15 to 30% with cases in which CPR is performed for 30 minutes or longer compared to cases in which CPR is performed for 10 minutes or less, even when there are short (< 6 minutes) arrest times. As predicted from Szmolensky's studies, if the arrest time is > 6 minutes, then the neurologic recovery rate is essentially zero if CPR lasts longer than 15 minutes.

"NEW CPR"

Efforts to augment the forward blood flow of SECPR have by and large produced few benefits. In an attempt to increase the pressures generated by sternal compression, simultaneous ventilations and compressions were attempted (SVC-CPR). This "new" CPR failed to effectively augment cerebral perfusion pressures because the greater pressures generated also caused corresponding increases in jugular vein and intracranial pressures, causing perhaps an even net negative effect in cerebral perfusion pressures.

Alternating abdominal compressions with sternal compressions (interposed abdominal compression or IAC-CPR), in an attempt to increase diastolic venous return, has at least produced greater cardiac outputs and cerebral perfusion pressures. However, the net incremental increase in cerebral perfusion pressures (about 5 to 10%) is not adequate to maintain neuronal integrity. In addition, this method can lead to hepatic injury and the promotion of gastric regurgitation. Therefore, IAC-CPR is not the answer.

OPEN CHEST CPR

Open chest cardiac massage was widely utilized within the hospital before the advent of closed chest cardiac massage in 1960. Open chest CPR produced excellent survival rates with viable brain function. In 1953, Stephenson reported 1200 cases of medical cardiac arrest treated with open chest CPR. In these cases, 28% of the patients were discharged alive from the hospital; 14% of the procedures were performed in the general hospital wards, with a 17% survival rate. In this study, massage of up to 2.5 hours could lead to recovery. The infection rate was low, even after thoracotomies were performed without sterile conditions.

Multiple studies have supported positive previous experiences (such as Stephenson's) with evidence of the hemodynamic superiority of open chest CPR (OCCPR). OCCPR can be relied upon to generate perfusion pressures and cardiac outputs of at least 20% of normal and even up to 80% of normal. There seems to be more blood flow going to the brain than the face during OCCPR. Microscopic studies of neurons in animals in which OCCPR had been maintained for hours have shown striking preservation of mitochondrial and cellular membranes and limitation of intracellular lactate, calcium, iron, and free fatty acid accumulation. All of these, as will be explained in the next section, probably mediate cellular injury in the postresuscitation syndrome.

More studies examining the efficacy of OCCPR for medical cardiac arrest patients not immediately resuscitated will almost surely be forthcoming. Two preliminary studies[17a] from San Francisco and from Phoenix have failed to show any appreciable improvement in survival or cerebral outcome, but these studies were limited by the late implementation of OCCPR. It is likely that OCCPR will occupy some niche in our resuscitation of the cardiac arrest patient — limited to in-hospital occurrences and after a short (e.g., 7 minutes) period of refractoriness of standard resuscitation measures.

EMERGENCY CARDIOPULMONARY BYPASS

Recent advances in technology have made feasible a new modality for emergently providing substantial cerebral flows through cardiopulmonary bypass (CPB). The heart-lung machine was originally developed for the provision of CPB, usually by venoarterial pumping of blood via an oxygenator, to enable open-heart surgery. CPB permits full control over perfusion pressure, flow, temperature, and composition of the perfusing fluid when used following elective circulatory arrests.

So far there has been little experience using emergency CPB without thoracotomy for the treatment of medical cardiac arrest, but several studies are now under way in laboratory animals. Safar and colleagues[17a] have conducted preliminary studies with CPB in dogs subjected to various situations of cardiac arrest. So far, their studies have shown that the controlled reperfusion and assisted circulation possible with CPB have led to good neurologic outcome after up to 15 minutes of normothermic total circulatory arrest and to restoration of spontaneous circulation after up to 20 minutes of cardiac arrest. They showed a clear superiority of CPB over external CPR and also over OCCPR in promptly restarting perfusion, even after very prolonged cardiac arrest.

Previously there were limitations of CPB: the requirement of thoracotomy, the time required for inserting a large-bore tube into the venae cavae and cannulating the femoral artery while the patient is being bounced around by external CPR, and the lack of availability of a small portable emergency pump oxygenator primed with plasma substitute. A portable emergency pump oxygenator is now available in commercial production. In addition, a new technique has been developed allowing institution of CPB through the percutaneous insertion of a long-bore, multiple-hole catheter via the femoral vein into the inferior and superior venae, a standard cannula into the femoral artery, and the portable membrane oxygenator.

Clinical feasibility trials of emergency CPB after prolonged cardiac arrest will no doubt be forthcoming and may actually be the topic or part of the topic for the third phase of the worldwide Brain Resuscitation Clinical Trials (BRCT III). In the future, it is very possible that some form of closed-chest emergency CPB with a portable apparatus primed with plasma substitute may become part of the emergency resuscitation armamentarium of many physicians for both in-hospital as well as prehospital use.

PATHOPHYSIOLOGY OF CEREBRAL ANOXIA: HEMODYNAMICS AND ORGAN INJURY

When circulation to the brain stops in a cardiac arrest, the patient loses consciousness within about 15 seconds. The EEG becomes isoelectric in 15 to 30 seconds, and agonal gasping followed by apnea and maximal pupillary dilation starts at 30 to 60 seconds. The brain uses up its oxygen stores in 10 seconds and its brain glucose and ATP in 5 minutes, and it is at the later time when brain tissue lactate concentrations are maximal. Multiple studies have linked the degree of brain injury not only to the degree of lactic acidosis that has been reached but also to the level of prearrest serum glucose. There is little doubt that hyperglycemia enhances brain cellular injury in sudden global anoxia.

If no reperfusion occurs, uniform tissue autolysis ensues, which probably starts in the brain after only 1 to 2 hours of no blood flow. When reperfusion is delayed after 5 minutes or more of cardiac arrest, it provokes multifocal reperfusion failure, which is proved to occur in the brain and in multiple other organs. Reperfusion triggers a complex series of events that in their full manifestation result in the development of miliary, multifocal necrotic lesions with inhomogenous distribution throughout the brain.

The No-Reflow Phenomenon

After a cardiac arrest, cerebral hemodynamics undergoes a predictable series of events for at least 5 minutes. This is followed by subsequent reperfusion. A period of transient increase in cerebral blood flow (reactive hyperemia) follows the period of no flow — the postischemic period of reperfusion with a normal blood pressure. After about 15 to 30 minutes, total cerebral blood flow declines to below normal values and almost ceases after about 1.5 to 2 hours. Coincident with this progressive decrease in cerebral blood flow is the progression of a massive increase in cerebral vascular resistance. This concurrent decrease in cerebral blood flow and increase in cerebral vascular resistance is the "no-reflow phenomenon" first described by Ames and colleagues in 1963.[18] It occurs independently of the intracranial pressure level.

The no-reflow phenomenon can occur unrelated to luminal and microcoagulation. Using follow-up electron microscopic studies, Chan and colleagues[19] have shown areas in which there was no evidence of fibrin or platelet thrombi in the microcirculation in brains observed to suffer from this phenomenon. The phenomenon probably represents a derangement in cerebral autoregulation in which massive diffuse cerebral vasospasm ensues; this is possibly also associated with platelet aggregation and, to a secondary degree, vascular stasis. As discussed in later sections, this phenomenon is probably calcium ion mediated and results from the high concentrations of thromboxane A_2, leukotrienes, and other vasoactive amines liberated from biochemical processes occurring both in the anoxic and in the reperfusion phases of arrest and resuscitation.

MECHANISMS OF NEURONAL INJURY DURING THE ARREST (NO-FLOW) PHASE

As mentioned above, once blood flow to the brain decreases to < 10% of the normal rate or ceases altogether — as in cardiac arrest — glucose and ATP, the energy stores of the brain, are rapidly depleted within about 5 minutes. The precipitous fall in energy rapidly reduces the cell's ability to maintain ionic gradients across the plasma membrane. Maintaining the very strictly regulated transmembrane potentials through constant ionic pumping is probably the most ischemic sensitive function of the cell. When this fails, excitable tissues depolarize. Sodium and calcium cascade into the cells and potassium and magnesium rush out. Extracellular fluid, of course, comes with the sodium, and intracellular and intraorganellular edema develops. When no blood flow persists, there is minimal net change in electrolyte content between the blood and the interstitial fluid. However, if some blood flow persists, marked ionic shifts occur from an equilibrium that establishes itself among intracellular, interstitial, and blood compartments.

The calcium concentration of the intracellular fluid (cytosol), mitochondria, and endoplasmic reticulum is normally fastidiously regulated by a very metabolically active (and ischemically sensitive) calcium/magnesium ATPase pump located in the membranes of the cell and the organelles. Under normal homeostatic conditions, a gradient of about 10,000:1 exists between extracellular and intracellular calcium. Calcium is also partially bound in membranes and is thought to function in maintaining structural integrity of at least the sarcolemma-glycocalyx complex of some cells.

Once the membrane pumps are disabled by the loss of energy substrates and calcium floods the cytosol, a remarkable sequence of destruction develops:

1. *Initial calcium entry:* Degeneration begins when membrane calcium, water, and ions flood the cell. The significant hypocalcemia that occurs in shock probably represents the effect of generalized calcium entry into all ischemic cells.

2. *Calcium sequestration:* The mitochondria and nuclei actively sequester the massive amounts of calcium in the cell.

3. *Prostaglandin production:* Once calcium floods the cytosol, it activates protein kinases and phospholipases (especially phospholipase A_2). These destructive enzymes digest the cellular membranes into free fatty acids (FFAs), the most important of which is arachidonic acid (AA) — the precursor of prostaglandins. FFAs are destructive to the cells. As detergents, they enter into cellular membranes and decrease the integrity of the membranes, causing further influx of calcium and water. They disrupt the membranes of the mitochondria and further reduce ATP synthesis.

4. *The role of thromboxane A_2:* The new high levels of AA now drive two basic pathways: the cyclooxygenase pathway, leading to the production of high levels of prostaglandins — the most destructive of which is thromboxane A_2 — and the lipoxygenase pathway, leading to the production of similarly high levels of leukotrienes, which have similar properties to thromboxane A_2. Thromboxane A_2 is particularly destructive in the setting of ischemia. It is a very potent vasoconstrictor and inducer of platelet aggregation and, thus, is a powerful thrombogenic substance. It is normally elaborated primarily by the platelets in their role of maintaining vascular homeostasis. Thus, in the setting of ischemia, the thromboxane A_2 (created in high levels from the membrane degradation) creates further ischemia through the inducement of intense vasoconstriction and platelet aggregation, the latter of which releases even more thromboxane A_2. This may very well be the explanation of the no-reflow phenomenon discussed above.

Another prostaglandin, prostacyclin (PGI_2), could have an important role in the ischemic process. Prostacyclin (along with PGI_3, produced through the trienoic pathway that, incidentally, is not inhibited by nonsteroidal antiinflammatory agents) is one of the body's natural antagonists of thromboxane A_2 and the leukotrienes. The prostacyclins are very potent vasodilators and inhibitors of platelet aggregation and, thus, serve a very helpful function in the setting of ischemia.

The problem arises in the setting of ischemia and anoxia. It has been demonstrated that the ischemic brain is deficient in the production of prostacyclins. The preferred pathway within the ischemic cells is toward the production of thromboxane A_2. This leads to the natural hypothesis that exogenously administered prostacyclins may be helpful in checking the no-reflow phenomenon.

5. *Hypoxanthine*: The hydrolysis of ATP leads to an accumulation of hypoxanthine. The increased calcium enhances the conversion of xanthine dehydrogenase to xanthine oxidase, which primes the neuron for the production of the oxygen free radical O_2^-, once oxygen is reintroduced during the reperfusion that occurs with resuscitation of normal blood flow.

NEURONAL INJURY AFTER PERFUSION IS RESTARTED: REOXYGENATION INJURY AND POSTRESUSCITATION SYNDROME

In the course of a "successful" resuscitation, perfusion is reestablished. After as little as 5 minutes of no blood flow to the brain, another sequence of destructive processes leading to cell death occurs in the neurons. (We have already seen one destructive reperfusion event — the no-reflow phenomenon.) These sequences of events are set up by the buildup of the various metabolites elaborated during the period of no flow and have been shown to be even worse if ischemia continues after the period of no flow (see the previous section, CPR and Trickle Perfusion). They are the basis of what Negovsky termed "the postresuscitation disease" or what Safar more appropriately calls the "postresuscitation syndrome."[17]

At the organelle level, the structure of ribosomes is maintained during complete ischemia but rapidly degenerates during reperfusion, producing prolonged severe disturbance of protein biosynthesis. Some membrane-bound enzymes lose activity with reperfusion. Diffuse homogeneous neuronal damage present during ischemia progresses to severe damage localized to certain areas of the cerebral cortex mentioned above (the development of miliary microinfarcts).

Postischemic cells are at particular risk during reperfusion because of decreased membrane integrity and compromised machinery of ATP generation. These cells may very well experience further decay of ionic gradients, which then equilibrate across the total circulating blood volume.

Massive cell swelling and calcium influx are observed during reperfusion. The destructive sequelae of increased calcium in the cells begun during the period of no flow are continued and potentiate other destructive sequences.

Calcium sequestration in the mitochondria is augmented during reperfusion. The reason for this is that the low oxygen content in the no-flow situation eventually stops electron transport. With more calcium being delivered to the membrane-damaged cells and energy available again, the calcium sequestration by the mitochondria grows. It takes energy for the mitochondria to pump calcium in, so the mitochondria use up all of their ATP; none is used in oxidative phosphorylation. Thus, in reperfusion, calcium acts like cyanide: It becomes a metabolic poison and can totally uncouple oxidative phosphorylation.

Free radical production. Free radicals are extremely reactive oxygen derivatives having a single electron in their outer electron shell. Free radicals are very damaging to cells and organelles and can irreversibly damage them by degrading membranes, proteins, and DNA. The events that occur during the no-flow state lead to the accumulation of substances that, combined with the reintroduction of oxygen to the cells, can lead to the elaboration of high levels of free radicals. These, along with calcium, are believed to be the mediators of the postresuscitation syndrome. The process, as postulated by Babbs and White,[20a] proceeds as follows:

1. During reperfusion/reoxygenation, the superoxide free radical, O_2^-, is produced in an excessive level through the xanthine oxidase system and through the effects of the leukotrienes on neurons. These overwhelm the body's natural defense against free radicals.
2. Free iron is released from ferritin during ischemia.
3. The iron catalyzes the conversion of O_2^- to the hydroxyl free radical (OH^-). The hydroxyl radicals attack proteins and lipid components of the lipid-rich brain, causing widespread lipid peroxidation chain reactions that alter molecular architecture.

Clinical observations of the postresuscitation syndrome have demonstrated two phases of neurologic injury: an *immediate phase,* in which patients either never wake up or have a neurologic deficit from the time they wake up, and a *delayed phase,* which usually occurs days after patients awaken from their arrest. It is currently thought that calcium is the primary mediator of immediate phase neurologic injury and that free radicals are responsible for the deficits developing during the delayed phase.

Safar and colleagues also have hypothesized a subsequent period of cerebral intoxication due to ischemic damage of extracerebral organs, such as a leaking gastrointestinal tract and hepatic failure, and also the potential for "intoxicated blood," made toxic and more viscous by stasis and interaction with other ischemic tissue. There is no documentation for the latter two factors, but it is not inconceivable that the blood may bring more calcium, more thromboxane A_2 from the platelets, more leukotrienes from the neutrophils, and other as yet unspecified "toxins" from ischemically damaged extracerebral organs. Free-glutamate release appears to add to neurotoxicity.

SUMMARY OF MECHANISMS OF BRAIN INJURY DURING ARREST AND REPERFUSION

Thus, there are specific hemodynamic, cellular, and biochemical events during cardiac arrest and the subsequent reperfusion period accompanying resuscitation that can cause brain injury. We have seen that there is a critical "threshold" of 35% of normal blood flow for neurologic function to continue and about 15 to 20% for the neurons to live (cellular viability). Only CPR that is begun right away and performed properly can provide 20% of normal cerebral blood flow. When blood flow to the brain stops, the ionic gradients break down; calcium rushes into the cells and begins a vicious series of destructive reactions leading to the production of thromboxane A_2, leukotrienes, and uncoupling oxidative phosphorylation in the mitochondria and, in whole, damaging cellular and organelle membranes.

Reperfusion can worsen the process and cause the postresuscitation syndrome, bringing in O_2 and more calcium, causing severe vasospasm (no reflow), which leads to the production of the extremely destructive free radicals O_2^- and OH^-, further poisoning the mitochondria.

Clinically, Safar and colleages divide the problem into four phases:

Phase I — Begins with the arrest and is the no-flow period, i.e., complete cerebral anoxia.

Phase II — Transient global (reactive) hyperemia lasting about 15 to 30 minutes.

Phase III — (If phase I is ≥ 5 minutes) delayed, prolonged global hypoperfusion beginning 30 to 90 minutes after the period of no flow and lasting 12 to 48 hours. This is the period of no reflow. The postresuscitation syndrome begins here. This period is also referred to as the period of "reoxygenation injury."

Phase IV — the period of "delayed concurrent postischemic hypoperfusion injury" in which patients subsequently develop neurologic injury 3 to 5 days after the insult (possibly free radical and/or prostaglandin mediated). This may also be the period in which "cerebral intoxication" by the blood and by blood-borne toxins from ischemically damaged extracerebral organs occurs. This period may result in resolution of neurologic deficits, continuation (persistent coma), or worsening (death).

BRAIN RESUSCITATION

It should now be clear that there exists a huge need to prevent or minimize the brain injury in patients who have had an episode of global ischemia from a cardiac arrest. The growing knowledge of the pathophysiology of ischemic and postresuscitation injury will enable more efforts at developing agents or methods that will aid in this aim.

Barbiturates

Barbiturates were among the first agents to show experimental amelioration of ischemic brain injury. Many of their properties proved to be potentially beneficial in cardiac arrest and the postresuscitation syndrome: reduction of cerebral oxygen demand, edema, seizures, improvements of cell energy charge, and cyclic adenosine monophosphate (AMP) stores and decrease in free fatty acid accumulation. Barbiturates have also been shown to be weak calcium-entry blockers. In addition, barbiturates have been shown by multiple investigators to be effective in ameliorating focal brain ischemic damage.

Initially barbiturates showed promise in improving the cerebral outcome from global ischemic insult in rhesus monkeys by Bleyaert and associates.[20] Subsequent studies showed conflicting results regarding the benefit of barbiturates in this situation. In light of this ambiguity, the first international randomized clinical trial of postresuscitation — the Brain Resuscitation Clinical Trial (BRCT I) — was organized in 1979 by Safar and associates to specifically examine the efficacy of thiopental loading in brain resuscitation.

BRCT I failed to show any statistically significant benefit of thiopental loading between control and treatment groups in the proportion of patients recovering with good neurologic function, occurrence of a persistent vegetative state, or mortality. The study did, however, demonstrate the safety of massive thiopental loading in these critically ill patients. Thus, massive thiopental loading probably does not work for brain resuscitation in the postarrest period but can be used safely in postresuscitation patients who have specific indication for its use, such as seizures, increased intracranial pressure, or sedation.

Another anticonvulsant, phenytoin, has shown promise for brain resuscitation. Aldrete[21] gave phenytoin at a dose of 7 mg/kg IV to 10 previously healthy patients suffering cardiac arrest during anesthesia who woke up with severe neurologic deficits (coma, fixed and dilated pupils, or posturing). They found that 9 out of the 10 recovered almost total neurologic function. In addition, studies have shown that phenytoin stabilizes neuronal membranes and ion fluxes, decreases cerebral oxygen consumption by approximately 40%, and prolongs the normal function of the neuron in conditions of hypoxia and ischemia. Phenytoin, of course, has its proven benefits as antiarrhythmic and anticonvulsant, both of which are of potential benefit in the postcardiac arrest patient. There seems to be nothing to lose and perhaps something to gain in the routine prophylactic (e.g., seizures and arrhythmias) use of phenytoin in therapeutic doses for the postresuscitation patient.

Calcium-Entry Blockers

The rationale for therapy with calcium-entry blockers after cardiac arrest rested on blocking the massive accumulation of this ion in the cytosol and mitochondria during and following ischemia. It was hoped that this would result in preservation of ATP synthesis, improved myocardial performance and cerebral perfusion, and decreased production of free radicals generated from the calcium-activated generation of free acids and arachidonic acid (and its by-products, thromboxane and leukotrienes). In addition, calcium-entry blockers have been shown to decrease platelet aggregation, increase red blood cell (RBC) deformability, directly cause vasodilation, and improve the myocardial oxygen supply/demand ratio.

Calcium-entry blockers (such as flunarizine) have been shown to prevent the delayed postarrest hypoperfusion syndrome in the brain when given to dogs after a 20-minute episode of normothermic cardiac arrest. The same beneficial effect has subsequently been shown for verapamil, magnesium sulfate, and lidoflazine.[22] It does seem that the calcium-entry blockers have a greater effect on cerebral vessels than on peripheral vessels because cerebral vascular muscle tone is more dependent on the entry of extracellular calcium.[23]

Given after cardiac arrest, calcium-entry blockers have been shown to improve both short- and long-term neurologic outcome in experimental global ischemic animal models. Multiple investigations have shown the effectiveness of lidoflazine in dogs submitted to cardiac arrest and the effectiveness of nimodipine in aortic occlusion in dogs and in the neck tourniquet model in monkeys.

One of the problems that exists is that, of the currently approved calcium-entry blockers, verapamil, the only one that can be given parenterally, can cause hypotension and atrioventricular blocks, reduce inotropy, and, in high enough doses, even induce electromechanical dissociation. Diltiazem matches the experimental lidoflazine in being less hypotensive than nimodipine or nifedipine and less likely to produce heart block than verapamil but cannot be given parenterally.

The promising experimental results in animals, combined with widespread clinical use of calcium-entry blockers after cardiac arrest and the lack of safety of some of these drugs, were the stimuli for the second phase of the Brain Resuscitation Clinical Trials (BRCT II).

Free-Radical Scavengers

If the current impressions of the pathophysiology of the postresuscitation syndrome are correct, then the use of free-radical scavengers should be helpful for cerebral resuscitation.[24] One of the experimental problems is that free radicals are evanescent and cannot be measured in vivo. One preliminary study of a combination of free-radical scavengers — mannitol, 1-methionine, tromethamine (THAM), magnesium sulfate, and dextran 40 — ameliorated neurologic injury to dogs with asphyxial cardiac arrest. A further study with the ion chelator deferoxamine and the free-radical scavenger superoxide dismutase minimized the no-reflow phenomenon and improved normalization of evoked potentials in dogs with an asphyxial arrest of 7 minutes. A further outcome study of deferoxamine in rats with cardiac arrest is also promising. Further study with deferoxamine and free-radical scavengers will doubtless be forthcoming in the near future.

Other Potential Brain Resuscitation Measures

There are a number of other experimental agents and methods that have shown some benefit or promise in ameliorating the brain damage of anoxia and the postresuscitation syndrome.

Indomethacin has been shown to be protective for cerebral blood flow after ischemia but only blocks the cyclo-oxygenase pathway of prostaglandin production and must be given before the insult to work effectively. Prostacyclin infusion during ischemia has shown uniform organ protection from ischemia in the brain, heart, liver, and kidney and remains to be corroborated in further studies. Prostacyclin may very well be a very useful agent to specifically block the no-reflow phenomenon and possibly to ameliorate blood-borne intoxication that is mediated by thromboxane and leukotriene.

The potentials for emergency cardiopulmonary bypass and emergency open heart cardiac massage have already been mentioned and remain to be either refuted or supported in the next few years. Other methods that show promise but have yet to be evaluated in clinically relevant animal outcome preparations include naloxone, dimethyl sulfoxide, hypothermia, osmotherapy, hemodilution, anticoagulation, allopurinol, ATP-MgCl$_2$, and various inhibitors of lactate generation.

In the long run, Safar will probably be proven correct for his prediction that because the postresuscitation syndrome is multifactorial, no single therapy is likely to achieve a breakthrough in ameliorating the postischemic-anoxic encephalopathy. More likely, each patient has more than one of the previously described pathophysiologic processes in various combinations and degrees. The most likely and successful approach to brain resuscitation in the future will be to minimize the arrest and CPR time with immediate resuscitation and, if the latter is not successful, then to immediately place the patient on cardiopulmonary bypass.

This procedure will be followed by a systematic process that will enable us to measure the relative role of each component in the postresuscitation syndrome and to "tailor" our therapy specifically to the various components of the syndrome active in each patient. Ideally, too, we will develop methods of determining the extent of permanent neurologic damage so that we will not pursue unreachable goals and continue to perpetuate the nightmare of patients with persistent vegetative states.

WHAT CAN BE DONE *NOW?*

Much of the above is experimental in nature and as yet cannot and should not be used on patients until their safety and efficacy have been proven or disproven to a reasonable degree. However, much can be accomplished with our current tools to prevent and ameliorate the brain damage associated with sudden cardiac death that is grounded in the knowledge of the known pathophysiology of global ischemia and the postresuscitation syndrome. A protocol for brain-oriented intensive care should be developed by every intensive care unit caring for the postarrest/postresuscitated patient. Safar and his associates have published their representative protocol in many sources. The basics of such brain-oriented intensive care should include the following:

1. Reperfusion with moderate hypertension initially after arrest with strict maintenance of normotension throughout the period of coma maintaining mean arterial pressure (MAP of 90 to 100 torr or normal systolic pressure for the patient). The moderate hypertension may already be induced by the epinephrine administered during the resuscitation. Almost needless to say, hypotension after resuscitation would be exceedingly disastrous and should be treated as aggressively as possible with fluids and pressors. Again, optimal fluid and pressure management may very well require hemodynamic monitoring. Important variables to carefully monitor include MAP, CVP or PCWP, UF, cardiac rhythm, temperature, and blood gases.
2. Controlled hyperventilation (arterial P_{CO_2} 25 to 35 torr). This will not only mitigate the brain acidosis and lower the intracranial pressure but can also redirect blood flow to ischemic areas by causing vasoconstriction of normal arterioles with shunting of blood to diseased areas (reverse steal).
3. Maintain and ensure oxygenation by scrupulous pulmonary toilet, prevention of aspiration, pulmonary emboli, and subsequent pulmonary edema of either cardiogenic or noncardiogenic cause. This may very well necessitate central hemodynamic monitor-

ing and low levels of positive end-expiratory pressure.

4. Immobilization (neuromuscular paralysis) if the patient is combative or not cooperating with the ventilator.

5. Sedation if needed.

6. Maintenance of normoglycemia. Both hypoglycemia and hyperglycemia may be harmful. In the ischemic state, hyperglycemia contributes to the tissue acidosis and under any condition can increase serum osmolality while hypoglycemia deprives the brain of necessary substrate for its existence. If there is little risk for rearrest, then the error should be on the slightly hyperglycemic side.

7. Seizures should be prevented at almost all cost, since seizure activity can increase brain metabolism by 300 to 400%, and this can be disastrous in the postarrest situation. As mentioned above, phenytoin is an attractive agent to use for this situation since it is safe, stabilizes membranes and ionic fluxes, is a cardiac antiarrhythmic, and may have some benefit in preserving the brain.

8. Hyperthermia should be treated to keep the supply/demand ratio at an optimum. Any possibility of sepsis should be pursued vigorously with appropriate cultures and sensitivities. The threshold for use of antibiotics should be low in these very unstable patients.

9. Maintaining the patient in metabolic balance. This includes monitoring and normalizing the serum electrolytes, magnesium, phosphorus, osmolality, and colloid oncotic pressure. Dialysis for postischemic acute tubular necrosis should be started early and performed aggressively.

10. The patient should be fed either parenterally or enterally.

11. Monitor the patient's clotting status, and watch for the onset of disseminated intravascular coagulation.

12. A nasogastric tube should be in place and prophylaxis for gastric stress ulceration should be instituted with bihourly antacids and either ranitidine or famotidine (avoiding cimetidine because of its central nervous system side effects and inhibition of the cytochrome-P_{450} system.)

PREDICTING NEUROLOGIC OUTCOME AFTER CARDIAC ARREST

It is important to be able to predict the eventual neurologic outcome of victims of cardiac arrest for many reasons. Brain dead, persistently vegetative, or severely impaired elderly patients are an extreme burden both emotionally as well as economically to their families and to society in general. Humanitarian reasons alone dictate that we discontinue life support for patients with brain death if the latter can be determined reliably and consis-

tently. Much attention has lately been given to the patient with a persistent vegetative state who is spontaneously breathing and has electroencephalographic activity. Although these patients are not brain dead, their chances of having a meaningful life are minimal. Long-term survival of these patients should be prevented with the use of "letting die" protocols (including the judicious withholding of antibiotics, surgery, pressors, and antiarrhythmics).

The first step in evaluating the prospects of postanoxic encephalopathy is to evaluate the severity and the duration of the ischemic insult. This can be estimated by determining what Safar calls the "total insult time" — estimate and total the duration of the following four periods: 1) any hypoxic time prearrest (from hypotension, hypoxemia, or anemia), 2) the arrest or down time (period of no flow), 3) the CPR time (duration of resuscitation), and 4) the duration of any hypoxic or ischemic time (hypotension, hypoxemia, anemia) post resuscitation. The total insult time is the sum of these four periods.

The criteria derived by the Harvard ad hoc committee for the determination of *brain death* (persistent coma, areflexia, and isoelectric or "flat" EEG at least 24 hours after the insult) are still the medical and legal standard. Early prediction of permanent *vegetative state* using absent midbrain reflexes and deep coma beyond 12 hours after cardiac arrest is possible but not 100% reliable. Teasdale and Jennett have shown that the Glasgow coma scale (GCS) has prognostic value after brain injury.[25]

In assessing the depth of coma and its outcome, the rapid recovery of eye and upper airway reflexes is a good prognostic sign. The absence of the oculocephalic (doll's eye) or oculovestibular (caloric) reflexes at 6 to 12 hours after the insult, continued coma, and pupillary nonreactivity are all poor prognostic signs. The recovery pattern over time is very important prognostically. Electrocortical activity recovers intermittently at first and then continuously and may normalize. The longest period of unresponsiveness followed by complete neurologic recovery has been 2 weeks after cardiac arrest and around 1 year after head injury.

There has been some promise in correlating the severity of the ischemic insult and degree of permanent brain damage after cardiac arrest with cerebrospinal fluid levels of the brain isotope of creatine kinase: CK-BB. This fraction has been shown to peak at 40 to 72 hours after the insult, presumably resulting from leakage of the enzyme from the damaged tissues into the cerebrospinal fluid (CSF). After cardiac arrest, if the CSF CK-BB levels are above 80 U/L, then the neurologic prognosis is expected to be poor. Levels above 20 U/L are definitely abnormal (normal levels being < 5 U/L).

EEG activity and evoked potentials have so far not proven reliable for predicting outcome, primarily because recovery patterns for the postarrest brain have not yet been established. Other methods measuring severe progressive reduction in cerebral blood flow and cerebral oxygen consumption are complex and expensive but a bit more reliable than the EEG. The former can be diagnosed by nuclear magnetic resonance (NMR) spectroscopy, global nonperfusion on the angiogram, multifocal severe hypoperfusion on cold xenon-enhanced computerized tomography (CT) scanning, and brain atrophy on NMR or CT scanning.

It is generally recommended that brain death should not be determined and certified until the resuscitated patient has had the benefit of post-CPR all-out life support. Decisions on "letting die" for patients in a persistent vegetative state after cardiac arrest should be postponed for about 1 week after arrest, and these should be made with a consensus of medical consultants in communication with the patient's family. The continued focus is on prevention of neuronal death. Other approaches are "nerve growth factor" and use of drugs to block the neuronal damage due to excitatory neurotransmitter release.[26]

CONCLUSIONS

Sudden death and postanoxic encephalopathy pose a continuing challenge to the clinician. A large portion of our elderly die daily from sudden cardiac arrest, and, perhaps worse, a smaller portion survive their sudden death to suffer lives of permanent disability or persistent vegetative states. The challenge before us begins with continuing to use and develop all available means to predict the patient who is at high risk of dying suddenly and to intervene on those factors we can modify to prevent death. Progress has been made on this front in risk factor identification and modification, antiarrhythmic development, electrophysiologic testing, measuring and treating the total ischemic burden of the heart, and implanting automatic cardioverters/defibrillators into the hearts of identified high-risk patients.

For the 25% of elderly patients with coronary heart disease whose first manifestation of that disease is sudden death, we have continued to determine the limits of the human brain. We now know that the brain can tolerate not 5, but more like 20, minutes of total anoxia, but our current methods of resuscitation still require us to begin CPR immediately and to restore normal perfusion within 8 to 10 minutes to ensure good brain recovery. If the period of arrest without CPR is > 5 minutes, then a series of destructive events occurs that terminates in a state of multiple miliary microscopic infarcts, which we term postanoxic encephalopathy.

Initial attempts at preserving and resuscitating the brain and, in the process, preventing postischemic encephalopathy, appear promising. The future of emergent cardiopulmonary bypass immediately instituted for the arrested patient, or open-chest cardiac massage, calcium-

entry blockers, free-radical scavengers, and general brain-oriented intensive care are all important beginnings in the quest to understand and treat this complex problem. Much study on these and other, as yet unknown, methodologies will surely be forthcoming.

REFERENCES

1. Kouwenhoven WB, Jude JR, and Knickerbocker GG: Closed-chest cardiac massage, JAMA 173:1064, 1960.
2. Kuller L: Sudden and unexpected non-traumatic deaths in adults: a review of epidemiological and clinical studies, J Chronic Dis 19:1165, 1966.
3. Kuller L, Cooper M, and Perper J: Epidemiology of sudden death, Arch Intern Med 129:714, 1972.
4. Linn BS and Yurt RW: Cardiac arrest among geriatric patients, Br Med J 2:25, 1970.
5. Cobb LA and Werner JA: Predictors and prevention of sudden cardiac death. In Hurst JW, editor: The heart, New York, 1982, McGraw-Hill Book Co, pp 599–610.
6. Norris M: Symposium on identification and management of the candidate for sudden cardiac death, Am J Cardiol 39:846–851, 1977.
7. Moss AJ: Prediction and prevention of sudden cardiac death, Ann Rev Med 31:1, 1980.
8. Spain DM, Bradess VA, and Mohr C: Coronary atherosclerosis as a cause of unexpected and unexplained death: an autopsy study from 1949–1959, JAMA 174:384, 1960.
9. Hinkle LE, Jr, and Thaler HT: Clinical classification of cardiac deaths, Circulation 65:457–464, 1982.
10. Mirowski M: The AICD: an overview, J Am Coll Cardiol 6:462, 1985.
11. Mirowski M et al: Mortality in patients with implanted automatic defibrillators, Ann Intern Med 98:585, 1983.
12. Echt DS et al: Clinical experience, complications, and survival in 70 patients with the automatic implantable cardioverter defibrillator, Circulation 71:289, 1985.
13. Luceri RM et al: The automatic implantable cardioverter-defibrillator: results, observations, and comments, PACE 1343–1348, 1986.
14. Marchlinski FE et al: The automatic implantable cardioverter defibrillator: efficacy, complications, and device failures, Ann Intern Med 104:481, 1986.
15. Eisenberg MS et al: Treatment of out-of-hospital cardiac arrests with rapid defibrillation by emergency medical technicians, N Engl J Med 302:1379, 1980.
15a. Tresch DD et al: Should the elderly be resuscitated following out-of-hospital cardiac arrest? Am J Med 86:145–150, 1989.
15b. Murphy DJ et al: Outcomes of cardiopulmonary resuscitation in the elderly, Ann Intern Med 111:199–205, 1989.
16. Safar P: Recent advances in cardiopulmonary-cerebral resuscitation, Ann Emerg Med 13(A):856, 1984.
17. Safar P: Cerebral resuscitation after cardiac arrest: a review, Circulation 74:IV138–153, 1986.
17a. Safar P: Cardiopulmonary cerebral resuscitation: a marvel for physicians and paramedical instructors, prepared for the World Federation of Societies of Anaesthesiologists, Philadelphia, 1987, WB Saunders Co.
18. Ames A et al: Cerebral ischemia, part 2: the no-reflow phenomenon, Am J Pathol 52:437, 1968.
19. Ames A III: Earliest irreversible changes during ischemia, Am J Emerg Med 1:139, 1983.
20. Bleyaert AL et al: Thiopental amelioration of brain damage after global ischemia in monkeys, Anesthesiology 49:390, 1978.
20a. Babbs CF: Role of iron ions in the genesis of reperfusion injury following successful cardio-pulmonary resuscitation: preliminary data and a biochemical hypothesis, Ann Emerg Med 14:777, 1985.
21. Aldrete JA et al: Phenytoin for brain resuscitation after cardiac arrest: an uncontrolled clinical trial, Crit Care Med 9:474, 1981.
22. Vaagenes P et al: Amelioration of brain damage by lidoflazine after 10 minutes ventricular fibrillation in dogs, Crit Care Med 12:846, 1984.
23. Braunwald E: Mechanism of action of calcium-channel-blocking agents, N Engl J Med 307:1618, 1982.
24. Bulkley GB: The role of oxygen free radicals in human disease processes, Surgery 94:407, 1983.

25. Teasdale G and Jennett B: Assessment of coma and impaired consciousness: a practical scale, Lancet 2:81, 1974.

26. Bircher N: Brain resuscitation. In Schwartz G et al, editors: Emergency medicine: the essential update, Philadelphia, 1989, WB Saunders Co.

SUGGESTED READINGS

Abramson NS et al: Neurologic recovery after cardiac arrest: effect of duration of ischemia, Crit Care Med 13:930, 1985.

Abramson NS et al: Randomized clinical study of thiopental loading in comatose cardiac arrest survivors, N Engl J Med 314:397, 1986.

Astrup J, Siesjo BK, and Symon L: Thresholds in cerebral ischemia: the ischemic penumbra, Stroke 12:723, 1981.

Baskin DS and Hosobuchi Y: Naloxone reversal of ischemic deficits in man, Lancet 2:272, 1981.

Bircher N and Safar P: Comparison of standard new closed chest CPR and open-chest CPR in dogs, Crit Care Med 2(5):384, 1981.

Bircher N, Safar P, and Stewert R: A comparison of standard "MAST"-augmented and open-chest CPR in dogs, Crit Care Med 8:147, 1980.

Cantadore R et al: Cardiopulmonary bypass for resuscitation after prolonged cardiac arrest in dogs, Ann Emerg Med 13:134 (abstract), 1984.

Chaing J: Cerebral ischemia. III Vascular changes, Am J Pathol 52:45, 1968.

Chandra N et al: Augmentation of carotid flow during cardiopulmonary resuscitation by ventilation at high airway pressure simultaneous with chest compression, Am J Cardiol 48:1053, 1981.

Respiratory Disorders

Problematic Pulmonary Syndromes

Stephen L. Demeter, M.D., F.A.C.P., F.C.C.P.
and Edward M. Cordasco, M.D., F.A.C.P.

Acute pulmonary disorders pose a special threat to the elderly, whose respiratory function is generally compromised as a result of changes in pulmonary physiology that accompany the aging process. Reduced pulmonary capacity in this age group is generally related to alterations in lung and chest wall compliance. With advancing age, the chest wall becomes increasingly stiff as the bony thorax becomes more rigid, and lung elastic recoil decreases. These changes lead to a decrease in the expiratory flow rate, forced vital capacity (FVC), and gas diffusion, as well as an increase in the closing volume (CV) and residual volume (RV). (See Table 18–1.)

Alveolar ducts and sacs enlarge progressively with age and may form cystic areas with dilation and disruption of adjacent walls and associated capillaries, without fibrosis. As a consequence, there are fewer alveoli and less total alveolar surface area for gas exchange. The degeneration of alveolar-septal membranes results in hyperinflation, or so-called senile emphysema, and is probably related to the diminished elastic recoil. It has been estimated that the normal individual would become disabled by emphysema at the age of 180 years. However, the rate of emphysematous progression is clearly influenced by both genetic/hereditary and environmental factors. Consequently, there are nonsmokers who develop crippling emphysema in the sixth and seventh decades as well as individuals who continue to smoke into their ninth and tenth decades without pulmonary complaints.

Despite the loss of elastic recoil, total lung capacity remains unchanged due to the opposing loss of chest wall compliance and weakened respiratory muscles. Variable increase in alveolar diameter and the tendency for distal airways to collapse leads to an increase in residual volume and reciprocal decrease in the vital capacity. Simply put, there is more "nonusable" structural air and less "usable" ventilatory exchanging air as one grows

Table 18–1   Changes in Pulmonary Function with Aging

Parameter	Direction of change
Spirometry	
Vital capacity	↓
Forced expiratory volume	↓
Maximum midexpiratory flow rate	↓
Total lung capacity	—
Residual volume	↑
Fuctional residual capacity	↑
Compliance	
Static muscle strength	↓
Elastic lung recoil	↓
Work of breathing	↑
Gas exchange	
Diffusion capacity	↓
Ventilation-perfusion inequality	↑
Alveolar-arterial oxygen gradient	↑
Arterial oxygenation	↓
Arterial carbon dioxide tension	—

From Zimert I: Working up the elderly patient: how far to go, Diagnosis 4:82, 1983.

older. This results in unventilated, dependent lung regions where perfusion is greatest, low ventilation-perfusion ratios ("wasted perfusion"), and hypoxemia.

Arterial oxygen tension (PaO_2) falls with age, but the arterial carbon dioxide tension does not change. These findings cannot be explained by age-related changes in diffusion capacity and probably are related to airway closure during exhalation. However, both central and peripheral chemoreceptor function declines with age, and elderly subjects have been found to have a diminished ventilatory response to hypoxic and hypercapnic challenge. Hereditary or genetic factors may also play a role. Multiple age regression formulae have been developed to calculate the expected PaO_2 in elderly patients. A simple nomogram to remember is that for a patient 70 years old, the expected PaO_2 is 70 torr, and in the range between 60 and 80 years old, the PaO_2 varies 1:1 inversely with age. Thus, for a 65-year-old patient, the expected PaO_2 would be 75 torr based on sea level measurements.

In summary, then, age-related changes in the respiratory system cause a diminution in function reserve of the lung parenchyma, respiratory muscles, and ventilatory control mechanisms, thereby predisposing the elderly patient to respiratory failure. (See Table 18–1.) In addition, pulmonary defense mechanisms decline with age, making infectious and autoimmune diseases of the elderly more common and more difficult to eradicate.

DYSPNEA

A frequent precipitating factor that brings the elderly patient to the emergency department, dyspnea is one of the most important symptoms of lung disease. Elderly patients report dyspnea as an uncomfortable sensation of breathlessness, which the emergency physician must distinguish from simple tachypnea (rapid breathing) or hyperpnea (increased ventilation). Because dyspnea is a subjective state, it is difficult to measure, and the factors responsible for it are poorly understood. Causes of dyspnea in the elderly, however, include virtually all conditions that result in significant functional impairment of either the respiratory (gas exchange and/or pulmonary mechanics) or the cardiovascular system (circulatory and/or cardiac function) as well as any hematologic abnormality that impairs oxygen delivery. Hysterical overbreathing, on occasion, can precipitate tetany in the elderly. On the other hand, persistent deep, panting respirations in an ill-looking elderly patient strongly suggest underlying metabolic acidosis. Finally, it is common for the relatives of elderly invalids to report "attacks of breathlessness," which, in fact, are periodic episodes of Cheyne-Stokes respiration — a very common condition in the elderly age group characterized by intervals of hyperpnea that alternate with intervals of apnea. Cheyne-Stokes breathing can come and go over a period of weeks or months without any noteworthy change in the patient's condition. Periodic breathing in the elderly probably results from coarseness of acid-base control. As with Cheyne-Stokes breathing, there is a link with cerebrovascular disease and congestive heart failure.

The emergency evaluation of the acutely dyspneic patient must be systematic and precise. The mode of onset, past history, concomitant symptoms, and clinical signs usually narrow the diagnostic possibilities. The patient may already carry a diagnosis of asthma, emphysema, or heart failure, which makes evaluation more straightforward. Further clues or confirmation are obtained from such tests as the chest x-ray (e.g., Figure 18–1), electrocardiogram (ECG), complete blood count (CBC), and arterial blood gases (ABGs). In patients with asthma or chronic obstructive pulmonary disease, use of a peak expiratory flowmeter can provide objective assessment of initial lung function and can be repeated to check response to therapy.

Cardiac and Pulmonary Status

It is not uncommon for the emergency physician to have difficulty determining whether dyspnea is secondary to pulmonary edema or acute respiratory failure. For example, an adequate history often is not readily available from agitated patients or their families. Heart rate, blood pressure, and respiratory rate may indicate the severity of the illness but are not very useful in the differential diagnosis. Too often, the patient with pulmonary edema exhibits extensive wheezing due to bronchial irritation from edema fluid and compression of airways by engorged peribronchial lymphatics. In addition, patients with impaired left ventricular function have bronchial hyperresponsiveness.[1-3] Similarly, the basilar rales of

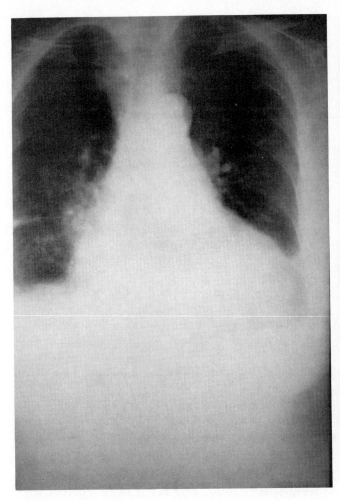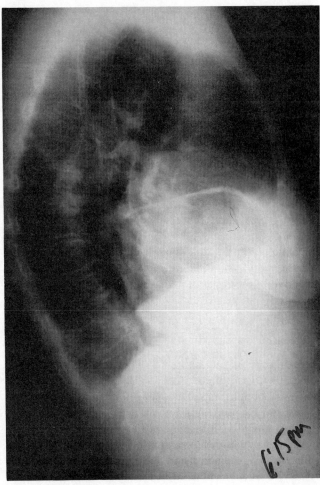

Figure 18–1 Congestive heart failure demonstrating cardiomegaly, cephalization of vessels, fluid accumulation in fissures, and perihilar fluffiness.

pulmonary edema may be mimicked by chronic pulmonary disease with bibasilar fibrosis. A checklist, such as the one in Table 18–2, is often useful in distinguishing one etiology from the other, but, at times, differentiation cannot be made until the patient is admitted to the intensive care unit (ICU), and a pulmonary capillary wedge pressure (PCWP) is measured with a Swan-Ganz (flow-directed) catheter.

Initial treatment of the dyspneic patient relies upon a number of modalities that vary according to the clinical setting and the patient's condition. In the emergency department, one of the most important objectives is to recognize impending or progressive respiratory failure and to intubate and provide mechanical ventilation early in the patient's course when needed.[4-7] Low-flow oxygen (e.g., 2 to 3 L/minute by nasal cannula; 24 to 38% Venturi mask) permits partial correction of hypoxia without great risk of respiratory depression, pending the results of ABG analysis. Administration of sedatives, especially if the patient is combative, restless, or confused, is contraindicated, since these signs may indicate hypoxia. Intravenous aminophylline (5 to 6 mg/kg over 20 to 30

minutes loading dose) may improve clinical signs and symptoms in both pulmonary and cardiac disease. The application of rotating tourniquets to the extremities effectively decreases cardiac preload in a readily reversible fashion. If the patient's blood pressure drops, hemodynamic correction quickly follows the release of the tourniquets. These therapeutic modalities can be safely instituted pending the results of ABGs and chest films.

Although the portable anteroposterior (AP) chest x-ray has notable deficiencies, overt congestive heart failure will generally produce interstitial or alveolar fluid accumulation. Small doses of intravenous morphine sulfate (2 to 4 mg slow push) and furosemide (20 mg if the patient is on oral furosemide therapy, 40 mg if the patient is on chronic furosemide therapy) can then be administered. In addition to the chest x-ray, an ECG must be obtained to assess cardiac arrhythmias or ischemic changes. Even without a history of chest pain, an ECG is mandatory to exclude the diagnosis of a myocardial infarction, which, in the elderly, frequently presents with acute dyspnea or dyspnea on exertion.

Table 18–2   Differentiation of Pulmonary and Cardiac Dyspnea

	Pulmonary	Cardiac
History	Industrial exposure; extensive tobacco use; recurrent respiratory infections; previous abnormal pulmonary function tests; daily cough-producing sputum, perhaps purulent	Previous angina, myocardial infarction, or rheumatic fever; previous evidence of abnormal cardiac function, such as an abnormal ECG, presence of a murmur, or cardiomegaly seen on film
Physical examination	Increased respiratory rate; increased thoracic AP diameter; clubbing; localized rales; rhonchi; evidence of consolidation	Increased respiratory rate; S_3 and S_4 gallops; diffuse or symmetrical rales; murmur
ECG	Low voltage; poor R wave progression; RVH	Old or recent MI; LVH except in mitral stenosis where RVH may be present
Chest pain	Increased pulmonary volume with large AP diameter and flattened diaphragms; localized consolidation; small heart; normal pulmonary vasculature	Normal pulmonary volume and diaphragm; cardiomegaly; pulmonary vascular redistribution; Kerley-B lines; interstitial or alveolar edema
Pulmonary capillary wedge pressure	Normal (< 12 mm Hg)	Elevated (usually > 20 mm Hg)
Pulmonary function tests	Markedly abnormal (restrictive or obstructive pattern)	Normal or mild abnormalities

Reprinted with permission from Alpert JS: Cardiac decompensation. In May HL, editor: Emergency medicine, New York, 1984, John Wiley & Sons. LVH = Left ventricular hypertrophy; RVH = right ventricular hypertrophy.

HEMOPTYSIS

Hemoptysis is a distressing and, potentially, life-threatening symptom that warrants immediate evaluation and treatment.[8] Massive hemoptysis producing more than 600 mL of blood per 24 hours or 1,000 mL over several days carries a 50 to 100% mortality and is an indication for emergency bronchoscopy and surgical therapy.[8] Causes of massive hemoptysis are summarized in Table 18–3. Actual incidence figures depend on the patient population studied. Nonetheless, among the most common causes in most series are chronic bronchitis, bronchiectasis, and bronchogenic carcinoma followed by tuberculosis, fungal infections, bacterial pneumonia, and abscess. Pulmonary embolism produces hemoptysis in approximately 30% of all cases of documented emboli associated with pulmonary infarction.[9] Interestingly, even with the advent of the fiberoptic bronchoscope, the cause of hemoptysis remains undiagnosed 5 to 15% of the time.

Diagnosis

The initial evaluation of hemoptysis is aimed at localizing the hemorrhagic site and quantifying the amount of bleeding and includes a detailed history, physical examination, and chest x-ray (Figure 18–2). The history is often invaluable, providing information regarding the duration and extent of bleeding, prior episodes of hemoptysis, and the presence of underlying cardiopulmonary disease or other disorders. For example, abrupt production of pure blood in the geriatric patient suggests vascular etiologies associated with carcinoma, pulmonary infarction, or rupture of a tuberculous aneurysm. As a rule, blood mixed with purulent sputum is indicative of an infectious etiology, such as pneumonia, bronchitis, or lung abscess. If the source of the bleeding is an intrathoracic structure, the patient may be able to localize the site of bleeding to the right or left lung (a tickling or bothersome irritation is sometimes experienced on the affected side).

The physical exam must exclude extrathoracic sources of bleeding from such structures as the nasal passages,

Table 18–3   Major Causes of Massive Hemoptysis

Infection	Tuberculosis
	Bronchiectasis
	Bronchitis
	Lung abscess
	Necrotizing pneumonia
	Mycetomas and other fungal infections
Neoplasm	Bronchogenic carcinoma
	Metastatic disease
	Bronchial adenoma
Cardiovascular disease	Mitral stenosis
	Arteriovenous malformation
	Pulmonary embolus/infarction
	Pulmonary vasculitis
Miscellaneous	Pneumoconiosis
	Swan-Ganz catheterization
	Coagulopathies
	Endotracheal foreign bodies
	Idiopathic hemoptysis

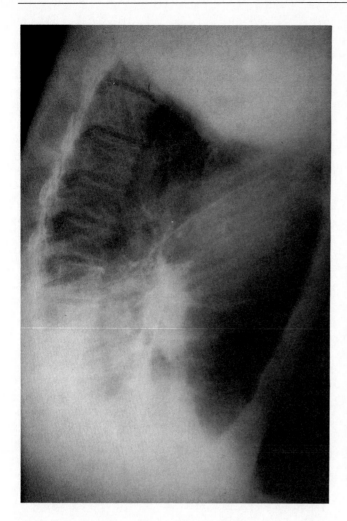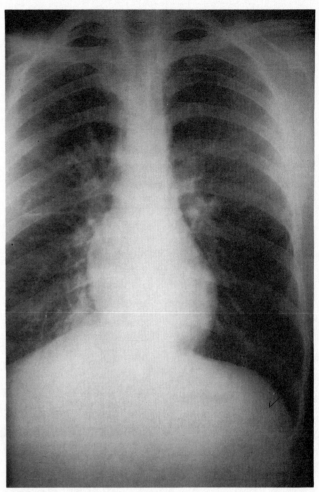

Figure 18–2   Sixty-year-old man with hemoptysis secondary to pulmonary vasculitis. Note the prominent interstitial pattern and fluid in fissures.

sinuses, and oropharynx. It is especially important to distinguish hemoptysis from epistaxis and hematemesis; as a rule, expectorated blood is usually bright red, frothy, has an alkaline pH, and is often mixed with sputum containing macrophages and white blood cells. Localized wheezing or rales suggests pulmonary disease that is confined to one side of the chest, a finding that is particularly useful when the chest x-ray is normal. Cardiac examination may reveal a murmur consistent with mitral stenosis. In addition, the presence and degree of respiratory compromise must be established. Asphyxiation from aspirated blood, rather than blood loss, is the major threat to life.

Initial laboratory investigation of hemoptysis should include a CBC, coagulation studies, type and crossmatch, ECG, ABGs, and spirometry. Sputum should be collected for routine bacterial, mycobacterial, fungal, and cytologic studies. The chest radiograph may suggest both cause and location of the hemoptysis; most acute inflammatory diseases (e.g., active tuberculosis, pneumonia, hemoptysis) will produce pulmonary infiltrates. In addition,

85% of neoplasms and most pulmonary emboli associated with infarction will show localized pulmonary lesions. However, findings on the plain chest x-ray may be misleading, particularly in patients who have generalized inflammatory conditions of the lung, and a negative chest x-ray is not uncommon.

Treatment

While conservative management may suffice for many cases of low-volume hemoptysis in the elderly, more aggressive measures are required for massive hemoptysis. The four goals of emergency therapy are to prevent asphyxiation, to provide respiratory support, to maintain vital signs, and to stop bleeding (See Figure 18–3).

The prevention of airway obstruction is of paramount importance. The patient should be placed immediately at bed rest in a slightly head-down, lateral decubitus position with the suspected site of hemoptysis oriented in the dependent condition. Continuous monitoring and admission to an ICU with constant nursing care and suction

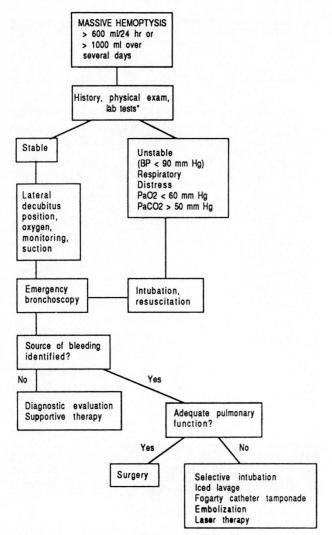

*Lab tests: complete blood count, coagulation studies, arterial blood gases, type and cross-match, ECG, chest x-ray, and spirometry

Figure 18-3 Treatment of patients with massive hemoptysis.

equipment at the bedside is recommended in all cases of massive hemoptysis. Supplemental oxygen is administered to maintain a Po_2 of approximately 60 mm Hg. Many patients will require endotracheal intubation. This permits a tracheobronchial toilet and use of mechanical ventilation with positive end-expiratory pressure (PEEP). PEEP not only may improve oxygenation but also, to the extent that it increases intrathoracic pressure, may provide a barometric tamponade to the hemorrhagic site.

Once an airway is established and the patient is properly positioned, coagulation status should be reviewed and abnormalities corrected. Vital signs are supported by administration of volume expanders and blood transfusion (hematocrit should be kept above 30). Severe cough may aggravate bleeding and must be controlled. All patients should undergo bronchoscopy to determine the exact location of the hemorrhage. We recommend use of a rigid, rather than a flexible, bronchoscope. Because it has a larger lumen, the rigid bronchoscope provides su-

perior suctioning, ventilation, and airway maintenance. In addition, rigid bronchoscopy allows for interventions, such as iced saline lavage or Fogarty catheter tamponade. Provided hemoptysis is not significant, flexible bronchoscopy may be used as an alternative to visualize the bronchial subdivisions. Either method will localize the site of bleeding in up to 90% of patients.

Following localization of bleeding, standard therapy for massive hemoptysis is thoracotomy and resection of the bleeding source. If the patient is inoperable (bilateral advanced pulmonary disease, unresectable carcinoma, or poor pulmonary function), there are alternative medical approaches. These include selective ventilation of the nonbleeding lung, endobronchial tamponade, laser therapy, or iced saline lavage. Recently, bronchial arteriography with selective vasopressin perfusion, Gelfoam embolization, or balloon occlusion has been proposed as a means of stopping massive inoperable bronchial bleeding.

ASPIRATION SYNDROMES

Aspiration of endogenous foreign material into the airway is an important cause of pulmonary morbidity and mortality in the elderly.[10] A high index of suspicion is important. In this regard, the emergency physician must be able to identify those elderly patients who are at risk for aspiration and then institute appropriate therapy. The mortality rate from aspiration in the elderly ranges from 40 to 70%, even with the best treatment regimens.

Conditions that predispose to aspiration in the geriatric patient include neurologic disorders affecting the level of consciousness, alcoholism, sedative-hypnotic drugs, and general anesthesia. The presence of a nasogastric, endotracheal, or tracheostomy tube may disrupt sphincter mechanisms that normally protect against aspiration. Gastrointestinal disorders, such as swallowing dysfunction (perhaps secondary to a stroke), gastroesophageal reflux, hiatus hernia, and obstructive lesions (such as esophageal strictures), or neurologic disease (such as amyotrophic lateral sclerosis), may cause recurrent aspiration. Finally, chronic aspiration of lipid materials can occur in many elderly patients who use mineral-oil or oil-based laxatives. These oily substances may pass through the pharynx and into the lungs without stimulating a reflex cough response.

Aspiration of oral secretions occurs with some regularity, even in normal individuals, but this is usually self-limited and of little clinical consequence. In the elderly, however, apsiration represents a debilitating and life-threatening problem. In general, it is useful to characterize aspiration syndromes (Table 18-4) according to 1) what is aspirated, 2) the frequency and volume of aspirate, and 3) the state of the patient's lower respiratory tract defense mechanisms.

Table 18–4 Aspiration Syndromes

Chemical pneumonitis (Mendelson's syndrome)
Hemorrhagic tracheobronchitis
Adult respiratory distress syndrome

Foreign body aspiration
Cafe coronary
Postobstructive atelectasis
Hemorrhagic pneumonia

Bacterial aspiration pneumonia
Pneumonitis
Abscess
Empyema

Exogenous lipoid pneumonia
Chronic bronchitis
Recurrent pneumonia
Bronchiectasis
Chronic interstitial fibrosis

Recurrent small-volume aspiration
Chronic persistent cough
Adult-onset asthma
Tracheobronchitis
Chronic interstitial fibrosis

Diagnosis

In 1946, Mendelson first described the natural history of a fulminant insult resulting from massive aspiration of gastric contents. Large, poorly localized aspirates, having a pH less than 2.5, are associated with greater injury and mortality. Initial pathologic changes include atelectasis, hemorrhage within the bronchial wall, marked interstitial and peribronchial edema, and areas of necrosis. The diagnosis may be difficult to prove unless the aspiration is witnessed or gastric contents are visualized directly in the airway or suctioned from an endotracheal tube. The most important clinical features of chemical pneumonitis are severe dyspnea (usually within 2 hours of the event), coughing, wheezing, unexplained rales, cyanosis, and, frequently, hypotension. Severe hypoxemia may also be present and occurs in association with a normal or low $PaCO_2$ and a wide alveolar-arterial oxygen difference. The alveolar-capillary membrane may be damaged, leading to exudation and, in severe cases, to adult respiratory distress syndrome (ARDS) (Figure 18–4). This is characterized by the production of frothy, nonpurulent sputum and a chest radiograph demonstrating diffuse, fluffy infiltrates. It is distinguished from cardiogenic pulmonary edema by low pulmonary capillary wedge pressures (PCWPs) and by the large volumes of fluids required for resuscitation.

Aspiration of large food particles may cause asphyxia and sudden death, the so-called cafe coronary. Aphonia is often a clue to the diagnosis. Smaller particles may

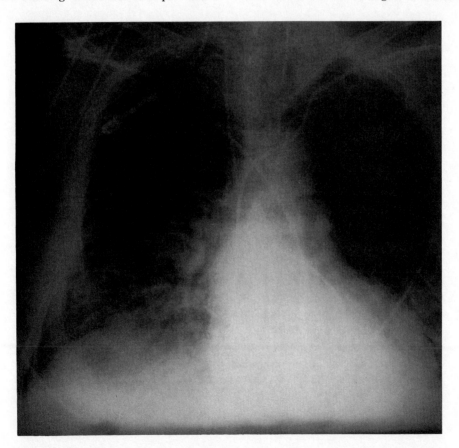

Figure 18–4 ARDS in a patient with chemical pneumonitis. Note the fluffy bilateral infiltrates without marked predilection for the hilar regions.

occlude small bronchi and result in dyspnea, wheezing, and postobstructive atelectasis. Hemorrhagic pneumonia may be seen in about 6 hours. This is followed by a widespread granulomatous reaction with macrophages and giant cells. The degree of injury (and mortality) is greater with larger volumes as in acid aspiration. In contrast to acid aspiration, pulmonary changes in food aspiration occur later, and intense bronchial transudation is not seen. The chest x-ray is normal in 80% of cases. In addition, the $PaCO_2$ is usually higher than in acid aspiration, with the degree of hypoxia similar in both syndromes.

Although chemical pneumonitis and mechanical obstruction usually cause acute symptoms, aspiration pneumonia is more insidious with symptoms occurring gradually several days after the initial episode of aspiration. Over 50% of patients with documented aspiration become infected. Pneumonitis, necrotizing pneumonia, abscess, and empyema are common sequelae. Symptoms often include fever, weight loss, and productive cough. Anemia and an elevated white blood cell count are frequent associated findings. The diagnosis is confirmed clinically by an x-ray and appropriate cultures. Areas of the lung most commonly involved depend on the patient's position at the time of aspiration: posterior segments of upper lobes if supine, lower lobes if erect. The bacteriologic findings in aspiration pneumonia reflect the flora of the oro-pharynx. Anaerobes and pneumococci are the most frequent pathogens in nonhospitalized patients; however, in hospitalized patients, gram-negative bacilli, primarily enteric organisms, are more common. In contrast, patients with chemical pneumonitis may develop secondary bacterial infections due to aerobic gram-positive and gram-negative organisms, such as *Staphylococcus aureus* and *Pseudomonas aeruginosa*.

Lipid aspiration, which can be caused by aspiration of mineral oil laxatives, nasogastric feedings, or petroleum jelly nasal preparations, is commonly overlooked in the elderly. Patients develop symptoms ranging from chronic bronchitis to recurrent lipoid pneumonias and pulmonary fibrosis. The chest x-ray reveals interstitial infiltrates or an inflammatory process (Figure 18–5). The diagnosis must be suspected on clinical grounds in any elderly patient with persistent lower respiratory complaints.

Recurrent aspiration of small amounts of oral feedings, liquid gastric contents, or formula feeding solutions may present with a variety of clinical pictures. Small airway disease may predominate with insidious onset of bronchorrhea, chronic cough, and adult-onset asthma. Recurrent pulmonary infiltrates in dependent lung segments or changes in the lower lung fields resembling miliary tuberculosis are common manifestations of repeated aspiration. If signs and symptoms are due to

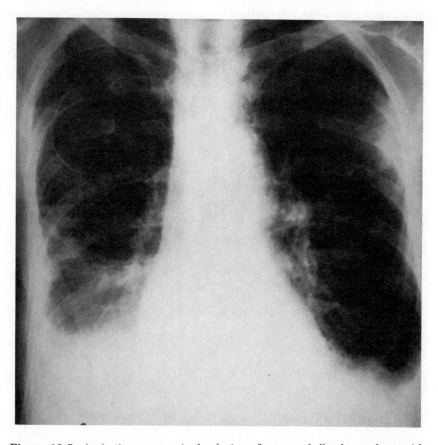

Figure 18–5 Aspiration pneumonia developing after a cerebellar hemorrhage with respiratory arrest.

aspiration of oral feedings, the diagnosis can be made by watching the patient swallow water. Glucose reagent strips can be used to rule out aspiration of formula feeding rich in glucose (aspiration has occurred if glucose > 25 mg/dL). Examination of the sputum may show sheets of pleomorphic gram-positive and gram-negative forms (rods, spirochetes, and fusiform bacteria) pathognomonic of mixed aerobic and anaerobic infection.

Treatment

The hallmark of therapy for aspiration syndromes in the elderly is primary prevention. Prophylactic measures should be instituted in all patients with a depressed level of consciousness, especially if the nasogastric tube has been placed. Such patients should be placed in the head-down position and may require prophylactic intubation for airway protection. The use of high-volume, thin-walled endotracheal and tracheostomy tubes may further decrease the risk of aspiration.

Once aspiration has transpired, treatment requires aggressive ventilatory support, fluid management, and general supportive care. The patient should be positioned in a left lateral decubitus position with the head down. Vigorous tracheal suction may be followed by bronchoscopy to remove particulate matter. Bronchial lavage is not helpful since the gastric acid is rapidly neutralized by tracheobronchial secretions. The early initiation of ventilatory support based on blood-gas determinations, along with the appropriate application of positive pressure ventilation, appears to be one of the most important modes of supportive care. Rapid intravenous fluid administration may be necessary to replace the "third-space" loss of intravascular volume into the injured lung. Fluid replacement should be guided by changes in central venous pressure, urine output, and frequent monitoring of vital signs. If cardiac failure is suspected, it may be necessary to monitor the PCWP in order to administer fluids safely and effectively.

Aerosolized bronchodilators and intravenous aminophylline are useful in treating bronchospasm associated with aspiration. The question of corticosteroid administration remains controversial. The prevalent attitude, however, is that steroids are of no benefit and may predispose the patient to more serious infection — especially with gram-negative organisms — or other complications.

Daily sputum cultures are indicated, and blood cultures should be taken if there are extensive lung infiltrates. Some centers believe that the patient should be monitored closely and antibiotics instituted only when there is clinical evidence of infection (i.e., purulent sputum, fever, leukocytosis, consistent Gram stain). Other institutions rec ommend empiric therapy in the high-risk patient. Once the decision is made to use antibiotics, an agent should be chosen that is effective against the most likely infecting organisms. Ampicillin-sulbactam (Unasyn), with its comprehensive coverage of anaerobes and efficacy against commonly implicated gram-negative organisms (excluding *Pseudomonas*), is an excellent initial choice for aspiration pneumonia. A third-generation cephalosporin is also a suitable choice when indicated.

Lesser degrees of aspiration may warrant a trial of conservative therapy. If the clinician suspects occult gastroesophageal reflux as the cause of a patient's chronic cough or new-onset asthma, the patient should be instructed to elevate the head of the bed on 8-inch blocks. Reflux may be treated with antacids, H_2 antagonists at bedtime, and nothing by mouth for 2 hours before bedtime. Formula feedings by nasogastric tube may need to be stopped and given parenterally.

PNEUMONIA

Pneumonia is the leading infectious cause of death in the geriatric age group (Figure 18–6). The elderly patient with pneumonia is more likely to develop bacteremia and such complications as empyema and meningitis. Furthermore, geriatric patients are susceptible to a number

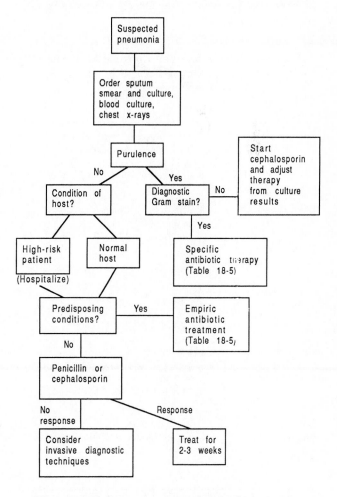

Figure 18–6   Treatment of acute bacterial pneumonia.

of respiratory pathogens (e.g., gram-negative bacilli) and are more likely to develop nosocomial pneumonia than younger hospitalized patients. In part, this is due to a breakdown of the body's immunologic defense systems. The prevalence of chronic disease, which further decreases immunity and impairs respiratory tract clearance, allows pharyngeal colonization by pathogens that may be aspirated into the lungs.

Appropriate management of the elderly patient with pneumonia requires selection of an antimicrobial regimen that is active against the pathogens most commonly encountered in the setting involved. An offending organism is isolated in only 57 to 74% of cases; therefore, many patients must be treated empirically. Specifically, antimicrobial selection depends upon whether the infection is community acquired or whether it was acquired in a chronic care institution (i.e., nursing home) or hospital. Each setting, in combination with associated host[12-16] conditions, predisposes to different etiologic agents. (See Table 18–5.)

Streptococcus pneumoniae (pneumococcus) is still the most common pathogen isolated in the elderly who live at home, causing 40 to 60% of cases in which a pathogen is identified. *Haemophilus influenzae* has emerged as a significant etiologic agent in the elderly and now represents the second most commonly isolated bacterium. This organism can be recovered from the oropharynx of healthy adults and from 60% of patients with chronic bronchitis. Oropharyngeal anaerobes are important bacterial respiratory pathogens in elderly patients with altered consciousness, swallowing disorders, alcoholism, and bronchogenic carcinoma. Other common bacterial causes of community-acquired pneumonia in the aged include *Staphylococcus aureus*, group B streptococcus, *Klebsiella pneumoniae*, and *Branhamella catarrhalis* (formerly known as *Neisseria catarrhalis*). Some of the "atypical" and viral pneumonias that do not respond to penicillin therapy are more common in elderly than in younger persons. Middle-aged and elderly men are prone to Legionnaires' disease, although it can occur in any age group. *Legionella pneumophila* has been reported with increasing frequency since its recognition in 1976. Its prevalence appears to be related to geographic area, and in England, it is considered to be the second most common cause of pneumonia. Influenza A is responsible for most viral pneumonias in the elderly. Pneumonias caused by *Mycoplasma pneumoniae*, parainfluenza virus, rhinovirus, and adenovirus are more common in younger people. Finally, while the overall incidence and mortality from infections with *Mycobacterium tuberculosis* has

Table 18–5 Recommended Empiric Antibiotic Regimens for Suspected Bacterial Pneumonia in the Elderly

Setting	Usual pathogens	Antibiotic therapy*	
		Not life threatening	Life threatening
Community	*Streptococcus pneumoniae,* mixed flora, *Haemophilus influenzae,* gram-negative bacilli	Ampicillin-sulbactam (Unasyn), pencillin G or ampicillin, first- or second-generation cephalosporin	Third-generation cephalosporin, ampicillin-sulbactam (Unasyn), or aztreonam plus aminoglycoside
Institution	Mixed flora, *Streptococcus pneumoniae,* gram-negative bacilli	As per community setting	Third- or fourth-generation cephalosporin, ampicillin-sulbactam (Unasyn), or aztreonam and trimethoprim-sulfamethoxazole plus aminoglycoside
Hospital (not immunocompromised)	Gram-negative bacilli, *Staphylococcus aureus, Streptococcus pneumoniae,* mixed flora	Third-generation cephalosporin plus aminoglycoside or ampicillin-sulbactam (Unasyn)	Maximum doses
Immunocompromised	As above plus *Legionella pneumophila*	Maximum doses: third-generation cephalosporin plus aminoglycoside plus erythromycin	Same: maximum doses trimethoprim-sulfamethoxazole

Modified from Bentley DW: Infectious disease. In Rossman I, editor: Clinical geriatrics, Philadelphia, 1986, JB Lippincott Co, p. 445.

*The antibiotic regimen(s) listed first are the drug(s) of choice; other choices are given in case of hypersensitivity or allergy to the first regimen.

been decreasing since 1900, the elderly now comprise the largest group with active infection. Onset is particularly insidious in the elderly, and diagnosis often requires a high index of suspicion.

Gram-negative organisms are the most common etiologic agents in pneumonia acquired by elderly persons in the nursing home or hospital. Mortality associated with gram-negative bacteria is estimated to be 50% despite appropriate antibiotic therapy. These nosocomial pneumonias are acquired by aspiration of oropharyngeal contents, bacteremic spread, and use of aerosolization equipment. While *Klebsiella pneumoniae* is the most common gram-negative organism to cause pneumonia in the elderly, *Pseudomonas aeruginosa, Serratia marcescens, Acinetobacter calcoaceticus,* and *Escherichia coli* are also important pathogens.

Diagnosis

Sir William Osler proclaimed that "in old age, pneumonia may be latent, coming on without chill; The cough and expectoration are slight, the physical findings ill-defined and changeable, and the constitutional symptoms out of proportion to the extent of the local lesion." The emergency physician must recognize that generalized, nonspecific deterioration in the geriatric patient's general level of health is frequently the first sign of pneumonia. In the elderly, the classic symptoms of cough, chest pain, productive sputum, and fever are often entirely absent and such nonpulmonary complaints as anorexia, lethargy, confusion, vomiting, malaise, dehydration, or inappropriate antidiuretic hormone secretion may dominate the picture. Moreover, the presence of an occult pulmonary infection, as well as acute myocardial infarction, should be evaluated in all elderly patients who present with confusion of acute onset.

Pneumonia in the geriatric patient is often characterized by physical findings that are nonspecific and, on occasion, confusing. For example, many elderly patients are too ill or too weak to cough effectively or to cooperate in the production of sputum. They may not be able to take deep inspirations, and breathing sounds on auscultation may be misleading because of pre-existing emphysema or chronic congestive heart failure. The two physical signs that are most sensitive, but least specific, are increased pulse rate and tachypnea. Mean temperature in elderly patients with bacterial pneumonia is 101 to 102° F. However, approximately 20% of elderly with community-acquired pneumonia are afebrile on admission to the hospital. Recording of postural changes in blood pressure and pulse rate is useful in assessing hydration and intravascular fluid volume. On further examination, the patient may have grunting respirations, sternal retraction, nasal flaring, decreased breath sounds, and localized rales. However, the presence of such findings is unreliable, and, therefore, patients should be x-rayed when their respiratory rate is 24 breaths/minute or higher.

Radiologic examination is useful in the elderly patient (Figure 18–7), although an infectious etiology and a specific etiologic agent must be demonstrated by other means. Lobar consolidation, cavitation, and large pleural effusions support a bacterial etiology, and infiltrates localized to the posterior segment of the right upper lobe or superior segments of the lower lobe suggest aspiration that occurred in the supine position. Necrotizing pneumonia with cavitation may suggest anaerobes, gram-negative bacilli, or *S. aureus* as likely pathogens. In cases where bilateral involvement is accompanied by a mixed interstitial-alveolar pattern, primary viral pneumonia should be suspected. Incomplete consolidation interrupted by air-filled spaces is likely to occur in the elderly patient with emphysema. Older patients also have delayed resolution of chest film findings, defined as incomplete clearing in 4 weeks.

If a chest x-ray of good quality fails to reveal a new pulmonary infiltrate, the diagnosis of pneumonia should be questioned. However, it should be stressed that the initial chest radiograph can be normal in the following conditions: 1) early stages of pneumonia, 2) endobronchial tuberculosis, 3) severe dehydration, and 4) neutropenic host with gram-negative pneumonia. Concomitant diseases that occur frequently in older persons can also severely limit the sensitivity and specificity of the chest radiograph. These disorders include obstructive lung disease, heart failure, atelectasis, pulmonary emboli, and lung cancer.

If pulmonary infection is suspected in the emergency department, the physician should obtain a representative sputum specimen for microscopic examination and culture. Unfortunately, a CBC is often of limited value, since the total white blood count can be quite variable. In general, however, most elderly patients with pneumonia will have a discernible left shift in the polymorphonuclear leukocyte count. Blood cultures are useful since they are positive in 15 to 25% of all cases and occasionally will be positive when a sputum sample is negative. There are no serologic tests generally available for tuberculosis and other common bacterial infections. If tuberculosis is suspected, several sputum specimens for acid-fast stains and mycobacterial cultures should be submitted. Anergy to intermediate purified protein derivative (PPD) may be present in 10 to 20% of elderly patients with active disease, although some of these patients have positive reactions to second-strength PPD.

The sputum Gram stain is of significant diagnostic value to the experienced observer. First, it is helpful in determining the validity of the specimen obtained so that the clinician does not waste laboratory resources and expense on unnecessary cultures. Finally, a valid sputum specimen provides an invaluable guide for initial antibiotic therapy, pending culture results and susceptibility testing.

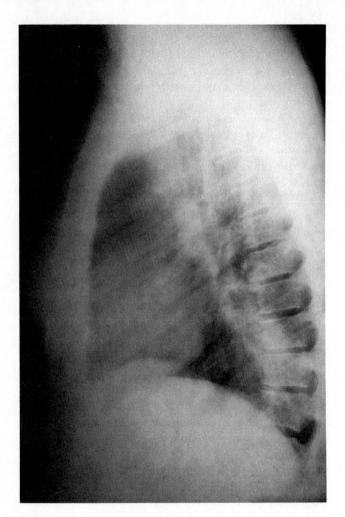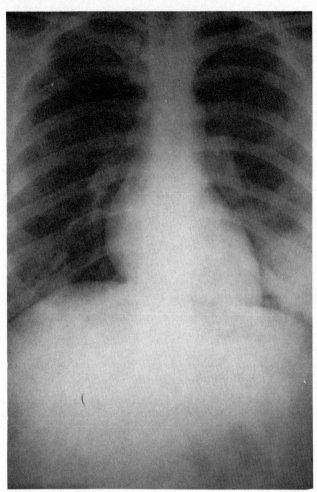

Figure 18–7 Pneumonia in the basal segment of the lower left lobe, not evident on auscultation.

If the patient cannot expectorate spontaneously, inhalational administration of a bronchodilator and a hypertonic saline aerosol may be effective. However, because many elderly patients with pneumonia are cognitively disabled, dehydrated, or debilitated, it is often difficult to obtain valid respiratory secretions. In certain critically ill patients — those with neutropenia, immunosuppression, etc., invasive procedures (transtracheal or endotracheal aspiration, fiberoptic bronchoscopy) should be considered. However, this subgroup of patients is subjected to considerable discomfort and risk of complications (e.g., bleeding). If a pleural effusion is present, thoracentesis should be performed to distinguish between sterile parapneumonic effusions and empyema. A pleural fluid pH of less than 7.20, the presence of bacteria by Gram stain, or a culture of the pleural fluid is an indication for thoracostomy tube drainage. Despite vigilance on the part of the emergency physician, errors in the diagnosis of bacterial pneumonia occur, and they include 1) failure to recognize the bacterial agent on sputum Gram stain, 2) overdiagnosis of pneumococcal pneumonia because of the prevalence of Gram-positive cocci universally present in saliva, 3) delay in the recognition of bacterial superinfection (e.g., staphylococcal superinfection of influenza), 4) failure to suspect bacterial agent in certain situations (e.g., *Klebsiella* in the nursing home patient), and 5) failure to recognize infection in the pleural space, central nervous system (CNS), joints, etc.

Indications for Hospitalization

It is virtually a clinical caveat that hospitalization is required for any patient over the age of 60 with pneumonia. Less aggressive, outpatient therapy is acceptable only if the patient clearly has unilobular pneumococcal pneumonia, is likely to be compliant, and has no underlying disease. If outpatient therapy is deemed to be appropriate, we treat with intramuscular procaine penicillin G (1.2×10^6 units) followed by oral amoxicillin (500 mg PO t.i.d), or erythromycin (500 mg PO q.i.d) for 10 to 14 days. Hospitalization is clearly warranted for any elderly patient who appears likely to be noncompliant with this outpatient antibiotic program.

Other factors that strongly influence the decision to admit elderly patients with pneumonia include 1) pre-existing systemic disease that can worsen or impede recovery (alcoholism, diabetes mellitus, obstructive lung disease, malignancy, uremia, malnutrition); 2) extrapulmonary extension (including the presence of a pleural effusion); 3) hypoxemia (PO_2 < 60 mm Hg or a significant change from baseline); 4) inability of the patient to tolerate or absorb oral antibiotics; and 5) sociologic reasons (lives alone). In addition, elderly patients with established or suspected high-morbidity pneumonias — multilobar, cavitary or necrotizing, aspiration, gram-negative, or staphylococcal pneumonias — should be triaged into the hospital.

High-risk and/or immunocompromised patients should be admitted to the ICU. This subgroup includes elderly patients who manifest signs of acute respiratory failure, confusion, or sepsis. Some studies suggest that older people who are seriously ill are not sent to the ICU as frequently as they should be. In hemodynamically compromised patients (e.g., congestive heart failure), central venous pressure monitoring or Swan-Ganz catheterization will be necessary to guide fluid management. ABGs should be monitored closely in all elderly patients. If the PaO_2 is less than 55 mm Hg and the $PaCO_2$ is over 55 mm Hg in the presence of acute acidosis, mechanical ventilation is indicated. Elderly patients will generally respond better to volume-cycled respirators, as frequent changes in pulmonary compliance can occur in the elderly patient.

Antibiotic Therapy

Rational antibiotic therapy for the aged patient with pneumonia should be guided by the clinical features, knowledge of the patient's environment prior to hospitalization, the presence of underlying disease, and a clear understanding of pathogens most likely to be involved. Microscopic evaluation of a Gram-stained sputum specimen remains the most helpful aid to the selection of initial antibiotic therapy.

When adequate sputum is not available, or when the establishment of a definitive microbiologic diagnosis appears unlikely, the antibiotic regimen is selected empirically based on epidemiologic patterns of geriatric pulmonary infections, host features, and the setting in which the pneumonia was acquired. Recommendations for initial treatment of suspected bacterial pneumonias are summarized in Table 18–5.

S. pneumoniae and mixed flora are responsible for about 80% of all community-acquired pneumonias. These infections are comprised of two or more respiratory pathogens, normal oropharyngeal commensals, or both. In general, they respond to therapy for pneumococcus, if this organism is identified on Gram stain. Penicillin G, ampicillin-sulbactam (Unasyn) 3 g IV q.6h., or a cephalosporin is the initial antibiotic of choice in this setting.

Clindamycin (300 to 600 mg q.6h. IV) can be substituted in those patients with a history of an anaphylactic reaction from either a penicillin or cephalosporin. Ampicillin-sulbactam has broad gram-negative and anaerobic coverage that makes it ideally suited to the treatment of aspiration in the elderly. In patients with life-threatening pneumonia, broad-spectrum antibiotic therapy is indicated with an aminoglycoside in combination with ampicillin-sulbactam or a third-generation cephalosporin. Occasionally, empiric antibiotic regimens will have to be modified to account for specific pathogens that are predictably associated with a specific disease state or underlying condition. For example, if the pneumonia occurs during an influenza epidemic, staphylococcal pneumonia is a possibility, and one of the semisynthetic penicillinase-resistant penicillins should probably be used. (See Table 18–6.)

In institutionalized or nursing home outpatients, the most frequent etiologic agents are mixed flora and *S. pneumoniae*. The initial choice of antibiotic is the same as that recommended for non-life-threatening community-acquired pneumonias. However, in moderately ill patients or life-threatening situations, the regimen must also include coverage against aerobic gram-negative bacilli (e.g., *Klebsiella pneumoniae*). Antibiotic therapy should include a third-generation cephalosporin with good anti-*Pseudomonas* activity, plus an aminoglycoside.

In hospitalized or chronically ill patients, staphylococci and/or gram-negative microorganisms are responsible for

Table 18–6 Epidemiologic Associations Between Predisposing Conditions and Pneumonia

Predisposing conditions	Organism(s)
Splenectomy	*Streptococcus pneumoniae*
Influenza	*S. pneumoniae, Haemophilus influenzae, Staphylococcus aureus*
Aspiration	Anaerobes, mixed flora
Pulmonary neoplasm	*S. pneumoniae, H. influenzae,* anaerobes
Atypical pneumonia	*Legionella pneumophila*
COPD	*S. pneumoniae, H. influenzae, L. pneumophila, Branhamella catarrhalis*
Neutropenia	*Pseudomonas aeruginosa,* enteric gram-negative bacilli, *S. aureus*
Contaminated respiratory equipment	*P. aeruginosa, Klebsiella pneumoniae*
AIDS	*Pneumocystis carinii*
Chronic alcoholism	*S. pneumoniae, H. influenzae, Klebsiella* species, *Legionella* species, *S. aureus,* anaerobes
Pulmonary alveolar proteinosis	*Nocardia asteroides*

a significant number of bacterial pneumonias. Empiric therapy in these patients should consist of a third-generation cephalosporin plus an aminoglycoside. In immunocompromised patients, maximum doses of each drug are required as well as erythromycin to include coverage of *Legionella pneumophila*. If *Pneumocystis carinii* is suspected, high intravenous doses of TMP-SMX should be added, especially if a diffuse interstitial pattern is present on chest films. Antibiotic therapy should be narrowed as soon as the pathogen is identified.

The anticipated response of bacterial pneumonias to antibiotic therapy is variable, but, in general, improvements in the chest x-ray are delayed and infiltrates may progress in the initial stages of appropriate treatment, making other clinical parameters more valuable for therapeutic monitoring early in the course (e.g., serial evaluations of Gram-stained sputum). If the patient responds to initial therapy and then deteriorates, the possibility of a superinfection or a complication of pneumonia such as empyema should be considered.

OBSTRUCTIVE PULMONARY DISEASE AND ACUTE RESPIRATORY FAILURE

Chronic obstructive pulmonary disease (COPD) represents one of the major geriatric health problems in the United States. It accounts for more than 44,000 deaths annually and is second only to heart disease as a cause of morbidity and mortality. The complications of both COPD and its therapy are life threatening in the elderly and must be dealt with rapidly and effectively.[7,17,18]

The term COPD refers to a wide variety of disease processes that have in common a reduced expiratory airflow. Most elderly patients with COPD fall into the major categories of asthma, chronic bronchitis, and emphysema. Many of these patients manifest an overlap syndrome made up of several or all of the components (e.g., chronic bronchitis accompanied by acute exacerbations of asthma). These diseases have unique characteristics that must be understood by emergency physicians who care for patients in respiratory failure.

Asthma is characterized by an increased responsiveness of the tracheobronchial tree to various stimuli and is manifested by diffuse narrowing of the airways. The narrowing varies considerably from time to time whether spontaneously or as a result of treatment, and pathology consists of airway smooth muscle hypertrophy and constriction, mucosal inflammation with edema, and mucous hypersecretion. Smooth spasm probably accounts for the rapidly reversible types of acute asthma, while inflammatory edema and mucous plugging of the airway account for more nonresponsive forms of the disease.

The term chronic bronchitis denotes a clinical syndrome characterized by recurrent bronchial hypersecretion clinically diagnosed by the presence of chronic productive cough with no other cause, such as infection, neoplasm, or cardiac disease. Hyperplasia and hypertrophy of the mucous glands in the submucosa of the large airways are often present. In contradistinction to asthma, mucosal edema in chronic bronchitis is hemorrhagic in nature, while smooth muscle spasm is less apparent. Patients with chronic bronchitis (also called "blue bloaters") have a low PaO_2 because of altered ventilation-perfusion relationships in the lung and because of hypoventilation. The latter leads to increases in arterial $PaCO_2$. Persistent obstruction and recurrent infection can lead to necrotizing changes in bronchial walls.

Emphysema is defined as an abnormal enlargement of the air spaces distal to the terminal bronchioles associated with the destruction of alveolar walls. The diffusion capacity of the lung for carbon monoxide is reduced, reflecting loss of functional alveolar capillary membrane available for gas exchange. Since collagen and elastic fibers are destroyed, the elasticity of the lung is reduced, and this leads to premature closure of small airways. The fact that both alveolar walls and capillary beds are destroyed together tends to keep the distribution of ventilation-perfusion relationships more normal. Cyanosis and edema are not usually found until late in the course of illness. Residual volume and total lung capacity are usually increased, giving the appearance of a barrel chest, which is hyper-resonant to percussion with faint breath sounds and a prolonged expiration (i.e., "pink puffer").

The typical "exacerbation of COPD" in the elderly results from acute airway infection, which accounts for about 55% of cases. Respiratory infections cause edema of the involved mucosa, increased bronchial smooth muscle irritability, and increased mucous secretion. Airflow is limited, work of breathing increases, and dyspnea ensues. The airway abnormalities lead to ventilation-perfusion imbalances, which can precipitate further hypoxemia, respiratory acidosis, hemodynamic deterioration, and cor pulmonale. A variety of other factors associated with acute decompensation of COPD are listed in Table 18–7. Any process that augments the obstruction to airflow, adds to the work of breathing, impairs gas exchange, and/or affects pulmonary vascular resistance may worsen the patient's symptoms.

Diagnosis

The diagnosis of COPD is confirmed by pulmonary function tests. A decrease in the ratio of forced expiratory volume in one second (FEV_1) to the FVC is its hallmark. Normal patients over 60 years old can expire at least 75% of their vital capacity in the first second (FEV_1/FVC = 75%). A ratio of FEV_1/FVC of 65 to 75% indicates mild obstruction, 50 to 65% is moderate obstruction, and less than 50% is severe obstruction. Measurement of lung volumes is less critical but often reflects hyperinflation and air trapping. Pulmonary function tests are important

Table 18–7 Indications for Mechanical Ventilation in COPD

1. Severe respiratory acidosis, hypoxemia, and altered mental status such that the patient cannot cooperate with conservative treatment

2. Failure of an aggressive treatment regimen to correct acidosis and hypoxia associated with increasing somnolence

3. Progressive respiratory muscle fatigue

4. Inability to expectorate copious secretions associated with progressive deterioration

5. Cardiopulmonary arrest

not only for diagnosis but also for quantitation of the severity of disease. Acute respiratory failure from COPD rarely occurs until FEV_1 is less than 1 liter and becomes increasingly likely as the FEV_1 falls below this value.

The diagnosis of COPD-induced respiratory failure is made on the basis of clinical presentation and the ABGs while the patient is breathing room air. A common definition is an arterial oxygen tension (PaO_2) less than 50 mm Hg and/or an arterial carbon dioxide tension ($PaCO_2$) greater than 55 mm Hg associated with a worsening of the patient's symptoms compared to his or her baseline condition. Uncompensated respiratory acidosis provides an additional clue for differentiating acute respiratory failure (ARF) from chronic respiratory failure. The increased $PaCO_2$ and widened alveolar-arterial O_2 gradient (> 40 mm Hg) reflect severe ventilation-perfusion mismatch (the major mechanism of abnormal gas exchange in COPD).

At the time of presentation, symptoms and signs of ARF are not dissimilar from the steady state but are usually more marked in degree, especially dyspnea at rest and the use of accessory respiratory muscles.

Respiratory alternans or paradoxical breathing with tachypnea and CO_2 retention indicates inspiratory muscle fatigue. Auscultation of the chest may demonstrate rales, rhonchi, wheezes, tracheal stridor, or absent breath sounds resulting from poor air movement. Cyanosis may be newly present or more pronounced. Pulsus paradoxus and tachycardia result from the increased work of breathing. A loud pulmonic component of the second heart sound, a parasternal heave, or tricuspid insufficiency may reflect elevated pulmonary artery pressures. Elevated neck veins, tender enlarged liver, and peripheral edema indicate cor pulmonale (Figure 18–8). In extreme cases, mental confusion, extreme anxiety, stupor, or coma may be present as a result of the profound hypoxemia and hypercapnia.

While emergency treatment is being initiated, a thorough search should be made for the precipitating cause of the respiratory failure. (See Table 18–8.) Sputum examination with Gram stain and culture, CBC, and electrolyte determinations should be done. A theophylline level is needed if the patient is taking such medication. The chest x-ray is seldom diagnostic; there is evidence of overinflation in 60% of patients, including a narrow and elongated heart shadow, flattening of the diaphragm, increased AP diameter, and accentuation of thoracic kyphosis. ECG changes are nonspecific but may include right ventricular hypertrophy, P-pulmonale, and low QRS voltage. The ECG is useful in the detection and monitoring of dysrhythmias associated with COPD.

TREATMENT

While the prospects of "curing" a patient of emphysema, chronic bronchitis, or asthma are poor, prompt institution of appropriate drug therapy in the emergency depart-

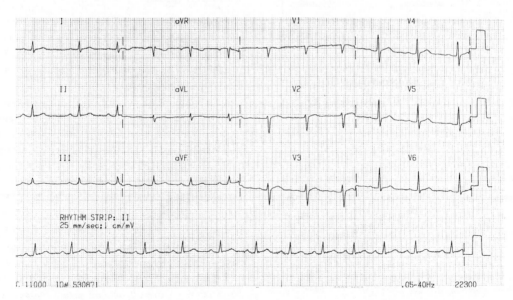

Figure 18–8 ECG from an 80-year-old patient with COPD. Note the low voltage and the right shift of P and QRS axis.

Table 18–8   Causes of Acute Decompensation in COPD

Common	Uncommon
Tracheobronchitis	Pneumothorax
Pneumonia	Pleural effusion
Aspiration	Chest wall injury
Lobar atelectasis	Neuromuscular
Pulmonary emboli	Toxic fumes
Bronchospasm	Abdominal problem affecting
Left ventricular failure	mechanics of breathing
Cardiac arrhythmia	Head injury affecting
Noncompliance with therapy	respiration
Adverse drug effects	Cerebral accident
Removal of hypoxic drive	Metabolic alkalosis
Surgery	Other systemic illnesses
	Electrolyte abnormalities
	($\downarrow K^+$, $\downarrow PO_4^=$, $\downarrow Mg^{++}$)

ment and adjunctive measures can keep the elderly patient from developing ARF. Therapy of COPD is aimed at correcting life-threatening hypoxemia, improving airflow, treating primary or secondary infection, and avoiding complications. About 75% or more of patients with COPD-induced respiratory failure can usually be managed conservatively, without an artificial airway or mechanical ventilation (Figure 18–9).

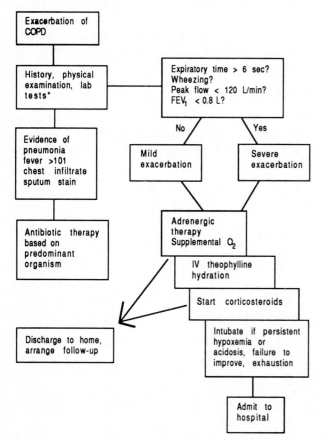

*Lab tests: spirometry, chest x-ray, ABGs, theophylline blood levels

Figure 18–9   Treatment of COPD.

Oxygen Therapy

The mainstay of therapy in respiratory failure is supplemental oxygen. An increase in inspired FIO_2 improves tissue O_2 delivery, decreases bronchoconstriction, and reverses the hypoxia-induced pulmonary hypertension. This reduces the afterload burden on the right ventricle and improves cardiac output. However, many patients rely on their hypoxic ventilatory drive for respiratory stimulation. High PaO_2 produced by overzealous use of supplemental oxygen can lead to hypercapnia with CO_2 narcosis and acidosis by shutting off the hypoxic drive.

After an initial arterial sample is drawn, 24% O_2 is administered by Venturi mask. The goal of O_2 therapy is to maintain the PaO_2 in the range of 55 to 65 mm Hg. Small increases in a PaO_2 below 60 mm Hg will produce large changes in arterial O_2 content. The Venturi mask may be changed to deliver 28% or 30% O_2 if necessary. Delivering oxygen by nasal cannula does not provide a flow that is adequately quantifiable. The breathing pattern of a critically ill patient is such that, with rapid shallow respirations, the O_2 delivered to the patient at 1 to 2 L/min by nasal cannula may actually be excessive (> 30%). ABGs must be repeated to monitor the response of supplemental O_2. Continuous ear oximetry or conjunctival oximetry may replace the need for repetitive arterial sampling.

The clinician should not be alarmed with the almost expected rise in $PaCO_2$ with oxygen administration. As long as the patient remains coherent, easily arousable, and does not develop profound acidemia (pH < 7.30), conservative treatment with the low-flow oxygen should continue.

Bronchodilators

Aminophylline and theophylline represent the cornerstone of oral bronchodilator therapy for the elderly asthmatic, bronchitic, or cardiac patient.[19,20] They are metabolized by the liver, and clearance is remarkably sensitive to hepatic dysfunction caused by disease (primary and hypoxia-induced) or low-flow states (congestive heart failure and propranolol-induced).

Complications of aminophylline include seizures, which may even occur at therapeutic levels, increased angina, palpitations, and arrhythmias. Nervousness and lack of sleep are also encountered in the geriatric population. Aminophylline toxicity in the elderly may also mimic chronic organic brain syndrome, multi-infarct dementia, and psychosis. Draw blood levels on patients who display a constellation of symptoms and who are taking an aminophylline preparation.

Certain drug interactions may precipitate aminophylline toxicity. Cimetidine and other liver-metabolized antibiotics (erythromycin, clindamycin) decrease excretion of aminophylline. Ephedrine and other sympathomimetic agents, in combination with aminophylline, may cause excessive CNS stimulation, precipitating bizarre behavior and sleeplessness.

Because of rapid onset of action and significant bronchodilator effects, beta-adrenergic agents and/or theophylline are initial agents of choice in ARF. Beta-adrenergic agents, given either subcutaneously or by inhalation (via nebulization), produce greater and more rapid bronchodilatation than intravenous aminophylline and, when used alone, are adequate therapy for most patients with mild to moderate obstruction. For patients with more severe degrees of obstruction ($FEV_1/FVC < 50\%$), a beta-adrenergic agent in combination with intravenous aminophylline is recommended.

Older nonselective bronchodilators, such as epinephrine and isoproterenol, have given way to new drugs with longer duration of action and more selective action on the bronchial tree (beta-2 adrenergic activity). In older patients and those with cardiovascular problems, we prefer to use a relatively beta-2-specific adrenergic agonist, administered via inhalation through nebulization. Albuterol (Ventolin, Proventil) is now available in this country as a nebulized solution (5 mg/mL) in doses of 2.5 to 5 mg every 20 minutes as needed ($\times$ 6 doses). Metaproterenol (Alupent, Metaprel) is marketed in a 5% solution for inhalation. Doses of 0.3 to 0.5 mL (15 to 25 mg) diluted in 2.5 mL normal saline may be given hourly for 3 to 4 doses, then every 3 to 4 hours thereafter. The duration of action for albuterol and metaproterenol is approximately 4 to 6 hours.

Intravenous aminophylline, which is 85% anhydrous theophylline, has been shown to improve airflow obstruction in chronic bronchitis and emphysema. Besides its specific effect on the airways, theophylline benefits the patient by augmenting the ventilatory response to hypoxia, increasing respiratory muscle contractility, and improving right and left ventricular performance. The therapeutic range of serum theophylline is 10 to 20 mg per liter. For the patient who needs immediate relief and who is not already receiving theophylline therapy, a loading dose (5.6 mg/kg ideal body weight) is necessary to promptly produce a therapeutic serum level. If theophylline monitoring is unavailable and the patient has been taking oral theophylline preparations at home, we recommend decreasing the loading dose by 50% or utilizing maintenance infusions alone. A simple nomogram for the maintenance infusion rate is 0.5 mg/kg per hour in patients over 65; 0.25 mg/kg per hour in elderly patients with liver or cardiac disease. Close monitoring of the serum theophylline concentration is essential since clearance in critically ill patients may fluctuate. Adverse effects of serum concentration above 25 mg per liter include cardiac arrhythmias and seizures.

A third method of bronchodilatation is the use of an aerosolized parasympatholytic, such as atropine sulfate. The mechanism of action of these drugs appears to be a blocking of the normal baseline cholinergic tone to the bronchial smooth muscle, thus resulting in bronchodilatation. Ipratropium bromide (Atrovent) is a derivative of atropine recently marketed in this country for inhalation treatment of patients with COPD. It has additive bronchodilating effects when combined with beta-adrenergic agonists and has fewer complications than atropine sulfate.

Corticosteroids

The benefit of corticosteroids in patients with COPD and respiratory failure is no longer considered controversial.[21,22] Some investigators note significant improvement in pulmonary function testing as early as 1 hour after intravenous administration, with peak effects in 4 to 8 hours. Although the exact mechanism of action is not well understood, there are many studies that demonstrate the rapid effect of the drug on inflammatory-cell populations, heightened sensitivity of the bronchial airways to beta-adrenergic stimulation, and inhibition of bronchoconstrictor substances.

The optimal dose of glucocorticoids has not been established, but most physicians give 0.5 to 1.0 mg/kg body weight methylprednisolone (or equivalent) initially and repeat every 4 to 8 hours, with tapering after results of pulmonary function testing improve. Others believe that higher doses (500 mg methylprednisolone) are required initially to overcome steroid resistance. Currently, it is our practice to administer 250 mg of hydrocortisone succinate as a slow bolus intravenously every 4 to 6 hours. Adverse reactions include hypokalemia, hypertension, hyperglycemia, muscle weakness, and psychological abnormalities, but these are rare when corticosteroids are used for a short time.

Optimal Corticosteroid Tapering Schedule Following Exacerbation of Asthma

Although corticosteroids have been known to be effective in the treatment of severe asthma for more than 30 years, no adequate data exist to help the emergency physician determine how rapidly steroids can safely be withdrawn in patients who have experienced an acute exacerbation of their illness. Published recommendations run the gamut, from a few days to several months, but controversy persists, with some experts claiming that rapid tapering of corticosteroid therapy is associated with a higher exacerbation and hospital readmission rate, while other experts claim that long tapering schedules place patients at risk for complications of long-term corticosteroid therapy.

Given the clinical importance, economic implication, and widespread use of this outpatient prescribing practice, the investigators[20a] conducted a randomized, double-blind, placebo-controlled trial to determine whether a long corticosteroid tapering following an exacerbation of asthma reduced the likelihood of re-exacerbation and/or readmission to the hospital.

Non-steroid-dependent adult men (n = 43) — hospitalized for asthma exacerbations and treated with steroids acutely during a 1-year period — were randomly assigned to corticosteroid tapering regimens of 1 or 7 weeks, following an 8-day course of high-dose corticosteroid therapy. Specifically, the short taper consisted of 7 days using daily prednisone doses of 45, 30, 25, 20, 15, 10, and 5 mg; the long tapering consisted of each of the above doses for 7 days each for a total of 7 weeks.

With respect to clinical deterioration for each dosage schedule, this study found no significant difference between the long-taper and short-taper groups in their rate of re-exacerbation (41% versus 52%) or readmission (22% versus 21%) during the 12-week study period. Failure was defined as a re-exacerbation of asthma requiring additional high-dose corticosteroid therapy during the 12-week study period. Patients who did not have a re-exacerbation during the 12 weeks were evaluated with spirometry, with no significant differences occurring between the two groups. Those patients who required mechanical ventilation for their initial hospitalization (n = 7) or who reported more than 2 days of worse than usual dyspnea during the 12-week period (n = 20) had high rates of re-exacerbation (86% and 80%, respectively). Confirming the clinical impressions of some experts, the results of this trial also indicate that more patients in the long-term taper group reported corticosteroid side effects (41% versus 14%), including weight gain, edema, easy bruising, and acne. Based on rigorous statistical analysis, the authors contend that their results provide reasonable certainty (90%) that a long taper does not result in a large reduction (50% or more) in re-exacerbations compared to a short taper. Moreover, they conclude that the relapse rate is high in this population regardless of the corticosteroid tapering regimen employed and that a long taper does not justify its routine use.

Corticosteroid therapy is pivotal to the management of exacerbations of asthma that fail to respond to conventional bronchodilator therapy. Curiously, despite the universal use of high-dose, short-course steroid therapy to treat this disorder, no previous studies have addressed the important question of how rapidly corticosteroid therapy should be withdrawn following an exacerbation. The value of conducting such a study is clear. If not associated with an increased readmission of treatment failure rates, the use of a short-term tapering schedule, because of its reduced likelihood of steroid-induced side effects, would have a significant clinical advantage over a long-term tapering regimen.

Based on this clinical trial, physicians can expect a short-term (7 days) tapering of prednisone therapy in adult men to be just as effective as a long-term (7 weeks) tapering regimen and to be associated with a significantly lower incidence of side effects. Although this recommendation will apply to large numbers of patients, three aspects of this study deserve comment. First, the patients receiving systemic corticosteroids at the time of initial exacerbation were excluded from the study. Second, most of the patients in this study were older men (mean age, 63 years) with histories of heavy smoking and abnormal spirometry, whose clinical picture would be considered consistent with COPD with a reversible component. This condition is frequently indistinguishable from asthma. Finally, those included in the study tended to have severe exacerbations as evidenced by the need for mechanical ventilation (16%) and high hospital readmission rates. These factors should be considered before extrapolating the results of this investigation to all outpatients with exacerbation of reversible airway disease.

Epinephrine

Asthma is a reversible but serious respiratory condition that still claims more than 2,000 lives annually in the United States. For the past 80 years, the rapid reversal of acute bronchospasm and hypoxemia associated with asthma using subcutaneous epinephrine has been confirmed by numerous investigators. Despite its efficacy, many physicians are reluctant to administer subcutaneous epinephrine to acute asthmatics 40 years of age or older, especially those with concomitant heart disease or a history of hypertension, because of the potent cardiovascular effects of the drug. A group conducted a study[20b] to determine whether the administration of subcutaneous epinephrine (0.3 mL, 1:1000) is associated with an increased risk of cardiovascular side effects — adverse hemodynamic consequences and arrhythmias — in patients more than 40 years of age as compared with patients younger than 40.

Conducting their prospective investigation in a large urban teaching hospital, these researchers administered three subcutaneous doses of 0.3 mL 1:1000 epinephrine 20 minutes apart to 95 adult asthmatics 15 to 96 years of age during 108 asthma exacerbations. Thirty-nine of the 108 episodes occurred in patients over the age of 40, 48.7% of whom were men. Patients were diagnosed as having an acute asthmatic attack if they had had an established history of reversible bronchospasm, dyspnea, or wheezing on presentation and if they had diminished peak expiratory flow rates. Individuals with a previous history of chronic obstructive lung disease, chronic bronchitis, or an acute myocardial infarction, as well as patients presenting with angina or those who had received epinephrine prior to admission, were considered ineligible. In addition, the use of aerosolized adrenergic agents was prohibited during the study period.

Heart rhythm and rate, blood pressure, respiratory rate, and clinical response were prospectively evaluated before, during, and after administration of epinephrine doses. The investigators found that initial systolic blood pressures were higher in the older than younger age group (146 ± 4.2 versus 130.6 ± 3.2 mm Hg), while the incidence of sinus tachycardia was not significantly different (49.3% older versus 59% younger) between the two groups. The only significant difference ($p < 0.0033$) between asthmatics in the two age groups occurred after the first dose of epinephrine when mean systolic blood pressure was observed to decrease by 9.5 ± 3.3 mm Hg in patients older than 40 years, while it increased 1.3 ± 1.9 mm Hg in the younger age group.

The authors noted there was no significant difference in the occurrence of ventricular arrhythmias between patients less than and older than 40 years of age, although isolated ventricular premature beats (VPBs < 10/hr) were observed after treatment in 11.6% of the younger patients and in 21.6% of those over 40 ($p > 0.05$). There were no adverse consequences from these ventricular irregularities. While atrial premature beats (APBs) occurred significantly more often in the older than younger age groups (32.4% versus 10.1%, $p < 0.05$), all atrial tachycardias resolved spontaneously without symptomatology or adverse cardiac consequences. Of special interest is the fact that mean systolic and diastolic blood pressures, heart rate, and respiratory rate decreased as bronchoconstriction was relieved and respiratory flow rates improved with epinephrine therapy in the older age group.

Clinical improvement was similar in each of the populations studied, with an average increase in peak flow rates of 47.1%, 24.5%, and 25.1% after the first, second, and third doses of subcutaneous epinephrine, respectively.

This study has important implications for the initial pharmacologic treatment of the adult asthmatic. A nonselective alpha- and beta-adrenergic agonist, epinephrine has long been considered standard therapy for acute asthma. It relaxes bronchial smooth muscle and constricts bronchial arterioles, reaching a detectable serum level within 5 to 10 minutes after subcutaneous injection and attaining peak blood levels between 20 to 40 minutes. Because of its chronotropic effect on the sinoatrial node and positive inotropic effect on the myocardium, however, epinephrine can increase myocardial irritability and oxygen consumption, thereby precipitating cardiac arrhythmias in susceptible individuals.

While many practitioners routinely use epinephrine to relieve asthma in the young adult and pediatric patient, the proarrhythmogenic potential of epinephrine has deterred its use in older adults, especially those with preexisting cardiac disease or hypertension. This is unfortunate, since subcutaneous epinephrine is a relatively inexpensive, easily administered, and efficacious bronchodilator. In the older age group, many experts advocate aerosolized, inhaled selective sympathomimetic agents, which, although just as efficacious as parenteral epinephrine, have been associated with fewer cardiovascular side effects. It should be noted, however, that the cost difference between injection and inhalation treatment is substantial. In most institutions, subcutaneous epinephrine 1:1,000 is approximately one third the cost of sympathomimetic inhalation therapy.

The result of this limited study suggests that use of subcutaneous epinephrine can probably be safely expanded to include selected asthmatic patients over 40 years of age, providing these individuals have not had a recent myocardial infarction and do not report anginal symptoms on presentation. The use of epinephrine in older patients with recent silent myocardial infarction or severe coronary ischemia as determined by ECG findings was not specifically evaluated in this study and, therefore, the safety of its use in this population remains questionable.

Mechanical Ventilation

Despite aggressive intervention therapy, a number of elderly patients with COPD will require mechanical ventilation. This decision should not be based exclusively on the degree of hypoxemia or hypercapnia, but on the patient's mental, acid-base, and physical status. Indications for intubation in COPD are summarized in Table 18–7. In general, however, the presence of acute respiratory acidosis unresponsive to initial pharmacotherapeutic measures is an absolute indication for emergency intubation.

By monitoring the patient, obtaining serial ABGs, and having the equipment and personnel to intubate and institute mechanical ventilatory support promptly, a decision can be deferred while other therapy is administered. While the ED physician may wish to avoid intubation in the elderly patient, allowing the situation to deteriorate can be disastrous.

There are several aspects of ventilator management that are unique to this subgroup of patients. At the time of intubation, most geriatric patients will be exhausted from the work of breathing. Respiratory muscles can be put at rest without the risk of disuse atrophy by assist-control or intermittent mandatory ventilation (IMV). The machine rate is set high enough to assume 60 to 70% of patient's ventilatory needs. At least 24 to 48 hours of continuous ventilator rest should be given before considering weaning procedures. Tidal volumes of 8 to 10 mL/kg usually are sufficient. To avoid air trapping, flow rates should be adjusted to allow adequate time for full expiration. In most cases, an inspiratory to expiratory time ratio of 1:2 to 1:3 is satisfactory, though the respiratory rate may have to be decreased to achieve this. The goal of ventilator therapy is not to normalize blood gas values.

The supplemental oxygen should be titrated to maintain an adequate PaO_2 level of at least 60 mm Hg but not so much that the ventilatory drive is suppressed. Patients with pre-existing CO_2 retention should be ventilated in such a manner as to return them to their baseline $PaCO_2$. Attempts to impose a normal $PaCO_2$ (i.e., 40 mm Hg) on these patients will cause alkalosis and may make it more difficult to wean the patient from the respirator. The baseline $PaCO_2$ can be determined from previous medical records or ventilating until a low normal pH is attained. The time spent on the ventilator should be kept as short as possible. Prolonged mechanical ventilation leads to problems with muscular dyscoordination, risks of barotrauma, infection, alteration in normal acid/base equilibrium, and a general decline in overall status.

PREVENTION OF COMPLICATIONS

A number of complications are so frequent in hypercapnic patients that strategies should be instituted from the outset to detect them early and, if possible, to prevent them. Some of the important complications include:

Arrhythmias
Infections
Pneumothorax
Cor pulmonale
Secondary erythrocytosis
Pulmonary embolism
Hypokalemia
Decreased phosphate
Peptic ulcer disease

Patients with acute or chronic respiratory failure are likely to develop cardiac arrhythmias. Perhaps the most important of these are multifocal atrial tachycardia, ventricular tachyarrhythmias, ventricular premature contractions, and atrial fibrillation. Specific drug therapy may be needed. The most frequent causes of arrhythmias in COPD patients are hypoxemia, hypokalemia, excessive use of sympathomimetic drugs, and digitalis toxicity. Fluorocarbons, the "inert" component of many aerosolized medications, are also arrhythmogenic.

Infection — either confined to the lungs or systemic — is a constant threat to the patient with ARF. Patients may present with infection as a precipitating cause for ARF, or they may develop it during hospitalization (nosocomial infection). Efforts to mobilize secretions are important and include hydration, intermittent positive pressure breathing (IPPB), and ultrasonic nebulization. Antibiotics should be used at the first sign of infection. (See Table 18–6.) The most common pathogens are *Streptococcus pneumoniae, Haemophilus influenzae,* and viral agents.

Pneumothorax may occur in patients with ARF who are not mechanically ventilated; but it appears to be substantially more frequent with positive pressure ventilation (barotrauma). This condition must be recognized early as it may prove rapidly fatal in these compromised patients. Sudden deterioration of the patient — or apparent "malfunction" of the respirator — may signal pneumothorax. In ventilated patients, the best safeguard is to avoid high ventilatory pressures or PEEP.

Patients with ARF may have elevated levels of antidiuretic hormone, decreased renal blood flow, and right-sided heart failure, all leading to increased extravascular lung water, which will respond to diuretics. Digitalis preparations appear to have little benefit in the routine treatment of cor pulmonale and right-sided heart failure. Unless some concomitant left ventricular failure is present, these agents should be avoided. Vasodilators might directly relieve pulmonary hypertension or improve function by causing afterload reduction; they also can reduce preload and worsen right ventricular function. At the present time, these drugs should not be considered as standard modes of therapy for the COPD patient with acute decompensation.

Immobilization, dehydration, right-sided heart failure, and erythrocytosis make patients with ARF especially susceptible to deep venous thrombosis and its complication, pulmonary embolism. Two strategies are available to the practitioner to reduce this complication: 1) monitoring of the lower extremities with impedance plethysmography and radiofibrinogen leg scanning and 2) administration of prophylactic "low-dose" heparin.

Electrolyte disturbances are frequent in the elderly and should be corrected. Chronic CO_2 retention and diuretic therapy lead to a hypochloremic alkalosis and potassium wasting by the kidney. Potassium preparations that do not include chloride are obviously of no value in treating this problem. Hypophosphatemia, which can occur after a few days of IV glucose therapy, can impair oxygen delivery to tissues through its effect on the oxyhemoglobin dissociation curve. Adequate nutritional support is essential during respiratory failure.

One common complication of ARF is gastrointestinal bleeding, usually caused by gastritis or frank ulceration of the stomach. Careful monitoring of hematocrit and stools for occult blood is indicated. Routine administration of antacids, H_2 antagonists, and/or sucralfate is now practiced in many critical care units.

PULMONARY EMBOLISM

Pulmonary embolism (PE) is a life-threatening cause of dyspnea that must always be considered in the elderly patient with shortness of breath.[9] Probably no acute cardiopulmonary disorder is more frequently misdiagnosed. Some 600,000 cases of symptomatic PE occur in the United States each year; PE is the contributing cause of death in 200,000 patients. As many as 70 to 90% of elderly patients dying in the hospital have PE at autopsy. The increased incidence of this condition reflects a number of factors associated with aging that predispose to thrombus formation, including immobility, congestive heart failure, venous disease, obesity, malignancy, hip trauma, and hypercoagulable states (Figure 18–10).

Diagnosis

In over 90% of patients, the clot originates deep in the venous system of the pelvis and thighs. Of these clots, 50% will embolize. Calf thrombi rarely embolize but extend into the thigh in about 15% of patients. Unfortunately, the clinical diagnosis of deep venous thrombosis of the lower extremities is extremely difficult and is missed in about one half of the cases.

The presenting symptoms of PE may be classic — pleuritic chest pain, dyspnea, tachypnea, and hemoptysis of sudden onset — or unusual, such as syncope and hypotension. The clinical picture largely depends upon the extent of vascular occlusion as well as on the patient's prior cardiovascular status. Because of poor collateral circulation, elderly patients are more likely to develop pulmonary infarction after PE, which may mimic some of the clinical manifestations of bacterial pneumonia. The frequencies of various symptoms and signs observed in the largest series with angiographically documented PE are shown in Table 18–9. Although the classic textbook picture is uncommon, patients generally have either dyspnea, chest pain, or tachypnea; the absence of all three symptoms makes the diagnosis of PE unlikely. Localized rales, rhonchi, wheezes, or a pleural friction rub is often seen. Other findings include unexplained fever, tachycardia, or an increased pulmonic component of the second heart sound.

Since symptoms and signs associated with PE are nonspecific, the ECG, chest radiograph, and ABG may help to increase or decrease the clinical suspicion of an embolus. The ECG is normal in more than one third of patients. The most common abnormalities are sinus tachycardia and nonspecific ST-T wave changes. Elderly patients with pre-existing cardiopulmonary disease are more likely to develop right-sided heart dysfunction with only a minor insult. Evidence of right heart strain

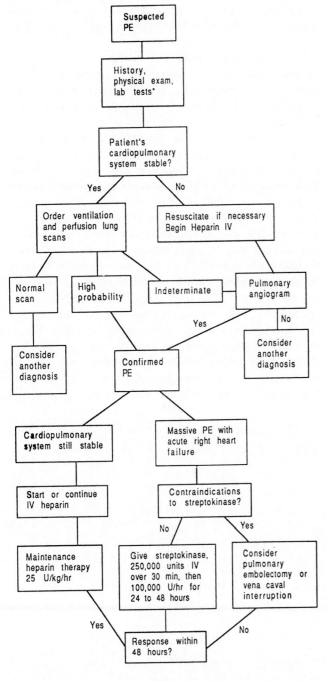

*Lab tests: chest x-ray, ECG, ABGs, plethysmography or other noninvasive test for DVT

Figure 18–10   Pulmonary embolism in elderly patients.

Table 18–9   Symptoms and Signs of Pulmonary Embolism

	Incidence (%)
Symptoms	
Dyspnea	84
Pleuritic chest pain	74
Apprehension	59
Cough	53
Hemoptysis	30
Sweats	27
Syncope	13
Signs	
Tachypnea (> 16)	92
Localized rales	58
Increased PO_2	53
Tachycardia (> 100)	44
Fever (> 37.8°C)	43
S_3, S_4 gallop	34
Thrombophlebitis	32
Murmur	23
Cyanosis	19

From Bell WR, Simon TL, and DeMets DL: The clinical features of submassive and massive pulmonary emboli, Am J Med 62:358, 1977.

includes the presence of right bundle branch block, right axis deviation, P-pulmonale and an $S_1Q_3T_3$ (S wave in lead 1, Q wave in lead 3, and an inverted T wave in lead 3) (Figure 18–11). Although the chest x-ray is frequently normal, areas of consolidation and atelectasis, usually located peripherally in the lower lung fields, can be seen. A pleural effusion, when present, is bloody in 65% of patients. Patients with massive emboli may present with a normal chest x-ray or exhibit an elevated hemidiaphragm, distended pulmonary arteries (Figure 18–12), or an area of decreased lung markings.

Laboratory studies have been of limited value as elevation of lactic dehydrogenase, SGOT, and bilirubin are not specific for pulmonary emboli. Arterial hypoxemia is common in elderly patients, especially in the presence of congestive heart failure and pneumonia. An acute decrease in arterial Po_2 unassociated with the usual conditions helps to suggest the diagnosis of pulmonary emboli. Even large emboli, however, can occur with relatively good preservation of arterial Po_2. In cases of COPD, in which PE may be particularly difficult to recognize, an unexplained respiratory alkalosis, particularly if the patient is a chronic CO_2 retainer, should always arouse suspicion of PE.

Although clinical and laboratory findings can strongly indicate pulmonary embolism, the diagnosis is confirmed only by special diagnostic procedures.[23] The lung perfusion seen is an extremely sensitive but nonspecific test for diagnosing PE (Figure 18–13). If the scan is normal, the diagnosis of an acute PE is excluded. The presence of perfusion defects is often difficult to interpret, especially in the presence of obstructive pulmonary disease, congestive heart failure, pneumonia, asthma, or carcinoma. Even the addition of a ventilation scan — to look for segmental areas of high ventilation-perfusion ratios — may not be helpful in the aged, especially those with coexistent respiratory disorders. In general, 10% of patients with a low probability scan, 30% of patients with a moderate probability scan, and 90% of patients with a high probability scan have a pulmonary embolism.

Since the major source of emboli is deep venous thrombosis of the leg veins, several methods have been developed to detect this condition. Doppler ultrasound, radioactive fibrinogen labeling, impedance plethysmography, and venography are most commonly used. Venography is the most specific but has the highest morbidity (Figure 18–14).

Pulmonary angiography remains the "gold standard" for diagnosing PE. The utilization of selective arteriography, accompanied by the recent addition of geometric magnification and oblique techniques, has significantly enhanced the diagnostic sensitivity of this test. Pulmonary vessels as small as 0.5 mm in diameter can be visualized. However, pulmonary angiography has a definite but low morbidity and mortality. Elderly patients with ventricular aneurysms, cardiomyopathies, or severe congestive heart failure are particularly prone to complications. Hockberger and Rothstein[25] have recommended the following indications for performing angiography: 1) when the ventilation-perfusion lung scan is of intermediate or low probability but the clinical picture is highly suggestive of pulmonary embolism, 2) when assessing patients at potential high risk for bleeding complications during anticoagulation therapy (e.g., recent cerebrovascular accident, active gastrointestinal bleeding), and 3) when managing unstable patients who are thought to be suffering from massive pulmonary emboli prior to the use of expensive and potentially hazardous fibrinolytic therapy or surgical embolectomy.

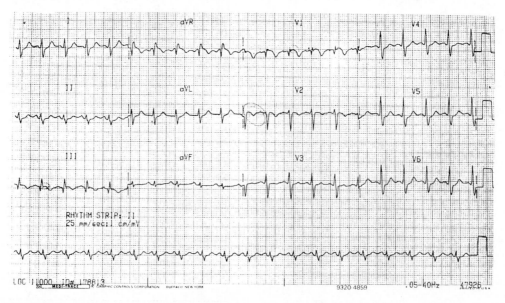

Figure 18–11 ECG revealing sinus tachycardia and bundle branch block. Note the $S_1Q_3T_3$ pattern. This patient succumbed shortly after this ECG to a massive saddle embolism.

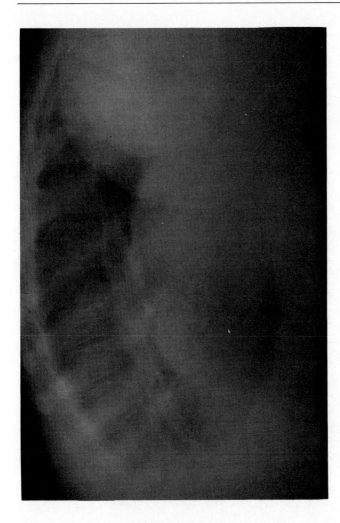
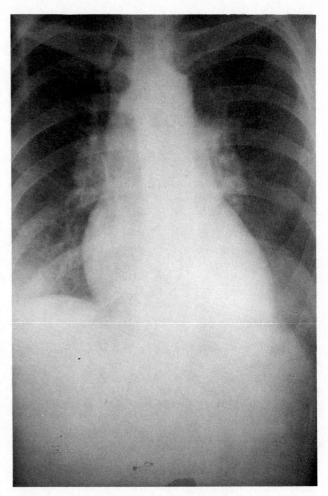

Figure 18–12 Acutely dyspneic patient with pleuritic chest pain. Note the mild cardiomegaly and prominent dilated pulmonary arteries. Distal oligemia confirms Westermark's sign. Bilateral pulmonary emboli were subsequently confirmed.

Treatment

Emergency treatment of acute PE includes cardiopulmonary stabilization and prevention of further embolization. Humidified oxygen, analgesics for pain, bed rest, warm soaks, and elevation for thrombophlebitis should be employed as soon as possible. In severe cases, continuous positive pressure oxygen may prove useful, particularly when pulmonary edema is present. Hemodynamic monitoring and support of the circulation as well as pulmonary vasodilators are necessary to prevent right heart failures. Aminophylline may prove useful if dyspnea is prominent or pulmonary edema is present.

Heparin continues to be the mainstay of therapy for the majority of patients with pulmonary emboli. Indeed, in the absence of any absolute contraindications (e.g., uncontrolled bleeding, hemorrhagic lesions, allergy to heparin, malignant hypertension), heparin therapy should be instituted immediately after a PE is suspected and before the diagnostic workup is completed. The drug's action begins immediately and can be reversed if a major com-

plication or the need for surgery arises. A loading dose of 5,000 to 15,000 units is given intravenously and is followed by a maintenance dose of 25 units/kg/hr by continuous infusion. If close monitoring of the patient is not possible, intermittent heparin therapy should be considered. In most patients with submassive PE, 5,000 to 7,500 units of heparin intravenously every 4 hours is adequate, but complications from bleeding are more common with this method. These regimens are then adjusted to maintain the activated partial thromboplastin time (A-PTT) at 1.5 to 2.5 times the control value, although rigid control may not be necessary. The goal of anticoagulation is the prevention of thrombus formation either in the diseased peripheral veins or in the lungs distal to the embolus. Heparin does little to hasten the resolution of existing thrombi.

In life-threatening pulmonary emboli, a decision has to be made between embolectomy and the use of urokinase or streptokinase thrombolytic therapy. Embolectomy has a 25% case fatality rate and is used much less frequently than in the past.[24] Thrombolytic agents provide the only

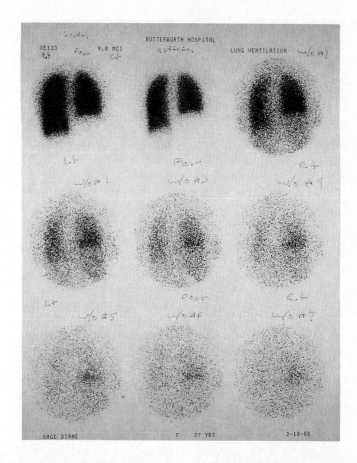

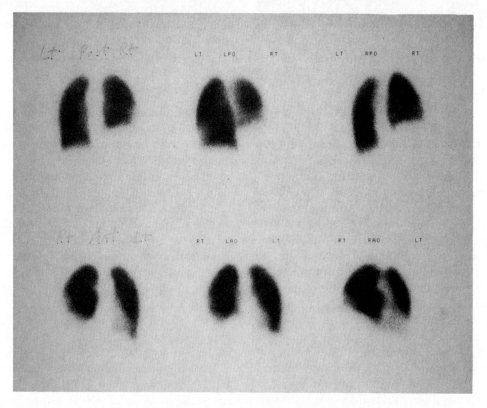

Figure 18–13 Ventilation/perfusion scans revealing a single large perfusion defect involving the lateral segment of the right middle lobe. Ventilatory pattern does not match, therefore constituting a V̇/Q̇ mismatch with high clinical suspicion of pulmonary emboli.

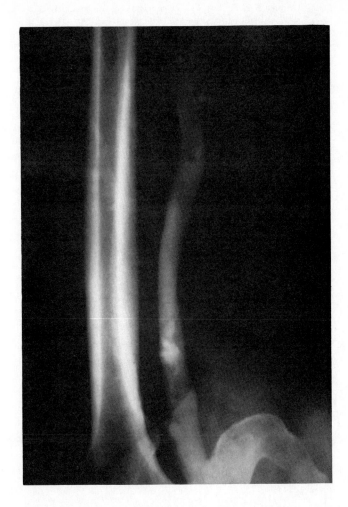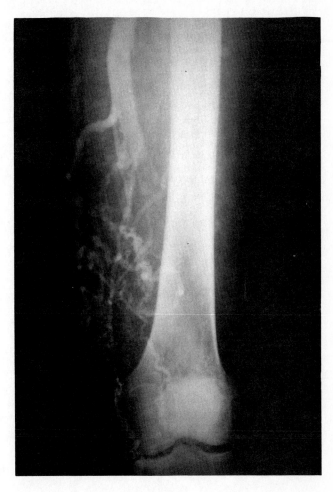

Figure 18–14 Thrombophlebitis of femoral vein with proximal reconstitution via collaterals. Irregularities can also be noted in the deep femoral vein.

medical means for directly lysing a formed thrombus. There is no demonstrable difference in the efficacy of the two drugs. However, streptokinase may be antigenic, and urokinase is approximately four times more expensive. Tissue plasminogen activator (TPA) appears to be very effective in the acute phase of pulmonary arterial occlusion and despite its very high cost, evidence is accumulating suggesting its effectiveness. The major indication for the use of thrombolytic therapy is in those patients with severe and persistent cardiorespiratory compromise (requirement for mechanical ventilatory support and/or hypotension after the first few hours of medical support and anticoagulation). These agents are given by bolus infusion into a peripheral vein. The incidence of major hemorrhage and intracranial bleeding is approximately twice that associated with heparin therapy, with the hemorrhage often occurring at the site of previous surgery or trauma.

REFERENCES

1. Cubanes LR et al: Bronchial hyperresponsiveness to methacholine in patients with impaired left ventricular function, N Engl J Med 320:1317, 1989.
2. Fishman AP: Cardiac asthma, N Engl J Med 320:20, 1989.
3. Gross NJ and Skorodin MS: Role of the parasympathetic system in airway obstruction due to emphysema, N Engl J Med 331:421–425, 1984.
4. Rosen RL: Acute respiratory failure and chronic obstructive lung disease, Med Clin North Am 70:895–907, 1986.
5. Moser KM: Acute respiratory failure with hypercapnia. In Moser KM and Spragg RG, editors: Respiratory emergencies, St. Louis, 1982, CV Mosby Co.
6. Mathews J: Chronic obstructive pulmonary disease. In Tintinalli JE, Rothstein RJ, and Krome RL, editors: Emergency medicine: a comprehensive study guide, New York, 1985, McGraw-Hill Book Co.
7. Francis PB: Acute respiratory failure in obstructive lung disease, Med Clin North Am 67:675–678, 1983.
8. Noseworthy TW and Anderson BJ: Massive hemoptysis, CMAJ 135:1097–1099, 1986.
9. Bell WR, Simon TL, and DeMets DL: The clinical features of submassive and massive pulmonary emboli, Am J Med 62:355–360, 1977.
10. Bynum LJ and Pierce AK: Pulmonary aspiration of gastric contents, Am Rev Respir Dis 114:1129–1136, 1976.
11. Reference deleted.
12. Garb JL et al: Differences in etiology of pneumonias in nursing home and community patients, JAMA 240:2169–2172, 1978.
13. Gleckman RA and Bergman MM: Bacterial pneumonia: specific diagnosis and treatment of the elderly, Geriatrics 42:29–41, 1987.

14. Horton JM and Pankey GA: Pneumonia in the elderly, Postgrad Med 71:114–122, 1982.

15. Rozas CJ and Goldman AL: Responses to bacterial pneumonia, Geriatrics 37:61–66, 1982.

16. Verghese A and Berk SL: Bacterial pneumonia in the elderly, Medicine (Baltimore) 62:271–283, 1983.

17. Bone RC: Treatment of respiratory failure due to advanced chronic obstructive lung disease, Arch Intern Med 140:1018–1021, 1980.

18. Davis AL: Managing the patient with advanced chronic obstructive pulmonary disease, part 1, Hosp Med 22:126–151, 1986.

19. Eaton ML et al: Efficacy of theophylline in "irreversible" airflow obstruction, Ann Intern Med 92:758–762, 1980.

20. Murciano D et al: A randomized controlled trial of theophylline in patients with C.O.P.D., N Engl J Med 320:1521, 1989.

20a. Ratto D et al: Are intravenous corticosteroids required in status asthmaticus, JAMA 260(4):527–529, 1988.

20b. Cydulka R et al: The use of epinephrine in the treatment of older adult asthmatics, Ann Emerg Med 17:322–326, 1988.

21. Klaustermeyer WB and Hale FC: The physiologic effect of an intravenous glucocorticoid in bronchial asthma, Ann Allergy 37:80–86, 1976.

22. Ellul-Micallef R and Fenech FF: Intravenous prednisone in chronic bronchial asthma, Thorax 30:312–315, 1975.

23. Tow DE and Simon AL: Comparison of lung scanning and pulmonary angiography in the detection and follow-up of pulmonary embolism: the urokinase-pulmonary embolism trial experience, Prog Cardiovasc Dis 17:239–244, 1975.

24. Thrombolytic therapy in thrombosis: a National Institutes of Health Consensus Development Conference, Ann Intern Med 93:141–144, 1980.

25. Hockberger RS and Rothstein R: Pulmonary embolism, Emerg Med Clin North Am 1:393–415, 1983.

Acute Asthma

Sandra M. Schneider, M.D., F.A.C.E.P.
and Steven E. Gentry, M.D.

Asthma is defined by the American Thoracic Society as "a disease characterized by an increased responsiveness of the trachea and bronchi to various stimuli and manifested by widespread narrowing of the airway that changes in severity either spontaneously or as a result of therapy."[1] This definition is often difficult to apply to the elderly. Because of normal physiologic changes associated with advanced age (discussed below), most elderly have fixed pulmonary deficits on which to superimpose the reversible airway obstruction of asthma. Asthma in the elderly is often diagnosed as chronic bronchitis or chronic obstructive pulmonary disease (COPD) even when asthma may coexist.

❑ Some components of this chapter that address the adult patient appear in Schwartz GR et al, editors: Emergency medicine: the essential update, Philadelphia, 1989, WB Saunders Co.

Good epidemiologic studies on the prevalence of asthma in the elderly are difficult to perform and, therefore, are fraught with error. However, available studies do emphasize that asthma is common in the elderly with or without fixed pulmonary obstruction. In one study in which patients were simply asked if they had asthma, a prevalence rate of 6 to 7% was found, and this held nearly constant from age 5 to over 70.[2] However, over 70% of the asthmatic patients over the age of 50 also gave a concurrent diagnosis of chronic bronchitis or emphysema. In the same study, all subjects were followed for 4 years, and new asthma developed in 1.4% of the population, regardless of age. The subjects over 40 who later developed asthma had a higher number of respiratory complaints on entry into the study.[2]

Another epidemiologic study looked at a randomly selected elderly population in Wales.[3] They found that 61% of this population had spirometric evidence of airway obstruction and that 41% of the population had a significant reversible component (i.e., asthma).

Although overall mortality is low (4,000 per year),[4] most deaths occur in the age group over 50.[5] In addition, morbidity is high with admission rates as high as 46% reported in this age group.[6]

PATHOGENESIS

The airways are innervated by both the sympathetic and parasympathetic nervous systems. They also are under the influence of a number of other mediators, the receptors for which line the entire bronchial tree. These factors working in combination set the bronchomotor tone of the airway at any given time and at any age. Viral respiratory infections, air pollutants, and other stimuli can heighten vagal tone,[7] thereby causing airway constriction in the larger airways, as well as increased secretion of mucus and dilation of the pulmonary vessels. The effects of alterations of sympathetic tone depend upon the type of adrenergic receptor that is stimulated.

Adrenergic receptors are divided broadly into two classes: alpha and beta. These in turn are divided into subclasses: α_1 and α_2, and β_1 and β_2. Stimulation of the β-receptors, which in the lung are predominantly β_2, results in bronchial smooth muscle relaxation and bronchodilation. Alpha stimulation, on the other hand, leads to bronchoconstriction.[7] Also, there may be other factors that are responsible for setting bronchomotor tone. For example, prostaglandin $PGF_2\alpha$ has a potent bronchoconstrictive action, while prostaglandin PGE_2 is a potent bronchodilator.[8]

The interaction of these multiple factors produces the bronchomotor tone. For example, one theory suggests there may be an abnormality in the number or function of the β-receptor allowing the α-receptors to override, leading to bronchoconstriction. Another theory suggests there is a hypersensitivity or an increased number of α-receptors, again, increasing their activity over the β-receptors, resulting in a tendency to bronchoconstriction. Use of drugs such as beta blockers may lead to bronchoconstriction in asthmatics but, interestingly enough, not in patients with normally responsive lungs.[7]

In addition to these factors, inflammation of the airway from environmental stimuli or infection may cause the development of airway edema and the emigration of inflammatory cells into the lumen of the airway. This inflammation may be associated with an increase in epithelial permeability, which precipitates a rush of fluid into the already compromised lumen. Stimuli felt to produce this type of reaction include cigarette smoke, nitrogen dioxide, and ozone.[9]

The acute asthmatic attack, then, is characterized by a combination of smooth muscle contraction of the airway, inflammation and edema within the airway wall, and increased secretion of mucus. The hypersecretion of mucus, in addition, leads to mucous plugs with small areas of atelectasis and hypoventilation. All of these mechanisms work to diminish the lumen of the airway, with resultant obstruction to airflow.

Asthma often is classified by the presence of a stimulus that reliably and repeatedly causes bronchospastic episodes. Extrinsic asthma is bronchoconstriction as the result of a specific allergen, usually airborne. In general the elderly have intrinsic asthma with no demonstrable stimuli.[3]

Many other stimuli also can precipitate acute bronchospasm. Respiratory infections are associated with asthmatic attacks in many individuals. Also, medications can contribute to bronchospastic disease. In the elderly, beta-blocking cardiac or glaucoma medications are most often implicated.[10] Also, analgesics such as aspirin and nonsteroidal anti-inflammatory agents may inhibit prostaglandin synthesis and in turn incite an acute asthmatic attack in a patient with reactive airway disease.[11,12] Environmental agents that may induce acute asthmatic attacks in susceptible patients include sulfur dioxide and metabisulfite, which are used to preserve foods and are commonly sprayed on food in salad bars and in restaurants. Sensitivity to this material is estimated to be present in up to 5% of asthmatics.[13,14] Certain food additives such as the Food and Drug Administration's (FDA) yellow no. 5 and azo dyes, which may be used in drugs, particularly in theophylline compounds, also have been reported to provoke asthmatic attacks.[15] Monosodium glutamate (MSG) has also been associated with precipitating asthma. Cigarette smoke is a potent cause of airway constriction, even in patients exposed only to "second-hand" smoke.[16] Despite a large number of anecdotal cases, one study failed to find a relationship between air pollution index and the rate of asthmatic attacks.[17]

Finally, psychologic factors may influence bronchomotor tone. Hyperventilation may induce an acute asthmatic attack.[18] In addition, factitious asthma may occur in patients with and without known psychiatric disease.

Effects of Aging

The physiologic changes that occur with advancing age contribute to the airway obstruction, and many previously compensated individuals become symptomatic in later life. Among the changes seen are changes in chest wall dynamics. Radiographic evidence of kyphosis is present in 68% of the elderly,[20] and this reduces chest wall expansion. There is increased rigidity of the chest wall due to calcification of the costal cartilages and generalized muscle stiffening.[21] This decrease in compliance leads to increased work in breathing.

Within the lung itself, there is a decrease in alveolar size and a subsequent decrease in total surface area.[21] Vital capacity decreases steadily from age 20, and the residual capacity increases by 68% by age 80.[21] Although there are no changes in airway resistance, elastic recoil decreases and lowers expiratory velocities.[21] Diffusion capacity falls 5 to 8% per decade beyond age 20.[22]

Many cardiac changes contribute to the fall in pulmonary reserve. Cardiac output decreases 1% per year from the third to ninth decade.[23] A generalized stiffness in both the heart and large vessels increases systemic and pulmonary vascular resistance,[22] which acting together produce a ventilation-perfusion mismatch and a decrease in arterial oxygen tension. Measured PO_2 falls 2.1 to 4.1 mm Hg per decade.[22]

The above factors all lead to a reduction of work capacity. In fact, the physical work capacity of the average 70-year-old is 50% that of the average 20-year-old.[21] Therefore, compensatory abilities are less, allowing the apparent emergence of previously quiescent or forgotten asthma.

CLINICAL PRESENTATION

The acute asthmatic presents with symptoms of dyspnea, coughing, and wheezing. In the young asthmatic, this presentation is classic and rarely missed. However, elderly patients may present with just cough and/or shortness of breath.[2] Many of these patients also produce copious amounts of sputum and are, therefore, classified as having chronic bronchitis. Other diagnoses may also present with cough and dyspnea, for example, congestive heart failure and occupational lung disease; these may also be concurrent illnesses.

Signs of severe life-threatening asthma that require prompt and aggressive therapy include inability to speak, change in mental status, and presence of cyanosis. Patients in very severe distress will usually sit bolt upright and will be diaphoretic.[24]

Pulsus paradoxus is another sign of severe asthma, but it should be noted that this sign may be absent in as many as 50% of acute life-threatening asthmatic attacks.[25,26] In addition, it disappears with only a minor alteration in airflow obstruction and, therefore, is not a particularly good monitoring tool.

As a rule, except for the above, history and physical exam correlate poorly with the patient's condition. There is no correlation between the duration of bronchoconstriction, or any other historical data, and the severity of bronchoconstriction as measured by pulmonary function tests.[27] Because there may be long periods of remission between attacks, a previous diagnosis of asthma may be dismissed or even forgotten.

Physicians perform poorly when asked to predict patients' clinical severity based on history and physical exam.[28] Indeed, one study suggests that the patients themselves are better predictors of their own flow rates than their physicians.[28]

Laboratory testing also has little relationship to clinical severity. White blood cell counts may show eosinophilia, or perhaps an increase in neutrophils due to either infection or intrinsic catecholamine release. Sputum samples may show signs of infection but do not predict the outcome of the asthmatic attack. Routine chest x-rays, although somewhat useful in children,[29] have been shown to be nearly worthless in most adults.[30] However, in the elderly they may differentiate congestive heart failure or pneumonia from acute bronchial asthma.

Arterial blood gases (ABGs) have been used repeatedly to assess the clinical status of patients with asthma. These tests are painful and often provide very little useful information. Many studies have now been performed that show poor correlation between the results of Po_2 or Pco_2 and pulmonary function testing.[31,32] Although it is true that an increase in Pco_2 correlates with a severe asthma attack and discloses a fatiguing asthmatic and the necessity for urgent intubation, generally this is more easily and quickly noted on the basis of physical examination and spirometry.

Transcutaneous systems now exist for monitoring of both Po_2 saturation and an estimate of Pco_2, which may eliminate the need for arterial puncture. However, abnormal vasoconstriction often is present in these patients[33] and may hamper the use of these instruments. Further data need to be collected.

The gold standard for assessing the severity of acute asthma is the pulmonary function test (PFT). Hand-held peak flowmeters and small spirometers are inexpensive and accessible to all emergency physicians. They are the best, easiest, and most appropriate way of assessing and monitoring the asthmatic patient. PFTs should be performed on all patients with acute bronchospasm who are capable of cooperating with the procedure. This should be done immediately upon entering the emergency department and thereafter at regular intervals (30 to 60 minutes) during therapy to the point of discharge. Spirometry may eliminate the need for ABGs and, therefore, the associated pain, discomfort, and expense. A second physician can then assess the patients' progress using the same guidelines and parameters. Ideally, spirometry should be followed daily on hospitalized patients.

The choice between the hand-held peak flowmeter and the bedside spirometer should depend primarily upon cost and individual circumstances. While the peak flow measurements are more effort related, a study by Nowak has shown very good correlation between peak expiratory flow rate (PEFR) and forced expiratory volume in one second (FEV_1).[34] It also has been shown that both of these parameters correlate well with symptomatology. At approximately 50% predicted FEV_1 and 45% predicted PEFR, all symptoms of acute bronchospasm are gone. All physical signs of bronchoconstriction are gone at an FEV_1 and PEFR of approximately 65% and 55% predicted, respectively.[27]

When evaluating PFTs, it is important to compare the values obtained from an individual patient to the values predicted for that patient. Factors such as age, height, and sex introduce substantial variability into PFT measurements. Using large population studies, a number of regression equations have been proposed to predict "normal" values for pulmonary function tests. In the elderly, it is preferred that "baseline" PFTs be used in assessing the severity of an acute episode.

TREATMENT

General Principles

For the most part, the treatment of acute bronchospasm in the elderly is similar to that of younger patients. Many of the agents used, however, have adverse effects that, although irritating and inconvenient in most patients, can be severely limiting in the geriatric population. Also, regimens employing several drugs often are necessary, with the resulting potential for detrimental interactions. Accordingly, great care must be taken to monitor for side effects and to adjust medication doses to prevent them. Finally, it must be recognized that many elderly patients presenting with bronchospasm also have some degree of underlying fixed obstructive lung disease. Although the goal of therapy in these patients still should be to improve airflow as much as possible, the response often is slower and less complete than that seen in younger patients.

Adrenergic Agonists

The most potent dilators of bronchial smooth muscle, and the agents with the most rapid onset, are the sympathomimetic drugs. Beta$_2$ receptors are the most common adrenergic receptors in the lung, and stimulation of these receptors causes relaxation of the bronchial smooth muscle with resultant bronchodilation. For this reason, agents that stimulate β_2-receptors ("beta-agonists") have become increasingly important in the treatment of asthma.

The prototype of the beta agonists, and the agent that has been in use for the longest time, is epinephrine. Although it is a component of a number of over-the-counter inhalers for asthma, epinephrine usually is administered by subcutaneous injection at the onset of therapy for an acute asthmatic attack. Unfortunately, epinephrine is not selective for β_2-receptors and, accordingly, causes a wide range of side effects. These include anxiety, tremor, nausea, and headache, as well as the potentially more dangerous manifestations such as tachycardia, hypertension, and arrhythmias. The prevalence of underlying cardiovascular disorders is high in the geriatric population,[35] making this group still more susceptible to these effects. Therefore, in this population parenteral epinephrine generally has been abandoned in favor of other agents that show greater specificity for β_2-receptors (Table 19–1).

Attempts to decrease adrenergic side effects have led not only to more specific agents, but to more selective methods of drug delivery. Inhalation of nebulized bronchodilator solutions, either by jet nebulizer or by metered dose inhaler (MDI), is an established, validated method for treatment of acute bronchospasm. Despite theoretical concerns regarding inadequate delivery of the medication to poorly ventilated portions of the lung, numerous studies have shown inhalation therapy with beta agonists to be as effective as parenteral administration.[36-38] Moreover, direct application of the agent to the airways allows the use of very small doses of medication, resulting in fewer adrenergic side effects while producing equipotent bronchodilation. For these reasons, inhaled beta agonists have become a mainstay of therapy for bronchospasm and are favored as the initial therapy for acute asthma in older patients with questionable cardiac status.[36-38] In addition, inhaled beta-agonists can be given on a routine basis for chronic therapy for bronchospastic disease.[39]

Although solutions delivered by jet nebulizer and properly administered MDIs appear to be equally effective in relieving bronchospasm, MDIs require significant patient effort and coordination. A number of spacers and mechanical devices (e.g., Inspriease) have been marketed to facilitate patient use of these agents. Nevertheless, jet nebulizers seem to be easier for patients to use in the acute setting. Also, many individual patients report greater symptomatic relief using jet nebulizers, making their routine use at home increasingly popular. Common preparations include metaproterenol, 0.2 ml of a 5% solution, isoetharine, 0.5 ml of a 1% solution, or albuterol, 0.5 to 1.0 ml of a 0.5% solution, brought to 2 ml with saline.

Table 19–1   Adrenergic Agents

Agent	Available forms	Pharmacokinetics (inhaled)		
		Onset (min)	Peak (min)	Duration (hr)
Nonselective				
Epinephrine	I, SC	5–10*	20	1
Ephedrine	O	60†	120–210	3–5
Beta-selective				
Isoproterenol	I, IV	5	5–10	1
Beta$_2$-selective				
Isoetharine	I	1–5	5–15	1–4
Metaproterenol	I, O	5–15	30–60	2.5–6
Terbutaline	I, O, SC	5–30	60–90	3–6
Albuterol‡	I, O, IV§	5–15	30–120	3–6

*Pharmacokinetics for subcutaneous administration.
†Pharmacokinetics for oral administration.
‡Also named "salbutamol" in Europe.
§IV form currently not available in the United States.
I = Inhaled; IV = intravenous; O = oral; SC = subcutaneous.

These may be repeated as often as every 30 to 60 minutes during the initial hours of therapy for an acute attack. For chronic therapy, MDIs are used with average doses of two puffs 2 to 4 times daily, depending on the agent used.

Theophylline

Probably no bronchodilator has engendered as much controversy in recent years as theophylline.[40] Originally the mainstay of bronchodilator therapy, many questions have arisen as to what role, if any, theophylline should play in the management of acute bronchospasm. Even the mechanism by which it works has been called into question. In the past, theophylline was thought to operate by inhibiting the enzyme phosphodiesterase, which breaks down intracellular 3' to 5' cyclic adenosine monophosphate (cAMP). High levels of cAMP cause smooth muscle relaxation, so inhibition of the metabolism of this compound results in bronchodilation.[41] Pharmacologic evidence has been presented, however, that is incompatible with this explanation.[42,43] Other theories have been proposed, including the operation of theophylline as an adenosine antagonist and the modulation of existing beta-adrenergic tone.[43-46] Nevertheless, each of these theories has inconsistencies, and a completely satisfactory explanation of the action of theophylline must await further investigation.[40]

In addition to its actions as a bronchodilator, theophylline has a number of other useful functions. These include increasing respiratory muscle contractility and resistance to fatigue, increasing respiratory drive, inhibiting mediator release, and increasing cardiac output and right ventricular function.[40] However, adverse effects also are seen, including nausea, vomiting, headache, sinus tachycardia, and, in toxic doses, confusion, seizures, and ventricular arrhythmias.[41] Moreover, the clearance of theophylline can be affected by a number of host factors, such as liver disease, smoking, congestive heart failure, and various medications.[43] Theophylline clearance also is related to the patient's age, with older patients generally metabolizing the agent more slowly.[43] For this reason, it is extremely important to monitor serum theophylline levels closely. A "therapeutic range" for theophylline concentration of 10 to 20 μg/ml generally has been accepted. However, both therapeutic effects and toxicity appear to be dose related, and there is considerable individual variation.[43,47,48] Thus, one patient may experience dose-limiting toxicity at a much lower level than another patient. Therefore, therapy should be individualized, with the goal of achieving the maximum theophylline concentration (within the therapeutic range) that does not cause undue toxicity. Considering the potential lability of theophylline clearance, however, in chronic therapy one might elect to maintain a lower level and, thereby, a larger margin of safety.

The role of theophylline in the emergency management of the severe asthmatic has been questioned. A number of reports have described an additive effect of theophylline when combined with adrenergic agents.[36,49] Other studies fail to support this finding, however.[37,50] The reasons for this inconsistency are unclear. The suggestion has been made that the variability may depend on the dose and potency of the beta-agonist used.[37] In any event, it is evident that the role of theophylline in the emergency treatment of acute bronchospasm still is in evolution. A reasonable approach is to initiate therapy with a beta-agonist, either parenteral (e.g., subcutaneous epinephrine) or inhaled (e.g., nebulized metaproterenol). If aggressive therapy with beta-agonists does not effect sufficient bronchodilation, theophylline can be added. Intravenous treatment with aminophylline, a water-soluble compound containing about 85% theophylline by weight, generally is preferred.

A number of protocols for intravenous aminophylline dosing have been described,[47,51] but as a rough guide, a loading dose of approximately 5 mg/kg is administered over 20 to 30 minutes. If the patient has been taking theophylline prior to admission, this loading dose is reduced by half. The availability of rapid measurement of blood theophylline levels in many laboratories simplifies this question, since patients with therapeutic levels need not receive a loading dose. As a rough guide, 1 mg per kg of aminophylline will raise the theophylline level by approximately 2 μg/ml. After loading, a maintenance dose of approximately 0.5 mg/kg/hour is given by continuous infusion. This is adjusted upward in children and smoking adults who are otherwise healthy and adjusted downward in patients with liver disease or congestive heart failure.[51] When switching a patient from intravenous to oral therapy, a slow-release formulation should be given in doses equivalent to those given intravenously, bearing in mind that theophylline is approximately 1.2 times as potent as aminophylline. If intravenous therapy was not used, relatively low doses of a slow-release formulation should be given initially. Once steady-state levels are attained, the dose can be adjusted to achieve a therapeutic level. Again, it must be emphasized that frequent blood theophylline levels are crucial in guiding therapy. Also, therapy with beta agonists should be continued. Theophylline should be considered a supplement to the sympathomimetics and not a replacement for them.

Steroids

Steroids have been used in acute bronchospasm practically since they were available for clinical use. In a report to the Medical Research Council by the Subcommittee on Clinical Trials in Asthma in 1956, 13 centers reported on the use of steroids in acute asthmatics.[52] By today's standards they used what would be considered low-dose cortisone therapy, a maximum of 350 mg per day for a maximum of 9 days. By the second day of therapy, the cortisone group began to show marked improvement over the group that received a placebo. However, these patients were monitored only on the basis of observation by the clinician, temperature, respiratory rate, and pulse.

Since that time, many authors have studied the efficacy of steroids in the treatment of asthma using more objective testing. Some studies have shown little or no effect,[53-55] while others have shown significant improvement with steroid therapy.[56,57] Many of these studies, particularly the negative studies, relied on a very small study population[53,55] or included chronic and refractory asthmatic patients as part of their patient population,[54,57] not immediately transferable to an acutely ill patient. Most recently, Littenberg and Gluck published a series on patients who received methylprednisolone, 125 mg, on admission to the emergency department, and then they monitored the effect on the subsequent admission rate.[6] Although no objective criteria were used in establishing the need for admission, their study showed a marked decrease in admission rate. In another study that used objective criteria and a standarized protocol and included a large number of older patients,[58] similar results were found. In both of these cited studies, the admission rate decreased by over 50% compared to a similarly treated population that received a placebo.

The time required to see the beneficial effect of steroids has varied among the many studies performed. Elluh-Micallef demonstrated a significant improvement in bronchospasm within 1 to 2 hours after steroid administration.[59] Other authors have found similar results.[60] The actual mechanism causing this early steroid action is not completely understood. Clinically, it appears that cortisol by itself produces no major change in airway obstruction. However, when given in conjunction with beta agonists, a significant improvement occurs in the FEV_1.[60]

In an animal model, hydrocortisone has been shown to potentiate the responses to epinephrine and norepinephrine.[61] It has been suggested that one action of cortisol is to unmask the β-receptor and potentiate the effect of the subsequent administration of beta-agonist drug.[60] Other possible actions of cortisol include an acceleration of mucociliary clearance and an improvement in ventilation-perfusion matching.[60]

Therefore, unlike traditional teaching, it appears that cortisol does have an early effect that can be of value even in the emergency department. The optimal dose for steroids still remains unclear. However, it is clear that early administration of some dose in excess of 125 mg of methylprednisolone together with beta-agonist medication will be beneficial in reducing the need for hospitalization and more intensive medical intervention.

The use of long-term steroid medication as an outpatient should not be initiated without careful weighing of the risk-benefit ratio. Objective improvement of airway obstruction following steroid therapy can be useful in justifying the inherent risks of steroids.

Anticholinergic Agents

Although anticholinergic agents in the form of stramonium cigarettes were perhaps the first bronchodilators used,[62] only in the last few years have they re-emerged as an accepted form of therapy for bronchospastic disorders. This undoubtedly is related to the relatively recent delineation of the role of the parasympathetic nervous system in regulating airway caliber.[63] Vagal efferent fibers enter the lung at the hilum and travel along the posterior walls of the airways, forming ganglia within and around the airway walls. Postganglionic fibers then supply structures within the airway walls, including smooth muscle and submucosal glands.[64] Stimulation of these vagal fibers causes increased levels of intracellular cyclic guanosine monophosphate (cGMP), which antagonizes the more familiar cAMP system and results in bronchoconstriction.[65,66] The degree of vagal tone affecting the airways can be modified through reflex arcs and central nervous effects, although it is not yet clear to what degree these factors contribute to clinical disease.[64] An important feature of the postganglionic fibers, however, is that they are largely cholinergic and thereby susceptible to intervention using cholinergic blockers.

The prototypic cholinergic blocker is atropine. Nebulized solutions of atropine have been used in acute bronchospasm, and substantial degrees of bronchodilation can be achieved.[67] Unfortunately, adverse effects have proven limiting. Atropine is absorbed well through the pharyngeal, gastric, and airway mucosa, and the resulting systemic distribution causes symptoms of parasympathetic blockade, including dry mouth, urinary retention, loss of visual accommodation, and tachycardia.[63] The development of newer agents, however, has eliminated this problem. Ipratropium bromide (previously known as Sch 1000) is a quaternary isopropyl derivative of atropine. It is absorbed very poorly through mucosal surfaces, and blood levels after its administration almost are undetectable.[65] Ipratropium is available as a metered dose inhaler that delivers 20 μg per actuation; the usual dose is 40 to 80 μg 3 to 4 times daily.

The role of ipratropium in the treatment of acute asthma is not yet clear. The onset of action is seen within seconds to minutes, but peak effects do not occur for 60 to 90 minutes.[68] In direct comparison to beta-agonists in acute bronchospasm, ipratropium does not cause any greater bronchodilation and may, in fact, be somewhat less effective.[69-71] The duration of action, however, is longer.[65] A more effective use for anticholinergic bronchodilators may be in combination with other agents. As described above, smooth muscle relaxation due to cholinergic blockade occurs through an entirely different pathway from that due to beta stimulation. This suggests that simultaneous use of the two classes of broncho-dilators may provide added benefit. Studies on this subject generally have supported this contention, but wide[69-74] variation in response exists between individual patients. However, older patients generally tolerate ipratropium well, and there is evidence to suggest that this population is particularly responsive to the agent.[75] Even if maximal bronchodilation does not improve, the addition of ipratropium to a drug regimen may permit the doses, and thereby the toxicity, of other agents to be reduced.

Cromolyn

Although not a bronchodilator or anti-inflammatory agent, cromolyn has been used in the prophylactic treatment of bronchospastic disease. Pretreatment with cromolyn has been demonstrated to prevent broncho-constriction caused by some, but not all, stimuli, making the indications for its use somewhat controversial.[66,76] Its role clearly is prophylactic, however, and its use is contraindicated in an acute asthmatic attack or status asthmaticus.[66] Originally, it was felt to exert its protective effect through the stabilization of mast cell membranes, thereby preventing the release of mediators following interaction of antigen with cell surface–linked antibody.[76] More recently, however, this mechanism has been called into question.[76] Cromolyn is absorbed poorly, making it necessary to deliver the medication topically. Until recently, the drug has been available only in the form of a gelatin capsule containing a finely divided powder that is inhaled using a special device (Spinhaler). This form of delivery may well account for some of the pharyngeal irritation of which patients often complain following inhalation.[66] In the past few years, however, an MDI has been marketed that simplifies use of the drug and may reduce this problem. The usual dose of cromolyn by MDI is two puffs (1600 μg) 4 times daily.

Other Therapy

In addition to pharmacologic intervention aimed at reversing airway obstruction, a number of other supportive measures are appropriate. All patients being treated for an acute asthmatic attack should receive supplemental oxygen. Many bronchodilator medications also cause some vasodilation, which partially can abolish hypoxic regulation of vascular tone. This can worsen the already impaired matching of ventilation and perfusion and, thereby, contribute to hypoxemia.[39] Additionally, many patients in acute bronchospasm are dehydrated. This dehydration can be caused by poor oral intake during the course of their attack and by inordinate water loss with hyperventilation. In older patients, the development of bronchospasm often is more gradual,[77] with less of a tendency toward dehydration. Also, many elderly patients

suffer from cardiac dysfunction.[35] Therefore, rehydration must be performed gently and with careful monitoring.

Antibiotics generally are not required during asthma attacks. Many episodes of bronchospasm are triggered by noninfectious causes, and most of those related to infection are virally induced.[78] Furthermore, asthmatics often are colonized chronically with potentially pathogenic bacteria without experiencing an increase in their symptoms.[78] However, clear evidence of bacterial infection does warrant treatment with antimicrobial agents. Such evidence would include characteristic infiltrates on chest radiographs and the presence of bacteria and polymorphonuclear cells in a gram-stained smear of sputum.

There have been several reports in the literature of patients experiencing cardiac arrhythmias during the treatment of their acute asthmatic attack.[79,80] Many of these arrhythmias are related to treatment with both beta-agonists and theophylline compounds. There is a distinct correlation between the age of the patient and the presence of these arrhythmias. Therefore, cardiac monitoring is indicated for patients in the geriatric age group.

A number of interventions are of questionable use during an asthma attack. There is no evidence that intermittent positive pressure breathing (IPPB), with either nebulized saline or bronchodilators, is helpful in acute asthma. In fact, it may contribute to hyperinflation, decrease the mechanical advantage of the diaphragm, induce barotrauma, and possibly increase mortality.[81] Inhaled steroids and cromolyn also are not indicated in acute asthma. These agents have no immediate advantage over other medications and may cause irritation of the airways and worsen bronchospasm. Finally, any medications, such as sedatives or anxiolytics, that decrease respiratory drive should be avoided.

Mechanical Ventilation

Mechanical ventilation should be considered in patients who display signs of severe, life-threatening bronchospasm (inability to speak, altered mental status) or in patients who have other signs of very severe asthma and appear to be increasing their bronchospasm despite institution of therapy. It should be noted that, besides simple support, mechanical ventilation provides little advantage for the acutely bronchospastic patient. Higher concentrations of inspired oxygen and decreased work of breathing can be attained, but little to no improvement in the actual bronchospasm and inflammation is achieved.

When using mechanical ventilation, one should use an appropriate endotracheal tube — one that is large enough to allow for suctioning in a volume-controlled ventilator. Very often, these patients generate very high peak pressures, so intensive care monitoring for possible pneumothorax is very necessary. Use of a mechanical ventilator, which more gradually attains peak flow, may be important in some asthmatics who develop very high peak pressures with normal ventilators.

Usually, heavy sedation and/or paralysis are necessary. These interventions increase chest wall compliance and eliminate discoordination between patient and ventilator breaths, thereby reducing airway pressures. Positive end-expiratory pressure (PEEP), sometimes at very high levels, has been useful in some patients.[82] As with any ventilated patient, all efforts at monitoring with ABGs, appropriate nutrition, appropriate volume status, and intensive drug therapy should be maintained.

As mentioned above, many older patients presenting with bronchospasm also have some degree of underlying irreversible chronic airway obstruction. Accordingly, clinical response in these patients may be limited. Because of the generally progressive course of chronic obstructive lung disease, some patients may eventually reach a point where even maximal therapy will not result in clinical improvement. To many of these patients, the institution of mechanical ventilation may represent prolongation of an already difficult existence. In such circumstances, caring physicians might serve their patients best by providing supportive care directed toward maintaining patient comfort. Aggressive medical therapy can be continued but within the bounds set by the patient. Obviously, such a course is appropriate only in end-stage, irreversible cases, and then only when the patient desires it, with full understanding of the consequences (see Chapter 1). Such decisions should be made by patients in consultation with their families and in nonacute settings, rather than urgently in the face of impending respiratory failure. Any patient desiring full medical support certainly should be entitled to receive it. However, many patients, when faced with the options, choose death in relative comfort to the prolongation of life by a mechanical ventilator.

ADMISSION CRITERIA

Asthmatics can be broken into two major groups: those responding rapidly to treatment and those responding more slowly. Those who respond rapidly tend to be younger, have a history of atopy, have attacks that last less than 24 hours before presentation, and require no maintenance steroids.[83] In general, the elderly respond more slowly regardless of previous therapy.[84]

There now are several sets of criteria by which one can predict early the need for hospitalization. The usefulness of these various indexes is dependent on the presence or absence of an observation unit in the emergency department and the length of time one can comfortably observe an acute asthmatic in each given area. In some settings, it is necessary to make an initial decision for hospital admission almost upon entry to the emergency department. Efforts to predict the need for hospital admission

have not been extremely good under these conditions. Studies have shown that ABGs and even PEFRs are poor indicators of hospital admissions.[85] An index established by Fischl, which took into account PEFR in addition to parameters found on physical examination, was marginally successful in predicting the need for hospitalization.[86] In some studies, pretreatment PEFR, or an FEV_1 less than 20% of the predicted normal rate, correlated with the need for subsequent hospitalization.[87]

A more appropriate tool is to look at the initial response to treatment. An initial improvement of 20% in either the PEFR or the FEV_1 correlated well with the final discharge in the patient.[87] Indeed, in one study, no patient with an initial PEFR above 30% predicted normal and more than a 20% increase in PEFR posttreatment required admission.[88]

We have set up a protocol in the emergency department of our hospital that allows for routine monitoring of patients using spirometry. All patients are treated with beta agonist or beta agonist and theophylline therapy, and PFTs are recorded every 30 minutes. As long as patients continue to improve their FEV_1 by at least 20% every 30-minute period, they are kept in the observation unit of the emergency department. They are considered as candidates for discharge at the point at which their PEFR or FEV_1 reaches 70% of the predicted or 70% of their normal baseline. At this point, they should be free of all physical signs and symptoms of acute bronchospasm. Those patients who fail to reach their targeted pulmonary function measure and fail to make substantial progress in any given 30- to 60-minute period are considered candidates for admission. By using this protocol, we have found that we can decrease the amount of time asthmatics spend in the observation area of the department and actually decrease the admission rate.[89]

It is very important in the care of asthmatics to note that when they are discharged, their bronchospasm is not completely corrected. Therefore, it is imperative that the intensive therapy that they initially receive be continued on an outpatient basis. This should include continuation of all forms of therapy (with the exception of the initial steroid dose) that were instituted. It is also important for the asthmatics themselves to understand that they have not yet reached their baseline and that it may take anywhere from 3 to 7 days to attain this level. Appropriate follow-up should be undertaken within this period to evaluate therapy and to adjust medication dosage (particularly theophylline). Patients with a history of atopy should be counseled carefully about re-exposure to the allergen. Patients with food allergies should be counseled about necessary food precautions in the future.

FATAL ASTHMA

It is prudent to review the fatalities associated with this disease. Asthma accounts for at least 4,000 deaths per year worldwide.[4] Most of these deaths occurred in patients over the age of 55.[5] In the United States, the mortality rate is somewhat lower than abroad but represents 1.3 deaths per 100,000 population.[4] Among the causes of death frequently listed is an adverse reaction to bronchodilators. This concern came from an observed increase in the number of deaths in the United Kingdom in the early 1960s that corresponded to the use of aerosolized bronchodilators. Several studies have concluded that this represents a very small or possibly even nonexistent problem.[4] A more likely cause of death is simply asphyxia secondary to refractory bronchoconstriction, due in large part to the need for more effective therapy. Other contributing factors may include sedation, the onset of barotrauma from high-pressure mechanical ventilation, hypersensitivity to drugs, or concomitant use of beta-blocking agents. There is a need to improve patient and physician knowledge about acute asthma. In addition, better medications with more efficacy and less toxicity are needed to decrease these mortality figures.

HORIZONS

Further understanding and research into the role of environmental and food substances in precipitation of asthma is essential. For example, an NIH study currently under way is evaluating monosodium glutamate as a stimulus.[90] Such studies are urgently needed. Another study has just revealed community outbreaks of asthma associated with soybean dust.[91]

Further studies are also needed on the substance VIP (vasoactive intestinal polypeptide), which is present in normal lungs, but was markedly deficient in the lungs of five patients who died from asthma.[92] This substance has a relaxant effect on airway smooth muscle and is believed to be important in regulating bronchial tone. This type of research opens up many therapeutic possibilities.

REFERENCES

1. American Thoracic Society: Definitions and classification of chronic bronchitis, asthma, and pulmonary emphysema, Am Rev Respir Dis 85:762, 1962.
2. Banerjee DK et al: Underdiagnosis of asthma in the elderly, Br J Dis Chest 81:23, 1987.
3. Dodge RR and Burrows B: The prevalence and incidence of asthma and asthma-like symptoms in a general population sample, Am Rev Respir Dis 122:567, 1980.
4. Benatar SR: Fatal asthma, N Engl J Med 314:423, 1986.
5. Burr ML et al: Asthma in the elderly: an epidemiological survey, Br Med J 1:1041, 1979.
6. Littenberg B and Gluck EH: A controlled trial of methylprednisolone in the emergency treatment of acute asthma, N Engl J Med 314:150, 1986.
7. Leff A: Pathogenesis of asthma, Chest 81:224, 1982.
8. Parker CW and Snider DE: Prostaglandins and asthma, Ann Intern Med 78:963, 1973.
9. McFadden ER: Pathogenesis of asthma, J Allergy Clin Immunol 73:413, 1984.
10. Schoene RB et al: Timolol induced bronchospasm in asthmatic bronchitis, JAMA 245:1460, 1981.

11. Margolis M and Mohan KK: Analgesic and asthma, South Med J 75:1239, 1982.
12. Szczeklik A and Gryglewski RJ: Asthma and anti-inflammatory drugs: mechanisms and clinical patterns, Drugs 25:533, 1983.
13. Baker GJ, Collett P, and Allen DH: Bronchospasm induced by metabisulphite-containing food and drugs, Med J Aust 2:614, 1981.
14. Jamieson DM et al: Metabisulfite sensitivity: case report and literature review, Ann Allergy 54:115, 1985.
15. Lee M et al: Tartrazine containing druge, Drug Intell Clin Pharm 15:782, 1981.
16. Dahms ET, Bolin JF, and Slavin RG: Passive smoking: effects on bronchial asthma, Chest 80:530, 1981.
17. Goldstein IF and Dulberg EM: Air pollution and asthma: search for a relationship, J Air Pollut Control Assoc 31:370, 1981.
18. Demeter SL: Hyperventilation syndrome and asthma, Am J Med 81:989, 1986.
19. Downing ET et al: Factitious asthma: physiological approach to diagnosis, JAMA 248:2878, 1982.
20. Edge JR et al: The radiographic appearance of the chest in persons of advanced age, Br J Radiol 37:769, 1964.
21. Zoller DP: The physiology of aging, Am Fam Physician 36:112, 1987.
22. Horvath SM and Borgia JF: Cardiopulmonary gas transport and aging, Am Rev Respir Dis 129:S68, 1984.
23. Brandfobrener M, Landowne M, and Shock NW: Changes in cardiac output with age, Circulation 12:557, 1955.
24. Breener BB: Position and diaphoresis in acute asthma, Am J Med 74:1005, 1983.
25. Carden DL et al: Vital signs including pulsus paradoxus in the assessment of acute bronchial asthma, Ann Emerg Med 12:80, 1983.
26. Jardin F et al: Mechanism of paradoxic pulse in bronchial asthma, Circulation 66:887, 1982.
27. McFadden ER, Kiser R, and DeGroot WJ: Acute bronchial asthma: relations between clinical and physiologic manifestations, N Engl J Med 288:221, 1973.
28. Shims CS and Williams MH: Evaluation of the severity of asthma: patients versus physicians, Am J Med 68:11, 1980.
29. Brooks LJ, Cloutier MM, and Afshani E: Significance of roentgenographic abnormalities in children hospitalized for asthma, Chest 82:315, 1982.
30. Findley LJ and Sahn SA: The value of chest roentgenograms in acute asthma in adults, Chest 80:535, 1981.
31. Martin TG, Elenbaas RM, and Pingleton SH: Use of peak expiratory flow rates to eliminate unnecessary arterial blood gases in acute asthma, Ann Emerg Med 11:70, 1982.
32. McFadden ER and Lyons HA: Arterial blood gases in asthma, N Engl J Med 278:1027, 1968.
33. Bouchier D and Dawson KP: Transcutaneous oxygen monitoring in acute asthma, Aust Paediatr J 20:213, 1984.
34. Nowak RM et al: Comparison of peak expiratory flow and FEV_1 admission criteria for acute bronchial asthma, Ann Emerg Med 11:64, 1982.
35. Harris R: Cardiovascular disease in the elderly, Med Clin North Am 67:379, 1983.
36. Rossing TH, Fanta CH, and McFadden ER: A controlled trial of the use of single versus combined-drug therapy in the treatment of acute episodes of asthma, Am Rev Respir Dis 123:190, 1981.
37. Fanta CH, Rossing TH, and McFadden ER: Treatment of acute asthma: is combination therapy with sympathomimetics and methylxanthines indicated? Am J Med 80:5, 1986.
38. Rossing TH et al: Emergency therapy of asthma: comparison of the acute effects of parenteral and inhaled sympathomimetics and infused aminophylline, Am Rev Respir Dis 122:365, 1980.
39. Webb-Johnson DC and Andrews JL: Bronchodilator therapy, N Engl J Med 297:476 and 758, 1977.
40. Jenne JW: Theophylline use in asthma: some current issues, Clin Chest Med 5:645, 1984.
41. Van Dellen RG: Theophylline: practical application of new knowledge, Mayo Clin Proc 54:733, 1979.
42. Taylor SM and Downes H: Bronchodilator mechanisms in bullfrog lung: differences in response to isoproterenol, theophylline and papaverine, J Pharmacol Exp Ther 223:359, 1982.
43. Bukowskyj M, Nakatsu K, and Munt PW: Theophylline reassessed, Ann Intern Med 101:63, 1984.
44. Fredholm BB, Brodin K, and Strandberg KB: On the mechanism of relaxation of tracheal muscle by theophylline and other cyclic

nucleotide phosphodiesterase inhibitors, Acta Pharm Toxicol 45:336, 1979.

45. Vestal RE et al: Effect of intravenous aminophylline on plasma levels of catecholamines and related cardiovascular and metabolic responses in man, Circulation 67:162, 1983.

46. Mackay AD, Baldwin CJ, and Tattersfield AE: Action of intravenously administered aminophylline on normal airways, Am Rev Respir Dis 127: 609, 1983.

47. Mitenko PA and Ogilvie RI: Rational intravenous doses of theophylline, N Engl J Med 289:600, 1973.

48. Vozeh S et al: Theophylline serum concentration and therapeutic effect in severe acute bronchial obstruction: the optimal use of intravenously administered aminophylline, Am Rev Respir Dis 125: 181, 1982.

49. Wolfe JD et al: Bronchodilator effects of terbutaline and aminophylline alone and in combination in asthmatic patients, N Engl J Med 298:363, 1978.

50. Siegel et al: Aminophylline increases the toxicity but not the efficacy of an inhaled beta-adrenergic agonist in the treatment of acute exacerbations of asthma, Am Rev Respir Dis 132:283, 1985.

51. Jusko et al: Intravenous theophylline therapy: nomogram guidelines, Ann Intern Med 86:400, 1977.

52. The British Medical Research Council: Controlled trial of effects of cortisone acetate in status asthmaticus, Lancet 2:803, 1956.

53. McFadden ER et al: A controlled study of the effects of single doses of hydrocortisone on the resolution of acute attacks of asthma, Am J Med 60:52, 1976.

54. Tamsdell JW, Berry CC, and Clausen JL: The immediate effects of cortisol on pulmonary function in normals and asthmatics, J Allergy Clin Immunol 72:69, 1983.

55. Tanaka RM et al: Intravenous methylprednisolone in adults in status asthmaticus: comparison of two dosages, Chest 82:438, 1982.

56. Fiel SB et al: Efficacy of short-term corticosteroid therapy in outpatient treatment of acute bronchial asthma, Am J Med 75:259, 1983.

57. Fanta CH, Rossing TH, and McFadden ER: Glucocorticoids in acute asthma: a critical controlled study, Am J Med 74:845, 1983.

58. Schneider SM et al: Mega dose methylprednisolone as initial therapy in patient with acute bronchospasm, J Asthma (in press).

59. Ellul-Micallef R: The acute effects of corticosteroids in bronchial asthma, Eur J Respir Dis 63(suppl 122):118, 1982.

60. Arnaud A and Charpin J: Interaction between corticosteroids and beta-agonists in acute asthma, Eur J Respir Dis 63 (suppl 122):126, 1982.

61. Kalsner S: Mechanism of hydrocortisone potentiation of responses to epinephrine and norepinephrine in rabbit aorta, Circ Res 24:283, 1969.

62. Gandevia B: Historical review of the use of parasympatholytic agents in the treatment of respiratory disorders, Post Med J 51(suppl 7):13, 1975.

63. Gross NJ and Skorodin MS: State of the art: anticholinergic, antimuscarinic bronchodilators, Am Rev Respir Dis 129:856, 1984.

64. Barnes PJ: Neural control of human airways in health and disease, Am Rev Respir Dis 134:1289,1986.

65. Rebuck AS, Chapman KR, and Braude AC: Anticholinergic therapy of asthma, Chest 82:55S, 1982.

66. George RB and Payne DK: Anticholinergics, cromolyn, and other occasionally useful drugs, Clin Chest Med 5:685, 1984.

67. Cavanaugh MJ and Cooper DM: Inhaled atropine sulfate: dose response characteristics, Am Rev Respir Dis 114:517, 1976.

68. Storms WW, DoPico GA, and Reed CE: Aerosol Sch 1000: an anticholinergic bronchodilator, Am Rev Respir Dis 111:419, 1975.

69. Ruffin RE, Fitzgerald JD, and Rebuck AS: A comparison of the bronchodilator activity of Sch 1000 and salbutamol, J Allergy Clin Immunol 59:136, 1977.

70. Elwood RK and Abboud RT: The short-term bronchodilator effects of fenoterol and ipratropium in asthma, J Allergy Clin Immunol 69:467, 1982.

71. Leahy BC, Gomm SA, and Allen SC: Comparison of nebulized salbutamol with ipratropium bromide in acute asthma, Br J Dis Chest 77:159, 1983.

72. Rebuck AS, Gent M, and Chapman KR: Anticholinergic and sympathomimetic combination therapy of asthma, J Allergy Clin Immunol 71:317, 1983.

73. Ruffin RE et al: Combination bronchodilator therapy in asthma, J Allergy Clin Immunol 69:60, 1982.

74. Bryant DH: Nebulized ipratropium bromide in the treatment of acute asthma, Chest 88:24, 1985.

75. Ullah M, Newman GB, and Saunders KB: Influence of age on response to ipratropium and salbutamol in asthma, Thorax 36:523, 1981.

76. Bernstein IL: Cromolyn sodium, Chest 87:68S, 1985.

77. Bellamy D and Collins JV: "Acute" asthma in adults, Thorax 34:36, 1979.

78. Hudgel DW et al: Viral and bacterial infections in adults with chronic asthma, Am Rev Respir Dis 120:393, 1979.

79. Emerman CL, Crafford WA, and Vrobel TR: Ventricular arrhythmias during treatment for acute asthma, Ann Emerg Med 15:699, 1986.

80. Josephson GW: Dysrhythmogenesis associated with the treatment of acute reversible airway obstruction, Ann Emerg Med 11:425, 1982.

81. Karetzky MS: Asthma mortality: an analysis of one year's experience, review of the literature and assessment of current modes of therapy, Medicine 54:471, 1975.

82. Qvist J et al: High-level PEEP in severe asthma, N Engl J Med 307:1347, 1982 (letter).

83. Benfiels GFA and Smith AP: Predicting rapid and slow response to treatment in acute severe asthma, Br J Dis Chest 77:249, 1983.

84. Smith AP: Patterns of recovery from acute severe asthma, Br J Dis Chest 75:132, 1981.

85. Kelsen SG et al: Emergency room assessment and treatment of patients with acute asthma: adequacy of the conventional approach, Am J Med 64:622, 1978.

86. Fischl MA, Pitchenik S, and Gardner LB: An index predicting relapse and need for hospitalization in patients with acute bronchial asthma, N Engl J Med 305:783, 1981.

87. Banner AS, Shah RS, and Addington WW: Rapid prediction of need for hospitalization in acute asthma, JAMA 235:1337, 1976.

88. Martin TG, Elenbaas RM, and Pingleton SH: Failure of peak expiratory flow rate to predict hospital admission in acute asthma, Ann Emerg Med 11:466, 1982.

89. Schneider SM: Effect of a treatment protocol on the efficiency of care by house officers to the adult with acute asthma, Ann Emerg Med 15:703, 1986.

90. Cohen S: Personal communication, NIH, 1989.

91. Anto JM, Sunyer J, and Rodriguez-Roison R: Community outbreaks of asthma associated with soybean dust, N Engl J Med 320:1097, 1989.

92. Ollerenshaw S et al: Absence of immunoreactive vasoactive intestinal polypeptide in the tissue from the lungs of patients with asthma, N Engl J Med 320:1244, 1989.

Infectious Diseases and Thermodysregulation

Thermoregulatory Disorders

Louis J. Perretta, M.D., F.A.C.E.P.

Disorders of temperature regulation are frequently encountered in elderly patients who come to an emergency department (ED). When environmental etiologies have been ruled out, temperature disturbances are usually a manifestation of a serious systemic disease. There are a wide variety of medical conditions that may affect an individual's ability to regulate core body temperature, leading to either hypothermia or hyperthermia. Not only are the elderly more likely to develop diseases that cause disturbances in temperature regulation, but a number of pharmacologic agents commonly prescribed for this subgroup have been shown to cause temperature disorders. The older individual also has a decreased ability to respond to environmental fluctuations in temperature, since many physiologic processes that maintain thermoregulatory homeostasis in younger individuals are impaired or absent in the geriatric age group.

This chapter will address the problem of hypothermia and hyperthermia in the elderly, highlighting both etiologies and impaired thermoregulatory mechanisms unique to this population.

PATHOPHYSIOLOGY OF HYPOTHERMIA

Hypothermia is defined as a core temperature less than 35°C. A number of disorders can predispose an individual to hypothermia by decreasing heat production, increasing heat loss, or interfering with the central or peripheral control of thermoregulation. Environmental exposure to cold, probably the most common cause of hypothermia, lowers core temperature by increasing heat loss.

Body temperature is closely regulated through a balance between heat production and heat dissipation. Metabolic activity in the heart and liver is responsible for the majority of endogenous heat production. Heat is subsequently dissipated at the body surface, with the skin accounting for 90% of heat loss and the lung contributing the rest. The thermal load is dissipated primarily through radiation cooling (70%) with a smaller amount given off by the evaporation of insensible perspiration. The preoptic nucleus of the anterior hypothalamus is the thermal control center, maintaining body temperature at a given set value.

When the core body temperature is elevated, the hypothalamus stimulates the autonomic nervous system to produce sweating and cutaneous vasodilation, both of which decrease core body temperature. Conversely, when core body temperature or skin temperature decreases, the hypothalamus conserves heat by producing cutaneous vasoconstriction. In addition, the hypothalamus can increase heat production by stimulating muscular activity in the form of shivering. The appreciation of cold at a conscious level induces the individual to exercise, wear more clothing, and move to a warmer environment. Exposure to heat influences the decision to remove clothing and move to a cooler environment. In addition, nonthermal stimuli, such as the consumption of alcohol or drugs, produce vasomotor changes that affect temperature regulation.

Epidemiology

Hypothermia in the elderly usually develops while the individual is indoors, with a fall in core body temperature resulting from cold surroundings, concomitant illness, or some combination of the two. In the United States, mortality data for hypothermia-associated deaths do not accurately reflect the true incidence of primary or secondary hypothermia in the elderly. In fact, it may be possible that some hypothermia deaths go unreported on death certificates because the physicians and/or coroners were unaware of exposure to the cold as a potential cause of death.[1] Mortality data from the National Center for Health Statistics show that the highest mortality rates for hypothermia occur in the elderly and that males are at a greater risk than females.[2] The mortality rate associated with hypothermia in the elderly is around 50%.[6]

In Great Britain, the problem of hypothermia in the elderly has been studied more extensively than in the United States. One survey found that 3.6% of all elderly patients admitted to the hospital had a temperature of less than 35°C.[3] In another study, it was shown that 10% of the elderly living at home have borderline hypothermia.[4] The fact that mortality in the winter months is seen mainly in the elderly has been attributed to underlying medical illness as well as a decreased ability to respond to a cold environment. In Great Britain, there was a correlation between environmental temperature and the number of cases of hypothermia. The characteristic profile of the elderly hypothermic patient is one living alone in a home or apartment that is poorly heated.

Etiology

In the elderly, three factors contribute to or can produce hypothermia: 1) physiologic predisposition, 2) environmental milieu, and 3) associated or underlying medical conditions.

Older individuals are less able to compensate for environmental heat loss than younger persons. A decrease in the basal metabolic rate in the elderly is primarily responsible for this thermoregulatory compromise. Consequently, winter is the most likely time of the year for accidental hypothermia in this population. In addition to the inability to compensate for a decline in body temperature, the elderly may also have a decreased ability to sense changes in ambient temperature. Several authors have shown that the elderly actually prefer temperatures that are lower than those preferred by younger people.[5-7] In addition, younger adults are able to notice a change in temperature of 1°F, while it is common for an older person to fail to notice changes in temperature of less than 3°F.[9,10] Thermal control is also related to total body water since water protects the body from thermal changes by acting as a buffer and heat reservoir.[11] Since total body water decreases with age, older people become hypothermic more quickly, because there is less body water to store heat.

The elderly are also less likely to develop tachycardia and increase their cardiac output in response to a cold stress. In many older individuals, this is exacerbated by a diminished vasoconstrictor response to cold, which is sometimes associated with orthostatic hypotension. In fact, one study has shown that individuals prone to orthostatic hypotension are at increased risk of developing hypothermia.[9] In addition to the diminished vasoconstrictor response, other problems related to the autonomic nervous system that lead to hypothermia include decreased shivering[8] and low resting peripheral blood flow.[11] Endogenous polyamines, such as spermidine and spermine, are known to cause hypothermia in animals. A recent study has demonstrated an association of low body temperature in the elderly with high levels of spermine.[12]

In addition to impaired thermoregulatory mechanisms, there are several environmental factors that contribute to the high incidence of hypothermia in the elderly. Fixed incomes, coupled with higher energy costs, help to explain why older people tend to keep the temperature in their homes and apartments lower. Damp and drafty dwellings, combined with old and/or poorly functioning furnaces, also contribute to cold environments.[13] Living alone is another factor that is associated with a high risk of hypothermia in the elderly, as is malnutrition, which can cause decreased fat stores. It has been shown that fat metabolism is the major form of energy production at low body temperatures.[14] Adequate energy intake in the elderly is important since it may actually protect against hypothermia.

A comprehensive list of medical conditions causing hypothermia in the elderly is shown in Table 20–1. Many patients with accidental hypothermia, especially older individuals, also suffer from severe concomitant illness. The associated condition may have contributed to the fall in body temperature or may be a complication of the hypothermia itself. Prompt recognition of associated medical problems in the older hypothermic patient positively influences the course of treatment and outcome.[15]

Medical Causes

In severe hypothyroidism, metabolic heat production is decreased and hypothermia usually results. Hypothermia is a common feature of myxedema coma,[16] which is primarily a disease of the elderly, and is precipitated by such factors as cold, infection, trauma, seizures, and drugs. Frequently, the coexistence of myxedema can be suspected when the body temperature fails to rise satisfactorily during rewarming of a hypothermic patient.[17] The presence of hypopituitarism can also precipitate hypothermia by decreasing metabolic heat production.[15]

In the elderly, shivering may be defective or absent, and older individuals are often forced to restrict heat-generating physical activity because of paralysis, parkinsonism, arthritis, or falls that may leave the individual immobilized. Inactivity predisposes to hypothermia by decreasing metabolic heat production. Living alone, recent bereavements, and social isolation are also associated with inactivity.[18]

Table 20–1 Medical Conditions Associated with Hypothermia in the Elderly

Increasing Heat Loss
Ethanol ingestion
Paget's disease
Dermal disorders
  Psoriasis
  Exfoliative dermatitis
  Burns
  Malnutrition

Decreasing Heat Production
Hypothyroidism/myxedema
Hypopituitarism
Starvation
Arthritis
Stroke
Parkinson's disease
Hypoglycemia

Interfering With Control of Thermoregulation
CNS pathology
  Stroke
  Subarachnoid hemorrhage
  Subdural hematoma
  Head trauma
  Wernicke's encephalopathy
  Parkinson's disease
Systemic diseases
  Uremia
  Hepatic failure
  Carbon monoxide poisoning

Other medical conditions associated with heat loss include dermal disorders, such as psoriasis and exfoliative dermatitis, which cause excessive heat loss through two possible mechanisms: increased peripheral blood flow and transepidermal water loss with evaporation. Paget's disease and malnutrition with lack of subcutaneous fat are also associated with increased heat loss and hypothermia.[15]

Central nervous system (CNS) disease can produce or contribute to hypothermia in the elderly by impairing central thermoregulation. Stroke, subarachnoid hemorrhage, subdural hematoma, tumor, head trauma, and Wernicke's encephalopathy have all been associated with hypothermia.[11] Low cardiac output, secondary to acute myocardial infarction, has been shown to cause thermoregulatory disturbances resulting in hypothermia.[19] Hypothermia has also been reported with severe infections, bacteremia, and sepsis. These patients have a significantly higher mortality than those with hypothermia associated with other conditions.[20] It has been shown that hypothermic patients with severe infection and bacteremia have an increased cardiac index and decreased systemic vascular resistance. Cardiac index is decreased, and systemic vascular resistance is increased in hypothermic patients without severe infection.[21] Infection may also cause central thermoregulatory or hypothalamic dysfunction, leading to hypothermia.[15]

Hypothermia is a well-known complication of diabetic ketoacidosis[22] and hypoglycemia.[23] There is evidence that the incidence of hypothermia in elderly diabetics, particularly women, may be higher.[24] Other systemic diseases that cause hypothermia via their effect on the hypothalamus include uremia, hepatic failure, and carbon monoxide poisoning.[11]

Hypothermia can be induced with drugs, many of which are commonly used by the elderly (Table 20–2). Ethanol causes hypothermia by inducing vasodilation, reducing shivering, and depressing central thermoregulation.[25] Hypothermia may be seen as a complication of acute Wernicke's encephalopathy, while phenothiazines and cyclic antidepressants such as imipramine act on the hypothalamus to inhibit shivering.[26] Benzodiazepines, barbiturates, and reserpine may lead to hypothermia by impairing centrally mediated vasoconstrictor response to the cold.[25]

Prognosis

Generally, hypothermia in the elderly carries with it a poor prognosis, since many of these patients have underlying medical illness and/or are on medications that predispose them to hypothermia. A recent study found ischemic heart disease to be the most prevalent underlying disease, but chronic renal failure, hypertension, and organic brain syndrome were also prevalent.[26a]

The mortality rate for hypothermia in the elderly is extremely high, with reports in the literature varying between 50% and 74%.[6,26a] This is in sharp contrast to the lower mortality rate seen with hypothermia in the young, emphasizing the importance of recognizing and treating the underlying medical conditions that might be present in the elderly. Infection is a common cause of hypothermia and was found to be the immediate cause in a vast majority of cases in one study. The infections seen included pneumonia and urinary tract infections as the most common (Table 20–3). It is for this reason that the initiation of antibiotic therapy should not wait for culture results. Although hypothermia deaths were associated with thrombocytopenia and hypoproteinemia, mortality rates were not affected by age, sex, degree of hypothermia, or whether patients developed hypothermia in or out of the hospital.[26a]

Presentation

Symptoms of hypothermia in the elderly are usually insidious in presentation and often develop over several days. Initial symptoms include diminished mental status,

Table 20–2 Pharmacologic Agents Causing Hypothermia

Phenothiazines	Ethanol
Antidepressants	Reserpine
Benzodiazepines	Barbiturates

Table 20–3　Causes of Hypothermia*

	In-Hospital (%) (n = 26)	Out-of-Hospital (%) (n = 28)
Infection		
Urinary tract	38	32
Pneumonia	31	21
Skin infection	4	7
Peritonitis	8	0
Gastroenteritis	0	7
Cholecystitis	4	0
Unknown source	0	4
Cerebrovascular accident	8	11
Terminal heart failure	8	7
Myxedema coma	0	4
Barbiturate overdose	0	4
Intestinal obstruction	0	4

Reproduced with permission from Kramer MR et al: Arch Intern Med 149:1521, 1989. Copyright 1989, American Medical Association.

*None of the differences between in-hospital and out-of-hospital cases are significant.

extremity stiffness, weakness, shivering, increased muscle tone, and hypertension. These last three symptoms are usually diminished or absent in elderly patients. Elderly patients may complain of feeling cold despite diminished cold perception. If core temperatures drop below 35°C, many patients no longer complain that they are cold. The elderly hypothermic patient frequently presents only with symptoms of confusion, uncooperativeness, and unresponsiveness. Consciousness becomes further impaired as the central temperature falls, eventually leading to coma. Other earlier and more subtle neurologic signs include slurred speech, ataxia, and extensor plantar responses.[27] Unfortunately, most signs and symptoms of hypothermia are nonspecific, and the only reliable way to make the diagnosis is by measuring core body temperature. This is difficult because most standard thermometers measure temperature in the range of 35°C to 42°C (95°F to 104°F). More accurate measurement of core body temperature can be made by a rectal, rather than oral, temperature, taken with a low-reading thermometer capable of measuring temperatures from 25°C to 40°C.[30]

Other signs of hypothermia include gastric dilatation, impaired hepatic function, decreased renal blood flow, and renal tubular dysfunction. The clinician may have difficulty distinguishing hypothermia from primary hypothyroidism. Obtaining TSH levels, which are raised in hypothyroid hypothermia and normal in primary hypothermia, will help distinguish between these two conditions.[28] Hypothermia will also tend to alter the oxygen dissociation curve so that less oxygen is given up to the tissues, thus leading to tissue anoxia.[29]

As temperature falls, cardiac dysrhythmias become common. These dysrhythmias include supraventricular tachycardias, atrial fibrillation, ventricular tachycardia, and ventricular fibrillation. In addition, heart block and asystole can occur, leading to cardiac arrest at tem-

peratures below 32.2°C. Ventricular fibrillation is the principal cause of death at core temperatures below 28°C.[31] A characteristic Osborn, or J, wave, which is a positive deflection in the left ventricular leads at the junction of the QRS and ST segments, occurs in one fourth to one third of all hypothermic patients.[11] The presence of a J wave (Figure 20–1) is neither pathognomonic nor prognostic. As the body temperature reaches 30°C, patients become hypopneic and hypotensive.

Treatment

Two methods are commonly used to treat hypothermia: slow, spontaneous rewarming and rapid, active rewarming. The treatment regimen selected depends upon whether or not there is a life-threatening complication of hypothermia. If such a complication exists, rapid, active rewarming should be utilized. It should be noted that rewarming alone is adequate treatment for environmental causes of hypothermia. However, when hypothermia is caused by an associated medical disease, rewarming may be inadequate unless the underlying disease is aggressively treated as well.

Slow, Spontaneous Rewarming

Slow, spontaneous rewarming is now recognized as the treatment of choice in the elderly. This is done without the use of external heat and is best accomplished by wrapping the patients in warm blankets in order to gradually raise the core temperature at a rate of 1°F per hour (0.5°C). The ambient temperature should exceed 21°C, and the air should contain a high amount of humidity. If the temperature fails to rise more than 0.5°F per hour, other causes of hypothermia such as myxedema crisis, hypoglycemia, and gram-negative sepsis may be present.[9] This rewarming technique presupposes that the patient is able to metabolically generate a sufficient amount of heat in order to spontaneously rewarm. When

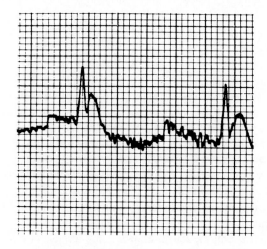

Figure 20–1　"Osborn," or J, wave.

there is no shivering, metabolic heat production may be insufficient to raise core temperature. Shivering could be absent because of core temperatures below 30°C, associated medical conditions, drug ingestions, or uncorrected hypoglycemia.

Rapid, Active Rewarming

Rapid, active rewarming, which involves a transfer of exogenous heat to the patient, can be accomplished by internal or external methods. Active rewarming is mandatory when there is cardiac instability and decompensation since defibrillation is rarely successful at temperatures below 28° to 30°C. Active rewarming is also indicated for patients with impaired CNS control of thermoregulation or when endogenous thermogenesis is insufficient. Examples of diseases that cause insufficient thermogenesis are hypopituitarism, adrenal insufficiency, hypothyroidism, and cerebral infarction.

Active external rewarming (AER) can be achieved by placing the patient in a warm bath or water. This method presents several problems: difficulty in monitoring patients, performing cardiopulmonary resuscitation (CPR), and forcing them to remain in a hemodynamically disadvantageous head-up position.[32] Other methods of external rewarming include plumbed garments that circulate warm fluids, water bottles, heating pads, and blankets.[33]

In the elderly, AER has been shown to be dangerous for a majority of patients, since the extensive vasodilatation that usually accompanies AER can result in hypotension and inadequate coronary perfusion.[27] In addition, dilation of peripheral and core vessels can result in sudden cooling of the core as well as a sudden exposure of the core to lactic acid.[8] This "after drop" can cause fatal arrhythmias. The reported mortality rate with AER is 60.3% as compared with a mortality rate of 44% when using slow, spontaneous rewarming in all age groups.[33]

Active internal rewarming (AIR) allows for active rewarming, while minimizing the possibility of rewarming collapse (after drop) in patients with core temperatures below 30°C. Techniques for AIR include mediastinal irrigation, peritoneal dialysis, hemodialysis, gastric irrigation, and extracorporeal blood warming. Rewarming through the airway with heated gases may prove to be a very effective means of core rewarming in the elderly.[34] In fact, airway rewarming, by inducing selective warming of the endocardium via pulmonary venous blood, may reduce the risk of ventricular fibrillation.[35] Slow rewarming is still the treatment of choice in elderly patients, using AIR with inhaled gases for severe cases, and extracorporeal rewarming for those patients in diabetic coma or with cardiac arrhythmias.[27]

Lastly, the association of ventricular fibrillation with orotracheal intubation in the hypothermic patient is worth mentioning. Although ventricular fibrillation has been described as a complication of intubation, there is no evidence showing this relationship in the setting of a normal arterial blood gas (ABG). It has been demonstrated that correction of hypoxia and acidosis prior to intubation will decrease the incidence of ventricular fibrillation in hypothermic individuals undergoing intubation.[36]

In treating hypothermia in the elderly, the clinician should investigate for the presence of associated medical conditions and treat those accordingly. In the elderly, hypothermia that does not occur in the presence of environmental cold or does not respond to slow, spontaneous rewarming should raise high suspicion for the presence of an associated medical illness.

HYPERTHERMIA

Hyperthermia, although less common in the elderly than hypothermia, is a serious problem with a high mortality rate. Hyperthermia can also be a manifestation of systemic illness. The raised body temperature is usually caused by exposure to excessive heat, impaired thermoregulatory reflexes, or the effect of circulating pyrogens.[37] Hyperthermia is defined as the presence of a temperature of at least 40.5°C for at least 1 hour.[38] Heat stroke is characterized by hyperthermia, along with severe CNS disturbances such as delirium, seizures, or coma. Hyperthermia and heat stroke are usually thought to be problems encountered in younger individuals undergoing physical exertion in the warm weather; however, the elderly are most likely to acquire heat illnesses during heat waves without exercise.[39]

Physiology

Increases in body temperature are more likely to occur in elderly patients, especially when high external temperatures continue for several days. As with hypothermia, impaired thermoregulation in the elderly may render them unable to control body temperature even in moderate environmental heat.[37] This situation can occur with hypothalamic dysfunction, spinal cord injury, skin lesions, or certain pharmacologic agents.

Normally, the earliest response to an elevated core temperature is peripheral vasodilatation, which increases blood flow to the skin so that heat can dissipate to the cooler external environment. When the ambient temperature exceeds 37°C, sweating is required for adequate heat dissipation.[40] Compared with younger individuals, the elderly show a higher threshold before sweating will occur for a given heat load.[37] In one study, 42% of elderly men and 62% of elderly women at home who were exposed to ambient temperatures of 46°C for a prolonged period of time failed to show sweat on the forehead as did younger subjects.[41] Cutaneous vasodilatation and sweating, which occur in response to heat stress, cause blood flow increases up to 20 times and result in decreased peripheral vascular resistance. This requires an increase in cardiac output and a high-output state. Elderly patients with impaired cardiovascular status may be unable to maintain sufficiently high cardiac output to lose heat, causing an increase in core body temperature.

Certain medical conditions, as well as pharmacologic agents, may inhibit sweating, increase motor activity, or impair cardiovascular status. These conditions, which will be discussed in a subsequent section, contribute to the development of hyperthermia. In addition, temperature elevations may be caused by circulating endogenous pyrogens that raise the body temperature by increasing the CNS thermoregulatory set point. Acclimatization, which is an adaptation of the body to heat stresses over several days to 2 weeks, may be limited in the older patient with congestive heart failure, arteriosclerotic cardiovascular disease, or other illnesses that impair the ability to sweat or increase cardiac output.[42]

Etiology

Heat illness or hyperthermia is a disease that encompasses a comprehensive spectrum from minor heat syndromes such as heat edema, heat cramps, and heat syncope to the most serious syndrome — heat stroke. Heat exhaustion, which can be be viewed as a precursor to heat stroke, is between the two poles of this spectrum. In addition to the usual heat syndromes, severe and prolonged fever in the elderly may be difficult or impossible to distinguish from hyperthermia.

Infectious Causes

As already mentioned, circulating endogenous pyrogens can cause fever by raising the hypothalamic set point. Infection usually causes release of pyrogens, but several other medical conditions have been associated with the release of endogenous pyrogens and subsequent temperature elevations (Table 20–4). Fever is often encountered with malignant disease, such as malignancy of the reticuloendothelial system, lung, liver, pancreas, kidney, and colon.[43]

Infection continues to be the most common cause of fever of undetermined origin (FUO) in the elderly, with abdominal abscesses, tuberculosis, and infective endocarditis being the leading causes.[44] Other common causes of FUO in the elderly include neoplasms such as lymphomas[45] or collagen vascular diseases. In one study examining FUO in the elderly, it was shown that giant

cell arteritis accounted for 16% of the cases.[46] Fever has also been associated with myocardial infarction, pulmonary embolus, and nontraumatic strokes.[47,48] Fever associated with strokes has been shown to be most commonly caused by underlying pulmonary infection.[49]

Pharmacologic Causes

There are many pharmacologic agents that can cause hyperthermia by 1) increasing muscular activity and heat production, 2) increasing metabolic rate, or 3) impairing heat dissipation (Table 20–5). Drugs that cause muscular hyperactivity include cyclic antidepressants and monoamine oxidase inhibitors. Drugs such as salicylates and thyroid hormones lead to hypermetabolism. Ethanol and phenothiazines impair thermoregulation, while anticholinergics, tricyclic antidepressants, and phenothiazines impair the body's ability to dissipate heat.[46] Diuretics, beta-blockers, and sympatholytic antihypertensive agents all impair cardiovascular compensation, which is necessary to prevent hyperthermia.

Environmental Causes

The majority of hyperthermia seen in the elderly, however, is usually environmental in etiology. Heat illnesses in the elderly are often seen during heat waves, especially when coupled with strenuous activity, a lack of air conditioning, or poor ventilation. These instances will be the major focus because they are the most common, often preventable, and usually readily treatable.

Presentation

There are several different types of heat illness that can present in the elderly. These can be divided into minor heat emergencies, which include *heat edema, heat cramps,*

Table 20–5   Pharmacologic Agents Causing Hyperthermia

Increased Muscular Activity
Amphetamines
PCP
Monoamine oxidase inhibitors
Cocaine
Tricyclic antidepressants
Halothane, succinylcholine ("malignant hyperthermia")
Antipsychotics, lithium ("neuroleptic malignant syndrome")

Increased Metabolic Rate
Salicylates
Thyroid hormone

Impaired Thermoregulation
Phenothiazines
Ethanol

Impaired Heat Dissipation
Anticholinergics
Antihistamines
Tricyclic antidepressants
Phenothiazines

Table 20–4   Medical Conditions Causing Fever/Hyperthermia

Infectious disorders	Neoplastic disease
Mechanical trauma	Vascular accidents
Crush injury	Immune disorders
	Collagen vascular disease

and *heat syncope*. The more serious heat emergencies include *heat exhaustion* and *heat stroke*.

Heat edema, which presents as swelling of the hands and feet, is especially common in the elderly. Many patients may present simply with pitting edema, which usually occurs in the first few days after exposure to a hot environment and is self-limiting, usually resolving after acclimatization occurs. It is important to distinguish heat edema from other (i.e., cardiac) causes of edema that are treated with diuretics, since administration of diuretics to elderly patients with heat edema will make them more likely to develop heat stroke.

Heat cramps are caused by salt depletion. The hyponatremia that results may interfere with calcium-dependent relaxation.[49] Patients with heat cramps usually develop painful but benign involuntary skeletal muscle spasms that occur in muscles after cessation of exercise.[50] This condition is more likely to occur in physically active individuals. Treatment of heat cramps includes oral fluid replacement with a solution such as Gatorade or intravenous saline if the patient is unable to tolerate oral fluids.

A variation of vasovagal syncope, *heat syncope*, is seen primarily in those who stand or work in the heat for a prolonged period of time. It is caused by arteriolar vasodilatation without compensatory tachycardia,[51] resulting in a pooling of the blood in the lower extremities. This condition is easily treated by postural changes, which involve elevating the feet or lowering the head. The use of support hose on the lower extremities to promote venous return may prevent heat syncope.[50]

Heat exhaustion is characterized by weakness, dizziness, nausea, or syncope due to excessive loss of both water and salt. This condition is classified as either hypernatremic (primary water loss) or hyponatremic (primary sodium loss).[49] Vague symptoms and signs complicate the diagnosis of heat exhaustion. The diagnosis is usually made after ruling out other underlying illnesses and identifying a precipitating factor, such as a broken air conditioner, poorly ventilated apartment, or the presence of a heat wave. Heat exhaustion and heat stroke should be considered in elderly patients who present with confusion and elevated temperature, especially during heat waves in which environmental temperatures exceed 95°F for more than 3 days. Hypernatremic heat exhaustion can occur in elderly bedridden individuals who are unable to communicate their thirst or are denied water intake.

Obtaining a rectal temperature is the only way of accurately measuring core temperature and subsequently being able to differentiate heat exhaustion from heat stroke. Studies have demonstrated that the presence of tachypnea alone can raise the average temperature difference (rectal versus oral) significantly.[52] In heat exhaustion, most patients will have temperatures of less than 39°C; they may even be normal. In addition, mental function is basically intact in these individuals with only slight confusion or irritability present.

Heat stroke occurs when the body's ability to dissipate heat becomes unable to compensate for the heat burden imposed by the environment, endogenous sources, or exertion. Heat stroke should always be suspected in patients with a history of heat exposure, temperatures greater than 41°C, and CNS manifestations such as delirium, psychosis, violent behavior, loss of consciousness, focal findings, and seizures. Two types of heat stroke are usually described: classical and exertional. Both types are true medical emergencies associated with a mortality rate ranging from 10 to 80%.[38-40]

Classic heat stroke typically affects the elderly during a heat wave. Most of these patients are older than 70 years[39] and may have underlying medical problems such as congestive heart failure, diabetes mellitus, alcoholism, or diuretic and anticholinergic use. Classic heat stroke develops over a period of several days during a heat wave in persons who are unable to take adequate fluids or move to a cooler environment. CNS manifestations are usually the first to appear and include confusion, bizarre behavior, seizures, and coma. Other neurologic abnormalities — such as dystonia, muscle rigidity, decerebrate posturing, and transient hemiplegia — may also be present, requiring careful differentiation from meningitis.[49] Sweating may be present or absent but is usually decreased in the elderly.[42,58] Patients with heat stroke have elevated rectal temperatures, sometimes greater than 41°C.

In addition to hyperthermia and CNS dysfunction, there are several other clinical manifestations of hyperthermia that may be life threatening. Shock and acidosis can result from the inability to maintain cardiac output in the presence of peripheral vasodilatation and dehydration. Hyperthermia may also impair cardiac output by causing myocardial necrosis, pulmonary hypertension, or both.[54]

Patients with heat stroke will also hyperventilate, at rates up to 60 per minute, in order to lose heat. The respiratory alkalosis that results can produce paresthesias, carpal spasm, tetany, and hypokalemia.[55] Abnormal bleeding, which results from thrombocytopenia or impaired synthesis of clotting factors, is frequently seen in patients with hyperthermia. Disseminated intravascular coagulation can result from activation of the coagulation system by direct thermal injury to vascular endothelium.[56] Muscle breakdown may also occur as a result of direct thermal injury, muscular hyperactivity, or tissue ischemia.[57] Renal failure can occur secondary to the shock state and dehydration as well as the aforementioned rhabdomyolysis. Cardiac arrhythmias may also occur in acute hyperthermia because of myocardial injury, acidosis, hyperkalemia, or hypokalemia. Hypokalemia is more common in elderly patients with classic heat stroke.[39]

Differential Diagnosis

Recognition of heat illness can be difficult in situations when there is no heat wave and the presentation is subtle. A high index of suspicion should always be maintained, and a rectal temperature should always be obtained. It is also essential that the physician consider other medical conditions that can present with significant temperature elevations.

A lumbar puncture can usually distinguish meningitis and encephalitis from heat stroke. Malaria, although rare in nonendemic areas, can be distinguished with a peripheral blood smear. Other diseases such as epilepsy, head trauma, cerebrovascular accidents, thyroid storm, diabetic ketoacidosis, and infection-sepsis can also mimic heat stroke. A careful history and laboratory findings help make the distinction, with initial SGOT, LDH, and CPK levels being high in heat stroke and normal or slightly elevated in the infectious or other diseases.[18]

Treatment

Cooling should be started immediately in patients with temperatures above 41°C, and this should take precedence over all other diagnostic measures. The two methods of cooling involve the use of ice water baths and evaporative cooling.

Evaporative cooling can be performed by moving air over a wet, disrobed patient. Patients should be suspended and warm water should be used in order to prevent shivering. This method is similar to the methods developed in Saudi Arabia, which have been shown to be very successful.[59,60] The use of ice water baths is impractical, is often dangerous, causes shivering, and makes monitoring and airway management more difficult. A specific tank for cooling has been developed but is not in widespread use.[61]

The airway may require protection, since coma, convulsions, and vomiting put patients at risk for aspiration. Patients with hyperthermia have high tissue-oxygen needs and require supplemental oxygen administration.

An intravenous (IV) line should be started, and fluid administration should be initiated. Fluid requirements are usually low in patients with environmental heat illness, and fluids should be administered cautiously. Elderly people should have Swan-Ganz catheterization prior to large amounts of fluid administration in order to avoid pulmonary edema. The fluid of choice is normal saline.

All patients with hyperthermia should be monitored for dysrhythmias and carefully evaluated for gastrointestinal (GI) bleeding. Shivering is best treated with diazepam or chlorpromazine, although chlorpromazine may cause hypotension and lower the seizure threshold.

In the elderly, prevention involves avoiding heat, reducing activity, and maintaining adequate hydration. It is important that the elderly adjust in their environment, so that they are away from direct sunlight and always maintain adequate ventilation. It should be stressed that cooling alone may not be adequate treatment for the elderly hyperthermic patient, since associated medical conditions may coexist. The physician should aggressively search for and treat these associated conditions.

REFERENCES

1. Rango N: Exposure related hypothermia mortality in the United States, 1970–79, Am J Public Health 74:1159, 1984.
2. Leads from the MMWR: Hypothermia associated deaths — United States 1968–70, JAMA 255(3):307, 1986.
3. Goldman A et al: A pilot study of low body temperatures in old people admitted to hospital, J R Coll Physicians Lond 1113:291, 1977.
4. Fox RH et al: Body temperatures in the elderly: a national study of physiologic, social, and environmental conditions, Br Med J 1:200, 1973.
5. Watts AJ: Hypothermia in the aged: a study of the role of cold sensitivity, Environ Res 5:119, 1971.
6. Horvath SM et al: Metabolic responses of old people to a cold environment, J Appl Physiol 8:145, 1955.
7. Kaag CL and Kountz WB: Stability of body function in the aged: effects of exposure of the body to cold, J Gerontol 5:227, 1950.
8. Kallman H: Protecting your elderly patients from winter's cold, Geriatrics 40(12):69, 1985.
9. Kurtz RS: Hypothermia in the elderly: the cold facts, Geriatrics 37:85, 1982.
10. Collins KJ, Exton-Smith AN, and Dore C: Urban hypothermia: preferred temperature and thermal perception in old age, Br Med J 282:175, 1981.
11. Matz R: Hypothermia: mechanisms and countermeasures, Hosp Pract 21(1A):45, 1986.
12. Restivo KM et al: Accumulation of polyamines and their weak association with lower body temperature in elderly convalescent patients, J Lab Clin Med 110(2):217–220, 1987.
13. Collins KJ, Easton JC, and Exton-Smith AN: Shivering thermogenesis and vasomotor responses with convective cooling in the elderly, J Physiol 320:76, 1981.
14. Stoner HB, Little RA, and Frayn KN: Fat metabolism in elderly patients with severe hypothermia, Q J Exp Physiol 68:701, 1983.
15. Maclean D and Emslie-Smith D: Accidental hypothermia, 1977, Philadelphia, J.B. Lippincott Co.
16. Treatment of myxedic coma, Lancet 2:768, 1956 (editorial).
17. Cooper KE: Temperature regulation and its disorders: hypothermia in recent advances in medicine, ed 15, London, 1986, Churchill Livingstone.
18. DeMonchaux C: Psychological factors in hypothermia, Social Science Research Council Report, 1975.
19. Doherty NE et al: Hypothermia with acute myocardial infarction, Ann Intern Med 101(6):797–798, 1984.
20. Lewin S, Brettman LR, and Holzman RS: Infection in hypothermic patients, Arch Intern Med 141:920, 1981.
21. Morris DL et al: Hemodynamic characteristics of patients with hypothermia due to occult infection and other causes, Ann Intern Med 102(2):153, 1985.
22. Gale EAM and Tattersal RB: Hypothermia: a complication of diabetic ketoacidosis, Br Med J 4:1387, 1978.
23. Molnar GW and Read RC: Hypoglycemia and body temperature, JAMA 227:916, 1974.
24. Neil HA, Dawson JA, and Baker JE: Risk of hypothermia in elderly patients with diabetes, Br Med J 293:416, 1986.
25. Wilson GM: Hypothermia in clinical medicine, Med Sci Law 9:231, 1969.
26. Irvine RE: Hypothermia in old age, Practitioner 213:795, 1974.
26a. Kramer MR, Vandijk J, and Rosin AJ: Mortality in elderly patients with thermoregulatory failure, Arch Intern Med 149:1521, 1989.
27. Brocklehurst JC: Textbook of geriatric medicine and gerontology, London, 1978, Churchill Livingstone.
28. Woolf PD et al: Accidental hypothermia: endocrine function during recovery, J Clin Endocrinol Metab 34:460, 1972.
29. MacNichol MW: Respiratory failure and acid base status in

hypothermia, Postgrad Med J 43:674, 1967.

30. Collins KJ: Hypothermia: the facts, New York, 1983, Oxford University Press.

31. Zell SC and Kurtz KJ: Severe exposure hypothermia: a resuscitation protocol, Ann Emerg Med 4:339, 1985.

32. Rosen P et al: Emergency medicine: concepts and clinical practice, St. Louis, 1983, The CV Mosby Co.

33. Reuler JB: Hypothermia: pathophysiology, clinical settings and management, Ann Intern Med 89:519, 1978.

34. Lloyd E: Accidental hypothermia treated by central rewarming through the airway, Br J Anaesth 45:41, 1973.

35. Lloyd E and Mitchell B: Factors affecting the onset of ventricular fibrillation in hypothermia, Lancet 2:1294, 1974.

36. Billen JP et al: Ventricular fibrillation during orotracheal intubation of hypothermic dogs, Ann Emerg Med 15:412–416, 1986.

37. Wollner L and Spalding JMK: The autonomic nervous system. In Brocklehurst JC, editor: Textbook of geriatric medicine and gerontology, ed 3, London, 1978, Churchill Livingstone.

38. Rosenberg J et al: Hyperthermia associated with drug intoxication, Crit Care Med 14(11):964, 1986.

39. Hart GR et al: Epidemic classical heat stroke: clinical characteristics and course of 28 patients, Medicine 61:189, 1982.

40. Olson KR and Benowitz NL: Environmental and drug induced hyperthermia, recognition and management, Emerg Med Clin North Am 2:459, 1984.

41. Foster KG et al: Sweat responses in the aged, Age Ageing 5:91–101, 1976.

42. Ellis FP: Heat illness, Trans R Soc Trop Med Hyg 70:402, 1976.

43. Kelleher JP and Sales JEL: Pyrexia of unknown origin and colorectal carcinoma, Br Med J 293(6):1475, 1986.

44. Kauffman CA and Jones PG: Diagnosing fever of unknown origin in older patients, Geriatrics 39(2):46, 1984.

45. Petersdorf RG and Beeson PB: Fever of unexplained origin: report on 100 cases, Medicine 40:1, 1961.

46. Esposito AL and Gleckman RA: Fever of unknown origin in the elderly, J Am Geriatr Soc 26:498, 1978.

47. Murray HW et al: Fever and pulmonary thromboembolism, Am J Med 67:232–235, 1979.

48. Rousseaux P et al: Fever and cerebral vasospasm in ruptured intracranial aneurysms, Surg Neurol 14:459, 1980.

49. Pizelonski MM et al: Fever in the wake of a stroke, Neurology 36:427, 1986.

50. Knockel JP: Environmental heat illness: an eclectic review, Arch Intern Med 133:841, 1974.

51. Stewart CE: Preventing progression of heat injury, Emerg Med Rep 8(16):121, 1987.

52. Beezer CB: Heat stress and the young athlete: recognizing and reducing the risks, Postgrad Med 76(1):109, 1984.

53. Tandberg D and Sklar D: Effect of tachypnea on the estimation of body temperature by an oral thermometer, N Engl J Med 308(16):945, 1983.

54. Rew MC, Bershas I, and Sefteh H: The diagnostic and prognostic significance of serum enzyme changes in heat stroke, Trans R Soc Trop Med Hyg 63:325, 1971.

55. Clowes GH and O'Donnell TF: Heat stroke, N Engl J Med 291:564, 1974.

56. Knochel JP: Dog days and siriasis: how to kill a football player, JAMA 233(6):513, 1975.

57. O'Donnell TF: Acute heat stroke: epidemiologic, biochemical, renal and coagulation studies, JAMA 234:824, 1975.

58. Gabow PA, Kaehny WD, and Kelleher SP: The spectrum of rhabdomyolysis, Medicine 61:141, 1982.

59. Schoenfeld Y and Odassin R: Age and sex difference in response to short exposure to extreme dry heat, J Appl Physiol 44:1, 1978.

60. Khogali M, Mustafa MK, and Gumaa K: Management of heatstroke, Lancet 2(8309):1225, 1982.

61. Weiner JS and Kohgali M: A physiologic body cooling unit for treatment of heatstroke, Lancet 1(8167):507, 1980.

Infections in the Frail Elderly

Stephen R. Jones, M.D., F.A.C.P.

In the early 1900s, our population had a pyramidal shape with a broad base of young and progressively diminishing numbers of older people. The projected shape for the year 2000 changes from a pyramid to a rectangle. This chapter will not discuss infections in the general population of the elderly since this group is too heterogenous. Instead, infections in the frail and vulnerable elderly will be defined and discussed. Because of the critical nature of sepsis in the elderly, this topic is discussed in detail in Chapter 22.

DEFINITION OF THE FRAIL ELDERLY

The frail elderly population is characterized by those individuals with functional impairment: immobility, incompetence (dementia), and/or incontinence. These are the impairments that move people from a low-support to a high-support living environment; from traditional housing to retirement housing, congregate housing, residential care; and, eventually, perhaps to a skilled nursing facility (Table 21–1).

THE HIGH INCIDENCE OF INFECTION

The most common cause of transfer from the nursing home to the short-stay acute-care hospital is infection. Providing medical care to several nursing homes and operating a geriatric clinic for their hospital, Irvine et al.[1] compared the two populations. Twenty-seven percent of the patients they admitted to a hospital from nursing homes had infectious diseases; only 12% admitted from the community had infectious diseases. The most common infectious diseases of the frail elderly are pneumonia (lower respiratory tract infection), urinary tract infections, and skin and skin structure infections. Other studies have confirmed these observations.

Infections in such a frail population may lead to the *geriatric cascade*. For example, a simple viral respiratory tract infection may lead to a chest infection or pneumonia, which itself may lead to death. The toxic delirium from even a mild infection may lead to a fall and a hip fracture with immobility and then incontinence, pressure sores, or death. This is an extremely fragile group of individuals, and even a mild infection may lead to more serious infections or to coexisting morbid conditions that may lead to death.

PATHOPHYSIOLOGY
Host Defense Mechanisms

What is the pathophysiology of infection in this group of individuals? A number of physiologic variables decrease with age: cardiac index, glomerular filtration rate, vital capacity of the lung, renal plasma flow, and maximal breathing capacity.[2]

Table 21–1   Characteristics of Frail Elderly

Defined by functional impairment
    Immobility
    Incompetence (dementia)
    Incontinence

Infections are common
    Pneumonia
    Urinary tract infection
    Skin and skin structure

Infections lead to further morbidity and mortality (geriatric
    cascade)

Host defense mechanisms may be considered in three general groups: 1) factors that work at body surfaces (e.g., skin, mucous membranes, cilia in the lungs, the cough reflex), 2) extracellular fluid factors such as antibodies, complement, and other factors that are currently being elucidated daily such as interleukins, and 3) cellular factors such as fixed and mobile phagocytes. There is little conclusive evidence that humoral and cellular immunity are significantly diminished in the elderly. Most importantly, it is the defects in those factors operating at organ surfaces that are most important for the susceptibility of the frail elderly to infection (Table 21–2). These defects may include the following:

- Thinning of the skin occurs as one ages; pressure sores and trauma inflict more damage more easily.
- Decreased ciliary activity and decreased cough reflex occur in the lungs, which predisposes the elderly to infection in the lower respiratory tract.
- In the gastrointestinal tract, gastric acid is decreased, and gastric acid is responsible for destroying many gastrointestinal pathogens.
- Decrease in gut motility decreases clearance of pathogens.

Table 21–2   Pathophysiology of Infection

Host defenses
    Body surface factors impaired
    Extracellular fluid factors normal
    Cellular factors normal

Body surface factors
    Thin, fragile skin
    Decreased ciliary activity
    Decreased cough reflex
    Decreased gastric acid
    Decreased gut motility

Mechanical risk factors
    Pressure sores
    Indwelling urethral catheter
    Nasogastric tubes

Coexisting morbid conditions
    Soft tissue edema
    Pulmonary edema

In the immune system, the only thing that has been reliably and reproducibly demonstrated is a mild fall-off in the T-lymphocyte activity and some decreased production of lymphokines. This, however, has never been correlated in any meaningful way with increased infection in the elderly in the absence of disease (e.g., AIDS) or a condition involving immunosuppression (such as treatment for cancer).

Mechanical Risk Factors and Coexisting Morbid Conditions

A variety of mechanical risk factors operate at body surfaces and are important in the pathophysiology of infections in the frail elderly. Pressure ulcers predispose to cellulitis and perhaps then to bacteremia. Indwelling catheters and even condom catheters have been associated with urinary tract infections. Feeding tubes predispose to aspiration pneumonia. Soft tissue injury and wounds from immobility or movement of the patient by caregivers lead to cellulitis. Furthermore, a number of comorbid conditions exist in the elderly that predispose them to infectious diseases. Soft tissue edema — which may be the result of venostasis, congestive heart failure, or low albumin — may lead to cellulitis. Pulmonary edema, which may lead to pneumonia, may be the result of congestive heart failure or may be caused by acid aspiration.

MICROBIOLOGY

Two key points should be remembered about the microbiology of infection in this group:

1. The usual site-pathogen rules are valid (pneumococcus is the most common cause of pneumonia; *Staphylococcus* and *Streptococcus* are the most common causes of soft tissue infections; and aerobic gram-negative bacilli still cause urinary tract infections in the frail elderly as they do in the more healthy population.
2. A generalizable rule in the frail elderly is that with mucosal and skin surface alterations there is an increased risk for aerobic gram-negative bacillary colonization and infection.[3,4] For example, the oropharynx becomes colonized with aerobic gram-negative bacilli in up to 50% of frail individuals. This is a rare event in the healthy individual. Pressure ulcers become colonized with fecal bacteria and aerobic and anaerobic gram-negative bacilli.[5] Aerobic gram-negative bacilli are always the most common cause of urinary tract infections, but *E. coli*, the most common uropathogen in the general population, becomes less important; more exotic and antimicrobial-resistant gram-negative bacilli such as *Klebsiella, Enterobacter,* and *Proteus* species are isolated more frequently in the frail elderly.

EARLY RECOGNITION

The early recognition of the infection is important. However, the presentation of infection in the elderly may be subtle and nonspecific. This is more common in the frail elderly and the "old-old" over 75 years of age. Fever may be absent in as high as 25% of infections, and the first sign of infection in the elderly may be confusion or the inability to perform a function that was done easily in the past, such as toileting or urinary maintenance or fecal continence. A high index of suspicion is required for detection of infection in this group.

ETHICS

Medicine has been accused of overapplying technology and needlessly and perhaps thoughtlessly preventing the inevitable death of the frail elderly individual. William Osler is often quoted, "pneumonia may well be called the friend of the aged, taken off by it in an acute, short, often painless illness, the old escape those cold gradations of decay that make the last state of all so distressing."[15] In many situations the "last state of all" that causes distress often occurs in the intensive care unit or in an acute care ward.

Although an enormous amount of progress has been made in the ethical management of the frail elderly over the last decade, there is need for improvement. Courts and medical investigators have addressed the issue. In a study published in 1979, Brown et al.[6] studied two long-term care facilities and 190 episodes of fever and found that 109 of these patients were worked up and treated with antimicrobials (there was a 9% mortality). Another 81 patients were not worked up and not treated, and the majority of these patients died. This documents a standard of practice, that is, not every patient with a fever in a long-term care facility is evaluated and treated with antimicrobials.[7] This has been substantiated by a court decision. In 1978, in the Tennessee Court of Appeals, the court declared that antibiotics could be regarded as a heroic measure that could risk iatrogenic disease. More recently, the Presidential Commission for the Study of Ethical Problems in Medicine and Biomedical Research has stated that they found no particular treatments, including such ordinary hospital interventions as *antibiotics,* to be universally warranted. Nevertheless, the decision to forego particular life-sustaining treatment is not grounds to withdraw all care, especially when this care is needed to ensure patients' comfort, dignity, and self-determination. This is the dominant consideration in the care of the frail elderly.[8]

ANTIMICROBIAL USE IN LONG-TERM CARE FACILITIES

There are an enormous number of infectious diseases that are treated in nursing homes.[9] The first systematic review of this practice was published in 1987.[10] The findings of the two studies are similar. Many antibiotics are used inappropriately in nursing homes, and the reason for the misuse is that aerobic gram-negative rods are not well covered by empiric therapy. In many instances, this was not because of lack of knowledge on the part of practitioners, but because antimicrobial agents that are effective and easy to administer in the nursing home have not been available. Recently introduced antimicrobials possess many of the features that will make them acceptable for use in the nursing home. An important characteristic is effectiveness against aerobic gram-negative bacilli. One such new antimicrobial is aztreonam. It is given intramuscularly every 8 to 12 hours and is effective *only* against the aerobic gram-negative bacilli. A second group is the fluroquinolones — orally administered drugs that are effective against a broad range of pathogens.

SPECIFIC INFECTIONS

Three specific infections will be reviewed: urinary tract infections, pneumonia, and skin and soft tissue infections.

Pneumonia (Lower Respiratory Tract Infection)

Background

There are four fundamental factors associated with pneumonia and its special virulence in the frail elderly (Table 21–3). First, the prevalence of colonization of the oropharynx with aerobic gram-negative bacilli is high.[3,4] Surveys of normal individuals have shown these bacteria are isolated from the oropharynx in only 1%. In a survey of nursing home residents, the prevalence was 37% and, if bedridden, 50%. Colonization, coupled with the greater propensity for large-volume aspiration, make the frail elderly particularly prone to pneumonia and, especially, infection caused by aerobic gram-negative bacilli. The pneumococcus, however, still remains the most common cause of pneumonia in this group. *Haemophilus influenzae* is more common in older people than in healthy, younger people.[11,12]

If material is aspirated, the frail elderly are less likely to be able to clear the microorganisms. This is due to poor cough reflex, decreased ciliary clearance, and decreased clearance at the alveoli. Lastly, these individuals are less likely to respond against systemic effects (sepsis) of the invading bacteria.

Table 21–3 Factors Associated with Pneumonias

Pharyngeal colonization with gram-negative bacilli
Aspiration
Poor clearance of aspirated material
Poor systemic response to sepsis

The clinical features of pneumonia in the frail elderly include a more insidious onset of the infection (Table 21–4). Fever may be absent, and confusion may be the most prominent change. Chest pain is less common, and the cough may be weak or absent. The majority of patients produce minimal sputum. Raised respiratory rate is a useful clinical sign.[14]

Antimicrobial Choices

The recommendations for the empiric therapy of pneumonia in the frail elderly take into account several modifying variables: clinical severity, the predominant bacterium on the sputum Gram stain (if available), and the community or institutional microbiology.[14]

- If the pneumococcus is suspected:
  penicillin-G 600,000 U IM b.i.d.
- If aerobic gram-negative rods are suspected or cannot be excluded:
  cefotaxime 2 g IM/IV q. 8 to 12h.

  or

  ceftriaxone 2 g IM/IV q. 12h.
- If *Pseudomonas* is prevalent in the community or institution:
  clindamycin 600 mg IM/IV combined with *aztreonam* 1 g q. 12h.

  or

  imipenem/cilastatin 500 mg IV q. 8h.
- If *Legionella pneumophila* is suspected, add to the regimen chosen above:
  erythromycin 1 g PO/IV q. 6h.
- If *Staphylococcus aureus* is highly probable (i.e., there is strong evidence from the sputum Gram stain):
  nafcillin 2 g IV q. 4h.

(However, all of the above regimens provide satisfactory antistaphylococcal therapy.)

There are a variety of other choices that may be appropriate.

Urinary Tract Infections

Background

The prevalence of bacteriuria increases with age and is associated with advancing functional disability. This is often accompanied by the placement of urinary drainage devices.[16-19] The prevalence of asymptomatic bacteriuria is higher in the frail elderly than in a young and healthy population.[20-26] The incidence is roughly proportional to the degree of diminishment of self-care: 27% in a population living in residential care and 33% in an intermediate-care setting. Virtually each patient with an indwelling catheter is infected.

Although the frail elderly are under more intense medical scrutiny than the general healthy population, this is unlikely to entirely explain the greater prevalence of asymptomatic bacteriuria. The high prevalence is probably multifactorial: fecal incontinence with perineal and periurethral contamination, poor hygiene, inadequate emptying of the bladder, and past instrumentation. Immobility and fecal incontinence are the two major factors for infection (Table 21–5). Unlike in younger people, the presence of pyuria is not highly correlated with bacteriuria. In a population-based study in Finland, 47% of residents had pyuria, but only half of these had bacteriuria.[26]

Because of the recurrent acute-care hospitalizations of these patients, many have acquired a fecal flora containing uropathogens that are more resistant to antimicrobials than those isolated from the general population. These will include species of *Enterobacter cloacae, Serratia, Proteus, Providentia,* and *Pseudomonas.* For purposes of deciding which antimicrobial drug is appropriate, it is useful to classify patients into subgroups (Table 21–6).

Antimicrobial Choices

Asymptomatic. Although it has been suggested that the elderly with asymptomatic urinary infection die earlier than their noninfected cohorts, a recent randomized, controlled trial showed that therapy did not effectively provide a permanently sterile urine and had no effect on mortality.[21] This was true whether or not an indwelling catheter is present. Treatment of asymptomatic elderly with bacteriuria is not recommended.[22]

Symptomatic. Since bacteriuria is common, and the signs of infection are nonspecific in the frail elderly, the obvious dilemma frequently arises. The empiric treatment of a urinary tract infection is appropriate both when specific symptoms and signs are present or if nonspecific findings are due, with a reasonable probability, to a urinary infection. Because an indwelling catheter may be colonized with multiple bacterial species, some of which are not present in the bladder, the urine specimen for culture should be collected with a new catheter.

- If *Pseudomonas* is not likely:
  oral therapy possible:
  trimethoprim/sulfamethoxazole 1 tablet q. 12h.

Table 21–4 Clinical Features of Pneumonia

Insidious onset	Chest pain uncommon
Fever may be absent	Cough weak or absent
Delirium common	Sputum minimal or absent

Table 21–5 Factors Associated with Bacteriuria

Incontinence	Instrumentation
Immobility	Indwelling catheter
Residual urine in bladder	Condom catheters

Table 21–6 Urinary Tract Infection

Asymptomatic
  With Foley catheter
  Without catheter
Symptomatic
  Conventional urinary tract infection symptoms
  Subtle nonspecific symptoms

or

ciprofloxacin 500 mg PO q. 12h.
parenteral therapy required:
  cefotaxime 1 g IM/IV q. 12h.

or

ceftriaxone 1 g IM/IV q. 24h.

- If *Pseudomonas* is likely:
  oral therapy possible:
    ciprofloxacin 500 mg PO q. 12h.
  parenteral therapy required:
    aztreonam 1 g IM/IV q. 12h.

or

imipenem/cilastatin 500 mg IV q. 8h.

Skin and Skin Structure Infections

Background

The most common association of skin infections in the frail elderly are pressure sores. Pressure sores are graded I to IV (Table 21–7). Grades II through IV are associated with the loss of continuity of the epidermis. Grades III and IV allow ready invasion by local microbes. Grade IV is often associated with osteomyelitis. The ulcers are commonly colonized by fecal bacteria. The microbiology of pressure sores shows that the aerobic gram-negative bacilli (Enterobacteriaceae) are most commonly isolated but *Pseudomonas, Staphylococcus aureus, Streptococcus faecalis, Streptococcus pyogenes,* and anaerobic bacteria such as *Bacteroides fragilis* also are recovered frequently. When associated with bacteremia, any of these microorganisms may be present; however, the most common isolates are *Proteus* and *Bacteroides fragilis*.

Antimicrobial Choices

Colonization of the pressure sore should not be treated with systemic antimicrobials, and when local or generalized sepsis is associated with a pressure sore, the wide variety of bacteria present must be empirically treated. The following antimicrobial regimens are appropriate:

clindamycin 800 mg and *aztreonam* 1 g IV/IM q. 8 to 12h.

or

ampicillin-sulbactam 1.5–3 gm q. 6h. and *aztreonam* 1 g IV/IM q. 8 to 12h.

or

imipenem/cilastatin 500 mg IV q. 6h.

Table 21–7 Clinical Grades for Pressure Sores

Inflammatory response affected epidermis only
Shallow ulcer; inflammation of dermis
Ulcer through skin to subcutaneous fat
Ulcer through to fascia

OTHER INFECTIONS

A wide variety of other infections must also be considered in the frail elderly but are beyond the scope of this chapter. Covert infections must be suspected in the septic frail elderly before the infection reaches a catastrophic stage. They include covert intraabdominal septic processes such as a ruptured appendix or gangrenous cholecystitis.[27] Furthermore, infective endocarditis occurs disproportionately in the elderly.[28,29] This is probably due to turbulent flow over sclerotic heart valves. When infective endocarditis occurs in the elderly, its manifestations are more likely to be subtle and nonspecific than in the younger person. Tuberculosis is also more common in the frail elderly.[30] A variety of pulmonary and extrapulmonary presentations are possible.

In summary, infections are a common cause of morbidity and mortality in the frail elderly. Aberrant and subtle presentations and a high prevalence of aerobic and bacillary infections are important considerations in recognizing these infections and choosing therapy.

REFERENCES

1. Irvine PW, Van Buren N, and Crossley K: Causes for hospitalization of nursing residents: the role of infection, J Am Geriatr Soc 32:103–107, 1984.
2. Saltzman RL and Peterson PK: Immunodeficiency of the elderly, Rev Infect Dis 9:1127–1139, 1987.
3. Valenti WM, Trudell RG, and Bentley DW: Factors predisposing to oropharyngeal colonization with gram-negative bacilli in the aged, N Engl J Med 298:1108–1111, 1978.
4. Mackowiak PA et al: Pharyngeal colonization by gram-negative bacilli in aspiration-prone persons, Arch Intern Med 138:1124–1127, 1978.
5. Allman RM: Pressure ulcers among the elderly, N Engl J Med 320:850, 1989.
6. Brown NK and Thompson DJ: Nontreatment of fever in extended-care facilities, N Engl J Med 300:1246–1250, 1979.
7. Mott PD and Barker WH: Hospital and medical care use by nursing home patients: the effect of patient care plans, J Am Geriatr Soc 36:47–53, 1988.
8. The Hastings Center: Guidelines on the termination of life-sustaining treatment and the care of the dying, Bloomington, 1987, Indiana University Press.
9. Zimmer JG et al: Systemic antibiotic use in nursing homes, J Am Geriatr Soc 34:703–710, 1986.
10. Jones SR et al: Appropriateness of antibiotic therapy in long-term care facilities, Am J Med 87:499–502, 1987.
11. Garb JL et al: Differences in etiology of pneumonias in nursing home and community patients, JAMA 240:2169–2172, 1978.
12. Community-acquired pneumonia requiring hospitalization. Is it different in the elderly? J Am Geriatr Soc 33:671–680, 1985.
13. McFadden JP et al: Raised respiratory rate in elderly patients: a valuable physical sign, Br Med J 284:626–627, 1982.
14. Marrie JT, Durant H, and Kwan C: Nursing home-acquired pneumonia, J Am Geriatr Soc 34:697–702, 1986.
15. Berk SL: Bacterial pneumonia in the elderly: the observations of Sir William Osier in retrospect, J Am Geriatr Soc 32:683–685, 1984.
16. Warren JW et al: Fever, bacteremia, and death as complications of

bacteriuria in women with long-term urethral catheters, J Infect Dis 115(6):1151–1158, 1987.

17. Warren JW et al: A prospective microbiologic study of bacteriuria in patients with chronic indwelling urethral catheters, J Infect Dis 146(6):719–723m, 1972.

18. Breitenbucher RB: Bacterial changes in the urine samples of patients with long-term indwelling catheters, Arch Intern Med 144:1585–1588, 1984.

19. Rubin M, Berger SA, and Zodda FN Jr: Effect of catheter replacement on bacterial counts in urine aspirated from indwelling catheters, J Infect Dis 142(2):291, 1980.

20. Nicolle LE et al: Bacteriuria in elderly institutionalized men, N Engl J Med 309:1470–1475, 1983.

21. Nicolle LE et al: The association of bacteriuria with resident characteristics and survival in elderly institutionalized men, Ann Intern Med 106(5):682–686, 1987.

22. Boscia JA, Abrutyn E, and Kaye D: Asymptomatic bacteriuria in elderly persons: treat or do not treat? Ann Intern Med 106(5):764–765, 1987.

23. Boscia JA et al: Therapy vs. no therapy for bacteriuria in elderly ambulatory nonhospitalized women, JAMA 257:1067–1071, 1987.

24. Boscia JA et al: Lack of association between bacteriuria and symptoms in the elderly, Am J Med 81:979–982, 1986.

25. Warren JW et al: Cephalexin for susceptible bacteriuria in afebrile, long-term catheterized patients, JAMA 248(4):454–458, 1982.

26. Alling B et al: Aerobic and anaerobic microbial flora in the urinary tract of geriatric patients during long-term care, J Infect Dis 127(1):34:39, 1973.

27. Price FM, Kimbrough RC, and Jones SR: Gallbladder gangrene as evidence of catastrophic, covert gallbladder disease in the chronically ill and elderly, Medical Rounds 1:21–30, 1988.

28. Terpenning MS, Buggy BP, and Kauffman CA: Infective endocarditis: clinical features in young and elderly patients, Am J Med 83:626, 1987.

29. Robbins N, DeMaria A, and Miller MH: Infective endocarditis in the elderly, South Med J 73:1335–1338, 1980.

30. Stead WW and Lofgren JP: Does the risk of tuberculosis increase in old age? J Infect Dis 147:951–955, 1983.

SUGGESTED READINGS

Gorse GJ et al: Bacterial meningitis in the elderly, Arch Intern Med 144:1603–1607, 1984.

Kane RL, Ouslander JG, and Abrass IB: Clinical implications of the aging process. In Kane RL, Ouslander JG, and Abrass IB: Essentials of clinical geriatrics, New York, 1984, McGraw-Hill Book Co.

Sepsis

George R. Schwartz, M.D., F.A.C.E.P.

GENERAL CONSIDERATIONS

While bacteremic infections in any age group are serious, in the elderly they are more common and more frequently life-threatening. Esposito and his colleagues[1] found a case-fatality rate of 26% in patients 65 or older with bacteremic infection. Smith[2] reports that patients aged 65 and older make up about 50% of all people with septicemia. Of these people, one half have a severe underlying disease.

For this discussion, bacteremic infection and sepsis will be used interchangeably and are distinguished from a transient bacteremia without infection. However, in the elderly, even a transient bacteremia associated, for example, with dental work or medical instrumentation, may lead to more serious consequences such as endocarditis or abscess.

The alterations in immune function in the elderly have been discussed elsewhere in this book. These immunologic reductions are related to aging, the environment (e.g., malnutrition, alcoholism), and underlying diseases with the influences of each often difficult to separate. For example, the monocytes and macrophages undergo changes[3] in a variety of disease states associated with aging, such as diabetes mellitus. An overall trend toward decreasing immunologic reactivity in the aged is compounded by medications that may be used for treatment. For example, corticosteroids or anticancer chemotherapy medications can markedly reduce the normal defense mechanisms. Splenectomy also predisposes to sudden overwhelming septicemias particularly with the pneumococcus organism. While overall antibody response may be less in the elderly, immunization is still effective and will reduce mortality from infections such as influenza.[4] The immunologic deficiency in those over 80 has prognostic significance and underscores the need for early recognition and rapid treatment in this age group. When tests were made of cellular and humoral immunity in the elderly, those patients over 80 years of age who were hyporesponsive had a higher mortality rate over the subsequent 2 years than a similar group of octogenarians with more responsive immunologic systems.[5]

Smith[6] points out that the heightened sensitivity of the elderly to infection is not just related to decreasing immunologic function. He notes that there can be less ciliary activity in the respiratory tract, reduced digestive (and bacteria-killing) enzymes in the intestinal tract, and even reduced protection from natural barriers such as the skin.

Any sort of medical device or procedure heightens the risk of infection — from administration of a simple IV to placement of a urinary catheter or gastrostomy tube. With the heightened immunologic risk, a mild infection with bacteremia can rapidly progress to an overwhelming life-threatening infection with sepsis.

The overall approach to sepsis in the elderly is early recognition of the infection, identification of the source, suitable cultures for microorganism identification, and rapid institution of suitable antimicrobial agents.

Each of these areas is discussed below.

EARLY RECOGNITION

In the late nineteenth and early twentieth centuries, physicians began to increasingly describe a clinical "shock" syndrome associated with bacteria in the blood.[7,8] Because of the lack of effective treatment, such cases were almost uniformly fatal. The introduction of effective antimicrobial drugs has, of course, completely changed this situation but underscores the importance of early recognition since the shock syndrome is a late phenomenon and very difficult to treat even in a healthy younger person. With the decreased immunologic capability and less physiologic reserve in the elderly, early recognition is imperative to reduce mortality from sepsis. Recent findings of myocardial depressant substances causing early cardiac dysfunction in septic shock underscore the need for early treatment.[36]

CLINICAL MANIFESTATIONS

Reduced Fever

While fever and chills are characteristic symptoms of sepsis, the elderly patient may present with confusing symptoms. Rather than fever, the elderly patient may present with hypothermia. Smith[2] reports that 20 to 30% of elderly patients present atypically. He notes that fever is absent in 12% of the elderly versus only 4% in younger patients.

Gleckman and Hilbert[9] reported on 27 patients who had afebrile bacteremia. Of this group, 25 (93%) were 65 years or older.

The reduced fever response is associated with aging but can also result from medications used to treat underlying chronic diseases. For example, salicylates, corticosteroids, and other antiinflammatory agents can markedly reduce the fever response. In addition, a study we conducted at our emergency department demonstrated that oral temperatures were often inaccurate, and a rectal temperature is mandatory in the elderly when infection is suspected. Mouth breathing, tachypnea, low ambient temperature, and difficulty in placing the oral temperature gauge may all give a falsely low and misleading reading.

Mental Status Changes

Mental status changes are also more common in the bacteremic septic elderly person. With preexistent mental changes in older people, the deterioration due to sepsis may be masked. Also, with temperature elevation, symptoms of a recent stroke can be reproduced, and unless a detailed evaluation occurs, symptoms caused by sepsis can be misdiagnosed as "stroke." Sometimes the presenting symptoms may be unexplained confusion or nonspecific malaise. Anorexia, vomiting, and diarrhea are also common nonspecific signs. The value of taking blood cultures and having a high index of suspicion is stressed and, if there are signs of infection, beginning antibiotics presumptively is recommended.

Skin Lesions

Also be particularly aware of skin lesions in the elderly. Not only can they be a cause of a toxic shock–like syndrome,[10] but they can rapidly spread throughout nursing homes and hospitals.[11] Because of the readily treatable nature of these conditions (penicillin for *Streptococcus* infections, oxacillin or methicillin for staphylococcal along with adequate fluids, vasopressors, and supportive treatment), they must not be overlooked. Also, skin lesions such as the purpura associated with meningococcal infection, an ominous finding, could be ascribed in the early stages to easy bruisability. Diagnosing meninococcal sepsis early is essential since there are effective treatments early in the course of the disease (e.g., penicillin), but the prognosis can rapidly worsen as fulminant sepsis with hypotension develops.[34]

Decubitus ulcers or pressure sores are frequently found in the frail elderly, particularly those with neuromuscular diseases. When septicemia develops from decubiti, the mortality rate approaches 50%.[12] Because of the polymicrobial nature of this sepsis (*Proteus* sp., *E. coli, Klebsiella, Pseudomonas,* and gram-positive cocci), broad-spectrum antibiotic treatment is needed.[33]

OTHER EARLY SIGNS AND SYMPTOMS

The early signs of sepsis might refer to the source or infected organ. In one study of 190 febrile elderly patients, respiratory infections accounted for 58% and urinary tract infections for 15% — together almost 75%.[13] Respiratory symptoms (cough, sputum, chest pain) and urinary tract infection (UTI) symptoms (flank pain, dysuria) should alert the physician to check further if there is even the slightest suspicion of bacteremia.

Although the above study followed patients with fever, it must be stressed that the presentation of a septic elderly patient may be a hypothermic state.

Reviewing backward from a known septic state, Esposito and his colleagues[1] determined that the urinary tract led the list as a cause (34%), followed by the biliary system (20%), the respiratory system (13%), other abdominal infection such as diverticulitis or appendicitis

(8%), endocarditis (7%), and meningitis (4%). These categories will be covered in detail in subsequent sections.

The elderly patient with symptoms and signs of gallbladder infection, abdominal pain in the right upper quadrant, and tenderness must be evaluated for sepsis.

LATER SIGNS OF SEPSIS

Shock, hypotension, circulatory collapse, and intense vasoconstriction (early vasodilation) are ominous and require immediate aggressive resuscitation, fluids, and antibiotics. One main objective in the elderly is to diagnose and begin treatment prior to reaching this often preterminal state.

There is usually marked hyperventilation with a respiratory alkalosis and severe mental status changes early in this state. The mental changes (delirium) are partly due to the infection, and when the individual is in a shock state, they can be caused or increased by hypoperfusion. The persistent shock state may lead to hepatic impairment and renal failure, along with a marked acidosis.

The most common organisms responsible for bacteremic shock are *Escherichia coli, Klebsiella,* and *Streptococcus. Staphylococcus* is rising in importance. Broad-spectrum antibiotic coverage is essential until the culture is returned. The organisms are, of course, somewhat different, depending on the source of the infection. *E. coli* is the most common organism from biliary tract sepsis, while pneumococcus and *Klebsiella* are more common from the lungs, and *Streptococcus* and *Staphylococcus* are common from skin and soft tissue sources. If *Pseudomonas aeruginosa* is involved, newer antibiotics with anti-*Pseudomonas* activity are needed (e.g., piperacillin, mezlocillin, carbenicillin).

MENINGOCOCCAL SEPSIS

Meningococcal septicemia, although rare, deserves mention because this condition must be recognized early to reduce the high fatality rate. People over the age of 60 have double the mortality rate when compared to that of all age groups combined.[35] Fever, chills, weakness, nausea, vomiting, and headache are nonspecific signs. The skin rash, which is petechial in nature, should be searched for. There is usually a marked leukocytosis, although the presence of leukopenia and thrombocytopenia indicates a worse prognosis. Patients may progress to a severe shock state with marked hypotension. Once this state develops, mortality in all groups becomes 50% or greater, even with intensive treatment and suitable antibiotic use. Penicillin and ampicillin, sometimes combined with chloramphenicol, have been the antibiotic choices for the last two decades. Sulfonamide-resistant meningococci have rendered the sulfa drugs of less use in this disease, and their use as "first-line" treatment is no longer recommended unless combined with other antibiotics. Some authorities[37] recommend initiation of treatment with a third-generation cephalosporin (e.g., ceftriaxone).

LABORATORY EVALUATION

Standard tests that are available on an emergency basis can be very useful. Testing for electrolytes and blood urea nitrogen (BUN) is important for fluid replacement. The arterial lactate levels may indicate severity.

The complete blood count (CBC) may show leukocytosis or leukopenia in some cases. Usually the presence of leukopenia carries a poorer prognosis. Thrombocytopenia may be evident. Abnormal clotting factors compatible with disseminated intravascular coagulation are seen in about 10% of cases.[16] Abnormalities of bilirubin or hepatic enzymes point to the biliary system as the cause.

When neutropenia is present (often associated with treated cancer), the defenses are markedly impaired (particularly with a neutrophil count below 1000/mL). Infections in patients with neutropenia are usually bacterial with gram-negative rods being most common, followed by *Staphylococcus* as the most common gram-positive organism. There may be few or no local symptoms[15] and, in skin/soft tissue infections, almost no pus. Because of the common staphylococcal organisms, treatment while awaiting cultures should include an antistaphylococcal antibiotic.

Other laboratory examinations will reveal any skin lesions or organ system abnormality (e.g., liver enlargement, flank or biliary pain, cardiac arrhythmias or murmurs, central nervous system symptoms), which can help to focus the evaluation. The urine should be checked since it is so common a source, and there may be few symptoms. Sputum, cerebrospinal fluid, ascitic fluid, and any drainage should be cultured.

BLOOD CULTURES

Blood cultures are the cornerstones of evaluation and offer later guidance for treatment.

Three cultures at different times will give the highest positive yield in sepsis since bacteremia can be intermittent. *However, it is unwise to withhold antibiotics from a septic patient.* One blood culture must suffice and treatment must be started, recognizing that even if a negative culture is returned, there is a 20% chance it is in error. The greatest error, of course, is to allow the patient to remain untreated when sepsis is suspected. Antibiotic treatment should rapidly follow the culture (see p. 290). The easiest method of culture is to take 30 ml of blood from a single site and divide it into three culture bottles. Later, after treatment is initiated, further cultures may be taken. This may prove valuable if the organism is unusual or insensitive to the antibiotic chosen.

X-RAYS/SCANS

A chest x-ray can be important in the diagnosis of pneumonia or an occult malignancy. Clinical signs and symptoms should guide x-ray examination. Gallbladder studies may be indicated based on clinical symptoms, and computerized tomography (CT) and MRI scans can be useful if the central nervous system is involved or if an abscess is suspected.

Essential time should not be spent on time-consuming studies, however, in a septic elderly patient who requires, first, stabilization and treatment initiation, after which further testing may be done.

SOURCES OF INFECTION

The most common sources of infection leading to septicemia are:

1. Urinary tract
2. Gallbladder/biliary system
3. Respiratory system
4. Intraabdominal infection
5. Endocarditis
6. Meningitis

Each will be dealt with here only from the vantage point of sepsis with some caveats and tips. They are covered well in other chapters of this book.

Urinary Tract Infections

Indwelling catheters, recent instrumentation, prostate enlargement with obstruction, and pelvic relaxation are all risk factors for infection. For sepsis to develop, the kidney must generally be involved in infection (pyelonephritis), although urinary tract symptoms may be scanty.

When sepsis arises from the urinary tract, the leading organisms are E. coli, followed by Proteus, Klebsiella, and Pseudomonas.[17] A Gram stain of sediment can be helpful.

Suitable antibiotics are also discussed in Chapter 21. However, in general, when gram-negative rods are seen or suspected, an aminoglycoside (e.g., gentamicin) should be instituted, coupled with an agent for gram-positive cocci (e.g., ampicillin). Some of the newer antibiotics have been used as well as ceftriaxone (if Pseudomonas is unlikely). Discussion of the range of newer antibiotics is beyond the scope of this chapter but can be found in specific discussions throughout this book.

Septicemia from Biliary Tract Infection

As the second most common cause of sepsis in the elderly, biliary tract disease stands out because of the frequent need for surgery, although advances in antibiotics and supportive care have shown that good recovery can occur in some cases with only medical treatment.

Of 19 patients with sepsis due to bacterial cholangitis, 15 recovered without operation.[14] Five refused surgery, three patients were considered unacceptable surgical risks, two were uncertain diagnoses, and five were between 82 and 90 years of age and responded to treatment.

Of the 76 bacteremic episodes cultured, the organisms were E. coli (48%), followed by Klebsiella (22%), Streptococcus (15%), and Proteus (10%). Nineteen of the 76 episodes had more than two bacteria cultured — of which streptococci were found in 14 of the 19 as the second or third organism.

In biliary tract infection, an effective antibiotic combination has been gentamicin and ampicillin. As empiric therapy, this is recommended, although some authors suggest other choices such as the acylureidopenicillin antibiotics, for example, piperacillin or mezlocillin.[18] With the wide choice of suitable antibiotics now available, the clinician should become comfortable with use of a particular regimen.

Respiratory Tract Infections

The most common cause of sepsis arising from the respiratory tract is pneumonia. The usual causes and treatments for pneumonia are found in Chapters 18 and 21. There are usually preexistent lung diseases (e.g., COPD, emphysema) that predispose to infection. The organisms usually associated with community-acquired bronchopneumonia in the elderly are Streptococcus pneumoniae and Haemophilus influenzae,[19] although Klebsiella is seen more frequently in debilitated or alcoholic patients.

The physician should not overlook the occasional extremely severe Legionnaires' disease, however, caused by a gram-negative bacillus. (These require erythromycin or rifampin for antibiotic treatment.)

Sepsis due to pneumonia is complicated by marked respiratory impairment, which frequently requires advanced ventilator management, treatment of respiratory failure, and management of sepsis.

Pneumonia remains a major cause of death in the elderly. At an extended care facility, 41% of 1,696 postmortem examinations of those 65 or older showed evidence of terminal pneumonia, although as the primary cause of death pneumonia was only 15%.[20] Sepsis due to pneumonia can be fulminant and with the respiratory impairment can rapidly lead to death.

Antibiotic management depends on a Gram stain of the sputum. If there is a clear gram-positive diplococci pattern, penicillin is sufficient. If H. influenzae (small gram-negative coccobacilli) is involved, ampicillin is indicated. If there is concern about ampicillin resistance, a third-generation cephalosporin can be used. A mixed infection in a severely ill patient can usually be well treated with an ampicillin-gentamicin combination. (See also Chapter 21, p. 283, and Table 18–5, p. 242.)

In general, gram-negative bacteria play a minor role in community-acquired pneumonias. However, in institutional settings where the patient is bedridden, coliform bacteria and *Pseudomonas* are more common. Aspiration is also more frequent and the achlorhydria that may be found allows bacterial colonization of the stomach contents.

Klebsiella pneumoniae (Friedländer's bacillus) is more common in the debilitated and elderly and carries a high mortality rate (25 to 50%).

Intraabdominal Infection

The major considerations involve diverticulitis, intestinal perforation, appendicitis with peritonitis, and mesenteric ischemia and infarction.

In these cases, the condition may require surgical intervention (with perforation and appendicitis). However, diverticulitis may be treated with aggressive medical management unless perforation has occurred that necessitates surgery. Because of the anaerobic intestinal bacteria, preoperative antibiotic treatment should include clindamycin for *Bacteroides* infection in such cases of spillage of large bowel contents into the peritoneal cavity.

Bacterial Endocarditis

Valvular abnormalities are far more common in the elderly and result in a surface and crevices that can lead to endocarditis. The clinical picture is that of septicemia with an added finding of signs of embolization: petechiae in the subconjunctiva, subcutaneous hemorrhages in the hands, Osler's nodes, or Janeway's lesions. Embolism to the kidneys can result in hematuria. Central nervous system (CNS) emboli can cause confusion and paralysis.

Examination must focus on signs of emboli and careful listening for a cardiac murmur. Misdiagnoses are common but can be lethal since the development of septic shock rapidly leads to congestive heart failure.

Meningitis

Diagnosis of bacterial meningitis is easy in the febrile patient with a stiff neck and other meningeal signs and symptoms. In the elderly patient who may be confused, obtunded, or have a multisystem disease, the diagnosis is difficult, particularly when sepsis supervenes.

If specific organisms are seen in the CSF fluid (e.g., pneumococcal or meningococcal meningitis), treatment can be focused using high doses of penicillin. Ceftriaxone has become a widely used cephalosporin because of its wide-spectrum, low toxicity, and effective penetration of the cerebrospinal fluid.

Knowing the likely organism is of greatest importance in focusing specific therapy, as well as the clinician's experience with the newer antibiotics.

ANTIBIOTIC CONSIDERATIONS

Analyzing data from 207 patients, the bacteria most commonly causing sepsis are *E. coli* (43%), *Streptococcus pneumoniae* (17%), *Staphylococcus aureus* (10%), *Klebsiella pneumoniae* (7.7%), beta-hemolytic streptococci (7.2%), *Proteus* (5.3%), *Streptococcus viridans* (2.8%), and *Pseudomonas aeruginosa* (1.4%). This information may serve to guide presumptive therapy before culture results are available.

The enormous range and variety of antibiotics now available to the clinician can be confusing. Libke's work[37] can help clarify the field. Often, it is best to gain familiarity with a few antibiotics and know how to use them well. Then, if one is dealing with an infection outside of this range, it is easier to get a specific consultation from an infectious disease specialist.

Any physician who may be called to treat sepsis in an elderly patient should have a basic regimen he or she knows how to use and be prepared to institute treatment without delay. Many of the broad-spectrum, third-generation cephalosporins were designed as less toxic alternatives to the aminoglycosides. However, in severely ill patients infected by undefined organisms, many clinicians are reluctant to replace the ampicillin-gentamicin or cephalosporin-aminoglycoside combinations with which they have become familiar and which have demonstrated efficacy. Certainly, after culture and sensitivity reports become available, it is always prudent to select the narrowest spectrum, least toxic effective antibiotic.

In the emergency setting rapid decision must be made, often without the benefit of culture material or even Gram stains of infected fluids. In such cases the clinician must make some rapid assessments to determine the need for additional antibiotic coverage. For example:

1. Is *Pseudomonas* infection likely?
2. Could the infecting organism be a penicillin-resistant staphylococcus?
3. Is *Bacteroides* infection (most likely from intestinal spillage) a problem?
4. Is *Haemophilus influenzae* infection resistant to ampicillin likely?
5. Is there a possibility of *Legionella* sepsis (requiring erythromycin or rifampin)?
6. Is the patient immunocompromised or granulocytopenic due to preexistent disease, malnutrition, or possible treatment for cancer, an organ transplant, or another condition? In such cases anti-*Pseudomonas* treatment should be added.
7. Does severe renal or hepatic impairment mandate use of the least potentially toxic antibiotic available?
8. Does known allergy necessitate use of only certain antibiotic classes?

PATHOPHYSIOLOGY OF SEPTIC SHOCK: IMPLICATIONS FOR TREATMENT

Septicemic shock is due to the damaging actions of exotoxins and endotoxins on a cellular level. Microthrombus formation leads to tissue necrosis and hemorrhage. The kidney can be involved with cortical or tubular necrosis. Necrosis can also occur in the liver. The lungs undergo marked change with edema and increased permeability of cells. Hyaline membrane formation occurs. Respiratory failure may occur. The heart, intestines, and glands (pancreas and adrenal) can undergo hemorrhage and necrosis.

TREATMENT CONSIDERATIONS

The major cause of death in septicemia is shock, which raises the mortality rate in the elderly. One study showed a 60% mortality,[22] another greater than 70%,[23] and this figure increases with advancing age. The pathologic and physiologic changes of septic shock are well covered elsewhere.[24]

For this discussion, we need only focus on the essential need to reduce the damaging actions of exotoxins and endotoxins at a cellular level and to rapidly restore adequate perfusion and oxygenation to maintain the organ systems and maintain cardiac and pulmonary function and to correct the metabolic defects, primarily involving a severe metabolic acidosis. Septic shock can result in renal tubular necrosis, as well as adult respiratory distress syndrome (ARDS). Endotoxins may initiate disseminated intravascular coagulation.

Intensive intravenous fluid resuscitation with careful monitoring is critical. Avoid inotropic agents (e.g., dopamine) unless fluid resuscitation is unsuccessful. If used, dopamine is usually mixed as 400 mg in 500 mL of 5% dextrose and water, or saline solution, and the infusion is titrated. The physician should avoid vasoconstrictors (e.g., norepinephrine) since the profound vasoconstriction can reduce kidney and other organ flow.

Corticosteroids are of unproven benefit for this condition. However, it should be remembered that Addison's disease or acute adrenal insufficiency can be precipitated or worsened by the stress of infection. Naloxone has been used experimentally, but its benefit is unproved. The objective of these treatments is to correct the abnormalities in tissue perfusion so that cellular metabolism can be restored. However, the cornerstone of sepsis treatment must be to treat the infection.

The elderly patient may have preexistent renal or liver abnormalities, which can reduce excretion and metabolism. The reduced muscle mass requires adjustment in medication dosage. The presence of chronic biliary tract abnormalities or the acute biliary tract infection may also reduce hepatic metabolism. However, these considerations pale in comparison to the urgency with which sepsis must be addressed in the elderly patient. With mortality rates over 70% (and even higher in the over 80 group), focus must be on fluid resuscitation and intravenous instillation of appropriate antibiotics.

LEGIONELLA PNEUMONIA

This disease is probably far more common than realized. Often called Legionnaires' disease after the American Legion Convention at the Bellevue Stratford Hotel in Philadelphia (1977) where an outbreak was first recognized, the condition is more serious in the elderly. More than 50% of the deaths are in the over-60 age group.

Overall mortality may range from 16%[25] to 47%.[26] Bacteremia is present in almost 40% of cases,[27] and deaths are due to pulmonary insufficiency, sepsis, and circulatory collapse.[28]

The elderly are at higher risk since the condition has a predilection for patients with underlying pulmonary, cardiac, renal, or malignant disease.[29] Transplant patients are also at high risk, most likely due to immunosuppression.

The organism (*Legionella pneumophila*) lived in the stagnant water of the hotel's air conditioning system in the original outbreak but has since been found in aerosols from portable humidifiers. Tap water may be contaminated with the organism.[30] *This condition should be considered in the septic elderly patient because the mortality is high, bacteremia and sepsis are frequent, and diagnosis is difficult.*

A Gram stain of the sputum shows neutrophils but usually no organisms. Chest x-ray shows pneumonia, usually of one or two lobes, although a pleural effusion may be the only sign.[31] Blood tests are generally abnormal but nonspecific. There is an elevated white blood cell count, and serum sodium may be low.

Definitive diagnosis rests on specialized tests to detect the organisms. These include the following:

1. Direct fluorescent antibody (results available within a few hours when the lab is equipped).
2. Culture — *Legionella pneumophila* will not grow on standard bacteriology media (one of the principal reasons for the great puzzlement during the first carefully studied outbreak). Special media for culture are required.[32] Most laboratories are now equipped to detect this organism when requested. However, the geriatric emergency medicine practitioner must be alert to this possibility; with cultures of blood or other material, he or she should specifically ask for this analysis. Radioimmunoassay of the *Legionella* antigen in the urine is not widely available and involves delay.

Erythromycin given intravenously (1 g every 6 hours) is the treatment of choice in the severely ill *Legionella*-septic patient.

REFERENCES

1. Esposito A et al: Community-acquired bacteremia in the elderly: analysis of one hundred consecutive episodes, J Am Geriatr Soc 7:315, 1980.
2. Smith IM: Prevalence, diagnosis and treatment of infectious diseases. In Calkins E, Davis PJ, and Ford AB, editors: The practice of geriatrics, Philadelphia, 1986, WB Saunders Co.

3. Johnston RB: Current concepts: immunology monocytes and macrophages, N Engl J Med 318:12, 1988.

4. Howells CHL et al: Influenza vaccination and mortality from bronchopneumonia in the elderly, Lancet 1:381–383, 1975.

5. Roberts-Thompson IC et al: Aging, immune response and mortality, Lancet 2:368–370, 1974.

6. Smith IA: Host resistance impairment and protection against infection. In Calkins E, Davis PJ, and Ford AB, editors: The practice of geriatrics, Philadelphia, 1986, WB Saunders Co.

7. Brill NE and Libman E: Pyocaneus bacillaemia, Am J Med Sci 118:153, 1899.

8. Felty AR and Keefer CS: Bacillus coli sepsis: clinical study of 28 cases of bloodstream invasion by the colon bacillus, JAMA 82:1430, 1924.

9. Gleckman R and Hilbert D: Afebrile bacteremia: a phenomenon in geriatric patients, JAMA 248:1478, 1982.

10. Cone LA et al: Clinical and bacteriologic observations of a toxic shock–like syndrome due to *Streptococcus pyogenes*, N Engl J Med 317:3, 1987.

11. Ruben FL et al: An outbreak of *Streptococcus pyogenes* infections in a nursing home, Ann Intern Med 101:494, 1984.

12. Galpin JE et al: Sepsis associated with decubitus ulcers, Am J Med 61:346, 1976.

13. Brown NR and Thomson DJ: Non-treatment of fever in extended care facilities, N Engl J Med 300:1246, 1979.

14. Siegman-Ingra Y et al: Septicemia from biliary tract infection, Arch Surg 123:366, 1988.

15. Pennington JE: Fever, neutropenia and malignancy: a clinical syndrome in evolution, Cancer 39:1345, 1977.

16. Jacobs RA: Sepsis in adults. In Callaham M, editor: Current therapy in emergency medicine, St. Louis, 1987, CV Mosby Co.

17. Sanderson PJ and Denham MJ: Antibiotic practice in elderly patients. In Denham MJ, editor: The treatment of medical problems of the elderly, Baltimore, 1980, University Park Press.

18. Blenkharn JI and Blumgart LH: Streptococcal bacteremia in hepatobiliary operations, Surg Gynecol Obstet 160:139–141, 1985.

19. Garb JL et al: Differences in etiology of pneumonias in nursing home and community patients, JAMA 246:2169, 1978.

20. Gerber IE: Terminal pneumonia in the aged, Mt Sinai J Med 47:166, 1980.

21. LaForce FM: Hospital acquired gram-negative rod pneumonias: an overview, Am J Med 70:644, 1981.

22. Wardle N: Bacteremia and endotoxic shock, Br J Hosp Med 21:223, 1979.

23. Sheagren JN: Shock syndromes related to sepsis. In Smith LH and Wyngaarden JB, editors: Cecil review of general internal medicine, ed 3, Philadelphia, 1985, WB Saunders Co.

24. Williams RKT and Denham MJ: Septicemia and infective endocarditis. In Denham MJ, editor: Infections in the elderly, Lancaster, England, 1986, MTP Press, Ltd.

25. Galpin JE et al: Legionnaires' disease: description of an outbreak of pneumonia, N Engl J Med 297:1189, 1977.

26. Yu VL et al: Legionnaires' disease: new clinical perspective from a prospective pneumonia study, Am J Med 73:357, 1982.

27. Rihs JD et al: Isolation of *Legionella pneumophila* from blood using the BACTEC: a prospective study yielding positive results, J Clin Microbiol 22:422, 1985.

28. Band JD and Fraser DW: Legionellosis. In Braude AI, Davis CE, and Fierer J, editors: Infectious disease and microbiology, ed 2, Philadelphia, 1986, WB Saunders Co.

29. Kirby BD et al: Legionnaires' disease: report of 65 nosocomially acquired cases and a review of the literature, Medicine 59(3):188, 1980.

30. Kundsin RB and Walter CW: Legionella prosthetic-valve endocarditis, N Engl J Med 9:58, 1988.

31. Munder RR, Yu VL, and Parry MF: The radiographic manifestations of *Legionella* pneumonia, Semin Respir Infect Dis 2:242, 1987.

32. Vickers RM et al: Culture methodology for the isolation of *Legionella pneumophila* and other Legionellaceae from clinical and environmental specimens, Semin Respir Infect Dis 2:274, 1987.

33. Allman RM: Pressure ulcers among the elderly, N Engl J Med 320:850, 1989.

34. Swartz M: Meningococcal disease. In Wyngaarden JB and Smith LH, editors: Cecil textbook of medicine, Philadelphia, 1988, WB Saunders Co.

35. Anderson BM: Mortality in meningococcal infections, Scand J Infect Dis 10:277, 1978.

36. Dhainaut JF: Myocardial depressant substances as mediators of early cardiac dysfunction in septic shock, J Crit Care 4:1, 1989.

37. Libke RD: Use of newer antibiotics. In Schwartz GR et al: Emergency medicine: the essential update, Philadelphia, 1989, WB Saunders Co.

Metabolic, Endocrine, and Nutritional Disorders

Overview of Endocrine and Metabolic Emergencies

William L. Isley, M.D., Stephen Hamburger, M.D., and Gideon Bosker, M.D., F.A.C.E.P.

Metabolic disorders in the elderly constitute a special challenge for the acute care clinician. Signs and symptoms are frequently nonspecific or may suggest disease in a nonendocrine organ system. As a result, the physician may be tempted to attribute the patient's problems to the aging process or to cerebral or cardiac dysfunction. An appropriate index of suspicion is, therefore, the primary prerequisite necessary to diagnose metabolic disorders in the elderly.

Four specific factors complicate the assessment, diagnosis, and management of the geriatric patient with endocrine or metabolic dysfunction: 1) the normal aging process (a process which is still incompletely understood), 2) the presence of multisystem disease, 3) polypharmacy (often inappropriate), and 4) the patient's decreased ability to care for himself or herself. For example, simple chores such as drinking an adequate amount of water or preparing appropriate meals may be beyond the ability of the elderly patient, precipitating severe derangements in water

metabolism. These considerations are relevant to the discussion of metabolic and endocrine disorders in the elderly and readily differentiate approaches in caring for the geriatric age group in the same way that growth disorders and sexual precocity are unique to the pediatric population.

In this chapter, we will discuss major topics in acute care medicine including electrolyte disorders, thyroid dysfunction, and diabetes mellitus from a geriatric perspective.

DISORDERS OF SODIUM AND WATER METABOLISM

Alteration in kidney function, hormonal action, and thirst make the elderly susceptible to disorders of sodium and water metabolism. Kidney size and renal function decrease with advancing age. Since lean body mass also decreases, serum creatinine frequently does not rise. Therefore, a normal serum creatinine concentration may be observed despite a significant decrement in glomerular filtration rate. Concentrating ability and diluting capacity also decline with age. Moreover, the aged kidney conserves sodium less avidly. As a result, in the elderly, the ability to regulate the internal milieu is sufficiently compromised so that the limits of water and salt ingestion or deprivation tolerated in youth may cause extreme disability in the geriatric patient.

Alterations in hormonal action may also impair renal function. Plasma renin activity and aldosterone decrease with age, while renal responsiveness to vasopressin may decline as well. Volume-mediated release of vasopressin decreases with age, though the regulation of osmoreceptor-triggered antidiuretic hormone appears to be unaltered.[1]

Hypodipsia is often present in the elderly. Diminished thirst may lead to marked metabolic derangement despite unrestricted access to fluids. Drugs and limited access to water are the major exogenous factors that affect water and salt metabolism in the elderly. A list of drugs that may impair water excretion is given in Table 23–1. Water and salt homeostasis is also compromised by major organ disease, particularly cardiac dysfunction.

Hypernatremia

Although less common than hyponatremia, hypernatremia (a serum sodium concentration greater than 150 mEq/L) can present as a medical emergency.[10] Hypernatremia can result from solute overload (salt water drowning, sodium chloride ingestion) or free water loss (febrile illness, hot environment, respiratory infection, osmotic diuresis, postobstructive diuresis, dialysis, or diabetes insipidus). Acquired defects in vasopressin responsiveness (nephrogenic diabetes insipidus) from drugs, hypokalemia, or hypercalcemia should also be considered. Hypodipsia and inadequate access to fluids may compound the problem.

The patient may complain of thirst if he or she is alert, but a decreased sensorium is frequently present. Stupor, coma, or seizures can occur. The patient may appear dehydrated, though skin turgor and mucous membranes are more difficult to evaluate in the elderly.

Since hypernatremia is usually associated with some underlying disease, treatment of that disorder is of utmost importance. Mortality, particularly in acute hypernatremia, is high. The initial consideration should be

Table 23–1   Drugs That May Impair Water Excretion

Chlorpropamide	Tricyclic antidepressant agents
Narcotics	Phenothiazines
Nicotine	Clonidine
Anesthetics	Bromocriptine
Vincristine	Diuretics
Cyclophosphamide	Nonsteroidal antiinflammatory
Clofibrate	agents
Carbamazepine	

maintenance of the circulation with colloid or crystalloid to restore blood pressure. The fluid deficit can be estimated by the following formula:

$$\text{Water deficit} = (0.6 \times \text{observed body weight}) \times \left(1 - \frac{\text{desired serum sodium concentration}}{\text{actual serum sodium concentration}}\right)$$

One-half the fluid deficit should be replaced over 6 to 12 hours, with the remainder replenished over 24 to 48 hours. Maintenance fluids plus any additional that continue to be lost (skin, renal, respiratory, or gastrointestinal) should be considered when administering fluids. One-half normal saline is the fluid of choice.

Hyponatremia

The clinical picture of hyponatremia in the geriatric patient is nonspecific. Weakness, anorexia, nausea, muscle cramps, stupor, coma, or seizures may be the initial presenting symptoms. In extreme cases, focal neurologic deficit or seizures may occur.[2] Physical signs vary depending upon the volume status of the patient and the rapidity with which the hyponatremic state was achieved. In the elderly, skin turgor and mucous membranes may be difficult to evaluate. Inspection of the neck veins in the supine position is a better clinical assessment of the volume status of the patient. Symptoms are more pronounced when the serum sodium concentration is less than 130 mEq/L, especially when these levels occur acutely in less than 48 hours. Chronic or slowly progressive changes in the level of serum sodium are better tolerated, and neurologic symptoms may not occur until the abnormality is extreme. Most cases of hyponatremia do not require rapid correction. However, it is essential that patients with hyponatremia have appropriate diagnostic and therapeutic measures to prevent worsening of the clinical state.[3]

Serum sodium concentration is determined by total body sodium and total body water. Simply stated, there may be an excess of body water relative to sodium or a decrease in body sodium relative to water. Hyponatremia may be separated into three categories. Euvolemic hyponatremia is encountered when there is a mild increase in total body water with little or no change in total body sodium. A marked increase in total body water with a lesser increase in total body sodium occurs in hypervolemic hyponatremia. In hypovolemic hyponatremia, decreased total body sodium is accompanied by a less than proportionate decrease in total body water.

Occasionally, "pseudohyponatremia" can exist when the serum sodium concentration is actually normal but improper specimen collection (above an intravenous site), hypertriglyceridemia (grossly lipemic serum), a dysproteinemia, extreme hyperglycemia, or an unmeasured solute (alcohol, mannitol) causes the lab to report an abnormally low result. In the case of dilution by dextrose-containing intravenous (IV) fluids, all laboratory analytes except glucose will be determined to be low. A normal measured serum osmolality in the face of hyponatremia will point to pseudohyponatremia in triglyceride excess states and dysproteinemia. Serum osmolality will be high in patients with a large concentration of unmeasured solute or extreme hyperglycemia.

Clinical Presentation

A meticulous medical and, particularly, medication history is extremely important in evaluating the patient with hyponatremia. A history of kidney, liver, heart, thyroid, pituitary, or adrenal disease is very important. Diagnostic and therapeutic considerations relevant to the hyponatremic patient are listed in Table 23–2.

Hypovolemic hyponatremia results from water and salt losses from the gastrointestinal tract (vomiting or diarrhea), burns, "third spacing," diuretics, or primary renal salt-losing states.[4-7] Adrenal insufficiency can also present as hypovolemic hyponatremia. The patient with volume depletion and hyponatremia may manifest orthostatic hypotension, collapsed neck veins, and tachycardia. Urine output is decreased. The urine sodium concentration is quite helpful in determining the etiology of sodium depletion. Extrarenal fluid losses characteristically generate a low urinary sodium concentration (< 10 mEq/L), whereas renal losses are associated with a urine sodium concentration greater than 20 mEq/L. The urine sodium is variable in adrenal insufficiency.

Treatment of hypovolemic hyponatremia requires acute correction of the volume deficit. Restoration of tissue perfusion takes precedence over correction of the serum sodium concentration. The volume deficit is usually corrected with isotonic sodium chloride, though hypertonic (3% saline) solutions can be used in the patient with neurologic symptoms who has extreme hyponatremia,[8] in the range of 115 mEq/dL or less. During therapy, it is important to assess the volume status of the patient carefully. While uncommon in the elderly (except those previously treated with pharmacologic doses of glucocorticoids), adrenal insufficiency can present with vomiting and diarrhea. Corticosteroids should be administered if adrenal insufficiency is suspected. To screen the patient for adrenal insufficiency, obtain a serum specimen for determination of cortisol, administer cosyntropin (250 μg)

IV or intramuscularly (IM), and obtain another serum specimen for cortisol determination 60 minutes later. If need be, dexamethasone can be given during this test since it will not interfere with the cortisol radioimmunoassay. The stimulated cortisol value should equal or exceed 20 μg/dL. Noninvasive monitoring (orthostatic blood pressure, pulse changes, neck vein distention, urine output) is usually sufficient. Serum electrolytes should be periodically determined. Treatment of the underlying disorder is mandatory.

The patient with euvolemic hyponatremia exhibits neither edema nor extracellular fluid depletion. Diagnostic possibilities include hypothyroidism, adrenal insufficiency, acute water intoxication, and the syndrome of inappropriate secretion of antidiuretic hormone (SIADH). Acute water intoxication rarely leads to marked hyponatremia unless renal or cardiac compromise exists. However, the elderly may be more prone to this problem if they have received hypotonic fluids in the hospital environment. If there is no evidence of an endocrine disorder in euvolemic hyponatremia, SIADH is usually present. The causes of SIADH are listed in Table 23–3. Diagnostic criteria for making the diagnosis of SIADH include the presence of normal volume status (no edema, ascites, or hypotension); absence of renal, cardiac, hepatic, adrenal, or thyroid dysfunction; and a urine osmolality inappropriately concentrated for the serum osmolality. The urine sodium is inappropriately high. The measurement of plasma vasopressin levels is not necessary in the usual clinical setting.

Treatment consists of treatment of the primary disease process and restriction of fluids to 500 mL per day. In patients with central nervous system dysfunction, more rapid treatment may be necessary. Hypertonic saline may be administered while instituting a free water diuresis with a loop diuretic such as furosemide. Potassium repletion is necessary when loop diuretics are given. The rapidity with which normonatremia should be attained is debatable. Some authors suggest that central pontine myelinolysis may follow rapid correction of hyponatremia.[9] However, this disorder usually occurs in patients who are extremely malnourished, are alcoholic, or have other severe systemic diseases. A reasonable course is to increase the serum sodium concentration by 2 mEq/L per hour to a level of 125 mEq/L, and then more slowly thereafter. In the elderly adult with cardiovas-

Table 23–2 Diagnostic and Therapeutic Considerations in the Hypotonic Hyponatremic Patient

	Hypovolemia	Euvolemia	Hypervolemia
Step 1: Assess volume status of patient.			
Step 2: Control salt and water intake.	Administer saline	Restrict fluid*	Restrict fluid
Step 3: Assess major organs.	Gastrointestinal tract, kidney, adrenal glands, skin	Adrenal, thyroid glands	Heart, liver, kidney
Step 4: Measure urine sodium.	High = renal loss Low = nonrenal loss	If not elevated, reassess Step 1	High = renal disease Low = salt- and water-retaining disorder

*Neurologic signs and symptoms may require administration of hypertonic saline and furosemide.

Table 23–3 Conditions Associated with SIADH

Malignancy (particularly small cell carcinoma of the lung)

Pulmonary disease (cancer, tuberculosis, pneumonia, lung abscess, chronic obstructive pulmonary disease)

Central nervous system disease

Drugs (see Table 23–1)

Trauma

Stress

Psychosis

cular or renal disease, careful assessment of volume status of the patient is necessary. In chronic settings, demeclocycline or lithium can be used. These drugs induce a nephrogenic diabetes insipidus.

Hypervolemic hyponatremia occurs in patients with increased body water relative to sodium. The hallmark of this disorder is edema. These patients usually have long-term, sodium-retaining disorders such as congestive heart failure, cirrhosis with portal hypertension, nephrotic syndrome, or severe hypoalbuminemia from nutritional or gastrointestinal disorders. Patients with acute or chronic renal failure rarely manifest hypervolemic hyponatremia.

A low urine sodium concentration (less than 10 mEq/L) is present unless the patient has received diuretics or has primary renal disease. Patients with volume expansion and hyponatremia are usually asymptomatic due to the chronicity of their disease state. However, excessive water intake may lead to progression of the hyponatremia.

Treatment of hypervolemic hyponatremia is directed at the underlying disease state. The primary pathophysiologic condition may make treatment of hyponatremia difficult. However, avoidance of excessive water and salt intake may be all that is necessary. Inducing a free water diuresis with loop diuretics may be helpful.

DISORDERS OF POTASSIUM BALANCE

Potassium is the major intracellular cation. Normal regulation of potassium is dependent upon the renin-angiotensin-aldosterone system, insulin, plasma osmolality, rate of delivery of sodium to the distal tubule, and catecholamines. Total body potassium decreases with age. However, this is probably due to the decrease in lean body mass that occurs with aging. Thus, a true state of total body potassium depletion does not exist in the healthy elderly subject.

Serum potassium remains relatively constant throughout life. However, the aging-related decline in renal function, plasma renin activity, and aldosterone, plus the tendency for the elderly patient to be ingesting drugs that affect potassium homeostasis, make potassium balance more tenuous in the elderly. Inadequate potassium intake may rarely be a significant factor, par-

ticularly in hospitalized patients receiving intravenous fluids. Obligatory renal potassium loss occurs even in normal patients on a low potassium diet.

Pharmacologic agents associated with alterations in potassium homeostasis are listed in Table 23–4. These drugs are discussed further in the sections that follow.

Hyperkalemia

Hyperkalemia may produce no symptoms or nonspecific symptoms such as weakness. Major manifestations are cardiac and neurologic. Electrocardiographic findings progress from peaking of the T waves, to PR and QRS lengthening, to absence of P waves, to a merger of the QRS complex with the T wave to form a sine wave pattern. Ventricular fibrillation or asystole is imminent in this latter circumstance. Unfortunately, electrocardiographic changes do not necessarily correlate with serum potassium concentrations. Furthermore, a patient may develop ventricular fibrillation without previous changes in the electrocardiogram. Neurologically, an ascending flaccid paralysis may develop that can ultimately progress to respiratory failure.[11]

The physician's first task when confronted with an elevation of serum potassium in an asymptomatic patient is to ensure that true hyperkalemia exists. Hemolysis from the trauma of drawing blood is a common problem in the elderly. Extreme thrombocytosis and leukocytosis can also artifactually increase serum potassium. A plasma potassium determination (drawn in a heparinized tube) should be within 0.2 to 0.3 mEq/L of the serum potassium concentration.

Hyperkalemia can occur from excessive potassium intake, decreased potassium excretion, or potassium translocation from the intracellular to the extracellular space (Table 23–5). Salt substitutes or potassium supplements

Table 23–4 Drugs Affecting Potassium Homeostasis

Increased Potassium Intake
Potassium supplements

Increased Renal Potassium Loss
Diuretics
Penicillins
Amphotericin

Decreased Potassium Loss
Triamterene
Spironolactone
Amiloride
Beta blockers
Converting enzyme inhibitors
Prostaglandin synthesis inhibitors
Heparin

Increased Cellular Potassium Uptake
Beta-2 agonists

Decreased Cellular Potassium Uptake
Beta-2 blockers
Digitalis

Table 23–5 Causes of Hyperkalemia in the Elderly

Factitious (hemolysis, thrombocytosis, leukocytosis)

Increased input (potassium supplements, salt substitutes, cell breakdown states)

Decreased output (renal failure, inadequate distal tubular flow, Addison's disease, hyporeninemic hypoaldosteronism, tubulointerstitial disease, drugs)

Altered distribution (insulin deficiency, acidosis, hyperglycemia, aldosterone deficiency, beta blockers, succinylcholine, digitalis toxicity)

are common sources of extra potassium intake in the elderly.[12] Renal failure (more pronounced in acute than chronic), Addison's disease, hyporeninemic hypoaldosteronism (patients with mild renal failure and tubulointerstitial disease, frequently diabetes mellitus), drugs that interfere with the renin-angiotensin-aldosterone system (beta blockers, prostaglandin synthesis inhibitors, converting enzyme inhibitors, or heparin), medications that interfere with renal distal tubular potassium secretion (spironolactone, triamterene, or amiloride), obstructive uropathy, and amyloidosis all reduce potassium loss in the urine. Digitalis toxicity, beta-2 blockers, acute metabolic and respiratory acidosis, hyperosmolality, and cell breakdown states (hemolysis, gastrointestinal bleeding, and rhabdomyolysis) can result in hyperkalemia due to translocation of potassium to the extracellular space.

Treatment should be begun in any patient with a serum potassium concentration greater than 6 mEq/L, even in the absence of electrocardiographic abnormalities (Table 23–6). Obviously, discontinuation of offending drugs and relief of possible urinary tract obstruction is important.[13,14] Intravenous calcium can be given to counteract the effects of hyperkalemia on the heart. There may be some concern about giving calcium to the patient on digitalis, particularly if digitalis toxicity is a possibility. Some experts suggest administering calcium as a dilute solution over 20 to 30 minutes rather than as a bolus to minimize complications. Sodium bicarbonate administered intravenously will cause a shift of potassium to the intracellular compartment and stimulate potassium secretion by the kidney. The onset of action is approximately 10 minutes and the duration of effect is about 2 hours. Infusions of insulin and glucose will also stimulate potassium uptake by the cells. Ten units of insulin can be added to 500 mL of 5 to 10% glucose and

Table 23–6 Treatment of Hyperkalemia

10% calcium gluconate infusion	(10–20 mL IV)
Sodium bicarbonate	(50–100 mEq IV)
Insulin and glucose	(10 U regular insulin with 50–100 g glucose IV over 1 hour)
Sodium polystyrene sulfonate	(25–50 g PO or per rectum)
Loop diuretics	(40 mg furosemide IV)
Dialysis	

administered over 1 hour. The potassium-lowering effect should occur in 1 to 2 hours. Loop diuretics (furosemide, ethacrynic acid, or bumetanide) cause renal potassium loss. Sodium polystyrene sulfonate, a cation-exchange resin, can be used to remove potassium via the gut. It can be administered rectally (50 g of sodium polystyrene sulfonate mixed with 50 g of sorbitol added to 200 mL of 10% dextrose in water solution as a retention enema for 30 to 60 minutes) or given orally (25 g sodium polystyrene sulfonate mixed with 50 to 100 mL of 20% sorbitol taken every 3 to 4 hours). Peritoneal dialysis or hemodialysis can be used if necessary. If hyperkalemia recurs and the cause is not obvious, assessment of adrenal function and stimulation of the renin-angiotensin-aldosterone system with volume depletion maneuvers is in order. Patients with chronic hyporeninemic hypoaldosteronism are treated with mineralocorticoids or loop diuretics.[15]

Hypokalemia

Hypokalemia is frequently found in the elderly population, usually due to diuretic intake. Signs and symptoms of hypokalemia may include muscle weakness, cramps, pain, and paresthesias. Occasionally, smooth muscle function will be severely affected so that the patient will manifest urinary retention or bowel obstruction. Hypokalemia can mask the usual manifestations of hypercalcemia. Electrocardiographic manifestations include the presence of U waves, nonspecific ST-T changes, prolonging of the PR interval, and premature atrial and ventricular contractions and supraventricular tachycardia. Rarely, high-degree atrioventricular (AV) block or ventricular tachyarrhythmias may develop, especially in the patient with intrinsic heart disease or digitalis toxicity. Hypokalemic patients may have nephrogenic diabetes insipidus leading to polyuria and dehydration. Glucose intolerance may develop in the hypokalemic patient. Rarely, rhabdomyolysis can occur.

Etiologies for hypokalemia in the elderly include inadequate potassium intake, excessive potassium loss, and potassium translocation into cells. Causes of hypokalemia are classified by urine potassium concentration in Table 23–7. Dietary deficiency of potassium is probably a rare cause of hypokalemia. Excessive renal potassium losses occur in patients receiving diuretic therapy, those who have magnesium deficiency (hospitalized patients or patients on magnesium deficient diets), and those with hyperaldosteronism states (primary aldosteronism, Cushing's syndrome, congestive heart failure, renal artery stenosis, nephrotic syndrome). Gastrointestinal potassium losses can occur with vomiting and diarrhea, especially in laxative abusing patients or patients with colonic villous adenomas. Potassium translocation into cells occurs with insulin, beta-2 agonist therapy, and rapid cell growth states such as those found in treated pernicious anemia patients.

Table 23–7   Causes of Hypokalemia in the Elderly

Urine Potassium < 10 mEq/L
Altered distribution (alkalosis, beta-2 agonists, rapid cell growth states, stress, acute medical illness)
Dietary deficiency
Gastrointestinal loss (vomiting, diarrhea, fistulae)
Cutaneous loss (sweating, burns)

Urine Potassium > 10 mEq/L
Magnesium deficiency
Diuresis (drugs, osmotic, postobstructive, recovery phase of acute tubular necrosis)
Nonreabsorbable anions (penicillins)
Primary aldosteronism
Renal artery stenosis
Malignant hypertension
Renin-secreting tumors
Cushing's syndrome

Treatment of hypokalemia involves potassium chloride administration and therapy of the primary potassium-losing disorder if one exists. Patients with suspected magnesium depletion should have magnesium repletion since potassium supplementation may be ineffective until magnesium stores are replenished. Patients who tolerate oral potassium chloride can be given this medication as liquid or in one of the newer tablet forms. If the serum potassium concentration is less than 2.5 mEq/L, IV potassium chloride should be utilized. It is wise to give no more than 40 mEq potassium chloride in 1 liter of IV fluid over 60 minutes. *Patients with serum potassium concentration lower than 2 mEq/L should have cardiac monitoring while potassium repletion is carried out.* In extreme states of potassium depletion, more potassium can be administered through two different intravenous routes. Potassium chloride should not be given through central catheters due to the possibility of adverse effects on cardiac conduction.

THYROID DISEASE

Thyroid disease appears to be more common in the elderly. The presentation of thyroid disease in the geriatric patient is frequently not the "classic" picture noted in textbooks. Symptoms may be assumed to be related to the aging process. Furthermore, thyroid hormone excess in the geriatric patient may produce symptoms that suggest thyroid deprivation, while hypothyroidism may present with a picture more likely to be associated with hyperthyroidism in youth. A high suspicion of thyroid dysfunction is appropriate in the ailing elderly patient.[16-18]

Hyperthyroidism

Hyperthyroidism in the elderly may present in such a fashion that the examiner has no suspicion of thyroid disease. The "classic" presentation of an anxious, sweating, wide-eyed female with a goiter is not the usual presentation in geriatric medicine. Frequently, manifestations of hyperthyroidism in the elderly suggest a non-endocrine organ disease process. Specifically, weight loss may suggest malignancy or gastrointestinal disease, mental status changes may point to central nervous system dysfunction, or tachyarrhythmias or heart failure leads to an extensive cardiac evaluation. Hyperthyroidism in the elderly may present with a change in mental status, weight loss, congestive heart failure, or tachyarrhythmias. Lethargy and constipation, symptoms usually associated with hypothyroidism, may be present. Occasionally, none of the "classic" signs and symptoms of thyrotoxicosis will be present. The patient without such findings and in a depressed or apathetic mood is said to have "apathetic thyrotoxicosis" of the elderly.[19]

The elderly patient with hyperthyroidism frequently does not have an enlarged thyroid gland. If a goiter is present, it may be small. Cardiovascular manifestations of hyperthyroidism are especially important in the elderly. The stress of hyperthyroidism added to preexisting heart disease may be particularly dangerous. Patients may present with tachycardia, widened pulse pressure, a hyperdynamic precordium, and a systolic murmur. "High output" heart failure may be present. Atrial fibrillation is a not uncommon presentation of hyperthyroidism, particularly in the elderly. Occasionally, embolic phenomena may occur in patients with atrial fibrillation.

Graves' disease is the most common cause of hyperthyroidism in the elderly. Other etiologies include toxic multinodular goiter, solitary toxic nodule, and iodine-induced thyrotoxicosis. Exogenous iodine may be derived from contrast materials utilized in radiographic diagnostic procedures or in medications such as amiodarone, an antiarrhythmic agent.

The physician must have a low threshold for suspicion of thyroid disease in the elderly patient. Changes in weight, mental status, or cardiovascular status in the elderly should prompt the examiner to consider the diagnosis of hyperthyroidism. Failure to make a correct diagnosis in these patients in a timely fashion may make treatment of the manifestations of the disease ineffective. Furthermore, common diagnostic and therapeutic maneuvers may place the patient with unrecognized thyrotoxicosis at risk for thyroid storm, a situation with catastrophic potential. Patients treated with beta blockers may have masking of the hyperadrenergic signs and symptoms of thyrotoxicosis. Thus, the elderly patient treated with these agents may be even less likely to have any of the "classic" signs and symptoms of hyperthyroidism.

The diagnosis of hyperthyroidism can be made by direct measurement of serum free T_4 (FT_4) or an approximation of this measurement such as the free thyroxine index (FT_4I). The free thyroxine index is obtained by multiplying the total serum thyroxine value (T_4) by some measurement of hormone-binding capacity (resin T_3 uptake, T_3 uptake binding ratio, thyroid hormone binding ratio). This result is a dimensionless number, but it correlates well in most instances with actual free thyroxine concentrations. In a minority of cases, the results of the FT_4 or FT_4I will be normal, but the diagnostic suspicion will be so high that the measurement of serum T_3 will be indicated to consider the possibility of "T_3 toxicosis." An elevation of the serum free T_3 index (FT_3I), derived in an analogous fashion to the serum FT_4I, indicates hyperthyroidism. However, "T_4 toxicosis" (FT_4I elevated while FT_3I normal) is much more common than "T_3 toxicosis," especially in the elderly or severely ill patients. A thyrotropin releasing hormone (TRH) stimulation test may be useful in borderline cases to diagnose hyperthyroidism. However, a "flat" TRH test may not always indicate frank hyperthyroidism, particularly in older male patients, patients with multinodular goiters, patients with severe nonthyroidal illness, and patients treated with dopamine. A normal TRH test rules out hyperthyroidism, however. Rarely, a hyperthyroid patient who is severely ill may have normalization of both serum T_4 and T_3 values until he recovers from his nonthyroidal illness. TRH stimulation tests in these cases are uninterpretable. Serial measurement of thyroid hormones is the only sure means of definitively making this diagnosis in the severely ill patient.

Newer technology using immunoradiometric techniques for measuring thyrotropin (TSH) may be helpful for screening for hyperthyroidism. In particular, this methodology may be helpful in differentiating low TSH concentrations from normal TSH values. A low TSH value would be indicative of hyperthyroidism. However, severe nonthyroidal illness may also result in suppression of TSH. Therefore, in very ill patients, low TSH values by immunoradiometric assay may not always indicate hyperthyroidism.

Hyperthyroid patients may have abnormalities in liver function tests, anemia, granulocytopenia, impaired glucose tolerance, or hypercalcemia. All these abnormalities are nonspecific.

In patients without nodular goiters, Graves' disease can usually be differentiated from other forms of hyperthyroidism by the radioactive iodine uptake (elevated in Graves' disease). Radioactive iodine is the definitive treatment for all elderly patients with thyrotoxicosis due to autonomous function of the thyroid gland. Thyroid storm after administration of therapeutic doses of radioactive iodine is a rare occurrence but more likely in the elderly. Rendering the patient euthyroid with antithyroid drugs (prophylthiouracil or methimazole) prior to radioactive iodine therapy may be necessary in patients at high risk for thyroid storm. In iodine-induced thyrotoxicosis, beta-blockers may be utilized until the patient recovers.

Thyroid storm is fortunately a rare manifestation of hyperthyroidism. It occurs when extreme manifestations of hyperthyroidism coexist with fever, tachycardia out of proportion to the fever, and central nervous system dysfunction. Since elderly patients frequently have fewer of the classic signs and symptoms of hyperthyroidism, hyperpyrexia with mental confusion in the elderly should suggest the possibility of thyroid storm.[20]

A precipitating factor of thyroid storm must always be vigorously pursued. Infection should be considered the culprit until proven otherwise. Treatment includes blocking hormonal release (iodides, glucocorticoids), inhibiting hormonal synthesis (antithyroid drugs), blocking conversion of thyroxine to triiodothyronine (propylthiouracil, glucocorticoids), and alleviation of the hyperadrenergic state (beta blockers). Antithyroid drugs should be given prior to iodine.

Hypothyroidism

Hypothyroidism may occur in 6 to 7% of the elderly female population. Goitrous and nongoitrous forms exist, though of special note are patients with previous radioactive iodine treatment of hyperthyroidism or thyroid surgery who have been lost to follow-up.

Patients may be relatively asymptomatic or have many nonspecific symptoms. The nonspecificity of the signs and symptoms of hypothyroidism frequently lead to a failure to make this diagnosis. Classic symptoms include weakness, lethargy, weight gain, dry skin, cold intolerance, hoarseness, constipation, and paresthesias. Textbook signs include dry and coarse skin, coarse hair, periorbital edema, bradykinesia, peripheral edema, delayed relaxation phase of the deep tendon reflexes, and bradycardia. However, the elderly may present with weight loss, nonspecific musculoskeletal complaints, congestive heart failure, evidence of bowel obstruction, anemia, carpal tunnel syndrome, or altered mental status (psychosis, dementia, depression, coma, or seizures). Hyponatremia due to inability to excrete free water may compound the neurologic picture.

A diagnosis of primary hypothyroidism is usually made when the patient has an elevated serum TSH concentration. Although some patients with an elevated TSH will have quite normal FT_4 or FT_4I values and be relatively symptom free (a setting sometimes called "subclinical hypothyroidism"), it is our bias that all patients with consistent elevations of serum TSH should be treated with thyroid hormone. Causes of permanent hypothyroidism in the elderly include previous ablative therapy (surgery and radioiodine) and chronic thyroiditis. In the recovery phase of nonthyroidal illness and in the course of self-limited diseases such as subacute and silent thyroiditis, mild increases in serum TSH usually return to normal in a matter of weeks and do not require treatment.

Two aspects of hypothyroidism are of special concern to the clinician treating the geriatric population. Due to the high incidence of coexisting coronary artery disease in the elderly, the treatment of hypothyroidism must be approached with care. Geriatric patients with marked or long-standing hypothyroidism should have their thyroid replacement therapy initiated at a relatively small daily dose of thyroxine (0.025 mg). Increases in the thyroxine dose (by 0.0125 to 0.025 mg) every 2 to 4 weeks until full replacement (approximately 0.075 to 0.125 mg) is achieved allow for a gradual increase in myocardial oxygen demand. Angina occurring in the setting of thyroid hormone replacement should be treated with aggressive medical therapy and discontinuation of the thyroid hormone. It should be remembered that while the serum half-life of thyroxine is approximately 1 week, the biologic half-life is much longer.

Myxedema coma is a rare but dreaded complication of hypothyroidism.[21] It usually occurs in elderly patients during winter months. Intercurrent illness or exposure is usually related to metabolic decompensation. Known precipitants of myxedema coma are listed in Table 23–8.

Altered mental status and hypothermia are the hallmarks of myxedema coma, though one fifth of reported patients have normal temperatures. A normal temperature may indicate bacterial infection in these patients. The majority of comatose, hypothermic patients will not have myxedema coma. However, the physician must always consider myxedema coma as a possibility in this clinical situation since it is a readily treatable disorder.

The physician considering the diagnosis of myxedema coma should question the patient's family or acquaintances carefully about a previous history of Graves' disease (frequently the manifestations of remote hyperthyroidism may be remembered by the family), radioactive iodine treatment, thyroid surgery, or thyroxine therapy. Inquiry should be made as to symptoms suggestive of hypothyroidism.

The classic signs and symptoms of hypothyroidism may or may not be present in the patient with myxedema coma. Assessment of the neck for a surgical scar is certainly important. Temperatures below 80°F have been reported, so thermometers that measure temperatures

Table 23–8   Precipitating Factors for Myxedema Coma

Infection
Drugs (phenothiazines, barbiturates, narcotics, anesthetics)
Respiratory failure
Congestive heart failure
Cerebrovascular accident
Trauma
Exposure to cold
Gastrointestinal hemorrhage
Metabolic disturbances (hypoglycemia, hyponatremia,   hypoadrenalism)
Surgery
Seizures

below 94°F should be used. Shivering is not seen in patients with myxedema coma. Patients with profound hypothermia are less likely to survive than those patients whose body temperature is near normal. Myxedematous patients may present in shock. Since hypothyroidism decreases the sensitivity of central nervous system respiratory centers to hypoxic and hypercarbic drives plus predisposes the patient to airway obstruction and respiratory muscle weakness, the patient may be in profound respiratory distress. Goiters are infrequently seen in patients with myxedema coma. The patient may have pleural or pericardial effusions or ascites. Signs of bowel obstruction may be present. Localizing neurologic signs may also be seen.

Laboratory tests may reveal hyponatremia or hypoglycemia. Rarely, hypercalcemia is seen. Leukocytosis may not be present despite overwhelming infection. Acid-base balance is dependent upon the perfusion and ventilation status of the patient. Cerebrospinal fluid protein concentrations can be increased. Cardiac enzymes may be elevated with increases in the specific cardiac fraction of creatinine phosphokinase (CPK). Hypothyroidism may cause decreased voltage and nonspecific changes in the electrocardiogram. The physician should be especially alert for signs of infection (particularly respiratory).

Myxedema coma is a clinical diagnosis. Due to the high mortality of this disorder, the clinician does not have the luxury of waiting for the results of laboratory tests to definitively diagnose hypothyroidism. Prior to initiation of therapy, serum should be obtained for the measurement of serum TSH and FT_4I or FT_4. Adrenal reserve should be evaluated with a cosyntropin stimulation test, though corticosteroids are usually given. Reversible corticotropin (ACTH) deficiency can occur in primary hypothyroidism due to hyperplasia of the pituitary thyrotropes.

Treatment of myxedema coma (Table 23–9) includes 1) extensively searching for an underlying cause, particularly infection, and treating empirically if necessary; 2) warming the patient passively; 3) securing and maintaining the airway and adequately ventilating the patient; 4) supporting the blood pressure with fluids (the patient may be poorly responsive to sympathomimetic agents); 5) glucocorticoids (hydrocortisone 100 mg intravenously every 8 hours); and 6) L-thyroxine 300 to 500 mg

Table 23–9   Treatment of Myxedema Coma

Treat underlying cause
Passively warm patient
Treat hypotension with fluids
Use pressors, if needed, cautiously
Secure the airway and mechanically ventilate if necessary
Hydrocortisone 100 mg IV q.8h.
Thyroxine 500 mg IV followed by
  a) 100 mg thyroxine IV qd or b) 25 mg triiodothyronine
  IV q.6h.

intravenously followed by either 100 mg L-thyroxine IV daily or 25 mg L-triiodothyronine IV every 6 hours. If sympathomimetic agents are used in conjunction with L-thyroxine, the patient may be at greater risk for cardiac arrhythmias. Continuous cardiac monitoring is indicated in these patients.

Glucose-containing solutions are usually given to these patients. It is controversial whether profoundly myxedematous patients should be treated only with thyroxine. Some experts believe that triiodothyronine should be given since severely ill patients have a block in the conversion of T_4 to T_3. Triiodothyronine therapy normalizes some metabolic parameters more rapidly than thyroxine treatment in hypothyroid patients. However, no commercially available parenteral preparation of triiodothyronine is available. If the physician chooses to use this medication, an aqueous solution suitable for intravenous administration must be prepared. This can be done by dissolving 100 mg of L-triiodothyronine in 1 mL of 0.1 normal sodium hydroxide and diluting with normal saline. Nonspecific binding to plastic tubing can be prevented by adding albumin. The solution must be passed through a millipore filter for sterilization. In this author's opinion, thyroxine is probably adequate treatment.

Since myxedematous coma patients have alterations in mental status, the part that hyponatremia, particularly when profound, may play in depressing the sensorium is problematic. A free-water diuresis can be induced by the administration of a potent loop diuretic such as furosemide. If the patient has seizures and severe hyponatremia, hypertonic saline and furosemide should be given. Potassium replacement will be necessary if diuretics are administered. Central venous monitoring may be necessary if hypertonic saline is given.

Since hypothyroidism affects drug metabolism, alterations in drug pharmacokinetics should be considered.

TYPE II DIABETES MELLITUS

Type II (noninsulin dependent) diabetes mellitus occurs in approximately 4% of the elderly population. Decreased ability to care for self, living alone, intercurrent illness, decline in renal function, and polypharmacy all may place the patient at risk for marked diabetic decompensation. When such derangement occurs, the outcome may be catastrophic.

Hyperglycemic Hyperosmolar Nonketotic Coma (HHNK)

Hyperglycemic hyperosmolar nonketotic coma (HHNK) is a dreaded complication of noninsulin dependent diabetes mellitus with a mortality of 20 to 50% in many series.[22-27] The patient presents with altered mental status (lethargy, stupor, coma, or seizures). A not infrequent presen-

tation is a comatose, aged patient who is brought by relatives or friends to the emergency department after not being seen for several days. If the patient is able to give a history, he or she may relate profound polydipsia and polyuria. A previous history of diabetes mellitus may be lacking. As the name implies, ketosis is minimal, so tachypnea and sweet-smelling breath are absent. Signs of dehydration are usually present. The patient may be hypothermic. Urinary retention and gastric distention may occur. Virtually any focal neurologic sign is possible in the hyperosmolar patient. Mental status correlates inversely in a rough fashion with plasma osmolality.

Extreme hyperglycemia leads to a shrinkage of the intracellular compartment to maintain the extracellular compartment. This shift of water apparently leads to the plethora of neurologic symptoms and signs seen in HHNC. The patient should be assumed to have an infectious process until proven otherwise.

The plasma glucose concentration is usually greater than 600 mg/dL, resulting in marked hyperosmolality. The glucose level reaches such elevations due to the inability of the kidney (due to renal disease or volume contraction from the preceding osmotic load) to "dump" the excess glucose in the urine. The osmotic diuresis is self-perpetuating as glucose elevation causes more dehydration, and fluid loss raises plasma glucose concentration further. Hyperosmolality also suppresses endogenous insulin release, further worsening the hyperglycemia.

Ketosis is minimal in these patients, presumably due to sufficient insulin activity to suppress ketogenesis, though hyperosmolality itself may inhibit ketone production. The patient may be mildly acidotic, however, due to lactic acidosis (poor perfusion) or renal insufficiency.

The serum osmolality can be approximated as follows:

$$2 \times ([Na^+] + [K^+]) + \frac{[glucose]}{18} + \frac{[BUN]}{2.8}$$

where serum sodium (Na^+) and potassium (K^+) are measured in mEq/L, and glucose and BUN in mg/dL.

The measured serum sodium concentration may be depressed due to osmotic shifts of water into the extracellular space and sodium loss in the urine.

Hemoconcentration may lead to elevation of the hematocrit. BUN and creatinine concentrations are increased, consistent with prerenal azotemia.

Therapy for this disorder is outlined in Table 23–10. Free water deficits are massive, ranging from 6 to 18 liters. Approximately half the fluid deficit should be replenished over 12 hours with the rest replaced over the next 24 hours. Maintenance fluids and those continuing to be lost should be considered in determining fluid therapy. Considerable debate exists concerning proper fluid therapy. Perfusion should be restored with normal saline (usually 1 to 2 liters or until the patient no longer has a marked orthostatic drop in blood pressure). Most authorities recommend half-normal saline as the fluid of

Table 23–10   Treatment of Hyperglycemic Hyperosmolar Nonketotic Coma

Restore blood pressure with normal saline.
Look vigorously for underlying cause and treat.
One-half normal saline at approximately 250 mL/hr. Add dextrose when blood sugar reaches 300 mg/dL.
Insulin 10–25 IV bolus, followed by 5 U/hour IV constant infusion. Increase if no response in plasma glucose concentration.
Potassium with potassium chloride and potassium phosphate.
Monitor blood sugar, renal function, and potassium.

Table 23–11   Predisposing Factors for Hyperglycemic Hyperosmolar Nonketotic Coma

Infection
Burns
Insulin withdrawal
Drugs (steroids, diuretics, beta-blockers, phenytoin, phenothiazines, azathioprine, diazoxide, glycerol)
Pancreatitis
Cerebrovascular accidents
Dialysis
Heat stroke
Hypothermia
Parenteral hyperalimentation
Myocardial infarction
Gastrointestinal hemorrhage
Surgery
Excessive carbohydrate intake
Unknown

choice after blood pressure is stabilized. Glucose should be added to the IV when the serum glucose reaches 250 to 300 mg/dL. Potassium should be given as needed. Although hypophosphatemia and hypomagnesemia are not often clinically significant, administration of potassium phosphate and magnesium sulfate is not harmful as long as the patient has adequate urine output. With magnesium sulfate use, however, constant monitoring is essential to avoid excess. The volume status of the patient should be closely monitored. Occasionally, central monitoring will be required. A constant regular insulin intravenous infusion should be utilized after an initial bolus (10 to 25 units). Some HHNK patients will be very sensitive to insulin and may respond to doses as low as 3 to 5 units per hour. Other patients will require larger doses. It is wise to start at approximately 5 units per hour and increase or decrease the rate as necessary. Since experimental data suggest that cerebral edema may occur if the plasma glucose is lowered quickly from

300 mg/dL to normal in those patients, it is wise to lower the glucose concentration slowly once this level is reached.

A vigorous search for the cause of the metabolic derangement is in order (Table 23–11). If no obvious precipitant is found, broad-spectrum antibiotic coverage may be considered after appropriate cultures have been taken.

The marked metabolic abnormalities seen in these patients are often fully reversible with appropriate treatment. Sometimes the diabetes requires only diet or oral agents as therapy once the complicating factors that led to HHNK are eliminated.

Rapid and Systematic Assessment of Metabolic and Acid-Base Disorders

Metabolic problems in the elderly are frequently encountered within the province of the emergency department. The manifestations of such disorders are legion. In cases of acute renal or pulmonary failure, ingestion of toxins, and diabetic coma, the nature of the metabolic derangement can frequently be diagnosed from the history, physical examination, and laboratory data base. However, when a metabolic disturbance is expressed as a focal neurologic lesion, coma, seizure disorder, cardiac arrest, myopathy, or nonspecific symptom complex, the diagnosis may be much more difficult. In such cases, if a systematic approach to metabolic problems is not employed, the disease may go undiagnosed and, hence, untreated.

To ensure rapid institution of appropriate therapy for derangements of metabolic homeostasis, the emergency physician must be familiar with myriad disorders and be able to distinguish among them using a paucity of quickly available laboratory data.

Metabolic Emergencies: Importance of Early Diagnosis

Metabolic derangements can serve as diagnostic clues to the presence of the following:

1. Toxic ingestions
2. Hemodynamic compromise
3. Respiratory failure
4. Postictal states
5. Others (SIADH, Addisonian crisis, hypothyroidism, etc.)

Therapeutic decisions depend upon rapid diagnosis:

1. Choice of IV fluids
2. Oral therapy
3. Dextrose therapy
4. ETOH therapy (i.e., in ethylene glycol ingestion)
5. Insulin therapy
6. Others (dialysis, hemoperfusion with charcoal, etc.)

Disposition and triage of patients depends upon early recognition of the nature and severity of metabolic disturbance:

1. ICU, CCU versus dialysis
2. Invasive versus noninvasive monitoring

Clinical Conditions: Metabolic Problems in the Elderly

Metabolic disorders in the emergency department include the following:

1. Shock (lactic acidosis, rhabdomyolysis, hyperkalemia, hyperphosphatemia, alcohol or drug ingestion, respiratory alkalosis, or acidosis)
2. Cardiopulmonary arrest (hypokalemia or hyperkalemia, lactic acidosis, hypocalcemia in electromechanical [EM] dissociation, etc.)
3. Seizures (hyponatremia, hypocalcemia, hypomagnesemia, hypoglycemia, hyperosmolar states, rhabdomyolysis, etc.)
4. Coma (diabetic or alcoholic ketoacidosis, hyperosmolar nonketotic coma, hyponatremia, hypoglycemia, hyperammonemia, etc.)
5. Respiratory failure (hypercapnia, CO_2 narcosis, etc.)
6. Toxic ingestion (methanol, ethylene glycol, paraldehyde, ethanol, etc.)

Emergency Department Battery (EDB)

The emergency department battery (EDB) is a conceptual, quasialgorithmic scheme that is intended to guide the emergency department physician in the diagnosis and evaluation of acute metabolic emergencies in the geriatric patient.

The EDB framework (EDB-6, EDB-9, EDB-15, EDB-18, EDB-20 — number represents how many lab tests are included in the battery) is organized in hierarchical fashion to facilitate the diagnosis of increasingly complex and/or unusual metabolic derangements. The laboratory tests in the EDBs include only those available on a STAT basis.

EDB-6 = Na, K, Cl, CO_2, Glucose, BUN

This is the minimal and initial diagnostic data base for the evaluation of metabolic disorders in coma, seizures, acute renal failure, nonketotic hyperosmolar coma, prerenal azotemia, high anion gap (i.e., organic acid) acidoses, adrenocortical insufficiency, toxic ingestions, and in nonspecific presentations.

NOTE: The EDB-6 is almost always used in conjunction with other lab tests (especially ABGs) in order to fully elucidate the exact nature of a metabolic disturbance. Creatinine is usually measured to assess renal function.

EDB-9 = EDB-6 + pH, PCO_2, PO_2

The EDB-9 is needed for nearly all of the entities listed under EDB-6 plus all cases of suspected mixed acid-base

disorders, respiratory distress, as well as for nonmetabolic disorders such as asthma, pulmonary embolism, and pulmonary edema.

EDB-15 = EDB-9 + U_{Na}, U_{Cl}, $U_{ketones}$, $U_{glucose}$, U_{osm}, P_{osm}

The EDB-15 is needed for many of the conditions listed under EDB-6 and EDB-9, as well as for the *complete* and *rapid* evaluation (or confirmation) of diabetic ketoacidosis, alcoholic ketoacidosis (false negative nitroprusside reaction for ketones is common), and SIADH (syndrome of inappropriate ADH can easily be diagnosed as U_{osm} is inappropriately concentrated with respect to P_{osm}). It is also needed for distinguishing acute tubular necrosis (ATN) from prerenal azotemia and a differentiating "saline-responsive" versus "saline-resistant" (U_{Cl}) metabolic alkalosis. Finally, it is needed as a clue (P_{osm}) to the presence of ETOH, methanol, or ethylene glycol ingestions.

EDB-18 = EDB-15 + Ca, PO_4, Mg

This EDB is used for many of the conditions listed under other EDBs (i.e., DKA, ETOH withdrawal, renal failure, etc.) and especially when myoirritability (i.e., positive Chvostek's or Trousseau's syndrome), EM dissociation, rhabdomyolysis (i.e., elevated PO_4 and decreased Ca), lactic acidosis (elevated PO_4), starvation, metastatic cancer (elevated Ca), cardiomyopathy, or hypophosphatemia is present or suspected.

EDB-20 = EDB-18 + U_{Cr}, P_{Cr}

This EDB is used for renal disorders, assessment of volume status, and in other conditions when a renal failure index (RFI) may be helpful.

Diagnostic Tools For Rapid Evaluation of Metabolic Disorders

Arterial Blood Gas Interpretation

Table 23–12   Nine Categories of Acid-Base Disturbance as Defined by the PCO_2 and Bicarbonate Levels

PCO_2	Bicarbonate (mEq/L)		
	< 21	21–26	> 26
> 45	Combined metabolic and respiratory acidosis	Respiratory acidosis	Metabolic alkalosis and respiratory acidosis
35–45	Metabolic acidosis	Normal	Metabolic alkalosis
< 35	Metabolic acidosis and respiratory alkalosis	Respiratory alkalosis	Combined metabolic and respiratory alkalosis

BUN/Cr Ratio

When ratio > 15:1, this suggests *prerenal azotemia* (i.e., dehydration or prerenal hypoperfusion on some other basis).

Use of the Renal Failure Index (RFI) and Fractional Excretion of Sodium FE_Na

$$RFI = \frac{U_{Na}}{U_{Cr}/P_{Cr}} \; ; \; FE_{Na} = \frac{U_{Na}/P_{Na}}{U_{Cr}/P_{Cr}}$$

If RFI < 1: prerenal causes

If RFI > 1: ATN, vascular or postrenal causes

Interpretation of Urinary Electrolytes

U_{Na}. In general, a healthy (i.e., non-ATN) kidney is able to conserve sodium. Therefore, in the oliguric patient (anuria is seen almost *only* in postrenal *obstruction*) who has an elevated BUN and Cr, a *prerenal* picture will be characterized by a low U_{Na} (i.e., < 20 mEq/L), whereas the ATN picture will be characterized by high U_{Na} (i.e., > 40). NOTE: Diuretics can make a prerenal picture look like ATN because they increase U_{Na} excretion (in such cases use RFI or FE_{Na} to refine diagnosis).

U_{Cr}. In general, a healthy kidney is able to concentrate creatinine (Cr) in the urine, whereas a diseased (i.e., ATN, etc.) kidney will excrete Cr at about the same concentration as it is in the plasma.

Therefore, a *prerenal* picture is characterized by:

$$U_{Cr}/P_{Cr} > 20:1$$

whereas an ATN picture is characterized by:

$$U_{Cr}/P_{Cr} = 1:1$$

U_{Cl}. Value lies in distinguishing among etiologies in metabolic alkalosis. *Volume contraction* (i.e., nasogastric suction, diuretic therapy, dehydration) alkalosis will be characterized by avid NaCl reabsorption, and, therefore, the U_{Cl} will be low (i.e., < 10 mEq/L).

Metabolic alkalosis caused by *hyperadrenal* states (i.e., increased serum cortisol and/or mineralocorticoids that cause increased Na for K and H^+ exchange distally) is usually characterized by U_{Cl} > 10 mEq (Table 23–13).

U_{osm}. In general, a diseased kidney will not be able to concentrate well, and so in the oliguric patient with elevated BUN and Cr, an isosmotic urine suggests ATN, and a concentrated urine (i.e., >550 osm) suggests *prerenal* causes. Also, the U_{osm} is probably the most important test for ascertaining the diagnosis of SIADH. If the $U_{osm} > P_{osm}$ in the patient who is severely hyponatremic and hypoosmolar, this virtually confirms the diagnosis of SIADH. Actually, any U_{osm} that is not maximally dilute (i.e., 50 to 85 mOsm/L) in a patient with hyponatremia and hypoosmolarity is suggestive of SIADH.

Table 23–13   Value of the Determination of Urinary Chloride Concentration in the Differential Diagnosis of Metabolic Alkalosis

Saline responsive (U_{Cl} < 10 mEq/L)	Saline resistant (U_{Cl} > 10 mEq/L)
• Loss of gastric secretions (i.e., vomiting or nasogastric suction) • Diuretic therapy	• Primary aldosteronism • Cushing's disease • Adrenocorticotropic–hormone (ACTH) producing tumors • Severe potassium depletion • Steroid therapy

Serum Osmolality

Serum osmolality can be both calculated and measured. If calculated:

$$S_{osm} = 2 \times Na^+ + Glucose/18 + BUN/3$$

where serum sodium (Na^+) is measured in mEq/L, and glucose and BUN in mg/dL.

If measured:

$$S_{osm} \text{ CALCULATED } S_{osm}$$

then molecules (i.e., other than Na, BUN, and glucose) with significant osmotic properties are present in the serum. In general, these might be ETOH (a 25 mOsm difference between calculated and measured serum osmolality would be compatible with an ETOH level of 100 to 120 mg/dL), methanol, ethylene glycol, or mannitol. Therefore, patients whose serum osmolality cannot be explained by ETOH level should be suspected of having ingested one of the above-mentioned toxins.

Winter's Formula

Winter's formula is a quick way to measure appropriateness of respiratory response (i.e., hyperventilation or hypoventilation) to a metabolic disturbance.

As a rule:

If $PCO_2 = 1.5$ (total serum CO_2) + 8.3, appropriate respiratory compensation is present.

If $PCO_2 < 1.5$ (total serum CO_2) + 8.3, then a primary respiratory alkalosis is superimposed on metabolic disturbance.

If $PCO_2 > 1.5$ (total serum CO_2) + 8.3, then a primary respiratory acidosis is superimposed on metabolic disturbance.

Bypassing Henderson-Hasselbalch Equation

A simple method reported that allows you to *estimate* serum bicarbonate (HCO_3^-) concentration from the arterial blood gas (ABG) values, pH, PCO_2 is shown in Table 23–14.

Table 23–14   Estimating Bicarbonate Ion Concentration

| Range | $[HCO_3^-]/P_{CO_2}$ estimate | Examples | |
		$[HCO_3^-]/P_{CO_2}$ from pH	Estimated $[HCO_3^-]$
Severe acidemia (7.00 > pH)	0.20	if pH = 6.89 $\dfrac{[HCO_3^-]}{P_{CO_2}} = 0.02$	$[HCO_3^-] = 20\%$ of P_{CO_2}
Mild — moderate acidemia (7.00 ≤ pH ≤ 7.40)	(pH − 7) + 0.20	if pH = 7.25 0.25 + 0.20 = 0.45 $\dfrac{[HCO_3^-]}{P_{CO_2}} = 0.45$	$[HCO_3^-] = 45\%$ of P_{CO_2}
Alkalemia (pH > 7.40)	2[(pH − 7) − 0.10]	if pH = 7.60 0.60 − 0.10 = 0.50 2 × 0.50 = 1.00 $\dfrac{[HCO_3^-]}{P_{CO_2}} = 1.00$	$[HCO_3^-] = 100\%$ of P_{CO_2}

From Kamens DR et al: Circumventing the Henderson-Hasselbalch equation, JACEP 8:462, 1979.

Anion Gap

$$Na^+ - (Cl^- + HCO_3^-) = AG$$

NOTE: This is one of the most important diagnostic tools to measure for the evaluation of acute metabolic emergencies.

The anion gap is a calculation of diagnostic convenience. There is, of course, no true anion gap since positive and negative charges in the blood must be equal. However, the principal cation of the blood, sodium (Na), exceeds the sum of the principal anions, chloride and bicarbonate, by about 12 ± 2 mEq/L in normal persons. The additional, or so-called unmeasured, anions include albumin (which is an anion at physiologic pH) and other metabolites such as sulfate, phosphates, and small amounts of organic acids. When metabolic acids are generated and added to the body fluid, the hydrogen ion of the acid destroys bicarbonate, and if the anion associated with the proton (i.e., hydrogen) is any other than chloride, the sum of chloride and bicarbonate must fall, thereby increasing the anion gap.

Differential Diagnosis of Elevated and Reduced Anion Gap

The most important thing about the anion gap is for the emergency physician to get into the habit of using this simple and revealing calculation on a routine basis. Failure to employ this diagnostic tool may allow any of the following to go undetected:

1. Organic acidoses
2. Toxin-induced acidoses
3. Severe alkalemia
4. Mixed acid-base disturbances

A reduced anion gap may also be an important finding and is frequently the first clue in the ED that cirrhosis, lithium toxicity, hypercalcemia, hypermagnesemia, or multiple myeloma is present (Table 23–15).

Anion Gap and Alkalemia

NOTE: This is a relatively new, but relevant, discovery.

$$\text{Anion gap} = Na^+ - (Cl^- + HCO_3^-) = AG$$

When investigating the cause of an elevated anion gap (AG), the ED clinician routinely seeks evidence for the presence of lactic acidosis, ASA ingestion, advanced renal failure, methanol, paraldehyde, or ethylene glycol ingestion, diabetic ketoacidosis (DKA), or alcoholic ketoacidosis.

Table 23–15   Differential Diagnosis of Metabolic Acidosis

Normal anion gap (hyperchloremic)	Increased anion gap
Gastrointestinal loss of HCO$_3$ • Diarrhea • Ureterosigmoidostomy • Anion-exchange resin • Small bowel drainage	**Increased acid production** • Diabetic ketoacidosis • Lactic acidosis • Starvation • Alcoholic ketoacidosis • Inborn errors of metabolism
Renal loss of HCO$_3^-$ • Carbonic anhydrase inhibitors • Renal tubular acidosis (RTA)	**Ingestion of toxins** • Salicylate overdose • Paraldehyde poisoning • Methanol ingestion • Ethylene glycol ingestion
Miscellaneous • Dilutional acidosis • Hyperalimentation acidosis	**Acute or chronic renal failure**

Frequently, however, consideration is not given to the possibility that changes in unmeasured anions, originating from plasma proteins, may have contributed to the increase in anion gap. It is now well established that increases in unmeasured anions may result from alkalemia-induced elevations in the net negative charge of plasma proteins.

Anion Gap, Serum Proteins, and Alkalemia

$$AG = Na^+ - (Cl^- + HCO_3^-)$$

The anion gap largely reflects organic sulfates, phosphates, and negatively charged serum proteins, of which albumin is the most important.

Alkalemia
$$Albumin - H \rightarrow Albumin^- + H^+$$

$$Albumin^- \uparrow \rightarrow \uparrow \ ANION \ GAP$$

Anion Gap: Some Pearls

Recognize that a *normal measured serum* HCO_3^- does *not* mean that there is not a *metabolic acidosis* present. If there is a preexisting metabolic alkalosis (i.e., vomiting, diuretics, ETOH'ism, metabolic compensation for respiratory acidosis, etc.), the serum HCO_3^- will be elevated *at first* and then can *fall to a normal range* (or perhaps lower) in the presence of a superimposed metabolic acidosis.

The presence of a preexisting metabolic alkalosis can be detected using the AG.

$$\Delta AG = AG \ (calculated) - AG \ (normal, i.e., 12)$$

$$\Delta HCO_3^- = HCO_3^- \ (expected - i.e., 24 \ mEq) - HCO_3^- \ (measured)$$

If:

$$\Delta AG > HCO_3^-$$

suspect a metabolic acidosis that has been superimposed on a preexisting metabolic *alkalosis.*

Anion Gap: Extended Data Base (i.e., further lab workup in ED)

Extended Data Base for Evaluation of Elevated Anion Gap

1. DKA: urine ketones, serum ketones, serum K^+, serum PO_4, glucose, lactate level, ABG
2. Alcoholic ketosis
   - Urine ketones (but note that the nitroprusside reagent, Acetest, may be entirely negative because this kind of acidosis is characteristically a B-OH butyric acidosis; serum ketones are usually positive)
   - Glucose (especially important, since this syndrome may be accompanied by hypoglycemia, i.e., hypoglycemic ketoacidotic coma)
   - Urine glucose (almost always negative in this kind of ketoacidosis)
3. Lactic acidosis
   - Lactate level, K^+; may need to draw CN^-, methemoglobin, or carboxyhemoglobin level for "unexplained" cases of lactic acidosis
   - In cases of quickly resolving LA, consider generalized motor seizures as likely etiology and initiate workup as needed
4. Salicylate overdose: salicylate level, ABGs, and lactate level (if acidosis is very severe; salicylates may uncouple oxidative phosphorylation and lead to LA)
5. Ethylene glycol ingestion: blood level, serum osmolality, urinalysis, and renal workup
6. Methanol: blood level, serum osmolality
7. Paraldehyde
8. Alkalemia: work up various etiologies

Low Anion Gap: Differential Diagnosis

Causes of Low Anion Gap

1. Reduced concentration of unmeasured anions
   - Dilution
   - Hypoalbuminemia
2. Systematic underestimation of serum sodium
   - Hypernatremia (severe)
   - Hyperviscosity
3. Systematic overestimation of serum chloride
   - Bromism
4. Retained nonsodium cations
   - Paraproteinemia
   - Hypercalcemia, hypermagnesemia, lithium toxicity

Anion Gap and Metabolic Acidosis

Lactic Acidosis (Most Common Cause of Elevated AG)

Causes

1. Inadequate oxygen delivery
   - Cardiac arrest
   - Shock states
   - Profound anemia
   - Hypoxemia
2. Failure to utilize oxygen
   - Phenformin
   - Ethanol
   - Diabetic ketoacidosis
   - Leukemia and lymphoma
   - INH overdose
3. Others
   - Hepatic cirrhosis
   - Pregnancy
   - Pancreatitis
   - Seizures
   - CRF

Case Presentations

Lactic Acidosis Presenting as Respiratory Problem

A 70-year-old white male presents to the emergency department with a depressed LOC. He appears to be in moderate respiratory distress. Vital signs reveal that BP = 105/70, R = 22, Temp = 37.5°C, and HR = 120. Cardiac exam reveals an S_3, and a pulmonary exam reveals diffuse rhonchi and rales bilaterally, posteriorly. A history of COPD is obtained. Initial lab data include ABG:pH = 7.25, P_{CO_2} = 57, P_{O_2} = 52. (A medical resident is called to see the patient and makes a "diagnosis" of acute respiratory failure with respiratory acidosis.) Additional lab values are returned to the ED: Na = 136, Cl = 90, HCO_3^- = 25, K = 4.0, BUN = 40, Cr = 1.6. (Anion gap elevated = 21.) Elevated AG suggests that metabolic acidosis is the primary metabolic derangement. Lactic acid is drawn and elevated (10.6 mmol/L) (Figure 23–1). The patient is treated with diuretics and morphine for cardiac failure (low output state) and pulmonary edema, which a chest x-ray confirms. Repeat tests of blood gas shortly after treatment show pH = 7.35, P_{CO_2} = 54, P_{O_2} = 60, and HCO_3^- = 30. This represents the levels of the patient's baseline state (i.e., chronic respiratory acidosis with metabolic compensation).

In summary, this is a case in which the acidosis resolved with treatment directed at low output failure rather than at the respiratory system.

ALSO NOTE:

Δ AG = 21 – 12 = 9
Δ HCO_3^- = 24 – 25 = (–1)
Δ AG > ΔHCO_3^- giving a clue to the presence of preexisting metabolic alkalosis

Severe Acidosis and Hyperkalemia

An 80-year-old white male, who is taking digoxin and diuretics, is brought to the ED with severe SOB, tachypnea, and mental confusion. Vital signs: Temp = 38.2°C, HR = 110, RR = 28, and BP = 180/105. The physical exam reveals a dehydrated, dyspneic patient, with rhonchi and rales at the right lower lung base. A chest x-ray reveals an infiltrate, and an ECG strip shows occasional focal PVCs. The patient is started on 3 L O_2 and the following EDB results are returned: pH = 7.16, P_{O_2} = 60, P_{CO_2} = 54, Na = 135, Cl = 108, CO_2 = 21, K = 7.1, BUN = 90, Cr = 2.2, U_{Na} = 48, U_{Cr} = 118, U_{osm} = 440, anion gap = 8.

$$\text{RFI (Renal Failure Index)} = \frac{U_{Na}}{U_{Cr}/P_{Cr}} = \frac{48}{118/2.2} = .94$$

Because the RFI was less than 1 (and also because the BUN/Cr was greater than 20), the patient was presumed to have prerenal azotemia; 2 amps (110 mEq) of $NaHCO_3$, 25 U regular insulin, and 1000 ml $D_{10}W$ (i.e., 100 g glucose)

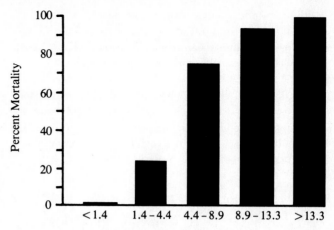

Figure 23–1 Relationship with mortality — the prognostic significance of initial arterial lactate concentration in 52 patients with shock from various causes is shown. The mortality in patients with a lactate level of 1.4 to 4.4 mmol/L (22%) was significantly less than when the lactate levels were between 4.4 and 8.9 mmoles/L (78%). (From Perets DI: Ann NY Acad Sci 119:1133, 1965.)

were administered in the ED. The patient improved clinically and repeat EDB revealed that K = 5.9, pH = 7.28, P_{O_2} = 60, and P_{CO_2} = 50.

NOTE: This patient has a primary hyperchloremic (non-AG) metabolic acidosis superimposed on a chronic respiratory acidosis (presumable second-degree COPD). In distinguishing among the causes of the acidoses, it is important to note the following:

1. That a P_{CO_2} = 54 will not explain a pH = 7.16
2. That while an HCO_3^- = 21 does not "immediately" suggest a significant metabolic acidosis, it is compatible with this diagnosis if you assume that a patient has a chronically elevated HCO_3^- (35 to 40 mEq) as a compensatory response to a chronic respiratory acidosis

CONCLUSION: Do not assume normal measured serum HCO_3^- rules out.

The RFI (calculated from values obtained in the ED) was useful in ascertaining that this patient's elevated BUN, Cr, and potassium, as well as the oliguria and metabolic acidosis, were on the basis of a prerenal azotemia rather than ATN. Once this had been determined, a sodium load ($NaHCO_3$) could be administered without much fear of fluid overload. CONCLUSION: Obtaining urinary diagnostic indices in the ED can be quite helpful in deciding initial fluid therapy and can frequently anticipate or rule out the necessity for dialysis.

Respiratory Acidosis in Pulmonary Edema

A 65-year-old white male with a previous history of CHF presents to the emergency department with a CC: SOB. Vital signs: BP = 180/100, R = 24, Temp = 37°C, and HR = 115. Physical exam reveals bibasilar rales and an S_3 gallop. ABGs are drawn at the time of admission, and the patient is subsequently given 6 mg morphine sulfate IV. Initial (i.e., pretherapy) ABGs return: pH = 7.27, P_{CO_2} = 52, P_{O_2} = 64 (anion gap from EDB-6 is WNL). Patient improves dramatically and repeat gases show pH = 7.36, P_{CO_2} = 38, P_{O_2} = 79.

COMMENT: When hypercapnia and acute respiratory acidosis are caused by alveolar edema and broncho-constriction secondary to LV failure, administration of MS — despite the fact that it is a respiratory depressant — is usually safe and effective.

Metabolic Derangement Presenting as Cardiac Arrest

A 68-year-old white male with a previous history of CAD collapses suddenly at home, without a prodrome of chest pain, nausea, or diaphoresis. He is taking digoxin and diuretics but no K supplementation. The patient is successfully resuscitated by the paramedics, who have intubated him and given him 1 amp of $NaHCO_3^-$ about 30 minutes before arrival at the emergency department. The patient was cardioverted from ventricular fibrillation to NSR and started on a lidocaine drip by the paramedics. Upon admission to the ED he is perfusing well: BP = 120/70, Resp rate (artificial ventilation), and HR = 86. ECG reveals old AMI with multifocal PVCs. First lab data to return are ABGs: pH = 7.62, P_{CO_2} = 30, and P_{O_2} = 160 (50% F_{IO_2}). Calculated serum bicarbonate is 31 mEq/L. On the basis of combined primary metabolic and respiratory alkalosis, the patient is presumed to be hypokalemic and volume contracted, probably secondary to diuretic therapy. Therefore, 10 mEq KCl is added to IV to run over observation period (45 minutes) in ED. EDB-6 returns 30 minutes after arrival and shows: Na = 139, Cl = 90, CO_2 = 30, K = 2.9, BUN = 37. Cr = 1.1, AG = 18 (lactate not measured). The patient's frequent PVCs respond to KCl therapy.

COMMENT: The ED physician who thinks quickly can recognize that metabolic alkalosis in the arrest patient might be the first tip-off of a volume contraction, hypokalemic metabolic alkalosis. If the ventricular arrhythmia appears refractory to suppressive therapy, quick administration of KCl may be warranted. This patient's elevated AG probably reflects alkalemia rather than acidosis. The elevated BUN/Cr ratio argues convincingly for prerenal azotemia that, in this case, was probably induced by diuretic therapy.

Necessity of Measuring Anion Gap in Mixed Acid-Base Disorders

A 65-year-old white female presents to the emergency department after four days of heavy alcohol ingestion and persistent vomiting. On admission she is confused, lethargic, and responds to questions inappropriately. There is no odor of alcohol or ammonia. ABGs reveal

pH = 7.52, P_{CO_2} = 28, and P_{O_2} = 90. Based upon this data, the medical intern in the ED makes a "diagnosis" of acute respiratory alkalosis. The EDB-6 returns and reveals a BUN = 28, Cr = 2.3, Na = 129, Cl = 78, K = 3.0, and a diagnosis of acute respiratory alkalosis with incomplete metabolic compensation. The ED resident is called to see the patient. He calculates the AG (26), which suggests an organic acidosis. Serum lactate is measured (elevated 13.9 mmoles/L), urinary ketones = 1+, and serum ketones positive 1:8.

COMMENT: What initially appeared to be a simple respiratory alkalosis is actually a complicated, mixed acid-base disturbance requiring urgent therapy. This patient had both a primary respiratory and metabolic alkalosis (secondary to vomiting) and superimposed upon these were alcoholic ketoacidosis and alcohol-induced acidosis (Figure 23–2). This patient resolved all her metabolic derangements with the vigorous administration of D_5NS and KCl.

NOTE: The initial measured serum bicarbonate (HCO_3) was 25 mEq/L (i.e., within the normal range), despite a significant lactic acidosis and ketoacidosis. How is this explained? Presumably, there was a significant primary metabolic alkalosis (secondary to vomiting, as explained above), which raised the bicarbonate to 35 mEq/L, a value that was then titrated down into the normal range by the presence of these two organic acids.

Hypothermia, Hypoglycemia, Hypotension

A 63-year-old white female with a history of metastatic breast cancer presents to the ED with an altered mental status and CC: weakness, nausea, and abdominal pain. PE reveals BP = 88/50, R = 26, HR = 110, and Temp = 35.4°C. The rest of the exam is noncontributory. The patient is observed in the ED and EDB-6 returns: glucose = 38 mg/100 mL, BUN = 34, Na = 132, CO_2 = 22, Cl = 100, and K = 49. The patient is given 50 mL of 50% $D_{50}W$ as well as volume replacement with 0.9NS with significant improvement in level of consciousness and slight increase in body temperature. A complete EDB-18 is collected: ABGs show pH = 7.48, P_{CO_2} = 82. Ca, PO_4, and Mg are WNL. U_{Cl} = 20 mEq, U_{Na} = 40, U_{ket} and U_{glu} are negative. U_{Cr} = 30, P_{Cr} = 1.1 (RFI greater than 1). The patient is admitted to medical wards where, within the next 18 hours, she has two more episodes of profound, sudden hypoglycemia, as well as persistent hypotension. She has two cardiac arrests and finally dies despite vigorous therapy.

COMMENT: At autopsy, this patient had an empty sella syndrome, with no remnants of pituitary tissue. Despite persistent hypotension (secondary to NaCl loss because of hypocortisolism), repeat bouts of hypoglycemia (also a result of inadequate glucocorticoids), and excessive urinary Na and Cl losses, the diagnosis of Addisonian crisis was not made. This patient expired be-

Ketone Metabolism

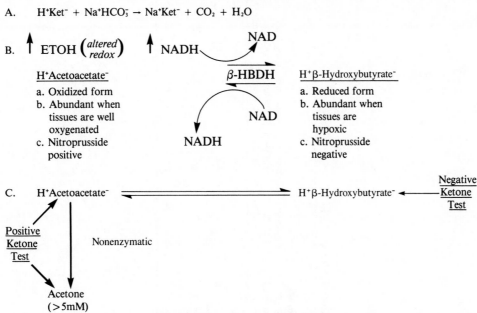

A. $H^+Ket^- + Na^+HCO_3^- \rightarrow Na^+Ket^- + CO_2 + H_2O$

Figure 23–2   Ketone metabolism.

cause steroids were never included in her therapeutic management.

Metabolic Disturbance Presenting as Focal Neurologic Lesion

A 70-year-old black female with CRF and AODM, who is taking oral hypoglycemia medication, is brought to the emergency department with a markedly depressed mental status and left-sided hemiparesis. PE reveals vital signs: Temp = 35.8°C, R = 24, P = 110, BP = 212/118. Neurologic exam demonstrates a profound left-sided hemiparesis, expressive aphasia, and the presence of a Babinski's reflex on the left. Initial diagnostic impression in the ED is intracerebral hemorrhage (hypertensive). EDB-6 returns: glucose = 26 mg/100 mL and otherwise normal electrolytes. Patient's entire neurologic deficit resolves after administration of 50 mL of 50% glucose IV.

COMMENT: Focal neurologic lesions (deficits and seizures) can result from metabolic derangements.

Metabolic Disturbance Presenting as Focal Neurologic Lesion

An 83-year-old black male with a history of oral hypoglycemic use and AODM is admitted to the emergency department with a depressed LOC and dense right-sided hemiparesis. VS reveals BP = 160/80, HR = 120, Temp = 38.2°C, and R = 26. The initial diagnostic impression is left middle cerebral artery thromboembolic infarction. EDB-6 returns: glucose = 1190 mg/100 mL; remainder of studies are consistent with diagnosis of nonketotic hyperosmolar coma. The patient is treated with insulin, hydration, and appropriate electrolyte replacement. Neuro-

logic status returns to baseline, including complete resolution of hemiparesis. (See Table 23–16.)

Mixed Metabolic Derangements

A 66-year-old white male alcoholic is brought to the emergency department comatose and diaphoretic. Vital signs are Temp = 36.2°C, R = 22, HR = 120, BP = 120/70. Cardiac and lung exam are noncontributory, but abdominal exam reveals hepatomegaly. The patient is given 200 mg thiamine IV and 50 mL $D_{50}W$, and quickly regains consciousness. EDB-6 (drawn before therapy) reveals glucose = 39, BUN = 6, Na = 139, K = 5.2, Cl = 100, CO_2 = 20. The initial diagnostic impression is hypoglycemia secondary to depleted hepatic glycogen stores. Despite glucose therapy, the patient's mental status remains somewhat unclear. Reassessment of the problem shows an AG of 19, suggesting organic acidosis. ABGs show pH = 7.28, P_{CO_2} = 35, P_{O_2} = 85; urine ketones = 2+, and serum ketones are positive at 1:4. Lactate, salicylates, and serum osmolality are WNL. The patient has hypoglycemic alcoholic ketoacidotic coma.

Acute Hyponatremia

A 68-year-old white male with a previous psychiatric history and mild hypertension (recently started on a thiazide diuretic) is brought to the ED in a postictal state after having had two generalized seizures. The paramedic described the seizures as beginning at the left arm, moving to the left leg, and then generalizing. Dilantin loading is started in the ED (at 25 mg/min), but despite this the patient has another seizure. EDB-18 returns with the following results: Na = 116, K = 2.8, CO_2 = 30, Cl = 80, BUN = 28; ABGs show pH = 7.52, P_{CO_2} = 100;

Table 23–16 Laboratory Summary of Nondiabetic Alcoholic Patients with Hypoglycemic Ketoacidotic Coma

Case	Arterial pH	Serum Acetest for ketones	Urine Acetest for ketones	Serum glucose (mg/dL) Initial	Discharge	Serum bicarbonate (mEq/L) (normal 24-30) Initial	Discharge	Lactic acid, arterial (mEq/L) (normal 0.5-1.5)	Serum β-hydroxybuty-rate (mEq/L) (normal<.05)	Anion gap (Na + K - [Cl + HCO$_3$])	Serum bilirubin (mg/dL)	Serum insulin (μU/mL)	SGOT (1U/L) (normal<17)
1......	7.16	+	+	25	105	14	21	2.6	9.8	27	1.0	..	55
2......	7.18	+	+	21	120	15	20	2.3	..	21	0.8	3	40
3......	7.23	–	–	27	125	17	24	..	7.3	22	0.7	..	35
4......	7.19	–	–	21	110	13	22	2.2	8.5	29	1.1	5	30
5......	7.18	+	+	19	105	15	23	2.4	5.9	24	0.9	2	31
Mean....	7.19	..	..	23	..	15	..	2.4	7.9	25	0.9	3	38

From Platia EZ and Hsu TH: Hypoglycemic coma with ketoacidosis in nondiabetic adults, West J Med 131(4):272, 1981.

P_{O_2} = 100; Ca, PO_4, and Mg are WNL. U_{Na} = 6, U_{osm} = 420, $Serum_{osm}$ = 245. On the basis of hyponatremia and inappropriate urinary concentration in the face of serum hypoosmolality, a diagnosis of SIADH is made (Figure 23–3). Because of continued seizures, 3% saline and diuresis with 20 mg of furosemide are initiated (Table 23–17).

SOME "CLINICAL PEARLS" FOR METABOLIC EMERGENCIES

1. Refractory ventricular fibrillation: Consider hypokalemia.
2. Diuretic therapy in a patient with altered mental status: Consider hyponatremia with/without SIADH.
3. Diuretic therapy in a patient with muscle weakness: Consider hypokalemia.

   Complications and side effects of diuretic therapy
   - Volume depletion
   - Hypokalemia, hyperkalemia
   - Hyponatremia (SIADH)
   - Acidosis, alkalosis
   - Hyperuricemia
   - Carbohydrate intolerance
   - Hypercalcemia
   - Hypersensitivity reactions
   - Gastrointestinal disorders

4. Hypothermia may be the first clue to the presence of hypoglycemia.
5. Hypothermia in combination with hypoglycemia and hypotension (in the nonexposed patient): Consider Addisonian crisis.
6. Hypothermia in combination with bradycardia and hyponatremia: Consider hypothyroidism.
7. Decreased anion gap in a patient with carcinoma: Consider hypercalcemia.
8. Hyperphosphatemia in a patient with shock: Consider superimposed lactic acidosis.
9. Hypocalcemia, hyperphosphatemia, and hyperuricemia in a patient with crush injury, muscle aches, or after strenuous exercise: Consider rhabdomyolysis.

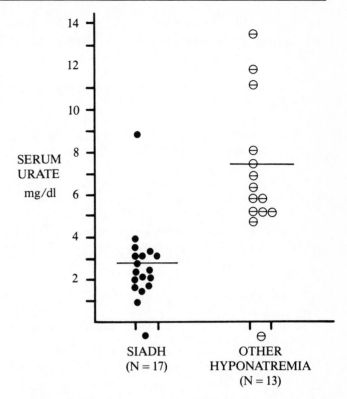

Figure 23–3 Serum concentrations of urate in each patient during hyponatremia.

Table 23–17   Differential Diagnosis of Hyponatremia with Normal Hydration

	Inappropriate ADH secretion	Hypo-pituitarism	Hypothyroidism	Diuretic-induced	Chlorpropamide-induced	Polydipsic vomiting
Creatinine clearance	Normal or ↑	Normal or slightly ↓	Normal or slightly ↓	Normal or slightly ↓	Normal or ↑	Normal or ↓
Serum K	Normal	Normal	Normal	↓	Normal	↓
Serum HCO_3^-	Normal	Normal	Normal	↑	Normal	↑
Urine Na^+	↑	↑	↓	↑ Early ↓ Later	↑	↓
Urine osmolality	↑	↑	↑	↑ Early ↓ Later	↑	↑
Metapyrone response	Normal	↓	Normal	Normal	Normal	Normal
H_2O load response	↓	↓	Delayed	Normal	Delayed	Normal
Correction	H_2O restriction	Cortisol	Thyroid	Withdraw diuretics or ↑ K^+ intake	Withdraw chlorpropamide	NaCl, KCl, and H_2O restriction

10. Increased anion gap in a patient with elevated serum osmolality: Consider ETOH ketoacidosis, ethylene glycol, methanol, or paraldehyde ingestion.
11. Focal neurologic lesions in the diabetic: Consider both nonketotic hyperosmolar states and hypoglycemia.
12. Acidosis and hypercapnia in patients with COPD: Remember the acidosis may represent an underlying and potentially correctable *metabolic acidosis* — you have to look for it!
13. Unexplained symptom complex consisting of neurologic, hematologic (thrombocytopenia, decreased O_2 delivery by RBCs, etc.), cardiac (cardiomyopathy), and/or respiratory (failure) disturbances in ETOH abusers, diabetics, and starved individuals: Consider hypophosphatemia.

REFERENCES

1. Detroyer A and Demaret JC: Clinical, biological, and pathogenic features of the syndrome of inappropriate secretion of antidiuretic hormone, Q J Med 45:521, 1976.
2. Arieff AI: Hyponatremia, convulsions, respiratory arrest, and permanent brain damage after elective surgery in healthy women, N Engl J Med 314:1529, 1986.
3. Nairns RG: Therapy of hyponatremia: does haste make waste? N Engl J Med 314:1573, 1986.
4. Ashraf N, Locksley R, and Arieff AI: Thiazide-induced hyponatremia associated with death or neurologic damage in out-patients, Am J Med 70:1163, 1981.
5. Lye M: Electrolyte disorders in the elderly, Clin Endocrinol Metab 13:377, 1984.
6. Miller M and Moses A: Drug-induced states of impaired water excretion, Kidney Int 10:96, 1976.
7. Levine JA: Heatstroke in the aged, Am J Med 47:25, 1977.
8. Ayus OC, Olivero JJ, and Frommer JP: Rapid correction of severe hyponatremia with intravenous saline solution, Am J Med 72:43, 1982.
9. Sterns RH, Riggs JE, and Schochet SS: Osmotic demyelination syndrome following correction of hyponatremia, N Engl J Med 314:1535, 1986.
10. Ross EJ and Christie SBM: Hypernatremia, Medicine (Baltimore) 48:441, 1969.
11. Williams ME, Rosa RM, and Epstein FH: Hyperkalemia, Adv Intern Med 31:265, 1986.
12. Sopko JA and Freeman RM: Salt substitutes as a source of potassium, JAMA 238:608, 1977.
13. Ponce SP et al: Drug-induced hyperkalemia, Medicine (Baltimore) 64:357, 1985.
14. Battle DC, Arruda JAL, and Kurtzman NA: Hyperkalemic distal renal tubular acidosis associated with obstructive uropathy, N Engl J Med 304:373, 1981.
15. Tuck ML, Sambhi MP, and Levin L: Hyporeninemic hypoaldosteronism in diabetes mellitus, Diabetes 28:237, 1979.
16. Campbell AJ: Thyroid disorders in the elderly: difficulties in diagnosis and treatment, Drugs 31:455, 1986.
17. Harvard CWH: The thyroid and ageing, Clin Endocrinol Metab 10:163, 1981.
18. Hurley JR: Thyroid disease in the elderly, Med Clin North Am 67:497, 1983.
19. Thomas FB, Mazzatein EL, and Skillman TG: Apathetic thyrotoxicosis: a distinctive clinical and laboratory entity, Ann Intern Med 72:679, 1970.
20. Tibaldi JM et al: Thyrotoxicosis in the very old, Am J Med 81:619, 1986.
21. Senior RM and Birge SJ: The recognition and management of myxedema coma, JAMA 217:61, 1971.
22. Arieff AI and Carroll HJ: Nonketotic hyperosmolar coma with hyperglycemia: clinical features, pathophysiology, renal function, acid-base balance; plasma-cerebrospinal fluid equilibria and the effects of therapy in 37 cases, Medicine (Baltimore) 51:73, 1972.
23. Arieff AI and Carroll HJ: Cerebral edema and depression of sensorium in nonketotic hyperosmolar coma, Diabetes 23:525, 1974.
24. Carroll P and Matz R: Uncontrolled diabetes mellitus in adults: experience in treating diabetic ketoacidosis and hyperosmolar nonketotic coma with low-dose insulin and a uniform treatment regimen, Diabetes Care 6:579, 1983.
25. Gerich JE, Martin MM, and Recant L: Clinical and metabolic characteristics of hyperosmolar, nonketotic coma, Diabetes 20:228, 1971.
26. Gordon EE and Kabudi UM: The hyperglycemic hyperosmolar syndrome, Am J Med Sci 271:253, 1976.
27. Khardori R and Soler NG: Hyperosmolar hyperglycemic nonketotic syndrome, Am J Med 77:899, 1984.

SUGGESTED READINGS

Adrogue HJ and Madias NE: Changes in plasma potassium concentration during acute acid-base disturbances, Am J Med 71:456, 1981.
Arieff AI: Effects of water, acid-base, and electrolyte disorders on the central nervous system. In Arieff AI and DeFronzo RA, editors: Fluid, electrolyte, and acid-base disorders, New York, 1985, Churchill Livingstone.
Arieff AI, Llach F, and Massry SG: Neurologic manifestations and morbidity of hyponatremia: correlation with brain water and electrolytes, Medicine (Baltimore) 55:121, 1976.
Bagdade JD: Endocrine emergencies, Med Clin North Am 70(5):1111–1128, 1986.
Bennett MH and Wainwright AP: Acute thyroid crisis on induction of anaesthesia, Anaesthesia 44(1):28–30, 1989.
Bennett WR and Huston DP: Rhabdomyolysis in thyroid storm, Am J Med 77(4):733–735, 1984.
Berl T et al: Clinical disorders of water metabolism, Kidney Int 10:117, 1976.
Davis P and Davis F: Hyperthyroidism in patients over the age of 60 years, Medicine (Baltimore) 53:161, 1974.
DeFronzo RA: Hyperkalemia and hyporeninemic hypoaldosteronism, Kidney Int 17:118, 1980.
DeFronzo RA, Bia M, and Smith D: Clinical disorders of hyperkalemia, Annu Rev Med 33:521, 1982.
Evangelisti JT and Thorpe CJ: Thyroid storm—a nursing crisis, Heart Lung 12(2):184–193, 1983.
Fulop M and Hoberman HD: Alcoholic ketosis, Diabetes 24:785, 1975.
Gilliland PF: Endocrine emergencies: adrenal crisis, myxedema coma, and thyroid storm, Postgrad Med 74(5):215–220, 225–227, 1983.
Hamburger S and Rush D: Alcoholic ketoacidosis—a review of 30 cases, J Am Med Wom Assoc 37:106, 1973.
Harrington JT and Cohen JJ: Clinical disorders of urine concentration and dilution, Arch Intern Med 131:810, 1973.
Howton JC: Thyroid storm presenting as coma, Ann Emerg Med 17(4):343–345, 1988.
Knochel JP: Hypokalemia, Adv Intern Med 30:317, 1984.
Kreisberg RA: Diabetic ketoacidosis: new concepts and trends in pathogenesis and treatment, Ann Intern Med 88:681, 1978.
Nicoloff JT: Thyroid storm and myxedema coma, Med Clin North Am 69(5)1005–1017, 1985.
Reed J and Bradley EL III: Postoperative thyroid storm after lithium preparation, Surgery 98(5):983–986, 1985.
Rush DR and Hamburger SC: Endocrine metabolic emergencies, South Med J 77(2):220–226, 1984.
Sheehy SB: Metabolic and endocrine emergencies, JEN 11(1):49–52, 1985.
Smith JD, Bia MJ, and DeFronzo RA: Clinical disorders of potassium metabolism. In Arieff AI and DeFronzo RA, editors: Fluid, electrolyte and acid-base disorders, New York, 1985, Churchill Livingstone.

Hyperosmolar Hyperglycemic Nonketotic Coma (HHNK)

David Rush, Pharm.D., **and Stephen Hamburger,** M.D.

Pathogenesis

Pathophysiology

Diagnosis

   Clinical presentation

   Laboratory examination

Management

   Supportive therapy

   Fluid and electrolyte therapy

   Normalization of the intermediary metabolism

   Avoidance of complications

   Diagnosis and treatment of the precipitating event

The clinical syndrome of diabetes mellitus encompasses several medical emergencies, the most prominent of which are diabetic ketoacidosis (DKA) and hyperosmolar hyperglycemic nonketotic coma (HHNK).[1] HHNK has become a frequently recognized complication of diabetes mellitus. Although HHNK was initially described nearly a century ago, awareness of this syndrome has increased in recent years. Despite increased recognition of this syndrome, which is characterized by pronounced hyperglycemia, hyperosmolality, and dehydration in the absence of ketoacidosis, the mortality rate remains significantly higher than that of DKA even in patients of comparable age. Many fatalities are attributable to a delay in diagnosis and initiation of appropriate therapy.

PATHOGENESIS

Although pathogenetic mechanisms in the syndrome of HHNK have not been completely elucidated, interest in its pathogenesis has focused on the lack of significant ketosis and depressed sensorium. Ketone bodies are normally produced by the liver in proportion to the circulating levels of free fatty acids (FFA) that act as substrate. Several reports have revealed that the FFA levels in HHNK are either normal or less than those found in DKA, implying a defect in lipolysis. Lipolysis depends on many variables, including the circulating levels of insulin, growth hormone, and cortisol, all of which may modulate the release of FFA from adipose tissue. Although the circulating levels of insulin have been found to be similar in patients with HHNK and DKA, growth hormone and cortisol, lipolytic hormones, have been found to be significantly lower than in patients with DKA. These results suggest that in some patients with HHNK the low levels of FFA and lack of ketosis might reflect the lower activity of lipolytic hormones. Other mechanisms for the lack of ketosis in this syndrome have been postulated. It has been suggested that severe dehydration might be antiketogenic resulting in low plasma FFA levels and ketone production, while in vitro studies have revealed that hyperosmolality inhibits the release of pancreatic insulin to glucose and FFA production from adipose tissue. Depressed sensorium in HHNK is correlated with the plasma osmolality. Nearly stuporous or obtunded patients have a plasma osmolality of at least 350 mOsm/kg, whereas patients with a plasma osmolality of less than 350 mOsm/kg usually are more alert. Sensorium does not correlate with the glucose concentration or the pH of either cerebrospinal fluid or plasma.

PATHOPHYSIOLOGY

Metabolic abnormalities, including osmotic shifts and renal response mechanisms, determine therapeutic strategies in patients with HHNK (Figure 24–1). The fundamental derangements in HHNK include a relative lack of insulin and a relative excess of antiinsulin hormones including growth hormone, cortisol, and glucagon (Table 24–1). The net result of the interaction of these hormones

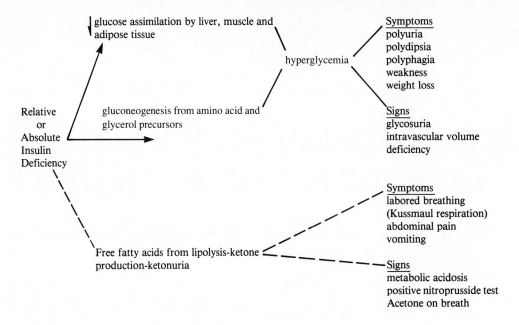

Figure 24–1 Pathophysiology of hyperosmolar, hyperglycemic nonketotic coma (HHNK). In HHNK the broken lines are suppressed.

is excessive production and underutilization of glucose, which results in pronounced hyperglycemia. Total body water generally represents about 60% of body weight with two thirds of water being intracellular and one third being extracellular. As the plasma glucose elevates, water moves from the intracellular fluid to the extracellular space until osmotic equilibrium is achieved. Thus pronounced hyperglycemia results in the loss of water from the intracellular fluid, which produces intracellular dehydration and concomitant albeit transient expansion of the extracellular fluid. These fluid and electrolyte shifts have diagnostic and therapeutic implications. As the plasma glucose rises, the renal threshold for glucose reabsorption is surpassed, resulting in glycosuria. Generally, the higher the glucose, the greater the renal excretion of glucose. Glycosuria causes an osmotic diuresis by inhibiting the reabsorption of water, which results in increased urine flow. With respect to loss of electrolytes, the osmotic diuresis in patients with HHNK is approximately 50 mEq sodium/L, while urinary potassium losses are about the same. The osmotic diuresis produces a water loss that is in excess of sodium losses, resulting in a hyperosmolar state and an intracellular

water depletion in most patients with HHNK. In addition, the loss of sodium leads to depletion of extracellular fluid volume. Much of the hyperglycemia in the patient with HHNK results, in part, from decreased renal excretion of glucose as well as decreased cellular uptake. As the extracellular fluid volume becomes depleted, the glomerular filtration rate decreases, thus dampening the normal renal escape mechanism for glucose.[2] Thus, a vicious cycle occurs:

1. The higher the plasma glucose, the more pronounced the depletion of extracellular volume.
2. The glomerular filtration decreases.
3. Less glucose is excreted in the urine.
4. The plasma glucose become more elevated.

A similar circumstance has been shown to occur in patients with DKA where much of the hyperglycemia is secondary to impaired excretion of renal glucose. In addition to the urinary loss of sodium, potassium, and water, other electrolytes including magnesium and phosphate have also been found to be depleted in patients with HHNK. In most instances, patients with HHNK have more pronounced volume depletion and higher plasma glucose levels than patients with DKA because of a longer duration of symptoms before therapy is initiated.

DIAGNOSIS

Clinical Presentation

HHNK occurs mainly in the elderly patient[3,4] with an average age of 60 years, although a case in a 9-month-old child has been reported.[5] The condition occurs with equal frequency in men and women. Prior to onset, many pa-

Table 24–1   Metabolic Effects of the Antiinsulin Hormones

	Insulin release	Muscle glucose uptake	Glucone- ogenesis	Lipolysis
Glucagon	↑	↓	↑	↑
Growth hormone	↑	↓		↑
Glucocorticoids	↑	↓	↑	↑

tients have no history of diabetes mellitus. Moreover, those with diabetes usually have been well controlled with diet or hypoglycemic agents. Although symptoms usually develop over a few days to a week unless an acute precipitating event is the cause, HHNK has occurred within several hours following peritoneal dialysis or major surgery. Symptoms reflect the osmotic diuresis and include polyuria, polydipsia, and occasionally polyphagia. Patients with HHNK generally have a longer history than do patients with diabetic ketoacidosis. Neurologic abnormalities are common. Unlike uncomplicated diabetic ketoacidosis, seizures are frequent in HHNK and occur in approximately 15% of patients. Focal signs characteristic of thromboembolic cerebral infarction are common as part of the initial presentation and frequently resolve with successful therapy. Indeed, in many cases, the admitting diagnosis is "cerebrovascular accident," which results in delay of the correct diagnosis and management of HHNK. Consequently, any comatose patient should have a screening test for glucose in blood and in urine so that delay in the diagnosis of HHNK is prevented. Not all patients with HHNK are comatose; half are either obtunded or stuporous, while a small percentage are alert.

INTERCURRENT ILLNESSES ASSOCIATED WITH HHNK

Infection, particularly pneumonia
Cardiovascular

- Myocardial infarction
- Cerebrovascular accident
- Gastrointestinal bleeding

Miscellaneous

- Pancreatitis
- Excessive carbohydrate intake
- Surgery
- Dialysis

DRUGS ASSOCIATED WITH HHNK

- Diuretics (particularly thiazides, chlorthalidone, furosemide)
- Glucocorticoid steroids
- Propranolol
- Immunosuppressive agents
- Dilantin (phenytoin)
- Diazoxide

CLINICAL FEATURES OF HHNK

- Average age is approximately 60 years old

- Equal frequency in men and women

- Majority of patients have no history of mild adult-onset diabetes mellitus

- Majority of patients have intercurrent illness

- Many patients have been on diabetogenic drugs

- Symptoms of polyuria, polydipsia, and polyphagia reflect osmotic diuresis

- Physical examination shows evidence of marked volume depletion and mental obtundation

---

Laboratory Examination

The diagnosis of HHNK is easily made once the syndrome is considered. No rigid criteria have been set but a laboratory diagnosis may be defined as:

1. Glycosuria of 3+ or 4+ without ketonuria
2. Extreme hyperglycemia usually greater than 600 mg/100 mL
3. Negative or minimally positive nitroprusside test (Acetest) (i.e., no greater than 2+ reaction when plasma is diluted 1:1 with water)
4. Serum osmolality greater than 350 mOsm/kg

In the absence of an osmometer, the approximate plasma osmolality may be calculated by using the formula:

$$\text{Osmolality (normal} = 285 - 300 \text{ mOsm)}$$

$$= 2\,[\text{serum Na}^+] + \frac{\text{blood glucose}}{18} + \frac{\text{blood urea nitrogen (BUN)}}{2.8}$$

In any given series, the individual values for blood glucose and plasma osmolality vary widely. In one large series, the mean blood glucose was 1166 mg/100 mL (standard deviation ± 306), and the mean plasma osmolality was 384 mOsm/kg H_2O (standard deviation ± 27).

Initial studies should include a complete blood count, electrolytes, blood urea nitrogen, creatinine, urinalysis, and arterial blood gases. Interpretation of the serum sodium must take into account the "pseudohyponatremia" induced by hyperglycemia; for every 100 mg elevation of glucose above 100, the serum sodium is reduced by

---

Physical examination usually reveals extensive evidence of extracellular fluid volume depletion. Relative or absolute hypotension and tachycardia are present in the majority of patients. Skin turgor is usually poor, but the value of this sign is difficult to assess in elderly patients. Many individuals also have a precipitating illness such as gastroenteritis or myocardial infarction. In addition, the use of certain drugs (e.g., thiazide diuretics, diphenylhydantoin, and glucocorticoid steroids)[6] has been associated with the onset of HHNK. Hospital procedures such as peritoneal dialysis or hemodialysis, hyperalimentation, and the use of mannitol have also produced HHNK.[5,7,8]

LABORATORY FINDINGS IN HHNK

- Glucose usually greater than 600 mg/100 mL
- Osmolality greater than 350 mOsm/kg
- Nitroprusside test usually negative
- Serum sodium usually normal to elevated
- Serum potassium normal to low
- BUN and creatinine and BUN/creatinine usually elevated

1.6 mEq/L. Knowledge of this relationship is important in determining the water deficit in such a patient. Elevated triglyceride levels might result in factitious hyponatremia. A normal or increased plasma osmolality coupled with a low serum sodium suggests this possibility. Many of the initial studies reflect marked intravascular dehydration. The hemoglobin and hematocrit are commonly elevated and return to normal with adequate fluid replacement. The BUN and creatinine are characteristically elevated as in the BUN/creatinine ratio (normally 10 to 1). With adequate treatment, the BUN and creatinine will return toward normal.

Many patients, even after successful therapy, will have residual impairment of kidney functions. Patients with HHNK have a total body depletion of potassium that is secondary to the osmotic losses in the urine and gastrointestinal tract. Unlike patients with diabetic ketoacidosis, patients with HHNK are uncommonly hyperkalemic. In one series, approximately 12% of patients with HHNK had hyperkalemia initially, whereas almost 30% had initial potassium levels below 4.0 mEq/L. In a series of patients studied by Arieff and Carroll, the mean initial values for BUN, creatinine, serum sodium, and potassium were 95 mg/100 mL, 5.6 mg/100 mL, 144 mEq/L, and 5.0 mEq/L respectively. The "normal" serum sodium, in spite of extreme hyperglycemia, reflects the tremendous loss of body water that occurs in patients with HHNK.

Metabolic acidosis is not infrequent in this syndrome and, as defined by a serum bicarbonate level of less than 21 mEq/L or an arterial pH of 7.35 or less, occurs in 40 to 60% of the patients. Slight lactate elevations are frequent but do not account for the majority of cases of metabolic acidosis. Renal failure accounted for several.[9] The cause for the metabolic acidosis is unknown in the majority of cases in HHNK, and, in most patients, it is probably multifactorial. A baseline electrocardiogram should always be obtained to identify a painless myocardial infarction. Appropriate bacterial stains and cultures should be done to rule out an infection.

MANAGEMENT

Supportive Therapy

The correction of HHNK encompasses four areas:

1. Replacement of fluid and electrolyte deficits
2. Normalization of the intermediary metabolism
3. Avoidance of complications
4. Diagnosis and treatment of the precipitating event

All patients should have a complete and up-to-date flow sheet (Figure 24–2), which will eliminate uncertainty about previous therapy and will indicate how the patient responds to various treatment modalities. If possible, central venous pressure lines and urinary catheters should be avoided to minimize the risk of a superimposed infection. If necessary, however, a Swan-Ganz catheter is preferred to a central venous pressure line. Gastric aspiration is useful for persistent vomiting or gastric atony. If the patient is unconscious, a cuffed endotracheal tube will help avoid aspiration pneumonia.

Fluid and Electrolyte Therapy

Fluid therapy in patients with HHNK is controversial. Most authors recommend normal saline while others prefer replacement with 50% normal saline, providing the patient is not clinically hypotensive or oliguric. Initial therapy is best determined by the clinical presentation of the individual patient. Regardless of the treatment chosen, careful monitoring is required to determine progress and changes in fluid replacement. Total body water loss in patients with HHNK has been estimated to average 24% with approximately 50 mEq/L of sodium and potassium lost from osmotic diuresis. These losses reflect an average 8 mEq/kg and 6 mEq/kg, respectively. Thus, most patients who presented with HHNK have marked clinical evidence of sodium depletion (relative or absolute hypotension, tachycardia, oliguria, and poor skin turgor), and require rapid correction of the sodium deficit with normal saline. Each patient is an individual, and the amount of normal saline required will differ. Most individuals with HHNK are elderly; as a result, sodium overload must be carefully avoided. Those patients who, upon initial presentation, do not have evidence of sodium depletion may be treated with 50%

Time	CLINICAL PARAMETERS				LABORATORY PARAMETERS						TREATMENT PARAMETERS		
					Blood					*Urine*	*Fluids*		*Insulin*
	Blood Pressure	Pulse	Urine Output	Physical Exam	Na⁺ / Cl⁻	K⁺ / CO₂⁻	pH / HCO₃⁻	BUN / Glucose		Glucose / Ketones	Type / Volume		Type/Dose/Route

Figure 24–2   Sample flow sheet for hyperosmolar hyperglycemic nonketotic coma.

normal saline. If this is done, careful and continuous monitoring of intravascular volume is necessary. Replacement with hypotonic fluids, along with simultaneous lowering of the plasma glucose by insulin, may induce hypotension and oliguria due to the movement of water from the extracellular to the intracellular space. Replacement of sodium deficit with normal saline results in a slower drop in the plasma osmolality. The average loss of water is approximately 75 to 100 mL/kg of body weight. The free water deficit may be calculated by the following formula:

$$H_2O \text{ deficit} = 0.6 \times BW_{kg} \left(1 - \frac{140}{[Na_{obs}]}\right)$$

Although several assumptions are made in this formula, it is adequate for the initiation of treatment. It is important to realize that the above formula does not take into account the ongoing urinary and nonurinary losses of fluid and electrolytes. Thus, replacement of free water must accommodate losses that have already taken place. Generally, replacement of the water deficit is accomplished by D_5 50% normal saline or 5% dextrose as the plasma glucose approaches 250 mg/100 mL. As the patient becomes more alert, water may be taken by mouth. Too rapid correction of the water deficit may result in water intoxication with cerebral edema. Moreover, extreme caution is advisable in those patients who present with a low plasma osmolality because removal of the osmotic effect of glucose by insulin therapy or use of hypotonic fluids may also cause water intoxication.

Total body potassium losses are probably higher in HHNK than in diabetic ketoacidosis; thus, the mean initial potassium in HHNK is lower. Potassium replacement, with the chloride or phosphate salt, is generally indicated as part of initial treatment. Contraindications to early potassium replacement include electrocardiographic evidence of hyperkalemia, known hyperkalemia, and probably oliguria. Careful monitoring of the potassium levels is required because electrocardiographic evidence of hyperkalemia is nonspecific.

Normalization of the Intermediary Metabolism

There has been a shift to the use of low-dose insulin therapy in the treatment of HHNK. The main goal of insulin therapy is to return carbohydrate metabolism to normal. Hyperglycemia in HHNK reflects three conditions:

1. Underexcretion of glucose by the kidney
2. Overproduction of hepatic glucose
3. Peripheral underutilization of glucose

Studies have shown that circulating insulin levels of approximately 200 mU/mL are sufficient to inhibit gluconeogenesis and to produce almost maximal glucose uptake by adipose tissue and muscle. This concentration of insulin may be achieved by intramuscular or intravenous administration. An initial injection of 20 units of regular insulin followed by 10 units per hour, given into the deltoid muscle, will result in a sufficient circulating level to reverse HHNK and cause a predictable fall in plasma glucose (approximately 80 to 100 mg of glucose per hour assuming adequate volume repletion). Satisfactory results have been shown in the treatment of HHNK with an intravenous loading dose of 5 to 10 units of regular insulin followed by a continuous infusion of 7 to 12 units per hour. Benefits of low-dose insulin include less hypokalemia, decreased incidence of delayed hypoglycemia, and less empiric dosing. Use of subcutaneous insulin is discouraged as this route depends heavily on the adequacy of intravascular volume. If there is any doubt about the practicality of the use of continuous infusion of insulin in a given hospital, the intramuscular route is the treatment of choice. It is important to realize that no matter how the insulin is given, it is only part of the total management of the patient with HHNK.

Avoidance of Complications

Although there are many potential fatal complications of HHNK, two are of importance and deserve mention:

1. Cerebral edema
2. Vascular thrombosis

Cerebral Edema

While cerebral edema is uncommon, it is a potentially fatal complication of HHNK. This complication should be suspected when clinical and biochemical improvement is followed by deterioration in cerebral function. Elevation of the intraocular or cerebrospinal fluid pressure (with or without papilledema) strongly suggests this possibility. Although no treatment is of proven benefit, hypotonic solutions should be stopped and hypertonic saline or mannitol begun in hope of reversing the process. In studies in animals with diabetic ketoacidosis, cerebral edema is uncommon when the plasma is not lowered rapidly to below 250 mg/100 mL.

Vascular Thrombosis

In several series of patients with HHNK, a high frequency of vascular occlusions has been noted. In many, the occlusions involve the mesenteric arteries and are overlooked clinically. Whether the occlusions precipitate the HHNK or are a complication of it (possibly secondary to extreme dehydration) is not known. Arterial thrombi may be a complication of the HHNK since they tend to become evident hours or days after the onset of the coma. Irrespective of cause or effect, vascular occlusions occur in a high frequency of patients with HHNK, and prompt recognition is extremely important.

Diagnosis and Treatment of the Precipitating Event

Approximately one half of patients with HHNK have a severe concurrent illness. In many, this is an infection, with bronchopneumonia being especially common. Some will have more than one complicating illness. Moreover, patients with HHNK may develop complications during therapy. These may be related to age or to the comatose state. Since many deaths are due to complications, it is crucial that these be recognized early and treated vigorously.

REFERENCES

1. Braaten JT: Hyperosmolar nonketotic diabetic coma: diagnosis and management, Geriatrics 42(11):83–88, 1987.
2. Butts DE: Fluid and electrolyte disorders associated with diabetic ketoacidosis and hyperglycemic hyperosmolar nonketotic coma, Nurs Clin North Am 22(4):827–836, 1987.
3. Kitabchi AE and Murphy MG: Diabetic ketoacidosis and hyperosmolar hyperglycemic nonketotic coma, Med Clin North Am 72(6):1545–1563, 1988.
4. Malone JK et al: The hyperglycemic hyperosmolar syndrome, Indiana Med 81(9):766–768, 1988.
5. Emder PJ, Howard NJ, and Rosenberg AR: Non-ketotic hyperosmolar diabetic pre-coma due to pancreatitis in a boy on continuous ambulatory peritoneal dialysis, Nephron 44(4):355–357, 1986.
6. Fujikawa LS, Meisler DM, and Nozik RA: Hyperosmolar hyperglycemia nonketotic coma: a complication of short-term systemic corticosteroid use, Ophthalmology 90(10):1239–1242, 1983.
7. Sypniewski E Jr, Mirtallo JM, and Schneider PJ: Hyperosmolar, hyperglycemic, nonketotic coma in a patient receiving home total parenteral nutrient therapy, Clin Pharm 6(1):69–73, 1987.
8. Seki S: Clinical features of hyperosmolar hyperglycemic nonketotic diabetic coma associated with cardiac operations, J Thorac Cardiovasc Surg 91(6):867–873, 1986.
9. Wood ML et al: Fetal rhabdomyolysis associated with hyperosmolar diabetic decompensation, Diabetes Res 8(2):97–99, 1988.

Myxedema Coma

David Rush, Pharm.D., and Stephen Hamburger, M.D.

GENERAL CONSIDERATIONS

The state of profoundly reduced metabolism due to thyroid deficiency is associated with a high mortality rate and is a medical emergency. Hypothyroidism is highly variable in its clinical presentation, and, not uncommonly, symptoms may be so mild that patients are normally active. Myxedema coma, the most serious manifestation of hypothyroidism, has a mortality rate that approaches 50%, despite institution of appropriate therapy.[1-3] Intercurrent illness accounts for much of this poor prognosis, and most cases with significant morbidity and mortality occur in the debilitated elderly patient who is oversedated and exposed to cold.[4-6] Frequently, medical personnel may fail to recognize the steady deterioration of a patient in whom thyroid replacement has been suspended. Finally, prolonged and unexplained unconsciousness after general anesthesia may be the first indication of severe thyroid deficiency in an elderly patient.

ETIOLOGY

Myxedema coma may be primary from thyroid disease, secondary from pituitary disease, or tertiary from disorders of the hypothalamus[7] (Table 25–1). Most cases of myxedema coma occur either in patients with long-standing autoimmune disease of the thyroid or in patients rendered hypothyroid by surgical or radioiodine therapy for Graves' disease. Approximately 4% of patients with hypothyroidism will have pituitary insufficiency as the cause of their hormone deficiency. Recognition of secondary or tertiary hypothyroidism may play a crucial role in the management of myxedema coma. Intrinsic thyroid disease includes destruction of the gland from an autoimmune process (Hashimoto's thyroiditis), an inherited enzymatic defect in hormone biosynthesis, administration of goitrogenic drugs, or administration of iodide to an individual with a defect in organic binding of iodide. The most common causes of hypothyroidism are autoimmune destruction of the gland or radioactive therapy for Graves' disease.

CHARACTERISTICS OF MYXEDEMA COMA

- Majority of patients are women
- Majority of patients are elderly
- Majority of cases occur in winter months
- Majority of cases occur after hospitalization
- Majority of cases are associated with stressful events or intercurrent illness

---

Patients with myxedema coma are usually elderly females[3,4] who have a long-standing history of hypothyroidism. The condition is more frequent in winter months with the majority of cases being associated with a stressful event or intercurrent illness, especially infection. In one review, almost 80% of the patients were female with half between the ages of 61 and 70 years, and over 90% of cases occurred in the winter months. Of note is that many cases of myxedema coma occur in patients hospitalized for other conditions. Use of certain drugs such as general anesthetics, phenothiazines, narcotics, and tranquilizers has been implicated in the production of myxedema coma in such patients. Excessive intake of free water resulting in hyponatremia may also play a role in the onset of the coma.[8]

Table 25–1 Etiology of Hypothyroidism

Thyroid insufficiency (primary)	Pituitary or hypothalamic insufficiency (secondary or tertiary)
Idiopathic	Tumors
Autoimmune (Hashimoto's thyroiditis)	Infiltrative disease (sarcoidosis)
Radioactive iodine therapy of Graves' disease	
Surgical therapy of Graves' disease	
Congenital enzymatic defect in thyroid hormone biosynthesis	

COMMON INTERCURRENT ILLNESSES IN MYXEDEMA COMA

- Infection
- Anemia
- Heart failure
- Ascites
- Pleural and pericardial effusions
- Seizures
- Aspiration
- Inappropriate drug therapy (dosage or frequency)

DIAGNOSIS

Clinical Presentation

Myxedema coma is a systemic disorder. In many patients, symptoms of hypothyroidism are present for several years and are vague in onset. Earliest complaints usually include fatigue, weakness, muscle cramps, and intolerance to cold. (See Table 25–2.) Paresthesias, weight gain, menstrual disturbances, constipation, hoarseness,[9a] hearing disturbances, and personality changes are also clinical aspects of fully developed hypothyroidism. These symptoms, along with a family history of previous thyroid disease or use of radioactive iodide for hyperthyroidism, strongly suggest the diagnosis. It is not uncommon to obtain a history of discontinuation of thyroid hormone therapy. Neurologic symptoms are common in myxedema coma; 25 to 50% of patients will develop grand mal seizures. Patients may even have, paradoxically, frank psychotic symptoms termed "myxedema madness."[9]

Table 25–2 Clinical Symptoms and Signs of Hypothyroidism

Symptoms	Signs
Cold intolerance	Sparse body hair
Fatigue	Puffy eyelids
Weakness	Dry skin
Weight gain	Yellow tinge to skin
Constipation	Pallor
Hoarseness	Large tongue
Muscle cramps	Delayed deep tendon reflex

With respect to the physical examination, hypothermia is frequent as is a systolic blood pressure of less than 100 mm Hg. Bradycardia is common. The patient is usually an elderly, obese female with yellowish dry skin and hyperkeratosis around the elbow and knees. Ecchymoses may be secondary to a diminished platelet count and increased capillary fragility. An enlarged tongue, puffy eyes, and scant body hair, particularly on the scalp and eyelids, are common. Thyromegaly is uncommon, but a surgical scar on the neck is frequent. The thorax may reveal an underlying pneumonitis or pleural effusion.[10] Cardiomegaly is frequent and is secondary to a pericardial effusion in approximately one third of patients. Abdominal distention caused by ascites,[11] paralytic ileus, or urinary retention is not uncommon. Fecal impaction is frequent. Most patients are comatose and deep tendon reflexes are markedly delayed. Differentiation of primary versus secondary or tertiary hypothyroidism is clinically difficult. Clues to this distinction are listed in Table 25–3.

Although few patients with hypothyroidism develop myxedema coma, all patients with this condition are hypothyroid. Myxedema coma does not occur without a relative or absolute deficiency of thyroid hormone, although there has been a recent case report of a patient in whom the serum thyroxine level was normal. Whether or not thyroid hormone deficiency alone may result in myxedema coma has been debated. Although this has been suggested, most patients also experience a stressful event[15,16] or intercurrent illness concurrent with the onset of myxedema coma. The following pathophysiologic derangements are commonly seen:

- Hypothermia
- CO_2 narcosis
- Hyponatremia
- Hypoglycemia
- Hypotension
- Intercurrent illness

Table 25–3 Differential Clues of Primary Versus Secondary or Tertiary Hypothyroidism

Primary (thyroid disease)	Secondary (pituitary) or tertiary (hypothalamic disease)
More common	Symptoms of increased
History of thyroid operation	intracranial pressure
Family history of thyroid disease	(headache, nausea, vomiting)
No evidence of other hormone deficiencies	Visual field defects
Surgical scar on neck	Evidence of other hormone deficiencies
Sella turcica normal	Sella turcica abnormal
Thyroid antibodies positive in autoimmune thyroiditis	Serum TSH normal or low
Serum TSH increased	

Hypothermia

Hypothermia is found in approximately 80% of fully developed cases of myxedema coma. It is probably the result of a decrease in the basal metabolic rate and production of thermal energy. It is so frequent that a normal temperature should suggest a complicating infectious process.

CO_2 Narcosis

The importance of CO_2 retention in the pathogenesis of myxedema coma was described in 1960. In a group of 26 patients with hypothyroidism, Wilson and Bedell found reductions in maximum voluntary ventilation, carbon monoxide diffusing capacity, and ventilatory responses to breathing carbon dioxide. In addition, the obese members of this group had small vital capacities and abnormally low maximal airflow rates. Varying degrees of hypercapnia were found. However, some of the patients' pulmonary function studies had returned to normal after thyroid hormone replacement. The cause of the pulmonary disturbance in myxedema coma is multifactorial.[9a] It has been shown that the patency of the airway may be negatively affected by extreme swelling of the tongue causing respiratory embarrassment. Myxedematous infiltration of the respiratory muscles with a resultant restrictive pattern of pulmonary function is thought to be contributory to the hypoxemia and hypercapnia. Obesity is known to worsen this type of respiratory problem. Also, the interaction of hypothyroidism and low pulmonary surfactant levels might play a causal role in pulmonary dysfunction. Abnormal response to carbon dioxide inhalation indicates an abnormality in central respiratory regulation in myxedema coma. Lastly, the effect of pleural effusions, ascites, paralytic ileus, and intercurrent pulmonary infection may contribute to the dysfunction seen in myxedema coma. It is of crucial importance to realize that individuals with hypothyroid problems are most sensitive to the respiratory depressive effects of certain drugs, including the phenothiazines, narcotics, and general anesthetics. Doses should be reduced, and dosing intervals may need to be prolonged because of delayed absorption and slowed metabolism and excretion. The dose of morphine should routinely be decreased one third to one half the normal analgesic dose; the respiratory rate should be closely monitored. Because patients with myxedema coma may have abnormal pulmonary function, baseline arterial blood gases should be obtained at the onset of therapy; the effect of hypothermia on arterial blood gases should be taken into account. For each decrease of $1°C$, arterial pH rises by 0.015, while P_{CO_2} (mm Hg) decreases by 4.4% and P_{O_2} (mm Hg) decreases by 7.2%. The percent change is in reference to the value measured at standard $37°C$.

Hyponatremia

Although the total body sodium space is expanded, hyponatremia is a frequent finding in myxedema coma. Several observations have led to the conclusion that this is dilutional and secondary to the impairment of water excretion. Patients with myxedema coma have been shown to have a marked reduction in the excretion of free water loads. A phenomenon such as this might be explained by the inappropriate secretion of an antidiuretic hormone. In rare instances, cortisol deficiency might contribute to the hyponatremic state. Decreased water delivery to the distal diluting segment of the nephron has also been thought to contribute to the hyponatremia. Pseudohyponatremia may also occur in myxedema coma secondary to the frequent elevation of the plasma triglycerides. Patients with pseudohyponatremia should have a normal plasma osmolality, however, compared to the low plasma osmolality seen in true hyponatremia. Whatever the mechanism, coma and seizures may occur secondary to a low serum sodium, especially at levels below 110 to 115 mEq/L. Thyroid hormone replacement is needed for full correction of the hyponatremic state.

Hypoglycemia

Hypoglycemia is uncommon in myxedema coma unless the deficiency of thyroid hormone is secondary to a pituitary or hypothalamic defect. In this circumstance, adrenal insufficiency may coexist. Intravenous glucose solutions are indicated in the treatment of myxedema coma; however, excessive free water can worsen a preexisting hyponatremia. Caution must be used with glucose replacement in hypoglycemia.

Hypotension

Severe myxedema coma is frequently associated with marked hypotension. Most of these patients will respond to thyroid hormone therapy; others will respond to adequate volume expansion with saline-containing solutions. If still hypotensive, vasopressor therapy may be necessary. Due to their synergistic effects on the myocardium, caution must be exercised in the concomitant use of vasopressor and thyroid hormone therapy. Cardiovascular monitoring during treatment is mandatory.

Intercurrent Illness

Thyroid hormone deficiency in the absence of associated stress or intercurrent illness is an uncommon cause of myxedema coma. Most patients have an intercurrent illness with infection being the most frequent. Infection accelerates the metabolic disposal and fractional clearance of both thyroxine and triiodothyronine. During acute infections, the thyroid may have a lag period in its compensatory response to these changes in hormone levels.

Thus, the increased hormone utilization and decreased hormone production incline the patient toward myxedema coma.

Laboratory Examination

The patient in whom hypothyroidism is suspected may have a number of electrolyte or radiographic abnormalities. A determination of serum electrolytes, glucose and blood urea nitrogen (BUN), a complete blood count (CBC), as well as serum thyroxine (T_4), triiodothyronine (T_3), T_3 resin uptake ratio, and thyrotropin (TSH) should be made prior to initiation of therapy. Urinary electrolytes and urinary osmolality may be helpful when hyponatremia is present, while an electrocardiograph (ECG) and chest x-ray should be obtained in all suspected cases of myxedema coma.

Laboratory procedures may be divided into diagnostic and corroborative tests (Table 25–4).

Diagnostic Tests

Tests of diagnostic nature include T_4 and serum triiodothyronine (T_3) levels. The T_3 resin uptake ratio should be obtained to identify potential thyroxine-binding protein abnormalities. Thyroid antibodies should be determined. These are most prevalent and highest in Hashimoto's (autoimmune) thyroiditis. The determination of serum TSH is crucial as it will be elevated in primary hypothyroidism and inappropriately normal or low in pituitary (secondary) or hypothalamic (tertiary) hypothyroidism. Thyroid scans and uptake have no role in the diagnosis of myxedema coma.

Corroborative Tests

Corroborative tests are used to assess the impact of thyroid hormone deficiency on organ system function. For example, the electrocardiogram in myxedema coma classically shows sinus bradycardia, low voltage, diffuse T-wave changes, and a prolonged Q-T interval. The chest x-ray frequently reveals cardiomegaly and a pleural or pericardial effusion. Effusions in myxedema coma usually are transudates. Anemia occurs in approximately half of the patients and is ordinarily normochromic normocytic. Occasionally, patients will have an iron deficiency anemia or be deficient in folate or B_{12}. Leukocytosis is frequently absent in spite of a stressful event or intercurrent illness. Muscle enzymes such as creatinine phosphokinase (CPK), oxaloacetic transaminase (SGOT), and lactic dehydrogenase (LDH) are frequently elevated. Isoenzymatic patterns usually reveal these enzymes to be skeletal in origin and not from myocardial muscle. Replacement with thyroid hormone rapidly restores normal enzyme levels. The cholesterol and triglyceride concentrations usually are elevated due to delayed catabolism. Plasma glucose is normal in the majority of patients; if it is low, however, pituitary, hypothalamic, or primary adrenal insufficiency is suggested. Hyponatremia is a frequent finding. Occasionally, this is secondary to the elevated triglyceride concentration, which is termed "factitious hyponatremia or pseudo-hyponatremia." Serum carotene levels, which cause the yellowing of the skin, are raised. Hypoxemia, hypercapnia, and respiratory acidosis are common findings on arterial blood gas measurement. Cerebrospinal fluid protein and pressure may be markedly elevated. Serum cortisol levels usually are normal, but a normal level might be "inappropriately" low in the stressful state. The production of cortisol and its peripheral degradation are decreased in myxedema coma. Urinary metabolites of cortisol are reduced. Skull x-rays occasionally show an enlarged or eroded sella turcica.

MANAGEMENT

Treatment for myxedema coma may be divided into that of the complicating illness and that of the thyroid hormone deficiency. It is important to realize that therapy must be initiated on the basis of clinical judgment.

MAJOR COMPLICATIONS IN MYXEDEMA COMA
- Hypothermia
- Respiratory acidosis
- Hyponatremia
- Hypoglycemia
- Hypotension

Supportive Therapy

Hypothermia

Measures must be taken to ensure heat preservation by passive methods (i.e., external rewarming with blankets). Active rewarming of hypothermic patients is potentially dangerous; peripheral vasodilation, circulation collapse, and death have occurred. Thyroid hormone replacement will slowly return the body temperature to normal.

Table 25–4   Laboratory Tests in Myxedema Coma

Diagnostic tests	Corroborative tests
• Serum T_4, T_3	• ECG
• T_3 resin uptake	• Chest x-ray, skull films
• Thyroid antibodies	• Arterial blood gases
• Serum TSH	• CBC
	• SGOT, CPK, LDH
	• Cholesterol, triglycerides
	• Glucose
	• Electrolytes
	• Cortisol

CO_2 Narcosis

Measurement of arterial blood gases is compulsory in patients with myxedema coma. Hypoxemia, hypercapnia, and respiratory acidosis will often be found. Oxygen supplementation and assisted ventilation are frequently needed, the latter often for long periods.

Hyponatremia

Hyponatremia usually responds to thyroid hormone replacement and water restriction. Severe hyponatremia (below 110 mEq/L) or hyponatremia associated with seizures, however, requires the judicious administration of hypertonic saline with or without furosemide therapy. Therapy may be discontinued with alleviation of hyponatremia-related symptoms or a serum of approximately 120 mEq/L. Since hypertonic saline is associated with congestive heart failure and furosemide therapy with decreased serum potassium levels, the patient and laboratory (i.e., urinary and serum electrolyte parameters) should be carefully monitored.[12]

Hypoglycemia

Glucose in intravenous fluids is recommended. Glucocorticoids are also helpful. Hydrocortisone, 300 mg per day in a continuous intravenous drip, should be adequate. Hypothalamic-pituitary-adrenal abnormalities in myxedema coma may last several weeks after thyroid hormone therapy is begun.

Hypotension

About half of patients in myxedema coma will be relatively hypotensive or in shock. Thyroid hormone replacement generally corrects the hypotensive state and, if not, cautious volume expansion will help. Vasopressor therapy must be administered with extreme caution since patients with myxedema coma are relatively unresponsive to such agents until adequate circulating levels of thyroid hormone are available. Simultaneous administration of pressor agents and thyroid hormones has been associated with myocardial irritability, and, as a result, cardiac monitoring is necessary.

Intercurrent Illness

Since most of the morbidity and mortality in myxedema coma is associated with the intercurrent illness and not thyroid hormone deficiency, it is critical to search for an underlying precipitating disease. Infection, particularly pulmonary, is the most common. Many signs of infection, such as fever, tachycardia, and leukocytosis, are masked in myxedema coma. A normal temperature is inappropriately high and should suggest an underlying infection.

TREATMENT OF COMPLICATING ILLNESSES OF MYXEDEMA COMA

Intercurrent Illness

1. Search vigorously for a clinically suppressed infection, realizing that a normal temperature in myxedema coma is inappropriately high.
2. Carefully search for other intercurrent illness associated with myxedema coma.

Hypothermia

1. Avoid external heat sources.
2. Cover with blankets.

Respiratory Acidosis

1. Monitor arterial blood gases.
2. Use respiratory support system if necessary.

Hyponatremia

1. Free water restriction usually sufficient.
2. If clinically needed, saline with the administration of furosemide.

Hypoglycemia

1. Use glucose in parenterally administered solutions.
2. Administer hydrocortisone sodium succinate (Solu-Cortef), 300 mg per day.

Hypotension

1. Usually responds to thyroid hormone replacement.
2. If needed, use vasopressor agents. Monitor cardiovascular system closely.

Thyroid Hormone Replacement

1. L-Thyroxine (T_4), 400 μg intravenously as a single dose, followed by 50 to 100 μg intravenously or 100 to 200 μg orally each day.
2. Triiodothyronine, 12.5 μg by nasogastric tube every 8 hours.

Thyroid Hormone Replacement

Because of few controlled studies, the best method of thyroid replacement remains controversial. While older literature emphasizes the advantages of T_3 (Cytomel) replacement, more recent reviews direct attention to T_4 (Synthroid) replacement. Much of the latter is attributable to the newer understanding of the sources of thyroid hormones in the blood. Although T_4 is secreted by the thyroid gland, approximately 50 to 80% of T_3 comes from the peripheral monodeiodination of T_4 to T_3. In addition, views on dosing patterns and route of administration remain clouded.[13,14]

Proponents of T_3 replacement therapy in myxedema coma cite its heightened metabolic activity, rapid onset of action, and short half-life. T_3 activity usually begins in 6 hours with a serum half-life of one day. Intravenous preparations of T_3 are not available commercially, so T_3 is usually given by nasogastric tube. Optimal dosage is not known; dosage ranges from 10 µg every 12 hours to 100 µg every 6 hours. A reasonable dose of T_3 is 12.5 µg every 8 hours. T_3 therapy has been complicated by angina, myocardial infarction, and cardiac irritability, especially when the agent is given intravenously.[13,14]

Recent studies have advocated the use of T_4 replacement because of its smoother effect and longer activity and because a portion is monodeiodinated to T_3 in the peripheral tissues. Studies have shown that approximately 500 to 700 µg of T_4 is required to restore a patient in myxedema coma to a low-normal euthyroid state.

The preferred route of administration is intravenous since oral and intramuscular absorption is variable. A single dose of 400 µg of intravenous T_4 followed by 50 to 100 µg intravenously or 100 to 200 µg orally each day seems to be an acceptable regimen. The initial dose may be decreased depending on the presence of restrictive factors such as cardiac disease. In a patient with angina or arrhythmias, the initial dose may be decreased to 300 µg intravenously. Although not as rapid as T_3, the activity of T_4 is not unreasonably delayed and cardiac toxicity is probably less. With this regimen, TSH levels begin to fall in 24 hours and usually will return to normal in 7 to 10 days. T_4 levels reach the normal range in 1 to 2 days.

REFERENCES

1. Bastenie PA, Bonnyns M, and Vanhaelst L: Natural history of primary myxedema, Am J Med 78(1)91–100, 1985.
2. Forester CF: Coma in myxedema, Arch Intern Med 3:734, 1963.
3. Gilliland PF: Endocrine emergencies: adrenal crisis, myxedema coma, and thyroid storm, Postgrad Med 74(5):215–220, 225–227, 1983.
4. McConahey WM: Diagnosing and treating myxedema and myxedema coma, Geriatrics 33:61, 1978.
5. Payne NR: Emergency care of the patient with myxedema coma, JEN 12(6):343–347, 1986.
6. Senior RM et al: The recognition and management of myxedema coma, JAMA 217:61, 1971.
7. Perlmutter M and Cohn H: Myxedema crisis of pituitary or thyroid origin, Am J Med 36:883, 1964.
8. Sterling FH, Richter JS, and Gianpetro AM: Inappropriate antidiuretic hormone secretion and myxedema: hazards in management, Am J Med Sci 253:697, 1067.
9. Nicoloff JT: Thyroid storm and myxedema coma, Med Clin North Am 69:1005–1017, 1985.
9a. Stahl N and Leiberman A: Acute upper airway obstruction due to myxedema and upper airway abnormalities, J Laryngol Otol 102:733–734, 1988.
10. Wilson WE and Bedell GM: The pulmonary abnormalities in myxedema, J Clin Invest 39:42, 1960.
11. Kinney EL, Wright RJ, and Caldwell JW: Value of clinical features for distinguishing myxedema ascites from other forms of ascites, Comput Biol Med 19(1):55–59, 1989.
12. Hantman D et al: Rapid correction of hyponatremia in the syndrome of inappropriate secretion of antidiuretic hormone: an alternative treatment to hypertonic saline, Ann Intern Med 78:870, 1973.
13. Holvey DN et al: Treatment of myxedema coma with intravenous thyroxine, Arch Intern Med 113:89, 1964.
14. Ridgway EC et al: Acute metabolic responses in myxedema to large doses of intravenous L-thyroxine, Ann Intern Med 77:549, 1972.
15. Kirk SJ, O'Kane HO, and Morton P: Coronary artery surgery and myxoedema, Br Heat J 58(6):674–675, 1987.
16. Nee PA et al: Hypothermic myxedema coma erroneously diagnosed as myocardial infarction because of increased creatine kinase MB, Clin Chem 33:1083–1084, 1987.

Hyponatremia and Hypernatremia

David Rush, Pharm.D., and Stephen Hamburger, M.D.

HYPONATREMIA

Disorders involving alteration of body sodium content or the sodium concentration in body fluids are common in the practice of geriatric medicine. The clinical picture is usually nonspecific and requires collaboration with laboratory findings. Clinical assessment of extracellular fluid volume, measurement of both serum and urine sodium, and osmolality is essential for diagnosis.

The normal value for serum sodium ranges between 135 to 146 mEq/L. Maintenance of serum sodium within a narrow range, approximately 2 mEq/L, occurs on a daily basis. Symptoms are more common when the serum sodium is less than 130 mEq/L or greater than 150 mEq/L, especially when the changes in serum sodium are acute. In contrast, slowly progressive or chronic changes in serum sodium are more tolerable, and symptoms may not occur until the abnormality is extreme.

Determination of serum osmolality by direct measurement and by calculation is necessary for appropriate evaluation. The normal serum osmolality ranges between 286 to 294 mOsm/kg of H_2O. Serum osmolality is calculated as follows:

$$\text{Serum osmolality} = 2(\text{Na}^+) + \frac{\text{glucose (mg/100mL)}}{18} + \frac{\text{BUN (mg/100mL)}}{2.8}$$

Normal serum osmolality in a hyponatremic patient indicates either pseudohyponatremia or the presence of osmotic substances other than sodium. Variations between measured and calculated serum osmolality are indicative of osmotic substances being present other than sodium, urea, or glucose (e.g., mannitol, glycerol, methanol, or ethylene glycol).

Etiology
Pseudohyponatremia

Pseudohyponatremia exists in the presence of hyperlipidemia or extreme hyperglobulinemia (multiple myeloma, Waldenstrom's macroglobulinemia, etc.). The abnormality in such cases is related to the amount of plasma that is occupied by the lipids or the proteins. Osmolality remains normal in this setting.

Hyponatremia with Decreased Total Body Sodium

This condition is characterized by a sodium deficit that exceeds the water deficit, resulting in a low serum sodium and manifestations of contracted extracellular volume. Such manifestations include orthostatic hypotension, tachycardia, dry mucous membranes, flat neck veins, poor skin turgor, and recent weight loss. Urine sodium values can be very helpful in determining the origin of the loss. A urine sodium of less than 10 mEq/L is indicative of a nonrenal source of sodium and water loss. The gastrointestinal tract is the most likely origin. However, the accumulation of fluid in a "third space" secondary to an intraabdominal process, massive burns, or severe muscle trauma must be considered. In contrast, a urine sodium of greater than 20 mEq/L, in the presence of normal renal function, suggests that the source of sodium and water loss is the kidneys. Diuretic excess, adrenal insufficiency, and salt-losing nephropathies are possible etiologies.

Diuretic-Induced Hyponatremia

Diuretic-induced hyponatremia is usually associated with hypokalemia. The etiology of diuretic-induced hyponatremia includes excessive sodium and water losses resulting in hypovolemia with secondary stimulation of an antidiuretic hormone by volume receptors. This results in true and dilutional hyponatremia. The potassium deficit may contribute to the hyponatremia by an intracellular shift of sodium in exchange for potassium, since this type of hyponatremia is partially corrected by potassium administration alone.

Hyponatremia associated with an osmotic diuresis results from obligatory natriuresis by the osmotic forces, even in the presence of volume contraction. Patients with diabetic ketoacidosis, mannitol therapy, and urea diuresis may have significant losses of sodium in the urine.

Adrenal Insufficiency

The hyponatremia of adrenal insufficiency is usually associated with hyperkalemia and prerenal azotemia. The increased renal losses of sodium and water result in hypovolemia with secondary stimulation of antidiuretic hormone. This results in a true sodium deficit and dilutional hyponatremia.

Renal Insufficiency

Hyponatremia associated with chronic renal insufficiency and extracellular volume depletion may result from salt restriction and excessive use of diuretics. Excessive losses of sodium are also common in these patients when vomiting or diarrhea is present.

The salt-losing tendency or "salt-losing nephropathy" is seen in a variety of tubulointerstitial diseases of the kidney, even in the absence of renal insufficiency.

Hyponatremia with Increased Total Body Sodium

In this type of hyponatremia, a low serum sodium is associated with an expanded extracellular volume and, frequently, with edema. This is seen in cirrhosis of the liver, congestive heart failure, nephrotic syndrome, and acute and chronic renal failure. Water retention exceeds sodium retention, resulting in the so-called "dilutional hyponatremia." The decrease in free water clearance or water retention in these disorders is multifactorial. There is a decreased delivery of glomerular filtrate to the diluting segment of the nephron and stimulation of antidiuretic hormone by a decreased effective intravascular volume. The urine sodium is usually less than 20 mEq/L, except in patients with acute and chronic renal failure whose urine sodium values may exceed this level.

Hyponatremia with Normal Total Body Sodium

A low serum sodium associated with a clinically undetectable increase in extracellular fluid volume is the hallmark of this condition. The water retention results in "dilutional hyponatremia." Characteristically, edema is absent, and urine sodium values approximate the daily sodium intake.

Hyponatremia associated with hypothyroidism is poorly understood. Proposed mechanisms include a decrease in cardiac output with stimulation of antidiuretic hormone and abnormal urinary dilution secondary to a distal tubule defect. Hyponatremia associated with adrenal insufficiency is due to an increased sodium loss in the urine; however, the defect in water excretion may contribute to the severity of the hyponatremia. Glucocorticoids may play a part in the etiology of the low serum due to their role in the maintenance of the impermeability of the collecting duct epithelium to water.

Administration of a variety of drugs, in addition to diuretics, can cause hyponatremia. Such agents include chlorpropamide (Diabinese), narcotics, carbamazepine (Tegretol), barbiturates, clofibrate (Atromid-S), vincristine, nicotine, isoproterenol, and tolbutamide. The mechanism of action is frequently due to the stimulation of antidiuretic hormone release. In addition, chlorpropamide enhances the action of the circulating antidiuretic hormone. Aspirin and indomethacin, both prostaglandin synthetase inhibitors, have been shown to enhance the action of antidiuretic hormone. Prostaglandins normally counteract the effect of antidiuretic hormone via a negative feedback system. Acetaminophen has been shown to enhance the action of antidiuretic hormone. The mechanism remains unknown. Cyclophosphamide (Cytoxan) can cause a defect in renal water excretion that seems to parallel excretion of an active metabolite of the drug. Lastly, oxytocin may cause hyponatremia by stimulation of vasopressin action.

SIADH

Hyponatremia associated with the syndrome of inappropriate antidiuretic hormone secretion (SIADH) is largely a diagnosis of exclusion. This syndrome should be considered if the following criteria are met:

1. Normal renal, adrenal, and thyroid functions
2. Absence of edema and intravascular volume deficiency
3. Urine osmolality inappropriately high compared to the low serum osmolality
4. Urine sodium values that approximate the daily sodium intake

This syndrome has been associated with a variety of benign and malignant disorders, such as central nervous system disorders, pulmonary disease, and certain malignancies, primarily lung cancer.

Diagnosis

Clinical Presentation

A detailed history and physical examination are pertinent in the evaluation of the hyponatremic patient. Special attention should be given to a history of diuretic use, vomiting, diarrhea, heart disease, renal disease, and liver disease. A careful drug history is equally important.

The physical examination should be geared to determination of the extracellular volume status of the patient. Evaluation of the neck veins, mucous membranes, skin turgor, and orthostatic blood pressure is helpful.

Signs and symptoms of hyponatremia range from lethargy and muscle cramps to multiple central nervous system symptoms, including seizures. The severity of symptoms is dependent on the rate of development and the severity of hyponatremia. Electroencephalographic changes may also be present but are nonspecific. (See Table 26–1.)

Laboratory Tests

Electrolytes, blood urea nitrogen (BUN), and urinary electrolytes and osmolality should be drawn.

Management

The treatment of hyponatremia is dependent upon the following:

1. The severity of signs and symptoms
2. The course — acute versus chronic
3. The underlying disease process

In the presence of pronounced central nervous system manifestations (such as seizures), hypertonic saline or mannitol should be administered, regardless of the etiology of the hyponatremia. These agents are used to produce an osmotic gradient. Extreme caution is necessary to avoid fluid overload by the hypertonic saline solution, especially in cardiac patients and in the elderly.

Correction of the hyponatremic state should be gradual to avoid serious complications. Diagnosis of the under-

Table 26–1   Signs and Symptoms of Hyponatremia

Thirst	Restlessness
Impaired taste sensation	Confusion
Anorexia	Delirium
Nausea/emesis	Muscle twitching
Muscle cramps	Coma
Abdominal cramps	Hemiparesis ⎫
Depressed sensorium	Ataxia ⎬ Chronic
Weakness	Babinski's reflex ⎭
Lethargy	

lying disease process is essential for appropriate management. Drugs known to cause hyponatremia should be discontinued and hormonal replacement considered in the thyroid- or adrenal-deficient patient.

In hyponatremic patients who are both salt and water depleted, replacement with isotonic saline is recommended to replace volume and sodium to a normal level. In patients with an excess of total body sodium and water, restriction of both salt and water is recommended. Sodium intake should be decreased to 2 g per 24 hours for moderate to severe sodium excess. A water restriction of 800 to 1200 ml/24 hours is usually sufficient.

In euvolemic patients, such as those with the syndrome of inappropriate secretion of antidiuretic hormone, therapy depends on the severity and chronicity of the disease. Rapid correction is achieved by administration of a loop diuretic combined with the use of hypertonic saline. This method is effective in correcting the serum sodium to a near-normal range by inducing a diuresis with simultaneous replacement of urinary sodium and potassium. Therapy includes administration of intravenous furosemide, 1 mg/kg of body weight initially, followed by subsequent doses to produce negative fluid balance and replacement of urinary sodium and potassium by 3% normal saline and potassium chloride. The desired negative water balance can be calculated as follows:

$$\frac{\text{Desired negative water balance}}{\text{(L)}} = \frac{\text{(total body solute)} \times \text{(1 L)}}{\text{desired plasma osmolality}}$$

where mOsm of total body solute = (total body water) × (plasma osmolality)

and total body water = (wt. in kg) × (60% or 70%)

Restriction of water intake to replace insensible losses only is adequate in the milder forms.

Drug therapy is recommended when the underlying cause is uncorrectable or when the syndrome of inappropriate secretion of antidiuretic hormone is not readily reversible. Demeclocycline and lithium interfere with the peripheral action of antidiuretic hormone. Demeclocycline in a dose of 1200 or 2400 g per day is preferred over lithium. Side effects include a high incidence of photosensitivity and a decrease in renal function, especially in patients with liver disease. Diphenylhydantoin, through its central action on antidiuretic hormone, may prove effective in SIADH secondary to central nervous system disorders.

HYPERNATREMIA

General Considerations

Although less common than hyponatremia, hypernatremia, which is defined as a plasma sodium concentration greater than 150 mEq/L, can present as a medical emergency. As a rule, pathophysiologic disturbances that cause renal or gastrointestinal water losses do not result in hypernatremia unless there is a disturbance in thirst or the individual is unable to drink or obtain water. Thus, hypernatremic emergencies are most commonly seen in the very young and the very old.

In the emergency setting, the main clinical manifestations of hypernatremia are neurologic and include confusion, stupor, or coma. Occasionally, focal neurologic deficits may be present; in those patients who have undergone a profound osmotic diuresis, signs and symptoms of volume depletion may dominate the clinical picture.

Etiology

Hypernatremia with Decreased Total Body Sodium

In this condition, the water loss exceeds the sodium loss, resulting in an elevated serum sodium level and serum osmolality. Hyperosmolality of the extracellular fluid stimulates the thirst mechanism and an antidiuretic hormone release. Failure to respond to thirst is common in the elderly and in patients with cerebrovascular diseases. Clinical manifestations of hypovolemia are usually prominent and associated hemoconcentration may be present, evidenced by an elevated hematocrit, total protein, serum albumin, and BUN. In children, metabolic acidosis is usually present, as well as hypocalcemia, which may be symptomatic. Hyperglycemia occurs in 50% of infants with hypernatremia. Sources of hypotonic fluid losses include the gastrointestinal tract, profuse sweating, and renal losses such as with hyperglycemia, mannitol administration, chronic renal failure, and postobstructive diuresis (urea). Urine sodium and osmolality vary according to the etiology. Extrarenal losses are associated with a urine sodium less than 20 mEq/L and a high urine osmolality. Renal losses are usually associated with a low, normal, or high urine sodium and osmolality.

Hypernatremia with Increased Total Body Sodium

This type of hypernatremia is characterized by an increased total body sodium that exceeds the total body water. When this problem exists, it is most likely iatrogenic in origin. This form of hypernatremia is seen in patients receiving large amounts of sodium bicarbonate during cardiopulmonary resuscitation or lactic acidosis, abortion induced by hypertonic saline, induction of emesis with saline, hemodialysis or peritoneal dialysis, hypertonic infant formula, heat stroke, and sea water drowning. Mild hypernatremia can exist in patients with hyperaldosteronism and Cushing's disease.

Hypernatremia with Normal Total Body Sodium

In this setting, the hypernatremia is associated with water loss without significant sodium loss. This form of hypernatremia is seen in patients with central or nephrogenic diabetes insipidus who fail to respond to thirst stimulation, due to either abnormal thirst response or lack of water. This form is also seen in febrile illnesses in the elderly and in heat stroke where there is an increased insensible loss. In the former, the urine will have an elevated osmolality with a variable urine sodium concentration. If the water loss is renal in origin, both the urine osmolality and sodium concentration may be variable.

Essential hypernatremia is a rare entity, usually associated with a hypothalamic lesion. These patients have an abnormal thirst response to an elevated serum osmolality. An antidiuretic hormone is present, although, in some of these patients, vasopressin release is stimulated more by volume depletion as opposed to hyperosmolality.

Diagnosis

Clinical Presentation

A detailed history and physical examination are essential for evaluation of the patient with hypernatremia. A history of systemic disease may be pertinent, especially as related to a recent hospitalization for a central nervous system disorder or renal disease. Information regarding recent exposure to extreme heat or symptoms of infection or stroke are important.

The physical examination should emphasize evaluation of the patient's volume status. Evidence of head trauma, stroke, or severe infarction should be sought. The signs and symptoms of hypernatremia are varied, ranging from restlessness alternating with lethargy to seizures. The deleterious effects of hypernatremia are related to the rapidity of development of the abnormality. The cerebrospinal fluid may be xanthochromic due to secondary capillary rupture.

Laboratory Tests

Electrolytes, BUN, and blood glucose should be drawn. Renal evaluation should include urinary osmolality and electrolytes. Serum osmolality should be calculated and measured.

Management

In general, complete correction of the hyperosmolality should be accomplished over a 48-hour period in order to avoid the development of seizures due to hypotonicity. In the presence of shock, colloid fluid should be given to keep the systolic blood pressure at an adequate level. It must be remembered that most plasma preparations are high in sodium content. After the fluid deficit is estimated, fluid replacement should be instituted. An estimation of the total amount of water deficit can be made by the following formula:

$$H_2O \text{ deficit} = 0.6 \times BW_{kg}(1 - \frac{140}{[Na_{obs}]})$$

where BW_{kg} = body weight in kilograms

In all cases, hypotonic fluids are of prime importance. In patients that also have sodium depletion, normal saline preparations should be given to replete intravascular volume, and the hypotonic fluids should be administered. Special attention must be given to the possible increase in osmolality by dextrose solutions.

If the patient is severely acidotic, sodium bicarbonate must be given with extreme caution. Serum electrolytes should be measured frequently as well as the serum osmolality. After large volumes of fluid, potassium levels may decrease and should be replaced as needed. Finally, the treatment plan must be modified to accommodate each patient based on the underlying disease.

SUGGESTED READINGS

Clifford DB: Hyponatremia and the brain, Am Fam Physician 38(3):119–124, 1988.

Laureno R and Karp BI: Pontine and extrapontine myelinolysis following rapid correction of hyponatraemia, Lancet 1:1439–1444, 1988.

Peces R, Ablanedo P, and Alvarez J: Central pontine and extrapontine myelinolysis following correction of severe hyponatremia, Nephron 49(2):160–163, 1988.

Rossi MF and Cadnapaphornchai P: Disordered water metabolism: hyponatremia, Crit Care Clin 3(4):759–777, 1987.

Hypokalemia and Hyperkalemia

Stephen Hamburger, M.D.

HYPOKALEMIA

General Considerations

Hypokalemia may present as a life-threatening medical emergency in the elderly patient. While gradual potassium depletion due to gastrointestinal losses, poor intake, or diuretic therapy may be asymptomatic, with moderate to severe depletion, neuromuscular symptoms (including skeletal muscle weakness or paralysis) may predominate. Although moderate potassium depletion rarely affects cardiac function or rhythm, severe or rapid reduction in serum potassium levels may cause cardiac arrest. Potassium deficiency enhances the cardiac toxicity of digitalis preparations. In patients who have had cardiac arrest, refractory ventricular arrhythmias should suggest the possibility of underlying potassium depletion and hypokalemia.

Hypokalemia is usually defined as serum potassium less than 3.5 mEq/L. (See Table 27–1.)

Etiology

1. Hypokalemia due to a shift of extracellular potassium is seen in various conditions. Both metabolic and respiratory alkalosis are usually associated with a low serum potassium level. Administration of glucose alone or glucose with insulin may be associated with hypokalemia. Glucose administration to diabetics with the syndrome of selective hypoaldosteronism may cause elevation of serum potassium rather than hypokalemia. Serum potassium should be monitored closely in diabetics who receive large doses of hypertonic glucose for suspected hypoglycemia.

2. Hypokalemia is a prominent feature in familial periodic paralysis.

3. Decreased total body potassium produced by increased renal losses of potassium is the most common cause of hypokalemia. Enhanced delivery of sodium and water to the distal nephron, induced by all diuretics including osmotic diuresis, is associated with significant hypokalemia. Potassium-sparing diuretics are the exception. Both proximal and distal renal tubular acidosis (RTA) are associated with hypokalemia. Diagnosis of RTA is suspected when hypokalemia is associated with metabolic acidosis, especially when diarrhea is excluded.

4. Drug-induced hypokalemia is seen with administration of large doses of carbenicillin or penicillin. Increased delivery of the poorly absorbable anions of these drugs to the distal nephron induces kaliuresis.

5. Ingestion of large amounts of licorice or its derivative, carbenoxolone, or occasionally chewing tobacco, is associated with hypokalemia.

6. Hypokalemia is a common feature with syndromes associated with mineralocorticoid hyperactivity. Metabolic alkalosis and hypertension are usually concomitant findings. Hypertension is characteristically absent in patients with Bartter's syndrome and those receiving diuretics.

Table 27–1   Causes of Hypokalemia

Internal Imbalance	External Imbalance	
Metabolic or respiratory alkalosis	Decreased intake	*Secondary*
Insulin or glucose administration	Increased loss	• Bartter's syndrome
Familial periodic paralysis	1. Renal loss	• Edematous states
Barium poisoning	• Diuresis	• Oral contraceptives
	Osmotic diuresis	• Renin-producing tumors
	Diuretics	• Renal artery stenosis
	• Acid-base disorders	• Malignant hypertension
	Renal tubular acidosis	*Miscellaneous*
	Metabolic alkalosis	• Liddle's syndrome
	Metabolic acidosis	• Hypercalcemia
	(chronic)	• Magnesium deficiency
	• Drugs	• Acute monocytic or
	Carbenicillin, penicillin,	myelocytic leukemia
	licorice, carbenoxolone,	2. Gastrointestinal loss
	acetazolamide	• Gastric fluid loss
	Mineralocorticoid hyperactivity	• Intestinal fluid loss
	Primary	• Villous adenoma
	• Primary aldosteronism	• Laxative abuse
	• Nonaldosterone	3. Skin losses
	mineralocorticoids	• Excessive sweating
	• Licorice, tobacco chewing	
	• ACTH-producing tumors	
	• Cushing's syndrome	

7. Hypokalemia is occasionally seen in association with magnesium deficiency, acute monocytic or myelomonocytic leukemia, and hypercalcemia.

8. Hypokalemia due to gastrointestinal losses of potassium is also common and may result from vomiting or gastric suction. The associated volume depletion, metabolic alkalosis, and secondary hyperaldosteronism contribute to the renal losses of potassium.

9. Severe hypokalemia occurs with protracted diarrheal states, especially with cholera and watery diarrhea hypokalemia syndrome associated with non–beta-islet cell hyperplasia.

10. Villous adenomas of the colon are occasionally associated with hypokalemia. Surreptitious use of laxatives or cathartics may present the physician with a diagnostic dilemma.

11. Severe sweating in a hot climate may contribute to significant losses of potassium.

Diagnosis

Clinical Presentation

The diagnosis of hypokalemia can usually be suspected from the clinical history. Neuromuscular complaints, weakness, and frank paralysis are suggestive of hypokalemia. Elderly patients on potassium-wasting diuretics are prone to hypokalemia as are alcoholics who have decreased intake combined with diuresis secondary to decreased antidiuretic hormone (ADH) production. Patients whose potassium deficiency is caused by surreptitious use of diuretics or laxatives or who have psychogenic, self-induced vomiting (bulimia) will rarely volunteer an accurate history. On physical examination, patients with lowered serum potassium levels may have decreased skeletal motor power or decreased or absent deep tendon reflexes.

EVALUATION OF PATIENTS WITH HYPOKALEMIA OR HYPERKALEMIA

1. Repeat laboratory test is mandatory to exclude error or hemolysis of blood sample.
2. Detailed medical history concerning prescribed and over-the-counter drugs and dietetic habits is very informative.
3. Complete physical examination is needed to evaluate body fluid status (edema, volume depletion) and arterial blood pressure.
4. Basic laboratory evaluation should include complete blood cell count, arterial blood gases, and renal function tests.
5. The renin-aldosterone profile and adrenal functions should be assessed when specifically indicated.

Electrocardiographic Manifestations of Hypokalemia

Supraventricular tachycardia and ventricular ectopic beats are relatively common with severe hypokalemia, especially in patients receiving digitalis therapy. The most frequently encountered electrocardiographic (ECG) changes, however, are S-T segment depression, flattened

T-waves, and appearances of a U-wave. Unexplained refractory ventricular tachycardia or fibrillation in patients with cardiac arrest may be due to hypokalemia.

Management

Correction of hypokalemia requires replacing potassium deficits with potassium supplements and identifying and correcting the underlying process responsible for hypokalemia. The serum potassium level may serve as a rough guide for estimating the total body potassium deficit, especially when more accurate measurements are not available. The total body potassium deficit may range between 100 and 150 mEq when the serum potassium is decreased by 1.0 mEq/L and between 400 and 600 mEq when the serum potassium is decreased by 2.0 mEq/L, especially in the absence of severe acid-base disorders.

Parenteral potassium administration should be restricted to severe hypokalemia or when oral intake is not possible.

Patients with severe life-threatening hypokalemia (i.e., who have a serum potassium less than 2.5 mEq/L and are taking a digitalis preparation) should have their serum potassium restored to normal as soon as possible. Short-term potassium chloride infusion up to 40 mEq per hour is permissible with cardiac monitoring and frequent vital signs, as well as frequent serum potassium determinations. Renal function must be known and great caution exercised to avoid hyperkalemia. Patients receiving more than 10 to 20 mEq/L intravenously should be monitored closely; the rate of administration and the concentration in the infusion fluid should be individualized depending on the clinical condition of the patient. Potassium chloride salt is the preferred preparation, especially when metabolic alkalosis is present. When hypokalemia is associated with metabolic acidosis as in renal tubular acidosis, potassium administration should precede or accompany alkali therapy.

Potassium supplements should be used with caution in patients with decreased renal function or diabetes.

Surgical intervention may be necessary for adrenal adenomas or renal artery stenosis.

Prostaglandin inhibitors, such as indomethacin, may be useful in the management of Bartter's syndrome.

HYPERKALEMIA

General Considerations

Disorders involving potassium homeostasis are relatively common in the practice of medicine. Hyperkalemia, which is defined as a serum potassium exceeding 5.5 mEq/L, is a potentially life-threatening medical emergency. Early recognition is essential and can reduce cardiac morbidity and mortality. Rapid institution of therapy can return potassium levels to a safe range and can prevent serious cardiac arrhythmias.

Overall understanding of the mechanisms involved is essential for appropriate diagnosis and management. Total body potassium averages between 50 and 55 mEq/kg of body weight. More than 95% of total body potassium is intracellular. The high gradient between the intracellular and extracellular potassium is maintained by an energy-dependent mechanism. The relationship between the intracellular and extracellular potassium is influenced by many factors. Insulin and the acid-base state of body fluids are the two more important factors in the internal regulation of potassium. The external balance of potassium, or the regulation of total body potassium, is maintained by a balance between the intake and excretion of potassium. Renal excretion contributes to more than 85% of the daily potassium intake. Renal excretion of potassium is altered by factors that influence the secretion of potassium in the distal nephron. The gastrointestinal tract excretes 10 to 15% of potassium. (See Table 27–2.)

Etiology

1. Pseudohyperkalemia is an in vitro phenomenon that is observed in hemolyzed blood samples or with disorders associated with extremely elevated white cell or platelet count. Prolonged use of a tourniquet may lead to elevated potassium levels in the blood sample.

2. Redistribution can also induce hyperkalemia. Hyperkalemia secondary to both acute metabolic or respir-

Table 27–2   Causes of Hyperkalemia

Pseudohyperkalemia	Severe leukocytosis
	Severe thrombocytosis
	Hemolysis of blood sample
Increased Total Body Potassium	Excessive intake
	Renal insufficiency
	Decreased mineralocorticoid activity (adrenal insufficiency, selective hypoaldosteronism)
	Drugs
	• Potassium-sparing diuretics
	• Potassium-containing antibiotics
	• Digitalis overdose
	• Prostaglandin inhibitors
	Distal tubular defect
	• Sickle cell anemia
	• Postrenal transplant
	• Systemic lupus erythematosus
Redistribution	Acute metabolic acidosis
	Acute respiratory acidosis
	Cationic amino acid administration
	Hyperkalemic familial periodic paralysis

atory acidosis is due to extracellular shift of potassium. The inverse relationship between blood pH and serum potassium is influenced also by the concentration of sodium bicarbonate in the extracellular fluid, by the responsible acid (mineral versus organic acid), and by the degree of renal dysfunction.

3. Administration of cationic amino acids, such as arginine hydrochloride, may lead to hyperkalemia by an external shift of cellular potassium.

4. Hyperkalemia may be associated rarely with a form of periodic familial paralysis.

5. Drug-induced hyperkalemia is common in the presence of renal insufficiency. Potassium-sparing diuretics, potassium-containing nonsteroidal antiinflammatory drugs, such as indomethacin, and massive overdose with digitalis may be responsible.

6. Hyperkalemia is a serious complication in acute renal failure. Life-threatening, severe hyperkalemia may occur in oliguric patients or those with increased catabolism, such as rhabdomyolysis. Significant hyperkalemia is unusual in the steady state of chronic renal failure. Factors such as systemic acidosis, prolonged constipation, and excessive intake, however, may cause hyperkalemia in chronic renal failure.

7. Hyperkalemia seen in sickle cell anemia, renal transplantation, and systemic lupus erythematosus is due to distal tubular defect in potassium secretion.

8. Hyperkalemia is a common finding in patients with generalized adrenal insufficiency as in Addison's disease. Hyperkalemia due to selective hyperaldosteronism is, however, more commonly encountered than the generalized form of adrenal insufficiency. Diabetics and those with chronic interstitial renal diseases are especially at risk.

Diagnosis

Clinical Presentation

As a rule, the most prominent manifestations of hyperkalemic emergencies occur in the heart. Occasionally, however, moderate to severe elevations in serum potassium can have striking effects on the peripheral muscles. Ascending muscular weakness may occur and, in some cases, may progress to flaccid quadriplegia and respiratory paralysis. Usual cranial nerve function is preserved.

Laboratory and Electrocardiogram Examination

A variety of ECG changes are encountered when the body's serum potassium rapidly rises above 5.5 mEq/L. The following changes are seen with increasing hyperkalemia:

- Peaked T waves
- Shortened QT interval
- Decreased P wave amplitude

- Widened P wave and QRS complexes
- Absence of P wave and sine wave
- Ventricular fibrillation and cardiac arrest

Management

Management depends on the severity of hyperkalemia, rate of development, and presence of ECG changes. Calcium salt infusion is lifesaving and recommended for severe hyperkalemia, for example, serum potassium higher than 7.0 mEq/L, especially in the presence of significant ECG changes. Calcium administration counteracts the neuromuscular effects of hyperkalemia. The onset of action is within minutes and lasts only for 30 minutes. Solutions available for use include calcium gluconate (10 mL of 10% solution contains 90 mg calcium) or calcium chloride (10 mL of 10% solution contains 360 mg calcium). Administration of calcium salts should be done with continuous monitoring of ECG.

Hyperkalemia should also be treated by enhancing potassium shift into the intracellular space. Intracellular potassium shift is best achieved by intravenous infusion of either hypertonic glucose and insulin or sodium bicarbonate. Hypertonic glucose is usually administered as 500 mL of 10% solution with 10 units regular insulin to prevent hypoglycemia. Sodium bicarbonate administration is achieved by infusion of 44 mEq of sodium bicarbonate ampules intravenously as needed. The onset of action is within 20 to 30 minutes and lasts only for a few hours.

Reduction in total body potassium is best achieved by increasing fecal excretion using ion exchange resin or by dialysis. Sodium polystyrene sulfonate (Kayexalate), an ion exchange resin, removes about 1 mEq potassium for each one gram. Kayexalate is given either orally or rectally as retention enema. Orally, 15 to 20 g in 30 mL of 70% sorbitol solution should be given and repeated as necessary. In general, hemodialysis is more effective in removing potassium than peritoneal dialysis.

Treatment of hyperkalemia usually requires a combination of the aforementioned modalities.

Hyperkalemia due to mineralocorticoid deficiency is managed by either the administration of Florinef, 0.05 to 0.2 mg daily, or by giving loop diuretics coupled with decreased potassium intake.

SUGGESTED READINGS

Adlinger K and Samaan N: Hypokalemia and hyperkalemia, Ann Intern Med 87:571–573, 1977.

Cohen J: Disorders of potassium balance, Hosp Pract pp 119–128, Jan 1979.

Linshaw MA: Potassium homeostasis and hypokalemia, Pediatr Clin North Am 34(3):649–681, 1987.

Nardone D: Hypokalemia and hyperkalemia, Ann Intern Med 82:54–57, 1975.

Patrick J: Assessment of body potassium stores, Kidney Int 11:476–490, 1977.

Weisberg LS, Szerlip HM, and Cox M: Disorders of potassium homeostasis in critically ill patients, Crit Care Clin 3(4):835–854, 1987.

Acute Nutritional Emergencies

George R. Schwartz, M.D., F.A.C.E.P.

This chapter will focus on four aspects of food-related factors in geriatric emergency medicine. The first is malnutrition and vitamin deficiency syndromes. These may actually account for acute presentations, and it is certain that physicians are underdiagnosing the presence of these conditions as both immediate contributors and background factors.

With ready access to vitamins, some of our elderly population have, on the other hand, vitamin excess syndromes, which may be easily mistaken for other diseases. When patients are asked what medications they are taking, rarely will vitamins be mentioned. This information must be requested, and it is worthwhile to habitually include this question after the initial question about medications. Also, certain supplements, such as L-tryptophan, are considered benign by many people, who take 1 to 4 g per day for sleep or other disorders. However, an eosinophilic myalgic syndrome has been reported, and there is now increased attention to what had been previously considered a "harmless supplement."

The third category involves basic difficulties in regulation of water that can lead to severe psychotic symptoms, convulsions, coma, and death. These factors can readily be overlooked.

Finally, it is important to focus on food toxicities as a source of acute symptoms — e.g., sulfites, monosodium glutamate (MSG) — and classic food poisoning by exotoxin and bacterial infection. These latter two groups may rapidly cause severe electrolyte disorders and dehydration, which place excessive strain on the reduced physiologic reserve and can cause serious morbidity or death.

MALNUTRITION AND VITAMIN DEFICIENCY SYNDROMES

Elderly patients frequently consume less than the "minimum daily requirement" of many vitamins,[1-8] and the symptoms that may result are frequently ascribed to other causes. Malabsorption, poor dentition, hypochlorhydria, and decreased intestinal secretions further tend to reduce absorption. Drugs and/or medications may also interact with nutrients.

As the mean age of the elderly population increases, these problems will tend to increase, despite some simple partial solutions (e.g., dental work, hearing aids, visual aids). Many of our elderly, either living independently or in institutions, are in states of malnutrition.

It is well known that severe chronic malnutrition is accompanied by marked physical and psychologic changes: apathy, emotional instability, retardation, memory impairment, and even psychotic illness. Some of our elderly are experiencing undiagnosed symptoms of these types.

Much of what we know of malnutrition has involved prisoners who have volunteered for studies, such as with Terris and Goldberger's classic studies on pellagra in the early years of the twentieth century.[9] Prisoners of war provided an unfortunate human testing ground for chronic malnutrition.[10]

One of the most unique books in the annals of medicine and a book extremely difficult to read without great emotion is the scientific reports of hunger disease prepared by Jewish physicians in the Warsaw ghetto in 1940.[11]

The Nazi troops had sealed several hundred thousand people off from the outside world, determined to starve their prisoners to death. Amidst this evil catastrophe, a group of physicians decided to undertake a careful investigation of the clinical, metabolic, and pathologic consequences of starvation. One physician survived to recover the manuscript and prepare it for publication so that the group's last wish before death was accomplished, *non omnis moriar* — "I shall not wholly die."

The relevance of this work in the present day, aside from the deep historical significance, is to demonstrate what may occur clinically in particularly vulnerable groups. Even in populations where the general standard of nutrition is high, there are people prone to malnutrition — the mentally ill, the aged, alcoholics (particularly elderly alcoholics), as well as those with chronic gastrointestinal disease and malabsorption. Some of these patients will present with acute signs and symptoms; others will remain in the shadowy background as "preexistent" conditions unless they are recognized by the acute care physician or nurse.

One recent example clarifies this "background." In June, 1988, Dr. Lindenbaum and his colleagues published a remarkable study which demonstrated neuropsychiatric disorders caused by cobalamin deficiency (vitamin B_{12}) in the absence of anemia or macrocytosis.[12]

What made this study particularly important was the wide range of symptoms — paresthesias being most common, followed by ataxia, memory loss, weakness, and fatigue. With some of the patients, the diagnosis was not made for years because of the absence of anemia. This study revealed that 40% of the 141 patients had no anemia or macrocytosis; 25 of the 40 patients were 60 or older (63%). This study underscores this concept of underdiagnosis of hypovitaminosis syndromes, despite our sophisticated medical care system.

In the late twentieth century, we should not be making the same mistakes that were made in the late eighteenth century. James Lind first published "A Treatise on the Scurvy" in 1753.[13] In this work, he clearly showed the benefits of using lemons and oranges to prevent scurvy, which had been responsible for millions of deaths. Yet, 100 years later ships were still sailing out without a supply of lemons and returning with scorbutic sailors, after having buried others at sea. It took almost 50 years for the British navy to take notice of his findings. Lind was very bitter at the time of his death, feeling he had failed to convey his important conclusions.

When deficiency syndromes do arise, replacement of a single vitamin is inadequate since we are dealing with problems with the entire diet (including, usually, protein and trace minerals) as well as possible other problems already mentioned (e.g., malabsorption, poor dentition, depression, medications, alcoholism).

The symptoms and signs in Table 28–1 represent "full-blown" syndromes. These conditions do not suddenly appear. Instead, there is a slow and insidious progression, although severe stress or infection may rapidly precipitate some signs or symptoms. Profound deficiencies may also occur in patients maintained for a considerable time on intravenous fluids particularly after surgery for a gastrointestinal disorder.

Many chronic conditions (e.g., Wernicke's encephalopathy, dementia) will not respond well to dietary change since the physiologic failure has given way to permanent anatomic change through deterioration and

Table 28–1 Signs and Symptoms of Vitamin and Nutritional Deficiency

Protein-Calorie Malnutrition	Thiamine Deficiency
Pallor	Peripheral neuropathy
Fatigue	Paresthesias
Coldness	Weakness, muscle tenderness
Inanition	Mental confusion
Contractures	Memory changes
Anemia	Beriberi heart disease (severe cardiac failure)
Impaired immunity	Wernicke's encephalopathy
Hypoproteinemia and edema	Footdrop, wristdrop
Hypotension	Decreased deep tendon reflexes
Autonomic nervous system hyporesponsiveness	Pulmonary and peripheral edema
Organ wasting (including heart)	

Niacin Deficiency	Ascorbic Acid Deficiency
Dermatitis*	Petechial hemorrhage
Mental confusion	Follicular hyperkeratosis
Gastrointestinal disturbance (e.g., pancreatic disorders)	Aching limbs
Depression	Bleeding or swollen gums
Lethargy	Joint effusions, hemorrhages
Diarrhea	Dyspnea
Weight loss	Edema
	Neuropathy
	Depression
B₁₂ Deficiency	Confusion
Anemia (macrocytic)	Ocular hemorrhages
Myelopathy	Coiled hairs, hair loss
Peripheral neuropathy	Dry eyes
Optic atrophy	Abdominal colic
Impaired vibration sense	
Ataxia	**Folic Acid Deficiency**
Footdrop	Macrocytic anemia
Fatigue, difficulty concentrating	Diarrhea
Exaggerated deep tendon reflexes	History of chronic medication (anticonvulsant use)
Paresis, paresthesias	Anorexia
Limb pain, cramps	Irritability
Disorientation and mental confusion	Confusion
Depression	Dementia
Memory impairment	Depression

*Hyperkeratotic hyperpigmentation on backs of hands, elbows, and neck.

cell death. Similarly, chronic calcium deficiency in the elderly can lead to widespread osteoporosis and, although not easily reversed, treatment should certainly begin with calcium and estrogens as needed for women.

Despite the resistance of some symptoms, others may clear rapidly when the deficiency is corrected. For example, the confabulation and disorientation of Korsakoff's psychosis may respond to thiamine within hours. Ocular abnormalities are present in over 90% of cases (nystagmus, sixth nerve palsies, sluggish pupils) and will similarly respond very rapidly, although nystagmus may be permanent.[14] The emotional abnormalities (anxiety, insomnia, later depression, some psychosis) usually respond well. Ataxia, on the other hand, takes a month or two for maximum resolution, and one fourth to one half of the patients will have ongoing balance difficulties. The confusion states take weeks to clear, and some memory loss remains unless treatment is started immediately after a short illness.

While the water-soluble vitamins will rarely cause problems in excess, marked abnormalities have occurred from excess vitamins A and D.[15] Table 28–2 illustrates the vitamin A, D, and E syndromes of deficiency and excess. Some older people might take, or their guardians might provide, an excessive amount of vitamins in a well-meaning attempt to strengthen bones or increase vision.

Table 28–2   Vitamin A, D, and E Syndromes

Hypovitaminosis A

Symptoms:
  Associated with malabsorption, diarrhea, gastroenteritis, or protein deficiency with infection
  Night blindness
  Conjunctival xerosis
  Corneal xerosis, ulcers
  Keratomalacia (leading to blindness)
Treatment:
  If eye lesions are occurring, treatment is urgent. An intramuscular injection of 100,000 units of water-miscible vitamin A will rapidly restore vitamin A levels. Oral supplementation is adequate in most cases. Oil-based vitamin A should not be given parenterally.

Hypervitaminosis A

Symptoms:
  Headache
  Malaise, anorexia
  Vomiting
  Pleural effusion, ascites
  Possible papilledema in adults
  Alopecia
  Weight loss
  Dermatitis
  Skeletal pain
  Liver enlargement, cirrhosis
Laboratory Findings:
  Elevated vitamin A levels
  Hypercalcemia
  Abnormal liver function tests
  Bone resorption on x-ray in chronic cases
Treatment:
  Simply eliminating the excessive vitamin is usually satisfactory. However, with hypercalcemia, normal saline intravenously over several days is effective.

Vitamin D Deficiency

  May be associated with decreased intake or can be related to anticonvulsant medications (e.g., hydantoins, barbiturates)
Symptoms:
  Bone pain
  Hyperparathyroidism
  Senile osteomalacia and fractures
  Muscle weakness
Laboratory Findings:
  Low-serum vitamin D level (< 10 ng/mL), hypoparathyroidism, hypocalcemia

Vitamin D Intoxication

Symptoms:
  Metastatic calcification
  Hypercalcemia
  Renal insufficiency
  Anorexia
  Anemia
  Dermatitis
Laboratory Findings:
  Elevated serum calcium, increased calcium in urine
  Serum vitamin D elevated (usually above 50 ng/mL)
  X-ray evidence of periosteal thickening or metastatic calcification
  Urine may show proteinuria
  ECG may show arrhythmias
Treatment:
  Fluids, saline diuresis
  Stop vitamin D intake
  Treat severe hypercalcemia with calcitonin or mithramycin
  Cholestyramine orally (8 g b.i.d.) may aid in decreasing hypercalcemia*

Vitamin E Excess

Long-term excess can cause:
  Nausea
  Vomiting, gastrointestinal upset
  Weakness and fatigue
  Creatinuria
  Visual blurring
Evaluation:
  Blood levels (normal 0.5 to 2.0 mg/dL)
Treatment:
  Simple discontinuance†

---

*See Jibani M and Hodges NH: Prolonged hypercalcemia after industrial exposure to vitamin D, Br Med J 290:748, 1985, for more information.
†See Bierie JG, Corash C, and Hubbard US: Medical uses of vitamin E, N Engl J Med 308:1063, 1983, for more information.

WATER INTOXICATION SYNDROMES

Endocrine alterations in the elderly are well addressed in Chapters 23 and 26. However, some mention of water-related syndromes is appropriate here.

Episodic water intoxication, which is characterized by profound hyponatremia and diverse neurologic signs ranging from ataxia to irreversible coma, occurs in patients with chronic psychiatric disorders.[16] The cause of the polydipsia is unclear although the prevailing view is that it is somehow related to the psychosis and dementia with cognitive dysfunction.

This condition has a marked abnormality in renal water excretion, probably due to increased sensitivity to the antidiuretic effects of vasopressin as well as to enhanced vasopressin secretion at a lower osmotic threshold.

Some elderly patients present with a similar electrolyte profile (e.g., hyponatremia), and this syndrome must be considered. Conditions that may mimic this include (1) polydipsia accompanied by excessive salt depletion through sweating or diuretics or (2) an inappropriate antidiuretic hormone (ADH) associated with an underlying condition such as cancer, chronic pulmonary infections, or central nervous system lesions or secondary to some drugs (e.g., vincristine, nicotine, narcotics, clofibrate, carbamazepine).

Water intoxication is diagnosed by taking a careful history along with evaluating laboratory tests that demonstrate low serum and urine sodium and low specific gravity. The presentation may be acute with seizures, coma, trismus, or opisthotonos.[17] The x-ray may show pulmonary edema, and computerized tomography (CT) scan can show cerebral edema and symmetric compression of the ventricles.

Treatment

Respiratory impairment must be treated with intubation or a ventilator if needed. Fluid restriction is commonly ordered. Saline solution infusion can result in a slow clearing of symptoms, but if symptoms are refractory or life threatening, hypertonic saline may be given cautiously. The basic condition is water excess, and too rapid administration of hypertonic saline can be dangerous.[18] Nairns[19] suggests raising the serum sodium 2 mEq/L per hour to a level of 120 to 130 mEq/L.

FOOD POISONING

Food poisoning assumes much greater importance in the elderly since dehydration and electrolyte imbalance, which are caused by profuse diarrhea or a period of intense vomiting, can more easily precipitate a lethal arrhythmia or cause mental changes, confusion, and severe hypotension in older patients, as well as leading to renal failure.

For example, one outbreak of *Escherichia coli*–associated hemorrhagic colitis is particularly illustrative.[20]

In this situation, 55 of 169 residents of a nursing home were affected. Of the residents, older age and previous gastrectomy increased the risk of acquiring the infection. Of the 55 affected residents, 19 died (35%) from the following causes: hemolytic-uremic syndrome (12 patients), acute colitis (1), cardiorespiratory failure (1), and nonspecific causes (5). This study also highlights the increased susceptibility in the elderly — 55 of 169 residents versus 18 of 137 staff members — and the much higher morbidity and mortality. Of the total, 35% of the residents died from their infection, whereas none of the staff died.

The high mortality underscores the need to admit elderly patients with infectious colitis into the hospital since these diseases are far more serious in such patients. The so-called "benign self-limiting" food poisoning can be lethal in the already physiologically compromised elderly patient.

"Food poisoning" following the ingestion of certain foods has multiple etiologies.

It may be caused by bacterial toxins that are ingested preformed or that are elaborated in the intestine by bacteria contaminating the particular food. For example, the ingestion of food (such as salads, ham and other cold meat products, and cream-filled desserts) contaminated with enterotoxin is responsible for staphylococcal food poisoning. Botulism, staphylococcal food poisoning, cholera (*Vibrio cholerae*), and food poisoning from *Clostridium perfringens* and *Bacillus cereus* are considered true intoxications, since clinical illness is produced in each case by a toxin.

Food poisoning may also be caused by a direct *infection* or invasion of the intestine by bacteria, as classically occurs in *Salmonella* food poisoning following ingestion of contaminated food — particularly poultry, milk and dairy products, egg products, and water. Other causes of food poisoning by direct bacterial infection include shigellosis (bacillary dysentery), *Campylobacter fetus* (enteritis), *Streptococcus faecalis,* and *Yersinia enterocolitica.*

E. coli produces gastroenteritis both by elaboration of an enterotoxin, as the cause of *E. coli* "traveler's diarrhea," and by direct bacterial invasion. Furthermore, in certain bacterial infections, it is unclear whether the acute gastrointestinal symptoms are caused by toxin or by direct infection, as with *Vibrio parahaemolyticus.*

Food poisoning may also be caused by viruses and protozoa, such as *Entamoeba histolytica,* the etiologic agent in amebiasis, and *Giardia lamblia.* Food poisoning produced by marine organisms, plants, and mushrooms is discussed later in this chapter. Food poisoning may also occur from toxic contaminants (PCBs, heavy metals, radioactivity), from natural toxic substances (e.g., akee fruit), or from toxic substances added to foods (e.g., MSG or sulfites).

Botulism

Botulism is a serious disease caused by the toxin elaborated by the spore-forming anaerobic bacillus

Clostridium botulinum. The toxin is generally conceded to be the most poisonous substance yet discovered. As an example of its toxicity, as few as 950 molecules of toxin can be lethal for white mice, and the amount of toxin that can cause human death has been estimated to be between 0.1 and 1 μm of toxin. The toxins are good antigens, but natural immunity in people rarely occurs because the lethal dose is less than that needed to elicit antibody production. Botulism is considered to be a rare disease, and outbreaks must be reported to the Centers for Disease Control (CDC) in Atlanta, Georgia.

From 1899 to 1977, 766 outbreaks involving 1,961 cases were reported in the United States. There were 99 deaths. The Canadian experience from 1919 through 1973 was reported by Dolman.[21] He found 62 authenticated outbreaks involving 181 persons, with 83 deaths. The incidence of fatality has been substantially reduced over the past two decades from greater than 60% to less than 20%. This reduction is primarily because of better respiratory care of victims, though it is possible that milder cases are being recognized. Prompt administration of antitoxin is probably also a factor.

There is good reason to suspect that botulism is far more common than is generally realized and is underdiagnosed, particularly in the elderly. The diagnosis is difficult to make, particularly in isolated cases. One analysis of eight cases of botulism caused by contaminated smoked fish showed that the attending physicians failed to reach the diagnosis initially in each instance.[22] An outbreak of botulism occurred in New Mexico in 1978, and more than half the affected group were not correctly diagnosed initially in the emergency department. Since death may occur rapidly from respiratory paralysis, cases unassociated with a large outbreak are likely to be unrecognized, especially in older people with preexistent disease. The mode of death appears natural. Conversely, since there is a range of disease — from very mild (associated with only a slight headache and perhaps some malaise and nausea) to lethal — very mild weakness may never come to medical attention.

Mode of Toxin Action

The action of the toxin prevents the release of the neurotransmitter acetylcholine at the neuromuscular and other cholinergic junctions. The *C. botulinum* toxin is protein in nature, and there are at least seven immunologically distinct types. In human beings, almost all disease results from the types identified as type A, type B, and type E, though there have been recent reports of a type F. It is impossible to determine in the acute situation the type of toxin involved in a case of botulism. As a result, the initial treatment requires use of a trivalent (A, B, and E) antiserum, which will be described in more detail in the section on treatment.

Geographic Considerations

Despite the difficulty in differentiating toxin type, some epidemiologic information is of interest and might perhaps have increasing relevance in the future. Of the outbreaks reported in the United States, approximately 40% were tested for type of toxin; 26% were type A, 7.8% were type B, and 4.2% were type E. Although outbreaks were reported from 44 states, 5 states (California, Oregon, Washington, Colorado, and New Mexico) accounted for more than half the cases. This may relate to the altitude, particularly in Colorado and New Mexico. A large part of these two states has an altitude greater than 5,000 feet, with a resultant reduction in the temperature at which water boils. At 5,000 feet, water boils at approximately 95°C (203°F) — as compared with 100°C (212°F) at sea level. Any chef can tell you this difference is important in food preparation. At 10,000 feet, water boils at about 90°C (194°F). Temperature makes a substantial difference when it comes to killing spores of *C. botulinum* in foods. A large-scale test demonstrated that type A and type B spores can be totally destroyed by boiling for 6.5 hours at 100°C. At 95°C, the time required for killing spores is doubled (13 hours). Using a pressure cooker can make a substantial difference. Heating to 120°C (248°F) resulted in spore death within 3 minutes. Although spores are resistant to heat, toxin is readily inactivated by heat. Boiling for 5 minutes, even at high altitude, ensures destruction of the toxin.

More than 90% of reported botulism outbreaks caused by type A occurred west of the Mississippi River. Two thirds of the reported type B outbreaks occurred in eastern states. Most of the type E outbreaks in the United States occurred in Alaska or in the Great Lakes region. No type A or type B has been reported from Alaska.

Types of Food Implicated

Botulism is much more likely to result from home-processed foods — particularly those that are smoked, pickled, or home-canned — than from commercially processed foods.[23] Despite the widely publicized outbreaks that have resulted from commercially prepared foods, of 766 outbreaks in the United States over a 78-year period,[24] only 66 could be traced to commercial foods.* Home-canned vegetables (e.g., tomatoes, beans) have been frequently implicated. If the pH of the food is lower than 4.5, toxin formation is unlikely though there have been some reports of toxin production from pickled herring kept at a pH of 4 to 4.2. Cases have been reported from smoked fish, ham, and other meats. The word botulism actually arises from the Latin *botulus*, which means sausage. In Alaska, a recent outbreak involved

---

*The CDC reports have been confusing in this statistic. In a report by a CDC representative in 1969, the statement appears that "since 1910 . . . only a few outbreaks have been ascribed to commercially prepared foods." In a 1977 report, the figure is given of 66 such outbreaks. This seems larger than "a few." No definitions of "commercially prepared foods" are given that might account for this apparent difference.

Case 1. A middle-aged man in good health had a complete dinner at a buffet one evening when he was traveling. He slept well that night and the next day decided to return to his home town by automobile. As he was driving, he noticed his eyes were "more tired than usual." By approximately 6 PM (24 hours after ingestion), he noticed he had some blurring of vision and a slight staggering of gait. He went to bed that night feeling generalized malaise and weakness, and at 5:30 AM (35.5 hours after ingestion), he awakened with nausea and vomiting. At that point, he had difficulty speaking, poor respirations, and generalized weakness. He went to a hospital emergency department, and the initial suspicion was that he had suffered a stroke. However, the next day his condition was recognized as botulism.

Examination showed an obese man with a slight tachycardia of 108, normal temperature, and normal blood pressure. His extraocular muscles showed weakness of the third, fourth, and sixth cranial nerves, and his deep tendon reflexes were decreased. His arterial blood gases showed a PO_2 of 55, a PCO_2 of 25, and pH of 7.48. His white blood cell count was 7,000, with 36 segment cells and 36 bands.

Over the next 24 hours, he had progressive respiratory difficulty and required intubation and later tracheostomy and ventilator support. Initial treatment included penicillin, 4 million units per day for 1 week, and he received 2 ampules of multivalent antitoxin. Subsequently, the type of *C. botulinum* toxin was identified as type A.

After a stormy hospital course, he began to improve and was discharged after 3 months of hospitalization. Five days after discharge from the hospital he was found dead in a chair. The cause of death was officially listed as cardiovascular disease, though the postmortem examination was inconclusive.

Case 2. An older man had eaten at a banquet somewhere between 6 and 8 PM. The next morning, at approximately 3 AM, 8 to 9 hours after the meal, he began to experience blurred vision that progressed to double vision. By early morning, he had slurred speech and swallowing problems, and he was stumbling. Emergency department personnel suspected that he had had a stroke. Subsequently, as the word spread about a local botulism outbreak, the diagnosis was established. Over the next 12 hours (18 to 30 hours after ingestion), he had increasing respiratory distress and was intubated and put on ventilator treatment. At this time, he had diffuse weakness (proximal muscles weaker than distal). He also was constipated and had urinary retention. His initial treatment was 4 million units of penicillin per day for 5 days, and one vial of multivalent antitoxin intravenously and another intramuscularly. He was discharged after 2 months. However, more than 6 months later, he still had some muscle weakness and occasional difficulty in swallowing.

Neurologic signs and symptoms develop within 1 to 2 weeks following a wound that has been contaminated with *C. botulinum*. The wound is usually one that has significant tissue injury, such as an open fracture, crush injury, or amputation. In all three of the recent cases, treatment with cephalosporin antibiotics failed to be prophylactic against the colonization of the bacteria in the wound. Wounds infected with *C. botulinum* may appear quite innocuous, without induration, crepitus, or lymphadenopathy. The neurologic picture is indistinguishable from that which occurs following ingestion of the toxin, and treatment with antitoxin is advised as soon as this rare syndrome is suspected. Perhaps physicians should inquire as to previous wounds when investigating patients with neurologic complaints. Unlike cases of food-borne botulism in which a certain amount of toxin is ingested, wound botulism results in an ongoing production of toxin. Delays in diagnosis may make a substantial difference in the clinical course.

The two cases above illustrate the difficulty of diagnosing food-borne botulism and its possible serious outcome.

Clinical Signs and Course

The following facts have been noted concerning botulism outbreaks:

1. In many outbreaks, initial cases are incorrectly diagnosed as flu, viral syndrome, or stroke. Early recognition and diagnosis are most difficult. It is important to note that in neither of the preceding cases was the correct diagnosis made on initial physician contact.

2. Symptoms usually appear within the first 24 hours

stored beaver tail and beaver flippers. The incidence of botulism appears to be higher among Eskimos because of their storage method, and ingestion of uncooked seal and whale meat.

Spoilage of the food may be obvious, but relying on gross signs is inadequate because of the lethality of very small amounts of the toxin. Although toxin-containing foods are the principal cause of the clinical syndrome of botulism, wound botulism has been reported in association with soil-contaminated deep wounds suitable for growth of the anaerobic *C. botulinum*.

Wound Botulism

The syndrome of botulism following infection of a wound by *C. botulinum* was first reported in 1943.

but may be delayed as long as 48 hours or even longer than 72 hours. My experience with a local outbreak exhibited a range of 8 to 80 hours for patients to develop initial symptoms.

3. Earliest symptoms involve vague malaise, headache, weakness, dizziness, blurred vision, and sometimes dry mouth.*

4. Progression is variable, but, most commonly, initial symptoms appear, and in severe cases, progression over the subsequent 6 to 8 hours leads to respiratory paralysis. Of 34 cases studied locally, 11 required mechanical ventilation. Botulism can be mild; symptoms may rarely progress beyond nausea and mild visual problems, or perhaps fatigue. Mild cases usually clear in 1 week.

5. An important early symptom is blurring of vision. Patients usually do not complain of classic diplopia. Instead, they say, "Everything is blurred," or "I can't get the image into focus," or "My eyes are tired or wandering."

6. Progression of more severe cases includes increasing problems with vision, slurred speech, dryness of mouth, diffuse weakness, difficulty in swallowing, and difficulty in walking, usually described as "staggering." The rapidity of the course is highly individual over a 24-hour period. Most significantly, the sensorium and intellectual functioning remain intact, and memory is not impaired. The neurologic symptoms are usually bilateral and symmetric and are motor, not sensory. The cerebrospinal fluid is normal.

7. Nausea and vomiting may occur, but large studies have demonstrated that in only 30 to 40% of cases of botulism were nausea and vomiting prominent. With detailed questioning, nausea was found as a symptom in 60 to 70% of patients. In contrast, visual difficulty was reported in more than 90% of the patients. Constipation and urinary disturbance were found in less than 50% of the patients. The visual disturbance results from abducens nerve palsy.

8. More severe cases show early third cranial nerve involvement. Pupils may become fixed and dilated.

9. *As a general rule, the earlier the onset, the more severe the case.*

Clinical Differentiation

In the elderly patient, early cases are difficult to diagnose as are mild cases that do not progress. No laboratory test can readily be used to diagnose botulism in the emergency department. Common conditions that figure in the differential diagnosis include Guillain-Barré syndrome, cardiovascular accident or transient ischemic attack, tick paralysis, heavy metal poisoning (particularly lead), psychiatric conditions, drug abuse, alcohol intoxication, or untoward reaction to medication — anticholinergic

type, myasthenia gravis, phenytoin toxicity, atropine poisoning, encephalitis, carbon monoxide poisoning, electrolyte abnormalities, and amyotrophic lateral sclerosis.

Diagnosis rests on clinical grounds. Confirmation comes from observing botulism in a mouse (sensitive to 900 molecules) that has been injected with toxin from the patient's serum or with the suspected food. It is worthwhile to test for toxin even weeks after the onset of clinical illness because of the high sensitivity of the mouse to the toxin as well as the reports of circulating toxin even 2 weeks after onset. *C. botulinum* and toxin also may be identified in the patient's feces.

Put all specimens in *leak-proof* containers, and remember that the *C. botulinum* toxin is the most powerful toxin known. In case of a spill, neutralize the specimens with a strong alkaline solution if available. Suitable specimens may include serum, stool, vomitus, food samples, food containers, or wound material. The specimens should be refrigerated. Label carefully! Include, in particular, any drugs the patient is taking. Call the CDC for further information.

Medical Treatment

Immediate care. Immediate attention must be given to airway and respiratory function. When deaths occur initially, they almost always result from respiratory paralysis. Careful gastric lavage should be performed. Emesis can be initiated if there is a good gag reflex. In addition, charcoal should be instilled through the tube after emesis and lavage. A cathartic is unlikely to be helpful but can be used and may speed the flow of the charcoal. Similarly, colonic enemas can be used.

If there is difficulty with breathing and arterial blood gases and if vital capacity deteriorates or initially shows hypoxia, hypercapnia, or a measurement of less than 100 mL, a tracheostomy should be considered. Certainly, with borderline cases, a trial of ventilatory assistance can be instituted prior to any surgical procedure. In the large 1977 Michigan outbreak of type B botulism, the presence of ptosis, dilated and sluggishly reacting pupils, and paresis of the medial recti was associated with the need for artificial ventilatory support in 8 of 11 patients. These aspects of third nerve dysfunction became apparent after approximately 12 hours. Tracheostomy is best performed as a slow, careful procedure under ideal conditions, since a ventilator may be necessary for months.

Antitoxin therapy. Trivalent antitoxin is available from the CDC and should be administered to all patients with suspected botulism. Each vial of equine antiserum contains 7,500 IU of type A, 5,500 IU of type B, and 8,500 IU of type E antitoxins. One to two vials are administered intravenously initially and again in 4 hours. One vial of antiserum may be given intramuscularly in 24 hours; repeated injections may be indicated, depending on the clinical condition. Desensitization may be necessary because the antitoxin is a horse serum derivative. In cases of

---

*In the largest series of botulism patients from a single outbreak (in Michigan, 1977), dry mouth was found in all those affected, and 86% had difficulty with focusing or diplopia. This outbreak was type B in origin.

known reactions to horse serum, 100 mg of hydrocortisone can be injected prior to the use of antiserum. Allergic reactions can be treated with antihistamines or steroids, or both. Of 30 patients in the 1978 New Mexico outbreak who received antitoxin, one developed serum sickness.

Penicillin. Penicillin is indicated in the management of patients with wound botulism, because this form of botulism is caused by active infection with *C. botulinum*. Since botulinum food poisoning is usually caused by toxin and not by the organism, penicillin probably serves no role in management of these patients; however, it is often used on an empiric basis and may occasionally treat a *C. botulinum* intestinal infection.[25] Penicillin therapy is usually continued for 1 week.

Guanidine hydrochloride. Guanidine hydrochloride has been used experimentally to chemically compete with the toxin. No dramatic results have been observed with guanidine, and its use is no longer routinely recommended.

Respiratory function. Continued meticulous maintenance of respiratory function is a most important aspect of treatment. A patient's improvement is best followed by a periodic assessment of vital capacity and arterial blood gases *off* ventilatory support. In cases of preexisting pulmonary disease, the baseline state may require estimation.

Hospitalization. In severe cases, patients may be hospitalized for as long as 3 to 6 months. Weaning from the ventilator may be difficult. With long-term hospitalization, release from the hospital must follow a graded rehabilitation program. Muscle wasting, lack of conditioning, orthostatic hypotension, and syncope frequently follow prolonged bed rest and muscle inactivity. There may be some minor dysphagia or malaise 6 to 12 months after the onset of illness.

Food Poisoning Caused by Microorganisms
Shigellosis

The *Shigella* species are aerobic, gram-negative, nonmotile bacteria. There are four main species, all of which can cause human disease. Asymptomatic carriers are common.

When bacillary dysentery occurs, the cause can be the ingestion of as few as 200 organisms. If a "suboptimal" number of bacteria are ingested, or if there is some immunity, an individual can have a subclinical infection or a nonsymptomatic carrier state. The range of clinical illness is very broad.

Although the condition is found more often in the tropics, it is endemic throughout the world. Epidemics have been traced to a variety of foods contaminated by feces, but, most commonly, milk, eggs, and dairy products are implicated.

The incubation period is usually about 48 hours; however, it may be as short as 8 hours, or symptoms can be postponed for a week. It appears that there is some small intestinal colonization, but the large intestine is the

preferred area. Bacterial growth depends on factors of immunity and existing flora, as well as the number of *Shigella* organisms. Usually, within 1 week after recovery, the organism is not found in the feces.

Occasionally, sequelae are reported, including neuropathy, arthritis, and skin eruptions. Sepsis in the acute stage is rare, but serious.

SYMPTOMS AND SIGNS OF SHIGELLA POISONING

1. Severe diarrhea: mucous, bloody stools
2. Abdominal colic and tenderness
3. Tenesmus
4. Fever to 40°C (104°F) and malaise
5. Pain often relieved by defecation
6. Bowel sounds active and high pitched
7. Possible syncope and hypotension with *Shigella dysenteriae;* if this species is responsible for the illness, it usually is more severe
8. Outpouring of polymorphonucleocytes into the intestines and stool; sometimes sheets of white blood cells can be seen microscopically
9. Rise in fever and white blood cell count
10. Hypotension and circulatory collapse (more common in the elderly)

Diagnosis. Table 28–3 shows a differential diagnosis of shigellosis with a comparison of amebic dysentery. The following features are helpful in diagnosis:

1. Stool culture
2. A rise in serum agglutinin titer in 50% of the cases — however, not useful in diagnosis or treatment because of the delay
3. White blood cell count usually greater than 10,000 with a left shift

Treatment. For management of shigellosis, give supportive treatment by preventing dehydration and maintaining electrolytes. The diarrheal condition is usually self-limited. However, shock with dehydration and acidosis may occur, requiring intensive treatment.

Antibiotics are useful in moderate to severe cases for shortening the clinical course. *Possible choices* include *ampicillin*, 1 g intravenously every 6 hours in severe cases; otherwise, ampicillin 500 mg orally 4 times daily for 5 days. This has been the accepted treatment for the past 8 to 10 years. However, drug-resistant strains have resulted. Thus, selection of an antibiotic is more difficult. *Other choices* include *cephalothin* or its derivatives, 1 g 4 times a day. *Chloramphenicol* was the old standby, but risk of toxicity and bone marrow suppression has made it a less desirable choice.

Antidiarrheal agents (e.g., diphenoxylate hydrochloride and atropine [Lomotil], paregoric, or opiates) must be used cautiously because they may prolong the clinical

Table 28–3   Acute Differentiation of Shigellosis from Amebic Dysentery in Elderly Patients*

Amebic dysentery	Shigella
Usually slower in progression with mild to moderate diarrhea	Rapid onset often with severe explosive diarrhea with cramps and tenesmus
Temperature usually less than 101°F	Temperature usually more than 101.5°F (though hypothermia may be present)
Usually moderate symptoms that tend to wax and wane (only rarely presenting with a fulminant course with explosive diarrhea)	Rapid dehydration can lead to hypotension and shock (which is the reason for the estimated 10 to 20% mortality rate in the elderly)
Blood in stool on microscopic examination	Gross blood in stool
Fecal smear shows mononuclear cells and trophozoites	Fecal smear shows many leukocytes
Other systemic manifestations outside of the gastrointestinal tract (e.g., amebic liver abscesses, lung abscesses, central nervous system [CNS] symptoms, intestinal perforation, peritonitis)	Some systemic manifestations (e.g., meningitis, pyelonephritis, and osteomyelitis) have been reported but are rare. Other manifestations — e.g., arthritis or Reiter's syndrome — occur days to weeks after the acute syndrome. Abdominal pain is common, however.

*A therapeutic trial with antibiotics is necessary if shigellosis is suspected since the mortality is so much higher in the elderly.

course. Nonproductive tenesmus would be the best indication for using such agents.

For amebic colitis, antimicrobial therapy is needed — usually metronidazole followed in 1 week by diiodohydroxyquin (to eradicate cysts). (See Table 28–3.)

Geriatric patients often require hospitalization and intensive treatment.

Salmonellosis

The salmonellae, named for Dr. Salmon who described them in 1885, are gram-negative motile bacteria. The most common form of salmonella-induced human disease is the syndrome of *Salmonella* gastroenteritis. The range of gastroenteritis can be mild to severe, with the latter being associated with abdominal pain, colitis, and signs of a systemic inflammation (fever, elevated white blood cell count, malaise, and so on).

Typhoid fever is caused by *Salmonella typhosa* and differs from the common gastroenteritis primarily by its severity, prolonged course, and hematogenous dissemination of the bacillus with accompanying diffuse manifestations. A persistent carrier state can result.

The primary reservoir is the vertebrate intestine, and the passage is from person to person by fecal contamination of foodstuffs. Most commonly, meat, poultry, dairy, and egg products have been implicated. However, other items, including creamy foods and prepared salads, have been implicated. Sterilization of contaminated foods is not always achieved by cooking, especially in large stuffed turkeys and in cooked eggs. The disease may also be transmitted by pets, since salmonellae can cause disease in animals. Dogs, cats, birds, and turtles have been commonly implicated.

To produce clinical disease in humans, at least 100,000 to 1 million bacteria of the nontyphoid salmonellae are usually required. To achieve these levels, a growth medium (i.e., food) is necessary, because simple contamination usually does not involve transfer of so many organisms. Subsequently, intestinal multiplication occurs. The need for a "minimum dose" makes direct fecal-oral transmission uncommon and in the United States water-borne transmission is uncommon because of overall water sanitation.

The clinical disease results from an infection. There appears to be no production of toxin. Thus, prevention must focus on overall sanitation and identification of asymptomatic carriers. Prevention is important not only in terms of human comfort but also in view of studies that have demonstrated that salmonellosis costs at least $500 to $1,000 per case for diagnosis, treatment, and follow-up, and unquestionably more in the elderly.

Because *Salmonella* bacteria are killed at a pH level of 2, the use of an antacid may increase susceptibility, as will conditions of reduced stomach acidity (including subtotal gastrectomy, vagotomy, and gastroenterostomy). It was noted that mortality was higher also in *E. coli* colitis in those who had achlorhydria.

Salmonella gastroenteritis is a reportable infectious disease. Estimates have been made that the incidence reported by the CDC (10 cases per 100,000 population) represents one tenth to one hundredth of the actual incidence. The incidence is highest in the summer.

Increased intercountry tourism, as well as intercountry trade involving foods, has resulted in increased risks of acquiring *Salmonella* gastroenteritis. There are more than 2,500 species of *Salmonella,* some of which are found in one country and not in another. Mass tourism tends to make a more uniform distribution (one of the aspects of a "world community"). The largest outbreak of *Salmonella* food poisoning in recorded history occurred in the United States in March, 1985. This situation demonstrates the impact of large companies with wide food distribution. More than 14,000 cases were reported (almost all confirmed) with at least four associated deaths. The source was a large dairy, and contaminated low-fat milk was the vehicle for transmission of the *Salmonella typhimurium*. Lawsuits involving at least $100 million have been filed.

Some epidemiologists believe *Salmonella* infections are increasing, in part, because of the widespread use of antibiotics in animal feed and the development of drug-resistant bacteria.[26] These can be passed widely by contaminated beef or chicken.

Although most acute symptoms subside within 2 to 5 days, occasionally a prolonged course of weeks occurs. Death from *Salmonella* gastroenteritis is uncommon and occurs primarily in infants and the aged and persons with severe underlying disease.

SYMPTOMS AND COURSE OF SALMONELLA POISONING

1. General incubation period is 8 to 48 hours.
2. Complaints of general malaise, headache, mild abdominal pain, and fever of 37.78° to 38.33°C (100° to 101°F) are common initially.
3. Despite some nausea and vomiting that may occur, major symptoms are cramps and diarrhea; tenesmus is common and may help in diagnosis.
4. Rarely, bloody diarrhea is present; shigellosis and amebic dysentery are more often associated with bloody stools.
5. Occasionally, abdominal symptoms are so severe as to suggest appendicitis or some other acute intraabdominal process.

Although arbitrary divisions have been made between "gastroenteritis" and the systemic disease "typhoid fever," the division may not be clinically clear-cut. *Salmonella* bacteria other than *S. typhosa* (the cause of typhoid fever) may produce gastrointestinal symptoms, as well as sustained fever, and even positive blood cultures. In addition, it is possible to be infected by *Salmonella* bacteria and have few gastrointestinal signs and symptoms but manifest chills, fever, anorexia, and even some hepatosplenomegaly. Spiking fever, headache, abdominal cramps, and rose spots on the torso are useful diagnostically.

The presence of bacteremia may result in a localized internal abscess, and even endocarditis, septic arthritis, or osteomyelitis can occur. Such severe infections usually show striking signs and a marked leukocytosis, though in typhoid fever leukopenia occurs after the first 1 to 2 weeks. The elderly are much more susceptible to endocarditis due to preexisting valvular disease.

Diagnosis. Diagnosis and differentiation from shigel-losis, enterotoxic *E. coli,* and amebic dysentery may be difficult. Other less common causes of acute diarrheal disease, such as that produced by *Vibrio parahaemolyticus* or viral agents, can also cause difficulty in diagnosis.

Clinically, definitive diagnosis rests on isolation of the organism from the stool. If the contaminated food is available, it can be cultured. Excretions from pets can be tested as well if they appear to be possible sources.

A fecal smear may show inflammatory leukocytes but, usually, somewhat less than with shigellosis and amebic dysentery. Bloody diarrhea is uncommon in *Salmonella* enterocolitis.

If there are systemic signs, blood cultures may show bacteremia. Although immunologic tests of various titers may show increases, the time delays usually render such tests of limited value.

Treatment. The cornerstone of treatment is prompt correction of dehydration and fluid and electrolyte imbalances. Intravenous fluids are often necessary, depending on clinical symptoms.

Antimotility agents (e.g., Lomotil and similar agents) that inhibit activity of the bowel substantially may also increase the severity of the disease. Experimental animals pretreated with antimotility agents showed increased susceptibility to *Salmonella* infection. If symptoms are severe and no contraindications are present, a low dose of morphine or atropine can be used to partially relieve symptoms.

In cases of limited *Salmonella* gastroenteritis, the use of antibiotics does not appear to be generally helpful. In fact, there is some evidence that the excretion of the organism occurs for a longer period of time after antibiotics have been used.

If the patient shows high fever, chills, or other evidence of severe systemic infection, antibiotics are indicated. Chloramphenicol (50 to 60 mg/kg/day in 4 to 6 doses) has been used, but because of toxicity, ampicillin (100 to 200 mg/kg/day in 4 divided doses) is recommended. Third-generation cephalothin derivative antibiotics have also been used successfully. The course of antibiotics is for 10 days to 2 weeks. In cases in which there is evidence of an abscess, endocarditis, osteomyelitis, or other evidence of persistent internal infection, antibiotics may have to be continued for 4 to 6 weeks, and surgical drainage may be needed.

Enteropathic E. Coli (Traveler's Diarrhea)

Method of acquisition. Dairy and meat products or contaminated water are common vehicles for infection. There is some suggestive evidence that bismuth salicylate may be effective prophylactic therapy against traveler's diarrhea (30 to 60 mL every 4 hours). However, this may increase susceptibility to other forms of food poisoning. In addition, other prepared foods (salads, sauces) may harbor bacteria from fecal contamination. A general rule is to eat cooked foods shortly after preparation and to wash and peel raw fruits and vegetables thoroughly.

Symptoms and course of illness. Acute diarrhea may begin 8 to 12 hours after ingestion of contaminated food or water, though there may be a delayed onset of up to several days. Common symptoms include abdominal cramps, tenesmus, and profuse watery diarrhea, though there is a wide range of clinical illness.

There appear to be two types of *E. coli* associated with food poisoning. One type does not produce a toxin, and symptoms result from intestinal infection. The other type is more commonly associated with the epidemic diarrhea of travelers, and this type does produce an enterotoxin. In the latter type, symptoms result from infection as well as from the effect of the toxin upon the colon. In general, *E. coli* produces a clinical disease that is usually milder than *Salmonella* disease or shigellosis, but in severe cases it may be indistinguishable from them. In fact, one strain of *E. coli* can cause severe hemorrhagic colitis and produce a toxin similar to one produced by *Shigella dysenteriae.* This is the type associated with high institutional mortality, e.g., in nursing homes.[20]

E. coli is of particular concern in the aged, who have limited tolerance to an electrolyte imbalance because of their overall condition, an underlying illness, or the taking of medications that can affect electrolytes (e.g., diuretics).

Diagnosis. Diagnosis may be possible by isolating the organism in food or water and by culturing a stool. Serologic diagnosis through testing for rises in titer against *E. coli* can be done, but such tests are not readily available. Smear of stool is important. Polymorphonucleocytes can be present, though usually less than with shigellosis. Bloody diarrhea is also less common, but has been associated with severe outbreaks.

Treatment. Supportive treatments are generally satisfactory for mild cases. Moderate to severe cases require antibiotic treatment and intensive fluid and electrolyte stabilization. The disease generally lasts in its acute form for only 2 or 3 days. However, nonspecific symptoms and malaise usually continue for at least 1 week.

Doxycycline (100 mg orally per day) has shown a demonstrable benefit when used prophylactically. Doxycycline or tetracycline should be used in severe cases when there is evidence of high fever. Bactrim (trimethoprim-sulfamethoxazole) has also been used successfully. In the usual case, however, the disease is treated effectively with clear liquids and intravenous fluids if the diarrhea is severe enough to produce dehydration or electrolyte imbalance. The over 80 age group is at much higher risk, and must be hospitalized for aggressive treatment.

Other causes of traveler's diarrhea. While *E. coli* is the most common cause, traveler's diarrhea may also be caused by other microorganisms including rotavirus (up to 10% of cases), *Salmonella* or *Shigella* (15 to 20%), and parasites (0 to 5%). Rotavirus infection is generally self-limiting.

G. lamblia infection generally occurs days to weeks after the exposure and is characterized by foul-smelling, watery stools. A stool smear and culture will help in diagnosing this parasite. This condition is usually not severe, but it occasionally requires treatment with metronidazole (250 mg 3 times daily for 5 days). Quinacrine may also be used.

E. histolytica is a parasite that invades the mucous membranes of the intestines, resulting in ulcerations, hemorrhage, and diarrhea. In severe cases, the parasite may cause perforation of the intestines or may invade other organs, particularly the liver or lung. Diagnosis rests on physical examination, stool examination, and possible liver function tests and liver scan. Treatment of confirmed cases is mandatory and should include metronidazole and iodoquinol.

C. Perfringens Conditions

C. perfringens is a nonmotile, gram-positive, spore-forming rod. Disease is caused by growth of bacteria and toxin formation. It is now considered to be one of the most common types of food poisoning.

Method of acquisition. Meat and poultry products are commonly implicated, as are gravies and creamy (dairy or mayonnaise-containing) foods.

Symptoms and course of illness. Because large numbers of organisms (usually greater than 10^6 organisms per gram) are generally necessary to cause significant disease, most food poisoning resulting from *C. perfringens* is relatively mild. The incubation period is more than 8 hours and usually less than 24 hours. The disease is associated with cramps and diarrhea. Diarrhea is generally not as profuse as that found with *Shigella, Salmonella,* or *E. coli*; characteristically, it is not bloody. There may be mild nausea, but vomiting is uncommon.

Diagnosis. Diagnosis is made by detection of the organism in food and stool.

Treatment. Symptomatic therapy is generally all that is required.

B. Cereus Conditions

B. cereus is a slightly curved gram-positive rod found singly and in chains. The organism is motile. Disease arises from infection and some toxin production.

Method of acquisition. Food, particularly meat, dairy, and poultry products, has been discovered to be contaminated with this organism. Dried foods (e.g., mixes, potatoes) may be contaminated. Growth does not ordinarily occur until hydration.

Symptoms and course of illness. Average incubation period is 8 to 12 hours. Average duration of illness is approximately 24 hours. Symptoms in order of magnitude are diarrhea, abdominal cramps, nausea, and vomiting. Fever is generally absent or is below 37.78°C (100°F).

Treatment. Supportive therapy with intravenous fluids is usually sufficient even for relatively severe cases. Antinauseants may be given. There is no evidence that antibiotics are of value.

Cholera

Cholera is caused by *V. cholerae,* a curved, motile, gram-negative rod. This condition is included because it can be rapidly fatal. Fortunately, however, it is rare in the United States at this time. During worldwide cholera pandemics, the United States has had many cases (e.g., 150,000 deaths in 1832 and 1849 and 50,000 deaths in 1866). In the United States, cholera is still endemic along the Gulf Coast with cases being reported particularly from Texas and Louisiana, where association with contaminated water and seafood has been found. While uncommon, this disease poses a great threat to the elderly due to the massive, rapid fluid-electrolyte shifts.

Method of acquisition. In the epidemic form, the *Vibrio* organisms are usually water-borne or come from seafood. Person-to-person transmission is usually in the nonepidemic form. Occasionally, it may come from a restaurant in which a worker is infected. Food can also become contaminated, particularly when "night soil" (human excrement) is used as a fertilizer.

Symptoms and course of illness. The illness develops usually within 8 to 48 hours after ingestion. With it comes a severe enteritis associated with passage of copious amounts of non-foul-smelling diarrhea usually containing mucus and occasionally blood. The disease arises in association with an exotoxin that causes a severe disorder of the intestinal tract and results in marked intestinal secretions. Frequently, the first stool is more than 1,000 mL with a characteristic appearance of "rice water." The symptoms arise directly from the gastrointestinal fluid and electrolyte losses. Prostration and a shocklike state may occur rapidly. The patient may die within 12 to 24 hours if intravenous fluids or oral electrolytes are not provided. The illness characteristically lasts 1 to 7 days. With adequate fluid and electrolyte repletion, recovery is rapid. Hypokalemia is a particular problem in those older people taking diuretics.

Diagnosis. Clinical suspicion of cholera is important, particularly in endemic or epidemic areas. Persons with decreased stomach acidity (because of surgical operations and antacids) are at higher risk. Also, those with type O blood are at higher risk for unknown reasons.

The organism may be identified by culture, and one may look for the organisms on a Gram stain slide. At medical centers familiar with cholera, a fluorescent antibody technique may identify the organism positively within 1 hour.

Treatment. The patient in a shock state must be treated with intravenous fluids. Oral fluids may be used when intravenous fluids are not available. A glucose-containing electrolyte solution may be given orally.

Generally, acidosis, severe potassium losses, and dehydration occur. Those experienced in treating cholera use weight as a measure of dehydration and consider the case to be severe if there is greater than a 10% body weight loss and mild if the loss is less than 5%.

In severely ill patients, the use of tetracycline has caused a highly significant reduction in total stool volume and duration of diarrhea and has resulted in a more rapid disappearance of the organism from the stool. The dose administered should be approximately 1 g of tetracycline by mouth initially, then at least 500 mg every 6 hours for a total of 3 days. The usual stool composition per liter in adults is sodium (135 mEq), potassium (15 mEq), bicarbonate (45 mEq), and chloride (100 mEq).

Cholera may be prevented by cooking all foods thoroughly, boiling water, and immunization, which seems to offer up to 75% protection for up to 18 months. Even when clinical disease develops, cholera appears to be less severe in the vaccinated patient.

Campylobacter Enteritis

Method of acquisition. Raw milk most frequently has been implicated in the transmission of *Campylobacter* enteritis.

Diagnosis. Diagnosis rests on isolating the organism (*Campylobacter fetus* subspecies *jejuni*) from a fecal specimen.

The common symptoms include diarrhea (in more than 90%), abdominal pain (in more than 80%), frequently with fever, headache, nausea, or vomiting. Bloody diarrhea is less common, but blood in the stool is present in about one fourth of cases.

Treatment. Treatment is supportive but must include identifying and stopping the offending food. In elderly patients, this ordinarily benign, self-limiting condition may develop into a severe illness, and tetracycline, sulfamethoxazole (Bactrim), or erythromycin should be used along with intravenous fluid therapy.

Listeriosis

Caused by the gram-positive bacillus *Listeria monocytogenes,* listeriosis can result in septicemia and meningitis as well as focal infectious symptoms. Milk and cheese products have been increasingly involved in its spread throughout the population. There is an increased susceptibility in immunocompromised patients. Ampicillin is usually the antibiotic of choice in treatment. Recent outbreaks (1985) may indicate an increasing problem.[27]

Staphylococcal Food Poisoning

Enterotoxic staphylococci are found widely on the skin and mucous membranes of many individuals. Most staphylococci (a gram-positive, clustered coccus) cannot elaborate this particular toxin.

When foodstuffs are contaminated, a lack of refrigeration and a warm environment are ideal conditions for bacterial growth and toxin elaboration. Foods usually implicated are those with a high fat content such as creamy cakes, custards, creamed soups, mayonnaise, and so on. However, cases resulting from meat products have also been reported. Milk has been rarely implicated. The ideal food as a culture medium is pancake batter, which has a pH close to 7, a high moisture content, and is frequently left without refrigeration for hours. Also beware of turkey stuffing and the "too-beautiful" cooked and dressed turkey too large to fit into a refrigerator and handled by many persons during its preparation.

Staphylococcal food poisoning is common. The toxin is preformed and is remarkably "heat stable." Therefore, even if food is subsequently cooked, a period of hours is necessary for toxin destruction. In fact, in one test, autoclaving for 15 minutes did not result in substantial reduction in potency.

There are at least four different types of toxin, but all may be elaborated by the same organism and, with minor variation, all have the same unfortunate effect.

Symptoms and course of illness. Symptoms usually begin within ½ hour to 6 hours after ingestion and may begin slowly or violently. Severe nausea and vomiting are common. The affected individual vomits repeatedly, then has dry heaves and may even vomit blood — probably representing a vomiting-induced Mallory-Weiss syndrome. After vomiting, abdominal cramps may become severe and diarrhea may develop. However, the diarrhea is usually relatively mild, and the individual scarcely notices this symptom.

Patients appear markedly "gray" and severely ill. Severe dehydration can result, and intravenous therapy must be started. Although the acute stage usually lasts less than 12 hours, many patients complain of severe nausea and malaise for 1 to 2 days. Hospitalization is often needed.

Milder cases do occur and may not be diagnosed as staphylococcal food poisoning unless a careful history is taken.

Initial studies were conducted with paid volunteers. Despite increased pay, few, if any, said they would volunteer again. Thus, current studies are done with primates, but monkeys are far less susceptible than humans. Toxin is not formed in appreciable amounts below 12.78°C (55°F) or above 48.89°C (120°F). If the food is acidic, toxin is produced very slowly, depending on temperature and acidity. If there is contaminated food with a pH of 7, or greater than 30% moisture content, appreciable amounts of toxin are produced in 4 ½ hours at 32.22°C (90°F). Given the same food, but changing the temperature, the same amount of toxin was produced in 10 hours at 18.33°C (65°F) and in 9 hours at 46.11°C (115°F). *Thus, the conclusion is that to prevent staphylococcal food poisoning, "keep it hot, keep it cold, or eat it within 2 hours."* Frequently, institutions such as nursing homes must prepare large quantities of food in advance, increasing the risk.

Simple diagnosis can be made by a Gram stain of the suspected food, which will show abundant staphylococci if contaminated (although this, of course, is not a test for the toxin). A culture can verify type, but the time period necessary for culturing renders the findings primarily of scholarly interest.

Treatment. To manage a staphylococcal food poisoning, give intravenous fluids. To prevent retching, use 10 mg compazine intramuscularly. Also, propantheline bromide, 15 mg or 30 mg intramuscularly, is effective. Medications that reduce stomach acid secretion are also useful such as H_2 blockers (e.g., cimetidine or ranitidine). Monitor electrolytes and urine output.

Fatalities have been reported because of mineral imbalance and dehydration. In the elderly, the severe retching may worsen existing heart disease, and myocardial infarction has been reported.

Since the disease is caused by a preformed toxin, antibiotics are of no value. No suitable antitoxin is available for routine use.

Physicians should document their findings carefully since many restaurant outbreaks result in legal action.

Although the acute stage generally is over within 2 days, weakness and malaise can often last for weeks.

Trichinosis

The worm *Trichinella spiralis* enters the body through pork or other meat that has been inadequately cooked. For many reasons, the United States does not routinely inspect for trichinosis, although an enzyme assay being developed will allow such testing in the future — a necessity for exporting pork to many countries.[28]

Trichinosis in humans causes weakness, swelling, and muscle pain along with general malaise and a low-grade fever. The duration of the acute illness is usually 3 weeks, although chronic indolent cases have been reported as well as rapidly developing cases leading to death.

According to the CDC, only 60 cases were reported in 1984. Autopsy studies have demonstrated that up to 4% of Americans harbor *Trichinella* worms in their muscles. Thus, very few cases are actually diagnosed. Symptoms are usually ascribed to "flu." The condition is rarely progressive. More often, the worms become encapsulated and do not cause later clinical disease. The risk of having trichinosis increases with age.

Shellfish-Associated Food Poisoning

Shellfish may be associated with typhoid fever, hepatitis, cholera, *Campylobacter* gastroenteritis, *V. parahaemolyticus* infection, and viral gastroenteritis. Of the latter type, the most common cause at this time appears to be the Norwalk virus. One study demonstrated widespread outbreaks of clam- and oyster-associated gastroenteritis with the Norwalk virus implicated as the cause.

Of 103 outbreaks affecting 1,017 persons in New York State, the most common symptoms were diarrhea (84%), nausea (52%), abdominal cramps (58%), and vomiting

(30%). Illness lasted only 48 hours in most people but up to a week in a minority. There is no specific treatment. The elderly are the group at highest risk for serious morbidity and mortality from shellfish ingestion. Cooking thoroughly reduces the risk and steaming for at least 4 to 6 minutes after the shell opens will reduce the number of cases dramatically. Elderly people should be advised to have their shellfish "well done."

Food Additives

There are well over a thousand food additives generally recognized as safe (GRAS), most of which are benign. Certain substances may trigger reactions in sensitive people. For example, sulfites are commonly added to fruit and vegetable salads and to potatoes to prevent darkening. Acute attacks of asthma have been triggered by such substances.* Another substance that is widely used is MSG, which acts as a flavor enhancer. Depending on dosage, many people will develop tingling, flushing, diaphoresis, nausea, vomiting, or headache. Some more sensitive individuals respond with behavioral changes including anger and depression. Asthma, chest pain, arrhythmias, balance difficulties, and diarrhea are also common symptoms.[30]

The subject of additives is generally beyond the scope of emergency medicine unless reactions occur that bring people to emergency facilities.

However, when outbreaks of food poisoning or food reactions occur, the emergency facility is often in the best position to detect early "epidemics." It is prudent then to be in touch with the CDC through their reports and the state health department. When there are occasional toxicities (e.g., heavy metal contamination, polychlorinated biphenyls [PCBs]), special testing can be initiated in the emergency department.

Food Poisoning Caused by Chemicals Naturally Present in Foods and Plants

As has been previously discussed, the difference between what is therapeutic and what is toxic may be just a question of dosage. Foods are composed of many chemical substances that are essential for life, such as carbohydrates, proteins, minerals, and vitamins. However, many foods contain chemical substances that are part of their nature but that do not appear to be involved in nutritional processes. In many cases, the chemicals exert modest effects, and even ingestion of large quantities will not exert apparent toxic effects. For example, lettuce contains the chemical lactucin, which exerts sedative effects when it is concentrated. Another example is spinach, which has a high oxalic acid content; however, even with larger ingestions, which might produce feelings of

malaise and bloating, a spinach overdose would only rarely present as a clinical problem. Conversely, there are common foods that can cause severe poisoning because of their being underripe, because too much has been eaten, or because the patient has been taking a pharmacologic agent that interacts in some way with a chemical or chemicals in a food. For example, the "vomiting sickness" of Jamaica has been traced to eating the unripe akee fruit. The toxic substance has been termed "hypolycin" because it acts to rapidly lower blood sugar.

The common potato plant ordinarily has leaves that contain belladonna-type actions. When some potatoes are unripe, belladonna poisoning can occur. In fact, deaths have been linked to eating potatoes. Even recently there have been outbreaks. Dr. Mary McMillan and Dr. S.C. Thompson reported on 78 cases of potato poisoning in 1979. Symptoms included severe circulatory impairment in three who needed hospitalization.[31]

Occasionally, outbreaks can also occur from glands of animals inadvertently allowed to remain in the food. For example, one large outbreak of thyrotoxicosis occurred among residents of southwestern Minnesota and adjacent areas of South Dakota and Iowa. The cause was ground beef prepared from neck trimmings containing large amounts of bovine thyroid hormone. Of these 121 cases, almost 25% were in patients over age 60.[32]

Alcohol is an example of toxicity of a common food in which overdosage may be lethal. However, there are many more. Severe toxicity with sympathomimetic effects can come from an overdose of nutmeg because of the content of myristin, and a prized fish of Japan called "fugu" contains a toxin that exerts cholinergic effects. Overdose can cause cholinergic poisoning.

As an example of food-drug interactions, the presence of tyramine in aged cheese, pickled herring, Chianti wine, and some other aged foods can cause hypertensive crises in patients who are taking monoamine oxidase inhibitors for treatment of depression.

Plant Poisonings

The number of plants that can exert toxic actions is vast. For purposes of emergency treatment, it is useful to identify the major type of chemical actions caused by the poisoning. Table 28–4 identifies common plants and their chemical actions. Table 28–5 offers symptoms and signs associated with plant intoxications, and Table 28–6 was prepared by the Food and Drug Administration (FDA) to alert health professionals and consumers to some herbal remedies that can be dangerous.

Mushroom Poisoning

Although the *Psilocybe* mushroom has gained notoriety, and poisoning from ingestion of these mushrooms can induce severe vomiting, abdominal cramps, and marked hallucinations, the poisoning is relatively benign because of a large tolerance of the body to psilocybin. The mush-

---

*Because of their dangers, sulfites were removed from the "GRAS" list for use in restaurants and salad bars in August of 1985.

Table 28–4 Chemical Actions of Some Poisonous Plants*

Digitalis-like; cardiotoxic
  Foxglove
  Oleander
  Lily-of-the-valley
Atropine-like; anticholinergic
  Jimsonweed
  Larkspur
  Nightshade
  Tomato and potato leaves, green potatoes
  Mandrake
  Henbane
Sympathomimetic; pressors
  Ephedra (Mormon's tea)
  Mistletoe
  Nutmeg
LSD-hallucinogenic effects
  Yohimbe
  Morning glory seeds
Parasympathetic (cholinergic)
  Poinsettia
Strychninelike
  Hemlock (conium fruit)
  Water hemlock (cicutoxin)
Nicotine effects
  Wild tobacco
  Tree tobacco
  Indian tobacco
  Cultivated tobacco made into tea

*Sometimes used in herbal teas and prescribed by folk healers for symptoms in the elderly.

room *Amanita muscaria* has also been eaten for its hallucinatory effects, and the Vikings were said to have consumed them prior to going into battle because of the rage-like reaction induced. With overdose, muscarine causes parasympathomimetic symptoms that occur usually within 30 minutes after ingestion and cause profuse salivation, lacrimation, bradycardia, and other cholinergic responses. Treatment involves atropine, which can be given at a dose of 0.5 to 1 mg intramuscularly or intravenously (when symptoms warrant). This dose can be repeated every 30 minutes.

Important questions in the assessment of mushroom poisoning are the following:

1. When were the mushrooms eaten? When did symptoms appear (time course)? Rationale: Symptoms that begin immediately or within the first hour usually herald a relatively minor poisoning. Emesis, charcoal, and a cathartic should be used. Delayed symptoms are characteristic of the amatoxin-containing mushrooms. The nature of the symptoms may indicate seriousness of the ingestion (e.g., hallucinations, muscarinic effects, sweating, delirium).
2. How many mushrooms were eaten? What types were they? Rationale: If different types were ingested, it is difficult to arrive at identification by symptoms. In addition, of course, there is a dose-related effect.

3. Did anyone who ate the mushrooms not get sick? Rationale: People often blame mushrooms because of the widespread awareness of their toxicity, whereas another food poisoning or virus might be the cause of symptoms.
4. Did the patient consume alcoholic beverages? Rationale: Some mushrooms have a disulfiram-type effect with added alcohol. As with Antabuse, there can be extreme nausea, vomiting, and headache.

The most severe mushroom poisoning comes from those containing peptide toxins (phallotoxins or amatoxins). They can be deadly at low doses. Symptoms may be delayed several hours to as long as 24 hours after ingestion. Severe abdominal pain, diarrhea, and vomiting are present. Amatoxins cause liver, brain, and renal tubule cell injury, which may lead to death. Early treatment consists of the following:

1. Supportive treatment, with monitoring of vital signs and urine output. Renal failure may occur. Urine output must remain high. Early diuresis may be necessary.
2. Large doses of steroids have been used empirically.
3. Hemodialysis or peritoneal dialysis should be used early, when available, because of the small molecular size of the peptide toxins. Dialysis may have substantial benefit if used early.
4. Penicillin, chloramphenicol, and sulfamethoxazole have been used in animals to decrease binding of the toxin to albumin. This might be of value if dialysis is used subsequently. Also, thioctic acid (50 to 150 mg every 6 hours) has been used in Europe but has not been well tested.

If severe poisoning has occurred, all these measures should be instituted as early as possible, along with activated charcoal and catharsis.

The characteristic course has been divided into three stages: 1) the first 24 hours (acute symptoms), 2) some remission (24 to 36 hours), and 3) severe stage (with clinical liver damage, renal failure, and seizures), which can lead to death in up to 80% of cases.

A specimen of the ingested mushroom can prove valuable in identification. For quick emergency department testing, rub some of the mushroom cap over newsprint and allow to dry. A drop of concentrated hydrochloric acid is applied to the paper. A bluish-green color indicates amatoxins. The mushroom should then be sent for chemical analysis. A negative "newsprint" test does not mean that amatoxins may not be present. Only a positive test is useful.

Miscellaneous Food Poisoning

Table 28–7 summarizes some other food poisonings and their treatment.

Table 28–5. Signs and Symptoms of Common and/or Serious Plant Intoxications*

	Dieffenbachia/Philodendron	Colchicum/Gloriosa	Euphorbia/Hippomane	Actaea/Anemone/Ranunculus	Convallaria/Digitalis/Nerium	Aconitum	Solanum	Pieris/Rhododendron/Veratrum	Conium/Laburnum/Nicotiana/Sophora	Cicuta	Taxus	Gelsemium	Brugmansia/Datura	Amaryllis/Narcissus/Wisteria	Ilex	Abrus/Ricinus	Prunus	Phytolacca	Podophyllum	Karwinskia
Mouth and Throat																				
Burning/irritation	++	++	D	++	+	+	D	+	+											
Increased salivation	+		D	++		+		D	+	+	D									
Dry mouth											+	+	++							
Dysphonia/dysphagia	+		D			±						+	+							
Gastrointestinal tract																				
Nausea		+			+	±		D	+	+				+	+	DD				
Vomiting		+	+	+	+	±	D	D	+	±	D			++	++	DD	D	++	+	
Diarrhea		++	+	+	+		D	D	+					±	±	DD		D	+	
Abdominal pain		++	++	+	+		D	D			D			+			D	+		
Decreased bowel sounds									+				++						±	
Cardiovascular																				
Tachycardia													+							
Bradycardia					+			++			D									
Arrhythmias					±	++					D									
Conduction defects					++															
Hypertension													+							
Hypotension								++			D									

Table continues on next page.

Table 28–5. – cont'd.

	Dieffenbachia/Philodendron	Colchicum/Gloriosa	Euphorbia/Hippomane	Actaea/Anemone/Ranunculus	Convallaria/Digitalis/Nerium	Aconitum	Solanum	Pieris/Rhododendron/Veratrum	Conium/Laburnum/Nicotiana/Sophora	Cicuta	Taxus	Gelsemium	Brugmansia/Datura	Amaryllis/Narcissus/Wisteria	Ilex	Abrus/Ricinus	Prunus	Phytolacca	Podophyllum	Karwinskia
Nervous and Neuromuscular																				
Dizziness				±		+		+	+		+	+								
Weakness/lethargy				±		+			+		D						D			
Syncope				±																
Delirium/psychosis				±										+						
Tremors/convulsions				±				D±	+			±					D±		±	
Depression/coma								D	+								D±			
Headache								+	±				+							
Paresthesias						++														
Muscle weakness/paralysis		±						D	+		+	+					D±		±	DD
Visual																				
Mydriasis						+			±			+	+							
Visual disturbances						+		D					+							
Cutaneous																				
Increased sweating								+	+								D	++		
Dry skin							+						++							
Flushing/rash											D		+							
Cyanosis											D						D±			
Miscellaneous																				
Hyperthermia													+							
Painful/bloody micturition				+																

*Key: + = Commonly occurs; + + = pronounced or persistent; ± = occasionally reported; D = delayed onset; DD = occurs significantly.

Table 28–6   Common Dangerous Herbal Remedies

Botanical name of plant source	Common names	Remarks
Arnica montana L.	Arnica; arnica flowers; wolfsbane; leopard's bane; mountain tobacco; flores arnicae	Aqueous and alcoholic extracts of the plant contain choline, plus two unidentified substances that affect the heart and vascular systems. Arnica, an active irritant, can produce violent toxic gastroenteritis, nervous disturbances, change in pulse rate, intense muscular weakness, collapse, and death.
Atropa belladonna L.	Belladonna; deadly nightshade	Poisonous plant that contains the toxic solanaceous alkaloids hyoscyamine, atropine, and hyoscine.
Solanum dulcamara L.	Bittersweet twigs; dulcamara; bittersweet; woody nightshade; climbing nightshade	Poisonous. Contains the toxic glycoalkaloid solanine; also solanidine and dulcamarin.
Sanguinaria canadensis L.	Bloodroot; sanguinaria; red puccoon	Contains the poisonous alkaloid sanguinarine and other alkaloids.
Cytisus scoparius L.	Broom-top; scoparius; spartium; Scotch broom; Irish broom; broom	Contains toxic sparteine, isosparteine, and other alkaloids; also hydroxytyramine.
Aesculus hippocastanum L.	Buckeye; aesculus; horse chestnut	Contains a toxic coumarin glucoside, aesculin (esculin). A poisonous plant.
Acorus calamus L.	Calamus; sweet flag; sweet root; sweet cane; sweet cinnamon	Oil of calamus, Jammu variety, is a carcinogen (causes cancer). FDA regulations prohibit marketing of calamus as a food or food additive.
Heliotropium europaeum L.	Heliotrope	A poisonous plant. It contains alkaloids that produce liver damage. Not to be confused with garden heliotrope (*Valeriana officinalis* L.).
Conium maculatum L.	Hemlock; conium; poison hemlock; spotted hemlock; spotted parsley; St. Bennet's herb; spotted cowbane; fool's parsley	Contains the poisonous alkaloid conine and four other closely related alkaloids. Often confused with water hemlock (*Cicuta maculata* L.). Not to be confused with the conifer hemlock, hemlock spruce, etc. (*Tsuga canadensis* L. Carr.).
Hyoscyamus niger L.	Henbane; hyoscyamus; black henbane; hog's bean; poison tobacco; devil's eye	Contains the alkaloids hyoscyamine, hyoscine (scopolamine), and atropine. A poisonous plant.
Exagonium purga (Wenderoth) Bentham. *Ipomoea jalapa* Nutt, and Coxe. *Ipomoea purga* (Wenderoth) Hanye. *Exagonium jalapa* (Wenderoth) Baillon.	Jalap root; jalap; true jalap; jalapa; Vera Cruz jalap; high John root	A large twining vine of Mexico, this plant has undergone many name changes. The drug is a powerful, drastic cathartic. Purgative powers of jalap reside in its resin. In overdoses, jalap may produce dangerous hypercatharsis.
Datura stamonium L.	Jimsonweed; datura; stamonium; apple of Peru; Jamestown weed; thornapple; tolguacha	Contains the alkaloids atropine, hyoscyamine, and scopolamine. Illegal drug for nonprescription use. A poisonous plant.
Convallaria majalis L.	Lily of the valley; convallaria; may lily	Contains the toxic cardiac glycosides convallatoxin, convallarin, and convalamarin. Poisonous plant.
Lobelia inflata L.	Lobelia; Indian tobacco; wild tobacco; asthma weed; emetic weed	A poisonous plant that contains the alkaloid lobeline plus a number of other pyridine alkaloids. Overdoses of the plant or extracts of the leaves or fruits produce vomiting, sweating, pain, paralysis, depressed temperatures, rapid but feeble pulse, collapse, coma, and death.

Prepared by the Food and Drug Administration, Washington, D.C.

Table continues on next page.

Table 28–6 — cont'd

Botanical name of plant source	Common names	Remarks
Mandragora officinarum L.	Mandrake; mandragora; European mandrake	The plant is a poisonous narcotic similar in its properties to belladonna. Contains the alkaloids hyoscyamine, scopolamine, and mandragorine.
Podophyllum peltatum L.	Mandrake; May apple; podophyllum; American mandrake; devil's apple; umbrella plant; vegetable mercury	A poisonous plant, it contains podophyllotoxin, a complex polycyclic substance, and other constituents.
Phoradendron flavescens (Pursh.) Nutt. *Viscum flavescens* (Pursh.)	Mistletoe; viscum; American mistletoe	Poisonous. Contains the toxic pressor amines β-phenylethylamine and tyramine.
Phoradendron juniperinum Engelm.	Mistletoe; viscum; juniper mistletoe	May be poisonous. Little is known about its properties.
Viscum album L.	Mistletoe; viscum; European mistletoe	Poisonous. Contains the toxic pressor amines β-phenylethylamine and tyramine.
Ipomoea purpurea (L.) Roth.	Morning glory	Contains a purgative resin. In addition, morning glory seeds contain amides of lysergic acid but with a potency much less than that of LSD.
Vinca major L. and *Vinca minor* L.	Periwinkle; greater periwinkle; lesser periwinkle	Contains pharmacologically active, toxic alkaloids such as vinblastine and vincristine that have cytotoxic and neurologic actions and can injure the liver and kidneys.
Hypericum perforatum L.	St. Johnswort; hypericum; klamath weed; goatweed	A primary photosensitizer for cattle, sheep, horses, and goats. Contains hypericin, a fluorescent pigment, as a photosensitizing substance.
Euonymus europaea L.	Spindle-tree	Violent purgative.
Dipteryx odorata (Aubl.) Willd. *Coumarouna odorata* (Aubl.) and *Dipteryx oppositifolia* (Aubl.) Willd. *Coumarouna oppositifolia* (Aubl.)	Tonka bean; tonco bean; tonquin bean	Active constituent of seed is coumarin. Dietary feeding of coumarin to rats and dogs causes extensive liver damage, growth retardation, and testicular atrophy. FDA regulations prohibit marketing of coumarin as a food or food additive.
Euonymus atropurpurea Jacq.	Wahoo bark; euonymus; burning bush; wahoo	The poisonous principle has not been completely identified. Laxative.
Eupatorium rugosum Houtt. *E. ageratoides* L.f. and *E. urticaefolium*	White snakeroot (also called snakeroot, righweed)	Poisonous plant. Contains a toxic, unsaturated alcohol called *tremetol* combined with a resin acid. Causes "trembles" in cattle and other livestock. Milk sickness is produced in humans by ingestion of milk, butter, and possibly meat from animals poisoned by this plant.
Artemisia absinthium L.	Wormwood; absinthium; absinth; absinthe; madderwort; wermuth; mugwort; mingwort; warmot; magenkraut; harba absinthii	Contains a volatile oil (oil of wormwood) that is an active narcotic poison. Oil of wormwood is used to flavor *absinthe,* an alcoholic liqueur illegal in this country because its use can damage the nervous system and cause mental deterioration.
Corynanthe yohimbe Schum. *Pausinystalia yohimbe* (Schum.) Pierre	Yohimbe; yohimbi	Contains the toxic alkaloid yohimbine (quebrachine) and other alkaloids.

Table 28–7   Other Food Poisonings and Their Treatments*

Name	Food involved	Symptoms/signs	Treatment
Chinese restaurant syndrome (MSG syndrome)	Monosodium glutamate	Flushing, diaphoresis, weakness, headaches, pruritus, lethargy, depression, hypotension, arrhythmias, asthma, balance difficulties, vomiting	No specific treatment; IV fluids as needed
Cyanide poisoning	Pits from apricots, cherries, cassava, unripe millet, bitter almonds	Metabolic poisoning, loss of consciousness, cyanosis, convulsions	Amyl nitrite, oxygen
Cycad poisoning	Cycad starch and leaves (eaten in Philippines, Malay)	Neurologic symptoms, weakness, paresthesias	No specific treatment
Diascorism	Toxic yam with diascorine	Convulsions, deaths have occurred	Anticonvulsants
Ergotism	Grain with ergot fungus	Hypertension, vasoconstriction, CNS symptoms	Vasodilation by amyl nitrite inhalation or papaverine infusion
Favism	Fava bean	Glucose-6-phosphate dehydrogenase deficiency (inherited) produces hemolysis, severe anemia	Supportive: monitor urinary output, transfusions as needed; deferoxamine may arrest hemolysis
Fish poisoning (ichthyosarcotoxism) (ciguatera toxin)	Ciguatera (sea bass, snapper, barracuda)	Fish usually good as food contains a toxin that causes weakness, paresthesia, GI symptoms, hypotension, and, in fatal cases, respiratory paralysis (probably formed due to ingestion of dinoflagellate by the fish)	Gastric lavage, respiratory support as needed; charcoal
	Puffer fish	Far Eastern fish contains a neurotoxin that can cause paralysis (tetrodotoxin) and death	
	Tuna, mackerel, mahi mahi, (scromboid)	Bacteria act on histidine in flesh, producing a toxin with GI symptoms; headache and allergic manifestation (histamine-like)	Antihistamines, cimetidine, supportive and symptomatic treatment
Hemagglutination	Castor bean, partially cooked bean flakes, kidney bean flour, legume seeds	Nausea, vomiting, respiratory impairment, anemia; deaths reported from castor beans	No specific treatment
Lathyrism	Some beans, peas	Muscular weakness, partial paralysis, spinal cord impairments	No specific treatment
Licorice poisoning	Licorice	Weakness, myopathy, hypokalemia	IV treatment for fluid-electrolyte imbalance
Paralytic shellfish poisoning	Mussels and clams, usually along Pacific coast June to October — associated with "red tides"	Paresthesias, neurologic symptoms, respiratory paralysis	Supportive, particular attention to respiratory function
Sulfite sensitivity	Added to foods as antioxidant, found in mixes, wines	Asthma, urticaria	Bronchodilators
Tartrazine (Yellow dye #5) sensitivity	Orange-yellow colored foods	Urticaria, asthma, anaphylaxis	Supportive and symptomatic

*Of the food poisonings listed, the fish and shellfish contain poisons generally not present in a dangerous amount (the puffer fish is an exception). Ergotism is due to a fungus contaminant. In contrast, yam poisoning, cyanide poisoning, hemagglutination reaction, cycad poisoning, lathyrism, and favism result from chemicals that are natural constituents of the foods.

REFERENCES

1. Hughes RE et al: Clinical manifestations of ascorbic acid deficiency in man, J Clin Nutr 24:432, 1971.
2. Hessov IB and Elsborg L: Nutritional studies on long-term surgical patients with special reference to the intake of vitamin B12 and folic acid, Int J Vitam Nutr Res 46:427, 1976.
3. Morgan AG et al: Nutritional survey in the elderly, Int J Vitam Nutr Res 43:465, 1973.
4. Roos D: Neurological symptoms and signs in a selected group of partially gastrectomized patients with particular reference to B2 deficiency, Acta Neurol Scand 50:719, 1974.
5. Vir SC and Love AHG: Nutritional evaluation of B groups of vitamins in institutionalized aged, Int J Vitam Nutr Res 47:213, 1977.
6. Gupta KL, Dworkin B, and Gambert SR: Common nutritional disorders in the elderly: atypical manifestations, Geriatrics 43:87–97, 1988.
7. Munro HN: Nutrition and the elderly: a general overview, J Am Coll Nutr 3:341–350, 1984.

8. Morley JE: Nutritional status of the elderly, Am J Med 81:679–695, 1986.

9. Terris M and Goldberger ON: Pellagra, New Orleans, 1964, Louisiana State University Press.

10. Helweg-Larsen P et al: Famine disease in German concentration camps: complications and sequels, Acta Psychiatr Neurol Scand [Suppl] 83, 1952.

11. Winick M, editor: Hunger disease: studies by the Jewish physicians in the Warsaw ghetto, New York, 1979, John Wiley & Sons.

12. Lindenbaum J et al: Neuropsychiatric disorders caused by cobalamin deficiency in the absence of anemia or macrocytosis, N Engl J Med 318:26, 1988.

13. Lind J: A treatise on the scurvy, ed 3, London, 1772, S Crowder, D Wilson, G Nicholls, T Cadell, T Becket, & Co.

14. Victor M, Adams RD, and Collins GH: The Wernicke-Korsakoff syndrome, Oxford, 1971, Blackwell Scientific Publications.

15. Goldman JM, Ahn Y, and Wheeler MF: Vitamin D and hypercalcemia, JAMA 254:1719, 1985.

16. Goldman MB, Luchins DJ, and Robertson GL: Mechanisms of altered water metabolism in psychotic patients with polydipsia and hyponatremia, N Engl J Med 318:7, 1988.

17. Eisbruch A, Lweinski U, and Djaidett M: Severe opisthotonos and trismus associated with water intoxication, J R Soc Med 77:158, 1984.

18. Gill G: Treatment of hyponatremic seizures with intravenous 29.2% saline, Br Med J 292:625, 1986.

19. Nairns RG: Therapy of hyponatremia: does haste make waste? N Engl J Med 314:1573, 1986.

20. Carter AO et al: A severe outbreak of *Escherichia coli* 0157:H7: associated hemorrhage colitis in a nursing home, N Engl J Med 317:24, 1987.

21. Dolman CE: Human botulism in Canada (1919–1973), Can Med Assoc J 110:191, 1974.

22. Koenig MG et al: Type B botulism in man, Am J Med 42:208, 1967.

23. Gangarosa EJ: Botulism in the United States, 1899–1967, J Infect Dis 119:308, 1969.

24. Centers for Disease Control: Botulism in the United States, 1899–1977: handbook for epidemiologists, clinicians and laboratory workers, Atlanta, Georgia, May 1979.

25. Chia JK et al: Botulism in an adult associated with food borne intestinal infection with *Clostridium botulinum,* N Engl J Med 315:239, 1986.

26. Holmberg SD et al: Drug resistant *Salmonella* from animals fed antimicrobials, N Engl J Med 311:617, 1984.

27. Fleming DW et al: Pasteurized milk as a vehicle of infection in an outbreak of listeriosis, N Engl J Med 312:404, 1983.

28. Kolata G: Testing for trichinosis, Science 227:621, 1985.

29. Morse DL et al: Widespread outbreaks of clam and oyster associated gastroenteritis, N Engl J Med 314:678, 1986.

30. Schwartz GR: In bad taste: the MSG syndrome, Santa Fe, 1988, Health Press.

31. McMillan M and Thompson JG: An outbreak of suspected solanine poisoning in schoolboys, Q J Med 48:227, 1979.

32. Hedberg CW et al: An outbreak of thyrotoxicosis caused by the consumption of bovine thyroid gland in ground beef, N Engl J Med 316:993, 1987.

Surgical, Traumatic, and Abdominal Disorders

Surgical Emergencies:
An Overview

Gideon Bosker, M.D., F.A.C.E.P., and John W. Grigsby, M.D., F.A.C.E.P.

Falls
  Common injuries resulting from falls
Other surgical emergencies
  Preoperative preparation

The diagnosis and treatment of surgical emergencies in the elderly present significant challenges for the emergency department physician. Poor clinical histories may make it difficult to elucidate an occult surgical problem, and, moreover, many histories in the elderly may not fit a classic pattern for many acute surgical conditions. The diagnosis of surgical emergencies in the elderly may also be difficult because, frequently, diseases are accompanied by nonspecific symptoms and signs. Clinical presentation in the elderly is often less obvious, and the presence of multiple organic and/or functional problems may obscure the primary illness. Frequently, multiple problems coexist, and symptoms due to complications of the primary surgical illness may be the most prominent feature of the clinical presentation. As a result, the overall approach to the diagnosis of surgical emergencies in the elderly must be aggressive.

FALLS

Falls in the elderly represent the greatest single cause of accidental death and are responsible for more than 50% of all accidental deaths in this population. In those over the age of 65, deaths from falls are more common than fatalities from all other accidents combined, with an annual prevalence rate of 30 to 40%. Falls are twice as common in females as in males until the age of 75, after which the frequency is similar. Falls are also mentioned as a contributing factor in 40% of nursing home admissions.[1]

The initial care of the elderly patient who has a fall includes the following: 1) allay anxiety, 2) thoroughly ex-amine acute injuries, 3) treat emergency conditions such as hypotension or hemorrhage, and 4) search, meticulously, for the underlying cause of the fall, which may be extrinsic or intrinsic. Approximately 40% of all falls are due to some extrinsic factor in the environment. Most occur in the bathroom or near the bed. Falling causes physical insecurity in the elderly and, therefore, promotes recurrence. With proper instruction and reorganization of the physical environment, most falls can be prevented. Extrinsic causes such as inappropriate footwear, scatter rugs, or poor lighting represent preventable causes.

A number of intrinsic causes of falls should be considered at the time of presentation in the emergency department. Changes associated with the aging process may give rise to an altered or unstable gait and predispose the elderly to falls. It is not uncommon for spinal, subcortical, and cortical reflexes that maintain posture to alter with age and result in stooped, broad-based gaits, shuffling, or swaying — all of which can predispose older people to postural instabilities and falls. Mental confusion, which may or may not be associated with dementia, and faulty judgment are also risk factors. Orthostatic hypotension, sometimes associated with medications (antihypertensives, diuretics, hypnotics, antidepressants, etc.) or inadequate nutrition and hydration are intrinsic factors that may be responsible for falls. In many patients over the age of 65, vasoactive reflexes are slow to respond, and a 20 mm Hg drop in blood pressure may occur in up to 25% of the healthy elderly. Finally, increased muscle mass in the lower extremities, diminished vascular resistance, and increased venous pooling can predispose the elderly to orthostatic hypotension and presyncopal or syncopal attacks that may culminate in a fall.

It is estimated that approximately 25% of all falls in the elderly are associated with an acute change in cardiac rhythm, which may be either supraventricular or ventricular in origin. Vertebrobasilar insufficiency should be considered when a fall has occurred in a patient who gives a history of hyperextending or reaching over the head. Dizziness due to labyrinthitis, occult blood loss (due to chronic peptic ulcer or diverticulitis), medications, or depression may also give rise to falls in this susceptible subgroup. Transient ischemic attacks involving the basilar system and undiagnosed epilepsy may also be responsible for injuries associated with falls. A number of different conditions that may cause syncope should be considered including vasovagal syncope, cough syncope, micturition syncope, and defecation syncope. Finally, tumors, endocrine disturbances, and changes in medications or in nutrition that cause electrolyte disturbances, such as hypoglycemia or hyponatremia, may be responsible for falls in the elderly.[2]

Common Injuries Resulting from Falls

A number of different organ systems may be involved in injuries resulting from falls. Head trauma, cervical spine trauma, blunt chest or abdominal trauma, and orthopedic trauma (pelvic fractures, femoral fractures, humeral fractures, radioulnar fractures, etc.) are the organ systems most often involved.

Falls account for more head injuries in the elderly than motor vehicle accidents and are associated with significant morbidity and mortality.[3] Head trauma is more serious in the elderly than in the young, because the elderly brain is shrunken and the tamponade effect is minimized. Neurons cannot withstand the same degree of injury, perhaps due to an intolerant cellular metabolic status. As a result, older patients show less favorable recovery from head trauma than the young. The incidence of subdural hematomas is greater in the elderly. Epidural hematomas are rare in the elderly, although when they do occur, they may have a high morbidity and mortality. Frontal blows to the skull are the most common cause of direct injuries, while blows to the occipital, temporal, and parietal regions can cause direct and contrecoup injuries. The most common sites of cerebral contusion are the inferior surfaces of the frontal and temporal lobes. Fractures of the skull are associated with a higher incidence of cerebral contusion, while subdural hematomas are more commonly observed without fractures. Subdural hematomas are more common after occipital trauma than frontal trauma.

Initial evaluation of the elderly patient who has sustained a fall, and who has head trauma, includes stabilization and the basic ABCs. The first hour is the most critical, and approximately half of those with blunt head trauma have systemic problems that predispose to further brain damage. Hypoxia, hypotension, hypercapnia, or anemia should be diagnosed and treated appropriately. A crosstable lateral x-ray of the cervical spine is required to evaluate the possibility of cervical spine injury. The possibility of airway obstruction should have been evaluated before this. In cases involving multiple trauma, there should be a diligent search for both external sites of bleeding. Once the patient's vital signs are stabilized, a complete neurologic exam should be performed. The level of consciousness should be assessed and the presence of focal neurologic deficits should be noted. Inspection of the scalp may give the exact location of skull trauma; the presence of subconjunctival hemorrhage and periorbital ecchymosis suggests a fracture at the base of the anterior cranial fossa. Bleeding or leakage of cerebrospinal fluid from the nose or ear is often associated with a basilar skull fracture. Diagnostic tests that can be performed in the emergency department include a skull x-ray, computerized tomography (CT) scan, and cervical spine x-rays. A spinal tap is contraindicated in acute head trauma. Treatment in the emergency department usually consists of fluid restriction and diuretics (furosemide 20 to 40 mg IV, mannitol 1 to 2 mg/kg over ½ hour, and hyperventilation, for P_{CO_2} less than 25).

In elderly patients who remain comatose for more than 12 hours, the mortality is 50% in the 60 to 70 age group and 60% in those over the age of 71. Only 25% of patients age 80 or over who are actively rehabilitated return to normal. As a rule, mental ability is restored less in the elderly than in young patients with head trauma; maximum mental recovery occurs at 6 months after resolution of coma.

Blunt Trauma to the Chest or Abdomen

On occasion, significant blunt trauma to the chest may result from a fall. Osteoporosis makes rib fractures especially common, and a small percentage may be accompanied by pneumothorax or hemothorax. Not surprisingly, chest trauma can result in early pulmonary decompensation in the elderly victim. Morbidity and mortality rates are higher in those who have sustained pneumothorax or hemopneumothorax. When blunt chest trauma due to falls is accompanied by hypotension, secondary to blood loss, caution must be exercised with fluid therapy, since overaggressive volume repletion may lead to pulmonary edema in those with underlying cardiac disease. Minor thoracic injuries in the elderly can present with significant symptoms and signs and, commonly, produce sequelae requiring therapy. For example, a rib fracture may predispose the individual to pneumonia, and minor injuries tend to incapacitate because of pain. The home environment must be carefully evaluated before discharging the elderly patients with blunt chest trauma for independent care.

Orthopedic Injuries

Orthopedic injuries comprise the largest class of surgical complications resulting from falls.[4] The elderly frequently have decreased bone density, unstable gait, or underlying neurologic illnesses that predispose them to falls and, consequently, to bony injury. Elderly females have a greater incidence of spinal osteoporosis than males. Areas most affected by osteoporosis among the long bones include the distal radius and the neck of the femur. The lumbosacral spine, also susceptible to osteoporosis, is especially prone to compression fractures. As a rule, early treatment and rehabilitation of orthopedic injuries in the elderly is imperative, with appropriate surgery usually recommended in the first 24 to 48 hours.

Pelvic fractures are the third leading cause of death in motor vehicle accidents and have a mortality rate of 15 to 20% in the elderly population. Because they are sometimes "silent," pelvic fractures must be suspected in all falls occurring in the elderly, as well as in automobile versus pedestrian accidents in this population. Lower urinary tract injuries occur in about 15 to 30% of all pelvic fractures, and neurologic injuries occur in about 17%.

Open pelvic fractures are accompanied by a mortality rate that exceeds 50%. Hemorrhage is the most significant complication, and life-threatening intramuscular bleeding can occur over a few hours. Blood loss can be extraperitoneal or retroperitoneal, and treatment consists of stabilization, including reduction and immobilization of fractures, blood replacement, use of military antishock trousers (MAST) when appropriate, use of angiography for localization of bleeding, and, on occasion, operative repair of major arterial/venous injuries.

A *hip fracture* is the most common orthopedic injury in the elderly patient who has fallen. The incidence is 1% in the 65-year-old age group and 2% in the 85-year-old age group. The female to male ratio is 2 to 1, and many studies have reported a 50% mortality in the first year among all patients sustaining hip fractures. About 70% of hip fractures occur in private homes and gardens, 20% occur in public places, and 10% occur in residential institutions. Contributing causes include osteoporosis and osteomalacia. Evaluation of the patient who is suspected of having a hip fracture is straightforward. The affected extremity is usually externally rotated and abducted and appears foreshortened. There is pain in the hip or anterior pelvis, and, on occasion, pain can be referred to the knee. Intertrochanteric fractures of the hip are most common, followed by subcapital, transcervical, and subtrochanteric. A diligent search must be made for associated pelvic fractures. Standard evaluation includes a CBC, electrolytes, BUN, glucose, urinalysis, and x-ray of the pelvis and chest. Treatment in the emergency department includes analgesics, proper positioning (slight flexion of hip and support of the knee), splinting as necessary (Hare Thomas half-ring), and surgery as early as possible with optimum results being obtained in the first 24 hours.

Humerus fractures usually result from the force of a fall that is absorbed in the deltoid area. Surgical neck fractures are most common, and presentation includes pain and tenderness in the shoulder with significant loss of motion.[5] Radial nerve palsies may occur with midshaft humeral fractures. Brachial plexus injuries should be sought when a proximal humeral fracture is accompanied by hyperextension of the arm. Impacted fractures usually require a sling and progressive range of motion, while disimpacted fractures require a surgical procedure.[6] Early motion is mandatory to prevent stiffness of the shoulder joint.

A *Colles' fracture* is seen in falls that occur on the outstretched dorsiflexed hand. A Colles' fracture is characterized by a "dinner-fork" deformity, a fracture of the metaphysis of the distal radius with dorsal angulation of the distal fragment, and fracture of the ulnar styloid. Initial treatment includes an analgesic, ice, elevation, and splinting. Closed reduction is the treatment of choice.

OTHER SURGICAL EMERGENCIES

Accurate diagnosis and proper evaluation and triage of surgical emergencies represent two of the most difficult but important parts of emergency care for the elderly population. Diagnosis of surgical conditions in the elderly patient may be difficult and complex, and, frequently, a single diagnosis will not explain the entire clinical picture.[7] Due to altered mental status or confusion associated with surgical emergencies, the elderly patient may be unable to give a history, and, when mental confusion is present, the history that is given may be misleading. Over 30% of elderly sick patients have emotional disturbances that unfavorably alter their perception of their acute illness. In addition to the fact that surgical emergencies in the elderly frequently present with unusual symptoms and signs, there is a high complication rate associated with the initial presentation. Some of these complications, such as sepsis, are difficult to recognize and require a high index of suspicion. There is also a higher incidence of an iatrogenic cause for surgical emergencies.

The diagnosis of *acute abdomen* always presents a challenge, especially in the elderly patient. The emergency department physician must consider, in addition to common abdominal diseases, a retroperitoneal process, genitourinary disease, or intrathoracic disease to explain abdominal symptoms. Obtundation and confusion with or without shock are common presentations of acute surgical abdominal emergencies. The most common causes of the acute abdomen in the elderly include cholecystitis, intestinal obstruction, and appendicitis.

Acute pancreatitis is the most common nonsurgical cause of abdominal pain in the elderly. Functional bowel disease is another common cause of gastrointestinal symptoms. Differential diagnosis of the acute abdomen in the elderly includes cholecystitis and biliary disease, small bowel obstruction, large bowel obstruction with or without volvulus, diverticulitis, appendicitis, pancreatitis, peptic ulcer disease with or without perforation, mesenteric occlusion, and functional bowel disease.

Among elderly patients with *biliary disease*, 80% of them present with complications such as cholecystitis, cholangitis, and pancreatitis. Cholecystitis in the elderly is accompanied by a higher risk of empyema, gangrene, or perforation of the gallbladder with resultant peritonitis. Patients at high risk include those with atherosclerotic heart disease, diabetes, and immunodeficiency. Cholangitis may present as septicemia with shock, with or without signs of abdominal disease. Gallstones are found in about one third of all geriatric patients; in one third of patients with painless jaundice, the cause is gallstones. The diagnosis cholecystitis may be difficult since the disease may present with nonspecific complaints of flatulence, dyspepsia, intolerance of fatty food, bilious attacks, and vague chronic right upper quadrant pain or discomfort. Nausea and vomiting, while common in the younger population, are not seen frequently in the elderly with cholecystitis. A rare form of cholecystitis present in the elderly is emphysematous cholecystitis, which is caused by gas-producing organisms. Pain is more severe, and the patient appears more toxic. Diagnosis with abdominal ultrasound is the most reliable method. Patients who are afebrile or unable to keep down food or liquids should be hospitalized.

Small bowel obstruction in the elderly can be of two types: mechanical or paralytic ileus. Mechanical small bowel obstruction usually presents with pain, distention, nausea, and vomiting, followed by obstipation. Adhesions resulting from previous surgery are the most common cause of small bowel obstruction. Hernias are present in about 50% of those with small bowel obstruction. Femoral hernias are more common in women than in men, but indirect hernia is the most common type in both sexes. Other causes of small bowel obstruction include malignancy, volvulus, and, rarely, gallstone ileus. The latter, although representing less than 1 to 2% of all cases with small bowel obstruction, should be considered in the female patient with no abdominal scars whose x-ray shows air in the biliary tract fistula. Paralytic ileus may be accompanied by symptoms similar to those seen in mechanical obstruction, but usually the pain and vomiting are less severe. Causes include drugs (narcotics, anticholinergics), abdominal sepsis, ischemia, electrolyte imbalance, ureteral stone, urinary tract operations, and fractures of the lumbosacral spine.

Symptoms of *large bowel obstruction* include abdominal cramps, change in bowel habits, presence of blood in the stool, distention, and nausea and vomiting. Malignancy is the major cause of large bowel obstruction in the elderly, and bowel cancer is the most common malignant tumor in this population. Two thirds can be diagnosed by sigmoidoscopy. Other causes of large bowel

obstruction include adenomatous polyps, fecal impaction, strictures secondary to colitis, volvulus, diverticulitis, and gynecologic tumors.

Colonic disease in this population may be misleading, since the incidence of constipation is not a direct result of aging — i.e., altered physiology. The factors provoking constipation in this age group are nonspecific and include inadequate fluid intake, laxative abuse, dementia, anal disease, neurologic disease, and electrolyte imbalance. Volvulus is an abdominal emergency, with 85% of the cases occurring in the sigmoid colon and 15% at the ileocecal junction. Volvulus is a twisting of the intestine around its mesentery. More commonly seen in males, volvulus presents with acute abdominal pain, obstipation, and rapid distention with signs of toxicity. Vomiting may be an early symptom, and in some patients, diarrhea may be the most prominent symptom.

Diverticulosis is present in 40% of patients over the age of 70 in the United States. One half of these patients have at least one episode of diverticulitis, which presents as discomfort or pain, usually in the left lower quadrant. It may be accompanied by rebound tenderness, constipation or diarrhea, and fever, with or without blood in the stool. There is a high incidence of complications from diverticulitis in the elderly, including abscess, obstruction, perforation with peritonitis, and severe colonic bleeding.

Although *appendicitis* can occur in the elderly population, the symptoms and signs are more vague than in younger patients.[8] There is frequently a delay in making the diagnosis. An underlying disease that may obscure the clinical picture is present in one half of elderly patients with documented appendicitis. The average duration of symptoms is much longer, and the disease may present with unusual features, such as femoral hernia sac or right lower quadrant abscess, though these are rare. The average stay in the hospital for the elderly before diagnosis is 24 hours, which increases the chances of complications. In those patients finally shown to have appendicitis, an incorrect diagnosis at the time of presentation was observed in one third of cases. Intestinal obstruction, cholecystitis, and diverticulitis were the most common mistaken diagnoses. If the diagnosis was suspected, 8% of the patients could have been operated on earlier. The postoperative complication rate (pneumonia, wound infection, etc.) is estimated to be 50%.

Pancreatitis is the most common nonsurgical cause of abdominal pain in the elderly. Its incidence increases with age, and it is often secondary to other disorders of the gastrointestinal tract, including cholecystitis and posterior wall gastric ulcer, as well as drug complications. Presentation usually includes atypical abdominal pain, with or without radiation to the back. Nausea and vomiting may or may not be present. Moreover, up to 10% of cases of pancreatitis in the elderly present without pain. Additionally, a small percentage of patients present with unexplained hypotension, altered mental function, or atypical pain referred to the chest.

A *peptic ulcer with perforation* is much more common in the elderly population than in the other age groups. Fifty percent of all cases present for the first time in the elderly population and are usually accompanied by complications (bleeding, perforation, etc.). Symptoms include atypical or vague pain and, while pain is the most prominent feature of the clinical picture, weight loss, vomiting, and anorexia are also common. Males predominate 2 to 1; the ratio of duodenal to gastric ulcer is 2 to 1 in the elderly versus 10 to 1 in the younger age group. There is a 20 to 30% fatality rate due to bleeding and a 10 to 20% fatality due to perforation. An operation in those with peptic ulcer disease and perforation may be delayed due to the reluctance of the elderly to leave home and go to the hospital, poor communications with their family doctor, reluctance of the family doctor to send an elderly patient to the hospital, atypical physical signs, or a reluctance to operate on high-risk patients unless absolutely necessary.

Mesenteric occlusion, especially when underlying cardiovascular disease is present in combination with atrial fibrillation, should be considered in elderly patients who present with an acute abdomen.[9,10] The presence of congestive heart failure or a recent myocardial infarction predisposes to mesenteric occlusion. Mesenteric vascular ischemia is manifested by food avoidance, postprandial abdominal pain, weight loss, and diarrhea, with or without rectal bleeding. Usually seen in elderly patients with ischemic disease and peripheral vascular disease, mesenteric occlusion may be exceedingly difficult to diagnose since the presence of nonspecific symptoms and the sudden onset of abdominal pain, distention, nausea, and vomiting can easily be confused with bowel obstruction. On occasion, mesenteric occlusion may present as unexplained vascular collapse without any signs of abdominal symptomatology. Medications such as digitalis and thiazide diuretics may have a role in nonocclusive mesenteric infarction and in some series are responsible for up to 50% of cases. Mortality rate is 80 to 90%, and the definitive surgical procedure should be performed within the first 8 hours of the clinical presentation. A high index of suspicion, early angiography, and rapid surgery are the key to successful treatment.

Functional bowel disease in the elderly is the most common cause of symptoms referable to the gastrointestinal tract. Generally, functional bowel disease is a diagnosis of exclusion and cannot be made until an accurate history and physical, radiologic exams, proctosigmoidoscopy, stool exam, and other laboratory studies have been completed. Symptoms include constipation, diarrhea, gaseous distention, cramping abdominal pain, mucus in bowel movements, general malaise, nausea, and fatigue. Contributory factors include physical fatigue, dietary indiscretion, use of laxatives and enemas, emotional problems (depression, boredom, etc.), fear of disease, and a lowered standard of living.

In patients with signs of *peritoneal irritation*, such as absent or diminished bowel sounds, rigidity, or rebound tenderness, hospitalization is required and parenteral antibiotics should be administered for nearly all patients with possible abdominal infections. Antibiotic selection should provide aerobic and anaerobic gram-negative rod coverage. Although a combination of clindamycin and an aminoglycoside has been used to provide antimicrobial coverage, these two drugs have well-known inherent risks and side effects with their usage. Clindamycin may result in the development of pseudomembranous colitis, whereas gentamicin and tobramycin may prove dangerous in patients with preexisting renal compromise and, in the frail elderly, in general. Metronidazole may be substituted for clindamycin as another choice for therapy against anaerobic organisms.

Based on its spectrum of coverage, low toxicity, and ease of administration, ampicillin-sulbactam (Unasyn) (1.5 to 3.0 g every 6 hours) may be the safest, most efficacious antimicrobial agent to initiate for the treatment of diverticulitis, especially in the nonimmunocompromised elderly patient. The drug's comprehensive anaerobic coverage, which includes *Bacteroides fragilis,* as well as its broad gram-negative coverage, is well suited to the mixed anaerobic-aerobic infections encountered in diverticular inflammation and perforation, as well as other abdominal and pelvic infections. In one study comparing ampicillin-sulbactam (Unasyn) to a combination of clindamycin plus gentamicin, a better bacteriologic outcome with equivalent cure rates and earlier discharge from hospital was seen in the Unasyn-treated group. Finally, the use of a single antimicrobial to provide both anaerobic and aerobic coverage would seem advantageous in the elderly patient who is prone to interdrug toxicity.

Preoperative Preparation

Preoperative preparation of the patient who requires an operative procedure for an acute surgical emergency includes full evaluation of the cardiovascular system, the respiratory system, the gastrointestinal system, and the genitourinary system, as well as a general assessment of nutritional status and neurologic function. Congestive heart failure in the elderly patient may be insidious and may include little more than weakness, lethargy, confusion, and mild dyspnea. Arrhythmias are common in this population; 10 to 15% of the elderly are admitted with atrial fibrillation, and 4% have aortic stenosis or other congenital valvular lesions. Symptoms and signs of the presence of coronary artery disease should be sought as the incidence of a painless myocardial infarction is high in this population. The respiratory system should be evaluated to exclude the presence of pneumonia or life-threatening respiratory disease. Underlying gastrointestinal problems may include disorganized esophageal motility, which predisposes to aspiration, the presence of gastric and duodenal ulcers (present in 10% of the elderly), colonic diverticula (60% of the elderly), and biliary disease (over 30% of the elderly have gallstones). The presence of infections and urinary tract obstruction should be excluded, fecal impactions should be removed, and the presence of prostatic hypertrophy should be noted. Azotemia should be corrected before surgery, if possible. About 15 to 30% of elderly patients develop acute organic brain syndromes after surgery. Stress due to fever dehydration, trauma, sepsis, or pain produces temporary mental disorder. Preexisting conditions are made worse by hospitalization and anesthesia. Elderly patients need meticulous postoperative support for at least 24 to 48 hours in an intensive care unit following an emergency surgical procedure. Postoperative problems that must be sought with vigilance include hypotension, hypothermia, pneumonia, thrombophlebitis and thromboembolism, acute renal failure, postoperative delirium, postoperative sepsis, and fluid and electrolyte disorders. Attention to these aspects of the postoperative course will significantly reduce morbidity and mortality in the elderly population.

REFERENCES

1. Tinetti ME and Speechley M: Prevention of falls among the elderly, N Engl J Med 320:1055, 1989.
2. Chipman C and Sarant G: What does it mean when a patient falls? Geriatrics 36(10):101–111, 1981.
3. Greer M: Emergency evaluation of head injuries in the elderly, Geriatrics 34:73–84, 1979.
4. Kallina C: Morbidity and mortality in elderly orthopedic patients, Surg Clin North Am 62:297–300, 1982.
5. Rose S et al: Epidemiologic features of humeral fractures, Clin Orthop 168:24–30, 1982.
6. Neer C: Displaced proximal humeral fractures, J Bone Joint Surg 51:1077–1089, 1970.
7. Vowles K: Geriatrics: "surgical traps in the elderly," Br J Hosp Med 26:454–458, 1981.
8. Yusuf MF and Dunn E: Appendicitis in the elderly: learn to discern the untypical picture, Geriatrics 34:73–79, 1979.
9. Singh RP and Lee STJ: Acute mesenteric vascular occlusion: a review, Int Surg 65:231–234, 1980.
10. Sachs SM, Morton JH, and Schwartz SI: Acute mesenteric ischemia, Surgery 92:646–653, 1982.

SUGGESTED READINGS

Bangs C: Caught in the cold, Emerg Med 14:29–40, 1982.
Besdine R: Accidental hypothermia: the body's energy crisis, Geriatrics 35:51–59, 1979.
Callaham M: Heat illness, Consultant pp. 59–62, August 1980.
Coakley D, editor: Acute geriatric medicine, Littleton, MA, 1981, PSG, Inc.
Goldfrank L: Heat stroke, Hosp Phys pp. 24–35, August 1980.
Goldfrank L and Kinstein R: Emergency management of hypothermia, Hosp Phys pp. 47–52, August 1980.
Hurtz K: Hypothermia in the elderly: the cold facts, Geriatrics 37:85–93, 1982.
Kager L: A randomized controlled trial of ampicillin plus sulbactam vs. gentamicin plus clindamycin in the treatment in intraabdominal infections: a preliminary report, Rev Infect Dis 8(suppl):S583–S588, 1986.
Kolavowski A and Gunter L: Hypothermia in the elderly, Geriatr Nurs pp. 362–365, Sept 1981.
Linn BS, Linn MW, and Wallen N: Evaluation of results of surgical procedures in the elderly, Ann Surg 195:90–96, 1982.
Pieper R, Kager L, and Nasman P: Acute appendicitis: a clinical study of 1018 cases of emergency appendectomy, Acta Chir Scand 148:51–62, 1982.
Weiss M and Lesnick GJ: Surgery in the elderly: attitudes and facts, Mt Sinai J Med 47:208–214, 1980.

The Acute Geriatric Abdomen

Richard Caesar, M.D., F.A.C.E.P.

The acute geriatric abdomen poses what is arguably one of the most treacherous and challenging
diagnostic dilemmas facing the emergency physician. In fact, the gastrointestinal system, an arena

noted for nebulous complaints and neglected symptomatology, is the site of many processes which demonstrate
our relative underappreciation of atypical presentations
of common diseases in the elderly and their need for special diagnostic evaluation. For example, persistent nonspecific problems in this population can degenerate
precipitously into a variety of acute — and, sometimes, life-threatening — abdominal conditions. And in
the present health care system, it is primarily the emergency department physician to whom geriatric patients
present with these problematic abdominal conditions.

Sudden onset of abdominal discomfort in an elderly patient usually generates a complex and extensive differential diagnosis. Consider the case of the 80-year-old
gentleman who presents to the emergency department
with severe epigastric pain, fever, and vomiting. Are his
previously documented gallstones (present in up to one
half of individuals 80 years of age or older) responsible
for his symptoms? If so, is the stone causing acute
cholecystitis at the cystic duct, or has it descended to the
ampulla of Vater and precipitated biliary pancreatitis? At
what point in the patient's course should a surgical consult be obtained? Will a serum amylase determination
tell the whole story? Should an abdominal ultrasound
examination be performed? Perhaps the stones, which
have been present for 30 years, are only red herrings and
the patient, who has been on prednisone and ibuprofen,
is presenting his peptic disease for the first time with a
penetrating ulcer, as do 50% of patients in this age group.
Can gastrointestinal hemorrhage be ruled out merely because there is no blood in the emesis? The patient, who is
also in rapid atrial fibrillation, cannot recall if he has
ever had an irregular pulse before, yet his condition
demands we consider impending small bowel infarction,
secondary to embolization of left atrial thrombus to the
superior mesenteric artery. Each of these myriad conditions can present with the original constellataion of
complaints that include epigastric pain, fever, and vomit-

ing, and each condition can progress to mental obtundation and shock. But the same presentation can also be seen with gastroenteritis in the 80-year-old patient for whom a diagnostic laparotomy will be decidedly unhelpful.

Complexity and contradiction are the hallmarks of acute abdominal pain in the geriatric patient. Consider the 70-year-old woman, a local politician, whose only documented medical problems have been chronic constipation and a few right-sided colonic diverticula, discovered on a previous barium enema. In the emergency department, she presents with 3 days of right lower quadrant pain, bloating, fever, and nausea. What is the source of her abdominal pain? Rupture of a previously benign diverticulum, which has now produced a pericolic abscess? Has she had these symptoms too long (3 days) to consider appendicitis, or was her appendix removed with her partial hysterectomy 36 years ago? Or have the anticholinergic affects of her recent antidepressant use (during the recent election) combined with her chronic constipation to produce a sigmoid volvulus? The negative plain film will rule out the volvulus but not, as it turns out, the incarcerated femoral hernia which has turned gangrenous and will soon generate septic shock. The emergency specialist, without the luxury of time, must consider multiple simultaneous conditions in an unstable patient and decide which, if any, are responsible for the patient's acute symptomatology.

CLINICAL PRESENTATION

Emergency medicine physicians with experience in clinical geriatrics readily acknowledge the bewildering array of obstacles to proper diagnosis and treatment in this age group. This patient population is composed of notoriously poor historians. Dementia, in particular, obscures time-honored symptoms, putting the clinician at a considerable disadvantage. Furthermore, the elderly present atypically with common problems or nebulously with more obscure pathology. The older patient, for example, is far more likely to have undergone previous laparotomy. The resulting adhesions and other forms of scarring not only increase the likelihood of intestinal obstruction but alter the three-dimensional relationships of intraabdominal structures. Consequently, signs and symptoms in these patients can deviate from classical patterns.

Abdominal musculature in the elderly is thin, atrophic, and reacts with less splinting, guarding, or palpable spasm than in the younger patient. As a result, objective findings seen in younger patients are often absent in the elderly. Beneath that musculature, the omentum is likely to be both smaller and less likely to seal off an acute abdominal process. Consequently, the sequelae of intraperitoneal contamination with pus, blood, or bile occurs earlier and more frequently. In response to such inflammation, the elderly patient's temperature and

leukocyte count may rise later and to a lesser degree, depriving the clinician of still more critical objective data. Finally, age is associated with atherosclerosis of the intraabdominal vasculature and a more tenuous splanchnic circulation, thereby predisposing to perforation and gangrene, particularly involving the appendix, gallbladder, or small intestine.

The elderly present with a greater *number* of complaints. Consequently, signs and symptoms have a propensity to blend and superimpose upon one another, until teasing apart specific complaints becomes an exercise in frustration. In this setting, physicians tend either to ignore certain details or force simplistic categories onto the facts. Compounding this already difficult scenario is our basic knowledge that elderly physiology, with diminished recuperative powers, offers us little room for missed diagnoses.

Given that elderly patients are often poor and misleading historians and that their acute abdominal complaints can suggest an intimidating variety of both trivial and life-threatening pathology, it is not surprising that geriatric patients with abdominal pain consume a disproportionate amount of time and resources in the emergency department. Comparing lengths of stay in the emergency department of elderly (over 65 years) versus younger patients, and categorizing major complaints into shortness of breath, chest pain, and abdominal pain, Baum and Rubinstein[1] observed that the discharged geriatric patient with abdominal pain was the *single most time consuming of all emergency room visitors,* with almost 2½ hours spent, on average, in the department. Furthermore, despite well-documented higher admission rates for elderly (47%) versus the nonelderly (18%), when these patients *were* discharged from the emergency department their recidivism rate was nearly twice as high (29% versus 15%) as younger patients with identical complaints.

BILIARY TRACT DISEASE IN THE ELDERLY

Cholecystitis

The incidence of stones within the gallbladder (cholelithiasis) and within the common bile duct (choledocholithiasis) — as well as inflammation of the gallbladder (cholecystitis) — increases significantly with each decade of life.[2] Various studies report that after age 50, there is approximately a 5% increase in the incidence of cholecystitis with each decade of life, ranging from a 25% incidence during the sixth decade to greater than 55% during the eighth decade. In one large Swedish study, one fourth of all patients over the age of 70 who presented with an acute abdomen were found to have cholecystitis.[3] The incidence of common bile duct stones roughly doubles during the same period. With age, the level of biliary cholesterol increases, raising the lithogenic index of bile and making the development of stones more likely.

In addition, the elderly are more prone to a variety of biliary tract *complications*. In one study of patients over the age of 65 with documented biliary tract stones, 80% eventually presented with complications. As a result, gallbladder disease has become the most common condition requiring laparotomy in individuals over age 60. Interestingly, among the general population, females with biliary tract disease outnumber males by a 2 to 3:1 ratio. In those over the age of 65 years, however, the incidence of biliary tract disease in males and females is almost identical.

Signs and symptoms of cholecystitis in the elderly are variable. The elderly patient with acute disease will most often complain of epigastric or right subcostal pain radiating to the back or right shoulder. If the pain subsides after several hours, the diagnosis of biliary colic *without cholecystitis* may be entertained. Pain, fever, and vomiting that persist usually indicate the presence of acute cholecystitis. In the elderly, fever and leukocytosis may be delayed, although signs of peritoneal irritation (percussion tenderness, rebound and/or involuntary guarding over the epigastrium or right upper quadrant) may actually occur earlier in the natural history of the disease. If complications, such as gangrene or perforation, develop, the patient may present with hypotension and frank septic shock.

At the more benign end of the spectrum of presentation are recurrent episodes of transient uncomplicated cystic duct obstruction — usually the result of multiple smaller calculi — which present with vague and less specific symptomatology. Frequently, the history is characterized by little more than subjective complaints of eructation, flatulence, relative anorexia, or mild fatty food intolerance; these symptoms may be accompanied by poorly localized upper abdominal or flank discomfort. Peptic disease, occult malignancy, right lower lobe pneumonia, variant angina, and upper urinary tract disease must be ruled out before the biliary tree is targeted for examination.

If asymptomatic biliary tract stones are documented, usually with abdominal ultrasound, the dilemma for the clinician is how best to manage the elderly patient with minimally symptomatic or so-called silent gallstones. Several factors should be kept in mind. First, the presence of a single large gallstone is associated with a substantially higher risk of complications than is so-called biliary gravel, or multiple small stones. Second, complications such as gangrene and/or perforation occur much more rapidly after the onset of initial symptoms in the geriatric population, mandating emergent rather than elective surgery. It should be noted in this context that in the case of *elective* cholecystectomy, age alone is associated with only a negligibly increased mortality. However, in the emergent surgical setting, advanced age becomes a significant risk factor.

In the largest study (Table 30–1) of its kind, Margiotta[4] reviewed 137 cases of patients over the age of 70 undergoing cholecystectomy and divided them into elective and emergent surgical groups. There was a 60% greater rate of complications among the emergent cholecystectomies, and an almost fourfold greater mortality rate in the elderly (12.5% versus 3.8%).

The presence of either diabetes mellitus or significant obesity significantly increases the risk of complications and should incline the clinician toward surgical consultations sooner rather than later. Indeed, diabetics manifest twice the incidence of biliary tract stones than do nondiabetics and sustain nearly twice the mortality rate secondary to complications resulting from rapid tissue necrosis.

The mainstay of emergent diagnosis of acute cholecystitis in the emergency department has become abdominal ultrasound examination. A positive ultrasound generally depicts dilated bile ducts, which are the most prominent of the localized inflammatory changes. However, if the patient with acute cholecystitis presents early enough in the course of the disease, there may be cystic duct obstruction without any evidence of dilatation of more distal ducts. In this setting, nucleotide scanning procedures such as HIDA or PIPIDA will delineate obstruction of the cystic duct and the diagnosis can be made promptly (see Table 30–7).

Table 30–1 Pathology in Elective (n = 78) and Emergency (n = 59) Cases of Cholecystectomy in the Elderly

	Elective	Emergency	Total
Pathology	n (%)	n (%)	n (%)

Acute
  Necrotizing
  Suppurative
  Hemorrhagic
	8 (10.0)	32 (54)	40 (29.5)

Acute and chronic	14 (18)	11 (19)	25 (18.5)
Total Acute	**22 (28)**	**43 (73)**	**65 (48)**
Subacute and chronic			
Chronic/fibrosing	56 (72)	16 (27)	72 (52)

Indications for prompt surgery in the asymptomatic geriatric patient with documented gallstones include the following:

1. Single large stone
2. Diabetes mellitus
3. Obesity
4. Immunosuppressive illness
5. History of pancreatitis
6. Possible common bile duct involvement
7. Absence of significant concomitant disease

These recommendations represent a general *reversal* of attitudes toward gallbladder surgery in the elderly. Rather than viewing the elderly as somehow too fragile for surgery or as a group for whom laparotomy should be postponed until a near-terminal precarious moment, it has been shown that the older population fares just as well as their younger counterparts under controlled (i.e., elective) conditions.[5] When definitive surgical treatment, however, is delayed in an otherwise appropriate operative candidate, complications become increasingly likely. Finally, while recognizing that age alone should not deter consideration of operative intervention, it should be noted that recent advances in *nonsurgical* management of biliary lithiasis extend the range of clinical options for these patients. Specifically, the combined utilization of bile acids (ursodeoxycholic and chenodeoxycholic acids) with extracorporeal shock waves (lithotripsy) has been successful in selected cases. For any elderly patient who is judged a poor operative candidate, these alternatives as well as others (e.g., stents for common bile duct stones) should be kept in mind by both the primary and consulting physicians.

Perforation of the Gallbladder

Because elderly patients are more prone to atherosclerotic vascular disease they are also more susceptible to perforation secondary to ischemic changes within the gallbladder wall. Whereas the gallbladder may take weeks to rupture after the onset of obstructive symptoms in the younger patient, perforation in the elderly may occur as early as 3 to 4 hours after the onset of symptoms. Generally, perforation is a condition limited to elderly males, in which mortality rates between 15 and 25% are reported.[6] Sequelae of perforation include bile peritonitis, cholecystoenteric fistula with or without gallstone ileus, and generalized abscess formation. Surgical intervention in this condition is mandatory.

Gallstone Ileus

Gallstone ileus (Figure 30–1) is a dramatic but relatively uncommon complication of perforation in which a large stone erodes through the gallbladder wall and migrates into the adjacent small bowel. The stone, which is

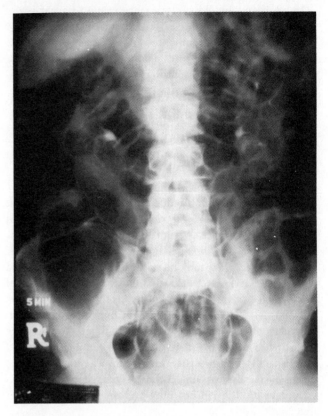

Figure 30–1 Enlarged small bowel loops associated with mechanical obstruction precipitated by gallstone ileus at the ileocecal valve.

usually at least 2.5 cm in size, moves distally and eventually causes mechanical small bowel obstruction at the ileocecal valve or at a more proximal narrowed site. The condition can be diagnosed on plain film of the abdomen if the characteristic triad of air in the biliary tree, gallstone in the intestine, and evidence of small intestinal obstruction is present. For reasons that are unclear, gallstone ileus is more common among women and, in one study,[7] was the etiology for 20% of intestinal obstructions in female patients over the age of 65. Only half the patients with gallstone ileus have previously documented biliary stones. Treatment consists of operative removal of the stone and repair of the cholecystoenteric fistula.

Emphysematous Cholecystitis

Emphysematous cholecystitis (Figure 30–2) is another complication that is felt to be secondary to severe vascular compromise within the gallbladder wall where compromised tissue permits growth of *Clostridium perfringens* or other gas-producing anaerobic organisms. The gallbladder appears as a distended radiolucent cavity on the abdominal plain film, which is often the only diagnostic procedure necessary to confirm the diagnosis. Gas may also be visible and will appear in the gallbladder lumen, wall, or pericholecystic soft tissue and ducts. Emphysematous cholecystitis occurs in only 1% of

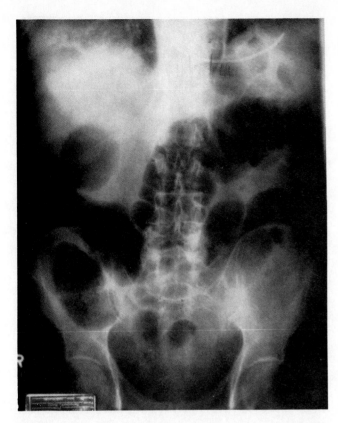

Figure 30–2 Collection of air in the right upper quadrant is characteristic of emphysematous cholecystitis.

Cholangitis and Empyema

The surgical literature describes the physical findings of ascending cholangitis with the so-called Charcot's triad: right upper quadrant pain, spiking fever, and jaundice. By definition, *ascending* (i.e., nonobstructive) cholangitis arises retrograde from the intestinal tract, producing infection of the common, cystic, and hepatic ducts. A separate and far less common entity, *suppurative* cholangitis, results when the gallbladder obstructs secondary stone, stricture, or neoplasm and then fills with frank pus. These patients will usually rapidly go on to septic shock.[9]

The microbiology of biliary infections includes both aerobes and anaerobes. Among aerobes, *Escherichia coli*, *Klebsiella* species, *Enterobacter* species, and enterococcus predominate. The major anaerobes are *Bacteroides fragilis* and *Clostridium*. Pure aerobic and mixed aerobic-anaerobic infections occur in about equal frequencies, while purely anaerobic infections are seen rarely.

When cholangitis (Figure 30–3) is suspected in the emergency department, fluid support and antibiotic therapy (see previous section) should be initiated promptly. Particular attention must be paid to coagulation studies since a significant percentage of patients with either suppurative or nonsuppurative cholangitis develop disseminated intravascular coagulopathy. Definitive treatment may include endoscopic papillotomy to decompress and drain the duct prior to cholecystectomy. In skilled

all patients with cholecystitis and is 5 times more common in males. The diagnosis should be suspected in any diabetic male with symptoms referable to the biliary tree. If the diagnosis is made in the emergency department, a surgical consult must be obtained and antibiotic therapy should be started immediately. Several adjunctive regimens are effective, including the following: an aminoglycoside (for gram-negative aerobes) in combination with clindamycin HCl (Cleocin HCl), 300 to 600 mg every 6 hours; or ampicillin-sulbactam, 1.5 to 3.0 g every 6 hours in combination with aztreonam.

The expanded spectrum penicillins such as ampicillin-sulbactam (Unasyn), ticarcillin, mezlocillin, and piperacillin are also active against gram-negative aerobes and anaerobic bacteria and have the additional advantage of covering enterococcus as well. However, their gram-negative spectrum (i.e., *Pseudomonas*) is not as complete as that of the aminoglycosides, which should be used in combination in the immunocompromised individual or when *Pseudomonas* or *Serratia* species are likely pathogens. A third-generation cephalosporin may be used as a substitute for aminoglycosides in a patient with compromised renal function. Once antibiotics are begun, emergent surgery should be performed unless otherwise contraindicated. Mortality rates of 15% (approximately four times that of uncomplicated acute cholecystitis) have been reported with this complication.[8]

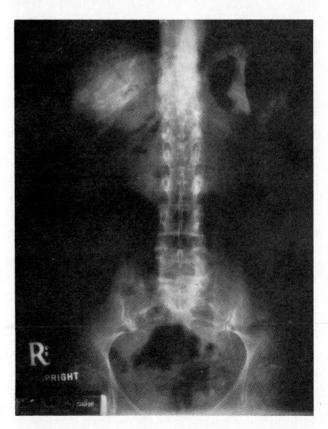

Figure 30–3 Cholecystoenteric fistula with air in the biliary tree.

hands, papillotomy is quick and may be performed without the risks of general anesthesia, allowing time for hemodynamic stabilization prior to surgery in the emergent setting.

Acalculous Cholecystitis

Any condition that predisposes to stagnation or concentration of bile predisposes to acalculous cholecystitis,[10] including prolonged narcotic use, dehydration, or low-flow hemodynamic states, such as congestive heart failure. Common in males over 65, acalculous cholecystitis frequently presents as a complication of an unrelated insult, such as a major trauma, burns, or septicemia. Because of its association with other serious pathology and its predilection for older patients, acalculous cholecystitis has a higher mortality rate (6.5%) than the more common calculous variety (4%). Surgical treatment is mandatory unless otherwise contraindicated.

PEPTIC ULCER DISEASE

Peptic ulcer disease should never be far from the top of the differential diagnosis in elderly patients who present with upper or midabdominal pain,[11] with or without evidence of gastrointestinal bleeding. Too often, clinicians rely on a previous history of peptic ulcer disease before making the diagnosis. In the elderly, however, an acute abdominal event is oftentimes the first manifestation of this condition.

Among all age groups, 10% of patients with peptic ulcer disease will present with an acute surgical abdomen as their *initial* manifestation of this condition. In the elderly, 50% of patients will present in this manner, of which 35 to 45% will present with a rigid, boardlike, quiet abdomen (with or without signs of shock) as their first and only manifestation of peptic disease. Consequently, while it may have taken the patient 60 or 70 years to *develop* this disease, once manifest, the acuity is high as is the incidence of complications. One series reports a bleeding or perforation rate of 31% in patients between the ages of 60 to 64 and 76% in patients 75 to 79 years of age.[11] Frank hemorrhage accounts for up to two thirds of the complications of peptic ulcer disease, with perforation (Figure 30–4) and outlet obstruction comprising the remainder of cases.

In the general population, the ratio of duodenal to gastric ulcer approaches 10:1. Among the elderly, however, it declines to 2:1. This relative increase in gastric ulceration has significant consequences. While accounting for only one third of all ulcers documented in this age group, gastric ulceration accounts for over two thirds of ulcer-related mortality in this same group. Part of this morbidity and mortality associated with gastric ulcers may be attributed to the relative lack of specificity of

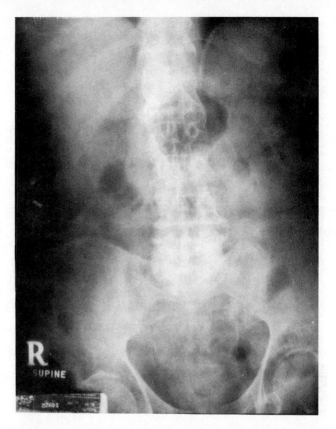

Figure 30–4   Air in the lesser sac indicates perforated gastric ulcer.

symptoms over prolonged periods of time. For example, in the elderly, mild nausea with gradual weight loss may predominate over more specific symptoms of pain or bleeding. The elderly population is especially prone to erosions of the superior aspect of the cardia, simulating angina or reflux disorders and further delaying diagnosis. Ulcers of the cardia are more likely to generate low-grade chronic blood loss than their duodenal counterparts.

Elderly patients with peptic ulcer disease are more likely to be on steroidal or nonsteroidal antiinflammatory agents, which compromise the gastrointestinal mucosa. One large study of elderly patients who expired in the hospital revealed a fourfold greater death rate from peptic ulcer/upper gastrointestinal hemorrhage in patients taking nonsteroidal antiinflammatory drugs (NSAIDs) than those who did not.[12] Additional investigations have demonstrated that NSAIDs can mask symptoms of preexistent peptic disease, thus delaying diagnosis and increasing morbidity and mortality. Some elderly patients who have *already* been diagnosed with peptic ulcer disease may be on chronic cimetidine (Tagamet) therapy. This medication, through its inhibition of the P-450 cytochrome oxidase system, may increase the serum levels of a number of other medications, including anticonvulsants (Dilantin, Tegretol), beta-blockers, theophylline, benzodiazepines, and Coumadin. Most experts feel ranitidine or famotidine to be preferable to cimetidine as an H_2 blocker in the elderly because of the aforementioned drug interactions.

MECHANICAL BOWEL OBSTRUCTION

The elderly individual is statistically more likely to have undergone a laparotomy than his younger counterpart and, consequently, more likely to develop postoperative adhesive scarring. Adhesions may become a problem relatively soon after surgery (weeks or months) or, in a more insidious fashion, with symptoms manifesting themselves many years after the offending surgery. As with all age groups, adhesions are the most common etiology for bowel obstruction in the elderly. The majority can be treated conservatively, with bowel rest, nasogastric suction, and hydration. However, a significant percentage will not resolve spontaneously and must undergo surgical lysis of adhesions, thus contributing to a vicious cycle of adhesion formation-obstruction-laparotomy with surgical "take-down" of adhesions, and renewed scarring. In addition to iatrogenic adhesions, the relative laxity of the bowel wall with advancing age predisposes these patients to herniation, which is often complicated by intestinal incarceration and strangulation. One British series found one third of patients over the age of 75 who presented with an acute abdomen to have some combination of strangulated hernia with intestinal obstruction.

With the exception of adhesive scarring in males, inguinal hernias (Figure 30–5) are the most common etiology for bowel obstruction in the geriatric population. Indirect inguinal hernia occurs when intestinal structures pass through the internal inguinal ring and through the inguinal canal. This space is created from failure of fusion of the processus vaginalis after the testis has descended into the scrotum. Because indirect inguinal hernia is most common from infancy through middle age, it is frequently overlooked as an etiology for bowel obstruction in the aged. With advancing years, however, increased intraabdominal pressure and dilatation of the internal inguinal ring allow the hernial sac to enter the previously empty peritoneal diverticulum.

Among elderly males, *direct* inguinal hernia is a more frequent cause for obstruction. This results from protrusion and occasional incarceration of intestinal contents within Hesselbach's area, owing to gradual weakening of the transversalis fascia. Direct inguinal hernias are uncommon in older women, in whom the *femoral* variety accounts for up to one third of hernias in this population. Femoral hernias descend through the femoral canal, beneath the inguinal ligament, and present as a palpable mass at or above the inguinal ligament itself.

Signs and symptoms of bowel obstruction are not distinctive or unique in the geriatric population. If the obstruction is complete, diffuse colicky abdominal pain, distention, nausea, vomiting, and eventual obstipation are usually present. "Rushes" and "tinkles" may be auscultated during resistance to peristalsis. Typical x-ray findings include increased small bowel gas (Figure 30–6) with multiple air/fluid levels scattered throughout the intestinal lumen proximal to the obstruction. Thumb printing, which represents edema of the bowel wall, may also be evident. Air/fluid levels among areas of the small bowel are much more specific and diagnostic than when

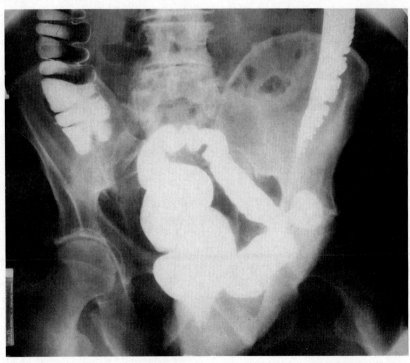

Figure 30–5 Femoral hernia.

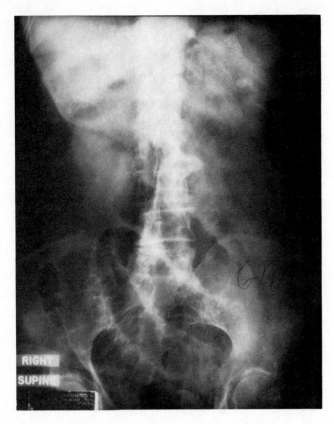

Figure 30–6   Small bowel obstruction.

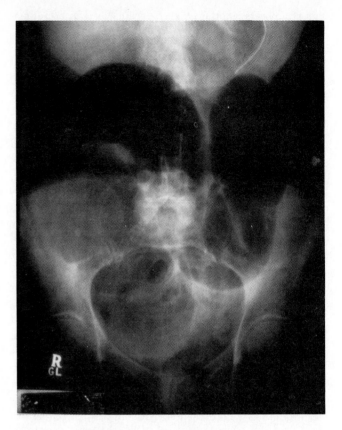

Figure 30–7   Sigmoid volvulus.

seen in the colon. If blockage is prolonged and distal, feculent emesis may ensue and if decompression is not accomplished promptly, particularly in the elderly, viscous rupture with peritonitis may occur and free air will be evident on the upright or decubitus plain film.

Obstruction of the *large intestine* is more likely to be partial and intermittent and to be associated with feculent emesis and heme-positive stools. Unlike small bowel obstruction, the most common cause of large bowel obstruction in the elderly is malignancy. Indeed, colonic cancer is the single most common cancer among the entire geriatric population. Colonic cancer represents 30% of all malignancies among males and 40% among females in the older age group. The left colon is by far the most common site with up to two thirds of all lesions within reach of the sigmoidoscope.

Volvulus

Volvulus (Figure 30–7) accounts for up to 10% of all cases of large bowel obstruction in those 60 years of age and younger and about 15% in the elderly.[14] The condition is characterized by rotation of a segment of bowel around the axis of its mesentery, a topologic derangement that compromises vascular supply and obstructs and causes distention of the involved lumen. Eighty-five percent of these cases involve the sigmoid colon, where *elongation* of

the affected region (so-called "redundancy") in the elderly predisposes them to this form of bowel obstruction. Fifteen percent of cases are cecal in origin and are characterized by a twisted, dilated cecum that is transposed or "flipped" over into the right upper quadrant on the plain film (Figure 30–8). A so-called bird's beak narrowing at one end of the dilated segment of bowel identifies the proximal portion of obstruction.

Both sigmoid and cecal varieties of volvulus are found more frequently in older patients. The former is more common in men, while the latter is equally common in both sexes. The reasons for this are unclear. In addition to advanced age, neurologic and/or psychiatric patients with neurologic and/or psychiatric dysfunction have a special predisposition for volvulus. It is speculated that use of psychiatric (typically anticholinergic) medication, deranged eating and drinking behavior, and little or no physical exercise play a role by producing chronic distention and elongation of the large bowel, thereby predisposing it to redundancy and eventual transposition on its mesenteric stalk. The usual presentation to the emergency department finds an elderly male transported from a psychiatric institution or other care facility with relatively abrupt onset of abdominal pain, colicky in nature, with persistence of pain between spasms, abdominal distention, and nausea and vomiting. There may be visible peristalsis and a palpable mass on abdominal exam.

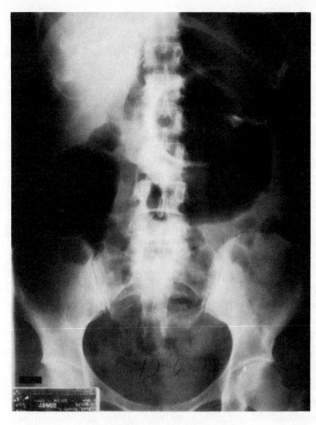

Figure 30–8 Sigmoid volvulus.

Treatment of cecal and sigmoid volvulus are markedly different. When volvulus involves the sigmoid, the distended lumen can usually be decompressed with the passage of a soft rectal tube (through a sigmoidoscope) with detorsion of the mesenteric axis. When the likelihood of peritoneal contamination is low, barium enema is often therapeutic. With recurrent episodes of sigmoid volvulus (which is seen in more than 50% of patients), partial colonic resection with anastomosis is generally preferred over detorsion and fixation. Cecal volvulus, on the other hand, invariably requires laparotomy, often with right hemicolectomy and ileocolonic anastomosis. Mortality rates, which vary from 25 to 40% in all first episodes of volvulus, are ascribed to a delay in diagnosis and underlying illness.

Constipation

In the context of catastrophic causes of intestinal obstruction, it is appropriate to discuss the vastly more prevalent, if less dramatic, condition of constipation among the elderly. In few other areas of clinical medicine are practitioners so overcome with therapeutic nihilism. It is almost as if aging universally brought with it the phenomenon of men and women going 4, 5, 8, or even 12 days with little or no bowel movement. Such nihilism generates inadequate history taking, errors in diagnosis, and considerable suffering, much of which can be ameliorated if not avoided entirely.

The following list of partially or completely reversible factors predisposing toward constipation in the elderly must be given serious consideration when approaching any patient with constipation, no matter how chronic the disturbance.

1. Medication side effect
   a. Anticholinergics (tricyclic antidepressant, antihistamines, antipsychotics)
   b. Narcotics
2. Poor fluid intake
3. Decreased fiber intake
4. Sedentary lifestyle
5. Depression/anxiety
6. Oral/dental disorders
7. Anorectal disorders
8. Reversible endocrinopathies
9. Iron and calcium intake
10. Neurologic disease
11. Laxative abuse
12. Hypokalemia

PANCREATITIS

Pancreatitis is the most common *nonsurgical* etiology for abdominal pain requiring hospitalization in the geriatric population.[15,16] Though not widely appreciated, its incidence increases with age, because the elderly are statistically (with exposure through time), pharmacologically, and histologically more vulnerable to all the following predisposing factors leading to pancreatitis:

1. Alcoholism
2. Biliary tract disease
3. Penetrating ulcer
4. Trauma
5. Drug reactions (thiazides, furosemide, estrogens, sulfonamides, tetracycline, and possibly steroids and procainamide)
6. Hypercalcemia
7. Carbon monoxide exposure
8. Hypothermia

Acute pancreatitis can be divided into clinical categories reflecting the underlying processes. In the elderly, as in the younger age group, interstitial (edematous) pancreatitis comprises 80 to 95% of cases, with hemorrhagic (necrotizing) pancreatitis (Figure 30–9) comprising 5 to 15%. Presentation includes epigastric pain, penetrating in nature, accompanied by low-grade fever, nausea, vomiting, and signs of volume depletion. But even in the presence of extensive inflammation, the elderly (as they do with cholecystitis) present at one end or the other of the clinical spectrum. Signs and symptoms

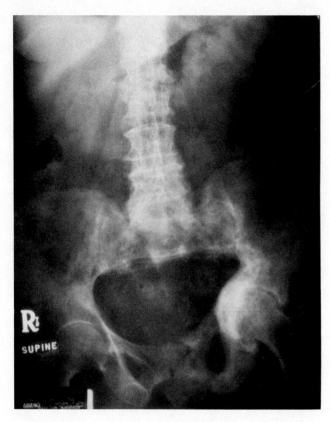

Figure 30–9 Necrotizing pancreatitis (with air in the pancreas).

of the geriatric patient with acute pancreatitis may be nonspecific, poorly localized, with the patient ill but not in acute distress. There may be anorexia for 1 or 2 days, upper or midabdominal pain, mild nausea, and little else. At the other extreme, some patients will present with agonizing epigastric or chest pain, hypotension, and shock. A certain subpopulation, estimated at 10%, arrives without complaint of pain or emesis but simply with unexplained hypotension and altered mental status. The relatively early onset of hemodynamic collapse in acute pancreatitis, which may even be associated with transient ST and T-wave changes on electrocardiogram (ECG), may be related to so-called myocardial depressant factor (MDF) elaborated by the inflamed or ischemic pancreas. Interestingly, geriatric females are affected significantly more frequently than are males.

Diagnostically, hyperamylasemia has been the cornerstone of clinical evaluation, but the nonspecificity of this enzyme elevation in the setting of a fragile, elderly patient compromised its diagnostic usefulness.[17] For example, hyperamylasemia can be seen in pneumonia, renal insufficiency, peptic disease, mesenteric vascular compromise, and other disorders. However, on occasion, the *magnitude* of hyperamylasemia is more specific and quite helpful, as in biliary pancreatitis where enzyme elevation may be five to ten fold greater than normal, well above the range of elevation seen in the other dis-

orders just mentioned. The ratio of amylase-to-creatinine clearance is also helpful. A value of greater than 5% (in the absence of diabetic ketoacidosis) is diagnostic of pancreatitis. While seen in a variety of other gastrointestinal disorders, the so-called sentinel loop (essentially a localized region of paralytic ileus) is also frequently associated with pancreatitis.

An area of mystery and relative controversy concerns the *pulmonary* complications of pancreatitis in *all* age groups.[18] Simple hypoxemia is the most common complication. In the elderly, however, the incidence of objective findings on chest x-ray ranging from small areas of basilar atelectasis to effusions, infiltrates, and frank pulmonary edema, is significantly increased and the severity of radiographic changes directly related to the degree of pancreatic inflammation. The pulmonary edema of acute pancreatitis in the geriatric population usually begins 2 to 3 days after the initial presentation and appears to be associated with serum triglyceride elevation. Consequently, once the diagnosis of acute pancreatitis in the elderly patient has been confirmed, careful observation of respiratory status is critical. Serial chest x-rays, blood gases, and prompt ventilatory assistance are often necessary to prevent rapid decompensation. Mortality rates for the initial presentation of acute pancreatitis are 15% in patients under 50 years of age, 30% in the 50- to 70-year old group, and 40% in patients over age 70. Interestingly, however, one study of 268 patients in Britain demonstrated that while mortality from pancreatitis was increased in the elderly, these deaths were generally secondary to associated illnesses that were prevalent in this age group. When only deaths due to complications of acute pancreatitis were analyzed, mortality rate was not significantly different between young and older patients.

APPENDICITIS

Appendicitis represents one geriatric abdominal emergency in which life-threatening disease can present with minimal symptomatology. For this and other reasons, clinicians have traditionally maintained an insufficient index of suspicion for appendicitis in the geriatric patient.[19] Reasons for this are clear. In the normal course of aging, the appendix typically involutes, and appendectomies in patients over age 60 account for only 8% of all those performed. (This figure is partially misleading, as a significant number of patients may have had incidental appendectomies as part of previous laparotomies in their younger years.) Geriatric patients with acute appendicitis still account for between 5 and 7% of all acute abdominal emergencies in this age group. Because of a low index of suspicion, however, significant delays in diagnosis have been found to be four times as common in patients in their seventh decade as compared to those patients in the fourth decade of life. Moreover, appendiceal perforation is more common in the elderly as compared to the general population.

Approximately 40 to 50% of geriatric patients going to laparotomy with acute appendicitis are incorrectly diagnosed preoperatively. These diagnostic errors, which lead to perforation of the inflamed appendix, are due primarily to the relative lack of both magnitude and specificity of the signs and symptoms in this subgroup (Table 30–2).

The patient, for example, may ascribe his or her discomfort to ongoing problems such as constipation and may have treated himself or herself with enemas for hours or even days prior to presentation. In addition, anatomical changes caused by previous surgery may produce unusual patterns of symptomatology; for example, the appendix may rupture into an inguinal or femoral hernial sac, or be anatomically relocated due to adhesive scarring from previous surgeries. A recent California study of 94 elderly patients with appendicitis reflects the problematic aspects of this condition both to the patient, who must decide to obtain treatment, and to the physician, who must make the diagnosis and arrange prompt surgery. In 83% of patients, more than 24 hours elapsed between the *onset* of symptoms and initiation of surgery, while in 53%, more than 48 hours had elapsed (Table 30–3). As expected, the incidence of complications (perforation, gangrene, abscess) (Figure 30–10) increased dramatically with delayed treatment. All 4 deaths were in patients greater than 80 years of age who had perforated after a surgical delay of greater than 24 hours.

A Mount Sinai Hospital study[19a] elucidated the variety of diagnoses with which the patients with appendicitis were *incorrectly* admitted. Errors in diagnosis ranged from metastatic colon cancer and intestinal obstruction to incarcerated inguinal hernia and PID. As in the California study, the New York group demonstrated roughly twice the incidence of both perforation and abscess formation in the elderly.

Table 30–2   Acute Appendicitis in the Elderly Population at the Mount Sinai Hospital (1974–1984)

Physical exam	Controls 20–60 yrs (n = 56)	60 + yrs (n = 70)
Abdominal tenderness		
Right lower quadrant	86	77
Other	12	17
None	2	6
Rebound tenderness*	74	51
Rectal tenderness*	74	51
Guarding	81	66
Abdominal mass	13	22
Rectal mass	6	6
Abdominal distention*	40	63
Bowel sounds		
Decreased	49	58
Normal or increased	51	42

* p < 0.025. From Hirsch.[19a]

Table 30–3   Acute Appendicitis in the Elderly Population at the Mount Sinai Hospital (1974–1984) — Delay in Diagnosis and Treatment

	Controls 20–60 yrs (n = 56)	60 + yrs (n = 70)
Time with Symptoms Before Seeking Care		
< 12 hr	39	17
13–48 hr	43	40
> 48 hr	18	43
Time from Emergency Room to Operating Room*		
< 12 hr	80	58
13–72 hr	16	26
> 72 hr	4	16

* p < 0.025. From Hirsch.[19a]

For the clinician who, in the elderly, expects the 8 to 24 hours of epigastric or periumbilical pain, followed by localization to the right lower quadrant with fever and leukocytosis, lifesaving laparotomy will be dangerously delayed. This disease is frequently missed in the elderly because it is not uncommon for the pain to remain poorly localized in these patients. Rebound and involuntary guarding on abdominal exam are seen in only 50% of cases (Table 30–4). Such symptoms as constipation (rather than one to two episodes of diarrhea frequently found in younger patients) and abdominal distention are not uncommon; rigors and/or hypothermia signify progression to perforation (Table 30–5). As in most cases of sepsis among the elderly, a white count differential characterized by increased bands *without leukocytosis* is a poor prognostic sign. Finally, the presence of a hypochromic microcytic anemia with heme-positive stools in the setting of acute appendicitis in the elderly is highly indicative of appendicitis secondary to neoplastic obstruction.

Table 30–4   Acute Appendicitis in the Elderly Population at the Mount Sinai Hospital (1974–1984)

	Controls 20–60 yrs (n = 56)	60 + yrs (n = 70)
Tachycardia (pulse 100)	30	34
Temperature		
< 100°F	48	34
100–101°F	39	51
> 102°F	13	14
Average	99.9°F	100.2°F
WBC count		
< 10,000	12	13
10–20,000	79	76
> 20,000	9	11
< 10,000 and no left shift	2	3
Average	14,500	14,400

From Hirsch.[19a]

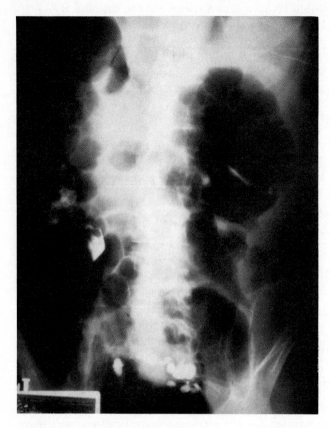

Figure 30–10 Periappendiceal abscess.

DIVERTICULAR DISEASE

Diverticulosis, defined as simple herniation of the bowel wall that does not violate the serosa, occurs in 50% of

Table 30–5   Acute Appendicitis in the Elderly Population at the Mount Sinai Hospital (1974–1984) — Perforation Rate

Pathology*	Controls 20–60 yrs (n = 56)	60 + yrs (n = 70)
Nonperforated	66	32
Perforated	34	68
Perforated with abscess	16	30
Perforated with generalized peritonitis	5	7

* $p < 0.001$. From Hirsch.[19a]

Americans over the age of 60, and increases thereafter. Most patients are asymptomatic, but they may experience constipation (as both a cause and effect of diverticular disease) and bloating with mild discomfort. Simple diverticulosis is an important cause of lower gastrointestinal bleeding, along with vascular ectasia and other arteriovenous malformations. The sigmoid colon is the area most commonly affected and is the only colonic segment involved in 65% of patients. Fifteen percent of patients with documented diverticulosis will have at least one episode of significant hemorrhage, which is generally not associated with pain and usually resolves spontaneously. Bleeding that fails to subside may be treated with vasoconstrictor agents instilled via selective mesenteric angiography. This method has been reported to be successful in greater than 90% of patients.

Although the condition can remain asymptomatic for years, with inflammation and/or violation of the outer (serosal) bowel surface, complications of diverticulosis ensue (Figure 30–11). Perforation may result in peritonitis

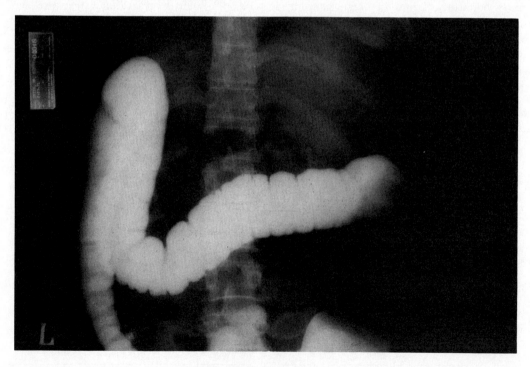

Figure 30–11 Diverticulitis.

or the contaminated area may be walled off by omentum, small bowel, or bladder, resulting in a pericolic abscess or chronic fistula formation. The abscess itself is not only a source of infection but may also cause bowel obstruction. In the early phase of diverticulitis, the presentation often consists of well-localized left lower quadrant pain exacerbated by defecation. Guarding on abdominal examination and, at times, a palpable mass (in the nonobese subject) will also be evident. Distal lesions may be palpable as a mass on rectal exam. Fever and leukocytosis of some degree are the rule, with the caveat, as in all potential abdominal catastrophes herein discussed, that the elderly patient may be unable to mount an elevated white count or fever, particularly in the face of overwhelming sepsis. On occasion, if the involved area is adjacent to the urinary bladder, pyuria and hematuria may result. Any suspicion of an inflammatory lesion in this setting rules out the use of barium enema, as contents under pressure may initiate or extend bowel rupture.

Clinical decisions regarding inpatient versus outpatient therapy for diverticulitis depend on the severity of the disease process. Stable patients without peritoneal findings at the younger end of the geriatric age spectrum can usually be sent home with enterically active wide-spectrum antibiotics (e.g., sulfamethoxazole and trimethoprim, amoxicillin), bed rest, liquid diet with stool softeners, and pain medication as necessary. Older patients who are more toxic and/or unable to take oral medications and fluids must be admitted for intravenous hydration while the bowel is placed completely at rest and they should receive parenteral antibiotic therapy (e.g., ampicillin-sulbactam [Unasyn] 1.5 to 3.0 g q. 6h. IV). Here again, most cases subside with conservative measures, but in the significantly ill patient who fails to respond within 24 to 36 hours or in whom abscess or fistula formation is suspected, temporary diverting colostomy with partial resection of the involved segment and eventual reanastomosis is generally recommended.

MESENTERIC VASCULAR OCCLUSION

Among the most age-specific gastrointestinal catastrophes is the acutely ischemic bowel secondary to mesenteric vascular occlusion or insufficiency. While this condition occasionally occurs in younger patients at risk for atherosclerotic cardiovascular disease, this is primarily a disease of the elderly, in whom risk increases with advancing age.[20]

When faced with the patient complaining of abdominal pain, there is a natural tendency to think diagnostically in terms of primary alimentary end-organ dysfunction. In this setting, the differential diagnosis will include hepatic, biliary, or primary gastrointestinal disease. Although this is appropriate, it should be stressed that when dealing with the elderly patient, a primary *vascular* etiology for abdominal pain (i.e., abdominal aortic aneurysm) (Figure 30–12) must always be entertained, both because of a greater statistical likelihood of occurrence in this age group and because of the dire consequences associated with a delay in diagnosis.

Etiologies for acute mesenteric ischemia include superior mesenteric artery embolus in about 30 to 35% of cases, superior mesenteric artery thrombosis in 10 to 15% of cases, and the "syndrome of nonocclusive ischemia" (NOMI) in about 40 to 50% of patients. These etiologies will be discussed separately, but it is useful to think of them collectively, since many features of their diagnosis and treatment are identical.

The patient with acute mesenteric ischemia usually is an elderly male who complains of diffuse abdominal pain, the severity of which is disproportionate to objective findings (i.e., severe discomfort with minimal physical findings). Often, there is a history of cardiovascular disease, such as recent myocardial infarction, congestive heart failure (or other "low flow states"), or atrial fibrillation. The abdominal pain is deep and visceral in nature; the patient may be doubled over and is usually very still. The difficulty in diagnosis stems from the fact that early in the ischemic process, often including the early stages of infarction, the clinician is presented with few objective

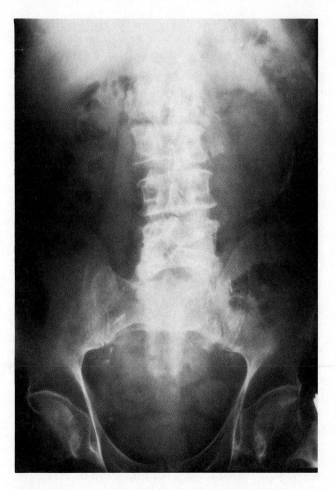

Figure 30–12 Calcified abdominal aortic aneurysm.

physical manifestations of concern. Besides the pain, abdominal distention and gastrointestinal bleeding may be the only findings until widespread bowel necrosis is well under way. Even these signs may be unreliable. In many patients, fever, rigors, nausea and vomiting, leukocytosis, and vascular collapse occur in varied but rapid succession. Laparoscopy, although useful for diagnosing transmural infarction, is not reliable for evaluating earlier stages of mucosal ischemia in which blood is shunted to the serosa and the normal intestinal appearance is preserved for the eye of the direct observer. Because of these diagnostic pitfalls, mortality figures for combined causes exceed 70%.

Acute Superior Mesenteric Artery (SMA) Thrombosis

Preexisting atherosclerosis is usually the setting for acute thrombotic obstruction in the mesenteric vasculature. The lesion typically forms within the first 2 cm of the artery's branch point from the aorta, where chronic turbulence of flow results in maximal plaque formation. Patients with thrombotic etiology for their vascular occlusion may report a history of postprandial "intestinal angina," usually upper abdominal in location, crampy in nature, and occurring 30 to 60 minutes after a meal.

SMA Embolus

Embolic occlusion, approximately twice as common as thrombotic occlusion, is most often seen in the elderly male with cardiovascular disease. Because of its acute angle as it takes off from the aorta, the superior mesenteric artery is well designed for harboring emboli, which most often originate from a mural thrombus in the left heart. Atrial fibrillation is an important risk factor. While these patients do not generally report a history of prior intestinal angina, they often have a history of previous embolic disease involving cerebral, iliofemoral, or other major arteries. It has been noted in one study that 20% of those patients presenting with SMA occlusion have been shown to have synchronous emboli in other arteries.

Syndrome of Nonocclusive Ischemia

In this condition, which probably accounts for as many as one half of all cases of mesenteric infarction, no specific obstructive lesion is discovered, but one or more of a variety of factors ultimately results in greatly reduced blood flow to the splanchnic bed. Hemorrhagic shock or hypovolemia from any cause can reduce flow to the mesentery where, in this setting, splanchnic vasoconstriction (to divert blood to heart and brain) compounds the problem. Similarly, patients with low output states from chronic congestive heart failure, recent myocardial infarction with reduced left ventricular func-

tion, and other primary cardiac causes are also at risk. Interestingly, because of more aggressive and sophisticated fluid resuscitation and monitoring of volume status along with more liberal usage of systemic vasodilators to unload the failing heart, this "low-flow" etiology appears to be declining in frequency.

Treatment

Elderly patients with mesenteric infarction, hemodynamic instability, and metabolic derangements are very poor operative candidates. Angiography, however, is a far less invasive maneuver and is being used with relative success both diagnostically and therapeutically in conditions associated with mesenteric ischemia. In a patient suspected of mesenteric occlusion, angiography will usually demonstrate the presence or absence of an obstructing lesion, define the lesion as an embolus, thrombus, or low-flow splanchnic constrictive state, and provide a vehicle for selective infusion of papaverine, a potent local vasodilator. It will demonstrate the presence or absence of adequate collateral vessels around an obstruction and provide the basis for a rational decision regarding eventual laparotomy with intestinal resection and arterial reconstruction. Beginning with Boley in the early 1970s[6,20] and his follow-up studies almost a decade later,[21] survival rates from combined causes incorporating the above protocol increased from 20% to greater than 50%, with 85% of the survivors requiring minimal or no intestinal resection and eventually returning to normal bowel function.

SELECTED ISSUES IN DIAGNOSTIC IMAGING

Technology is making increasingly sophisticated procedures more available for diagnosis of acute abdominal pain.[22-27] While we recognize that in 1989, the emergency department physician is not likely to order an endoscopic retrograde cholangiopancreatogram (ERCP) or to schedule lithotripsy, the *rationale* for such procedures and their role in the diagnosis and treatment of various conditions should be understood by any informed primary care physician. The emergency physician will often be consulted by patient and family on any of a variety of issues and may indeed decide, for example, in the setting of the acute abdomen, whether a surgeon or radiologist is the next clinician to be contacted. We have seen that for the geriatric patient with abdominal pain, diagnostic delay is not an uncommon source of increased morbidity and mortality. Thus, a potent argument can be made for earlier and *more complete* evaluation (including one or more imaging studies) within the emergency department setting. Merely admitting the elderly patient for "expectant observation," while waiting for his or her lab values or physical examination to drastically change, is no longer acceptable.

Imaging the Biliary System

Only in the past several years has ultrasonic evaluation of the biliary system emerged as part of the emergency physician's diagnostic armamentarium (Table 30–6). The most important change has been the development of real-time (as opposed to static) imaging capabilities, which can now orchestrate hundreds of thousands of ultrasonic tomograms in several planes into detailed and coherent images.

In evaluating patients with possible cholelithiasis or cholecystitis, a number of major and minor diagnostic criteria are defined sonographically. Complete nonvisualization of the gallbladder or the sonographic presence of gallstones are both considered major diagnostic criteria. The sensitivity of these major criteria is about 85%, while their specificity is greater than 95%. Minor diagnostic criteria include gallbladder wall thickening (greater than 4 to 5 mm), tenderness of the gallbladder when palpated during the examination (sonographic Murphy's sign), gallbladder enlargement (greater than 5 cm in any dimension), round gallbladder shape, and evidence of pericholecystic fluid. Of these, wall thickening appears to the most statistically reliable. More to the point, one study has demonstrated that the combination of a sonographic Murphy's sign in the presence of gallbladder enlargement on ultrasound was 99% predictive of "patients needing a cholecystectomy," regardless of the specific diagnosis.

In addition to its relative accuracy, advantages of ultrasound in this setting include rapidity of performance (5 to 15 minutes), minimal degree of preparation (ideally the patient should be NPO for 6 hours prior to the exam, but often adequate studies are obtained after shorter fasting periods), absence of any need for medication, absence of ionizing radiation, and relatively low cost (average cost $220). An important additional benefit of ultrasonography is its ability to evaluate the liver, pancreas, and kidneys within the same examination. The so-called screening abdominal ultrasound has been shown to detect nonbiliary causes of pain in the upper abdomen in 24 to 35% of patients without gallbladder disease.

Cholescintigraphy

Cholescintigraphy has not, traditionally, been within the province of the emergency department physician. Yet, 15 years ago the same statement could be made of diagnostic ultrasound and even computerized tomography (CT). Although less commonly considered in the emergency setting, the use of cholescintigraphy has become an increasingly valuable adjunct in the diagnostic evaluation of biliary pathology (Table 30–7). These radioactive scanning techniques (HIDA, PIPIDA, DESIDA) utilize radioisotopic-labeled technetium injected intravenously. After injection, the radioisotope is taken up by the liver and secreted, thereby visualizing hepatic and cystic ducts, the gallbladder, and common bile duct as well as the small intestine. When the original ultrasound has been nondiagnostic (because of obesity, inadequate preparation, or other reason), scintigraphy can often readily assess the patency of the biliary tree, particularly the cystic duct.

When the liver, hepatic duct, and common bile duct are visualized but the gallbladder is *not*, the diagnosis of acute cholecystitis can be made, usually implying the presence of a large stone within the cystic duct. When visualization of the gallbladder is merely delayed (greater than 1 hour), a diagnosis of chronic cholecystitis (usually multiple smaller stones and partial obstruction of the cystic duct) can be made. Finally, when the gallbladder is visualized but the common bile duct is *not*, and flow into the small intestine is delayed, a diagnosis of choledocholithiasis (usually a common bile duct stone) can be made. Sensitivities and specificities for the evaluation of acute cholecystitis by this method are generally greater than 90%. It should be noted that in alcoholic, severely ill, or other chronic fasting patients, as well as in patients with hepatitis and pancreatitis, the test is frequently falsely positive.

Table 30–6   Biliary Tract Ultrasound

Major diagnostic criteria
  Stone present
  Nonvisualization of gallbladder

Minor diagnostic criteria
  Wall thickening
  Sonographic Murphy's sign
  Gallbladder enlargement
  Round gallbladder shape
  Pericholecystic fluid

Advantages
  Accuracy
  Rapidity of performance
  Minimal preparation
  No ionizing radiation
  Other structures "screened"

Cost
  Average $220

Table 30–7   Cholescintigraphy

Purpose
  Assess status of biliary tract function

Indication
  Equivocal or nondiagnostic ultrasound

Criteria	Diagnosis
All ducts visualized but gallbladder not	Acute cholecystitis
Delayed visualization	Chronic cholecystitis
Gallbladder visualized Common duct not visualized Delayed flow into intestine	Choledocholithiasis

Cost
  $300 (not inclusive of radiologist's fee)

Ultrasound and Appendicitis

Until recent years, the emergency clinician evaluating appendicitis has had little support from diagnostic imaging. Plain films of the abdomen might show an appendicolith in a small minority of cases, indicating appendicitis in the appropriately symptomatic patient. But the sensitivity of plain films was unacceptably poor. Beginning in 1981 with initial case reports, this decade has generated improved technology and increasingly discriminating sonographic criteria for the diagnosis of appendicitis. These criteria include 1) visualization of a noncompressible appendix (an uninflamed appendix will not visualize on ultrasound); 2) the presence of fecaliths; and 3) maximal appendiceal diameter exceeding a certain length (6 mm is a figure currently used). With these kind of criteria, Jeffrey and colleagues[15] found the technique was 90% sensitive and greater than 96% specific with 94% accuracy. In another study, it was possible to distinguish gangrenous from phlegmonous appendicitis, and these varieties, in turn, from the more benign (or "catarrhal") appendicitis.

The advantage of an accurate, readily performed noninvasive screening technique is evident for any patient with possible appendicitis but especially for the elderly in whom this diagnosis is often made so belatedly. In light of the nonspecificity of symptomatology in these cases, where prompt surgery is curative and delay often fatal, a powerful argument can be made for the performance of a screening ultrasound exam on any patient over the age of 60 presenting with abdominal pain of uncertain etiology, especially when discharge from the emergency department is contemplated.

Ultrasonic Evaluation of the Pancreas

Diagnostic specificity in ruling in (or out) pancreatic disease in the elderly is a less critical matter than specificity in assessing the appendix or biliary tree. The decision whether to hospitalize the patient is based largely on the clinical presentation (e.g., hemodynamic status, degree of pain, tolerance of fluids and medications) rather than narrowly on the presence or absence of pancreatitis. Nonetheless, in the geriatric patient with abdominal pain, the process of ruling in pancreatitis as the etiology for abdominal symptomatology is valuable; once ruled in, surgery is rarely a consideration and further diagnostic procedures may be delayed pending clinical assessment and treatment of the patient's immediate condition.

The emergency department physician should not hesitate to consult with the radiologist to help explain abdominal pain or elevated enzyme levels. The advantage of ultrasound in the acute setting is its rapidity of performance, multidirectional imaging capacity, relative low cost, and accuracy in detailing the full length of the common bile duct. In this setting, the radiologist will describe a gland that is focally or diffusely enlarged (with edema) with more irregular margins and increased echogenicity. Biliary pancreatitis will reveal the presence of stones, while chronic disease may disclose pseudocyst formation.

While providing more extensive detail of pancreatic anatomy, there would appear to be little justification for "screening CT scans" in the setting just described. As a follow-up, either for inpatient or outpatient studies, CT is invaluable; however, in the evaluation of the patient with negative or equivocal ultrasonic findings, who has as yet undiagnosed abdominal pain, the decision whether to obtain immediate surgical consult, to admit, or to discharge the patient must be made on clinical grounds. The more definitive and higher resolution capacities of a CT scan and magnetic resonance imaging can generally be delayed.

CONCLUSION

Certain patterns emerge as recurrent themes in the diagnosis and treatment of the acute geriatric abdomen. Most prominent among these include the following facts:

- The elderly often present atypically in terms of anatomic location and duration of symptomatology.
- Symptomatology for a given entity within this population will range from benign nebulous complaints to obtundation, confusion, and shock.
- There is a need for an aggressive approach to *elective* surgery in selected cases, where prognosis is often comparable to that in younger subjects, but significantly worse under *emergent* conditions.
- Cholecystitis, intestinal obstruction, and appendicitis remain the most common etiologies for the surgical abdomen in the elderly; acute pancreatitis is the most common *nonsurgical* abdominal etiology for hospital admission.
- There is a need for a high index of suspicion for *vascular* etiologies for abdominal complaints in the elderly.
- Finally, with the regular use of ultrasonographic assessment and enhanced clinical skills on the part of emergency physicians, we will witness less often the tragic specter of elderly patients discharged from emergency departments suffering from mild or nebulous symptoms that are actually harbingers of impending abdominal catastrophe.

REFERENCES

1. Baum SA and Rubinstein Z: Old people in the emergency room: age related differences in emergency department use and care, J Am Geriatr Soc 35:398–404, 1987.
2. Crump C: The incidence of gallstones and gallbladder diseases, Surg Gynecol Obstet 53:447–455, 1979.
3. Fenjo G: Acute abdominal disease in the elderly: experience from two series in Stockholm, Am J Surg 143:751–754, 1982.

4. Margiotta DZ et al: Fragmentation of gallstones by extracorporeal shock waves, N Engl J Med 314:751–754, 1986.

5. Glenn F: Surgical management of acute cholecystitis in patients 65 years of age and older, Ann Surg 193:56–59, 1981.

6. Blake R and Lynn J: Emergency abdominal surgery in the aged, Br J Surg 63:956–960, 1976.

7. Day EA and Marks C: Gallstone ileus, Am J Surg 128:552–558, 1975.

8. Lygidakis NG: Incidence of bile infection in patients with choledocholithiasis, Am J Gastroenterol 77:12–17, 1982.

9. Pollock TW, Ring ER, and Oleaga JA: Percutaneous decompression of benign and malignant biliary obstruction, Arch Surg 114:148–151, 1979.

10. Long RN, Heimbach DM, and Carrico CJ: Acalculous cholecystitis in critically ill patients, Am J Surg 136:31–36, 1978.

11. Leverat M et al: Peptic ulcer in patient over 60: experience in 287 cases, Am J Dig Dis 11:279–285, 1966.

12. Griffin M et al: Non-steroidal anti-inflammatory use and death from peptic ulcer in elderly persons, Ann Intern Med 109:359–363, 1988.

13. Reference deleted.

14. Wertkin MG and Aufses AH: Management of volvulus of the colon, Dis Colon Rectum 21:40–45, 1978.

15. Hoffmann E, Perez E, and Somera V: Acute pancreatitis in the upper age groups, Gastroenterology 36:675–685, 1959.

16. Mallory A and Kern F Jr: Drug induced pancreatitis: a critical review, Gastroenterology 78:813–820, 1980.

17. Jam I et al: Elevated serum amylase activity in the absence of clinical pancreatic or salivary gland disease, Am J Gastroenterol 70:480–488, 1978.

18. Warshaw AL et al: The pathogenesis of pulmonary edema in acute pancreatitis, Ann Surg 182:505–510, 1975.

19. Wolfe W et al: Acute appendicitis in the aged, Surg Gynecol Obstet 94:239–247, 1952.

19a. Hirsch SB and Wilder JR: Acute appendicitis in hospital patients aged over 60 years (1974–1984), Mt. Sinai J Med 54(1):29–33, 1987.

20. Boley SJ et al: An aggressive roentgenologic and surgical approach to acute mesenteric ischemia. In Hyhus L: Surgery annual, New York, 1973, Appleton-Century-Crofts.

21. Boley SJ et al: Intra-arterial vasodilators and thrombolytic agents in experimental SMA embolus, Gastroenterology 82:1021, 1982.

22. Takada T et al: Ultrasound diagnosis of acute appendicitis, Int Surg 71:9–13, 1986.

23. Reid MH and Phillips HE: The role of CT and ultrasound imaging in biliary tract disease, Surg Clin North Am 61:787–825, 1981.

24. Martin K and Doubilet P: How to image the gallbladder in suspected cholecystitis, Ann Intern Med :722–729, 1988.

25. Jeffrey RB, Laing FC, and Townsend RR: Acute appendicitis: sonographic criteria based on 250 cases, Radiology 167:327–329, 1988.

26. Clark LR et al: Pancreatic imaging, Radiol Clin North Am :489–501, 1985.

27. Ungar JA: Acute care imaging techniques: a clinical approach. In Schwartz GR et al, editors: Emergency medicine: the essential update, Philadelphia, 1989, WB Saunders Co.

SUGGESTED READINGS

Cocco AE and Mendeloff AI: Effects of gastric irradiation in duodenal ulcer patients, Johns Hopkins Med J 126:61–68, 1970.

Fugiyama M et al: Change in lipid composition of bile with age in normal subjects and patients with gallstones, Hiroshima J Med Sci 28:23–29, 1979.

Hall A et al: Hernias of the abdominal wall. In Way L, editor: Current surgical diagnosis and treatment, East Norwalk, CT, 1977, Appleton & Lange.

Hauser S: Answers to questions on gallbladder disease, Hosp Med June:44–64, 1987.

Health and Policy Committee, ACP: How to study the gallbladder, Ann Intern Med 109:752–754, 1988.

Klein SR et al: Appendicitis in the elderly, Postgrad Med 83:247–254, 1987.

Lind CD and Scerda JL: Diagnosis: GI complaints in the geriatric patient, Hosp Med pp. 183–200, Oct 1987.

Lowenstein SR et al: Care of the elderly in the emergency department, Ann Emerg Med 15:528–535, 1986.

McInelly MJ, Turner MWB, and Miller H: Delay of diagnosis of hepatitis in the elderly, NY State J Med 87:126–138, 1987.

Phillips SL and Burns GP: Abdominal disease in the aged, Med Clin North Am 22(5):1213–1224, 1988.

Rinson JHC: The timing of biliary surgery in acute pancreatitis, Ann Surg 189:654–663, 1979.

Rossman I et al: Clinical geriatrics, Philadelphia, 1986, JB Lippincott Co.

Skander MP and Ryan FP: Non-steroidal anti-inflammatory medicines and pain-free peptic ulceration in the elderly, Br Med J 297:833–834, 1988.

Valdivieso V et al: Effect of aging on biliary lipid composition and bile acid metabolism, Gastroenterology 74:8871–8874, 1978.

Vartian CV and Septimus EJ: Intra-abdominal infections in the elderly: diagnosis and management, Geriatrics 41(2):52, 1986.

Rapid Recognition, Evaluation, and Management of the Acute Vascular Insult

Richard A. Yeager, M.D.

Acute arterial extremity ischemia

Ruptured abdominal aortic aneurysm

Aortic dissection

Thoracic aortic aneurysm

Acute mesenteric ischemia

Aortic graft-enteric fistula

ACUTE ARTERIAL EXTREMITY ISCHEMIA

Recognition and correct initial management of acute peripheral vascular insults in the elderly are essential to the practice of geriatric emergency medicine. Acute arterial ischemia of an extremity represents a relatively common vascular surgical emergency in the elderly population. In one large series,[1] the mean age of patients presenting with acute lower extremity ischemia was 66 years. Because cardiac emboli tend to flow to the lower limbs and because lower extremity atherosclerosis is prevalent in the elderly population, acute limb ischemia most often involves the lower extremities.

In the emergency setting, acute extremity ischemia is usually due either to arterial embolism or *de novo* thrombosis of a diseased artery.[1] In one series of 140 episodes of acute lower extremity ischemia, 71 (51%) were due to embolism and 69 (49%) were associated with arterial thrombosis. Cardiac sources account for approximately 80% of all peripheral arterial emboli. Patients most likely to have a cardiac origin for embolism include those with dysrhythmias, myocardial infarction, valvular heart disease, ventricular aneurysm, and congestive heart failure.

The differentiation between arterial thrombus and embolism to the lower extremities can be problematic, since many patients with lower extremity vascular disease also have concomitant cardiac disease, which can predispose to embolization.[2] In general, however, patients who have sustained acute arterial thrombosis of the lower extremities will have a previous history of claudication, whereas absence of ipsilateral pulses in combination with the presence of contralateral pulses usually suggests acute arterial embolization.

Other causes for acute limb ischemia include thromboembolic complications of aneurysm (subclavian, aortic, iliac, femoral, popliteal), as well as thrombosis of previously placed arterial bypass grafts. Aortic dissection should always be considered as a potential cause for acute limb ischemia. When all four limbs are cool and mottled, however, the patient is more likely to have a condition causing low cardiac output, rather than acute arterial occlusion.

Initial assessment of the patient with acute limb ischemia includes determination of peripheral pulses as well as Doppler systolic pressures. The degree of extremity ischemia depends upon the location of the arterial occlusion, status of collaterals, and the extent of clot propagation. With respect to physical findings, muscle and nerve tissues are generally more sensitive to ischemic insult than skin, with nerve fibers for proprioception and light touch the first to show evidence of impairment. *Paresthesias* and/or motor *paralysis* represent manifestations of severe limb ischemia that may be irreversible after 4 to 6 hours of vascular compromise. Other less ominous evidence for acute ischemia includes *pallor,* pulselessness, and *pain*. Firmness or muscle rigor usually indicates irreversible muscle damage. When this is suspected, the serum creatinine phosphokinase level can provide some objective measure of the amount of muscle death. If revascularization is performed in the presence of significant muscle death, reperfusion problems characterized by rhabdomyolysis, renal impairment, hyperkalemia, acidosis, and clotting abnormalities (i.e., disseminated intravascular coagulation [DIC]) may ensue. Consequently, some patients who present with advanced acute limb ischemia and muscle rigor are best managed by primary amputation. Additionally, limb perfusion can be so severely impaired that venous outflow is reduced enough to precipitate peripheral venous thrombosis. As a result, pulmonary embolism is another well-recognized complication — and, on occasion, the result of death — in patients with acute limb ischemia.

Emergency care of the ischemic limb includes application of a protective dressing and early surgical consultation, inasmuch as prompt assessment by the vascular surgeon will expedite patient management. With respect to underlying cause, a differentiation of embolism from thrombosis is of critical importance, since the preferred treatment for each condition is different. In addition to the clinical features, which help differentiate embolism from thrombosis, emergent arteriography will frequently provide diagnostically useful information (Figure 31–1).

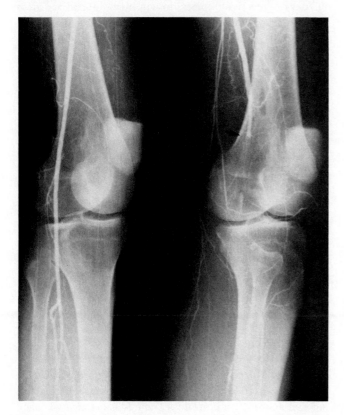

Figure 31–1 Arrow indicates left popliteal arterial embolus. Right side is normal.

Initial emergency intervention for patients with acute extremity ischemia is heparinization. Anticoagulation with heparin prevents clot propagation by affecting several sites in the clotting cascade. Heparin's primary action is to enhance endogenous antithrombin III, a naturally occurring antithrombotic agent. Antithrombin III inactivates factor Xa, thus inhibiting conversion of prothrombin to thrombin. This antithrombotic action ameliorates any associated arterial spasm by indirectly inhibiting the release of platelet factors and other products of thrombosis, which may have vasoconstrictive properties. An intravenous loading dose of 5,000 to 10,000 units of heparin is administered, followed by a continuous intravenous infusion to keep the activated partial thromboplastin time about two times the control value. Overall, the incidence of hemorrhagic complications with therapeutic heparin is about 6%, although elderly women are at higher risk for bleeding.

Operative intervention is usually required for patients with acute limb ischemia. Prompt surgical balloon catheter embolectomy is often employed for embolism, while thrombosis is usually managed by continued heparinization followed either by revascularization or amputation. Occasionally, when collaterals are adequate, heparinization alone will result in limb salvage. In one recent surgical series of acute lower extremity ischemia, overall limb salvage rate was 69%. Mortality was 11% for patients with embolism and 3% for patients with acute atherosclerotic thrombosis. Mortality is higher in patients with embolism, because of more serious underlying cardiac problems.

The role of thrombolytic therapy in acute extremity ischemia is still controversial.[3] Most experts believe that thrombolytic therapy has a role when a good surgical solution is lacking, as is the case in patients with thrombosis involving the distal tibial and pedal circulation. Furthermore, thrombolytic therapy may be appropriate when surgical intervention is relatively contraindicated, as in high-risk patients with recent myocardial infarction or other conditions that make surgical intervention problematic.

RUPTURED ABDOMINAL AORTIC ANEURYSM

Although successful operative management of ruptured abdominal aortic aneurysm was first reported in 1954, this vascular catastrophe remains a diagnostic challenge for the emergency practitioner. Mortality ranges from 25 to 50% in most recent series and, not surprisingly, atherosclerotic aneurysmal degeneration of the abdominal aorta occurs more commonly in the elderly. Mean age of patients with ruptured abdominal aortic aneurysm is about 70 years. In one large autopsy study,[4] one out of every 203 deaths was due to ruptured abdominal aortic aneurysm.

Forty-five percent of those aneurysms between 7.1 and 10.0 cm in diameter were ruptured at autopsy, compared to 25.3% of aneurysms 5.1 to 7.0 centimeters and 23.4% of those 4.1 to 5.0 cm in diameter. Clinical conditions linked to an increased rate of aneurysmal rupture include hypertension and obstructive pulmonary disease.

Because early diagnosis of ruptured abdominal aortic aneurysm is sometimes difficult, maintaining a high index of suspicion is essential.[5] Unfortunately, the classic diagnostic triad of acute abdominal or back pain, pulsatile abdominal mass, and hypotension is present in less than 50% of cases. It is important to recognize that the patient's pain can be referred to the flank, scrotum, or thigh. In addition, some patients present with little more than an acutely symptomatic groin mass. Complicating the diagnosis is the fact that, on occasion, a retroperitoneal hematoma will obscure palpable aortic margins, misleading the examiner to conclude that an aneurysm is not present. Obese patients are especially difficult to examine.

Although prior knowledge of an abdominal aortic aneurysm is diagnostically useful, this information is available in only about 25% of cases. Despite these limitations, the presence of acute abdominal or back pain associated with a pulsatile abdominal mass or prior history of an aneurysm is enough to establish the diagnosis and mobilize the surgical team. If the emergency physician waits for the development of hypotension, he or she has waited too long. Aortic rupture partially tamponaded by surrounding retroperitoneal structures is an unpredictable and unstable condition, and massive bleeding can occur at any time.

All too often, however, the patient presents to the emergency department in shock. Mortality rates are strongly influenced by the preoperative occurrence of shock and by delays in transporting the patient from the emergency department to the operating room. Death is usually due to early exsanguination, cardiac complications, or, in the late states, multiple organ failure. Advanced age has been linked to a higher mortality in some but not all series. The very elderly have survived ruptured aortic aneurysm surgery, so it would be a mistake to withhold operation using age alone as an exclusionary criterion.

As soon as the diagnosis of ruptured abdominal aortic aneurysm is suspected in the emergency department, the vascular surgical team should be mobilized. Large-bore intravenous cannulas and blood for type and crossmatching are mandatory. As a rule, time is of the essence and, consequently, performing additional tests such as a chest x-ray and ECG is not recommended when the presentation is obvious and the patient is unstable. Clearly, initial resuscitation of the patient should begin in the emergency department but more definite stabilization is better accomplished in the operating room where surgical control of the proximal aorta can be achieved. Initial

group O Rh-negative blood may be required in a few patients with profound shock prior to arrival of type-specific blood. As a rule, aggressive preoperative transfusion is discouraged since this may raise the blood pressure, which can contribute to further bleeding.

Not uncommonly, the physician examining a patient complaining of acute abdominal or back pain may be uncertain as to the existence of a pulsatile abdominal mass, especially when obesity or ill-defined aortic margins are present. If the patient is hemodynamically stable, a computerized tomography (CT) scan is recommended as the initial diagnostic procedure of choice. Although ultrasonography is preferred for the elective diagnosis and follow-up of patients with abdominal aortic aneurysm, in an urgent setting ultrasound examination is less definitive and, oftentimes, is hindered by overlying bowel gas. Furthermore, arteriography is time consuming and does not provide essential information for the management of the ruptured aneurysm. CT scanning, on the other hand, will accurately diagnose aortic aneurysm and can usually identify the presence of extraaortic blood or hematoma. False-negative CT scans can occur, however, and urgent surgery is recommended for any aneurysm patient with acute symptoms suggestive of rupture. For all practical purposes, mortality from untreated aortic aneurysm is 100%.

The most effective way to prevent death due to a ruptured abdominal aortic aneurysm is to repair the aneurysm electively prior to rupture. Mortality rates ranging from 1 to 4% are reported from recent elective series that have included high-risk patients. Once rupture occurs, the physician's ability to influence survival is dependent on early diagnosis and prompt surgical control of aortic bleeding.[6]

AORTIC DISSECTION

According to some autopsy studies, aortic dissection is a more common occurrence than ruptured atherosclerotic abdominal aortic aneurysm. In spite of its prevalence, however, aortic dissection is often misdiagnosed in the emergency department, usually because of a low index of suspicion on the part of the evaluating clinician. Complicating assessment is the fact that aortic dissection presents in myriad ways, many of which mimic other medical and surgical emergencies.

Categorization of aortic dissection has undergone some evolution but, at present, is quite straightforward. If the ascending aorta is involved, the dissection is termed "type A." If the ascending aorta is not involved, the dissection is termed "type B." This differentiation is of practical clinical importance, since the surgical approach for each type of dissection is different. Dissections are considered acute if they are less than 14 days old, whereas chronic dissections often present as aneurysms involving the thoracic aorta.

Aortic dissection in the elderly patient is usually associated with hypertension and acquired muscular degeneration of the aortic media, precipitated by the aging process. In one series, the mean age for patients with "type A" dissection was 49 years compared to 60 years for patients with "type B" dissection. The cardinal symptom of acute aortic dissection is sudden onset of severe pain in the anterior chest or interscapular region. Approximately 25 to 50% of patients will develop a new aortic diastolic murmur. In the majority of cases, the dissection originates as an intimal laceration, located either in the ascending aorta or in the proximal descending aorta. In 10% of cases, the intimal laceration is located in the aortic arch. Rarely, the dissection originates in the abdominal aorta. Proximal aortic dissection may result in aortic valvular incompetence, aortocardiac fistula, coronary arterial obstruction, pulmonary arterial stenosis, or aortic stenosis. Extension of the dissection into arterial branches of the aortic arch can produce arm or cerebral ischemia, whereas distal dissection can precipitate numerous and unpredictable alterations in end-organ and/or lower extremity blood supply. Impairment of blood supply to the spinal cord can result in paraplegia. Aortic rupture can also occur, leading to hemopericardium, hemothorax, hemoperitoneum, or hematoma formation in the mediastinum or retroperitoneum.

Because patients with aortic dissection usually present with acute chest pain, myocardial infarction must be considered in the initial differential diagnosis. In most cases of dissection, however, the electrocardiogram (ECG) will be normal or show evidence only of left ventricular hypertrophy. When retrograde dissection extends into the atrioventricular junction, however, conduction abnormalities may result. Furthermore, when dissection results in coronary arterial occlusion, an ischemic electrocardiographic pattern is evident.

Rapid assessment and prompt initiation of treatment is of paramount importance since untreated acute aortic dissection results in a 1% per hour mortality during the first 48 hours. As soon as the diagnosis of aortic dissection is considered, a cardiovascular surgeon should be called to assist in management. Aortic dissection is rapidly and accurately diagnosed by a CT scan utilizing intravenous contrast infusion. Conventional aortography is recommended by some experts to aid in surgical planning.

Once the diagnosis of acute aortic dissection is confirmed, emergency intervention should consist of blood pressure control (usually with sodium nitroprusside) and reduction of cardiac ejection velocity by beta blockade (either with intravenous propranolol or metoprolol). Level of consciousness, urine output, ECG, and systemic and pulmonary arterial pressures should be continuously monitored in an intensive care setting.

Experts agree that early surgical intervention affords the best chance of survival in patients with "type A" dis-

section. In addition, "type B" dissections complicated by progressive extension, occlusion of vital arteries, or rupture are treated by urgent operation. The presence of symptoms related to peripheral arterial occlusions should not distract surgical attention from the central problem of thoracic aortic dissection. Delayed elective surgery is often recommended in patients with "type B" dissection who initially are treated medically. Improved outcomes with operative intervention have provoked some experts to recommend urgent surgery for nearly all patients with acute dissection.

THORACIC AORTIC ANEURYSM

In 1953, DeBakey and Cooley reported the first successful resection of a thoracic aortic aneurysm with replacement grafting. During the past three decades, major advances have occurred in the surgical management of thoracic aortic aneurysm. Rupture of a thoracic aortic aneurysm is best prevented by elective surgical repair. Once rupture occurs, prompt recognition and appropriate operative management can produce a successful clinical outcome.

Thoracic aortic aneurysm occurs at an incidence of 5.9 new cases per 100,000 person-years. The two most common etiologies for thoracic aneurysm include aortic dissection and atherosclerosis. Atherosclerotic thoracic aneurysms are located predominantly in the descending aorta, while thoracic aneurysms due to dissection involve the ascending aorta slightly more often than the descending aorta. In one series, the mean age for patients with atherosclerotic thoracic aneurysm was 69 years, compared to 61 years for patients with thoracic aneurysms due to chronic aortic dissection. Other causes for thoracic aortic aneurysm include aortitis, cystic medial necrosis, congenital defects, syphilis, trauma, and bacterial infection.

Most elderly patients with ruptured thoracic aortic aneurysm can be diagnosed on the basis of the history, physical examination, and chest x-ray. Patients present with chest or back pain and chest x-ray evidence of a thoracic aortic aneurysm; tracheal deviation is not uncommon in patients with a rupture. Prior knowledge of a thoracic aortic aneurysm in a patient with acute symptoms raises the level of suspicion for rupture, although 70% of patients with rupture have no prior history of aneurysm.

Early involvement of the cardiothoracic surgeon is essential. When the diagnosis is in doubt and the patient is hemodynamically stable, the emergency CT scan with intravenous contrast is the diagnostic procedure of choice. Prompt blood replacement and emergency surgery give the patient the only chance for survival once rupture occurs. Although advanced age represents a risk factor for thoracic aneurysmectomy, elderly patients have survived emergent surgical repair of a rupturing thoracic aneurysm.

For ruptured aneurysms involving the ascending aorta, median sternotomy and total cardiopulmonary bypass are required. When rupture occurs with the more common descending thoracic aneurysm, a left thoracotomy and partial femoral-femoral bypass are often employed. Some surgical teams, however, have reported good results simply with descending thoracic aortic clamping and replacement grafting, avoiding femoral-femoral bypass or aortic shunting.

The most effective way to lower death rates from ruptured thoracic aortic aneurysms is to electively repair more aneurysms in patients who are surgical candidates. In one series of ascending thoracic aortic aneurysms treated surgically, in-hospital mortality was 60% for emergency operations as compared to 4% for elective repairs. Similarly, for descending thoracic aortic aneurysms, hospital mortality was 50% for emergency cases and 12% for elective procedures.[7]

ACUTE MESENTERIC ISCHEMIA

Although descriptions of mesenteric thrombosis have been recorded as early as the fifteenth century, it was Tiedemann's case report in the nineteenth century which first characterized the clinical problem. The contribution of Boley and coworkers[8,9] helped define the importance and frequency of acute mesenteric ischemia, which commonly occurs either as a result of superior mesenteric arterial occlusion or low-flow states in the mesentery. In the elderly, occlusion is precipitated by thrombosis of a diseased artery or an embolus originating, in most cases, from the heart. Nonocclusive causes for reduced blood flow include low cardiac output states as well as drug-induced mesenteric arterial spasm. Not surprisingly, acute mesenteric ischemia is predominantly a disease of the elderly. In one series, patients with nonocclusive mesenteric ischemia had a median age of 75 years, compared to 68 years for embolism and 77 years for arterial thrombosis. The reported frequency from a recent hospital series was one case of acute mesenteric ischemia every other month, with 38.2% of patients sustaining mesenteric thrombosis, 28.5% having embolization, and 28.5% with nonocclusive mesenteric ischemia.

Elderly patients with mesenteric ischemia classically present with sudden, severe midabdominal pain. Physical exam is oftentimes unremarkable, and this marked disparity between the patient's complaints and the physical exam is an important clinical clue to the diagnosis of acute mesenteric ischemia. Another group of patients present with abdominal distention or gastrointestinal bleeding. Leukocytosis is usually present, although the total leukocyte count may remain normal in the elderly patient with evidence only of a shift toward immature neutrophils.

With respect to metabolic activity, the mucosa is the most active layer of the bowel and, consequently, the most sensitive to ischemic insult. As a result, the earliest ischemic damage frequently involves the mucosal layer. Damage is microscopically apparent within 1 to 2 hours of occlusion. Fortunately, early ischemic injury to the mucosa and muscular layer is reversible. If flow is restored within a few hours, a regeneration process restores the intestinal wall. Progression to full-thickness involvement occurs after approximately 24 hours of low flow or occlusion. Once full-thickness involvement ensues, the patient usually manifests signs of peritonitis.

For the patient suspected of having early, acute mesenteric ischemia, mesenteric arteriography is the recommended diagnostic procedure of choice (Figure 31–2). Diagnosis of embolism, thrombosis, or nonocclusive mesenteric ischemia can usually be confirmed with this modality and appropriate therapy instituted. The goal of management is to promptly diagnose and then treat, thereby minimizing or preventing full-thickness bowel injury.

Surgical intervention often requires either mesenteric arterial embolectomy or bypass of a proximally thrombosed superior mesenteric artery. Patients with peritonitis require emergent laparotomy for bowel resection. Some authors recommend intraarterial vasodilators (i.e.,

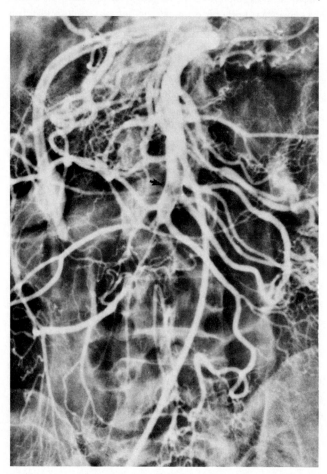

Figure 31–2 Arrow indicates superior mesenteric arterial embolus.

papaverine) for patients with nonocclusive mesenteric ischemia as well as for those with mesenteric arterial spasm secondary to embolism or thrombosis. Mortality rates, however, remain high, particularly in patients with either mesenteric arterial thrombosis or nonocclusive mesenteric ischemia. Moribund patients with terminal disease suspected of having mesenteric infarction are not appropriate for aggressive therapy.

AORTIC GRAFT-ENTERIC FISTULA

Aortic graft-enteric fistula is a dread condition, and successful emergency management is made even more difficult in the elderly patient with multisystem disease. Mean age of presentation is about 66 years. Graft-enteric fistula is a vascular emergency whose incidence seems to be declining, although the condition is not rare.[10,11] In one series of patients hospitalized with acute gastrointestinal bleeding, 3% had previously undergone abdominal aortic prosthetic graft placement. Of those bleeding patients with an abdominal aortic graft, 26% were ultimately found to have graft-enteric fistula. The large number of patients who have now undergone abdominal aortic grafting makes consideration of this diagnosis especially important.

Graft-enteric communication occurs when the overlying bowel erodes either at the level of the aorta-to-graft anastomosis or at some point along the body of the graft. A pseudoaneurysm at the aortic anastomosis is often, but not always, associated with the condition. The site of bowel involvement is usually either the distal duodenum or proximal jejunum. The classic bleeding pattern with graft-enteric fistula is a brief "herald" bleed followed by massive bleeding. This is not the common presentation, however, and any form of gastrointestinal bleeding in the patient with aortic graft surgery is suggestive of graft-enteric fistula. In addition, evidence of sepsis (fever and/or leukocytosis) often coexists. Some patients with graft-enteric communication never have clinically overt gastrointestinal bleeding.

Emergency management of the patient with significant hemorrhage includes aggressive resuscitation with attention focused on precise identification of a bleeding source. When nasogastric aspirate is negative for blood, sigmoidoscopy is performed to rule out anorectal lesions. In one series of patients with infrarenal aortic grafts and gastrointestinal bleeding, the most common cause for bleeding was graft-enteric fistula, followed by ischemic bowel and peptic ulcer disease. Preferred management of aortic graft patients with upper gastrointestinal bleeding includes prompt esophagogastroduodenoscopy. Endoscopy may be all that is required to diagnose graft-enteric fistula, but more likely than not will either identify or rule out other causes of upper gastrointestinal bleeding. If upper endoscopy does not identify an actively bleeding lesion and the patient is hemodynamically stable, an emergent CT scan is performed. Evidence of perigraft fluid or gas is compatible with a diagnosis of graft-enteric fistula. In addition, an anastomotic pseudoaneurysm identified on CT scan raises the index of suspicion for graft-enteric fistula. The selective use of arteriography also has a role, but it should be remembered that all testing modalities can give false-negative results for graft-enteric fistula. If no definite source for continued bleeding is identified, exploratory laparotomy is required as a diagnostic maneuver. Untreated graft-enteric fistula eventually results in mortality due either to sepsis or bleeding.

All patients with graft-enteric fistula are considered to have infected aortic grafts. Preferred operative management includes prompt aortic graft removal with bowel repair and extraanatomic bypass to preserve lower extremity blood flow. Surgical mortality with graft-enteric fistula is 35 to 50%. Many of these deaths are preventable with more prompt diagnosis and surgical intervention.

REFERENCES

1. Blaisdell FW, Steele M, and Allen RE: Management of acute lower extremity arterial ischemia due to embolism and thrombosis, Surgery 84:822, 1978.
2. Tawes RL et al: Acute limb ischemia: thromboembolism, J Vasc Surg 5:901, 1987.
3. Towne JB and Bandyk DF: Application of thrombolytic therapy in vascular occlusive disease, Am J Surg 154:548, 1987.
4. Darling RC et al: Autopsy study of unoperated abdominal aortic aneurysms: the case for early resection, Circulation 56(suppl 2):II–161, 1977.
5. Gerbode F: Ruptured aortic aneurysm: a surgical emergency, Surg Gynecol Obstet 98:759, 1954.
6. Donaldson MC, Rosenberg JM, and Bucknam CA: Factors affecting survival after ruptured abdominal aortic aneurysm, J Vasc Surg 2:564, 1985.
7. Moreno-Cabral CE et al: Degenerative and atherosclerotic aneurysms of the thoracic aorta, J Thorac Cardiovasc Surg 88:1020, 1984.
8. Boley SJ and Borden EB: Acute mesenteric vascular disease. In Wilson SE et al, editors: Vascular surgery: principles and practice, New York, 1987, McGraw-Hill, Inc.
9. Boley SJ, Brandt LJ, and Veith FJ: Ischemic disorders of the intestines, Curr Probl Surg 15:1, 1978.
10. O'Mara CS, Williams GM, and Ernst CB: Secondary aortoenteric fistula: a 20 year experience, Am J Surg 142:203, 1981.
11. Perdue GD et al: Impending aortoenteric hemorrhage: the effect of early recognition on improved outcome, Ann Surg 192:237, 1980.

SUGGESTED READINGS

Appelbaum A, Karp RB, and Kirklin JW: Ascending vs. descending aortic dissections, Ann Surg 183:296, 1976.
Bahnson HT: Thoracic aneurysms. In Sabiston DC Jr and Spencer FC, editors: Gibbon's surgery of the chest, Philadelphia, 1983, WB Saunders Co.
Bergan JJ and Yao JST, editors: Vascular surgical emergencies, Orlando, Fla, 1987, Grune & Stratton.
Bergan JJ et al: Nontraumatic mesenteric vascular emergencies, J Vasc Surg 5:903, 1987.
Bickerstaff LK et al: Thoracic aortic aneurysms: a population-based study, Surgery 92:1103, 1982.
Blaisdell FW: Use of anticoagulants in the ischemic lower extremity: an alternative perspective. In Kempczinski RF, editor: The ischemic leg, Chicago, 1985, Year Book Medical Publishers, Inc.
Bulkley GB, Haglund UH, and Morris JB: Mesenteric blood flow and the pathophysiology of intestinal ischemia. In Bergan JJ and Yao JST,

editors: Vascular surgical emergencies, Orlando, Fla, 1987, Grune & Stratton.

Crawford ES et al: Graft replacement of aneurysm in descending thoracic aorta: results without bypass or shunting, Surgery 89:73, 1981.

Crawford S et al: Infrarenal abdominal aortic aneurysm: factors influencing survival after operation performed over a 25-year period, Ann Surg 193:699, 1981.

Cronenwett JL et al: Actuarial analysis of variables associated with rupture of small abdominal aortic aneurysms, Surgery 98:472, 1985.

Dale WA: Differential management of acute peripheral arterial ischemia, J Vasc Surg 1:269, 1984.

DeBakey ME and Cooley DA: Successful resection of aneurysms of thoracic aorta and replacement by graft, JAMA 152:673, 1953.

DeSanctis RW et al: Aortic dissection, N Engl J Med 317:1060, 1987.

Gordon RD: Arterial thromboembolism. In Kempczinski RF, editor: The ischemic leg, Chicago, 1985, Year Book Medical Publishers, Inc.

Hoffman M et al: Operation for ruptured abdominal aortic aneurysms: a community-wide experience, Surgery 91:597, 1982.

Kapsch DN and Silver D: Anticoagulants (heparin, warfarin). In Wilson SE et al, editors: Vascular surgery: principles and practice, New York, 1987, McGraw-Hill, Inc.

Khaw H et al: Ruptured abdominal aortic aneurysm presenting as symptomatic inguinal mass: report of six cases, J Vasc Surg 4:384, 1986.

Lawler M Jr: Aggressive treatment of ruptured abdominal aortic aneurysm in a community hospital, Surgery 95:38, 1984.

Livesay JJ et al: Surgical experience in descending thoracic aneurysmectomy with and without adjuncts to avoid ischemia, Ann Thorac Surg 39:37, 1985.

McNamara JJ and Pressler VM: Natural history of arteriosclerotic thoracic aortic aneurysm, Ann Thorac Surg 26:468, 1978.

Meyer AA, Ahlquist RE, and Trunkey DD: Mortality from ruptured abdominal aortic aneurysms: a comparison of two series, Am J Surg 152:27, 1986.

Miller DC: Surgical emergencies of the thoracic aorta. In Bergan JJ and Yao JST, editors: Vascular surgical emergencies, Orlando, Fla, 1987, Grune & Stratton.

Miller DC et al: Operative treatment of aortic dissection: experience with 125 patients over a sixteen-year period, J Thorac Cardiovasc Surg 78:365, 1979.

Moore WS, editor: Vascular surgery, Orlando, Fla, 1986, Grune & Stratton.

Mulherin JL and Edwards WH: Improved survival after ruptured abdominal aortic aneurysm, South Med J 73:986, 1980.

Najafi H: Aortic dissection. In Sabiston DC Jr and Spencer FC, editors: Gibbon's surgery of the chest, Philadelphia, 1983, WB Saunders Co.

O'Hara PJ et al: Surgical management of infected abdominal aortic grafts: review of a 25-year experience, J Vasc Surg 3:725, 1986.

Ottinger LW and Austen WG: A study of 136 patients with mesenteric infarction, Surg Gynecol Obstet 124:251, 1967.

Pressler V and McNamara JJ: Thoracic aortic aneurysm: natural history and treatment, J Thorac Cardiovasc Surg 79:489, 1980.

Reilly LM et al: Gastrointestinal tract involvement by prosthetic graft infection: the significance of gastrointestinal hemorrhage, Ann Surg 202:342, 1985.

Roberts WC: Aortic dissection: anatomy, consequences, and causes, Am Heart J 101:195, 1981.

Smith GJ, Holcroft JW, and Blaisdell FW: Acute arterial insufficiency. In Wilson SE et al, editors: Vascular surgery: principles and practice, New York, 1987, McGraw-Hill, Inc.

Sorensen HR and Olsen H: Ruptured and dissecting aneurysms of the aorta: incidence and prospects of surgery, Acta Chir Scand 128:644, 1964.

Tribble CG, Christie AM, and Kron IL: Repair of thoracic aortic aneurysms in the elderly: are shunts necessary? J Vasc Surg 6:553, 1987.

Trout HH III, Kozloff L, and Giordano JM: Priority of revascularization in patients with graft enteric fistulas, infected arteries, or infected arterial prostheses, Ann Surg 199:669, 1984.

Wakefield TW et al: Abdominal aortic aneurysm rupture: statistical analysis of factors affecting outcome of surgical treatment, Surgery 91:586, 1982.

Weinbaum FI et al: The accuracy of computed tomography in the diagnosis of retroperitoneal blood in the presence of abdominal aortic aneurysm, J Vasc Surg 6:11, 1987.

Whittemore AD et al: Aortic aneurysm repair: reduced operative mortality associated with maintenance of optimal cardiac performance, Ann Surg 192:414, 1980.

Yeager RA et al: Aortic and peripheral prosthetic graft infection: differential management and causes of mortality, Am J Surg 150:36, 1985.

Yeager RA et al: Application of clinically valid cardiac risk factors to aortic aneurysm surgery, Arch Surg 121:278, 1986.

Yeager RA et al: Clinical spectrum of patients with infrarenal aortic grafts and gastrointestinal bleeding, Am J Surg 153:459, 1987.

Gastrointestinal Hemorrhage

Elizabeth London Rogers, M.D.

The diagnosis of gastrointestinal (GI) bleeding is obvious in the patient vomiting blood, passing black, heme-positive stools, or bleeding from the rectum. The diagnosis should also be considered in the elderly patient with a recent increase in angina symptoms, congestive heart failure, weakness, or dyspnea. The urgency and approach to managing the bleeding is dependent upon the site, rapidity, and continuance of the bleeding.[1]

The emergency management of GI bleeding involves a team approach. The first step — the rapid resuscitation and stabilization of the patient — is followed by diagnostic procedures to determine the cause. Therapy should then be directed toward the specific cause. Since there is increased mortality for all surgical procedures from delay and from deterioration of the patient's brain, kidney, liver, heart, and lungs, evaluation of the success of medical therapy must be made frequently in the first 24 to 48 hours. Surgery must then take place early if medical therapy is not succeeding.

UPPER INTESTINAL BLEEDING

Diagnosis

Bloody vomitus usually implies a lesion above the ligament of Treitz. The presence of "coffee ground" heme-positive material in the vomitus implies an upper intestinal bleed with acid present in the stomach. Melena, or black stool, occurs when there is more than 100 mL of blood coming from a lesion that is usually in the upper gastrointestinal tract; however, lesions as low as the descending colon can present with melena. Although bright red blood from the rectum is usually colonic in origin, the hyperperistaltic effect of blood may occasionally cause bright red bleeding from the rectum in patients with an active duodenal ulcer or variceal bleeds.

As soon as the patient comes into the emergency unit, an effort should be made to determine the significance of the bleeding (Table 32–1). Orthostatic hypotension is the earliest sign of volume depletion. A pulse greater than 100 is indicative of at least 20% loss in intravascular volume. Clinical shock occurs when the supine blood pressure decreases to less than 90/60, there is a decreased urine output, and the patient becomes confused. Myocardial ischemia with apparently painless myocardial infarction is frequent in the elderly but often unrecognized. Lactic acidosis due to decreased blood volume, uremia with BUN greater than 40, stress leukocytosis with white cell counts greater than 20,000, anemia of varying degrees, and hyperglycemia due to the gluconeogenesis of stress are also acutely seen with a significant bleed.

Step One — Stabilization

Once bleeding has been determined to be significant, the first and most important step is to stabilize the patient and to resuscitate if necessary. This should never be delayed for diagnostic tests because fluid and blood correction must occur early before renal, hepatic, or myocardial ischemia ensues. Stabilization (Table 32–2) involves the

Table 32–1   Signs of Significant Blood Loss

Orthostatic hypotension	Hematocrit < 28%
Pulse > 100	WBC 20,000
Decreased urinary output	BUN 40 mg/dL
Confusion	Lactic acidosis
Ischemia on ECG	

Table 32–2　Management of Acute Upper Intestinal Bleeding

1. Check for postural hypotension
2. Start IV with normal saline; type and crossmatch blood
3. Fluid and blood correction
4. Nasogastric aspiration
5. Gastroenterology, surgery, and radiology consultation
6. Determine cause of bleeding
7. Iced-saline or iced-water lavage
8. Administer H_2 blocking drops, sucralfate, prostaglandin inhibitors, or antacids to promote healing

Table 32–3　Causes of Upper Intestinal Bleeding

Most frequent	Historical clues
Duodenal ulcer	Previous history, typical ulcer symptoms but may be painless
Gastric ulcer	Dyspepsia atypical for ulcers
Gastritis	Trauma, sepsis, burns, ischemia, alcohol, aspirin, or NSAIDs in past 24–48 hours
Mallory-Weiss syndrome	Clear vomitus followed by bloody vomitus
Esophageal varices	Stigmata of chronic liver disease, patient need not be jaundiced

Less frequent	Historical clues
Esophagitis	Pyrosis and reflux symptoms
Stomal ulcers	Previous gastroenterostomy
Carcinoma (stomach)	Weight loss, early satiety, previous gastric surgery
Vascular	Telangiectasias on buccal mucosa

insertion of a large-bore intravenous catheter with instillation of normal saline or Ringer's lactate, packed cells, fresh frozen plasma, and plasma expanders as necessary. A nasogastric or Ewald tube is useful to determine the rapidity of blood loss, remove clots, and instill iced solutions for lavage. For the patient who is rapidly bleeding and cannot quickly be stabilized, nasotracheal intubation to prevent aspiration, a central venous line to better monitor volume status, and an arterial venous line to monitor blood pressure and pH may be necessary. At this time, there should be a consultation among the general physician, gastroenterologist, surgeon, and radiologist; successful care of the severe GI bleeder demands a team working effectively together from the beginning.

Determination of Cause

The major causes of rapid upper intestinal hemorrhage are peptic ulcer gastritis, esophageal varices, and the Mallory-Weiss syndrome. Information garnered from the history and physical examination may help in the diagnosis (Table 32–3).

After the pain is stabilized, diagnostic procedures should first consist of plain and upright x-rays of the abdomen to rule out perforation, obstruction, and small bowel ischemia. Endoscopy,[2] however, is the easiest, quickest, and most reliable way of determining the cause of the bleeding. It has a 70 to 95% success rate; is better than an upper GI x-ray series at visualizing the mucosal lesions of esophagitis, gastritis, and Mallory-Weiss syndrome; and can visualize the acutal bleeding site in patients who have more than one lesion. If bleeding is too brisk for adequate visualization by endoscopy, angiography may be useful. Angiography is most successful when bleeding occurs at a rate greater than 0.5 ml per minute. It has been reported successful in diagnosing 75 to 90% of brisk arterial bleeders and may pick up gastritis of the cardia missed by endoscopy.[3]

An upper GI series is best for the patient who has stopped bleeding or if an endoscopy has found no potential bleeding site. The finding of an abnormality by upper GI series does not necessarily mean that the site did

bleed; 20 to 50% of the patients who bleed and have varices seen on an upper GI series may actually be bleeding from other sources. Gastric analysis is not helpful in determining the cause of a bleed.

Therapy

Eighty percent of upper GI bleeders stop after iced gastric lavage, whether the solution used is saline, water, antacids, or Levophed.

Numerous drugs have been used with variable success. H_2 receptor antagonists, sucralfate, and antacids have been shown to be equally effective both in prophylaxis against stress gastritis and in healing chronic ulcers. Recent evidence indicates that intravenous H_2 blockers may be more useful than oral antacids or iced lavage alone in decreasing bleeding from acute gastritis. Anticholinergics should be avoided acutely as they increase tachycardia in already compromised patients. Prostaglandins, glucagon, somatostatin, and levarterenol are currently being investigated as potentially useful for the treatment of intestinal bleeding.

For those patients who do not stop bleeding after vigorous gastric lavage and intravenous cimetidine or other H_2 blockers, therapy specifically directed toward the cause should be undertaken. Emergency surgery should be performed on the patient with an ulcer who does not quickly stop bleeding in the hospital or whose bleeding is greater than 4 units in the first 2 hours or greater than 6 units over 24 hours. This is especially important for patients more than 60 years of age or those with gastric ulcers, associated medical disease, or continued or recurrent bleeding in the hospital.

In several institutions, alternative nonsurgical procedures are being developed that, with further refinement, may reduce the need for emergency surgery. These include endoscopic topical coagulation of ulcers with the use of laser beams or resins and angiographically placed catheters to instill vasoconstrictors or embolize discrete arterial bleeders.

For the patient with gastritis in whom intravenous H_2 blockers (e.g., cimetidine) and nasogastric lavage are unsuccessful, the addition of Levophed to the lavage or the administration of intravenous Pitressin may be useful. Surgery should be considered in the patient who has already bled 6 to 10 units and is not immediately stopping despite lavage, H_2 blockers, and vasoconstrictors. As vagotomy and pyloroplasty tend to decrease gastric bleeding only transiently, total gastrectomy is more effective, but this carries a 10 to 30% mortality, and few such patients ever lead a "normal" life subsequently.

For the patient with varices, it is important to maintain the central venous pressure at between 3 and 7 cm of water to ensure adequate intravascular volume and renal function without an increase in portal pressure. After acute stabilization, treatment of encephalopathy and the prevention of hypoxia, hypokalemia, and recurrent bleeds will determine the patients' chances of survival.

The two most common procedures used to stop variceal bleeding have significant mortality. The Sengstaken-Blakemore tube stops bleeding in 90% of cases but has a 10% mortality. It must be passed by an experienced person, otherwise, such complications as esophageal rupture, asphyxiation, and aspiration can occur. Intraarterial or intravenous Pitressin, at a dosage of 0.2 to 0.6 units per minute, has a high success rate in promptly stopping variceal bleeding. Complications of Pitressin usage, however, include infarcted bowel, fatal myocardial infarction, gangrene in local areas beyond the infusion, and the antidiuretic hormone action of vasopressin. Recent experience has been gained with the use of endoscopic sclerosing agents to sclerose the varices and with venous embolization of the bleeding varices to acutely stop bleeding. Both procedures are still in developmental stages but may be effective stop-gap measures.

If the bleeding cannot be controlled in 2 hours, and the patient is still hypovolemic despite vigorous management, or if bleeding persists beyond 10 units or beyond 18 hours, surgery should be considered, despite its acknowledged high morbidity. Surgical procedures used include transesophageal ligation of varices, esophageal transection, emergency mesocaval or portocaval shunt, and gastric devascularization.

LOWER INTESTINAL BLEEDING

Lower intestinal bleeding occurs less frequently than upper intestinal bleeding and presents most often as bloody diarrhea, blood around the stool or on toilet paper, or as occult bleeding. Seventy percent of life-threatening lower intestinal bleeds are due to diverticula, and 70% of these

diverticula are on the right side of the colon without inflammation. Common causes of massive lower intestinal bleeding include tumors, ischemic colitis, and arteriovenous malformations.[4,5]

Ischemic colitis is often painless and should be suspected in the elderly patient with hypotension, hypoxia, cardiac arrhythmia, or a history of digoxin administration.[6]

Arteriovenous malformations and angiodysplasias are found most often in elderly patients, especially those with aortic stenosis. Although most frequent in the cecum and ascending colon, they may be found in the jejunum, ileum, and stomach as well. Elective colonoscopy and angiography both result in moderate success in localizing arteriovenous malformations.

Infections that present with bloody diarrhea include shigellosis, amebiasis, and infections caused by *Campylobacter* species. Ulcerative proctitis and nonspecific proctitis can also be seen as a source of bloody stools in the elderly.

Although hemorrhoids are present in 50% of all people by age 50, they most frequently present with blood streaking rather than life-threatening bleeds. Polyps and tumors are also more likely to produce occult bleeding; however, bloody stools may be seen with larger lesions.

Intramural bleeding seen with bleeding diatheses, trauma, ischemia, vasculitis, and anticoagulant use should be suspected when there is evidence of "thumbprinting" on a plain film of the abdomen. A careful drug history is important because various drugs such as aspirin, enteric-coated potassium, and anticoagulants may be responsible for acute and chronic GI bleeding.[7,8]

After acute stabilization of the patient, the cause of bleeding should be determined. Proctosigmoidoscopy is useful to rule out bleeding hemorrhoids, tumors, or proctitis and to examine stool for ova, parasites, bacteria, and pus. Angiography is useful for briskly bleeding lesions. Colonoscopy is difficult to perform and interpret in an unprepared bowel and, therefore, will be of limited usefulness here. Barium enema should be performed only when one is sure that angiography will not be done or when angiography is negative.

Therapy

For the brisk bleeder, medical management consists of intravenous fluids and blood to stabilize the patient, followed by arteriographic therapy where available. Briskly bleeding diverticula, polyps, tumors, and arteriovenous malformations can be visualized by arteriography, and the bleeding can be controlled with intraarterial vasoconstrictors. If ischemic bowel disease is the cause of the bleed, intraarterial vasodilators may be of use in stopping the bleed in addition to correcting the hypoxia and underlying cardiovascular problems. If proctosigmoidoscopy is negative and arteriography is not available or not rapidly successful, emergency surgery is the procedure of choice when continued brisk bleeding is present.

For slower degrees of bleeding, elective colonoscopy may be useful after careful bowel cleansing. In addition to determining the cause, colonoscopic cauterization of bleeding sites and colonoscopic removal of polyps and some tumors can be achieved. Bleeding hemorrhoids are best treated by hemorrhoidectomy if bleeding does not spontaneously stop.

REFERENCES

1. Booker JA et al: Prognostic factors for continued or rebleeding and death from gastrointestinal haemorrhage in the elderly, Age Ageing 16(4):208–214, 1987.
2. Cooper BT and Neumann CS: Upper gastrointestinal endoscopy in patients aged 80 years or more, Age Ageing 15(6):343–349, 1986.
3. Moncure AC et al: Occult gastrointestinal bleeding: newer techniques and diagnosis and therapy, Adv Surg 22:141–177, 1989.
4. Avots-Avotins KV and Waugh DE: Colonic bleeding in the elderly, Clin Geriatr Med 1(2):433–443, 1985.
5. Berry AR, Campbell WB, and Kettlewell MG: Management of major colonic haemorrhage, Br J Surg 75(7):637–640, 1988.
6. Santos JC Jr et al: Angiodysplasia of the colon: endoscopic diagnosis and treatment, Br J Surg 75(3):256–258, 1988.
7. Caradoc L and Davies TH: Nonsteroidal anti-inflammatory drugs, arthritis, and gastrointestinal bleeding in elderly in-patients, Age Ageing 13(5):295–298, 1984.
8. Watson RJ, Hooper TL, and Ingram G: Duodenal ulcer disease in the elderly: a retrospective study, Age Ageing 14(4):225–229, 1985.

SUGGESTED READINGS

Eastwood GL: Endoscopic diagnosis and management of upper gastrointestinal tract bleeding, Adv Intern Med 30:449–470, 1984.
Roberts CM et al: Injection sclerotherapy for oesophageal varices in the elderly, Age Ageing 12(2):139–143, 1983.

Response to Trauma in the Elderly: Introduction and General Considerations

Daniel K. Lowe, M.D., and Donald D. Trunkey, M.D.

Organ system response and pattern of injury

    Musculoskeletal injuries

    Central nervous system injuries

    Chest/thoracic cage injuries

Management principles

    Prehospital phase

    Hospital phase

    Resuscitation

    Postresuscitation fluid shifts

    Infection

Trauma is not a common cause of death in the elderly. Only 2% of deaths after the age of 65 years are related to injuries. According to the National Center for Health Statistics, this represents over 30,000 deaths per year. For each year, over 140,000 deaths are related to injury for all ages so that the elderly patient group represents over 20% of the total trauma-related deaths. For ages 75 years and older, the death rate is higher than any other population group, including young males in their twenties. For the ages of greater than 85 years, the death rate is more than three times that of the 20- to 30-year-old age group.[1]

Not only does the elderly patient have a higher death rate from injury, but this population has a higher hospitalization rate and emergency department usage. Overall, the elderly group consumes over 30% of the trauma medical care resources.[18] Modern reimbursement methodologies using diagnostic related groups (DRGs) show a significant disparity in reimbursements for trauma patients with an average loss for severe injury of greater than $2,000 per case. Additional studies of reimbursements have shown that although patients over the age of 80 represent only a small percentage of all trauma admissions, they accounted for a significant reimbursement loss of approximately 17% in one study.[5]

The Major Trauma Outcome Study sponsored by the American College of Surgeons[7] compiled a review of 33,308 traumatized patients from 91 institutions over a 3-year period (1983 to 1985). These patients represent 0.3% of all injured patients in the United States, 1% of all trauma deaths, and 2% of all in-hospital deaths. The overall mortality in this extensive review was 10%. Patients over the age of 54, however, comprised 13% of the total population examined and showed a significant increased mortality rate. Patients over the age of 65 years comprised 8% of the study group and had a mortality rate of 17%.[7]

Epidemiologic data from these and other studies demonstrate that the elderly injured patient is a significant health care problem.

ORGAN SYSTEM RESPONSE AND PATTERN OF INJURY

Three mechanisms — falls, motor vehicle accidents, and burns — represent over 80% of the causes of accidental injury in the elderly. The effects of any mechanism of injury in this age group have a varied organ system response pattern. Overall, the general theory is that the elderly human exhibits a greater extent of injury per given amount of energy as well as a reduced capacity to recover. This theory has not been scientifically examined in the laboratory. A description of what does exist in the literature regarding responses to trauma in the elderly is oriented toward individual organ systems.

Musculoskeletal Injuries

The most frequently injured organ system in the elderly is the musculoskeletal system. In the 100 consecutive patients over age 70 years admitted to Harborview Medical Center, 77 patients (77%) had extremity or pelvic injuries, the most frequent site of injury, and 80% had multiple system trauma.[15] In contrast, the Rhode Island Hospital reported that in 63 elderly patients who survived a blunt trauma incident, musculoskeletal injuries occurred in only 25 patients (40%); overall multiple trauma was seen in 39 patients (62%).[14]

The Harborview series showed that musculoskeletal injury was equally present in survivors and nonsurvivors and could not be considered a factor contributing to mortality in the elderly. The quality of life following injury is a factor, however, and this series reported that 88% of the survivors did not return to independent living.[15] The high incidence of falls and musculoskeletal injuries in this elderly group of patients might contribute to the reported overall poor prognosis for independent living. In contrast, the series from Rhode Island reported that 89% of their elderly patients returned home after injury. In part, this may be attributed to the lower incidence of falls and subsequent musculoskeletal injuries seen in their group of patients.

The ultimate outcome goal of treatment following a serious injury in the elderly is return to preinjury function. Musculoskeletal injury seems to be a major factor most seriously challenging this outcome. The principles of management — "goals of patient care" — to achieve the best outcome are outlined by Brooker and Mandelbaum: 1) stabilization of the fracture, 2) optimal respiratory management, 3) minimize infection rate, 4) encourage union, 5) diminish complications of fracture, 6) early mobilization of the patient, and 7) maintenance of adequate nutrition.[16]

Avoiding Complications

Avoiding complications significantly alters the mortality and returns the function in this fragile group of patients. Therefore, the tendency may be to avoid any aggressive, particularly operative, approach in the patient with preexisting disease or cardiovascular instability. The frequent result is a longer hospitalization and, in the elderly particularly, a higher complication rate. Early stabilization of the fracture and mobilization of the patient result in optimization of respiratory function. Respiratory complications, which are the most significant cause of morbidity and mortality in the elderly injured patient, can then be avoided.[20]

Central Nervous System Injuries

Although central nervous system (CNS) injuries are much less frequent than musculoskeletal injuries in this age group, they have a much greater impact on recovery as well as ultimate outcome. In the Harborview series, 12 patients sustained CNS injuries with three deaths (25%); this is two times the incidence of CNS injury seen in survivors. This system injury was seen as a significant factor in the outcome, particularly when the patient required prolonged intubation.[15] In the Rhode Island Hospital series, CNS injury was seen as a major factor regarding functional outcome. In this review of elderly survivors from injury, a mild-to-moderate central nervous system injury (AIS 3 to 4) in this group resulted in more complications, longer hospital stay, and less functional recovery.[5]

In a series of 34 patients over age 65 with closed head injury and acute subdural hematomas, the outcome resulted in death in 25 patients (74%). The mechanism of injury was falls in 68% (23 of the 34 patients). Aggressive neurosurgical and critical care management was given to all patients, but the patients with good recovery were those with minor injuries, a near normal neurologic examination (Glasgow coma scale 13 to 15) and admission within 1 hour of injury.[3]

Spinal Injuries

Additionally, the elderly patient is at risk for spinal injury because of the chronic bony changes and resultant stiffening of the spine. Bony spurs may impinge into the spinal cord with even a minor force of insult and damage the cord. Certainly, the spinal stiffness increases susceptibility to fracture following trivial energy transfer. The osteoporosis in the elderly adds to the tendency to fracture. This combination of stiffness, spurs, and osteoporosis requires an increased level of suspicion in the elderly for the possibility of injury to the spine. The cervical spine must be evaluated by x-ray for even the most trivial of injuries in the elderly age group. In many cases, additional studies are indicated including flexion and extension films or CT scan to exclude injuries. Not only is the cervical spine at increased risk, but the thoracic and lumbar spine must be evaluated with a much higher degree of sensitivity because of an increased susceptibility for injury in this area as well.

Chest/Thoracic Cage Injuries

The bony changes associated with aging similarly affect the ability of the thorax to tolerate blunt trauma. The thoracic cage becomes brittle so that even minor forces of injury result in broken ribs. With the loss of thoracic wall integrity, there is an increased incidence of pulmonary contusion. Not only are the thoracic cage and lung at increased risk for injury from a lesser force insult than would cause damage in a younger person, but the aortic arch also has an increased susceptibility for disruption in the elderly. This is described as being secondary to a decrease in flexibility because of atherosclerosis associated with the aging process.

The thoracic cage and its contents are more susceptible to injury and to complications leading to increased morbidity and mortality. The leading cause of death in the elderly trauma patient after the first 24 hours is adult respiratory distress syndrome (ARDS).[20] More recent studies have confirmed the problem of respiratory complications in increased mortality associated with injury. A fivefold increase in ARDS was seen in a series of orthopedic patients where delay in operative repair was greater than 24 hours.[10] Increased age was not seen as a risk factor for infection in the major thoracic trauma patient as described in a series of 310 patients of whom 8 were over the age of 65 years. The mean length of stay in this group of 8 patients was 40 days, however, and a survival was seen in 7 patients. There was no obvious increase in infections in this group.[12] In the group of 100 patients at Harborview, thoracic injury itself was not considered a risk factor for increased mortality in the elderly. In the 15 nonsurvivors in this group of patients, 100% were intubated longer than 5 days and in 80% of the fatalities, pulmonary sepsis was a significant contributing factor.[15]

In summary, every organ system in the elderly patient tolerates injury poorly. With any given insult, the extent of injury is greater and the ability to recover is reduced compared to young people. Complications, primarily pulmonary, occur with a higher frequency and figure significantly in the outcome. The ability to return to preinjury function appears to be related to the injury pattern, aggressive surgical management, and avoidance of complications.

MANAGEMENT PRINCIPLES

Strict adherence to the principles of trauma care is most important in achieving a good outcome and return to preinjury function in the elderly patient. The pattern and extent of injury can only be altered in the preinjury phase by prevention measures. The clinician caring for the elderly trauma patient must pay attention to trauma management principles and avoid complications to get the best outcome. Adherence to these principles is required in all three phases of care: prehospital, initial assessment and resuscitation, and definitive care. Any significant deviation in any phase of care increases the risk for complication and will result in an increase in mortality or a decrease in the functional outcome.

Prehospital Phase

In the prehospital phase of injury care, the elderly patient presents the most significant challenge to the prehospital principle of "do no further harm." An elderly patient who is injured demands adherence to all of the principles of prehospital trauma care. Particular attention to immobilization is important because of the bony fragility and tendency to fracture. The elderly patient is more apt to have dentures or other materials in the mouth that must be removed to facilitate a patent airway. Oxygen supplementation is important in this group because of the increased incidence of vascular disease, particularly cardiac. Thermal protection should be considered as a high priority. Frequently, the elderly patient is hypothermic because of increased heat loss secondary to diminished subcutaneous fat reserves or delay in getting medical assistance. Attention to thermal protection is increasingly important in this age group because of the attendant myocardial irritability. Electrical monitoring of the heart should be done early in the management but should not delay getting the traumatized patient to a treatment facility. Stabilization in the field is not indicated for any patient with traumatic injuries. All prehospital treatments at the scene should be limited to less than 10 minutes. Most elderly trauma patients require admission to trauma facilities in an expeditious manner to reduce morbidity and mortality.

The prehospital team should communicate to the necessary trauma hospital the age of the patient and mechanism of injury. This advance notification will allow the trauma team to adequately prepare for assessment and resuscitation. Upon arrival, the trauma team needs to get a verbal report of the accident details and current status of the patient while the resuscitation commences. Additional details regarding past medical history, allergies, and medications need to be documented if available. Frequently, the hospital care team has access to this information through contact with family members and can relate this to the trauma team early in the assessment and resuscitative phase.

Hospital Phase

Priorities for assessment and resuscitation are the same for the elderly patient as with any trauma patient. A quick initial assessment of airway, breathing, and circulation should allow the physician to prioritize the resuscitation. Airway difficulties may occur because of dentures, which should be removed. The trauma team should be alert to the possibility of cervical spine injury because of the increased fragility in the elderly patient. A protected airway should be guaranteed. All elderly trauma patients should have supplemental oxygen therapy, preferably humidified. With any question of hypothermia, the provision of warmed and humidified oxygen can be used to aid in the rewarming process. Because of the increased frailty of the thoracic cage in the elderly, a careful assessment of respiratory capabilities should be done.

Management of shock and hemorrhage in accordance with established principles of trauma patient care should next occur. Close attention to core body temperature is a must in the elderly. Therefore, all solutions should be warmed to 30°C prior to administration. Warming blankets at room temperature must be utilized to reduce ongoing thermal losses. Cardiac arrhythmias can occur in any hypothermic patient during resuscitation, but the elderly patient is most susceptible because of intrinsic myocardial disease.

Resuscitation

Resuscitative measures in the elderly trauma patient should proceed according to standard protocols. Monitoring the response to treatments by physical assessment alone will frequently be misleading. Mental status may not necessarily improve because of an inadequate baseline. Peripheral perfusion may be impaired as a baseline as well. Heart rate may be abnormal because of intrinsic myocardial disease or the patient may be on medication such as a beta-blocking agent, which may limit heart rate response to hypovolemia. More subtle physical assessments such as tissue turgor, temperature, and pulse character all lack both sensitivity and specificity, particularly in the elderly patient.

The elderly trauma patient requires aggressive and early monitoring of the adequacy of resuscitation. Urinary output can be misleading because of the possibility of intrinsic renal disease. Certainly, all elderly male patients with moderate to severe trauma should be catheterized because of the high incidence of urethral outflow problems. Catheterization under these circumstances should be done with the usual precautions in patients with pelvic fractures and the resultant potential for urethral injuries at the bladder outlet. Patients with blood at the urethral meatus, boggy prostates on rectal examinations, and severe pelvic fractures should have cystourethrograms prior to catheterization.

Central venous pressure lines should be placed early in most elderly trauma patients because of the need for proper fluid management and for monitoring purposes. The lines should be placed on the same side as the thoracic cage injury, particularly if a tube thoracostomy has already been placed. Confirmation of the location and evaluation for pneumothorax is required. The large-lumen venous catheters are stiff, and the fragility of veins in the elderly can lead to venous disruption. Large-bore central venous lines can be utilized for fluid administration, but this should be done cautiously with cool to cold fluids or blood transfusions because of the potential to aggravate myocardial irritability. Conversion of the central venous pressure line to a Swan-Ganz catheter will increase the ability to monitor the patient with cardiovascular compromise. In the acute situation, particularly in the elderly patient, this can stimulate fibrillation and, therefore, should be avoided until the acidosis and hypothermia are significantly improved. The use of cardiotonic drugs in the elderly to improve myocardial

performance cannot be supported with scientific evidence of benefit. The potential chronotropic action of such agents can increase the left ventricular stroke work index to high levels, which may result in myocardial failure or ischemia. Although the practice of using a small dosage infusion of dopamine is common, the benefit is small and the risk is large — particularly if it delays shock resuscitation measures.

The initial assessment and resuscitation should proceed in an aggressive manner according to standardized protocols. During this time period will evolve the determination of the nature and severity of injury for each organ system as well as the response to the initial treatments. Plans for definitive care should necessitate input from family or other support people. Knowing the baseline medical and physical activity levels becomes important in making the best clinical decision for the patient. Aggressive management is indicated when such knowledge is unknown or is thought to be unreliable. When the clinical situation is thought to be hopeless or the baseline function of the patient is not good, aggressive management may not be indicated. Involvement of all pertinent family members in addition to documentation by living wills or other pieces of similar data will allow the most appropriate clinical decisions to be made. This can rarely be done in the acute setting. When in doubt, resuscitate.

Postresuscitation Fluid Shifts

Dependent upon the duration of shock, the peripheral capillary beds leak plasma in addition to the fluid sequestration and hematoma formation directly associated with tissue damage. With stabilization of the cardiovascular system, fluid reabsorption can begin as early as 24 hours and will maximize at 72 hours. Preparation for this fluid shift requires clinical attention, particularly in the patient with diminished cardiac reserve. The Swan-Ganz catheter measurements available during the early resuscitative phase will give several points on the patient's Starling curve.

Improvement in the patient's overall course can lead to such optimism that the monitoring may be discontinued early only to find that a sudden unexpected deterioration in the patient occurs. The fluid shifts may cause this deterioration and resultant cardiac failure. Prevention of this deterioration should occur as the known sequela of fluid absorption is well understood. Therefore, it is strongly recommended that elderly patients with significant peripheral fluid sequestration, as evidenced by weight gain, excess fluid requirements, and peripheral edema, be monitored by invasive catheters to properly monitor cardiac function during this vulnerable period. Consideration should be given to diuretic administration in such patients on the second through the fourth day following injury. Particular attention to electrolyte balance is necessary with the use of such agents. Cardiotonic agents may occasionally become necessary as well.

Infection

As has been previously discussed, the elderly traumatized patient is susceptible to pulmonary infection. Infection is a possibility in the respiratory system and elsewhere because of the immune system suppression. Judicious use of prophylactic antibiotics in trauma patients is similarly indicated in elderly patients. Careful attention to IV cutdown sites should occur, and they should be treated as open, infected wounds. All IVs placed in the initial resuscitative phase should be replaced in the first 24 hours because of increased risk of infection.

A most important consideration in the management of infection prevention in the traumatized patient is nutrition. The enteral tract is the most appropriate means by which to return to a normal nutritional state.[21] Major trauma patients should also be considered for parenteral hyperalimentation. Because of the increased frailty of the elderly trauma patient, nutritional considerations are very important and attention should be given to this early on in the course of even mild-to-moderate injuries. As soon as GI function returns, consideration should be given to enteral nutrition by a feeding tube.

REFERENCES

1. Baker SP, O'Neil B, and Karpf RS: The injury fact book, Lexington, MA, 1984, Lexington Books.
2. Waller JA: Injury control: a guide to the causes and prevention of trauma, Lexington, MA, 1984, Lexington Books.
3. Howard MA III et al: Traumatic intracranial hemorrhage in the elderly (Manuscript submitted for publication).
4. Russell MA et al: Chronic subdural hematoma mimicking transient ischemic attacks, J Trauma 25:113, 1985.
5. DeMaria EJ et al: Hospital costs and reimbursement in geriatric trauma patients (Manuscript submitted for publication, 1986).
6. Morris JA Jr et al: Pre-injury health as a determinant of outcome in the trauma patient (Manuscript submitted for publication, 1986).
7. Champion HR: The major trauma outcome study, American College of Surgeons Committee on Trauma.
8. Bongard FS et al: Geriatric burns: etiology, morbidity, and prevention (Manuscript submitted for publication, 1986).
9. Anous MN and Heinbach DM: Causes of death and predictors in burned patients more than 60 years of age. (Manuscript submitted for publication.)
10. Johnson KD, Cadambi A, and Seibert GB: Incidence of adult respiratory distress syndrome in patients with multiple musculoskeletal injuries: effect of early operative stabilization of fractures, J Trauma 25:375, 1985.
11. Schultz RJ et al: The role of physiologic monitoring in patients with fractures of the hip, J Trauma 25:309, 1985.
12. Walker WE et al: Patterns of infection and mortality in thoracic trauma, Ann Surg 201:752, 1985.
13. Schwab CW: The effects of trauma severity on hospital cost and its relationship to reimbursement under the prospective payment system: the short fall from DRGs for trauma care (Manuscript submitted for publication, 1986).
14. DeMaria EF et al: Aggressive trauma care benefits for the elderly (Manuscript submitted for publication, 1986).
15. Oreskovich NR et al: Geriatric trauma: injury patterns and outcome, J Trauma 24:565, 1984.
16. Mandelbaum ER and Brooker AF Jr: Trauma to the lower extremities. In Zytema GD, Rutherford RB, and Ballinger WF, editors: The management of trauma, ed 4, Philadelphia, 1985, WB Saunders Co.
17. Smith L: Injury in America: a continuing public health problem, Washington, DC, 1985, National Academy Press.
18. Mueller MS and Gibson RN: Age difference in healthcare spending, Soc Secur Bull 36:18, 1976.
19. Hogue CP: Injury in late life. I. Epidemiology, J Am Geriatr Soc 30:183, 1982.
20. Trunkey DD et al: Management of pelvic fractures in blunt trauma injuries, J Trauma 14:912, 1974.
21. Rolandelli RH et al: Enteral nutrition: advantages, limitations, and formula selection, J Crit Ill 3:93, 1989.

Evaluation and Management of Geriatric Trauma

Gerald B. Demarest, M.D.

Trauma is the fifth leading cause of death in the elderly, preceded by cardiovascular disease, stroke, and cancer. Although this group currently represents 11% of the population, it accounts for 25% of trauma fatalities or 24,000 deaths per year.[1] Until recently, knowledge regarding trauma care of this group has been sparse. The advent of gerontology as a specialty, the rapid growth of this group, and their disproportionate demands on health care and other social services have made it increasingly important to gain an understanding of the age-related factors involved in injury. On the average, elderly accident victims remain in the hospital twice as long as younger patients. Most of these events are the result of a complex interaction between changes of aging and hazards of the environment, particularly in the home, on the streets, and in hospitals or institutions.[2]

A significant accidental injury in a frail, elderly patient often leads to functional dependency, a decline in function of multiple organ systems, and, frequently, prolonged institutionalization or death. For these reasons, the prevention of accidents in elderly patients and optimal care of those who suffer injury are important responsibilities of the physician.[2]

Persons 65 years of age or older are less likely than persons in other age groups to be injured, but when they are injured, they are more likely to have a fatal outcome. For all injuries combined, population death rates are the highest in this group — at 166 deaths per 100,000 population for people age 75 to 84 years — compared with 64 deaths per 100,000 for people age 15 to 24 years. This is a reflection of this population's overall reduced intrinsic reserve and high risk for complications.[1]

Reported causes of injury and death in the elderly group have remained relatively constant during the last two decades as shown in Table 34–1. Falls are the leading cause of injury and death, accounting for 40% of fatalities.[5] One third of these are injuries to elderly pedestrians. House fires or ignition of clothing cause the majority of burn deaths in the elderly. Firearms, suffoca-

Table 34–1 Accidental Fatalities of Elderly Persons Aged 65 Years or Older and Causes (1981)

Falls	9,600 (40%)
Motor vehicle accidents	6,000 (25%)
Driver/passenger	4,000
Pedestrian	2,000
Fires, burns	1,700 (6%)
Firearms	1,200
Suffocation: ingested objects	1,200
Suffocation: mechanical	600
Poisoning: solid, liquid	400
Poisoning: gas	300
Other	3,000
Total	24,000

Source: Accident facts, Chicago, Illinois, National Safety Council, 1981.

tion, and poisoning make up the majority of the remaining fatalities in descending order.[1]

ETIOLOGY

Falls

In all age groups, falls represent the second leading cause of unintentional injury deaths in the United States and are exceeded only by motor vehicle related deaths. As a result of falls in and around the home, 10,000 individuals die annually and 7 million persons are injured.[6] In the elderly, falls are the largest cause of injury mortality and account for approximately 40% of deaths, though a decline in mortality rates for falls has been ongoing since 1978.[1] Most deaths from falls occur in persons aged 65 or greater.[7] Both the incidence and severity of complications as a result of falls increase steadily with age. The majority of elderly persons who fall do not die, but, as a result of falls, large numbers of emergency room visits and subsequent hospital admissions occur.

In the elderly, falls most commonly are a result of the accumulated effects of age and environmental hazards. Three times as many women as men are involved in falls that occur in the home.[7] Older people are stiffer and less coordinated and have gaits that are dangerous. Impairments in vision, hearing, and memory place them at high risk for environmental hazards that can cause falls.[8]

Acute changes in cardiac status account for as many as 25% of falls in the elderly. A relative decrease in cerebral blood flow is an important cause of falls. Orthostatic hypotension as a result of hypovolemic venous pooling, loss of muscle mass in lower extremities, and autonomic dysfunction are likely to induce this condition and the risk of fall. Syncope — the sudden unexpected loss of consciousness — is an important cause of serious falls. The causes of syncope include decreased cerebral blood flow from a variety of conditions as well as metabolic derangements, including hypoglycemia, hypoxia, and acid-base disturbances. Drop attacks are defined as sudden, unexpected falls without associated loss of consciousness or dizziness. This presents as a sudden flaccid weakness in the lower extremities and is usually attributed to transient vertebral-basilar artery insufficiency. This etiology should be considered if a patient falls when reaching for an object or hyperextending the head. Falls from dizziness or vertigo are extremely common. These symptoms are usually a reflection of one of the underlying etiologies previously mentioned, as well as vestibular dysfunction or the use of various drugs.

Drugs, including alcohol, are a cause or contributing factor in many falls. Especially important are sedatives, antihypertensives, diuretics, and hypoglycemic agents. Anemia, occult blood loss, transient ischemic attacks (TIAs), hypothyroidism, unstable joints, severe osteoporosis with spontaneous fracture, epilepsy, and electrolyte imbalance are other important causes of falls.

Motor Vehicle Accidents

Motor vehicle accidents account for 51,000 fatalities on our nation's highways annually.[9] Of these deaths, 4,000 individuals 65 years of age or older are killed as drivers or passengers. An additional 2,000 aged persons are killed as pedestrians.[9]

The elderly, with the exception of those with Alzheimer's disease, do not have higher crash rates than other age groups but do have substantially higher crash experiences per miles traveled when compared with middle-aged drivers if reported highway crashes per 100 drivers are examined.[10,11] While younger drivers are more likely to be involved in a serious single-vehicle crash of danger to themselves and their passengers, the elderly driver more often has a two-vehicle collision.[12,13] The very elderly are as likely to be involved in fatal crashes as young drivers, and this substantially exceeds the fatality experience of middle-aged drivers.[9] Once injured, the elderly driver is less likely to survive the injury.

There can be little doubt that the elderly pedestrian is ill equipped to deal with the hazards of the highway.[3] Studies show that pedestrian fatalities are comprised of three groups: preschool and elementary school children, middle-aged alcoholics, and the elderly.[14,15] As pedestrians, the elderly injured, 60 years of age or older, have a much higher mortality rate than other age groups both at the scene as well as those surviving long enough to reach the hospital.[16]

The effect of the aging process appears to have a major influence on the risk of injury and death in the elderly involved in motor vehicle accidents. Reduced ability to see or hear is an example. Several parameters of visual ability decrease markedly with age, including daylight acuity, glare resistance, and night vision.[3] The occurrence of medical conditions that alter attention and consciousness is of major importance as is alteration of judgment because of the onset of senile changes in the brain.[3] Finally, there is often decreased ability to implement appropriate actions once decided upon because of impairing medical conditions, including severe arthritis, emphysema, heart disease, and decrease in muscle mass, as well as other physical impairments.[3]

Burns

Exposure to fire or burns from contact with hot substances is the third leading cause of trauma deaths in the elderly, accounting for some 1,700 deaths annually.[9] One third of these individuals are fatally injured as a consequence of using alcohol and smoking in bed, or being caught in a building fire with exposure to heat and the toxic products of combustion. The majority of the remainder sustain injury and death by ignition of clothing or as a result of prolonged contact with hot substances. Factors associated with degenerative disease and physical impairment appear to contribute substantially to the overrepresentation of the elderly.[17] The elderly are more likely to be burned initially because of falls against hot surfaces, the inability to hold things without spilling them, and lesser sensitivity of nerve endings to substances that may be too hot. Because of physical infirmities, the elderly person who comes into contact with a hot surface or who is exposed to fire often is not able to remove himself until extensive damage has occurred. Once burned, preexisting cardiovascular, respiratory, and renal disease often makes it impossible for the elderly to overcome a serious but possibly survivable injury.[3]

CHARACTERISTICS OF THE ELDERLY TRAUMATIZED PATIENT

Cardiovascular Disease

Cardiovascular diseases in the elderly are complex, arising from a combination of changes associated with age-related disorders, acquired cardiovascular disease, and pathologic conditions unique to old age. Prolonged hemodynamic stresses and the biologic changes of aging over a lifetime produce anatomic, histologic, biochemical, and electrophysiologic changes that impair cardiovascular function and diminish cardiac reserve.[18]

The aged heart manifests a decrease in strength of contraction, cardiac output, speed and force of contraction, stroke volume, ventricular ejection fraction, left ventricle diastolic compliance and filling, and increased impedance to left ventricular ejection.[18]

Acquired cardiovascular diseases in the aged include ischemic heart disease usually secondary to atherosclerosis, orthostatic hypotension, cardiac dysrhythmias, TIAs, and congestive heart failure. The decreased inotropic response of the aged heart to catecholamines prolongs contraction, chronotropic, and vasodilation capacity. As a result, sudden major stress can precipitate cardiac dysrhythmias, heart failure, and sudden death.[18]

Osteoporosis

Osteoporosis affects an estimated 15 million persons, one third of whom have severe demineralization with vertebral fractures. Postmenopausal osteoporosis in women and senile osteoporosis in men are insidious in onset and generally follow a protracted course.[19]

The morbidity associated with osteoporosis is frequently disabling and sometimes devastating. In the United States, 80% of patients who sustain hip fractures do so as a result of preexisting osteoporosis. This fact accounts for 160,000 of these injuries per year. Annually, 2% of women and 1% of men aged 85 or older sustain femoral fractures.[20] Vertebral compression or crush fractures are a common disabling feature of advanced osteoporosis caused by collapse of demineralized vertebral bodies. These can occur in association with common activities such as bending and lifting or may be a consequence of the long-term effect of carrying the weight of the body upright. The overall effect of progressive osteoporosis in the elderly is unknown but is a significant factor in the occurrence and severity of fractures secondary to trauma and must certainly add to the morbidity and mortality associated with injuries.[19]

Pulmonary Characteristics

In old age, the lung has lost much of its elasticity due to losses of elastin. With this, a significant degree of alveolar dilatation occurs, described as senile emphysema.[21] Additionally, changes in the composition of collagen occur with an increased number of cross-links between subunits of collagen resulting in increased rigidity of structural tissue in the lung. This effect leads to a decrease in lung compliance and an alteration in gas exchange.

Aging has been related to a decrease in vital capacity (VC) and forced expiratory volume in one second (FEV_1), as well as a progressive reduction in arterial oxygen tension (PaO_2). Residual volume (RV), functional residual capacity (FRC), and closing volume (CV) all increase with age. The total lung capacity (TLC) and arterial CO_2 tension ($PaCO_2$) remain constant throughout life.[21]

With increasing age, a number of respiratory-dependent systems undergo alterations consistent with the aging process. Disordered patterns of breathing — including primary alveolar hypoventilation, sleep apnea syndromes, and Cheyne-Stokes breathing — may be a result of a combination of endocrinologic, neurologic, and circulatory disturbances that, with aging, predispose the elderly to these conditions.[21]

With age, reduced levels of consciousness, dysphagia, and disruption of the lower esophageal sphincter occur with increased frequency and predispose patients to aspiration and its consequences. Dyspnea is a subjective phenomenon and is related to an awareness of the need for increased respiratory effort. In aging, the progressive worsening of chronic heart disease, cardiomyopathies, and hypertensive states are all associated with left ventricular dysfunction that can lead to dyspnea.[21]

The incidence of pneumonia in elderly patients is increased, and these patients have more serious complications, debilitation, and associated illness. The frequency of pneumococcal pneumonia in the elderly is reported to be five to six times higher than in younger patients.[22] The occurrence of other gram-positive and gram-negative pneumonias in the elderly appears to be increased in hospitalized patients. *Klebsiella, Pseudomonas, Haemophilus,* and *Escherichia coli* are found more frequently in the elderly in nosocomial infection.[22] Lung diseases, other systemic illness, use of antibiotics, and debilitation with increased age have all been implicated as factors responsible for infection by these organisms.

Nutrition/Metabolism

One of the most significant factors influencing the onset of severity of age-associated diseases is nutrition. An elderly person's ability to obtain adequate nutrition may be impaired due to losses of income, mobility, relatives or friends, or even self-esteem.[23] Protein-caloric malnutrition is recognized more frequently among all hospitalized patients. Increased numbers of in-patient referrals for nutritional support services are for persons over age 60.[24]

Nutritional assessment tests — including percent ideal body weight, somatic protein mass, creatinine/height index (CHI), visceral proteins, absolute lymphocyte count, and measurements of cellular mediated immunity — have been described for a younger population. Many measurements commonly performed in nutritional assessment may be unreliable in the elderly due to various effects of the aging process. In developing norms for the elderly, careful subject selection will be necessary in order to exclude the presence of any acute or chronic disease state. Also, consideration must be given to the specific physiologic effects of the aging process.[25] The various effects of disease on blood proteins must be considered in nutritional assessment of the elderly including hepatic dysfunction, renal disease, and congestive heart failure. In addition, the acute stress of trauma, hypoxia, burns, and various carcinomas each can alter albumin synthesis. Finally, large numbers of immunologic abnormalities described in malnutrition have been documented in the elderly and have also been ascribed to the effects of aging.[26]

The caloric needs for men and women decline with age and are related to decreased metabolic rate, decreased activity levels, and reduction in the total mass of metabolically active cells.[23] Aged persons require fewer total calories but not less protein, vitamins, or minerals. Stressful environments and increased physical demands in trauma, infection, chronic disease, and altered gastrointestinal function may impair dietary nitrogen utilization. Clinical protein deficiencies can be correlated to fatigue, muscle weakness, tissue wasting, poor wound healing, and lack of energy.[23] The current RDA for protein is 0.8 g/kg of body weight. Studies have shown that this may not be an entirely accurate figure and that in conditions of stress higher levels of protein intake may be necessary.[26] It seems probable that in order to maintain nitrogen balance, the elderly may need more protein as their caloric intake is reduced. This need looms larger when one considers that illnesses common among the elderly can cause transient losses of body protein that will need to be replaced.[28]

Infectious Diseases in the Elderly and Senescence of the Immune System

The incidence and mortality rates for many bacterial infections are higher in the elderly. The explanation for this is twofold: associated predisposing illnesses and immunologic senescence. Bacterial pathogens such as gram-negative bacilli are more likely to occur in older patients. In addition, the diagnosis of bacterial infection in the elderly patient may be more difficult than in the younger patient. Finally, the underlying pathogenesis of a bacterial infection may differ in the elderly population when compared with a younger group.[29]

The treatment of bacterial infection in the elderly must take into consideration several factors. These include 1) the particular toxicity of some antibiotics in the elderly, 2) the fact that dosage based on creatinine clearance changes with age, 3) the existence of a larger variety of potential bacterial pathogens for most disease, making empiric therapy more difficult, and 4) the more fulminant course of many bacterial infections in the elderly patient.[29]

The immune system changes with age. The increased susceptibility of elderly patients to infections, neoplastic disease, and perhaps vascular injury may be a consequence of immune senescence.[30] With aging, cell-mediated and humoral immune response to foreign antigens is decreased, while the response to autologous antigens is increased. It has been suggested that autoantibodies and circulating immunocomplexes, which can damage tissues and organs, contribute to the pathologic changes that occur with age.[30] Whether immune senescence is a primary or secondary contributor to the pathobiology of aging, it is likely that increased knowledge of immune senescence and the ability to correct immune defects that occur in the elderly will offer the possibility for control of diseases of aging.

DIAGNOSIS AND TREATMENT
History and Physical Examination

As with all trauma patients, the principles of evaluation and treatment of the geriatric trauma victim include an initial evaluation of patient status regarding maintenance of the airway, breathing, and circulation. This is followed by management of acute life-threatening conditions, as they are identified, and then the performance of an in-depth history and physical examination. In the field or upon arrival in the emergency room, initial management principles should first focus on patency of the airway, adequacy and quality of breathing, and a rapid evaluation of intravascular volume status. Close, continuous monitoring of vital signs should be high on the list of priorities because of the elderly person's relative intolerance to shock and its effect. Establish large-bore peripheral intravenous catheters as a port for fluid resuscitation and transfusion access as well as a means of rapid medication administration. This also serves as a means of obtaining blood for diagnostic laboratory evaluation and type and crossmatching.

Along with the physical evaluation of the patient, an in-depth history should encompass pertinent information regarding the particulars of the injuring event, significant past medical history, medications, previous hospitalizations and surgeries, allergies, immunization status, as well as the determination of the time of the patient's last meal.

Neurologic evaluation in the form of level of consciousness and Glasgow coma scale assessment should be determined and recorded. This evaluation should be repeated at frequent intervals as a means of documentation in the evolution of a neurologic injury.

Radiographic studies routinely performed in the emergency room remain the same for the elderly patient as for all patients sustaining trauma. A cross-table lateral cervical spine film that visualizes all seven cervical vertebrae and the first thoracic vertebra should be undertaken in all patients who sustain injury to the head or neck. The importance of a high index of suspicion for risk of cervical spine injury in any patient who sustains head or maxillofacial trauma should be emphasized. Hyperextension injuries are significantly common in the elderly patient who falls forward and sustains injury to the forehead or face. Such hyperextension can "pinch" the cervical cord between the ligamentum flavum and posterior osteophytes that are especially common in the elderly population.[31] Patients who are comatose, or who are alert but have positive cervical spine findings, must be immobilized with a rigid collar or sandbags until a cross-table lateral radiograph clears them of injury.

Patients who manifest airway compromise and who are at risk for potential cervical spine injury should undergo airway control by intubation. This is accomplished through blind nasotracheal or oral intubation with an assistant holding axial traction and limiting head extension or flexion or, when this is not possible, by means of a cervical cricothyroidotomy.

Head Injuries

Subdural hematomas are nearly three times as frequent in the elderly as they are in younger patients, and the development of epidural hematomas is extremely rare.[32] While elderly patients have a higher incidence of subdural and intraparenchymal hematomas as a result of head trauma, they sustain relatively fewer severe cerebral contusions than do younger patients.[32] It is important to note that a subdural hematoma may present as a gradual neurologic decline. In fact, the fall for which the patient is being examined may be the result of a fall years ago.[32]

Except for specific indications, the routine use of head computerized axial tomography (CAT) scans has supplanted routine skull x-rays for patients with head injury. This modality provides rapid, accurate sequential cuts and gives detailed information on other structural damage of the brain and supporting elements. Indications for CAT scan generally include those individuals who present with loss of consciousness for periods of greater than 5 minutes or patients who present with a change in level of consciousness or lateralizing neurologic findings.

Chest Trauma

For the elderly patient who sustains significant blunt chest trauma, management principles remain the same. Normal workup of the elderly patient sustaining blunt chest trauma includes a routine anteroposterior (AP) chest x-ray. Because of the less elastic chest wall of the older person, blunt trauma is more likely to fracture several ribs or the sternum. These patients frequently present with soft tissue injury manifested by ecchymosis or hematoma formation. Crepitation or grating at the fracture site is a common finding. Too commonly, trauma from a fall or apparent insignificant blow will result in chest wall pain, revealing the occult hemothorax or pneumothorax. History of deceleration should alert one to the risk of thoracic aortic injuries and consideration for diagnostic aortography even without the presentation of widening of the mediastinum on the AP chest film or the older constellation of x-ray findings described in this clinical syndrome.

With superimposed medical disease and underlying intolerance to respiratory compromise, early arterial blood gas evaluation may give early indication of respiratory compromise in the high-risk patient. Low-dose supplemental oxygen by nasal cannula or face mask is frequently of benefit for the patient with minimal respiratory compromise but may be contraindicated in the patient with chronic obstructive pulmonary disease (COPD) and decreased CO_2 ventilatory drive. Early intubation should be considered for those patients manifesting respiratory failure by virtue of respiratory rates greater than 40 breaths per minute, PaO_2 levels less than 60 torr, and $PaCO_2$ levels above 50 torr.

Abdomen

The determination of the presence of significant intraabdominal injury requiring operative exploration in the elderly patient following blunt or penetrating trauma frequently presents as a diagnostic dilemma for the attending surgeon. The intolerance of this population to hypovolemic shock allows little margin for error in the determination of intraabdominal injury. A high index of suspicion should be accompanied by an aggressive approach in order to reduce the high morbidity and mortality rates in this population.

With blunt trauma, the most likely organs to be injured include (in order) liver, spleen, bladder, and kidney. Operative exploration is mandated by the following: 1) signs and symptoms of intravascular volume depletion without other obvious sites of ongoing blood loss outside the peritoneal cavity or retroperitoneal space, 2) obvious peritoneal irritation manifested by involuntary guarding, and 3) fractures of the pelvis and/or lower rib cage in which intraabdominal injury is strongly suspected.[33] For those patients in whom less obvious signs are present, the use of diagnostic peritoneal lavage and abdominal CAT scans have proven to be excellent adjunctive diagnostic measures for determination of significant bleeding or organ injury. These studies, along with an intravenous pyelogram (IVP) and cystourethrogram, as well as abdominal arteriography, are beneficial in elucidating the presence of injury in the otherwise stable patient.

Penetrating injuries follow a similar approach. Those patients with obvious ongoing blood loss, evisceration, or peritoneal irritation require exploration. Patients with less obvious symptoms because of head injury with a decrease in level of consciousness, paralysis, or under the influence of alcohol or drugs are managed in the following way: wounds of the anterior abdomen — nipple to pubis between anteroaxillary lines — are explored locally. Patients with hemo- or pneumothorax on AP chest x-ray or patients with penetration of the anterior fascia undergo diagnostic peritoneal lavage. Precautions of stomach and bladder decompression by placement of a nasogastric tube and Foley catheter, respectively, should be performed prior to placement of the lavage catheter in order to prevent injury to these structures. Operative exploration is mandated by 5 to 10 ml of nonclotting blood returned in the lavage catheter. If no blood is returned on aspiration, 1,000 ml of Ringer's lactate solution is infused, and the return is examined. Currently, there are controversies as to the absolute number of red cells in the returned lavage fluid that warrants exploration. Most centers utilizing this technique will explore patients with absolute red cell counts of 50,000 RBCs/μL or greater.[34] Spun lavage fluid hematocrits of greater than 2%, absolute white cell counts of 500 WBC/μL, evidence of bile, elevated amylase, and bacteria or food particles on laboratory evaluation also are indications for operative exploration.

Previous abdominal operative procedures represent an absolute contraindication to peritoneal lavage. Under these circumstances, consideration for a double contrast abdominal CAT scan evaluation of the abdomen as an alternative diagnostic modality should be undertaken.

The retroperitoneal abdominal structures continue to present a difficult anatomic area to ascertain as a site of injury. The genitourinary and vascular structures as well as the duodenum and pancreas may be evaluated by various adjunctive diagnostic studies including IVP, cystourethrogram, abdominal arteriography, ultrasonography, and abdominal CAT scan. Each may play a significant role in elucidating injuries that may have occurred in this region.

Fractures

Osteoporosis, which occurs with increasing age, is a condition that significantly increases the risk of fracture in the elderly patient. This risk mandates a careful examination of the bony structures of the extremities in all patients sustaining trauma. A careful history will lead to a high index of suspicion regarding fractures of the hip, shoulder, upper arm, and wrists. Examination of these areas, including neurovascular structures, will frequently lead to an early diagnosis of specific injury. The principle of early splinting and stabilization for prevention of further injury should be adhered to and will aid in reduction of morbidity and a more favorable result.

Colles' Fracture

The Colles' fracture is the result of a fall on an outstretched dorsiflexed hand. The injury is a fracture of the distal radius and occurs in the metaphyseal area. It is accompanied by the classic fracture at the base of the ulnar styloid that occurs approximately 60% of the time.[35] The "dinner-fork" deformity is frequently obviously manifested by swelling at the volar wrist and a dorsal depression deformity.

Evaluation should include testing of the median nerve and motor function of the finger flexors. Lateral and AP wrist films are mandatory and should visualize all carpal bones to rule out a more complex injury. The risk of concomitant injury at the elbow should be considered because of the nature of the cause. These fractures represent potentially complex injuries, and varying degrees of malunion are common.

Fractures of the Humerus

Fractures of the humerus are the result of inadvertent falls with absorption of the force on the deltoid area. The resultant injury is commonly a fracture of the surgical neck of the humerus (see Figure 42–2, p. 486). A similar fracture can occur due to a transmitted force through the humeral shaft when the blow is absorbed by an outstretched hand. Presentation is usually characterized by pain and tenderness in the shoulder or upper humeral area. A large ecchymosis may accompany the injury. Significant with these injuries is that of concomitant shoulder dislocation. These injuries should be confirmed by appropriate upper arm and shoulder x-rays.

Of major importance in evaluating fractures of the surgical neck of the humerus is the determination of whether the fracture is impacted or disimpacted. With impacted fractures, no fracture segment can be displaced more than 1.0 cm or angulated more than 45 degrees. When a patient has an impacted fracture, the arm can be moved gently hanging from the shoulder, waist bent 30 to 35 degrees without evidence of pain. Patients with disimpacted fractures will generally experience pain with any upper arm movement. Impacted fractures demonstrate no false motion of the humerus when the shoulder is rotated gently from a flexed elbow. Treatment of an impacted fracture is that of shoulder sling and progressive range of motion. In general, disimpacted fractures require hospitalization for surgery.

In the elderly, early mobilization with movement of the affected joint is important for the prevention of long-term joint stiffness and limitation in joint range of motion. Questions regarding the diagnosis of humeral fractures should be addressed by an orthopedic consultant.

Fractures of the Hip

The most common hip fractures seen in the elderly are those of the proximal femur. In general, these individuals are unable to walk. Because of significant pain, patients prefer not to be moved and are usually unwilling to sit even in a partially upright position. Pain from these injuries is localized to the area of the greater trochanter or anterior pelvis. Occasionally, hip fractures can present as pain referred to the knee.[36]

Isolated hip fractures do not usually present with hypovolemic shock, but determination of the patient's intravascular volume status should be made early with initiation of an intravenous catheter for fluid administration.

Pelvic fractures can be associated with marked blood loss and early shock. Early determination of intactness of neurovascular structures should be assessed and compared with the opposite extremity. Following initial management, appropriate x-ray evaluation includes affected hip and pelvis and both femoral necks and trochanters.

Fractures of the hip occur in one of four areas: subcapital, transcervical, intertrochanteric, and subtrochanteric (see Figure 42–1, p. 485). Intertrochanteric fractures are the most common followed by transcervical fractures.[37] The majority of these require operative fixation and, as such, make early orthopedic consultation mandatory.

SPECIAL OPERATIVE CONSIDERATIONS
Monitoring

Operative monitoring of body temperature has become routine. The elderly trauma patient is particularly susceptible to the deleterious effects of hypothermia, especially during long operative procedures with open body cavities and the attendant radiant and evaporative heat loss. This is compounded when large volumes of fluid and blood are given intravenously. Under these circumstances, the use of blood warmers for infused fluids, warming blankets, and external heat lamps in those severely injured patients when there is a drop in core temperature below 35°C is mandatory in order to avoid the development of bleeding diathesis and cardiac dysrhythmias.

Intraarterial pressure monitoring is currently in general use for all patients undergoing surgery for major trauma. The benefit of this type of monitoring is a continuous evaluation of systolic and diastolic pressure measurements as well as a port for access to arterial blood samples for measurement of arterial blood gas parameters.

In management of the geriatric trauma patient, the occurrence of superimposed disease states makes careful fluid resuscitation and monitoring mandatory, especially in cases of acute intravascular volume loss and shock. In addition to measurement of blood pressure, pulse, respiratory rate, electrocardiogram (ECG), and urine output, consideration for the monitoring of central venous pressure (CVP) measured at frequent intervals should be made for those patients receiving large volumes of fluid or those with a history of heart disease. The progressive CVP response to a fluid challenge is much more significant than that of isolated readings. A sharp rise in CVP with rapid infusion of fluids may indicate that the right heart cannot handle the load and infusion rates should be slowed. Those patients with low CVPs and hypotension should be considered hypovolemic and the fluid challenge should be continued. While usually accurate for fluid resuscitation, the response of CVP to fluid challenge becomes much less reliable in the face of sepsis, acute respiratory failure requiring positive pressure ventilation, or when preexisting cardiac or pulmonary diseases are present.[38]

For patients with severe coronary artery disease or those undergoing major operative procedures, consideration for placement of a Swan-Ganz pulmonary artery catheter for measurement of pulmonary wedge pressure

(PWP) should be undertaken. The pressure thus measured is the back pressure in the blood vessels in the lungs in a balloon-occluded artery and is a reflection of left ventricular function. A PWP reading of less than 10 torr suggests hypovolemia, whereas readings greater than 20 torr may indicate intravascular overload or left ventricular failure. As with the CVP, the progressive response of the PWP to a fluid challenge is more revealing than isolated readings.

Fluid Requirements

The geriatric trauma patient requires fluid and electrolyte replacement preoperatively and intraoperatively in amounts similar to those used for younger patients; however, several important considerations should be noted. These individuals have a blood volume similar to that of younger individuals, but even in mild disease states, hemoglobin content decreases and red cell fragility increases. Compensatory anemia is one of the most common disorders of blood volume encountered among geriatric patients. In addition, chronic hypovolemia is frequently found in this group of patients in which the disease states of malnutrition, chronic infection, malignancies of the GI tract, and metastatic neoplastic disease are common.

With aging, there is a progressive diminution in renal plasma flow and in glomerular filtration with a consequent decrease in renal function. Tubular function is decreased more than glomerular function, and the ability of the kidney to concentrate urine diminishes. These changes are frequently aggravated by chronic passive congestion secondary to myocardial insufficiency and result in impaired renal function and azotemia. The utilization of diuretics for control of hypertension or removal of intravascular volume in patients with congestive heart failure results in a depletion of serum potassium and other electrolyte abnormalities and should be monitored closely with frequent laboratory evaluation.

Initial Fluid Therapy and Transfusion Considerations

Isotonic electrolyte solutions are used for initial resuscitation. This type of fluid provides transient intravascular expansion and further stabilizes the vascular volume by replacing accompanying interstitial fluid losses. Ringer's lactate solution is the initial fluid of choice. Although normal saline is a satisfactory replacement, it has the potential for predisposing to hyperchloremic acidosis in the volumes administered to injured patients. This potential is enhanced in the face of impaired renal function. The initial fluid bolus is given as rapidly as possible. The usual dose is 1 to 2 liters. The patient's response is constantly monitored and observed during this initial fluid administration, and further therapeutic and diagnostic decisions are based on the observed response.

A small group of patients will respond rapidly to the initial fluid bolus and will remain stable. Such patients have generally lost less than 25% of their blood volume. No further fluid bolus or immediate blood administration is indicated in this small group of patients, but typed and cross-matched blood should be kept available. The largest group of patients will respond to the initial fluid bolus; however, as initial fluids are slowed, these patients begin to show deterioration in circulatory perfusion indices. In such cases, continued administration of fluid and blood is indicated. The response to blood administration should identify the patients who are still bleeding and require rapid surgical intervention. For those patients who show minimal or no response to initial fluid administration, the surgeon is faced with a dilemma. Either the initial diagnosis of hypovolemic shock is correct and rapid blood administration and early surgical intervention are needed to deal with exsanguinating hemorrhage, or the initial diagnosis of shock was incorrect and an alternative therapy should be undertaken. The central venous pressure is a useful tool in differentiating between these two groups of patients. Those with exsanguinating hemorrhage should have a low central venous pressure, and those with other causes of hypotension should have normal or high central venous pressure. For patients with transient response to initial fluid administration, or minimal or no response, with obvious active ongoing blood loss, consideration for transfusion is indicated. In these cases, fully crossmatched blood is preferable. Type-specific saline crossmatched blood can be provided by most blood banks within 10 minutes. Such blood is compatible within ABO and Rh blood types. Incompatibilities of minor antibodies may exist. Such blood is appropriate for patients with life-threatening shock situations. If type-specific blood is unavailable, type O blood is indicated for patients with exsanguinating hemorrhage. Cold blood is associated with a high incidence of myocardial arrhythmias and paradoxical hypotension. Blood should be warmed before and during massive transfusions.[39] Current controversies regarding transfusion and the risk of transmission of blood-borne disease (e.g., AIDS), as well as the physiologic effects of transfusion on the reticuloendothelial and immune systems, have raised many moral and ethical issues on the use of blood and blood products in the care of trauma patients.[40,41] To date, no satisfactory alternative has presented itself regarding the necessity of transfusion in the face of exsanguinating blood loss. Currently, a debate exists in the literature as to the optimal level of hemoglobin and hematocrit at which to maintain these patients without physiologic impairment.[42]

Length of Operation

As with all operative procedures, morbidity and mortality are directly related to the length of the procedure.

Though age, physical condition, injury type, and extent of operation represent important variables, the duration of an operative procedure in the injured geriatric patient should reflect only the time it takes to control the condition that threatens life.[43] Prolonged anesthesia linked with blood loss in a debilitated elderly patient predisposes to a state of shock that may become irreversible.[43] As with all trauma surgery, rapidity of control of blood loss, correction of life-threatening conditions, and meticulous attention to detail in as short a time interval as possible will lead to a better outcome and less risk of complications.

Indications for Noninterventional Therapy

Age by itself is never an absolute contraindicator for the surgical correction of a problem.[44] The moral and ethical issues of when to withhold operative therapy in the elderly trauma patient are complex and are based on several issues, including survivability, return of function, quality of life, and allocation of resources. Decisions regarding operative intervention as well as postoperative care optimally should include the patient, medical team, and family or responsible parties. The importance of these deliberations in such cases will serve several valuable functions: 1) ensure that the patient's self-determination is being respected, 2) seek to guarantee that medical intervention is serving the patient's best interest, 3) allow adequate resource allocation and equity considerations, and 4) reduce physician-nurse-family misunderstandings and discontent about resuscitation practices.[45]

For those patients who are competent, the decision for care is usually clear and easily arrived at, providing that the patient has received comprehensive information regarding the nature of the injury and a reasonable assessment of survivability. Unfortunately, in many cases, neurologic injury or the constellation of injuries has rendered the patient such that he is no longer an active participant. In these cases, the use of "Living Will" protocols for DNR (do not resuscitate) and the determination of brain death have been instituted in an effort to deal with these issues. Imbus and Zawacki[46] have utilized this approach in burn patients with such severe injuries that "survival is unprecedented." This protocol has been used with success in burn units and stands as a model in dealing with these issues, underscoring the importance with the elderly for preservation of dignity and quality of life and a concerted effort for self-determination.

POSTOPERATIVE CONSIDERATIONS
Intensive Care Unit

With the advent of more complex postoperative monitoring, the use of the intensive care unit (ICU) as a mode of therapy has gained widespread acceptance. The high technologic aspect of the care provided in this setting has allowed a much closer evaluation of the status of different systems on a minute-to-minute basis and has improved patient outcomes. This has not occurred without a price. Recent studies have reviewed the cost of outcomes of intensive care for ICU admissions of the elderly. In a 2-year study, conducted between 1977 and 1979, 44% of admissions to ICUs were for patients over 65 years of age and 21% were above 75 years.[47] Major interventions (i.e., intubation and mechanical ventilation) were more likely to occur in the elderly and occurred more frequently as the age increased. In medical ICUs the 1-year accumulated mortality for patients over 75 years was 44%. The average cost of hospitalization did not differ significantly in the survival groups of elderly at different age levels compared with nonsurvivors of the same age groups.[47]

ICU admissions for geriatric patients sustaining traumatic illness reflect an overall mortality of 15%. Oreskovich and Osler found that the Injury Severity Score (ISS) was not predictive of survival in the elderly injured. Major predictors were hypovolemic shock and central nervous system injury.[48]

In general, the ICU environment provides close observation of the elderly trauma patient in the postoperative period with monitoring and care of those systems at risk for acute change as a result of their traumatic illness, preexisting disease, or the consequence of operative intervention.

Pulmonary Complications

Respiratory complications are the most common and severe problems experienced in the postoperative geriatric patient. Risk factors that predispose these patients to respiratory complications include preexisting disease, emphysema, chronic obstructive pulmonary disease, history of heavy tobacco use, and the chronic effects of aging. In addition to ventilatory support, early mobilization, vigorous pulmonary toilet, chest physiotherapy with coughing and deep breathing, postural drainage, and the use of incentive spirometry all help reduce the risks of atelectasis and pneumonia. An early sputum culture will frequently give a clue to an impending pneumonia and may serve as a guide to future antibiotic therapy. Judicious use of narcotics, careful splinting with coughing, and nasogastric decompression all aid in reducing risks of pulmonary complications.

Mobility

There is no question that the early mobilization of the geriatric patient is of major importance in reducing the risk of pulmonary consequences in the postoperative period, including the risks of atelectasis, pneumonia, pulmonary embolus, and vascular problems. This is also beneficial in the reduction and prevention of skin breakdown and development of decubiti. Not enough can be said for the benefits of early mobilization in terms of the psychologic lift in the promotion of the "will to live" that is so important in this group. The fact that the patient is out of bed reinforces the idea that he or she is recovering and moving toward normal patterns of daily activity and improved mental status.

Nutrition

It can be said that of the major advances in surgical care in the past 20 years, the ability to provide adequate nutritional input to surgical patients has had a major effect in reducing morbidity and mortality. The provision of calories in the form of balanced substrates — including carbohydrates, proteins, lipids, vitamins, and trace elements — has resulted in an overall reduction of mortality and complications in the geriatric trauma patient. Of major importance following the initial period of stress in the postoperative patient is the determination of increased energy requirements. Increased energy expenditure is accompanied by humoral changes that serve both as mediators of the stress response and, in part, control the flow of energy and protein substrate to preserve effective circulating volume, critical organ function, and wound repair.[50] Whether or not nutrition is given enterally, peripherally, or in the form of central venous total parenteral nutrition will depend on the condition of the patient, ability to feed, severity of injury, and previous nutritional status. The consideration of a nutritional assessment consult can be of major benefit early in the patient's postoperative course for calculation of energy requirements and determination of the patient's overall nutritional status.[54]

Medications

The existence of concomitant medical illness affecting multiple organ systems in the aged makes the likelihood of medication usage high in the geriatric population. The activity of a drug in the body, whether therapeutic or toxic, depends on the dose, its frequency of administration, route of absorption, volume in which the drug is distributed, rate of metabolism, and route of excretion. The factors that determine the pharmacodynamics of a drug are also altered by the aging process. As people age, the proportion of body fat increases and lean body mass and total body water decrease. These changes may alter the distribution of a drug. Changes in perfusion as well as metabolic effects of aging on the liver and kidney may have profound effects on the breakdown and excretion of pharmacologic agents. Trauma, the stress response, shock, blood loss, and hypoxia may tend to potentiate the effect of any given drug. The careful elicitation of a medication history, especially by reliable friends and close relatives, may go a long way toward obtaining a complete drug history and preventing possible complications. It is important to carefully monitor drug usage in the perioperative period by clinical observations for toxic effects by plasma levels when possible and by ECG changes when appropriate.[51]

OUTCOMES
Return to Functional Levels

Studies concerning a return to functional levels as a result of trauma care in the elderly are controversial and varied. A 1984 study of injured elderly, 96% of whom were independent in their activities of daily living at the time of injury, revealed that following discharge only 7% of patients were independent at 1 year following injury and 72% required maintenance in a facility with full nursing care.[48] This is in contrast to DeMaria's review of a similarly injured elderly population in which 89% returned home by 1 year and 57% returned to independent living, at their preinjury functional level.[52] It is likely that the differences in these studies represent variables of individual patient populations, types of injury sustained, and modes of therapy instituted. It would seem, however, that significant numbers of elderly survivors of traumatic injury sustain long-term impairment as a result of their injuries and require the benefits of health care maintenance, far exceeding that needed for their younger, healthier counterparts.

Predictors of Outcome

Very little has been written to date regarding those markers or indices that can be used to determine outcome expectations of the traumatized elderly. The recent development of trauma scoring systems has added little toward determining those individuals who are likely not to survive. A national conference designed to evaluate the usefulness of various measures of severity of injury emphasizes the limitation of these indices when applied to the elderly, and this has been confirmed by others.[48,49,53] Osler utilized regression analysis to examine a data set comparing elderly and young trauma victims to determine the relative importance of several variables in predicting ultimate mortality.[49] Trauma score (TS), injury severity score (ISS), shock, Glasgow coma scale (GCS), age, ethnicity, and sex were examined. Shock and GCS were found to correlate strongly for demise in the geriatric population while ISS and TS were found to correlate in the younger control group. Thus, the physiologic response to injury (shock and GCS) seems predictive in the elderly while the extent of injury (ISS) is of greater importance in the young. Finally, markers of survival may be those aspects of previous medical illness. Though no specific studies have correlated survival with a history of preexisting diseases, one cannot help but believe that there exists a direct relationship between major preexisting medical illness and the likelihood of complications and risk for mortality with associated major trauma. Other predictors of outcome are likely to be the type and severity of trauma sustained, major neurologic injury, multiple system injury, presence of shock, respiratory compromise, and injury-promoting sepsis. All are likely to increase the risk for mortality in the elderly, as they do in all age groups of trauma patients.

REFERENCES

1. National Safety Council: Accident facts, Chicago, 1981, National Safety Council.
2. Snipes GA: Accidents in the elderly, Am Fam Physician 26:117–122, 1982.
3. Waller JA: Injury in the aged: clinical and epidemiological complications, NY State J Med 74:2200–2208, 1974.
4. Hogue CC: Injury in late life. I. Epidemiology, J Am Geriatr Soc 30:183–190, 1982.
5. Tinetti ME and Speachley M: Current concepts—geriatrics: prevention of falls among the elderly, N Engl J Med 320:1055, 1989.
6. Perry BC: Falls among the elderly: a review of the methods and conclusions of epidemiologic studies, J Am Geriatr Soc 30:367–371, 1982.
7. Chipman C and Sarant G: Falls and their consequences. II. In Schwartz GR, Bosker G, Grigsby JW, editors: Geriatric emergencies, Bowie, Md, 1984, RJ Brady Co.
8. Rubenstein LZ: Falls in the elderly: a clinical approach, West J Med 138:272–275, 1983.
9. National Safety Council: Accident facts, Chicago, 1983, National Safety Council.
10. Laur AR: Age and sex in relationship to accidents, Traffic Safety Res Rev 3:21, 1959.
11. McFarland RA, June GS, and Welford AT: On the driving of automobiles by older people, J Gerontol 19:190–197, 1964.
12. Waller JA and Goo JT: Highway crash and citation patterns and chronic medical conditions, J Safety Res 1:13, 1969.
13. Baker SP and Spitz WU: Age effects and autopsy evidence of disease in fatally injured drivers, JAMA 214:1079–1088, 1970.
14. Haddon W et al: A controlled investigation of the characteristics of adult pedestrians fatally injured by motor vehicles in Manhattan, J Chronic Dis 14:655–678, 1961.
15. Gerber SR: Cuyahoga court coroner's statistical reports, 1960–1970, Cleveland, Ohio.
16. Sklar DR, Demarest GB, and Osler TM: Increased pedestrian mortality among the elderly. (Manuscript submitted for publication.)
17. Barancik JI and Shapiro MA: Pittsburgh burn study, Pittsburgh and Allegheny City, Pennsylvania Environmental Health Program, Graduate School of Public Health, University of Pittsburgh, May 1972.
18. Harris R: Cardiovascular diseases in the elderly, Med Clin North Am 67:379–394, 1983.
19. Spencer H: Osteoporosis: goals of therapy, Hosp Pract 17:131–148, 1982.
20. Brocklehurst JC et al: Fracture of the femur in old age: a two-century study of associated clinical factors and the cause of the fall, Age Ageing 7:7–15, 1978.
21. Bradstetter RD and Kazemi H: Aging and respiratory system, Med Clin North Am 67:419–429, 1983.
22. Tillotson JR and Lerner AM: Pneumonias caused by Gram-negative bacilli, Medicine 45:65–76, 1966.
23. Reed LC and Eckert C: Enteral and parenteral nutritional support. In Handbook of geriatric emergency care, Baltimore, 1984, University Park Press.
24. Young EA: Nutrition, aging, and the aged, Med Clin North Am 67:295–313, 1983.
25. Mitchell CO and Lipschitz DA: Detection of protein-calorie malnutrition in the elderly, Am J Clin Nutr 35:398–406, 1982.
26. Chandra RK: Rosette-forming T lymphocytes and cell mediated immunity in malnutrition, Br Med J 3:608–609, 1974.
27. Gersovitz M et al: Assessment of the adequency of the current recommended dietary allowance for the dietary protein in elderly men and women, Am J Clin Nutr 35:6–14, 1982.
28. Munro HN: Nutritional requirements in the elderly, Hosp Pract 17:143–154, 1982.
29. Berk SL and Smith JK: Infectious disease in the elderly, Med Clin North Am 67:272–292, 1983.
30. Weksler ME: Senescence of the immune system, Med Clin North Am 67:263–272, 1983.
31. Cloward RB: Acute cervical spine injuries, Clin Symp 32:2–32, 1980.
32. Kirkpatrick JB and Pearson J: Fatal cerebral injury in the elderly, J Am Geriatr Soc 25:489–497, 1978.
33. Trunkey DD: Abdominal trauma in therapy in trauma, Burlington, Ontario, 1984–1985, BC Decker Inc.
34. Galbraith TA et al: The role of peritoneal lavage in the management of stab wounds of the abdomen, Am J Surg 140:60–64, 1980.
35. Dobyns JH and Linscheid ZL: Fractures and dislocations of the wrist. In Rockwald CA and Green DP, editors: Fractures, Philadelphia, 1975, JB Lippincott Co.
36. Devas M: Orthopedics. In Steinberg FU, editor: Care of the geriatric patient, ed 6, 1983, The CV Mosby Co.
37. Laskin RS, Gruber MA, and Zimmerman AJ: Intertrochanteric fractures of the hip in the elderly, Clin Orthop 141:188–195, 1979.
38. Tousaint GPM, Burgess JH, and Hampson LG: Central venous pressure and pulmonary wedge pressure in cited surgical illness: a comparison, Arch Surg 109:265–269, 1974.
39. American College of Surgeons: Shock. In Advanced trauma life support course instructor's manual, pp 170–191, 1984.
40. Aach RD and Kahn RA: Post-transfusion hepatitis: current perspectives, Ann Intern Med 92:539–546, 1980.
41. Feorino PM et al: Transfusion associated acquired immunodeficiency syndrome: incidence for persistent infection in blood donors, N Engl J Med 312:1293–1296, 1985.
42. Messmer K: Hemodilution, Surg Clin North Am 55:659–677, 1975.
43. Glenn F: Pre- and postoperative management of the elderly surgical patient, J Am Geriatr Soc 9:385–393, 1973.
44. Lichtenstein MJ and Billings FT: The management of perioperative medical problems in the aged. In Adkins RB and Scott HW, editors: Surgical care for the elderly, Baltimore, 1988, Williams & Wilkins Co.
45. President's Commission for Study of Ethical Problems in Medicine and Biomedical and Behavioral Research: deciding to forego sustaining treatment, Washington, DC, 1983, US Government Printing Office.
46. Imbus SH and Zawacki BE: Autonomy for burned patients when survival is unprecedented, N Engl J Med 297:308–311, 1977.
47. Campion EW et al: Medical intensive care for the elderly: a study of current use, costs and outcomes, JAMA 246:2052–2056, 1981.
48. Oreskovich MR et al: Geriatric trauma injury patterns and outcome, J Trauma 24:565–572, 1984.
49. Osler RM et al: Trauma in the elderly: four years experience. (Manuscript submitted for publication.)
50. Berarli L: Geriatric medicine, Med Clin North Am 1967:315–322, 1982.
51. Wilmore DW et al: Catecholamines: mediator of the hypermetabolic response to thermal injury, Ann Surg 178:180–653, 1974.
52. DeMaria EJ et al: Aggressive trauma care benefits of the elderly. Paper presented at meeting of the American Association for the Surgery of Trauma, Honolulu, Hawaii, September 1986.
53. Trunkey DD et al: Panel: current status of trauma severity indices, J Trauma 23:185–201, 1983.
54. Bone R: Providing nutritional support for critically ill patients, J Crit Ill 3:3, 1989.

Oncologic Emergencies in the Elderly

David M. Igdaloff, M.D.

SCOPE OF THE PROBLEM

Cancer is a disease with a particular impact on the elderly. At least 50% of all new cases of cancer (excluding nonmelanoma skin cancer) occur in people over 65 years of age. The reasons for this are not entirely known but probably relate to 1) the cumulative effects of random or environmentally induced genetic mutations, 2) the latency of possible viral inducers, 3) the temporal effect of tumor promoters following tumor initiators, 4) decreased immune surveillance with aging, and 5) changes in hormonal milieu with aging.

Whatever the mechanism, the impact of oncologic disease on health care for the elderly is significant and expected to grow. People over the age of 65 currently represent only 11% of the population. All cancer deaths occur in 58% of this same elderly population. By the year 2030, 18% of the population will be over age 65. Without a change in the current incidence and mortality of neoplasia, cancer in the elderly will have a major effect on the utilization and cost of health care resources.

While oncologic emergencies are not unique to elderly patients, peculiarities of the "aged host" have implications on presentation, recognition, and intervention. Decreased physiologic function with age decreases tolerance for small perturbations from baseline function. In addition, there is the potential for greater toxicity from treatment. Hearing and memory loss impede patients' understanding of their disease and its treatment. Also, there may be more difficulty expressing physical symptoms or emotional concerns. Coexistent illnesses more often complicate neoplastic disease in the geriatric patient. Psychosocial considerations particularly with relation to functional ability and requirements for care play an important role.

Patients may present with emergencies in three major contexts:

1. *Presentation of new cancer.* It is not at all unusual for previously undiagnosed cancer to present as an emer-

gency. This may be hemoptysis from lung cancer, bowel obstruction, or gastrointestinal (GI) bleeding from abdominal malignancy, mental status changes from metabolic derangement or anemia, or pathologic bone fracture. Due to the protean nature of malignant disease, virtually no organ system or symptoms complex is excluded when considering oncologic emergencies, and neoplasm must be considered in the differential diagnosis of multitudinous acute disorders.

2. *Complication of known cancer.* Patients with previously diagnosed cancer that may or may not have been treated may present emergently with complications related to tumor progression or metastases. In addition to the above-mentioned entities, this category often includes neurologic complications including seizure, altered level of consciousness, or focal neurologic deficit, as well as new or uncontrolled pain syndrome.

3. *Complication of treatment.* Effective therapy is available for many malignancies, and even advanced malignancies may be eradicated or at least palliated with currently available therapies. Unfortunately, these are often accompanied by toxicities that may mandate emergency intervention. The most significant entity in this category is infection secondary to neutropenia. Disturbances in GI mobility are another important group of disorders in this category.

Overview of Categories

Patients with either undiagnosed or previously diagnosed cancer, undergoing or not undergoing therapy, present emergently with problems related to one of the following major categories:

1. Functional impairment secondary to structural dysfunction
2. Metabolic and endocrine abnormalities
3. Hematologic abnormalities
4. Infection

Ethical Considerations

Before initiating treatment for oncologic emergencies, several factors need to be considered. Unfortunately, many elderly patients will die from cancer. In deciding whether to intervene in the natural history of the disease, the physician should consider what the natural history of the disease is, whether the patient has had prior treatment or not, the general condition of the patient, and the potential for cure or palliation. In patients with previously diagnosed cancer, the issues of intervention and life prolongation will often have already been dealt with by the individual and his or her family. Sometimes, only measures of comfort should be offered rather than specific medical intervention. In some localities, paramedical personnel may be obligated to initiate resuscita-

tive measures in patients with terminal malignancies who are being transported to acute care facilities. The attending emergency physician may be required to withdraw life support that has already been instituted. Family members, primary caregivers, and "living wills," if available, may aid in making such decisions.

SPECIFIC DISORDERS: FUNCTIONAL IMPAIRMENT SECONDARY TO STRUCTURAL DYSFUNCTION

Neurologic Dysfunction

Neoplasms involve the nervous system by direct extension, compression, metastases, metabolic effects, or by remote (paraneoplastic) effects. In 15 to 20% of patients with malignancy, a nervous system disorder will occur in the course of their illness. These disorders often present acutely and represent a significant number of cancer-related hospitalizations.[1]

Spinal Cord Compression

Spinal cord compression usually occurs as a late manifestation of malignancies that metastasize to bone, especially cancers of the breast, prostate, lung, and kidney. It is also seen in multiple myeloma and can be seen in tumors involving the prevertebral space, especially lymphomas. In the latter two neoplasms, spinal cord compression may, on occasion, be an initial manifestation of the disease. About 5% of patients with systemic cancer have spinal cord compression at autopsy.

Because of the anatomy of the vertebral column, clinical compression of the spinal cord is seen most frequently in the thoracic spine (about two thirds of the cases) with lumbar and cervical spine involvement less often. Pain is almost invariably present. Patients complain of central or radicular back pain that is aggravated by standing, recumbency, coughing, and sneezing. Sensory changes, including numbness or paresthesias, are commonly detected with motor weakness a later manifestation. Loss of rectal and bladder sphincter control is a late sign, except when there is cauda equina involvement, which is usually associated with perineal anesthesia. Early recognition of spinal cord compression is mandatory, because recovery of neurologic function is inversely related to the degree of impairment at the time of treatment.

Patients will often have percussion tenderness along the spine in the area of involvement. Neurologic deficits will be elicited, and pain may be exacerbated with neck flexion or straight leg raising. Plain x-rays of the spine are abnormal in 60 to 80% of patients. All patients suspected of having spinal cord compression should undergo emergency myelography to determine both the proximal and distal extent of tumor mass as well as other possible lesions. If a complete block is present, cervical or cisternal punctures are required to delineate the upper extent of the mass. Computerized tomography (CT) scanning with metrizamide may be helpful as an adjunct to myelography or in those cases in which it cannot be performed.

Treatment decisions are based on type of tumor, level of spinal cord involvement, rapidity of onset, clinical experience, and prior therapy. Immediate administration of dexamethasone (10 mg, then 4 mg every 4 hours) is usually instituted and may reduce peritumoral edema and offer temporary improvement in neurologic function prior to definitive treatment. Radiation therapy is most often utilized. Laminectomy will decompress the spinal cord and nerve roots, but it is often impossible to adequately remove the majority of the tumor, and postoperative radiation therapy should be administered. Systemic chemotherapy or hormone therapy should be used additionally in responsive tumors. Patients with autonomic dysfunction or paraplegia rarely improve after any treatment modality.

Intracranial Mass

Brain metastases may be the initial manifestation of an underlying malignancy, especially in patients with lung cancer. They may also be the first sign of recurrence following initial local or systemic treatment. They occur most frequently in relation to cancers of the lung, breast, and kidney and in sarcomas and malignant melanomas. Associated symptoms range from changes in personality or altered mentation to focal neurologic deficits and seizures. Headache may be absent but, when present, is often nocturnal and unrelenting. Protracted vomiting may be a prominent feature in some patients, especially those with posterior fossa involvement and/or an obstructive hydrocephalus, and may lead to exhaustive gastrointestinal investigations. Patients may present with a strokelike syndrome when there has been an acute hemorrhage into an occult metastasis.

Neurologic evaluation will reveal focal deficits, alterations in mental status, and possible papilledema. CT scan is the immediate procedure of choice. Administration of dexamethasone (10 mg immediately followed by 4 mg every 4 hours) and possibly mannitol if herniation is imminent is indicated prior to definitive therapy, which usually involves radiotherapy, although surgery may have a role in solitary metastases, obstructive hydrocephalus, and mass lesions of uncertain etiology. If the CT scan is negative, other causes for the neurologic changes must be considered.

Superior Vena Cava Syndrome[2-4]

Obstruction of the superior vena cava (SVC) is most often secondary to malignant neoplasms arising in or invading the mediastinum. The tumors most often responsible are bronchogenic carcinomas of the lung, accounting for 85%

NEUROLOGIC CHANGES IN CANCER PATIENTS

Metabolic
  Hypercalcemia
  Hyponatremia
  Hyperviscosity
  Uremia
  Hypoglycemia
  Hepatic failure
  Hypoxemia
  Anemia
  Polycythemia

Toxic
  Septicemia
  Drugs (steroids, narcotics, sedatives, metoclopramide, Indocin, etc.)
  Radiation

Meningitis
  Infectious
  Carcinomatous

Vascular
  Embolic (nonbacterial thrombotic endocarditis)
  Superior vena cava syndrome
  Hemorrhage from thrombocytopenia
  Disseminated intravascular coagulation

Other
  Opportunistic infection
  Paraneoplastic (multifocal leukoencephalopathy, etc.)

---

of cases, with lymphomas representing 10% of cases. The SVC syndrome is often the initial manifestation of disease. The vena cava is a soft-walled vessel and compression by tumor often remains clinically silent until critical or complete stenosis occurs. Intracaval thrombosis occurs in up to 50% of cases. The clinical presentation is often related to the rapidity of onset and the time for collateral vessels to develop. Venous return from the head, neck, thorax, and upper extremities is impaired leading to facial, arm, and tracheal edema. One may see neck and thoracic vein distention. There may be tachypnea and cyanosis. Vocal cord paralysis and Horner's syndrome may be associated findings. Eventually, altered levels of consciousness and focal neurologic deficits may develop secondary to brain edema and low cardiac output.

The clinical syndrome is usually easily recognized. Chest roentgenography will often demonstrate a right superior mediastinal mass. Contrast venography will demonstrate obstruction or thrombosis in the vena cava, but nuclear venography is generally as useful but with less potential morbidity.

Until recently, due to fears of hemorrhage, respiratory obstruction, and irreversible neurologic damage, it had been felt that diagnostic maneuvers carried a high risk in SVC obstruction, and that emergent or semiurgent radiation therapy should be administered prior to obtaining an histologic diagnosis. Several large published series have now demonstrated this not to be the case, and since many of the underlying tumors (small cell lung cancer, lymphoma) have specific therapies that are potentially curative, it is recommended that efforts should be made to make a timely tissue diagnosis prior to the institution of definitive therapy in most cases, including mediastinoscopy or thoracotomy if necessary. Ancillary measures such as diuretics, oxygen, phlebotomy, and elevation of the head of the bed may be effective in ameliorating symptoms in the interim.

Tracheal Obstruction

Obstruction of the trachea is a rare oncologic emergency that is part of the differential diagnosis of SVC syndrome. Lateral films of the chest and/or neck will allow assessment of the level and degree of tracheal obstruction. Immediate low tracheostomy may rarely be necessary in a severe case.

Hemoptysis

Minor hemoptysis may be an early sign of undiagnosed bronchogenic carcinoma. Massive hemoptysis is often a complication of advanced disease. Bronchoscopy is usually the diagnostic intervention of choice. If the bleeding can be lateralized, the patient should be kept with that side down to prevent aspiration of blood into the opposite lung. Emergency thoracotomy may be necessary, although for many patients massive hemoptysis is a terminal event.

Malignant Effusion
Pleural

Pleural effusion is one of the more common symptomatic manifestations of cancer. It often complicates lung cancer, breast cancer, lymphoma, as well as other tumor types and may be an initial manifestation of disease or the first evidence of disease recurrence. Excessive fluid accumulation may be related to pleural tumor implants, blockage of pleural lymphatics, or obstruction of lymph flow by mediastinal tumor. Effusion may occur concomitantly with SVC syndrome, pericarditis, or ascites.

Patients usually present with dyspnea. Pain is less common. Pleural effusion is detected by percussion and auscultation of the chest and confirmed radiographically. Lateral decubitus films confirm free-flowing fluid. Diagnostic and therapeutic thoracentesis should be performed. When dealing with malignant effusions, 1,000 to 2,000 ml can usually be safely removed. The fluid is usually exudative although cytology is positive in only 70% of cases. Pleural biopsy may be necessary. Long-term control may be achieved with effective systemic therapy or may require tube thoracostomy and injection of sclerosing agents such as tetracycline.

Pericardial

Although pericardial involvement by a neoplasm is rare and remains clinically silent in up to two thirds of those affected, recognition of malignant tamponade is an often missed but treatable oncologic emergency.[5] A high index of suspicion must prevail when considering pericardial abnormalities in the cancer patient. Lung cancer, breast cancer, and hematologic malignancies are the predominant causes. In newly presenting cases of pericardial tamponade, malignancy is the single most common underlying cause. Lymphatic and venous obstruction by a tumor as well as exudation from serosal implants result in excessive accumulation of pericardial fluid. The consequences are related to the rate of accumulation and the compliance of the pericardial cavity, as well as the myocardial mass and patient's blood volume. When hemodynamically significant, impaired diastolic filling of the heart occurs with compensatory tachycardia and increased peripheral vascular resistance. Subsequently, shock, cardiac arrest, and death occur without intervention.

Patients with symptomatic pericardial effusions complain of dyspnea, cough, and chest pain that may be relieved by leaning forward, orthopnea, and weakness. Alterations in consciousness and seizures may occur. On physical exam, one may detect tachycardia, jugular venous distention, pleural effusion, hepatomegaly, peripheral edema, and cyanosis. "Classic" findings of pulsus paradoxus, Kussmaul's sign, and pericardial rub are often absent. Echocardiography is the most useful test confirming the presence of a pericardial effusion. Chest roentgenograms and electrocardiograms are usually abnormal but nonspecific. Low voltage on electrocardiogram (ECG) is most often seen, with electrical alternans seen occasionally. CT scanning and right heart catheterization are additional useful tests in selected patients.

Acute pericardial tamponade is treated by withdrawal of fluid, most rapidly accomplished by pericardiocentesis. Intravenous fluid support, oxygen, and administration of sympathomimetic agents (particularly isoproterenol) can be used as temporizing measures. Positive pressure ventilation is contraindicated due to further impairment of venous return to the heart. Pericardiocentesis is safest when performed in a controlled environment (e.g., cardiac catheterization lab) with fluoroscopic and electrocardiographic guidance following confirmation of effusion by echocardiography. Fluid may be bloody in up to half of cases and should always be sent for cytology. Long-term management of pericardial effusions must be individualized and include intrapericardial sclerotherapy, surgical pericardiotomy, radiation therapy, and systemic chemotherapy.

Postirradiation pericarditis must be considered in the differential diagnosis of pericardial disease in the previously irradiated cancer patient. This may be an acute, inflammatory, effusive pericarditis occurring within months of radiotherapy that often resolves spontaneously or a chronic effusive-constrictive pericarditis that may occur up to 20 years after treatment.

Ascites

Accumulation of ascitic fluid most often complicates ovarian cancer but can be seen in carcinomas of the colon, pancreas, and stomach, as well as lymphoma, mesothelioma, and rarely other tumors. Patients may present with severe discomfort, anorexia, early satiety, and difficult respiration. Cytologic examination of the fluid is the basis of diagnosis. Peritoneoscopy may be necessary.

Large amounts of fluid can be removed by paracentesis when malignancy is the underlying cause of the ascites. One must be more cautious when fluid is secondary to liver disease, heart failure, or hypoalbuminemia.

Disturbances of Bowel Motility

Nausea/Vomiting

Nausea and vomiting is a common complaint of cancer patients and has numerous etiologies. It may be secondary to mechanical factors (see below) or hepatic infiltration by metastases. It may be seen with a number of metabolic abnormalities, including antineoplastic agents or analgesics. It may complicate radiation therapy of the abdomen. It may be a sign of increased intracranial pressure. A thorough history, physical exam, laboratory evaluation, and radiographs are necessary to differentiate among the various causes. Treatment should be directed by the underlying etiology.

Bowel Obstruction/Perforation

Obstruction of the gastrointestinal tract may be a presenting sign of primary bowel cancer or a manifestation of its recurrence. It may also be seen with other abdominal malignancies, especially ovarian cancer and, less often, other gynecologic, gastrointestinal, or urinary tumors. Nonmalignant causes may also account for bowel obstruction in the cancer patient. These include adhesions from previous surgery or complications of prior radiation.

Pain, nausea, vomiting, and obstipation are hallmarks of bowel obstruction. Occlusion of the bowel distal to a competent ileocecal valve can quickly lead to a closed-loop obstruction with subsequent perforation. Progressive pain and abdominal distention will be seen.

Supine and upright views of the abdomen should be obtained. If the patient is too ill for an upright film, a left lateral decubitus should be obtained. These will demonstrate air-fluid levels and dilated loops of bowel except with very proximal obstructions. Cecal dilatation greater than 12 to 14 cm should be considered a surgical emergency because of the risk of perforation. Free air may be seen on upright or decubitus films if perforation has already occurred.

Nasogastric intubation should be performed in the patient with bowel obstruction, and intravenous fluid and electrolyte administered. In cases of perforation, antibiotics to cover gram-negative enteric organisms and anaerobes should be instituted in addition. Some cases of obstruction will resolve with conservative therapy, while surgery may be necessary immediately or eventually in others.

Diarrhea/Constipation

Diarrhea in the cancer patient is most often a complication of therapy, either radiation or chemotherapy. Less often, it may be secondary to pseudomembranous colitis secondary to *Clostridium difficile* or humoral substances released by certain tumors. The history should help to differentiate among these etiologies.

In severe cases, the patient may exhibit signs of dehydration and electrolyte abnormalities may occur. Examination of the stool for white blood cells and *C. difficile* toxin may be helpful. Treatment is supportive with the use of antidiarrheals and replacement of fluid and electrolytes. Oral vancomycin or oral parenteral Flagyl can be used for pseudomembranous colitis.

Constipation, often already a problem in the elderly, may be exacerbated in the cancer patient by drugs and diminished food and fluid intake. It leads to discomfort as well as anxiety and may initiate an emergency room visit. It is important to rule out bowel obstruction, which can usually be done with the history, physical exam, and plain and upright films of the abdomen. The most common pharmacologic agents implicated in decreased bowel motility are the narcotic analgesics and the vinca alkaloids used in chemotherapy.

Prevention is the best treatment by ensuring adequate fluid intake and the use of stool softeners and laxatives such as magnesium hydroxide or senna preparations. Refractory cases may benefit from oral magnesium citrate or lactulose, enemas, or manual disimpaction when necessary. In the emergency room setting, reassurance and directions for a regular laxative program may be sufficient after acute obstruction has been ruled out.

Stomatitis/Esophagitis

Inflammation of the mucous membranes of the oral cavity and esophagus are usually temporary but often debilitating side effects of either chemotherapy or radiation therapy. Pain and dysphagia may be severe and may interfere with nutrition and hydration. Superinfection with *Candida* or herpes should be ruled out in susceptible patients.

Symptomatic treatment includes topical anesthetics or sucralfate. A solution containing equal parts of Mylanta, Viscous Xylocaine, and Benadryl Elixir is a soothing preparation that can be expectorated or swallowed. Parenteral hydration or nutrition may be required in severe cases. Acyclovir or anticandidal drugs should be added empirically in susceptible patients pending laboratory confirmation.

Obstructive Uropathy

Urinary tract obstruction may result from mechanical interference to the ureters or bladder outlet or from functional interference related to neurologic problems or pharmacologic interventions. The former may be related to primary or metastatic tumors to the retroperitoneum or pelvis. These most often include lymphoma, GI malignancies, lung cancer, bladder and prostate tumors, and gynecologic cancers. Neurologic problems may be secondary to spinal cord compression or pelvic nerve invasion. Offending drugs include narcotics, sedatives, and tricyclic antidepressants.

Although the onset of urinary tract obstruction may be insidious, with the diagnosis only established by laboratory or radiologic procedures, the patient may present with signs and symptoms of renal failure[6] (see below), pelvic or flank pain or mass, anuria, urinary incontinence, hematuria, or urinary tract infection.

Immediate intervention includes urethral catheterization to assess bladder residual volume in patients suspected of outlet obstruction or neurogenic bladder. Suprapubic cystostomy may rarely be necessary. Rapid decompression of the bladder should be performed cautiously because of the risk of bladder hemorrhage. Attention should be directed at correcting fluid and electrolyte abnormalities. Definitive treatment is dictated by the type and site of obstruction as determined with ultrasonography, intravenous and retrograde pyelography, and CT scanning.

Bone Pain and Pathologic Fracture[7]

Though rarely life threatening, primary or metastatic bone tumors contribute greatly to the morbidity of cancer patients by causing pain, immobility, and pathologic fracture. (Neurologic symptoms are discussed under spinal cord compression.) The vast majority of metastatic bone tumors are secondary to breast, lung, or prostate cancer and are usually identified early in the course of the illness. On the other hand, bone involvement in multiple myeloma may be a presenting complaint and manifest as an acute pathologic fracture.

Pain is the hallmark of cancer involving the skeleton. It is often localized and worse at night. Percussion tenderness at the site of involvement can often be elicited. Fracture occurs with advancing disease, most often in the weight-bearing bones of the femur, pelvis, and spine, but any bone can be affected. Hypercalcemia may coexist or be exacerbated by subsequent immobilization.

Radiographic examination will usually show lytic or mixed lytic and blastic changes once fracture has occurred. However, up to 50% bone loss must occur before plain radiographic changes are evident. Bone scanning with technetium-99m pyrophosphate is a highly sensitive imaging modality that should be employed early to identify skeletal involvement in those patients with malignancies at risk of metastasizing to bone. Alkaline phosphatase (and acid phosphatase in cases of prostatic cancer) is often elevated. Myeloma rarely causes bone scan abnormalities due to the pure lytic nature of the tumor (unless pathologic fracture has occurred). Compression fractures in the osteopenic spine of the elderly may be the first manifestation of myeloma and difficult to diagnose. One should look for coexistent anemia, renal failure, and protein abnormalities and carry a high index of suspicion. A needle or even an open biopsy may be necessary in difficult cases.

Once fracture occurs, surgical intervention is often necessary to maintain function and control pain unless the expected survival is very short (less than 3 months).[7] Expert orthopedic consultation should be obtained. Localized radiotherapy or systemic chemotherapy or hormone therapy will be useful for many patients following surgical fixation.

METABOLIC AND ENDOCRINE ABNORMALITIES[8,9]

Hypercalcemia

Hypercalcemia is the most common metabolic abnormality complicating malignancy, occurring in 10% of all cancer patients.[8,9] Furthermore, in hospitalized patients, neoplasia is the leading cause of hypercalcemia, accounting for 30 to 50% of cases. It is seen in solid tumors with or without bone metastases and in certain hematologic malignancies.

Breast cancer metastatic to bone accounts for up to 50% of cases of malignant hypercalcemia and is usually a late manifestation of disease. Tumors with osteoblastic metastases, such as prostate cancer, are rarely associated with hypercalcemia. In 10 to 40% of cases of hypercalcemia, there is no evidence of bone metastases. Epidermoid carcinoma of the lung, head, neck, and esophagus and adenocarcinomas of the kidney and liver are usually responsible. In these cases, hypercalcemia is mediated by the systemic effect of one or more humoral mediators.

Hematologic malignancies complicated by hypercalcemia include multiple myeloma and certain lymphomas.

Multiple myeloma heads the list, with up to 50% of patients developing hypercalcemia some time in their course. It is not unusual to see it as one of the initial manifestations of the disease, often in association with bone pain. Hypercalcemia appears to result from the production of the osteoclast-activating factor that stimulates bone resorption.

The clinical manifestations of hypercalcemia are related not only to the level of the serum calcium but also to the rate of its development. Its effects are most often seen in the neuromuscular, renal, gastrointestinal, and cardiovascular systems. One most often sees alterations in mental status such as fatigue, lethargy, and apathy. There may also be agitation, anxiety, or psychotic behavior. Alteration in consciousness progressing to stupor and coma are late signs. Polyuria and polydipsia are related to secondary changes in renal concentrating ability. This often results in dehydration, which further aggravates the hypercalcemia. Nephrocalcinosis may be seen, but nephrolithiasis, commonly seen in primary hyperparathyroidism, is rarely seen. Anorexia, nausea, vomiting, and abdominal pain are early signs, with obstipation and ileus occurring late. Increased gastric acidity may account for associated peptic ulceration. Pancreatitis, often seen in primary hyperparathyroidism, is uncommon in hypercalcemia associated with malignancy. ECG changes may be seen. Moderate elevation in the calcium shortens the systolic time interval and QT interval. As the calcium level increases, there is widening of the T wave, coving of the ST-T wave segment, and prolongation of the QT and PR intervals. Digitalis toxicity is potentiated by elevated levels of serum calcium.

Malignant hypercalcemia is easily differentiated from primary hyperparathyroidism. The former usually has a rapid onset with high serum calcium levels (75% > 14 mg/dL). There may be bone metastases with an elevated alkaline phosphatase, a normal or elevated serum phosphate and bicarbonate level, and a lower chloride level. Renal calculi, ectopic calcification, peptic ulcer, and obtundation are uncommon. PTH is normal or low. Primary hyperparathyroidism, on the other hand, has a more indolent course. The serum calcium is greater than 14 mg/dL in only 25% of cases. The serum bicarbonate and phosphate are normal or decreased, and the serum chloride is usually high (> 102 mmol/L). Bone x-rays show subperiosteal erosions in the hands. Serum PTH is high normal or high.

The treatment of hypercalcemia must be individualized. Aggravating factors should be removed when possible. These include dehydration, immobilization, calcium ingestion, vitamins A and D, thiazide diuretics, and certain hormones used in the treatment of breast cancer. The hallmark of treatment of hypercalcemia is forced hydration of the patient with saline. Monitoring of the central venous pressure may be required. Lasix or ethacrynic acid can be added to promote calciuresis once the intravascular volume has been repleted. Careful monitoring of the serum electrolytes is mandatory. With this intervention, the majority of patients will become symptom free within 2 to 3 days. Other measures including steroids, prostaglandin inhibitors, plicamycin (mithramycin), calcitonin, oral phosphates, and recently intravenous diphosphonates, as well as treatment of the underlying malignancy, are often added for longer term control.

Hyponatremia

Decreased serum sodium as a result of inappropriate secretion of antidiuretic hormone is most often seen as a result of small cell lung cancer. It may be aggravated by diuretic therapy and can be seen with certain antineoplastic drugs (e.g., cyclophosphamide, vincristine) as well as with morphine.

Patients may be asymptomatic, but as the serum sodium drops below 120 to 125 mEq/L, mental impairment sets in, progressing to seizures and coma with levels below 115 mEq/L. The diagnosis is suggested by the finding of an inappropriately high urine osmolality or sodium in the face of a low serum osmolality and nonexpanded extracellular fluid volume.

Nearly all cases related to small cell lung cancer respond to antineoplastic therapy. Severe cases should be treated with hypertonic saline infusion, possibly with the addition of a loop diuretic. In milder cases, fluid restriction may be all that is necessary. In refractory or relapsed cases, demeclocycline may be effective. It acts by inhibiting ADH at the renal tubule. Lithium can also be used but is more toxic and difficult to monitor.

Tumor Lysis Syndrome

Patients at risk of tumor lysis syndrome have rapidly proliferating tumors that are sensitive to antineoplastic therapy. These include undifferentiated lymphomas, acute leukemia, and, less often, small cell undifferentiated carcinoma of the lung. Following initiation of therapy, there may be rapid cell kill with release of intracellular substances into the bloodstream, including uric acid, potassium, and phosphate. This may result in acute renal failure, cardiac arrhythmias, hypocalcemia, and neuromuscular disorders.

Allopurinol should be administered prophylactically to patients at risk. In addition, alkaline diuresis may increase the solubility of uric acid and ameliorate renal failure but may aggravate hypocalcemia and tetany. Hemodialysis should be instituted early and may be lifesaving.

Renal Failure[6]

Uremia in the oncologic patient may be related to urinary tract obstruction (see above). It may also be related to intravascular volume depletion, nephrotoxic drugs (cisplatin, methotrexate, mitomycin-C, etc.), radiation therapy, paraproteinemia, uric acid (tumor lysis syndrome), hypercalcemia, or, less often, direct invasion of the kidney by tumors (most often lymphoma and leukemia). Symptoms include nausea, vomiting, lethargy, coma, and seizures. Oliguria or anuria may be present with signs of fluid retention. Congestive heart failure may be precipitated or exacerbated. The diagnosis is confirmed by laboratory evaluation. Bladder catheterization and renal ultrasound should be performed to rule out obstruction.

HEMATOLOGIC ABNORMALITIES

Venous Thrombosis and Pulmonary Embolism

Close to one quarter of all deep vein thrombosis occurs in patients with malignancy. In some, thrombosis may predate the diagnosis of malignancy by weeks or months. It may also be seen as a complication of therapy, particularly hormonal therapy with estrogens, antiestrogens, and progesterones. Classic symptoms of leg pain, swelling, and positive Homan's sign are unreliable. Usually, confirmation by phlebography is required although other methods (impedance plethysmography, ^{131}I fibrinogen scanning) may be helpful depending on the experience of the individual institution.

Patients with pulmonary embolism usually have tachypnea, with or without chest pain. Hypoxemia may be detected on examination of the arterial blood gases. VQ scanning of the lung may be diagnostic, although some cases may require pulmonary angiography.

Treatment is with anticoagulants. Thrombolytic therapy may be indicated in severe cases but has more risks. Some patients may require interruption of the inferior vena cava for lower extremity phlebothrombosis if anticoagulation is not tolerated or contraindicated.

Hyperviscosity

Increased blood viscosity is most often seen with plasma cell dyscrasias and Waldenstrom's macroglobulinemia but may also be seen secondary to paraproteinemias associated with other hematologic and nonhematologic malignancies as well as the result of erythrocytosis, either primary (polycythemia rubra vera) or secondary (as can be seen with hypernephroma, hepatocellular carcinoma, and certain other tumors, hypoxemia, etc.). Symptoms are related to circulatory disturbances from increased resistance to blood flow, especially in the nervous system and cardiovascular system. Neurologic findings range from headaches and vertigo to somnolence, stupor, and coma. Focal neurologic deficits can occur as well as seizures. Deafness may occur and peripheral neuropathies and myelopathies can be seen.

Cardiac failure can be precipitated, especially in the elderly. Disorders of hemostasis may also occur.

Physical signs are most readily appreciated on funduscopic exam where a characteristic "link-sausage" appearance of retinal veins is seen. Hemorrhages and exudates may be noted as well as visual impairment. Patients with erythrocytosis may have a characteristic ruddy complexion. Lymphadenopathy or splenomegaly may be present depending on the underlying disorder. Hematocrit and whole blood and serum viscosity are easily measured in the laboratory.

Plasmapheresis is the immediate treatment of choice for increased serum viscosity, when symptomatic, until the treatment of the underlying disorder (if any) has taken effect. Erythrocytosis should be controlled with phlebotomy to keep the hematocrit under 45 to 50%.

Anemia

Reduction of red cell mass commonly accompanies malignancy. It may be related to the suppressive effects of chronic disease on the bone marrow or as a consequence of chemotherapy or radiation therapy. Hemorrhage chiefly from the gastrointestinal tract is less often a factor. Anemia causes fatigue and weakness and can exacerbate neurologic or cardiac symptoms. Generalized or mucosal pallor may be evident. Many patients will tolerate a hemoglobin of 8.0 to 8.5 g/dL but some will require 10 g/dL. Transfusion therapy should be administered as necessary. Use of erythropoietin to stimulate bone marrow production is a promising approach in some cases.

Thrombocytopenia

Decreased platelet count occurs with marrow replacement by tumor, decreased production secondary to chemotherapy or radiation therapy, or increased consumption as seen in disseminated intravascular coagulation, sepsis, or less commonly immune consumption. It may occasionally be related to hypersplenism related to tumor involvement of the spleen (lymphoma and leukemia) or increased portal venous pressure.

Patients may complain of epistaxis or gum bleeding. More severe gastrointestinal hemorrhage may occur, and intracranial hemorrhage may be fatal. Petechiae may be noted, particularly on the lower extremities, but the oral mucosa, conjunctivae, and retina should also be examined. The diagnosis is confirmed by determining the platelet count. Other coagulation studies should be performed as indicated. In the absence of clinical bleeding, a platelet count above 20,000/μL is usually not associated with serious hemorrhage. Some patients may tolerate a count as low as 5,000/μL.

Treatment depends on the underlying cause. When there is a defect in platelet production, platelet transfusion is indicated to keep the platelet count above 10,000 to 20,000/μL. Random donor platelets do not need to be crossmatched or even type-specific. Each unit will normally raise the platelet count by 5,000 to 10,000/μL. Some patients, particularly those who have received multiple transfusions, may be refractory to random donor platelets. In this case, single donor or even HLA-matched single donor collections may be used, if available. In some refractory patients, epsilon-aminocaproic acid, an inhibitor of fibrinolysis, given orally or intravenously may be a useful adjunct to prevent or help control bleeding. In consumptive thrombocytopenias, treatment depends on treatment of the underlying cause.

Neutropenia

Neutropenia may be secondary to antineoplastic chemotherapy or radiation therapy and less often to bone marrow replacement by malignant disease. The greater the degree and duration of neutropenia, the greater the likelihood of supervening infection. Septicemia is uncommon with a granulocyte count greater than 1,000/μL. This risk greatly increases with an absolute granulocyte count under 500/μL and abruptly again under 100/μL.

Temperature elevation is the most prominent sign of underlying infection, although it may be normal or subnormal, particularly in the elderly patient. One may see changes in mental status or deterioration of functional ability in the patient presenting with acute sepsis (see Chapter 22). In addition to fever, there may be tachypnea or hypotension. In the absence of granulocytes, signs of acute inflammation may be reduced or absent. The skin and mucous membranes should be carefully inspected. Funduscopic exam may reveal evidence of fungal, viral, or protozoal infection. Pulmonary findings may be absent even with acute pneumonia. Catheterization of the bladder and digital rectal exam should be avoided in neutropenic patients, although both sites must be considered as likely sources of infection. Thrombocytopenia and/or disseminated intravascular coagulation may complicate septicemia.

Blood cultures should be obtained in any patient suspected of acute sepsis. In addition, urine, sputum, if any, and any suspicious skin or mucosal sites should be cultured. Chest radiographs should be taken routinely. Emergency bronchoscopy with washings and biopsies may be indicated in immunosuppressed patients with pulmonary infiltrates. If diarrhea is present, stool should be examined for *C. difficile* toxin, which may be the causative agent in granulocytopenic patients even without prior antibiotic therapy.

Infections in the granulocytopenic patient who has not been receiving antibiotics are usually bacterial and often secondary to gram-negative organisms. Broad-spectrum antibiotics should be instituted as soon as cultures have been obtained. With rapid institution of antibiotic therapy, without waiting for identification of the organism, mortality can be greatly reduced. Empiric drug or drug combination therapy must be tailored to the usual sensitivities of pathogens most often isolated in individual institutions. In addition to gram-negative organisms, including *Pseudomonas,* the gram-positive organisms *Staphylococcus aureus* and *Staphylococcus epidermidis* are seen not infrequently. Adjustments can be made once culture results are known. However, in 40 to 60% of febrile neutropenic patients, cultures will be negative, although clinical improvement will be seen with broad-spectrum antibiotic coverage.

INFECTION

Infection is not only one of the major complications of malignant disease, responsible for over 50% of all cancer deaths, but is also the most serious complication of cancer treatment. Susceptibility to infection in oncologic patients is related to both destruction of natural barriers by tumor invasion as well as immunosuppression secondary to the underlying disease, cachexia, and antineoplastic therapy. Infection associated with undiagnosed cancer is most often secondary to bronchial obstruction or bowel perforation. Infection and the neutropenic patient is discussed above. Opportunistic infection is another special problem in cancer patients. Both viral (herpes simplex or zoster) and fungal (*Candida*) infections often complicate the course of malignant disease. Empiric therapy is often indicated pending laboratory confirmation in patients clinically suspected of having these disorders.

REFERENCES

1. Delaney P: Neurologic emergencies in cancer patients, South Med J 74(7):825, 1981.
2. Ahmann F: A reassessment of the clinical implications of the superior vena caval syndrome, J Clin Oncol 2(8):961, 1984.
3. Likich JJ and Goodman R: Superior vena cava syndrome: clinical management, JAMA 23(1):58, 1975.
4. Perez CA, Presant CA, and Van Amburg AL III: Management of superior vena cava syndrome, Semin Oncol 5(2):123, 1978.
5. Press OW and Livingston R: Management of malignant pericardial effusion and tamponade, JAMA 257(8):1088, 1987.
6. Garnick MB and Mayer RJ: Acute renal failure associated with neoplastic disease and its treatment, Semin Oncol 5(2):155, 1978.
7. Colyer RA: Surgical stabilization of pathologic neoplastic fractures, Curr Probl Cancer 10(3):121, 1986.
8. Ebie N, Ryan W, and Harris J: Metabolic emergencies in cancer medicine, Med Clin North Am 70(5):1151, 1986.
9. Bruetman D and Harris JE: Oncologic emergencies. Part 2: metabolic complications, J Crit Ill 3:83, 1989.

SUGGESTED READINGS

DeVita VT Jr, Hellman S, and Rosenberg S, editors: Cancer, principles and practice of oncology, Philadelphia, 1982, JB Lippincott Co.
Glover DJ and Glick JH: Managing oncologic emergencies involving structural dysfunction, CA 35(4):238, 1985.
Kalia S and Tintinalli J: Emergency evaluation of the cancer patient, Ann Emerg Med 13(9):723, 1984.

Gynecologic Disorders

Matthew Montgomery, M.D., and William Cook, M.D.

Women are the largest consumers of health care. As our population ages, more women are in their postmenopausal years. Most of them have one third of their lives yet to be lived. Gynecologic problems during this period include largely disabling symptoms of the vulva and vagina and malfunction, herniation, and malignancy of the pelvic organs and tissues. While a good deal of medical and public attention is directed toward the reproductive system from adolescence through the perimenopausal years when this system serves well-recognized functions, much less is known about "normal" function and less is "expected" from the system in the older woman.[1]

Emergency department (ED) physicians must intervene and manage these patients appropriately in a timely manner, using the available historical, physical, and clinical information while operating within the constraints of their setting. Furthermore, both patient and medical colleagues expect the ED physician to have "the manual dexterity and skills of a surgeon, the analytic and synthetic ability of an internist, the calm and patience of a psychiatrist, the playfulness of a pediatrician, and the public relations skills of an administrator."[2]

The present chapter focuses on the consequences of declining estrogen production in postmenopausal women and on common gynecologic disorders and their treatment.

PHYSIOLOGIC CHANGES WITH AGING

As a woman goes through and passes the menopause, a series of changes take place in her body, some of which are related to a hypoestrogenic state and others to the general aging process. These changes vary considerably between individuals. Predictable anatomic changes include reduced vascularization, decreased fat content, thinning epithelial surfaces, and loss of tissue elasticity and tone.

Vulva

Atrophy of the vulva involves losing subcutaneous fat, graying hair, and thinning skin. The vulva becomes less prominent, the labia minora may appear proportionally larger, and Bartholin's glands atrophy, resulting in less lubrication. Clinically, the vulva may be found to have become pruritic and a source of irritation. Puckering of the vulvar tissue and of the introitus may make penile intromission exquisitely painful. Deflection of the penis anteriorly by a rigid perineum may create pressure on the urethral meatus, causing urethritis, local inflammation, and dysuria.[3] These changes become more severe with increasing age but may be attenuated by hormonal replacement.

Vagina

Vaginal atrophy may be characterized by thinning, pale, and sometimes friable mucosa. Decreased elasticity and increased submucosal connective tissue result in the gradual shortening and narrowing of the vagina with loss of its usual rugosity. There is decreased vascularity, and the tissues are more susceptible to inflammation and ulceration. The mucosa produces less glycogen and the flora colonizing the premenopausal female are reduced. This results in a more alkaline environment that is less resistant to infection. Progressive weakening of the vaginal wall and supporting structures also occurs, the result of which is an increased incidence of pelvic relaxation, cystocele, rectocele, and uterine prolapse.

Uterus

Atrophy is the dominant event occurring in the postmenopausal uterus. The corpus becomes smaller in relation to the cervix; the portio vaginalis of the cervix no longer projects into the vagina and the external os becomes flush with the vaginal wall. Colposcopic examination reveals withdrawal of the squamocolumnar junction of the cervix into the endocervical canal and may cause stenosis of the os. The covering squamous epithelium becomes thin and easily traumatized. Speculum examination may cause slight bleeding, which must be distinguished from pathologic hemorrhage.

The postmenopausal uterus tends to be small and firm. The lining of the endometrium loses its glandular character and becomes fibrous and hyalinized. Leiomyomas tend to atrophy, although they may still present problems.

Ovaries

Ovarian function begins to slowly decline early in life (about age 25). The ultimate consequence of this decline is the involution of the ovary from a follicle-rich, cyclic secretor of estrogen and progesterone to a stroma-rich, noncyclic, low secretor of androgen. This is followed by thinning of the cortex and a relative increase in the thickness of the medulla. Other structural features of the "aged" ovary, such as obliterative arteriolar sclerosis and surface epithelium cysts, indicate that obvious involution is admixed with persisting ovarian activity.[4]

PATIENT EVALUATION

History

The postmenopausal patient may present with an array of complaints; the most common gynecologic symptoms include vaginal bleeding, urinary complaints, pruritus vulvae, and pelvic pain. To gain the patient's confidence may be the most difficult obstacle in the history taking. Elderly women may be embarrassed or unwilling to undergo pelvic examination. A significant number may be unable to give a useful history of their obstetric and gynecologic experience. It is helpful if a relative or a close friend of the patient is available, but often this is not possible.

Fortunately, many elderly patients are fully alert and possess excellent recall. In obtaining the gynecologic history, parity, last menstrual period, and any previous gynecologic problems, including surgeries, must be

elicited. Also, any medications currently being taken, as well as estrogen used at any time, must be identified. Since vaginal bleeding is one of the most common complaints, it is very important to know that the bleeding is indeed vaginal and not actually hematuria or hematochezia.

Vaginal discharge may be due to infection, malignancy, foreign bodies, or trauma. Therefore, inquiries should be made about its color, consistency, and the presence of blood. Pessaries and certain douche solutions may be irritating to the vaginal mucosa and should be thought of as possible etiologic factors. Bloody mucoid discharge occurring postmenopausally may be due to carcinoma of the endometrium or cervix.

If the patient complains of pruritus, the history of incontinence, sexual activity, and hygienic measures may all be important. Broad-spectrum antibiotics frequently cause candidal vaginitis, vaginal discharge, and pruritus, and their use should be determined. Many of these patients will have tried a variety of home cures for their complaints, sometimes worsening the symptoms.

The review of symptoms is frequently of aid in establishing a gynecologic diagnosis or in the elimination of bowel or urinary tract disease. The proximity of bladder, uterus, and rectosigmoid and the inability of most elderly patients to pinpoint their symptoms make this survey worthwhile. Particular attention should be given to symptoms such as change in bowel habits, diminished appetite, alternating diarrhea and constipation, blood mixed with stool, tenesmus or pain with bowel movements, or change in the stool diameter. The gynecologist encounters sigmoid or rectal carcinoma all too often during surgery for a suspected ovarian cyst or myoma.[5] Consider ovarian cancer when no gastrointestinal cause can be found for nonspecific complaints such as dyspepsia, indigestion, gas, abdominal distention, flatulence, and slight anorexia.[6]

Sexual function in the geriatric patient is often overlooked during the history-taking process. It has been shown that the male is often sexually active into late life and that, theoretically, most women are capable of sexual activity all of their adult lives. With the anatomic changes that do occur in women, this sexual activity can be uncomfortable or painful. It can also be the source of vaginal bleeding, pruritus, dysuria, and other complaints. Taking a good sexual history along with a general medical history and social background is the best starting point for coping with these concerns.

How to take a comprehensive sexual history is well described by Munjack and Oziel.[7] Of course, it is not usual to obtain a full history on every woman with a gynecologic complaint. A few key questions should identify the elderly women who has sexual problems[4]:

- Are you sexually active?
- Is there any discomfort during intercourse?

- Has there been any change in your level of desire?
- Does your partner have any problems?

Often, taking such a history allows the clinician to identify a problem area that might be helped by medication or, more often, by education and simple counseling.[4]

Gynecologic Examination

The patient must be impressed with the fact that cancer of the genitalia or breast can occur at any age; for example, cancer of the ovary peaks in incidence at around age 77 to 80. Many older patients recognize that they have atrophic vaginal and vulvar tissue and resist a gynecologic examination that might be painful. Therefore, the physician must perform a thorough but gentle evaluation.

Begin the physical exam by palpating the cervical, axillary, and inguinal lymph nodes, noting any enlargement or tenderness. Next, examine the breasts, and teach the patient breast self-examination. After this, palpate the abdominal area very carefully, feeling for masses or abnormalities, particularly in the splenic, hepatic, and renal areas. An upper abdominal mass may suggest the presence of omental cake — the solid mass formed when the omentum is infiltrated with cancer, a sign of advanced ovarian disease. It may be palpated or detected by ballottement during the abdominal exam. Other signs of advanced ovarian disease are abdominal distention and ascites.[8]

During the pelvic exam, palpate all accessible organs; since there are no screening tests for many of the pelvic cancers, this is the only means of detecting abnormalities early. Begin with careful inspection and palpation of the vulvar area; too often it is ignored on the pelvic exam. Note any abnormal areas of skin including erythema, leukoplakia, ulceration, or masses. Next, observe and palpate the urethra, Skene's glands, and Bartholin's glands. A small vaginal speculum is recommended for the patient with an atrophic vulva and vagina. Lubrication may also aid in this procedure, although too much lubricant can interfere with a Papanicolaou (Pap) smear or wet mount. Complete vaginal and cervical examination is essential to rule out these organs as a source of symptoms (i.e., bleeding or pain). As you view the cervix and fornices, be sure to check the lateral vaginal fornix carefully for it can hide a small mucosal lesion. A Pap smear should be obtained from any abnormal areas visualized in the vagina or on the cervix. In taking Pap smears, be very careful about technique; improperly done smears probably contribute to at least half of the 10 to 35% false-negative rate generally reported.[9]

A careful bimanual examination is necessary to complete the pelvic evaluation. A patient on estrogen replacement may tolerate the usual examination without much difficulty. The atrophic vagina and vulva may, how-

ever, admit only one digit easily. Uterine size, shape, and mobility are all important factors to be evaluated. Also, the adnexal examination is very important, looking for any masses or abnormalities. Any enlargement in the ovaries is abnormal and will require further evaluation. In the woman more than five years postmenopausal, a palpable ovary is suspicious for neoplasia. A rectovaginal examination may yield additional information regarding the pelvic organs, including the rectum. At this time, the presence of hemorrhoids or other rectal pathology may reveal an alternative source of bleeding that was thought to be vaginal in origin.

A portion of the geriatric population is so severely debilitated physically or mentally that the examination becomes quite difficult. These patients may require several assistants to stabilize and aid in the examination. Occasionally, the condition will be so severe that the examination must be done in the left lateral position or under general anesthesia.

COMMON GYNECOLOGIC DISEASES IN THE GERIATRIC POPULATION

Vulva

Vulvar disorders rank among the most common gynecologic problems that primary care clinicians encounter. Common dermatoses — psoriasis, eczema, and seborrhea — may occur on the vulva. Other conditions not discussed in this chapter include Bartholin's gland infections, infected sebaceous cysts, molluscum contagiosum, condyloma, syphilis, and senile angiomas. In the geriatric age group, there is an increase in the incidence of diabetic vulvitis, hypertrophic dystrophy, and lichen sclerosus. Women with these lesions often present with complaints of burning, pruritus, or painful intercourse.

A thorough history, a gynecologic examination, and use of simple, available tests are the best way to establish a diagnosis and ensure accurate therapy. When the diagnosis is uncertain or the condition fails to respond appropriately to treatment, cross-consultation between gynecology and dermatology becomes important. Emergency physicians should remember that 1) chronic vulvitis can be a manifestation of many systemic diseases and 2) delay in diagnosis remains the major problem in management of vulvar cancer.[10]

Probably the most common inflammatory processes noted in the vulva are those associated with candidiasis. The elderly person with urinary incontinence exposes the vulvar zone to a constantly moist atmosphere, with subsequent skin maceration and infection. In addition, diabetes mellitus has a peak incidence among the older age groups and is highly correlated with candidiasis. Conversely, the patient may present with a chief complaint of vulvar irritation and a subsequent diagnosis of monilial vulvar vaginitis, which in turn provides a basis for the diagnosis of diabetes.[11]

Laboratory confirmation of monilial infections is by a 10% KOH smear of the vaginal discharge or vulvar encrustations. Miconazole cream or nystatin vaginal tablets are the most effective forms of treatment. Immediate vulvar relief can often be accomplished by the topical application of a 0.01% cortisone cream, either with or without supplemental nystatin, to the affected area. Trichomonal vaginitis may also trigger the onset of acute vulvar inflammation. Therapeutic success can usually be achieved with metronidazole.

The vulvar dystrophies represent a spectrum of disease ranging from atrophy to hyperplasia, with gross lesions of whitish-gray plaques, ulceration or cracking of skin, and symptoms of pruritus, dryness, and pain. Vulvar lesions may be localized or confluent, flat or elevated, and dusty red or gray white.[1] Heat, moisture, and scratching may further exacerbate the underlying condition. Stenosis due to atrophy of the vestibular mucosa may prevent coitus and often interferes with normal urination.

Treatment of vulvar dystrophy depends on the diagnosis that is made. It is axiomatic that any lesion that persists for 3 or 4 weeks should be biopsied. For atrophy of the vulva with persistent burning, application of 2% testosterone propionate (in petrolatum or unibase) is recommended.[3] This is applied 2 or 3 times daily for 6 weeks, then reduced to 2 times a week indefinitely. Pruritus and hyperplastic lesions may respond to topical steroid creams (especially fluorinated steroids), but their long-term use may result in further atrophy. It is extremely important to stress hygiene in all these patients if treatment is expected to work. Encourage the patient to wash with a mild soap, pat dry, then using a hand-held hair dryer to completely dry the vulva. This should be repeated 2 to 3 times a day until the symptoms are improved. Cotton underwear also allows good air circulation. Avoiding unprescribed or unrecommended ointments, lotions, creams, powders, and douches should be stressed.

The vulva is a common site of primary cancer and metastatic lesions, each of which requires an accurate diagnosis. Vulvar carcinoma represents 5 to 10% of all gynecologic cancers and occurs most frequently in the geriatric age group (mid-sixties on). The malignancy is associated with long-standing pruritus and is usually slow-growing and late-metastasizing.[1] The gross lesion may be a lump, mass, ulceration, or wartlike growth, and any suspicious lesion should be evaluated by a gynecologist or gyneoncologist. Epithelial dysplasia coexists with about 50% of invasive cancers and is considered by many oncologists to be a premalignant vulvar disease.[3] Lichen sclerosus, a very common vulvar dystrophy, is characterized by a thin parchment-type appearance of the vulvar area. About 5% of these lesions show various degrees of atypia; biopsies of suspicious areas should be taken liberally. Reddish lesions, indicative of Paget's disease, should arouse similar suspicion and should be referred for biopsy. Ulcerative and/or bluish lesions of the vulva may herald basal cell carcinoma and a tissue diagnosis is advisable.[11]

Vagina

Postmenopausal senile vaginitis, resulting from estrogen deprivation, is a diagnosis made when other pathology is ruled out, and the vagina has an atrophic appearance. It is the leading cause of postmenopausal bleeding. Other common symptoms include leukorrhea, urinary frequency and urgency, pruritus, and dyspareunia.[3] Without adequate estrogen support, the epithelium becomes highly susceptible to trauma and infection. The most common treatment is topical estrogen cream. One fourth of an applicator of estrogen cream is inserted into the vagina every fourth night until symptoms are relieved and then once or twice weekly as needed. Excess cream may run out of the vagina and cause a marked irritation around the vulva. Systemic estrogens also give relief of symptoms and may be more effective in advanced cases. Oral dosage is the equivalent of 0.625 to 1.25 mg of conjugated estrogen daily.

Infections with *Trichomonas vaginalis, Candida albicans,* and, occasionally, *Gardnerella vaginalis* may be superimposed on senile vaginitis. The diagnosis should be confirmed, and in addition to treating the senile atrophy, infection should be treated with appropriate agents. Venereal diseases (e.g., syphilis, chancroid) are seldom seen in this age group but must certainly be included in any thoughtful differential diagnosis. The elderly rape victim, who has not revealed an episode of sexual assault because of embarrassment, is a likely candidate for venereal disease exposure.[11]

Primary vaginal carcinoma is uncommon, accounting for less than 1% of gynecologic cancers. In one review, 70% of squamous cell carcinomas occurred in patients older than 50, and the peak incidence was between 60 and 70 years.[12] The most common sign of early vaginal cancer is painless vaginal bleeding, usually associated with a bloody discharge. These signs may be misdiagnosed as cervicitis or atrophic vaginitis in elderly patients. Patients with more advanced lesions will have pain, weight loss, and local swelling. Diagnosis can generally be made by visualization and biopsy. Radiation therapy is the usual method of treatment.[13]

Vaginal bleeding with an acute onset may be the result of trauma. Again, the atrophic changes make the vaginal wall more susceptible to tears and irritation. Primary repair is generally recommended but may need to be done under anesthesia. There are reported cases of such lacerations extending into the peritoneum or causing severe hematoma formation. Therefore, it is very important to have these complications ruled out on examination or with surgery.

Cervix

Chronic inflammation of the cervix in the geriatric patient may occur secondary to an atrophic cervix. This is usually associated with atrophic vaginitis and is best treated with an estrogenic cream. Cervicitis may also result from chronic irritation by pessaries, poor hygiene, or the changing vaginal flora. Frequent offending organisms include *Streptococcus,* coliform bacilli, *Candida,* and a wide variety of other organisms.[3]

While cervical malignancy occurs largely prior to the geriatric age period, significant numbers of invasive cancers can occur from ages 60 through 80 and beyond. Risk factors for dysplasia and carcinoma include early onset of sexual activity, multiple sexual partners, known infection with papilloma virus, prior history of untreated abnormal Pap smears, long intervals between Pap smears, and lower socioeconomic status.[14] A higher incidence of cervical cancer has also been noted in women married to men who have lost a previous wife to cervical cancer. Squamous cell carcinoma occurs in over 80% of cases, with adenocarcinoma comprising most of the remaining cases. Metastases and spread from other nearby organs to the cervix have been reported.

All symptoms of vaginal spotting, staining, discharge, or pain should be followed up by visualization of the cervix, obtaining a cytologic specimen, and referral for biopsy of any lesion. As stated earlier, the squamocolumnar junction of the cervix regresses higher into the endocervix with aging. It is essential to sample this junctional area where most cancers of the cervix originate. Cytologic sampling can be done by rotating a cotton-tipped applicator into the canal, then *rolling* it over a microscopic slide. Don't rub it over the slide, because this may force cells back into the cotton webbing. Obtain ectocervical specimens by gently scraping the ectocervical area with an Ayre spatula. Any blood or pus seen in the cervix must be evaluated for possible malignancy.

One should be aware that a cervical lesion *may not* be symptomatic, and a full viewing of the cervix and upper vagina should be part of any pelvic examination. Colposcopic examination by the gynecologist is also available for directed biopsy and assessment of suspicious areas. Benign tumors of the uterine cervix are uncommon with the exception of cervical polyps. In addition, several proliferative but nonspecific conditions may produce swelling of the cervix such as endocervical glandular hyperplasia.

Late symptoms of the disease include the development of pain referred to the flank or leg, which is usually secondary to the involvement of the ureters, pelvic wall, and/or sciatic-nerve routes. Some patients will complain of hematuria, dysuria, obstipation, or rectal bleeding due to bladder or rectal invasion. Persistent edema of one or both lower extremities as a result of lymphatic and venous blockage by extensive pelvic wall disease and distant metastasis are frequent manifestations of recurrent disease.[15]

Occasionally, a patient will present with significant bleeding from an ulcerative or exophytic cervical lesion. In most cases, the application of a vaginal pack impregnated with diluted epinephrine solution (1:500,000) or hemostatic agents such as Oxycel will control the bleeding. Treatment options for massive bleeding that is not controlled by packing include hypogastric artery ligation or embolization, high-dose radiation therapy, or cryosurgery.[14]

Uterine Corpus

The uterus usually reduces in size as age advances until the corpus and cervix become nearly equal. Leiomyomas usually shrink but will not disappear. If cystic degeneration occurs, the fibroids become calcified, producing a characteristic radiographic pattern of concentric rings of calcium. Any enlargement of the uterus or fibroid after menopause should be suspected of malignancy. Ultrasound may be helpful to determine whether a mass is adnexal or uterine, but it cannot determine if tissue is benign or malignant.[4]

Endometrial cancer is the most common malignancy of the female reproductive tract. The median age at the time of diagnosis is 61 years.[14] The strongest clinically identifiable risk factor is prolonged, continuous exposure of the endometrium to estrogen stimulation without the modifying effect of progestin or progesterone. Thus, conditions associated with continuous estrogenic status, such as polycystic ovary syndrome, theca granulosa cell tumors, and exogenous estrogen therapy, are definite risk factors.[16] Other risk factors include nulliparity, late menopause, diabetes, hypertension, and a family history of breast or ovarian cancer.[14,16] The overall mortality for endometrial cancer is less than 12%, primarily because there are distinct early warning signs.

About 80% of endometrial cancer patients have unexplained uterine bleeding. In postmenopausal women, the abnormal bleeding commonly takes the form of intermittent spotting or bleeding, which patients may term a "very light period."[16] Approximately 10% of patients also have cramping from uterine contractions as a result of material trapped behind a stenotic cervical os (hematometra). Infrequently, women with endometrial cancer will present with pulmonary symptoms or thrombophlebitis.[14]

Rule out all other possible causes for postmenopausal bleeding at this time (Table 36–1). The presence of blood dyscrasias, trauma, as well as prior treatment with estrogens, anticoagulants, and other medications should always be considered. As previously stated, the vagina and cervix are potential problem sources. On physical examination, the physician should carefully inspect the external genitalia, urethra, anus, vagina, and cervix for

Table 36–1   Common Causes of Postmenopausal Bleeding

Neoplasms
   Cervical and endometrial polyps
   Cervical carcinoma
   Uterine leiomyomas
   Adenomyosis
   Uterine carcinoma
   Ovarian tumors
Trauma
   Straddle injury
   Aggressive coitus
Systemic Causes
   Coagulation disorders
   Cirrhosis
   Hypothyroidism
   Anticoagulant therapy
Hypoestrogenic Atrophy
Hyperplastic Endometrium
   Exogenous estrogen administration
   Endogenous estrogen production (obesity, tumor)
Inflammation
   Endometritis
   Genital infections

lesions or atrophic changes that might produce bleeding. It is important to rotate the vaginal speculum to visualize the anterior and posterior vaginal walls so that lesions in these areas will not be missed. Carefully note the size, shape, and position of the uterus, as well as any induration or nodularity of the parametrium. A Pap smear should be performed to detect cervical abnormalities, but this should not be relied on to rule out endometrial pathology.

The cornerstone of the evaluation of postmenopausal bleeding is histologic sampling of the endometrium and endocervix. If there are no signs to suggest a significant loss of blood, the patient may be discharged with an immediate referral to a qualified gynecologist.

Ovary

There are no functional disorders of the ovary in the geriatric female and any enlargement has to be regarded as a neoplasm until proven otherwise. Of all ovarian tumors about 30 to 40% are malignant, accounting for almost half of the deaths from gynecologic cancer. Ovarian cancer affects all age groups, with the greatest frequency in those 50 to 70 years of age. The peak incidence is about age 77.

The poor prognosis is related to several factors: there is no detectable in-situ form of ovarian cancer; spread occurs rapidly by peritoneal implantation as well as vascular channels; and there are no early signs and symptoms. Routine vaginal cytology has not been effective in detecting preclinical ovarian carcinoma.[17]

The clinical manifestations of ovarian cancer suggest an advanced lesion. The most common presenting com-

plaint is abdominal swelling with either a large mass or ascites. Other manifestations include urinary tract complaints, idiopathic thrombophlebitis, vaginal bleeding, and cachexia. Reports from the literature indicate that a great number of women with ovarian cancer have vague abdominal complaints (e.g., dyspepsia, flatulence, nausea) for a long time before the diagnosis is made. Some of these women had a thorough workup, including a barium enema and gastrointestinal series, before a serious attempt at a pelvic examination was carried out.[3]

Physical findings that can alert you to a possible ovarian neoplasm are adnexal enlargement, fixation, or immobility; bilateral irregularity; and cul-de-sac nodularity on rectal/vaginal examination. The physician who performs a pelvic examination should be familiar with gastrointestinal, retroperitoneal, urinary, abdominal wall, and gynecologic pathology, which can present as a pelvic or adnexal mass (Table 36–2).

The ovary is unusual in that it is a common site of both primary and metastatic lesions. The breast and colon are the two most commonly encountered sites for primary cancer, and they should always be examined. Other sites that metastasize to the ovary include stomach, pancreas, endometrium, fallopian tubes, and cervix. Thus, further diagnostic measures (e.g., ultrasound) may be necessary before laparotomy, depending on the symptoms and signs.

Breast

The chief complaint of most patients with significant breast lesions is a lump or mass, and it is a presenting sign — and usually the sole manifestation — in 85 to 90% of cases due to malignancy. The five most common breast

Table 36–2   Causes of Adnexal Masses in a Postmenopausal Woman

Gastrointestinal
   Impacted feces
   Redundant or distended colon
   Appendiceal abscess
   Carcinoma of rectosigmoid
   Diverticulosis
Urinary
   Pelvic kidney
   Distended bladder
   Urachal cyst
Gynecologic
   Leiomyoma
   Endometriosis
   Ovarian cyst or neoplasm
   Uterine carcinoma
Retroperitoneal
   Neoplasm
   Abscess
Abdominal wall
   Hematoma of the rectal muscle
   Desmoid tumor

lesions of the female, which represent 90% of the conditions diagnosed on biopsy, include fibrocystic disease, fibroadenoma, intraductal papilloma, mammary duct ectasia, and cancer (Table 36–3). The breast may also be the site of contusions and lacerations secondary to trauma. A hematoma or subsequent fat necrosis may resemble a neoplastic process in the elderly female patient.[3]

Although neoplasms of the breast are treated by general surgeons, the emergency physician has an excellent opportunity to detect these lesions during the physical examination of elderly patients. Because mammary carcinoma is the second leading cause of death from cancer in women, every mass in the breast must be viewed with suspicion. Fixation, retraction, and asymmetry of the breasts, as well as discharge from the nipple, require further diagnostic study.[17] Other breast signs possibly associated with cancer include redness, dimpling, and underlying induration of the skin, perhaps accompanied by axillary lymphadenopathy, retraction, elevation, or eczema of the nipple.[18]

Distant metastasis occurs primarily via the bloodstream and usually is preceded by regional lymphatic metastasis. Organs commonly involved, in order of frequency, include lungs, bone, liver, adrenals, brain, and ovaries. Ten-year survival rates for patients with clinically palpable malignant lesions (1 cm in diameter or larger) are about 70% in the absence of lymph node involvement and about 38.5% with nodal involvement.[18]

Mammography (film mammography or xerography) is advocated in women with signs suggestive of breast disease, not only to assess the breast in question but to evaluate the other breast. This technique is also recommended as a routine measure in patients at high risk of breast cancer (Table 36–4). Definitive diagnosis is usually determined by incisional or excisional biopsy.

PELVIC RELAXATION

Pelvic relaxation refers to a group of anatomic, sometimes symptomatic, defects including uterine prolapse (descensus), relaxation of the anterior vaginal wall (urethrocele and cystocele), relaxation of the posterior

Table 36–3 Differential Diagnosis: Significant Breast Lesions

Carcinoma — solitary, unilateral, solid, hard, poorly defined, irregular, immobile, fixed, painless; may have a discharge, nipple retraction; skin changes common; enlarged axillary nodes

Cystic Disease — multiple, bilateral, tense or fluctuant, well defined, mobile, painful; may have a nipple discharge; no skin manifestations

Fibroadenoma — solitary, usually unilateral, solid, rubbery, well defined, freely mobile, painless; no discharge or skin lesions

Intraductal Papilloma — usually not a palpable lesion, painless; nipple discharge common; no skin lesions

Mammary Duct Ectasia — solitary, bilateral, solid, hard, poorly defined, irregular, slightly mobile, itching, burning; nipple discharge common; may have nipple or skin retraction; skin changes common in advanced disease

Table 36–4 Major Risk Factors Associated with Breast Cancer

Racial (e.g., Caucasian > other)

Geographic (e.g., United States > Japan)

Postmenopause or advanced age

High socioeconomic status

Familial history

Unmarried

Nulliparity or late first pregnancy

Previous breast cancer

Benign, inflammatory breast diseases

Adverse hormonal status (e.g., prolonged menstrual activity)

Obesity

wall (rectocele), and herniation of the peritoneum of the cul-de-sac (enterocele). Some form of pelvic relaxation occurs in a quarter of patients over age 60 and may be symptomatic in 10%.

The principal weakness is in the endopelvic fascia and the muscular levator sling. Traumatic (obstetric) stretching, occupational and unusual athletic endeavors, heredity, obesity, and postmenopausal attenuation all contribute in varying degrees to the development of pelvic relaxation.

The signs and symptoms depend on the combination and degree of anatomic defects. Uterine prolapse usually produces merely a sagging sensation in the pelvis. Under advanced conditions, the cervix may protrude from the introitus where it is subject to trauma, irritation, and secondary infection. Enteroceles and rectoceles generally are associated with varying degrees of tenesmus. Because this symptom complex develops so gradually and is associated with a high incidence of constipation in this population, its presence is usually elicited only on direct questioning.[11] Occasionally, a patient with a large rectocele may find it necessary to reduce the posterior vaginal wall manually in a backward direction to evacuate the rectum. The enterocele is subject to all the complications of hernias elsewhere in the body.

Cystoceles may be associated with increased urine retention and, thereby, a predisposition to chronic cystitis. As the competency of the proximal portion of the urethra diminishes, varying degrees of stress incontinence develop. The cystocele requires surgical repair if there are repeated bouts of cystitis or trigonitis, if the patient cannot empty her bladder adequately, or if the bladder protrudes to the vaginal introitus and causes an ulceration of the vaginal wall.[3]

A history and physical examination are usually sufficient to detect the cause of the patient's complaints if they are related to loss of pelvic structures. When the patient coughs, one is able to detect a marked descent of the urethra and/or bladder by depressing the posterior vaginal wall. A rectovaginal examination with the patient straining will generally confirm the presence of abdominal contents sliding into an enterocele sac. In the case of a simple rectocele, a finger inserted into the rectum should easily reach the apex of the mass bulging into the posterior aspect of the vagina. During the physical examination, it is important to determine whether or not extragenital disease (e.g., massive ascites, abdominal or pelvic tumors) may be contributing to pelvic organ displacement.[15]

The treatment of pelvic relaxation depends on the surgical correction of fascial and muscular defects. Pessaries are rarely used today, except for temporary replacement of a prolapsed uterus in the aged patient or the woman who is too sick to tolerate a surgical procedure. They may be associated with an increased incidence of vaginal carcinoma.[17]

OSTEOPOROSIS

Osteoporosis is a major public health problem in western societies. This condition afflicts 25% of "natural menopausal" women and 40 to 50% of "surgical menopausal" women not receiving estrogen replacement therapy. Osteoporosis represents a deficit in the amount of bone, not an abnormality of bone chemistry or mineralization (i.e., osteomalacia). It must also be distinguished from the asymptomatic physiologic bone loss occurring with age (i.e., osteopenia). Osteoporosis is a pathologic exaggeration of osteopenia, which in its early stages is asymptomatic but if left untreated progresses to a stage characterized by pain, deformity, and fracture.[19]

The patient at risk for osteoporosis is a postmenopausal woman who is slender and who has very fair skin and small bone structure. Other contributing factors include nulliparity, familial history,[21] poor diet, use of alcohol, calcium or vitamin D deficiency, smoking, lack of physical activity, and change in estrogen balance.[3,19] Study of osteoporotic bone has provided little insight into the pathogenesis other than an observed increase in bone resorption with normal or slightly decreased bone formation. Some women may also have a genetic tendency toward less bone mass.[21]

About 20% of all women suffer a hip fracture by the time they reach 90 years, brought on, in four cases out of five, by osteoporosis. Furthermore, about 25% of all white women over age 60 years suffer spinal compression fractures. The earliest fractures frequently involve the lower thoracic spine. With time, lumbar compression develops, and the patient may be left with chronic back discomfort due to spasm of the paraspinous muscles.[20] Osteoporosis is also associated with an increase in fractures of the distal radius.

The distinctive physical findings of osteoporosis are loss of height and deformity caused by fractures. Examine the patient's mouth; many women with osteoporosis have florid periodontal disease caused by loss of the alveolar bone that supports the teeth.[20] The presence of "thin" skin may also be indicative of early osteoporosis. The skin in some women appears to be transparent, indicating collagen breakdown paralleling similar changes in osteoporotic bone.[19]

The diagnosis of osteoporosis is basically one of exclusion in which the diminished bone density is not accompanied by any other metabolic abnormality. In uncomplicated osteoporosis, serum levels of calcium, phosphorus, and alkaline phosphatase are normal. The radiologic picture is one of uniform loss of bone density with cortical thinning and endosteal resorption. With increasing severity, progressive changes may be seen in the vertebrae. One sees increasing biconcavity of the end plates due to pressure of the nucleus pulposus. The anterior aspects of vertebrae collapse, which leads to wedging of vertebral bodies. In the femur, there is progressive loss of stress lines.[11]

Significant bone loss can be prevented or bone mass reestablished if therapy is commenced within 3 years after the menopause. Once osteoporosis is established, specific measures can be used to slow the rate. Therapy for established disease includes estrogens, androgens, fluoride, calcium supplements, vitamin D, calcitonin, and regular exercise.[19] Treatment should be carried out under continued supervision.

REFERENCES

1. Ryan KJ: Geriatric gynecology. In Bierman EL and Hazzard WR, editors: Principles of geriatric medicine, New York, 1985, McGraw-Hill Book Co.
2. Sklar DP: Problems in emergency medicine, Resident and Staff Physician 27:62–69, 1981.
3. Barber HRK: Geriatric gynecology. In Rossman I, editor: Clinical geriatrics, Philadelphia, 1986, JB Lippincott Co.
4. Barbo DM, editor: The postmenopausal woman, Med Clin North Am 71:1–149, 1987.
5. Kistner RW, editor: Gynecology: principles and practice, Chicago, 1986, Year Book Medical Publishers.
6. Barber HRK: Ovarian cancer. I, Cancer 29:341–350, 1979.
7. Munjack DJ and Oziel LF: Sexual medicine and counseling in office practice, Boston, 1980, Little, Brown & Co.
8. Williams TJ: Ovarian cancer: fewest signs, greatest challenge, Diagnosis 3:53–60, 1981.
9. Giuntoli RL and Mikuta JJ: Cervical cancer: regular office exams can stamp it out, Diagnosis 3:25–36, 1981.
10. Kaufman RL and Baker DP: Improving clinical diagnosis and management of vulvar diseases, Emerg Med Reports 6:153–159, 1985.
11. Reichel W, editor: Clinical aspects of aging, Baltimore, 1983, Williams & Wilkins Co.
12. Hilger RD: Squamous cell carcinoma of the vagina, Surg Clin North Am 58:25–36, 1978.
13. Jones HW: Vaginal cancer: common signs, uncommon cause, Diagnosis 3:71–85, 1981.
14. Houchbaum SR, editor: Obstetric and gynecologic emergencies, Emerg Med Clin North Am 5:399–641, 1987.
15. Romney SL et al, editors: Gynecology and obstetrics: the health care of women, New York, 1981, McGraw-Hill Book Co.
16. Dunn LJ: Endometrial cancer: increasing but highly curable, Diagnosis 3:39–50, 1981.
17. Wynn RM: Obstetrics and gynecology: the clinical core, Philadelphia, 1983, Lea & Febiger.
18. Leis HP: Diseases of the breast, AFP Family Pract Annual 23(s):57–71, 1981.
19. Notelovitz M and Ware M: Management of postmenopausal women. In Covington TR and Walker JI, editors: Current geriatric therapy, Philadelphia, 1984, WB Saunders Co.
20. Marcus R: Osteoporosis alert: clues to thinning bone, Diagnosis 7:60–68, 1985.
21. Seeman E et al: Reduced bone mass in daughters of women with osteoporosis, N Engl J Med 320:554, 1989.

Urologic Emergencies

Michael Kaempf, M.D., and Bruce Blank, M.D.

Urologic problems in the elderly are frequently encountered in the emergency department. They may not be the primary reasons for which the patients came to the emergency department, but often they are important in the evaluation and treatment of other diseases. This chapter will give a brief review of the more common urologic problems and the initial studies and treatments that can be initiated by the emergency department staff while awaiting urologic consultation.

Most urologic problems relate either to urinary tract infection, obstruction of urine, or a combination of both. Because most geriatric patients have other medical problems, prompt, accurate evaluation and treatment are imperative to prevent needless complications and prolongation of pain and suffering

A few studies can adequately assess the urologic status of an individual in an emergency department, and these can usually be done with a minimum of risk and expense to the patient. The most common tests are a urinalysis, urine culture and sensitivity, serum and urine electrolytes and creatinine, flat plate of the abdomen, abdominal pelvic ultrasound, and an intravenous pyelogram (IVP). Using these commonly available tests, prompt diagnosis of urologic problems can be made in over 90% of cases.

URINARY TRACT INFECTIONS

One of the most common presenting problems in the emergency department is acute urinary tract infection. Urinary infections become progressively more common in both males and females with age.

The most common presenting symptoms are urinary frequency, urgency, dysuria, and gross hematuria. Urinary tract infections are potentially more serious in males because of the frequently associated urinary obstruction and increased residual urine because of prostatic obstruction. Host resistance is also often lower in elderly patients, and their resistance to infection makes prompt treatment necessary.

Urinary infection is the most common cause of gram-negative bacteremia in the elderly patient, and the urinary tract must be evaluated adequately in any patient with an unknown source of fever and evident or apparent sepsis. Appropriate cultures should be taken, and broad-spectrum antibiotic coverage started as soon as possible while the workup continues for the source and site of the infection.

A KUB x-ray should be done to rule out calculus disease in any patient with a severe infection, and, if there is any question of a stone or if one is seen, an IVP or ultrasound should be done immediately to rule out urinary obstruction associated with the infection, since this often requires immediate surgery to relieve the obstruction.

URINARY OBSTRUCTION

Urinary retention should be suspected in any extremely ill elderly patient presenting at an emergency department. Most men over 60 will have some degree of bladder outlet obstruction, usually secondary to benign prostatic hypertrophy. Any severe illness can be complicated by urinary retention, and bladder emptying should be assessed on all patients who are obtunded or extremely ill. Overflow urinary incontinence, dribbling urine, urinary infection, or a palpable, distended bladder are the most common symptoms and findings in patients with urinary retention.

Initial treatment should be urethral catheterization and immediate decompression of the bladder. The practice of partially draining a markedly distended bladder is controversial. In the majority of cases, the catheter can simply be connected to a sterile catheter drainage bag without intermittent clamping and unclamping. Occasionally, in a very ill patient, release of a large intraabdominal volume can be associated with hypotension, but this is extremely uncommon.

Postobstructive diuresis must be watched for, and urinary output and vital signs should be monitored frequently after relieving the obstruction. Treatment of postobstructive diuresis includes adequate fluid volume replacement initially, with careful monitoring of the serum and urinary electrolytes to guide further fluid replacement.

Occasionally, difficulty in passing a catheter will be encountered, and this is most frequently due to urethral stricture. In most patients, when there is difficulty in catheterizing the bladder, adequate lubrication of the catheter and gentle, continuous pressure at the area of the external sphincter will usually overcome sphincter spasm. However, dangerous manipulation of the urethra should be avoided and urologic consultation obtained immediately if there are significant problems encountered passing a catheter in any patient. Suprapubic aspiration of urine can be done to obtain a specimen in a patient unable to void if there are initial problems in passing a catheter. Urethral dilation or passage of filiform catheters and followers should not be performed by anyone without extensive training and experience in these procedures.

Ureteral obstruction is usually caused by a ureteral calculus, but tumors of the bladder, ureter, and kidneys can also present with significant obstruction.

The most common presenting symptom of ureteral obstruction is flank pain, but often the pain may be diffuse and in the lower abdominal area, and differentiation between urologic, intraabdominal, and medical causes can be difficult at times. An IVP or ultrasound should be done in any patient with abdominal or flank pain and microscopic hematuria. If a stone or obstruction is seen on imaging studies, all urine should be strained since many patients will pass the stone after the diuresis associated with the intravenous contrast agent. As mentioned above, ureteral obstruction is much more serious if associated with concomitant urinary infection.

EXTERNAL GENITALIA
Urethral Prolapse

Prolapse of the distal urethral mucosa can present with pain, hematuria, urinary retention, or a palpable mass in an elderly female. It must be differentiated from carcinoma of the urethra, which is extremely rare.

Treatment is based on the primary presenting symptom. Occasionally, catheterization to relieve the obstruction is necessary, as well as excision of the redundant mucosa to prevent further episodes of bleeding or obstruction.

Paraphimosis

Paraphimosis (inability to return the foreskin distally from a retracted position to the normal anatomic position) and phimosis (inability to retract the foreskin proximally over the glans) are seen often in the elderly uncircumcised male, especially when hygiene is poor or the patient has a condom-type or indwelling Foley catheter.

Phimosis can cause severe inflammation of the glans and foreskin because of retained secretions and urine. Occasionally, the inflammation can be so severe as to cause urinary retention.

Treatment for phimosis involves local cleansing and antibiotics and occasionally a dorsal slit or circumcision if the phimosis is severe enough, but these are usually necessary in only the most severe cases.

Paraphimosis can usually be reduced by pushing the glans proximally with the thumbs while pulling the foreskin distally with the fingers. This should be done as soon as possible, since obstruction of the venous return from the glans can cause edema and necrosis. Often, an incision (under local anesthesia) through the constricting band can be done to facilitate reduction of the prepuce to its normal position. Circumcision should normally be done when the edema and inflammation have subsided to prevent further recurrence. Reduction of the foreskin after catheterization and proper hygiene can usually prevent paraphimosis associated with catheters. The nursing personnel must be given careful instruction on how to care for patients with condom catheters. Personnel must be careful to avoid penile injury, which can result from excessive constriction of the shaft with the proximal band of the condom sheath.

Priapism

Priapism (persistent, painful erection unrelated to sexual desire or stimulation) is uncommon in the geriatric population and should usually be treated by nonoperative measures since potency is often not a concern for the patient and spontaneous resolution is commonly seen.

The underlying cause is often idiopathic, but unsuspected systemic diseases should be looked for. Prostatic, bladder, testicular, rectal, kidney, and liver cancer have all been associated with priapism, as has leukemia. Many neurologic disorders and various hematologic diseases are also associated with priapism as are some medications such as phenothiazines, antihypertensives, and alcohol. Impotent men receiving intracavernous injections of papaverine or prostaglandins can also present with priapism.

Initial treatment should be conservative and usually will result in detumescence. Sedation, analgesia, and relief of urinary obstruction are important parts of priapism therapy. Aspiration and irrigation of the corpora cavernosa with a large-bore needle will cause the penis to become flaccid, but this procedure may need to be repeated. Surgical formation of a fistula between the engorged corpora cavernosa and corpus spongiosum should be reserved for those patients in whom potency is a major concern and the priapism has continued for more than 24 hours despite nonsurgical treatment. Treatment of other underlying systemic diseases should be initiated as soon as possible in conjunction with the above-mentioned treatment.

Scrotum

One of the most common causes of acute scrotal pain is acute epididymitis, which is often associated with lower urinary tract infection and bladder outlet obstruction. The presence of bacteriuria, pyuria, and dysuria with a reactive hydrocele and tender induration of the epididymis is usually associated with acute epididymitis, but differentiation from other potentially life-threatening conditions is necessary. Prehn's sign (positive if relief of pain is obtained by elevating the testes) and increased blood flow on Doppler examination or testicular scan are helpful in differentiating epididymitis from torsion of the testes and spermatic cord, which are uncommon in the elderly. Usually, there is a previous history of similar pain seen in torsion in the elderly.

Incarcerated or strangulated hernias often present with acute scrotal pain and swelling. Because of the extension of swelling into the inguinal area and history of previous hernia, the diagnosis is usually obvious. Reduction can sometimes be done in the emergency department while awaiting surgery.

Trauma to the scrotum can sometimes result in a hematocele and ruptured testes. The presence of severe ecchymoses and swelling with a history of trauma should make one suspect a hematocele. Surgical exploration should be done to drain the blood and suture the tunica albuginea to prevent further extrusion of seminiferous tubules and loss of testicular function.

The possibility of preexisting scrotal abnormalities such as testicular tumor or hydrocele also needs to be considered.

Pain referred into the scrotum can be seen with obstruction of the kidney or ureter that is usually associated with a normal physical examination of the scrotum.

Perineal infections are usually the result of urologic or anorectal disorders. Urethral strictures are the most common urologic cause of severe perineal infections, and usually there is a history of previous urethral stricture or urologic instrumentation or catheterization. Dissection along fascial planes (Buck's, Colles', and Scarpa's) explains the varying presentations and anatomic localizations of these infections. Occasionally, urinary cutaneous fistulae are seen, along with significant tissue necrosis. Assessment of the origin and extent of the infection are paramount in the treatment. Cultures should be obtained and the patient placed on broad-spectrum antibiotics as soon as possible. Frequently, surgical debridement with suprapubic urinary diversion is necessary to prevent significant morbidity.

TRAUMA

A complete urologic evaluation should be done in any multiply injured patient, because the urologic tract is often injured; unfortunately, urologic problems are often missed early in the care of severely injured patients.

Since many elderly men have a chronically large bladder volume, they are more susceptible to rupture of the bladder with blunt abdominal trauma. In any male with pelvic fractures or blood at the meatus, a urethrogram should be performed before urethral catheterization is attempted to document the integrity of the mucosa and prevent further damage if there is evidence of extravasation.

It is rare that a patient needs to be transferred to the operating room without adequate preoperative urologic evaluation.

SUMMARY

With a minimum of testing, adequate evaluation can be done in most elderly patients presenting to the emergency department to facilitate timely treatment and minimize further morbidity.

Diagnosis and Management of Prostate Disease in the Emergency Department

Gideon Bosker, M.D., F.A.C.E.P.

The broad and varied spectrum of prostate disease represents a unique diagnostic and management challenge to practitioners caring for both young and elderly male patients. The overwhelming majority of prostatic disease falls into three major categories: prostatitis,[1-3] benign prostatic hyperplasia (BPH),[4] and prostatic adenocarcinoma.[5,6]

As a general rule, diseases of the prostate present with symptoms that are very useful diagnostically. The voiding history, digital prostatic examination, and urinalysis are the basic data required for the practitioner to institute a systematic approach to assessment and treatment of prostatic disorders.

BPH is one of the most common medical problems faced by aging men. In the majority of cases, this condition is easily treated and rarely causes serious complications. Although the initial symptoms of benign prostatic enlargement are often the same as those for prostatic carcinoma — decreased force of urinary stream, hesitancy, straining to void, and postvoid dribbling — a physician performing a digital rectal examination can usually distinguish between the two disorders. Of those undergoing prostatic resection for BPH, 10% will have carcinoma.[7]

In the majority of cases, an adequate medical history and physical examination can help you to distinguish obstructive symptoms of the prostate from irritative symptoms. Obstructive symptoms are characterized by decreased force of the urinary stream, voiding difficulties, and urinary hesitancy. Urgency, dysuria, perineal discomfort, and pain at the head of the penis during or after voiding are the consequence of prostatic inflammation and are usually referred to as irritative symptoms.

When patients present with a combination of both irritative and obstructive symptoms, it becomes a challenge for the practitioner to distinguish between progressive inflammatory problems and obstruction caused by prostatic enlargement or carcinoma. A careful review of past symptoms and a thorough diagnostic evaluation will usually resolve this diagnostic dilemma.

The age of the patient is extremely relevant to the assessment of prostatic diseases. In prepubertal males, the prostate is poorly developed; as a result, prostatic disease is very rare. Any prostatic mass in this age group should be considered malignant until proven otherwise. Acute or chronic prostatitis can occur at any age following puberty but is most commonly seen in the 20- to 50-year-old age group. Benign prostatic enlargement and prostatic carcinoma are rare in patients younger than age 45. But, for reasons that are not well understood, a benign tumor often grows in the core of the prostate as a man ages. Most men over 50 will have some symptoms and 20 to 25% of men who reach the age of 80 will need surgery to correct the problem because of voiding difficulties.[8] In men less than 50 years old, BPH is much less common than prostatitis, urethral stricture, or neurogenic bladder disease. Hence, BPH must be a diagnosis of exclusion in this younger age group.

According to data from the National Center for Health Statistics, prostate surgery is the second most common operation in adult men (hernia repair being the first), with an estimated 367,000 prostate operations nationwide in 1986.[9] More than 75% of these procedures were among men 65 and over. Although prostatic cancer accounts for only a small minority of these cases, prostatic cancer is the second most common cancer in males in the United States and the third most common cause of male cancer deaths.[10] The treatment of prostatic cancer is complicated by the controversy concerning therapy for different stages of the disease. This will be discussed in later sections.

In 1990, an estimated 100,000 men in the United States will be diagnosed with prostatic cancer, and 26,100 deaths from the disease are expected to occur. The incidence and mortality of carcinoma of the prostate among blacks in the United States are almost twice those for whites. Despite numerous studies, no cause for this racial difference has yet been established.[8]

Age, of course, has a major impact on the incidence of prostatic cancer. The average age of prostate cancer patients at the time of diagnosis is 73 years. BPH also increases in incidence with age; although controversy persists, there is no indication that BPH is a necessary prerequisite or a proximate cause in the development of prostatic cancer. Nine out of ten prostate operations are transurethral resections.

Inflammatory diseases of the prostate are more common in the younger age group.[11,12] For many years, prostatitis and related diseases were classified according to a variety of characteristics, and only recently have definitions of chronic prostatitis, acute prostatitis, and prostatodynia been clearly established. Due to the difficulty of obtaining a clear diagnosis and the lack of successful treatment, particularly in chronic prostatitis, this urologic entity has been poorly understood and frequently relegated to the clinical wastebasket diagnosis of bacterial prostatitis. However, within the last 20 years, the contributions of many dedicated investigators have shed light on the diagnosis and treatment of this perplexing group of diseases.[13,14]

The purpose of this chapter is to review the recent advances in the classification, diagnosis, and treatment of various forms of prostatitis and prostate carcinoma.

GENERAL DIAGNOSTIC CONSIDERATIONS

Fortunately, the prostate is readily accessible to palpation by digital examination. Size, consistency, symmetry, the presence or absence of tenderness, and expressed prostatic secretions (EPS) should all be noted on the initial diagnostic evaluation (Table 38–1). For diagnostic purposes, the consistency and symmetry of the prostate gland are the most important physical characteristics. With prostatitis, the gland may be either firm or boggy. In acute prostatitis, areas of acute inflammation will be indurated and tender in comparison to uninvolved areas. On rare occasions, asymmetry of the gland can be caused by stones or abscess formation.

Benign prostatic hypertrophy is characterized by firm, uniform consistency and symmetry of the gland. In men over the age of 50, prostatic asymmetry is most commonly associated with prostatic carcinoma, and, for this reason, any patient in this age group with an unexplained asymmetric prostate should have a prostate biopsy. The usual diagnostic physical findings of prostatic carcinoma are areas of increased or asymmetric firmness, which can oftentimes be very subtle. Discrete palpable nodules and marked asymmetry constitute a more advanced form of the same lesion. In patients with prostatitis, tenderness will roughly be proportional to the extent and activity of the inflammatory process. Patients with BPH and carcinoma generally have little discomfort with digital palpation.

As far as laboratory examination, the amount, microscopic analysis, and cultures of EPS are critical in distinguishing among types of prostatitis.[15,16] Secretions can be expressed by milking the prostate digitally from its lateral to midline aspects and from the base toward the apex. As a rule, BPH and carcinoma produce only small amounts of nonspecific secretions.

PROSTATITIS

The definitive diagnosis of prostatitis is generally based on bacteriologic findings and examination of the EPS.[17,18] (See Table 38–2.) Both acute and chronic bacterial prostatitis are characterized by the presence of common urinary bacterial pathogens — most notably those of the

Table 38–1 Digital Rectal Examination in Prostatic Disease

	Prostatitis	BPH	Carcinoma
Size	Variable	Variable	Variable
Consistency	Boggy/irregular	Firm	Hard/irregular
Symmetry	Usually symmetric	Symmetric	Usually asymmetric
Tenderness	Often present	Absent	Absent
Secretions	Diagnostic	Not helpful	Not helpful

Table 38–2   Types of Prostatitis

Common	Uncommon	Suspected
Acute bacterial prostatitis	Gonococcal prostatitis	Prostatitis due to *Ureaplasma* pathogens (mycoplasmas)
Chronic bacterial prostatitis	Tuberculous prostatitis	Prostatitis due to *Chlamydia trachomatis*
Chronic calculous prostatitis	Parasitic prostatitis	Prostatitis due to viruses
Prostatodynia	Mycotic prostatitis	
	Nonspecific granulomatous prostatitis	
	• Noneosinophilic variety	
	• Eosinophilic variety	

Enterobacteriaceae group, including *Escherichia coli, Klebsiella pneumoniae, Proteus mirabilis,* and enterococci — that can be localized to the prostate. Symptoms of prostatitis can usually be attributed to acute or recurring cystitis. In nonbacterial prostatitis, urinary pathogens cannot be localized to the prostate. Signs of inflammation, however, can be found in the EPS. Prostatodynia is a common syndrome in which patients with complaints considered to be prostatic in origin produce secretion specimens that lack all signs of inflammation and culture positivity.

Patients with prostatitis will present with a number of symptoms referable to the prostate. They include dysuria, suprapubic pain, testicular pain, rectal fullness, urinary urgency, nocturia, and urinary frequency, pain in the inner thigh, and perineal pains or aches. Because all these symptoms may be attributable to entities other than prostatitis, there is a special need for accurate diagnosis on the basis of objective findings.

EXAMINATION OF EXPRESSED PROSTATE SECRETIONS (EPS)

Prostatic Localization Methods

Prostatic secretions are obtained by expression during transrectal massage. Because the EPS traverse the urethra during collection, contamination by urethral fluid always occurs. The criteria for abnormal prostatic inflammation are controversial, but most urologic specialists agree that the presence of more than 10 white blood cells per high-power field with clumps in the EPS is the standard measure of significant prostatic inflammation.[19]

The four-specimen collection for localization as described by Meares and Stamey is the standard procedure for the diagnosis and localization of bacterial prostatitis.[18] It is critical that the practitioner understand how specimens are collected according to this method for prostatic localization, since it is now considered the standard for evaluation of patients with irritative prostatic complaints. For the collection of all four specimens, it is essential that the patient be well hydrated. The VB_1 (or first-voided bladder) is collected by holding the sterile specimen container directly in front of the urethral

meatus. As the patient continues to void, the VB_1 culture tube is removed. After the patient has voided approximately 200 mL of urine, the second collection container (VB_2) is inserted into the stream and another 5- to 10-mL sample is collected. The patient is then instructed to stop voiding immediately.

After shaking any residual urine from the urethral meatus, you will instruct the patient to bend over. After wiping off residual drops of urine with a tissue, the prostate is then massaged while another collection tube is held in front of the meatus to collect the EPS. At the end of the massage, the last few drops of EPS can be collected by exerting gentle pressure on the bulbous urethra. Immediately after prostatic massage is completed, the patient is then instructed to void once more and the VB_3 is collected in a manner similar to the VB_1. After all the specimens are collected, they are refrigerated and should be plated by quantitative culture techniques within 1 to 4 hours after collection.

Interpretation of Cultures

The interpretation of the culture results from the four specimens collected depends on a comparison of the quantitative bacterial counts in each specimen. To clearly document cases of urethritis, prostatitis, or cystitis, the counts for the appropriate specimens must differ by at least one order of magnitude in order to be considered significant.

If the count of the VB_1 significantly exceeds the count of either prostatic specimen (EPS or VB_3), then urethritis or significant urethral colonization is present. If the count of either EPS or VB_3 significantly exceeds the count of the urethral specimen VB_1, then prostatitis is the diagnosis. If the count of the midstream urine specimen VB_2 significantly exceeds all other specimens, or all four aliquots show significant growth, then true cystitis or bladder infection is present (Figure 38–1).

In this event, the results cannot be interpreted with respect to the absence or presence of prostatic infection. The patient should be placed on an antibiotic regimen that will sterilize the bladder urine. The localization study should then be repeated in 4 to 5 days, when the bladder urine is sterile.

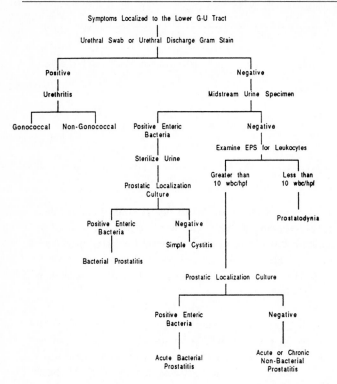

Figure 38–1 Flow diagram for the diagnosis of patients with prostatitis.

CLINICAL SYNDROMES

Acute Bacterial Prostatitis

Patients with acute bacterial prostatitis usually have severe symptoms related to the prostate as well as systemic signs of bacterial infection. The typical clinical presentation includes fever and chills, general malaise and myalgias, irritated and obstructive voiding symptoms (including frequency, urgency, dysuria, nocturia, hesitancy, and incomplete voiding), and low back pain with suprapubic and perineal discomfort.

On physical exam, you will note that the prostate is exquisitely tender and swollen, and you may be able to detect firm areas of induration. *Note: It is considered dangerous to perform vigorous prostatic massage in patients with acute prostatitis because of the risk of bacterial sepsis.* On examination of EPS, many white blood cells and lipid-laden macrophages are found and cultures of the prostatic fluid are uniformly positive for the infecting organism. Because the bladder urine becomes infected soon after development of acute bacterial prostatitis, the pathogen will appear in all four aliquots on lower tract localization cultures. In this case the culture should be repeated after a few days of antibacterial therapy so that a classic prostatitis pattern will become evident. While there is some controversy regarding this matter (because of the contraindication to prostatic massage at this point in the patient's course and because patients with acute prostatitis usually have a typical clinical presentation), it has been argued that lower tract localization cultures are not necessary to initiate appropriate empirical antibiotic therapy.

Most patients with acute bacterial prostatitis respond dramatically to therapy with antibiotics that normally do not diffuse into prostatic fluid from the bloodstream. It has been shown that cellular membrane barriers are altered in the acutely inflamed prostate and that acidic or basic antibiotics directed at the specific etiologic organism can be effective.

Most urologic consultants recommend empirical treatment with broad-spectrum antibiotics directed against gram-negative enteric pathogens. The patient should be treated with a parenteral aminoglycoside (Tobramycin, 3 to 5 mg/kg, intramuscularly) and a β-lactam antibiotic.[3] Parenteral therapy is continued until the patient is afebrile and then changed to an appropriate oral drug, usually trimethoprim-sulfamethoxazole (one DS tablet b.i.d.) for at least 4 weeks. If the patient is initially placed on oral therapy, it should be continued for at least 4 weeks.

Chronic Bacterial Prostatitis

In contrast to acute bacterial prostatitis, chronic bacterial prostatitis is not only difficult to diagnose and treat, but can vary widely in its clinical presentation.[1] Although on occasion chronic bacterial prostatitis develops in a patient with acute bacterial prostatitis, there is usually no history of prior acute attacks.

This condition is characterized by relapsing bacteriuria or cystitis, or both, with the same urinary pathogen. Unlike acute bacterial prostatitis, however, digital rectal examination of the prostate in these patients is usually normal. Prostatic calculi, when present, may be the cause of bacterial persistence and relapsing bacteriuria. When the lower tract localization techniques are used, it is apparent that chronic bacterial prostatitis is the most common cause of recurrent bladder infection in males.[3]

Classically, patients with chronic bacterial prostatitis will present with irritative voiding symptoms, including urgency, frequency, and dysuria, along with low back perineal and suprapubic discomfort. In contrast to acute prostatitis, however, chills and fever are absent unless there has been recent prostatic massage or urethral instrumentation. On physical exam, the prostate gland usually feels normal. Cultures may show infection in all four aliquots, or there may be significant numbers of bacteria in VB₃ or EPS exclusively, which is diagnostic for chronic bacterial prostatitis. Microscopic examination of the EPS shows increased numbers of white blood cells and the presence of lipid-laden macrophages. Although examination of the EPS cannot in itself distinguish between chronic and acute forms of bacterial prostatitis, it does rule out the nonbacterial form of prostatitis.

The most common organism associated with chronic bacterial prostatitis is *E. coli,* although infections with *Klebsiella, Enterobacter, Proteus, Pseudomonas,* and enterococci have also been documented.

Treatment

The treatment of chronic bacterial prostatitis is both problematic and controversial, and none of the antibiotic regimens currently recommended for the treatment of chronic bacterial prostatitis is ideal. The most commonly used and inexpensive agent, trimethoprim-sulfamethoxazole, has been shown to have a bacteriologic cure rate of approximately 40% after 90 days of therapy. A recent study compared carbenicillin with trimethoprim-sulfamethoxazole in 35 patients with bacterial prostatitis, most of whom had chronic bacterial prostatitis. Trimethoprim-sulfamethoxazole led to clinical improvement in 75% of patients but resulted in bacteriologic cure in only 40%, while oral carbenicillin led to clinical improvement in 89% of the patients and to bacteriologic cure in 74%.

In both groups, clinical improvement and cure rates were increased when the antimicrobials were given for 8 weeks instead of 4 weeks. These studies demonstrate that carbenicillin indanyl sodium is probably the most effective agent available at present for the treatment of chronic bacterial prostatitis and should be used as initial treatment for up to 8 weeks, if bacteriologic cure cannot be demonstrated at 4 weeks after initiation of therapy.[20] Erythromycin produced a cure rate of 88% in one study in patients who received 500 mg, 4 times a day, for 14 days. It should be considered along with trimethoprim-sulfamethoxazole as an alternate therapy to carbenicillin.[20,21]

Given the natural history of chronic bacterial prostatitis, it is apparent that even when the most appropriate antimicrobials are used, not all patients with this condition can be expected to undergo a bacteriologic cure. Consequently, there is a strong role for the use of suppressive therapy in patients with persistent bacteriuria. If recurrence occurs within 1 to 2 months after initial full-dose therapy has been completed, localization cultures should be repeated and a second course of curative antibiotic therapy initiated. If two or three attempts at cure are unsuccessful, suppressive therapy with low doses of trimethoprim-sulfamethoxazole should be given and further evaluation may be indicated. If the patient cannot be cured, suppressive therapy will usually provide protection against most symptomatic recurrences.

Patients who are refractory to medical therapy or harbor prostatic calculi[22,23] may benefit from radical transurethral resection of the prostate (TUR). Currently, most urologic specialists believe the overall cure rate of chronic bacterial prostatitis by TUR, as defined by lack of symptoms and negative follow-up localization cultures, is only about 33%.[11]

Nonbacterial Prostatitis

Nonbacterial prostatitis is the most common and difficult-to-treat variant of inflammatory prostatic disease. The typical presentation of nonbacterial prostatitis includes complaints of pain in the lower back, suprapubic area, testicles, groin, and, occasionally, the flank. Urinary symptoms are a prominent part of the initial presentation and include urgency, frequency, and dysuria. Unlike acute bacterial prostatitis, there is never a urethral discharge, and systemic signs of infection are absent. In addition, patients with nonbacterial prostatitis frequently complain of pain on ejaculation.

Physical examination will demonstrate a prostate that is normal in size, shape, and consistency, and there will be minimal tenderness. As is the case with other forms of prostatitis, the accurate diagnosis of this condition depends on the results of microscopic EPS examination and an accurately performed localizing culture. The EPS in nonbacterial prostatitis is almost identical to that in bacterial prostatitis, with increased numbers of white blood cells and lipid-laden macrophages. However, unlike the bacterial variance of prostatitis, localizing cultures in nonbacterial prostatitis are always *negative* in all four aliquots.

Since the hallmark of this condition is the lack of identifiable bacterial pathogens, many specialists have speculated that nonbacterial pathogens are the etiologic factors in this disease. On the basis of numerous studies, most investigators now believe that *Ureaplasma* and *Chlamydia* play an important role in nonbacterial prostatitis and are responsible for up to 15% of patients with chronic prostatic symptoms.

As a result, long-term antibiotic therapy with drugs used for bacterial prostatitis is not indicated in these patients. On the other hand, a short course of therapy with agents aimed at nonbacterial agents may be beneficial. One group recently demonstrated that tetracyclines are effective in reducing symptoms and decreasing the number of white blood cells in the EPS of patients with nonbacterial prostatitis. Erythromycin may also be used as an alternate agent. If short courses of therapy with these antimicrobials are unsuccessful, then further treatment is primarily symptomatic. Most urologists recommend a combination of sitz baths, prostatic massage, and pharmacologic therapy with agents such as antihistamines, benzodiazepines, and anticholinergics.[11,16]

Prostatodynia

This difficult-to-treat variant of prostatitis includes patients who exhibit no evidence of prostatic inflammation, either by physical examination or laboratory studies.[24] Most commonly, patients present with multiple complaints that include some combination of perineal pain or discomfort in the lower back, suprapubic area, and groin. On occasion, they may complain of a slow stream and urinary hesitancy. Dysuria, frequency, and systemic signs of infection are generally absent.

In a number of recent reports, there is a suggestion that many of these patients suffer from personality disturbances, with one demographic study indicating that emotional stress may be a large component of this syndrome.

On physical examination, the prostate is normal with no signs of tenderness to palpation. The diagnosis is made by finding no evidence of inflammation on microscopic examination of the EPS. Localization cultures for bacteria are negative for pathogens.

Due to the lack of evidence for inflammation in the prostatic fluid of this patient population, a noninfectious etiology for prostatodynia has been sought. Recent studies suggest that the syndrome may be caused by a primary voiding dysfunction and that a number of entities may be responsible. Urodynamic abnormalities have been found in patients with this condition.

Even before these recent studies, it had been empirically observed that alpha-adrenergic blockade with phenoxybenzamine improved symptoms in patients with prostatodynia. When long-term alpha-adrenergic blockade is indicated to alleviate symptoms, most urologists recommend prazosin.[11] Prazosin therapy may be started in daily divided doses of 2 to 3 mg and gradually increased to a maximum daily dose of 15 to 20 mg. Because many patients with prostatodynia have associated psychiatric disturbances, it may be that much of the therapeutic benefit observed with alpha blockade may, in fact, be due to a placebo effect, as well as reassurance that no significant pathology exists. Many of these patients may benefit simply from physician advice that encourages voiding on a regular schedule in a relaxed state of mind.

Benign Prostatic Hyperplasia

A universal and inevitable condition of aging men, BPH arises from the prostatic periurethral glands and stroma. As this tissue grows with age, the outer layers of prostatic glands are compressed and the prostatic urethra becomes obstructed to a variable degree. Interestingly, the size of the prostate gland on palpation has only a statistical relationship to the degree of obstruction. Moreover, the compressed outer layers of prostatic tissues form a convenient capsule for the adenoma. This allows surgical removal with minimal risk of loss of sexual function or continence. Finally, prostatic cancer usually arises from the so-called true prostatic glands, and they are not removed surgically in the procedure used to treat BPH. Thus, the risk of developing prostatic cancer is unchanged by an operation for BPH.

Presentation

Approximately 50% of all patients with BPH present with obstructive voiding symptoms that have progressed over a period of time to the point of being intolerable. The remaining patients present with complications. These include acute infection, gross hematuria, urinary retention,

renal failure, and an overflow type of urinary incontinence. Of all the voiding symptoms related to outlet obstruction, nocturia is one of the most common and is considered to be the *sine qua non* for the diagnosis of significant prostatic hypertrophy.

Diagnosis

The assessment of the patient with signs of urinary tract obstruction or voiding irregularity should include the history, physical examination, and appropriate blood and serum studies, including urinalysis, complete blood count (CBC), blood urea nitrogen (BUN), and creatinine. Intravenous pyelogram (IVP), cystoscopy, uroflow, and cystometric studies are then employed as indicated based on the results of initial studies.

A serum acid phosphatase should be drawn. An abnormal value will increase the chances of diagnosing an unsuspected metastatic prostatic carcinoma. An IVP or ultrasound examination should be performed on all patients whose history, physical examination, or laboratory studies suggest the possibility of significant urinary tract abnormality. A cystometrogram should be performed whenever there is a question of neurologic disease as a contributing factor in a patient with voiding dysfunction.

In patients who have urinary retention as the initial presentation, a catheter should be passed into the bladder. If the patient is difficult to catheterize, one should suspect a urethral stricture and a urologic consultation is indicated. Serum BUN and creatinine values are important to assess renal function. Patients with elevated BUN should be observed carefully after catheterization to prevent dehydration or hypokalemia resulting from a postobstructive diuresis. Finally, in the patient with a urinary tract infection, the infection should be cleared with appropriate antibiotics, and if symptoms persist or obstruction plays an important role, prostatectomy is indicated. If the obstruction resolves simply with antibiotic therapy, the patient should be evaluated for chronic bacterial prostatitis and treated accordingly.

When caring for the patient with BPH, it is important to determine whether or not to recommend surgery. In general, there are two definitive indications for surgery: 1) intolerable symptoms due to BPH and 2) evidence for harmful urinary tract obstruction.[25] With regard to surgical treatment, consider the patient's age, underlying medical conditions, and general health as well as the degree of symptomatology the patient is experiencing. For example, very mild symptoms due to BPH may progress, or they may remain stable for the lifetime of the patient. There is no way to accurately predict which will occur based on the initial presentation. Prophylactic surgery, therefore, is not warranted. A large postvoiding residual urine does not in itself create azotemia or threaten renal function. However, if the postvoiding residual urine is greater than 200 mL, early surgery is usually preferred to prevent progressive bladder decompensation. In these cases, you can expect surgery to eliminate the postvoiding volume and, therefore, reduce the chances of continuing recurrent infection.

Although the diagnosis of BPH is usually straightforward and substantiated on the basis of physical exam and laboratory tests, there are several pitfalls to be avoided in the diagnosis of clinical BPH. First, a number of drugs as well as undiagnosed diabetes mellitus are common causes of problematic urinary frequency and nocturia that are unrelated to the urinary obstruction of BPH. Second, if there is no history of voiding difficulty, one should be wary of diagnosing significant obstructive BPH on the basis of a single episode of urinary retention. Other causes should be sought. Acute alcohol intoxication as well as other acute central nervous system disorders can result in retention in the absence of mechanical obstruction. In addition, a number of over-the-counter cold remedies, as well as prescription drugs with anticholinergic side effects, can have profound temporary effects on the bladder and cause acute retention. Drugs in the elderly male most often implicated in bladder obstruction due to the anticholinergic syndrome include tricyclic antidepressants, antipsychotics, antihistamines, antidiarrheal agents, and antiparkinsonian drugs.

Treatment

Simple prostatectomy is the optimal therapy for all patients who have indications for treatment and can tolerate a general or regional anesthetic. Depending on the particular expertise of the urologic surgeon, transurethral, suprapubic, retropubic, or perineal prostatectomy may be recommended.[25] The overwhelming majority of cases are best treated by transurethral prostatic resection (TUR). Larger prostate glands are usually better treated by an open surgical procedure.

The safety of TUR is demonstrated by a mortality rate in a recent series that averages much less than 1%. Mortality rates increase, however, to the range of about 5%, when azotemia and other underlying medical diseases are present, and the patient is extremely old. In this high-risk group, the morbidity and mortality of TUR is substantially less than that seen with open surgical prostatectomy.

The incidence of life-threatening complications is low with any form of prostatectomy for BPH. Retrograde ejaculation is the rule rather than the exception in all forms of surgical therapy. Significant postoperative morbidity occurs in about 15% of patients. The most common postoperative complication is bleeding, which occurs in about 5% of patients and may be immediate or delayed. Acute epididymitis is the most common infectious complication and occurs in about 4% of patients. As a rule, hospitalization for bed rest and parenteral antibiotics are required for treatment.

Permanent incontinence is quite rare following simple prostatectomy, occurring in less than 5% of patients. Stress incontinence may persist for several weeks but should resolve as the external sphincter mechanism gradually accommodates to its new role as the exclusive mechanism for continence.

As far as sexual complications, loss of erectile potency can be anticipated in up to 50% of patients in whom the open perineal approach is used.

Although there is no obvious physiologic basis for developing impotence following simple prostatectomy using other techniques, there is an incidence of about 10% of impotence for the suprapubic-retropubic techniques and 5% for TUR. In those few patients who do develop organic impotence postoperatively and who are still sexually active, a number of prosthetic devices are available.

Urethral strictures will develop in less than 5% of patients within a year postoperatively. They are most common following TUR and can usually be handled by a single urethral dilation.

In summary, a TUR is the preferred method of prostatectomy for BPH unless the gland is extremely large. The uncomplicated TUR of the prostate will require a 3- to 5-day stay in the hospital. Most patients will require only one operation for BPH. However, true recurrence can occur in spite of adequate surgical removal. Most of these recurrences will occur 3 to 10 years following the initial operation. The incidence is less than 1% for any of the open techniques and about 5% following TUR.

PROSTATE CANCER

Methods for assessing and managing prostate cancer remain enigmatic and controversial despite significant advances in diagnosis, prognostication, and treatment.[26] Our growing fund of knowledge about how to best manage this disease is often undermined by unanswered fundamental questions about the course and consequences of both treated and untreated cancer of the prostate. In the emergency setting it is best to initiate referral if cancer is suggested or to treat the complications of diagnosed cancer. This discussion serves as necessary background information. Although, at present, it is not yet possible to define the optimal treatment for the varying stages of prostate cancer, there seems to be an increased focus on indicators such as tumor stage and grade in choosing a specific mode of therapy. In all cases, treatment must be individualized according to the needs of the patient.

Incidence

Age has a major impact on the incidence of prostate cancer. The disease is uncommon in men younger than age 50, with the incidence increasing sharply to more than

1,000 per 100,000 man years for American males age 85 and over. BPH also increases in incidence with age, and, although controversy persists, at present there is no indication that BPH is a cause of prostate cancer.

In light of the major impact of prostatic cancer on the male population in the United States and throughout the world, early diagnosis and effective local control are essential. Because localized prostate cancer rarely causes symptoms, routine rectal examination is considered to be the most effective method now available for detecting early disease. The majority of patients present with advanced disease. If all men 40 years of age and older were to undergo yearly rectal examination and ultrasound of the prostate, it is probable that there would be an increase in the diagnosis of localized, and potentially curable, prostate cancer.[10] Interestingly, young patients have a worse prognosis than older patients.

Diagnosis

A prostate nodule or area of induration is an indication for biopsy if the diagnosis of prostate cancer would mandate therapy in a particular patient. At present, transperineal needle and transrectal biopsy of the prostate are the most common methods used for obtaining tissue for diagnosis. TUR of the prostate has been reported to be the initial mode of diagnosis in a surprisingly high number of cases. Fine-needle aspiration of the prostate is also gaining wider use as a diagnostic method and indication for therapy for localized prostatic cancer. The reliability of this technique depends on the skill and experience of the urologic surgeon performing the aspiration. An accuracy rate of about 80% can be expected with the initial needle biopsy, and this percentage increases to about 90% with repeated attempts. Complications of this diagnostic procedure are bleeding and sepsis, both of which are rare when good technique is employed. While open perineal biopsy yields the most accurate diagnosis, it has the disadvantages of requiring general anesthesia as well as the concomitant risks of an open surgical procedure. Moreover, there is a 10% incidence of impotence postoperatively.

Once the histologic diagnosis of prostate cancer has been made, a staging workup is done in order to determine therapy. The usual procedures employed to determine the extent of the disease include acid phosphatase[28] bone scan or skeletal bone survey, computerized tomography, lymphangiography, and pelvic lymph node dissection.

Lymphangiography has a reported overall accuracy rate of 70 to 90% for detecting lymphatic nodal involvement from prostatic cancer.[6] Despite renewed controversy, lymphadenectomy is generally a diagnostic rather than a therapeutic procedure. CAT scanning has replaced lymphangiography as a staging method. Because bone metastases are present or eventually develop in 70 to 84% of patients with carcinoma of the prostate, bone scanning has become a critical staging procedure. The routine use of bone scans in staging followed the introduction of technetium-99m pertechnetate in the early 1970s. Recent studies have shown that bone scans are more accurate in demonstrating bone metastases than are skeletal surveys,[9] and changes on bone scan may precede those seen on conventional radiographs by up to 3 to 6 months.

It should be noted that while bone scans are highly sensitive, they have a low specificity. As a result, any pathologic condition that results in an increased blood flow to the bone — such as degenerative joint changes, old fractures, metabolic skeletal disorders, and Paget's disease — should be excluded if the bone scan is abnormal.

A new and promising technique for diagnosing and assessing the local extent of prostate cancer is transrectal ultrasonography, which can also be used to assess response to therapy.[29]

Stages

Following clinical evaluation of the patient with prostatic cancer, the disease is staged according to the criteria shown in Table 38–3. Stage A disease refers to incidental or clinically unsuspected prostate cancer that is found in tissue removed for apparently benign disorders. Stage A is subdivided into Stages A_1 (focal) and A_2 (diffuse or high-grade).

Stage A

The treatment of Stage A prostate cancer depends on the clinical distinction between A_1 and A_2 disease. For

Table 38–3 Staging System for Prostatic Cancer

The staging system (subject to minor variations) most often used in this country is as follows:

Stage A_1	Limited to prostate, microfocal, truly occult, sometimes called stage 0 — no clinical evidence of disease.
Stage A_2	Limited to prostate, clinically unsuspected, but diffuse, high-grade, or multifocal microscopic evidence of disease — no clinical evidence of disease.
Stage B_1	Limited to prostate — prostatic nodule is less than 1.5 cm. Normal acid phosphatase.
Stage B_2	Limited to prostate — prostatic nodule or palpable involvement of greater than 1.5 cm. Normal acid phosphatase.
Stage C	Local pelvic extension to periprostatic structures without metastases — palpable prostatic and periprostatic involvement. Normal acid phosphatase.
Stage D_1	Metastases only to pelvic lymph nodes. Acid phosphatase may or may not be normal.
Stage D_2	Metastases beyond pelvic lymph nodes, frequently to spine, pelvis, other bones. Acid phosphatase is elevated in 60 to 80%.

Stage A_1 no further therapy is generally indicated unless the grade of the tumor or the patient's age warrants further evaluation. A routine schedule of repeat palpation of the prostate and acid phosphatase determination at a 6-month level is considered adequate surveillance in most patients.

Some urologic specialists have suggested a policy of observation only for patients with Stage A_2 prostate cancer.[30] Although therapy is somewhat controversial, the adverse biologic potential for Stage A_2 prostate cancer strongly suggests that the treatment should be similar to that of a Stage B disease.[25]

The options for treatment of A_2 prostate cancer include radical prostatectomy, interstitial or external beam radiation, hormone therapy, and observation only. External beam radiation therapy has gained in popularity in recent years, while the rate of radical surgery for Stage A_2 disease has slightly declined.[26] Patients with debilitating illnesses or those over the age of 70 may be observed and started on hormonal therapy when indicated.

Stage B

Stage B prostate cancer is also divided into two stages: 1) Stage B_1, in which a nodule or area of induration is less than 1.5 cm confined to one lobe, and 2) Stage B_2, in which there is a nodule greater than 1.5 cm or an area of induration involving both lobes of the prostate. In Stage B disease, tumor size is a major indicator of lymph node metastases, which have been shown to occur in 18% of patients with small Stage B tumors and 34% in those with larger Stage B lesions.

The optimal management of Stage B prostate cancer is perhaps the most uncertain, if not the most controversial, issue in modern urologic oncology. This debate concerning treatment is based, in large part, on the poorly understood natural history of Stage B prostate cancer and, in part, on arguments concerning relative efficacies of surgery versus radiation therapy.

In general, most urologists recommend radical surgery or radical radiation after pelvic lymph node evaluation. Because removal of the tumor will result in cure if the malignancy is truly localized, radical prostatectomy appears, at present, to be the optimal approach to patients with true Stage B_1 lesions. In Stage B_2 lesions, the high incidence of nodal metastases and of microscopic residual tumor following radical prostatectomy makes surgery somewhat controversial. In these cases, radiation therapy — with its lower morbidity and mortality and its greater potential for eliminating locally invasive microscopic tumor — is considered the preferred treatment by many urologic surgeons and oncologists.

The likelihood of impotence and the risk of incontinence have probably had a major impact on the willingness of patients to undergo surgery, although it has been shown that impotence also occurs in a significant percentage of patients receiving external beam radiation to the prostate.[27,31] Not surprisingly, each therapeutic modality is accompanied by predictable complications and morbidity. Radical prostatectomy can produce erectile impotence in 50 to 90% of patients and some degree of incontinence in up to 10%. Urethral stricture will develop in less than 10%. The mortality rate in well-selected patients is about 1%.

Curative radiation therapy will produce impotence in only 50% of patients and, depending on the field size and dosage, will produce permanent inflammatory cystitis or proctitis in about 10%. Interstitial radiation by ^{125}I implantation of the prostate has also gained popularity in the treatment of localized disease. Controversy regarding the relative risks and benefits of surgery versus radiation therapy is unlikely to be resolved in the near future.

Stage C

Stage C prostate cancer is a locally advanced disease that poses a serious threat to the patient's survival. Studies suggest that the average life expectancy of patients with untreated Stage C disease is 2 to 3 years.[8]

The approach to patients with Stage C tumors is complicated by the fact that approximately 60% of patients actually have subclinical metastases at the time of presentation. Thus, the reported survival rate of 3 to 4 years is skewed by the significant number of patients who actually have Stage D disease initially. As a result, the role of radical surgery in Stage C disease is controversial.

Radiation therapy is now the most commonly recommended mode of treatment for Stage C prostate cancer. Actuarial survival rate of 62% at 5 years, 36% at 10 years, and 18% at 15 years has been reported.[6] While radical prostatectomy may be curative in a small percentage of patients with Stage C disease, there seems to be little enthusiasm for this approach among urologists.

In conclusion, a consistently effective means of controlling both local disease and the spread of distant metastases in Stage C disease does not seem to exist. Factors other than treatment should be the main determinants of clinical course and management.

Stage D

Stage D prostate cancer may be limited to pelvic lymph node involvement (Stage D_1) or be diffuse, particularly with bone or other distant metastases (Stage D_2). There is now a growing acceptance of the fact that pelvic lymph involvement in prostatic cancer indicates systemic disease, which is probably incurable by current surgical or radiotherapeutic techniques.[32,33] Within 3 years of diagnosis, about 50% of patients with positive pelvic nodes manifest progression of the disease, most notably with bone metastases, and 85% progress within 5 years. The average survival time for untreated Stage D_2 disease is probably less than 1 year.[34]

Stage D_1 disease, in which metastases are presumably limited to pelvic lymph nodes, presents a number of treatment options that would not generally be considered for Stage D_2 disease. As noted previously, however, there is now growing acceptance of the concept that nodal disease signifies systemic disease, which is incurable by current surgical and radiotherapeutic means. In a comparative study of radical prostatectomy, extended field irradiation, or delayed hormonal therapy in patients with Stage D_1 disease, the median survival time for all patients was about 40 months, and none of the pretreatment options prolonged survival. Although extended field irradiation is still sometimes employed for Stage D_1 disease, this study, as well as others, suggests that radiation therapy has little if any impact on the course of prostate cancer in the majority of patients with positive lymph nodes.[35]

A number of recent developments can be noted in the hormone therapy of prostate cancer. It has been well demonstrated that hormonal manipulation in prostate cancer is associated with dramatic palliative effects on the symptomatic patient suffering from Stage D disease. Moreover, whether or not hormone therapy significantly alters the survival of prostate cancer has also been questioned.

The usual methods employed in hormonal therapy are orchiectomy or oral estrogen administration, most commonly in the form of diethylstilbestrol (DES). (See Table 38–4.) Hormonal therapy is a medical castration that results from inhibiting pituitary release of LH. The recommended dose of DES is 1 to 3 mg per day. There is some evidence that the 1 mg dosage may be inadequate to completely suppress testosterone in some men while the possible cardiovascular side effects of DES are dose related and probably somewhat higher at the 3 mg daily dosage. Orchiectomy is a relatively simple and effective means of hormonal therapy and is the standard against which other types of hormone therapy have been judged. There is little if any evidence that the combination of orchiectomy and DES is superior to either method used alone. Leuprolide, an LH-RH antagonist, given by sub-

cutaneous injection, has been shown to be as effective as DES and is becoming a common alternative to DES therapy. Flutamide, an androgen blocker, is currently in clinical trials.

Although the majority of patients with metastatic prostatic cancer will respond to hormone therapy, the duration of response and cost of therapy are variable. (See Table 38–5.) Survival rates of 50% at 3 years and 10% at 10 years are generally reported. The prognosis for those patients who fail to respond to hormone therapy or whose tumors develop resistance to hormonal influence is extremely poor with average survival time of less than 1 year. At present, most studies show that chemotherapy does not improve survival in progressive Stage D disease.[36] Clearly, more clinical trials using chemotherapeutic agents are warranted.

Palliative Therapy

In the majority of patients with untreatable prostate cancer, appropriate analgesic use is the key to palliative treatment. Aspirin and other nonsteroidal antiinflammatory drugs are recommended for mild to moderate pain. For more severe pain, progressively stronger narcotic agents are generally necessary. When pain is severe and localized to a single area such as hips, pelvic bones, or lumbar spine, spot irradiation in a dosage of 3,000 rad usually offers prompt, long-lasting, and effective relief of pain. There are many factors involved in choosing the most appropriate treatment for the individual patient with prostatic cancer. Patient age and anticipated life expectancy, medical problems, sexual potency, potential complications of therapy, and, ultimately, consideration of

Table 38–4   Cost of Hormonal Therapy for a Month

Drug	Dosage	Cost/month
Diethylstilbestrol	1 mg t.i.d.	$ 9.65
Estinyl*	0.05 mg b.i.d.	19.00
Premarin†	10 mg/day	36.45
Stilphostrol‡	50 mg t.i.d.	83.20
TACE§	12 mg b.i.d.	26.50
Ketoconazole	400 mg t.i.d.	227.70

*Schering-Plough brand of ethinyl estradiol.
†Ayerst brand of conjugated estrogens.
‡Miles brand of diethylstilbestrol diphosphate.
§Merrell Dow brand of chlorotrianisene.

Table 38–5   Current Protocols of the National Prostatic Cancer Project of Patients with Prostatic Cancer Distant Metastases (Stage D_2)

Protocol number	Type of study patient	Treatments
1700	Newly diagnosed stage D_2	DES/orchiectomy or vuserelin acetate (LH-RH agonist) or DES/orchiectomy + methotrexate
2000	Newly diagnosed stage D_2	Leuprolide acetate + flutamide or leuprolide + placebo (double-blind study)
1500	Stage D_2, hormone failure, no pelvic irradiation	Methotrexate v doxorubicin + cyclophosphamide or cisplatin + 5-FU + cyclophosphamide
2400	Stage D_2, hormone failure with or without pelvic irradiation	Estramustine phosphate sodium (Emcyt) or flutamide

DES = diethylstilbestrol; 5-FU = 5-fluorouracil; LH-RH = luteinizing hormone–releasing hormone.

the quality of life with and without therapy must be considered to arrive at an appropriate combination of therapeutic modalities.

REFERENCES

1. Krieger JN: Prostatitis syndromes: pathophysiology, differential diagnosis, and treatment, Sex Transm Dis 11(2):100–112, 1984.
2. Meares EM Jr: Prostatitis, Annu Rev Med 30:279–288, 1979.
3. Ireton RC and Berger RE: Prostatitis and epididymitis, Urol Clin North Am 11(1):83–94, 1984.
4. Horton R: Benign prostatic hyperplasia: a disorder of androgen metabolism in the male, J Am Geriatr Soc 32(5):380–385, 1984.
5. Benson MC and Coffey DS: New concepts and controversies concerning prostate cancer, Prog Clin Biol Res 153:547–562, 1984.
6. Bahnson RR and Catalona WJ: Current management of prostatic carcinoma, Primary Care 12(4):795–813, 1985.
7. Huben RP and Murphy GP: Prostate cancer: an update, CA 36(5):274–292, 1986.
8. Whitmore WF Jr: Natural history and staging of prostate cancer, Urol Clin North Am 11(2):205–220, 1984.
9. Spirnak JP and Resnick MI: Clinical staging of prostatic cancer: new modalities, Urol Clin North Am 11:221–235, 1984.
10. Frame PS: A critical review of adult health maintenance. III. Prevention of cancer, J Fam Pract 22(6):511–520, 1986.
11. Orland SM, Hanno PM, and Wein AJ: Prostatitis, prostatosis, and prostatodynia, Urology 25(5):439–459, 1985.
12. Stamey TA: Prostatitis, J R Soc Med 74:22, 1981.
13. Segura JW, Opitz JL, and Green LF: Prostatosis, prostatitis or pelvic floor tension myalgia, J Urol 122:168, 1979.
14. Meares EM Jr and Barbalias GA: Prostatitis: bacterial, nonbacterial, and prostatodynia, Semin Urol 1(2):146, 1983.
15. Meares EM Jr: Prostatitis syndromes: new perspectives about old woes, J Urol 123:141–147, 1980.
16. Stamey TA: Prostatitis, J R Soc Med 74(1):22–40, 1981.
17. Meares EM Jr: Prostatitis and related diseases, DM 26(8):1–29, 1980.
18. Meares EM Jr and Stamey TA: Bacteriologic localization patterns in bacterial prostatitis and urethritis, Invest Urol 5:492, 1968.
19. Meares EM Jr: Prostatitis, Urol Clin North Am 2:3, 1975.
20. Thin RN and Simmons PD: Review of results of four regimens for treatment of chronic nonbacterial prostatitis, Br J Urol 55:591, 1983.
21. Meares EM Jr: Prostatitis: a review of pharmacokinetics and therapy, Rev Infect Dis 4(2):475–483, 1982.
22. Meares EM Jr: Infection stones of the prostate gland: laboratory diagnosis and clinical management, Urology 4:460, 1974.
23. Eykyn S, Bultitude MI, and Lloyd-Davies RW: Prostatic calculi as a source of recurrent bacteriuria in the male, Br J Urol 46:527, 1974.
24. Colleen S and Mardh PA: Studies on nonacute prostatitis: clinical and laboratory findings in patients with symptoms of non-acute prostatitis. In Davidson D, Dublin L, and Mardh PA, editors: Genital infections and their complications, Stockholm, 1975, Almquist and Wiksell International.
25. Whitmore WF: Disorders of the prostate. In Branch WT, editor: Office practice of medicine, Philadelphia, 1982, WB Saunders Co.
26. Chisholm GD: Treatment of advanced cancer of the prostate, Semin Surg Oncol 1(1):38–55, 1985.
27. Whitmore WF Jr: Irradiation and/or surgery: some areas of confrontation in urology oncology, Am J Clin Oncol 7:595–606, 1984.
28. Watson RA and Tang DB: The predictive value of prostatic acid phosphatase as a screening test for prostatic cancer, N Engl J Med 303:497, 1980.
29. Pontes JE et al: Transrectal ultrasonography of the prostate, Cancer 53:1369–1372, 1984.
30. Schmidt JD: Treatment of localized prostatic carcinoma, Urol Clin North Am 11:305–309, 1974.
31. Walsh PC, Lepor H, and Eggleston JC: Radical prostatectomy with preservation of sexual function: anatomical and pathological considerations, Prostate 4:473–485, 1983.
32. Donohue RE et al: Stage D1 adenocarcinoma of prostate, Urology 23:118–121, 1984.
33. Elder JS and Catalona WJ: Management of newly diagnosed metastatic carcinoma of the prostate, Urol Clin North Am 11:282–295, 1984.
34. Spaulding J: Carcinoma of the prostate in the elderly, Front Radiat Ther Oncol 20:133–138, 1986.
35. Catalona WJ and Scott WW: Carcinoma of the prostate: a review, J Urol 119:1, 1978.
36. Slack NH and Murphy GP: A decade of experience with chemotherapy for prostate cancer, Urology 22(1):1–7, 1983.

Ear, Nose, and Throat Emergencies

Lewis DeMent, M.D., F.A.C.E.P.

Elderly individuals with ear, nose, and throat (ENT) complaints present a complicated challenge to the emergency physician. The discomfort of itching and ear pain in a healthy 20-year-old swimmer may, in a 70-year-old diabetic, be the initial stages of fulminant malignant external otitis, which, if not recognized, can lead to profound morbidity and death. For emergency physicians, suspicions as to the cause of a complaint must be sharpened and focused. This will afford patients the best possible care; in the elderly with their complex past medical histories, one cannot be too thorough.

This chapter focuses on ENT disease processes that cause the elderly person to see an emergency physician because of pain, fear, or a sense of personal danger.

EAR INFECTIONS

Although usually not an immediately life-threatening disease, ear infections can cause a great deal of pain in any aged patient.

Otitis Media

In general, the older adult with acute otitis media has the same signs and symptoms as the young child — that is, ear pain, decreased hearing, and often fever. This usually follows an upper respiratory infection and is due to the lack of ventilation of the eustachian tube secondary to inflammation of the tube opening in the nasopharynx. It is thought that a vacuum develops in this closed system and then fluid is secreted into the middle ear, providing a rich medium for bacterial growth.

The physical findings include a red bulging tympanic membrane, lack of pain when the external ear is palpated, and possibly fluid visible behind the tympanic membrane. Pneumatic otoscopy usually reveals a tympanic membrane that does not move readily with air pressure. If the patient is in severe pain and if the tympanic membrane is bulging, myringotomy may be needed to provide comfort and to accelerate resolution of the process. Usually, the patient can be treated with oral antibiotics, analgesics, and decongestants for comfort. In adults, most of the infections are caused by *Haemophilus influenzae* or *Streptococcus pneumoniae,*[1] and penicillin or amoxicillin is the initial drug of choice. Rarely, suppurative complications can result even with antibiotic treatment, resulting in mastoiditis or even hydrocephalus.[37] Any marked worsening of otitis media should be evaluated for parenteral therapy. The CT scan or MRI can be very helpful in detecting sinus thrombosis.

Most cases of otitis media are bilateral in the setting of an upper respiratory tract infection (URI), although one ear may be affected more than another. However, in the older adult, the finding of a unilateral otitis media, especially in the absence of evidence of an URI, should alert the emergency physician to the possibility of a nasopharyngeal polyp or tumor as the cause of the eustachian tube dysfunction. Indirect nasopharyngeal laryngoscopy should be performed in an attempt to visualize the openings of the eustachian tube in the nasopharynx. Whether or not this procedure is successful in visualizing the abnormality, these patients need a thorough ENT examination. A benign cause should not be assumed.

External Otitis

In a like manner, external otitis is similar in all age groups. As the aging population increases and people are more active in their later years, even the typical swimmer's ear may be seen in the older adult. The signs and symptoms are severe pain when the pinna or tragus is pulled, a swollen external auditory canal, and possibly superficial hemorrhage and large amounts of necrotic debris lying in a mucoid discharge. The infection is often caused by relatively minor trauma such as hairpins, cleaning the ear, or exposure to excessive moisture.

Treatment consists of gentle cleaning of the canal with suction and placing a cotton wick through the stenotic canal so that medication will be effective in reaching the inner parts of the auditory canal. Often, a discharge from the canal will emit a foul odor typical for the common *Pseudomonas* infection.[1] Ear drops containing polymyxin-B, neomycin, and hydrocortisone used 4 times daily for a week will usually clear these infections, providing the patient has kept water out of the ear and avoided excessive attempts to clean the ear thereby causing further injury. Simple mucoid or keratin-containing drainage often responds to 2% acetic acid drops in the affected ear.

If small vesicles or furuncles are seen in the external canal,[2] they can be gently opened and then ointment or cream such as polymyxin-B, bacitracin, neomycin, or gentamicin can be used to help heal these areas. When the skin of the external ear becomes inflamed as in impetigo or cellulitis, then appropriate broad-spectrum antistaphylococcal and antistreptococcal systemic antibiotics are appropriate.

Malignant External Otitis

The same clinical picture of external otitis just described, or a chronic external otitis not responding to the usual treatment, or appropriate therapy in an elderly diabetic, should alert the emergency physician to a potentially fatal disease.

Malignant external otitis is a syndrome described by Chandler in the late 1960s.[3] This disease is almost exclusively seen in the elderly diabetic. On examination, the patient is found to have a chronic external otitis with granulation tissue present on the floor of the external auditory canal at the cartilage-osseous junction portion of the canal. With gentle probing, this tissue is found to be coming from a defect in the canal floor[3] and actually leads into the soft tissue at the base of the skull. There is tenderness behind the angle of the mandible although with little external ear pain. It is a poor prognostic sign when cranial nerve VII is involved.

When the debris is cultured, the results indicate a *Pseudomonas* infection. These patients rarely respond to the usual treatment for external otitis, and the infection tends to involve bone, cartilage, nerves, and blood vessels.

Aggressive therapy is directed to surgical debridement and systemic antibiotics (e.g., gentamicin IM 2 mL/kg/day and carbenicillin 24 g/day, 1 g IV given each hour) to attempt to prevent the tragic sequelae of mastoiditis, osteomyelitis, meningitis, brain abscess, and death.[3] In Chandler's series of 38 patients in 1972, there was a 38% mortality, but after the aforementioned antibiotic regimen was started, the death rate dramatically decreased.[3] Most patients require hospitalization for several weeks. The emergency physician must be aware of this syndrome to avoid perpetuating the typical conservative local therapy that usually cures external otitis but will only delay definitive therapy for this disease.

EAR TRAUMA

Trauma to the ear involves three anatomic areas: the external ear, the auditory canal, and the tympanic membrane or middle ear area. Most ear trauma in the elderly occurs as a result of falling, assaults, or auto accidents. However, there is also canal trauma, usually caused by the patient's attempt to clean the ear, and occasionally a tympanic membrane perforation caused by the same method or, more rarely, by hot metal or lightning striking.

Perforated Tympanic Membrane

Perforation of the tympanic membrane usually heals spontaneously and requires no surgical intervention. In the emergency department, a rough measure of the patient's ability to hear should be recorded, and the patient should be advised not to put any foreign material, including water, into the ear. The patient is referred to the ENT specialist for a thorough audiologic evaluation. It should be noted, however, that in the elderly a perforation caused by a blast injury requires less air pressure than in a younger person so that the elderly are more vulnerable to the blast effect.[5] Also, the injuries caused by lightning and molten metal often heal very slowly (if at all), and careful ENT follow-up is needed. Those patients whose perforation remains open for 3 months are considered for surgery. Only those patients with vertigo or perilymph leakage soon after the accident are explored early in the course of the disease.[5] Surgical intervention soon after a perforation may be needed in patients who have perilymph leakage or vertigo.[5]

Canal Trauma

Trauma to the external canal is usually a small abrasion or laceration, which can simply be cleaned and treated with a local antibiotic ointment. In the healing period, the patient should try to avoid getting water and other foreign material in the ear.

External Ear Trauma

Trauma to the external ear must be carefully evaluated to avoid complications. Lacerations to the skin of the outer ear can be cleaned and closed with small interrupted 6-0 nylon sutures. If, however, the cartilage is also injured, it should be closed with absorbable sutures and finally skin closed over it. Cartilage should not be left exposed; the risk of chondritis is high with resultant increased cosmetic deformity and possibility for chronic infection.

After the outer ear is sutured, fluffed gauze should be placed in the postauricular area and a turban-style bandage applied to prevent the ear from being collapsed and deformed. If a deforming hematoma is found, it should be evacuated with a needle or incision and the ear bandaged as described previously to prevent deformity (cauliflower ear).

NOSE INFECTIONS
Nasal Vestibulitis

Although not a medical emergency, the pain associated with anterior nasal infection can cause a person to seek immediate aid. The history is usually one of progressive tenderness to palpation of the tip of the nose, often following an upper respiratory infection or a spell of dry weather that causes formation of a great deal of crust in the nose. This subsequently becomes more bothersome and after picking the nose, the nose becomes very tender. These are often staphylococcal infections and can be treated by the patient by placing antibiotic ointment in small amounts in the nasal vestibule and applying intermittent moist heat to the nose. Resolution is usually effected in a few days. Advising the patient to use a lanolin-based ointment to prevent drying of the mucosa will help prevent future episodes.

Sinusitis

Paranasal sinusitis is usually a disease of young and middle-aged adults. Acute ethmoiditis is particularly more common in children[14]; however, the complications of sinusitis in the elderly adult can be severe. It has been noted that the elderly seek treatment later in the course of their disease than do younger people. In one study, the patients over 60 years of age had experienced severe symptoms for several months before seeing a physician.[15]

The more dangerous complication of acute or chronic sinusitis is cavernous sinus thrombosis.[14] The patient may have been treated for weeks or months for a chronic sinusitis and then abruptly have increased symptoms as the infection actually worsens.

To understand the clinical picture, one must recall the anatomy involved. Several veins — including the ophthalmic, angular, ethmoid, superior ophthalmic, and inferior ophthalmic — have direct valveless connections to the cavernous sinuses (Figure 39–1). Cranial nerves III, IV, VI, and the first two divisions of cranial nerve V along with the internal carotid artery pass through the cavernous sinus (Figure 39–2). Infections can travel intracranially through the veins, and once inflammation has begun, the sinus may become thrombosed, leading to the clinical syndrome causing the nerves to be affected.[14,15]

The signs and symptoms progress from the previous state of sinus fullness to facial edema as the venous drainage of the face becomes obstructed. Then there may be retinal swelling, decreased vision, and extraocular muscle paralysis as the cranial nerves are involved. Paresthesia or anesthesia of the first and second divisions of cranial nerve V then follow with frank meningitis and death close behind if not treated. The mortality rate continues to be in the 20% range even with modern antibiotic therapy.[14] In elderly debilitated or immunosuppressed patients, mucormycosis of the sinuses may cause a less toxic but otherwise typical picture of cavernous sinus thrombosis.[15]

Often, there is no material available for culture, and the patient must be treated empirically yet aggressively. The treatment involves hospitalization and massive intravenous doses of broad-spectrum antibiotics, including those capable of treating penicillin-resistant, staphylococcal infections. In addition, consideration should be given to anticoagulation if the patient's general condition allows.[14]

NASAL FRACTURE

Nasal fractures, the most common of all facial fractures,[16] occur frequently in older persons. Because falling spells and blackouts are common among the elderly, not to mention assaults and automobile accidents, nasal trauma is common.

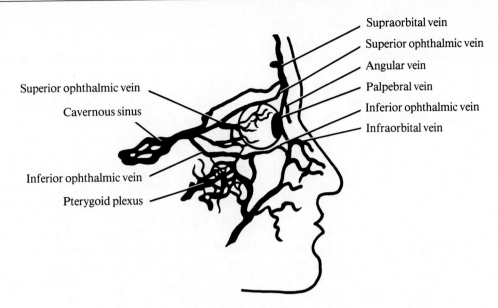

Figure 39–1 Venous drainage of middle third of face to cavernous sinus.

One of the duties of the emergency physician when examining a patient with a nasal injury is to completely evaluate the interior and exterior of the nose. The presence or absence of mucosal tears, septal deformities, or septal hematoma in particular should be evacuated because of the sequelae of septal necrosis, airway obstruction, and cosmetic deformity that may occur if the hematoma is not treated.[17]

The importance of the clinical expertise in recognizing nasal fractures is often undervalued. Unlike most bony trauma in the body, a fractured nose may be associated with a perfectly normal x-ray film. It has been said that the most important single factor responsible for missing the diagnosis of facial fracture is a dependence on x-rays and films to make the diagnosis.[16] The keys to making the correct assessment are observation, palpation, and discussion with the patient. The presence of nasal deformity, crepitus on palpation, ecchymosis, and epistaxis suggests the diagnosis. It is imperative to question these patients about past trauma since the patient could have a simple contusion of a previously deformed nose. One of the most important pieces of information to obtain is the patient's perception of the presence or absence of a new nasal deformity.

If there is a great deal of edema, then the reduction can wait 5 to 7 days and be accomplished by the ENT physician. If there is little edema and the patient is otherwise stable, then the emergency physician may wish to effect reduction prior to the increased swelling that usually occurs a few hours later.

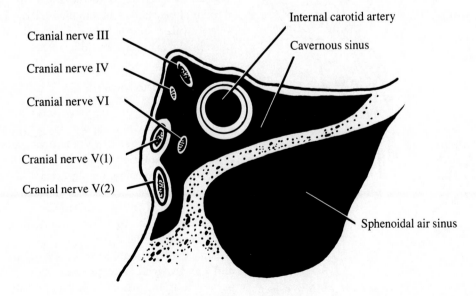

Figure 39–2 Anatomy of the cavernous sinus.

The treatment of a nasal fracture in an elderly person is not very different from the treatment in a younger person. The nose must be anesthetized sufficiently prior to reducing the fracture. This is accomplished by using either cocaine 5%[16] or topical lidocaine 4% with 1:1000 epinephrine on cotton pledgets placed in the nostrils. In addition, an external nasal block using lidocaine 1% or Marcaine ½% is performed.

Walsham forceps are used to realign the bony pyramid by disimpacting the bone (Figure 39–3). Then, Asch septal forceps are used to straighten the septum and, if displaced, replace it in the vomerian groove. Finally, the Salinger reduction instrument is used to further contour the tip of the nose.[16] Usually, most bleeding is stopped as the nasal structures are reduced to their correct anatomic positions. Packs are then used only if bleeding persists. A plaster splint can be taped to the nose to afford protection while vasoconstricting nose drops such as 25% phenylephrine hydrochloride can be used during the first 3 days to aid in shrinking intranasal edema to ease breathing.

EPISTAXIS

Treating the elderly patient who has epistaxis can be a very challenging and often frightening experience. A 75-year-old patient anticoagulated who is in shock with a posterior epistaxis can provide the most experienced emergency physician plenty of opportunity to use skills.

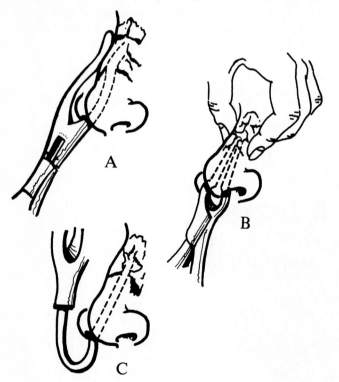

Figure 39–3 Closed reduction of nasal fractures. **A,** Walsham forceps. **B,** Asch septal forceps. **C,** Salinger reduction instrument.

Etiology

The etiology of epistaxis in the elderly is multifactorial. Anterior bleeding is often the result of local causes such as direct trauma, low relative humidity, recent upper respiratory infection with crust formations and mucosal drying, and minor trauma such as nose picking. The etiology of posterior bleeding, however, has been more difficult to understand. Hypertension and atherosclerosis are routinely seen in the elderly patient with epistaxis, which is often posterior in a branch of the sphenopalatine artery where it bends or where the vessel is contained in a bony canal in the inferior turbinate.[18] As the nasal arteries age, there is degeneration of the vessels characterized by a loss of muscle and its replacement in the tunica media vasorum with collagen. This had led to the idea that once these arteries bleed, they have less ability to contract and stop bleeding. There are, of course, more unusual causes of epistaxis, such as a person who had a ruptured internal carotid aneurysm that eroded through the paranasal sinuses and caused a near-fatal hemorrhage.[21]

Anatomy

To fully appreciate the clinical features of epistaxis, the vascular supply of the nose must be understood. Most patients with epistaxis have a bleeding site in the anterior part of the nasal septum known as Kiesselbach's plexus or Little's area — an area of convergence of several small blood vessels. In contrast, bleeding in the superior aspect of the posterior nasal cavity is usually from the anterior or posterior ethmoid arteries, and bleeding below the middle turbinate originates from branches of the sphenopalatine artery.[19] Another way of looking at the arterial distribution is to recognize that the area above the middle turbinate is supplied by the internal carotid artery while the area below the middle turbinate is supplied by the external carotid branches (Figure 39–4).

Approach to the Patient

The initial task in treating epistaxis is to quickly evaluate the patient's general hemodynamic stability. Is the patient vigorous? Has the patient had only an hour of intermittent anterior bleeding? Or is the patient weak, pale, and hypotensive, giving a brief history of bleeding all night? If there is any question, then the usual lifesaving measures of intravascular access, fluids, bloods, etc. are ordered. If the patient is stable, then an orderly approach can be undertaken.

Almost all patients with epistaxis are apprehensive, and the physician who proceeds calmly to reassure the patient that everything is under control will have an extra assistant at hand if the bleeding is indeed great. Time taken to softly explain each step in the treatment will

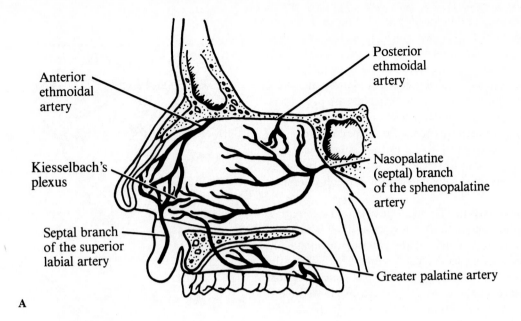

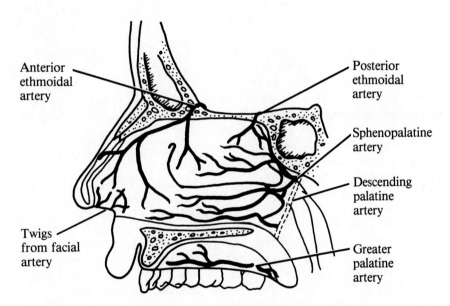

Figure 39–4 A, Septal blood supply. **B,** Lateral wall blood supply.

enhance a patient's cooperation so the procedures can be performed with skill and efficiency. If this rapport is established, sedatives are rarely needed. The patient and physician should be protected with aprons or gowns and the patient provided with facial tissue and an emesis basin.

Treatment

To effectively control nasal bleeding, the bleeding site must be found. To do this requires a cooperative patient, strong head light, suction equipment, and an organized approach to the nasal anatomy. The patient is instructed to blow out clots and pinch the nose closed and breathe through the mouth while the ENT instrument tray is readied. Suction is then used to clear the nose. To see the bleeding artery, a nasal speculum is inserted to open vertically in one naris, then the other. In the simplest case, a small vessel will be seen to bleed in the Kiesselbach's plexus.[18,19] The nasal mucosa is then anesthetized with a cotton pledget soaked in a half-and-half mixture of 4% topical lidocaine or 5% cocaine and 1:1000 epinephrine. After the excess anesthetic is squeezed from the cotton, the pledget is placed in the nostril; the patient is asked to pinch the nostrils closed for 3 to 4 minutes and breathe through the mouth. Obtaining full anesthesia if cocaine is used may require waiting 10 minutes.

When the cotton is removed, one can usually see small (feeder) vessels leading to the vessel that is bleeding. These are touched lightly with a silver nitrate stick, and then a new pledget is inserted. This sequence can be repeated until the main bleeder is bleeding slowly; it too can be cauterized with the silver nitrate stick. Often having an assistant hold the speculum while the physician applies suction and cautery simultaneously works well. In some cases, electrocautery is required and seems to cauterize more quickly. In the unusual case of a persistent septal bleeder, a small piece of oxidized cellulose or absorbable gelatin sponge soaked in thrombin can be applied to the bleeding site to aid in the hemostasis. Large packs of these agents are to be avoided because they tend to become large and boggy masses and difficult to remove later.

Anterior packing. If, when the septum is examined, no bleeding site is found, the next most likely site is the anterior or posterior ends of the inferior turbinate laterally.[19] These areas can be best located by watching the suction tubing as a Frazier suction tip is gently inserted along the floor of the nose. A return of bright red blood gives a clue to the location of the bleeder. If the bleeder appears to be along the anterior aspect of the turbinate, it too may be cauterized (if seen) but otherwise an anterior pack is needed.

To prepare for anterior packing, a cotton pledget soaked with the anesthestic agents previously described should be inserted deep into the nose. While waiting for the anesthetic to take affect, the pack itself should be prepared. A most effective pack is ¼ inch or ½ inch petroleum jelly gauze 6 feet long. An antibiotic ointment such as polymyxin B, bacitracin, neomycin, or gentamicin should be applied to the gauze since the incidence of sinusitis is increased with packs in place.

The anesthetic pledget should then be removed. The petroleum jelly gauze is inserted into the nose, starting with a loop about 4 inches from the end of the gauze (Figure 39–5). This prevents the end of the gauze from being aspirated into the throat. Each loop is successively applied until the entire pack is in place. Most nostrils readily accommodate 6 feet of packing.

When the anterior packing does not suffice or when it is apparent that the bleeding is coming from a truly posterior part of the nasal cavity, then a posterior pack is needed. The term "posterior pack" actually implies the combination of a posterior choanal pack and an anterior pack as previously described.

Posterior packing. Although balloon catheters[19] have been used to control posterior bleeding, unless there is an extreme sense of emergency, a well-placed lambs' wool pack is probably more effective. It is during the placement of the posterior choanal pack that the rapport with the patient will be most appreciated. These packs are uncomfortable and, at best, give the patient a feeling of suffocation. It is very important to encourage the patient to breathe slowly through the mouth while the pack is placed. Asking the patient to avoid biting the physician's fingers is a worthwhile precaution.

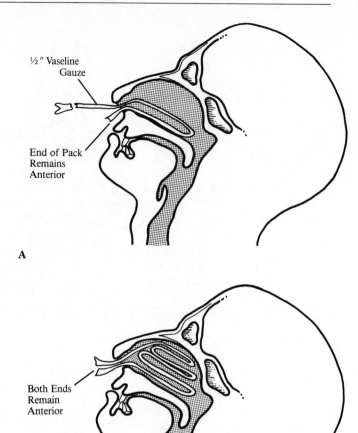

Figure 39–5 **A,** First step in anterior nasal pack procedure. **B,** Completing anterior nasal pack. (Based on drawings by Lewis DeMent, M.D., F.A.C.E.P.)

Again, the first step is anesthesia. The anterior nose is anesthetized as previously described. The oral pharynx and uvula can be sprayed with benzocaine to help retard the inevitable gag reflex.

A small rubber catheter is then placed through the nostril on the affected side and grabbed with forceps as it passes the uvula, bringing the end of the catheter through the mouth[19] (Figure 39–6). This is a natural pause in the procedure, and the patient can briefly rest while the two-string end of the lambswool pack is tied to the catheter. Then, while asking the patient to open the mouth wide, to not bite the physician's fingers, and to breathe through the mouth, the lambswool is placed behind the uvula with the fingers on one hand while the other hand pulls the catheter with the two strings through the nose. Again, a natural pause is present so the patient can rest. The bleeding is now controlled because the physician can simply hold the pack by the two strings and pinch the nostrils, causing effective anterior-posterior tamponade. The anterior pack is then placed and the two strings tied over a roll of gauze, causing no

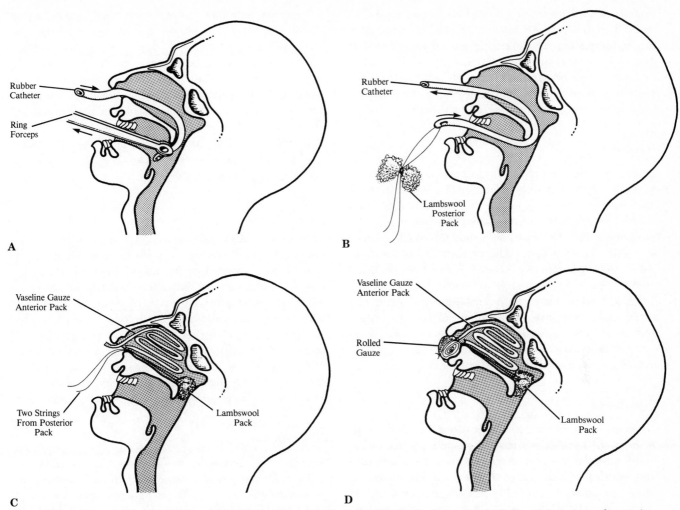

Figure 39–6   Posterior pack. **A,** Step 1: Passing rubber catheter. **B,** Step 2: Placing lambswool pack. **C,** Step 3: Anterior and posterior packs in place. **D,** Step 4: Securing packs. (Based on drawings by Lewis DeMent, M.D., F.A.C.E.P.)

pressure on the alae or columella. The remaining string dangling beyond the uvula is cut off at that level and will later facilitate removal of the pack.

Patients who have a posterior pack placed are at an increased risk for sinusitis,[19] and their general misery and potential for having life-threatening hemorrhage necessitate their hospitalization. Additional attention should be given to those patients who have chronic lung disease and a low PO_2 since the patient's PO_2 often decreases with a posterior pack in place.[20] A thorough in-hospital workup is then done to rule out a coagulation disorder or occult nasopharyngeal pathology.

In some patients, epistaxis may still be present after the unilateral anterior-posterior pack. The other nostril should then be packed in an anterior-posterior fashion, and most bleeding will then stop. An occasional patient may have to go to surgery rather urgently to have a vessel ligated if a bilateral anterior-posterior pack does not control the bleeding.

A patient who arrives in the emergency department after nasal bleeding has stopped presents an interesting therapeutic question. Should the nose be cauterized or packed even though not bleeding? In many patients who bleed from the septum, a small pimple-like area on the septum will be seen. This is usually the artery that bled, and it should be cauterized.

If no septal site is found, the question of packing remains. After the physician explains the packing procedure, most patients, providing they are medically stable and have an adequate home situation, elect to go home and return if the bleeding recurs. This approach seems to make sense because it is very difficult to confidently prevent recurrences by packing a nose when it is not bleeding.

An older patient who has experienced epistaxis should have a thorough ENT examination. Although simple anterior bleeding may be present, the patient should be evaluated to be certain that the bleeding does not represent the early signs of systemic disease such as leukemia or signs of local disease such as nasopharyngeal cancer.

THROAT

It is not that the treatment of acute throat problems differs so much from younger people, it is the heightened awareness that potentially dangerous causes in the elderly, if overlooked, can have tragic consequences. Most throat complaints in the elderly person are related to difficulty in swallowing and pain. Although many of these symptoms may be chronic and annoying, some may be acute or prompt a visit to the emergency department because of their progressively worsening nature.

Infection

In general, throat infections are less common in the older adult than in the child or middle-aged person. Although pharyngitis may still be present in the elderly, and an occasional patient with epiglottitis may be encountered,[22] an expanded differential diagnosis should be considered such as diphtheria, Ludwig's angina, candidiasis, and pharyngitis associated with leukopenia. These more unusual causes of pharyngitis must be considered because the elderly are more likely to be debilitated or immunosuppressed and to have serious chronic underlying disease such as diabetes or leukemia. These diseases usually require more treatment and follow-up care than most common causes of pharyngitis in the younger person.

Diphtheria

Although usually thought of as a disease of children in years past, diphtheria strikes the adult population as well.[23] Once an epidemic is started in an area, a significant number of older persons will usually be affected. During an epidemic from 1972 to 1975 in Seattle's "Skid Road" area, 11% of the cases and carriers were over 60 years old.[24] Recognizing the early cases in an epidemic can be a significant problem because the most common initial symptom is a sore throat[25] even before the telltale "dirty" pharyngeal membrane develops.

Diphtheria immunizations are effective for approximately 10 years, but many older persons are not immunized. Since the mortality rate continues to be in the 10% range, a high index of suspicion is warranted.[25] Cardiac failure, otitis media, vocal cord paralysis, adrenal insufficiency, and pneumonia are a few of the complications that are known to occur, so early recognition is paramount. Antibiotics (penicillin and erythromycin) will clear the body of the organism, but the mainstay of treatment is 40,000 to 100,000 units of antitoxin that are given intravenously after a scratch test is performed to check for antitoxin sensitivity.[23,25]

Ludwig's Angina

Ludwig's angina often occurs in the presence of poor oral hygiene in elderly debilitated men.[26] Infection spreads through minor traumatic lesions or infected teeth through the floor of the mouth and, by definition, involves sublingual and submaxillary spaces bilaterally.

These patients have a brawny cellulitis of the floor of the mouth, which tends to push the tongue upward. Because there is a danger of upper airway obstruction, these patients should be admitted to the intensive care unit. Pharyngeal cultures should be obtained prior to starting the patient on intravenous broad-spectrum antibiotics, including an aminoglycoside and a penicillinase-resistant penicillin. If a respiratory arrest occurs, a cricothyrotomy may have to be performed because routine tracheal intubation is often impossible because of the massive hypopharyngeal edema.[27]

Candidiasis

Candidiasis, which is usually seen in infants, may be seen in the elderly patient who has been on antibiotics or is immunosuppressed or debilitated from other chronic disease.[23] Even though the pain may not be severe as in other causes of pharyngitis, it nevertheless interferes with eating and swallowing. Candidiasis is recognized by the white cheesy patches on the oral and pharyngeal mucosa that, when scraped off, reveal an erythematous base. The initial treatment consists of stopping antibiotics and starting nystatin suspension 4 times a day and, of course, searching for any underlying disorder.

Neutropenia

Almost any hematologic disorder that results in neutropenia can cause a severe sore throat secondary to local bacterial invasion. These patients often appear ill and febrile and have cervical adenitis. Agranulocytosis caused by medications must also be kept in mind in addition to primary hematologic disorders. The patient tends to deteriorate rapidly unless antibiotics are started quickly.[23] (See Chapter 35.)

Peritonsillar Abscess (Quinsy)

The presence of a peritonsillar abscess must be recognized because the usual treatment for pharyngitis with antibiotics will not suffice. The typical history is one of persistent sore throat, odynophagia, and ear pain after antibiotic treatment.[28] On examination, the peritonsillar area is swollen and tends to push the uvula to the opposite side. Although this entity tends to occur in young and middle-aged adults, in the elderly patient this abscess may be superimposed on a tumor or, in rare cases, an internal carotid aneurysm.[29] It takes little imagination to appreciate the horror and chaos associated with an inadvertent incision and drainage of the internal carotid artery in the emergency department.

Incision and drainage should be performed in the emergency department only if a definite nonpulsatile, fluctuant abscess is present and assistance is available to aid in suctioning the patient. In most cases in the elderly, an ENT physician should be consulted and the patient admitted to the hospital. Abscesses that are not completely drained or that are treated late in their course may progress to peripharyngeal or retropharyngeal abscesses, which may be fatal if not treated.[23,28]

Cancer

A normal mouth and throat examination in the presence of sore throat symptoms should alert the physician to thoroughly evaluate the hypopharynx for malignancy. The common squamous cell cancers of the larynx are noted for causing the symptoms of pain on swallowing, hoarseness, and referred pain in the ear. This diagnosis should especially be considered in a chronic smoker or an alcoholic.[23] Any progressive sore throat, especially one that has persisted 2 or 3 weeks or recurred following antibiotic therapy, should be considered to represent a malignancy until proven otherwise. It is also rather characteristic of cancer that the throat pain may be transiently improved with antibiotic therapy and intensified by ingestion of citrus juices.[23] In a smoker who has a progressive history of a lump in the throat, the examiner must prove that a supraglottic tumor (typically squamous cell type) does not exist.[23,25]

Foreign Bodies

Foreign bodies in the pharynx and esophagus are common in the elderly population. Often, poor eyesight contributes to the problem; the person has difficulty seeing small objects such as fish bones. There may be trouble in mastication in general and less sensation in the mouth because of the presence of dentures, causing small objects to pass into the throat initially unnoticed.[23]

Problems that are seen in the emergency department usually are related to pharyngeal or esophageal foreign bodies. With the exception of chronic aspiration syndromes or acute "cafe coronary" presentations, foreign bodies that lodge in the glottis or trachea or are otherwise aspirated usually are expelled by the patient or found later when the patient develops pneumonia or other respiratory symptoms.

Pharyngeal

Small, sharp objects usually stick in the tonsils, tongue, or periepiglottic area in the vallecula or piriform sinuses.[23] Patients usually can localize[30] foreign bodies that lie above the cricopharyngeus, and it is mandatory to adequately view these periepiglottic areas when a patient complains of a localized pain. On occasion, a foreign body can be seen in a tonsil simply by looking into the patient's mouth. Usually, however, either indirect laryngoscopy or direct laryngoscopy with a strong headlight and a large mirror to adequately visualize the hypo-

pharynx will be required. When a foreign body is seen, it can be grasped with a long clamp and removed.

If a thorough examination reveals no foreign body, then the examiner may wish to use plain x-ray films to find a foreign body if it is known to be opaque.[23] If the patient is otherwise asymptomatic, the pharynx may have been only scratched, and the patient will improve in 24 to 48 hours. If no improvement is noted, then more investigation will be needed.

Esophageal

Although serious hemorrhage does not usually occur with esophageal foreign bodies, esophageal obstruction and esophageal perforation with mediastinitis are known complications.[31] There are also more severe but unusual complications, such as fatal hemorrhage from an esophageal foreign body that erodes into the aorta.[32] Esophageal foreign bodies usually become impacted at the cricopharyngeus, in the upper one third of the esophagus, or at the gastroesophageal sphincter. Although local pain that increases with swallowing accompanied by hypersalivation is the classic triad for the diagnosis of an esophageal foreign body, the presence of hypersalivation alone after an episode of difficulty correlates highly with the presence of an esophageal foreign body.[33] An elderly patient who is drooling or hypersalivating after eating should be suspected of having at least a partially obstructing esophageal foreign body.

If the history suggests an object that is radiopaque, such as a metal pin, plain x-ray films may reveal the location of the foreign body. This can then be removed by direct visualization during the esophagoscopy. If the history is one of choking on a bolus or food, then glucagon may be tried.[34] A dose of 1 mg is given intravenously and the patient observed for a few minutes. Being a smooth muscle relaxant, glucagon lowers the tone of the lower esophageal sphincter and allows the impacted bolus to pass into the stomach. If this treatment is not successful, then esophagoscopy may be required.

In general, when a skilled endoscopist is available, there is little need to do a barium swallow if clinical signs of obstruction are present because the barium tends to make the foreign body harder to see during esophagoscopy.[23] The use of a barium swallow is better left to elucidate suspected motility problems and dysphagia. In this case, the irritating foreign body, such as a small piece of bay leaf, may not cause an esophageal obstruction but might catch a swallowed barium-coated cotton ball, showing up well on the x-ray film during fluoroscopy.

LARYNGEAL TRAUMA

Fracture of the larynx usually occurs in the setting of an assault from a direct blow to the throat or in an automobile accident as the neck strikes the dashboard or steering wheel. The diagnosis is made from the history and clinical findings of hoarseness, subcutaneous emphysema, stridor, hemoptysis, and often a flattened thyroid cartilage. A problem for the emergency physician then becomes how to protect an airway that may be already partially obstructed or may at any time become fully obstructed.

This is one of the few times in airway management when tracheal intubation is probably not the best initial choice. Some physicians feel that the airway may be compromised further by attempting to intubate the patient.[23,25] The sense of urgency the emergency physician feels may be the best guide. If the patient is not in severe distress, then a more controlled but urgent tracheotomy may be a safer approach. This procedure is usually performed under local anesthesia by an ENT physician. Of course, if a patient is in immediate danger, intubation may have to be the first choice. The anatomy is usually distorted enough that a cricothyrotomy is not a good option. In more minor cases, if a fractured larynx is suspected, an ENT specialist should evaluate the patient promptly because if surgery is required, the patients who have their surgery in the first 24 hours have fewer subsequent problems with breathing and speaking.[25,36]

REFERENCES

1. Walike JW: Management of acute ear infections, Otolaryngol Clin North Am 12:439–445, 1979.
2. Farmer HS: A guide for the treatment of external otitis, Am Fam Physician 21:96–101, 1980.
3. Chandler JR: Pathogenesis and treatment of facial paralysis due to malignant external otitis, Ann Otol Rhinol Laryngol 81:648–658, 1972.
4. Chandler JR: Malignant external otitis, Laryngoscope 78:1257–1293, 1968.
5. Griffin WL: A retrospective study of traumatic tympanic membrane perforation in a clinical practice, Laryngoscope 89:261–281, 1979.
6. Feldman H: Sudden hearing loss: a clinic survey, Adv Otorhinolaryngol 27:40–69, 1981.
7. Morrison AW: Acute deafness, Br J Hosp 19(3):237–242, 1978.
8. Wilson WR et al: The relationship of idiopathic sudden hearing loss to diabetes mellitus, Laryngoscope 92:155–160, 1982.
9. Mattox DE: Medical management of sudden hearing loss, Otolaryngol Head Neck Surg 88:111–113, 1980.
10. Lindeman RC: Acute labyrinthine disorders, Otolaryngol Clin North Am 12:375–387, 1979.
11. Clemis JD and Becker GW: Vestibular neuronitis, Otolaryngol Clin North Am 6:139–155, 1973.
12. Heyman A et al: Report of the Joint Committee for Stroke Facilities. XI. Transient focal cerebral ischemia: epidemiological and clinical aspects, Stroke 5:275–287, 1974.
13. Garner JT and Jacques S: Positional vertigo and bruit: a surgical emergency, West J Med 127:414–416, 1977.
14. Yarington TC Jr: Sinusitis as an emergency, Otolaryngol Clin North Am 12:447–454, 1979.
15. Sheffield RW, Cassisi NJ, and Karlan MS: Complications of sinusitis, Postgrad Med 63:93–101, 1978.
16. Schultz RC and deVillers YT: Nasal fractures, J Trauma 15:319–327, 1975.
17. Jordan LW: Acute nasal and septal injuries, Eye, Ear, Nose and Throat Monthly 53:508–512, 1974.
18. Lingeman RE: Epistaxis, Am Fam Physician 14:79–83, 1976.
19. DeWeese DD et al: From a to z in nosebleed control, Patient Care, pp. 66–83, 1978.
20. Lin YT and Orkin LR: Arterial hypoxemia in patients with anterior and posterior nasal packings, Laryngoscope 89:140–149, 1979.
21. Polcyn JL: Epistaxis from rupture of aneurysm of internal carotid artery, JAMA 213(5):876, 1970.
22. Lindquist JR: Acute infections of supraglottis in adults, Ann Emerg Med 9(5):256–259, 1980.
23. Cody DTR: Diseases of the ears, nose and throat, Chicago, 1981, Year Book Medical Publishers Inc.
24. Pedersen AHB: Diphtheria on skid road, Seattle, Washington, 1972–1975, Pub Health Rep 92:336–342, 1977.
25. Boies LR Jr: Boies' fundamentals of otolaryngology, Philadelphia, 1978, WB Saunders Co.
26. Meyer BR, Lawson W, and Hirschman SZ: Ludwig's angina: case report with review of bacteriology and current therapy, Am J Med 53:257–262, 1972.
27. Rosen P et al: Emergency medicine: concepts and clinical practice, ed 2, St Louis, 1987, The CV Mosby Co.
28. Muller SP: Peritonsillar abscess: a prospective study of pathogens, treatment and morbidity, Ear Nose Throat 57:439–444, 1978.
29. Henry RC: Aneurysm of internal carotid artery presenting as a peritonsillar abscess, J Laryngol Otol 88:379–384, 1974.
30. Haglund S et al: Radiographic diagnosis of foreign bodies in the esophagus, J Laryngol Otol 92:1117, 1978.
31. Norberg HP and Reyes HM: Complications of ornamental Christmas bulb ingestion: care report and review of literature, Arch Surg 110:1494–1495, 1975.
32. Singh B et al: A fatal denture in the esophagus, J Laryngol Otol 92:829, 1978.
33. Allen T: Suspected esophageal foreign body: choosing appropriate managment, JACEP 8(3):101–105, 1979.
34. Glauser J, Lilja GP, and Greenfeld B: Intravenous glucagon in the management of esophageal food obstruction, JACEP 8:228, 1979.
35. Olson NR: Surgical treatment of acute blunt laryngeal injuries, Ann Otol Rhinol Laryngol 87:716–721, 1978.
36. Leopold DA: Laryngeal trauma, Arch Otolaryngol 109:106–111, 1983.
37. Isaacman DJ: Otitic hydrocephalus: an uncommon complication of a common condition, Ann Emerg Med 18:684, 1989.

Arthritic and Connective Tissue Disorders

Joint, Bone, and Connective Tissue Disease in the Elderly

Donald A. Wiens, M.D., F.A.C.E.P.

Rheumatic disorders are endemic in the elderly population. At any given time, about 40% of people over age 70 have back and/or other peripheral joint complaints. This percentage continues to increase with age and generally is higher in females than in males.[1,2]

Most patients have chronic progressive arthritic disorders, for which a diagnosis is already known and, consequently, the disposition in the emergency department may involve only symptomatic care and relief. Other patients may present with articular disorders for which rapid, accurate diagnosis and treatment can provide both significant relief of joint pain and prevention or reduction of future disability. Joints, like any other organ system with chronic disease, can develop acute disorders that indicate a flare of their underlying disease or a new disorder that is distinct from their underlying pathology. Awareness of joint disease patterns can prevent misdiagnosis of extraarticular and nonarticular disease as an articular disorder.[3]

Arthritis is defined as a pathologic alteration of structure and function in the tissues of the joints, and arthralgia is joint pain without physical or radiographic findings. Causes of arthritis and arthralgias are multiple, and detailed classifications to categorize the many arthritic conditions exist.[4] However, the joint itself, including synovial fluid, synovium, cartilage, and subchondral bone, has a limited means of expressing pathology and a systemic evaluation will allow accurate diagnosis and recognition of emergent disorders and complications.

HISTORY

The history should detail whether the symptoms are acute, subacute, or chronic. Also to be considered in the geriatric patient is whether this is an acute flare-up of a chronic joint problem. A history of systemic symptoms can be helpful in making the diagnosis. The presence of fever and chills is important as well as the more protean symptoms of malaise, fatigue, or poor appetite. Simply asking patients what diagnoses they have been given by their primary care physicians is often helpful in determining a chronic arthritic problem. Obtaining any history of recent trauma to the affected area, even if this trauma seems very slight, is useful. Also, a review of current medications and past therapy of similar conditions may be helpful in directing current treatment. Signs or symptoms of multiple joint involvement or a remote site of infection are also important to determine as is a review of other chronic medical problems. Many commonly used medications are relatively or absolutely contraindicated with other underlying organ disease. This will be discussed in further detail later in this chapter.

PHYSICAL EXAMINATION

During the physical examination, special attention should be paid to the patient's temperature, and to ocular, cardiac, and dermatologic findings. The examination of the affected joint or joints should include palpation of the overlying skin, skin temperature, skin color, and the presence or absence of palpable pain and swelling. The evaluation of swelling should determine whether this is the fluctuant feeling of an effusion or abscess, the doughy sensation of palpating synovial thickening, or of bony hardness. Range of motion of the affected joint or joints should be evaluated identifying motion with or without pain. Determine the distal tendon function, especially in patients presenting with problems of the fingers and wrists. Clues to chronicity may involve extensor tendon rupture, bony thickening, and muscle atrophy (especially in the muscle groups proximal to the affected joint) and should be sought.[2,3]

Diagnostic studies include radiographic, joint fluid analysis, and pertinent blood tests. The x-ray of the affected joint should be evaluated for the presence of an effusion, disruption, or destruction of the joint spaces, evidence of extraarticular or intraarticular calcifications, and subchondral bony changes. The subchondral bony changes can include bone thickening, osteophyte formation, and cystic degeneration. Also to be kept in mind in the geriatric patient with chronic joint disease and underlying osteoporosis are fractures following either minimal or almost no trauma. An exacerbation of back or neck pain can imply a compression fracture in the lumbar or thoracic spine, and a sudden increase in joint pain following very minor injuries can indicate a pathologic fracture in an already weakened extremity bone.

The analysis of joint fluid should be considered in any geriatric patient presenting with new onset of a painful, swollen joint and also should be considered in patients having a sudden flare of joint symptoms, even if an underlying diagnosis such as osteoarthritis or rheumatoid arthritis is known. Table 40–1 shows joint fluid findings in certain disease patterns.

Blood tests may or may not be helpful, and many that are eventually diagnostic would not be available on a timely enough basis to be useful in an emergency room (ER) disposition. A complete blood count (CBC), a uric acid rate, and a sedimentation rate are readily available from most laboratories. These tests rarely in and of themselves are diagnostic except perhaps for an elevated uric acid. Many other special tests exist, such as rheumatoid factor, ANA titers, and complement studies, but it would be a unique ED where these were available quickly.

OSTEOARTHRITIS

Osteoarthritis is the most commonly diagnosed joint disorder in the elderly population. If radiographic criteria are used, which include joint space narrowing, bony sclerosis, cyst formation, and osteophyte formation, the prevalence of osteoarthritis by age 70 approaches almost 100%. The number of people in this age group with func-

Table 40–1   Joint Fluid Findings

	Color	Clarity	Viscosity*	WBC	RBC	Crystals	Bacteria	% Glucose†
Normal	Straw	Clear	High	0–200	0	—	—	100
Traumatic	Amber/ bloody	Hazy	High	200–2000 75–90% PMNs‡	Many	—	—	100
Degenerative joint disorders	Straw	Slightly hazy	High	–1000 20% PMNs	0–few	—	—	100
Gout and pseudogout	Yellow/ milky	Cloudy	Medium	15,000 50–75% PMNs	0–few	Present	—	90
Rheumatoid arthritis	Yellow Green	Cloudy	Medium to low	20,000 50–75% PMNs	0–few	—	—	75
Septic	Gray	Cloudy	Low	50,000+ 90% PMNs	Few	—	Present§	50
Inflammatory	Straw	Cloudy	Medium	15–20,000 50–75% PMNs	Few	—	—	75–90

*Easily done with a drop of fluid between gloved fingers.
†As percent of serum level.
‡Polymorphonuclear leukocytes.
§Gram stain often negative.

tional loss, or symptomatic osteoarthritis, at any given time is less than half of this percentage.[3,4]

Primary Osteoarthritis

Osteoarthritis is divided into primary osteoarthritis, in which a precipitating cause of the arthritis is unknown, and secondary osteoarthritis, in which an initiating factor or factors can be discerned. Osteoarthritis should be thought of as a "final common pathway" rather than a discrete clinical entity. Most patients have primary osteoarthritis. This is a disease of aging and is more prevalent symptomatically in females than males. It is a disease of all races, and obesity has been felt to be a risk factor although recent studies have weakened this proposition.

Secondary Osteoarthritis

Secondary osteoarthritis has numerous underlying etiologies. These can be broken down into three major categories: mechanical disorders, congenital or developmental disorders, and systemic diseases. Trauma is the leading mechanical factor for development of secondary osteoarthritis. This includes fractures that enter into the joint space with disruption of the joint surface, postoperative degeneration, and major injury to the supportive structures of a joint, such as collateral ligament rupture of the knee or third-degree ankle sprains. Septic arthritis, especially if a delay in diagnosis and treatment occurs, will lead to extensive joint damage and, eventually, degenerative arthritic changes. Osteoarthritis often follows other arthritides such as gout or rheumatoid arthritis.

Less Common Causes

Aseptic necrosis also has a mechanical etiology. The alcoholic, diabetic, or chronic steroid therapy patient is at risk for this form of secondary osteoarthritis. Congenital and developmental abnormalities usually affect the hip. Congenital hip dislocation, Legg-Perthes disease, and slipped capital femoral epiphysis may cause one third to one half of cases of hip osteoarthritis. Numerous systemic diseases can also lead to joint degeneration. These include numerous rare inborn errors of metabolism or more common diseases such as diabetes and sickle cell anemia. In general, any systemic disease that can decrease joint blood flow, deposit abnormal metabolites, or affect peripheral nerve function and position sense will lead to joint degeneration.

Presenting Symptoms and Examination

The usual presenting complaint in osteoarthritis is joint pain. A typical history of the affected joint is pain with use and relief with rest. This pain is usually aching. This will progress to chronic pain including nocturnal joint pain with exacerbation from activity. The etiology of chronic pain is felt to be some combination of periosteal elevation and damage by osteophyte formation and possibly microfractures in areas of weakened cystic bone. Morning joint stiffness that relieves rapidly with use is the second cardinal symptom of osteoarthritis.[2]

The historical pattern that helps differentiate osteoarthritis from other arthritides is the above presentations of pain. The disease is insidious and usually takes months to years to develop. There are no systemic symptoms associated with osteoarthritis unless an underlying secondary disorder is causing these symptoms. Osteoarthritis is usually monarticular in its early presentation. The cervical and lumbar spine, hips, knees, and the interphalangeal joints of the hand are the usual involved joints in more established disease. This should be contrasted with rheumatoid arthritis, which usually has a more rapid polyarticular onset with systemic symptoms present in more severe disease. The joints commonly involved in rheumatoid arthritis are the wrist, elbows, ankles, and feet, which are uncommon joint sites in osteoarthritis.

The physical examination depends on the joints involved. Again, the hands are common sites of osteoarthritis. The distal interphalangeal joints are the most frequent site with bony thickening on the posterior joint surface being present. This bony sclerosis seen on the distal interphalangeal joints is known as Heberden's nodes. The proximal interphalangeal joints are also affected with the same pattern of posterior joint bony hypertrophy. This produces what is known as a Bouchard's node. The other hand site that is affected with some frequency in osteoarthritis is the first metacarpal phalangeal joint. Despite dramatic radiographic changes of bony thickening and joint destruction, most patients maintain fairly good hand function and little or no pain with hand use except in very advanced disease.

The presence of a warm, tender joint and/or an effusion with x-ray changes of osteoarthritis may be osteoarthritis but should suggest the possibility of a secondary joint process such as gout or infection. Involvement of the wrist, elbow, or shoulder is uncommon in osteoarthritis, as mentioned, unless prior joint trauma has occurred. Arthritic symptoms in these areas should suggest rheumatoid arthritis or an extraarticular pathology. Osteoarthritis of the hip is often secondary. Initially, there is little limitation of motion, and patients will present with pain that is perceived either in the hip, buttocks, or groin. Progression of disease in the hip will lead to an antalgic gait. This is an asymmetrical gait characterized by a shortened weight-bearing phase of the affected hip. The knees are frequent sites of osteoarthritis because of constant load-bearing trauma during ambulation. Involvement of the knee can lead to some of the most severe functional impairment seen in osteoarthritis. Involvement of the spine, at least by radiographic criteria, is present in almost 100% of adults age 70 or greater. Again, fewer than half of these patients will be symptomatic with this. The presenting symptoms of vertebral involvement include the insidious onset of pain, usually most prominent in the morning and with the development of stiffness.

Cervical Spondylitic Myelopathy

An uncommon but important to recognize complication of cervical osteoarthritis is a disorder known as cervical spondylitic myelopathy. This disorder is characterized initially by nonspecific complaints such as heaviness or numbness in the hands and feet. Later symptoms include increasing difficulty with ambulation, falls, and the development of bowel and bladder incontinence. The physical examination will reveal a reduction of cervical range of motion and often will show pain radiating down the arms and back with head flexion and extension. Spasticity in extremity muscle groups is seen in advanced disease, and often the most important and relevant early physical finding is brisk or very hyperactive tendon reflexes.[5,6]

The etiology of this disorder is impingement on the posterior spinal cord by osteophytes formed on the vertebral bodies. The patient at most risk for developing cervical spondylitic myelopathy is a patient with an underlying spinal stenosis and osteophyte formation. Lateral cervical spine films are an aid in making this diagnosis. Determination should be made of the canal spacing. This can be done by measuring the distance from the posterior aspect of the vertebral body to a point where the laminae of the spinous process fuse. Normal adults should show a distance of approximately 16 to 18 mm. In cervical spondylitic myelopathy, this distance measures between roughly 10 and 14 mm, and osteophyte formation is present.[7,8] Physical findings that suggest upper motor neuron disease and canal narrowing on x-ray should lead to at least a presumptive diagnosis of this disorder. The relevance of early recognition of cervical spondylitic myelopathy is that referral to an orthopedist for performance of either a decompression procedure or a stabilization procedure may prevent or delay the development of a wheelchair-bound incontinent elderly patient.[9,10]

Vascular Syndromes

Vascular syndromes can occur in elderly patients with severe osteoarthritis and osteophyte formation. The vascular foramina for the vertebral arteries sit lateral to the mass of the vertebral body in the cervical spine. Osteophyte impingement in the foramina can cause vertebrobasilar insufficiency. Symptoms of this include syncope or near syncope, drop attacks, or the presence of cranial nerve symptoms such as diplopia, dysarthria, or bilateral visual field defects. These symptoms may be positional and can be reproduced by cervical range-of-motion maneuvers. In the lumbar spine, a cauda equina syndrome can develop. This should be suspected in patients who develop aching pain in the low back or in the legs. Paresthesias, especially after exertion, can occur as this syndrome progresses.

Treatment Considerations

The treatment of uncomplicated osteoarthritis complaints is symptomatic. The affected joints should be put at rest and a mild to moderate-strength antiinflammatory medication prescribed. The most frequently used drugs are Indocin, Naprosyn, or Motrin. In the elderly patient (especially those with cardiac disorders or underlying renal disease, or those taking diuretics), medications such as Clinoril or Feldene may be safer to use than other nonsteroidal antiinflammatory drugs. Referral should be made for follow-up with the patient's internist or rheumatologist. Patients presenting with neurovascular complaints are a special management problem. Many of these conditions have developed over a long period of time and result in a fixed deficit that will not be amenable to surgical correction. Some patients, especially if diagnosed early, will respond to surgical decompression or fixation procedures and significant future impairment can be prevented.[6,8,9]

Caveats in Diagnosis

A caveat to bear in mind with the diagnosis and treatment of osteoarthritis is that it is a chronic, gradually progressive disease, usually without marked acute inflammatory joint symptoms. An acute, inflamed joint and an acute or subacute onset of polyarticular disease should be diagnosed as osteoarthritis very cautiously. Almost all elderly patients will show evidence of vertebral and hand radiographic changes consistent with osteoarthritis. Many will not have symptoms to go with these changes. An acute flare-up of disease involving these sites with appropriate radiographic findings still may not be osteoarthritis, and other syndromes causing pain in these areas should be considered. Finally, osteoarthritis rarely causes thoracic symptoms. Patients presenting with symptoms of pain referable to the thoracic spine often turn out to have disorders other than osteoarthritis. Mediastinal, vascular, gastric, and pancreatic pathology should always be kept in mind in elderly patients presenting with complaints referable to the thoracic area despite x-ray evidence of osteoarthritic changes in the thoracic spine.

RHEUMATOID ARTHRITIS

Rheumatoid arthritis is a systemic disease of all mesenchymal tissues that most frequently manifests as a joint disorder. It has an incidence of 1 to 2% in adult populations. Onset can be seen in childhood (juvenile rheumatoid arthritis), frequently in the twenties and thirties, and, occasionally, new onset of disease can occur up to the eighties or nineties. The prevalence again is higher in females. In most cases, rheumatoid arthritis is a progressive disease, and pain symptoms along with functional loss proceed with aging. The onset of disease can be gradual and chronic but also can occur acutely as a polyarticular inflammatory process with systemic symptoms of fever, malaise, painful adenopathy, splenomegaly, and occasionally with pleural and pericardial disease. This disorder is known as Still's disease and can occur up into the seventh, eighth, and ninth decades but is usually associated with a younger population.[11,12]

The suggested pathogenesis of rheumatoid arthritis is by rheumatoid factor. This is an immune globulin that can be of the IgM, IgG, or IgA class. This immune globulin is specific for complexing with the constant portion of IgG (the Fc fragment). The formation of rheumatoid factor–IgG complexes allows activation of the complement and the initiation of inflammatory synovial and joint disease. The systemic complications, which include vasculitis, rheumatoid nodule formation, and pleural and pericardial disease, probably occur by a similar mechanism. Interestingly, diseases that generate a chronic antigenic challenge, such as chronic infections like tuberculosis, subacute bacterial endocarditis, or hepatitis, and diseases of the collagen vascular class can produce positive rheumatoid factor titers.[13,14]

In the geriatric patient, the presentation may be acute or subacute symmetrical polyarticular disease. Fever is often present, and there has been a prodrome of malaise and fatigue. These patients are often quite ill and may end up needing to be admitted to the hospital to achieve initial control of their disease.[15] The presentation is often less clear, and, occasionally, the diagnosis is made after a workup of a fever of unknown origin. The more usual presentation in the elderly with new onset rheumatoid arthritis is a gradual monarticular or pauciarticular disease with few systemic symptoms, often following minor trauma. The differentiation between this and simple posttraumatic arthritis can be difficult especially since rheumatoid factor titers will probably be negative early in the disease. Laboratory findings are often not helpful. In acute severe disease, there is a leukocytosis, an elevated erythrocyte sedimentation rate (ESR) often in the range of 50 to 80, and positive rheumatoid factor. In milder disease, the only laboratory abnormality may be an elevated ESR. This should be contrasted with osteoarthritis in which the sedimentation rate will be normal unless other underlying disease is present that would elevate this. Analysis of synovial fluid may need to be done to differentiate a septic joint from a joint affected with rheumatoid arthritis. This differentiation may be difficult since there is some overlap with infectious arthritis in joint fluid findings as far as showing a very elevated white blood count in the range of 50,000 to 70,000 with a polymorphonuclear lymphocyte predominance. Secondary to metabolic activity of the leukocytes, the glucose level may also be low — a feature found in the septic joint as well. A further complication is that a septic joint may not show organisms on initial Gram stain. A helpful early clinical clue is that the joint inflamed from rheumatoid arthritis, even with effusion present, probably should not show redness.[14-16]

Radiographic findings in rheumatoid arthritis, especially early in the disease course, usually will show soft tissue swelling and, occasionally, some osteoporosis along the joint surface. This may be best seen where the synovium reflects onto the joint capsule. As the disease progresses, subchondral cyst formation and bony erosion are more prominent. Osteoporosis will often occur in advanced rheumatoid arthritis. Joint space narrowing and subluxations are common in more advanced disease as extensive joint destruction occurs.

Most elderly patients who present to the emergency department will have an established diagnosis of rheumatoid arthritis and are presenting with joint pain as a complication of a secondary joint disorder on top of, or with systemic complications of, rheumatoid arthritis. A systematic evaluation of specific joint sites should confirm the underlying diagnosis and reveal complications of rheumatoid disease.[12,16]

Examination of the hands is helpful in differentiation with osteoarthritis. The wrists and the metacarpophalangeal joints are most frequently involved in rheumatoid arthritis as opposed to more distal joint involvement in osteoarthritis. The "boutonniere" deformity, which is prominent over the dorsal surface of the metacarpophalangeal joints, occurs in rheumatoid arthritis. Marked bony destruction eventually leading to ulnar deviation of the wrist and prominence of the ulnar styloid occurs in advanced disease with rheumatoid arthritis. The extensor tendons of the wrists and fingers are involved and weakened as they cross the inflamed synovium and hypertrophied bone tissue. Extensor tendon rupture can follow very minimal trauma or even be spontaneous in rheumatoid arthritis. This should be suspected in patients presenting with acute loss of wrist and finger function from their baseline. For best results in tendon rupture, these should be repaired soon, ideally within several days from the injury. The knee joint is commonly affected in rheumatoid arthritis. A large amount of synovial surface area in the joint capsule makes the knee a common site of disease. Early physical findings are loss of complete extension and laxity of supportive ligaments. Diagnosis at this point and early physical therapy can help retard development of debilitating flexion contractures. Chronic effusion combined with the elevation of intraarticular pressure, developed during long periods of standing and ambulation, leads to the formation of posterior protrusion of the joint capsule — Baker's cyst. The patient often will not present until this ruptures. Symptoms of acute Baker's cyst rupture are a painful swollen calf with tenderness to palpation and often a positive Homans' test. Differentiation obviously must be made in this case with deep venous thrombosis. The cervical spine is often severely affected in rheumatoid arthritis. Extensive anatomic changes may be present within a few years of disease onset. Marked subluxations can occur generally in the area of C1 to C6. These usually do not produce cord symptoms, but minimal trauma can lead to fracture or further subluxations with cervical cord injury.

Atlantoaxial Subluxation

Atlantoaxial subluxation occurs in at least 10% of established rheumatoid arthritis patients and probably more than this. The cruciform ligament holds the dens in check anteriorly, and the alar ligaments attach laterally and restrict rotation and transverse motion of the dens. Bony destruction and ligamentous involvement with development of laxity in these structures predispose to subluxations of the dens. Bony destruction can also produce vertical subluxation of the odontoid. These entities can be diagnosed radiographically.

In determination of atlantoaxial subluxations, the distance between the anterior surface of the dens and the ring of the atlas is measured. This should not exceed approximately 2.5 mm in normal individuals. Flexion and extension views may bring out subluxation more clearly. Vertical subluxation can be measured by drawing a line from the upper surface of the hard palate down to the caudal portion of the occiput when viewing the lateral cervical spine film. This is called McGregor's line. If the occiput protrudes approximately over 4 to 4.5 mm above this line, vertical subluxation exists. Either anatomic abnormality of vertical subluxation or atlantoaxial subluxation can lead to pressure on the medulla or the upper cervical cord by the odontoid.[10,15]

This can produce an entity called basilar impression.[16a] The clinical presentation of this syndrome consists of upper motor neuron signs of spasticity and hyperactive reflexes, ataxia, and lower cranial nerve signs, such as hoarseness, difficulty swallowing, or deviation on tongue protrusion. Anterior cord symptoms such as position and vibratory sense deficits may occur. More caudal invagination of the cord produces symptoms of neck pain, headaches, and pain and weakness predominantly in the arms. Again, early recognition of the disease and early surgical decompression can prevent significant impair-

ment in these lesions. In the presence of atlantoaxial subluxation, minor head or neck trauma can produce severe injury or death by acute high cervical cord or medullary damage. Maneuvers such as firm hyperextension of the neck to facilitate intubation can guarantee an unsuccessful resuscitation.

Rheumatoid Nodules

Rheumatoid arthritis is a disorder of all connective tissue and causes disease discrete from articular sites. Rheumatoid nodules occur in approximately 20 to 30% of patients with rheumatoid arthritis. The usual location is near the olecranon process or the proximal forearm. These are rarely relevant in the emergency department setting, except as diagnostic aids. Occasionally, they can present as a problem due to a breakdown of the nodule and development of skin ulcerations. If a rheumatoid nodule occurs over a weight-bearing area, such as the sacrum in a bedridden patient, breakdown and extensive decubitus formation will occur with a subsequent risk of systemic infection.[11-13]

Complications

Vasculitis may develop in patients with rheumatoid arthritis. There is a predilection for males who have had long-standing and more severely progressive disease. Clinically and pathologically, the vasculitis is similar to periarteritis nodosa. Initial manifestations may be small skin ulcerations or areas of gangrene on the tips of fingers or toes, as seen with digital artery involvement. Peripheral neuropathies may develop as the blood supply along the nerve, the vasa nervorum, is involved. The presence of these symptoms and the occurrence of chest pain should be approached cautiously with suspicion of ischemic cardiac disease entertained. Mesenteric artery involvement can occur leading to mesenteric insufficiency or acute bowel infarction. Treatment is directed to specific symptoms. High-dose steroid therapy may be helpful if secondary complications, especially of cardiac or intestinal origin, occur.

Ocular complications are usually one of three types. These are episcleritis, iritis or uveitis, or keratoconjunctivitis sicca. Episcleritis refers to superficial inflammation of the sclera. In rheumatoid arthritis, this is due to a localized vasculitis of the sclera and conjunctiva. This is usually seen as a localized conjunctival injection that can be quite tender if palpated through closed eyelids. Treatment with oral salicylates and steroid ophthalmic drops will usually give relief. Unfortunately, episcleritis in rheumatoid arthritis is often recurrent. In some cases, this may reflect a rheumatoid nodule of the sclera, and a severe complication is breakdown of the nodule and acute rupture of the globe with leakage of vitreous humor. Scleritis or uveitis also occurs. This can occur gradually or may occur acutely. Acute onset is often part of a generalized systemic disease flare, known as Still's disease. These patients show painful red eyes with a miotic pupil. Treatment for this consists of steroid drops and a mydriatic, and consultation with an ophthalmologist. A mydriatic is important not only for pain relief for the patient but also for the prevention of posterior synechia — a common complication of this disorder. Keratoconjunctivitis sicca occurs in up to 10% of rheumatoid arthritis patients. This is due to lacrimal gland changes in chronic disease. The patient may complain specifically of dry eyes but usually presents with a history of a scratchy feeling in the eyes or a mild foreign body sensation. Schirmer's test is confirmatory of this disorder. Treatment is symptomatic only and usually consists of administering a dilute saline solution such as Ocean or a methylcellulose solution. This is important to prevent corneal abrasions and damage from chronic dryness.

Pulmonary and cardiac complications can occur from vasculitic disease and ischemic cardiac disease. With involvement of the pericardium, pericarditis and pericardial effusions develop, although this is frequently subclinical. An acute tamponade from a rheumatoid effusion is an extremely rare entity, but chronic mild congestive symptoms can occur with large effusions. Pleural effusions occur and can become large enough to cause respiratory symptoms. Differentiation from other more acutely serious causes of effusion is important.[10-14]

Patients with rheumatoid arthritis also are more susceptible to infections. This is probably due to the disease itself and possibly also due to the treatment regimens these patients undergo, which include steroids and sometimes other immunosuppressive medications. A rare complication, known as Felty's syndrome, is the presence of severe leukopenia and splenomegaly in rheumatoid arthritis patients. Infectious complications, until splenectomy is done, are very common in this condition. Hematogenous spread of infection into damaged and scarred joint tissue leads to septic joints in these patients. As mentioned earlier, be especially careful ascribing a hot, red, painful joint in the rheumatoid patient to just a flare-up of rheumatoid disease without very carefully ruling out septic origin for the change in joint symptoms.

GOUT AND PSEUDOGOUT

Gout and pseudogout are examples of secondary arthritis as is rheumatoid arthritis. The joint symptoms are one facet of an underlying systemic disease process. Gout and pseudogout are arthropathies induced by inflammatory reaction in the joint space to crystal formation.

Gout is a frequent cause of monarticular joint pain seen in the emergency department. In more severe cases, gout may present as a polyarticular disease though this is unusual. A gouty arthritis occurs when uric acid crystals in the joint space are phagocytized by polymorphonuclear (PMN) lymphocytes. An acute syndrome evolves as the PMNs degranulate and release the chemical mediators of inflammation. The urate crystals get into the joint space following minor trauma with dislodgement from tophaceous deposits in the synovium, or they can crystallize spontaneously in the synovial fluid when levels of uric acid reach saturation point. Gout occurs when elevated uric acid levels (usually 7 mg/100 mL or higher) persist over a long period of time or short higher elevation occurs. The etiology of this is from specific enzyme defects that lead either to overproduction of the purines (adenine and guanine) or, more commonly, to underexcretion of uric acid by the kidneys. In susceptible individuals, decreasing the glomerular filtration rate increases the likelihood of attack. This can be seen during the development of kidney disease from any cause, dehydration, hypovolemia, worsening cardiac disease, and institution of or increasing diuretic therapy. Alcohol binging is also a common precipitant.

The clinical presentation is usually quite dramatic. If this is early in the course of disease, the patient will complain of a very rapid onset of severe monarticular pain and the development of redness and swelling in the affected joint. This often occurs at night and the most common site of involvement is the first metatarsal phalangeal joint, which is known as podagra. If sufficient inflammation is present, there may be also complaints of systemic symptoms of malaise and low-grade fever. Occasionally, there can be multiple joint involvement, though this usually occurs in later and more progressive disease. In long-standing disease, tophi, which are nodules formed by uric acid crystals in the tissue and foreign body reaction, may be felt. These typically occur over the helix of the ear. These occur in other sites as well, sometimes causing confusion with a rheumatoid nodule.

In the acute setting, the important differentiation is with the septic joint. This is done by joint aspiration, which in gout will reveal crystals, often seen inside the PMNs. If a polarizing microscope is available and a red filter present, differentiation from calcium pyrophosphate crystals can be done. Uric acid crystals are yellow if viewed parallel with a red filter and turn blue when the filter is rotated perpendicular to the slide. Calcium pyrophosphate crystals show a reverse pattern. The clinical laboratory should be able to make this determination of birefringence. X-ray findings are usually limited early in the disease. Soft tissue swelling may be present. More advanced disease or a joint that has been attacked in the past by gouty arthritis often will show a fairly characteristic punched out bony lesion with a sclerotic margin. The only pertinent lab test to be done in the ER is to obtain a uric acid level and synovial fluid analysis if the diagnosis is not clear.

More severe disease with gout can occur when multiple joints are involved. Repeated attacks will lead to destruction of the involved joint, and excessive urine excretion of uric acid will lead to the formation of uric acid stones.

Treatment depends on the severity of the disease and complicating factors, if any are present. For uncomplicated disease, indomethacin or another nonsteroidal antiinflammatory drug is effective treatment. Again, caution should be used in patients with underlying renal disease, concurrent diuretic use, or history of heart failure and coronary artery disease. In these patients, sulindac or piroxicam may be a better choice of drugs. Standard treatment in the past has been the use of colchicine. Colchicine generally works best if used early in the course of an attack. The dose given is 0.5 mg by mouth, repeated each hour until either the attack is broken, gastrointestinal (GI) symptoms override further use of the drug, or a total of 6 mg is given. Colchicine can also be given intravenously (IV). The dose given IV is 2 mg. Colchicine is very destructive to tissue if extravasation occurs and should only be given in a well-placed intravenous site. The solution also should be diluted 10:1 with normal saline. If colchicine is to be used, the dosage should be reduced in patients with renal failure. Given this way, there is usually a dramatic relief in 1 to 2 hours for most episodes of gouty arthritis.

A more extensive polyarticular disease should be managed as an inpatient both for control of symptoms and reduction of uric levels, which generally are very high in patients with multiple joint involvement. Treatment with drugs that reduce uric acid levels should not be started during an acute flare. A sudden reduction in serum uric acid will solubilize existing synovial deposits. This can lead to reformation of these crystals in the joint spaces or in the kidney.

Uric acid nephrolithiasis occurs occasionally. As noted above, this occurs commonly after initiation of treatment to reduce uric acid levels. Clues to this diagnosis are symptoms of stone disease in a susceptible patient. Unless rimmed by calcium, a uric acid stone should be radiopaque on plain film and intravenous pyelogram (IVP). Treatment should be started with hydration and diuresis concurrently. If the urine is acidic, this causes further precipitation of the uric crystals. Along with hydration, and if not contraindicated, alkalization of the urine with sodium bicarbonate should also be instituted.

Pseudogout, or chondrocalcinosis as known in the European literature, is a secondary arthritis caused by release of calcium pyrophosphate crystals into the joint space. It is very uncommon under the age of 50 and increases in prevalence as aging continues. The presentation is variable. There is often antecedent minor or moderate trauma to the joint. In the most acute form, there is development over several hours to one day of an extremely painful joint with effusion and erythema. The course may be more indolent with gradual progression of pain, swelling, and development of effusion, or intermittent flare-ups, over a period of days or weeks. The

pathogenesis is the presence of calcium pyrophosphate crystals in the articular cartilage or menisci of the joint. Trauma, which often can be very trivial, can cause a disruption of crystals and release these into the joint. The free crystals of calcium pyrophosphate can incite a phagocytosis by PMNs with subsequent degranulation and initiation of inflammatory joint response, similar to that seen in gout.

It is doubtful that calcium pyrophosphate concentrates in joint fluid in sufficient amounts to cause supersaturation and spontaneous precipitation. The probable etiology is release of preformed crystals into the joint from cartilage. Pseudogout is found in association with diabetes, hypoparathyroidism, and metabolic disorders that lead to renal disease; specific cause and effect of any of these diseases with pseudogout is unclear. It is also unclear whether the presence of pseudogout can be used as a marker of other underlying diseases.

In the acute form, as a monarticular hot joint, distinction must be made from an infectious etiology. No specific blood tests are helpful and joint fluid is needed if there is any doubt in the diagnosis between pseudogout, gout, or a septic joint. Analysis will reveal crystals both free in the synovial fluid and in PMNs. Their appearance may be similar to uric acid crystals and polarized microscopy with a red compensator will need to be employed to differentiate between the two disorders. Pseudogout has a predilection for the knee, making acquisition of joint fluid uncomplicated in typical cases. The articular cartilage in the wrist and symphysis pubis are other sites of involvement.

The diagnosis rests on joint fluid studies, if aspiration is done, and radiographic evidence. The radiographic appearance acutely will show effusion in the joint and normal subchondral bone if other underlying bony disorders or joint disorders are not present. Often early, and always late, calcification in the articular cartilage and meniscus of the knee, if the knee is the affected joint, will be present. Late in the disease, areas of bony erosion, in a sort of punched out pattern similar to gout, can be seen. Treatment is similar to treatment used in gout. If not contraindicated, nonsteroidal antiinflammatory drugs will give relief. Colchicine has been used occasionally and has been found to be effective but results are inconsistent. Clinoril and Feldene may be safer alternatives to use than Indocin.

SEPTIC ARTHRITIS

Septic arthritis is the most serious disorder in the category of inflammatory joint disease. Missed or delayed diagnosis has dire consequences for restoration of joint function. Septic arthritis is often thought of in terms of hip infections in children or as a complication of intravenous drug abuse or gonococcal infection in younger adulthood. However, between 25 and 30% of patients with septic arthritis are in the geriatric age group. The presentation in the elderly is similar to their younger counterparts. Rapid onset of pain, effusion, erythema, and pain with motion occurs. Systemic symptoms of fever, chills, and malaise are usually present early in the disease course. However, palpable warmth and erythema can be difficult to detect in deep joint infections such as the hip or vertebra.[16,17]

A frequent concomitant to septic arthritis in the elderly is underlying joint diseases.[17,18] Osteoarthritis and rheumatoid arthritis are common associated conditions. Septic arthritis has been found more commonly in rheumatoid arthritis even though this is a less common disorder than osteoarthritis. It has been suggested that rheumatoid arthritis patients, as well as being more susceptible to joint infections, are more susceptible to infections in general. This is probably a result of host defense defects and associated use of immunosuppressive agents. As mentioned earlier, a red, warm, swollen joint in a chronic rheumatoid arthritis or osteoarthritis patient or a disproportionately inflamed joint in a generalized rheumatoid arthritis flare should be considered to be of infectious etiology. Other predisposing factors to developing infection are often present in the elderly. Corticosteroid use for systemic illness is frequently present. Diabetes mellitus is a predisposing factor. As in any age group, generalized debilitation and alcoholism are risk factors. A history of recent injection of the joint should be sought, and previous surgery, such as a prosthetic joint, should be determined.

The diagnosis rests on history, examination, and joint fluid analysis. The white cell count is high with a predominance of polymorphonucleocytes. The glucose level is usually less than 50% of serum levels, and the Gram stain is frequently negative. One small study found organisms on the Gram stain in less than 20% of aspirated joints that were eventually culture proven to be infected. Obviously, joint fluid culture should be done and blood cultures done as well. Hematogenous spread is the most common etiology for joint infections in the elderly patient. Occasionally, direct seeding from a wound or overlying skin infection occurs. In hematogenous spread, the underlying disease is often obvious, such as acute sepsis or pneumonia. The possibility of subacute bacterial endocarditis should be considered. The urinary tract is a common focus, and a urinalysis should always be done as part of the workup of a septic joint unless the cause is obvious. Radiographic study will show effusion early and often signs of underlying joint pathology. Bony destruction occurs only as a late finding. Adjacent osteomyelitic changes should be looked for both as a precipitating cause of the septic joint and as a late complication.

Treatment in the emergency department includes making a diagnosis, initiating proper cultures, and starting antibiotic therapy. In the non–hospital-acquired infec-tion, *Staphylococcus aureus* is the predominant pathogen. In the elderly, gram-negative organisms occur, especially in the immunocompromised patient. Initial therapy, pending cultures, should be an antistaphylococcal penicillin or cephalosporin plus an aminoglycoside.

DRUG REACTIONS AND INTERACTIONS

Antiarthritic drug therapy is complicated by side effects of the drugs used and interactions with other medications also in use. Alterations in absorption, distribution, and hepatic and renal excretion make the elderly more susceptible to drug toxicities. The presence of underlying diseases and often the use of multiple medications predispose them to other drug interactions. All these combine to increase complications of drug use in the elderly.[19,20]

Antiarthritic drugs can be classed as analgesics, anti-inflammatories, antigout, and a category entitled third-line agents, which consists of disease-modifying drugs. This section is meant to be a very brief review of the most commonly used drugs, and the earlier chapter on drug complications in the elderly should be referenced for further information. Propoxyphene is a commonly used analgesic. Respiratory depression is its most common serious side effect. This can be especially severe in the presence of other sedatives, such as benzodiazepines, narcotics, or alcohol. Codeine has well-known GI complications, and the elderly may perceive constipation as a high morbidity complication. Extreme caution should be used with either of these drugs in individuals with severe chronic obstructive pulmonary disease, especially of a chronic bronchitic pattern. Aspirin is the most commonly used nonsteroidal antiinflammatory drug. Salicylates have the problem of prolonging their own plasma half-life as the concentration increases. In the elderly, especially with hearing loss, tinnitus is often absent as an early warning sign of impending toxicity. Minimal increase in dosage or minimal decrease in renal function can rapidly lead to toxicity in the elderly. Acutely, symptoms in the elderly are the same as aspirin toxicity in any age group, including fever, lethargy, and hyperventilation. Chronic toxicity is common in the elderly also, and symptoms include apathy, lethargy, confusion, and, often, the presence of noncardiogenic pulmonary edema. Phenylbutazone has an increased risk of aplastic anemia and probably should not be used in the elderly.

Indomethacin has several potential side effects. Increased risk of GI blood loss contraindicates its use in ulcer disease. Several cardiovascular side effects occur. Indomethacin blocks the antihypertensive effect of beta-blocking drugs. Indomethacin also increases sodium and water retention through a renal mechanism contraindicating its use both in kidney disease and congestive heart failure. Indocin has been shown to reduce coronary artery blood flow, indicating caution in prescribing indomethacin to any geriatric patient, especially those with underlying heart disease. Other nonsteroidal antiinflammatory drugs should be used cautiously in patients with ulcer disease and certainly not at all in active ulcer disease or in patients with renal disease. (All the nonsteroidal antiinflammatory drugs will worsen fluid retention in renal disease.) Allopurinol is a xanthine oxidase inhibitor. If the decision to start this drug is made in the emergency room, the physician should be aware that interaction with other purine analog-type drugs such as 6-mercaptopurine or azathioprine could lead to severe and rapid development of toxicity due to inhibition of metabolism and breakdown by xanthine oxidase.

ISCHEMIC NECROSIS OF BONE

Ischemic necrosis of bone is an uncommon disorder and often underdiagnosed early in its course. This is frequently seen in children involving the epiphysis of the hip, which is known as Legg-Calvé-Perthes disease, or in other epiphyses under a plethora of eponymic labels depending on the site. Civil engineering projects and scuba diving contribute to ischemic necrosis of bone in the adult population.[21] Ischemic necrosis of bone occurs in the elderly population as well, commonly in association with certain drug therapies or underlying diseases. The initial event is occlusion of the arterial supply or obstruction of venous outflow in the bone. Most commonly, only the cancellous bone is involved. If the periosteum is spared by virtue of an alternate blood supply, there may be no perception of pain or other symptoms until extensive destruction of bone has occurred. Initial symptoms are fairly well-localized pain on active use or weight-bearing of the affected site. Pain at rest and at night occur in approximately 50% of the cases. Direct vascular trauma, either arterial or venous, accounts for many cases. Numerous medical disorders are also associated. Systemic lupus, alcoholism, long bone fractures elsewhere with fat embolus, and rheumatoid arthritis are all risk factors for ischemic necrosis of the bone. A disorder such as asthma, polymyalgia rheumatica, or renal transplantation (probably through the mechanism of concomitant steroid use) is also a risk factor. The pathogenesis is bone marrow ischemia, which leads to cell changes and edema, resulting in an elevated bone marrow pressure that leads to further ischemia and ultimate necrosis of bone. Steroid medication use is commonly associated with this disease. The mechanism is believed to be from hypertrophy of intramedullary lipocytes with secondary vascular occlusion from an increased bone marrow pressure.[21]

Radiographic changes are classed into four stages. The first is either abnormal bone or a faint osteoporosis. Next seen are areas of patchy osteoporosis and osteosclerosis; sclerosis is more prominent if the process occurs over a load-bearing site. A radiolucent crescent may appear that represents a fracture line in the damaged bone. The final stage is obvious destruction of bone and resorption. The hip is the most common site affected followed by the shoulder and knee. If this disorder can be suspected based on history of appropriate pain, associated risk factors, and hopefully early and minimal radiographic findings, appropriate diagnostic referral can be made. Initial workup consists of scintigraphic imaging and, in rare cases, determination of bone marrow pressure and interosseous venography.

The emergency room disposition should consist of putting the affected site at rest and appropriate referral. Early diagnosis may allow treatment and salvage of the affected site, preventing late pathologic fractures, joint destruction, and the need for joint replacement.

PATHOLOGIC FRACTURES

A pathologic fracture is defined as a fracture involving abnormal bone. A classic example of this is the elderly female with severe osteoporosis who has a minor fall sustaining a hip fracture.[22] Numerous other diseases will lead to pathologic fractures, and any elderly person sustaining a fracture after no or minimal trauma should be suspected of an underlying disease process.[22,23]

Diseases that lead to pathologic fractures are broken up into five major categories: systemic disease affecting bone metabolism, benign primary bone disease, malignant primary bone disease, metastatic carcinoma to bone, and a miscellaneous category.

Systemic skeletal disease in the elderly is common. Osteoporosis is almost universal in elderly patients. Paget's disease and osteopetrosis occur also, and, as in osteoporosis, treatment of the underlying disease is difficult or impossible. However, disorders of hypoparathyroidism, renal osteodystrophy, and osteomalacia may present a radiographic appearance similar to osteoporosis and be at least partially correctable. Along with treatment of the presenting fracture, evaluation can begin in the emergency department. Serum calcium, phosphorus, alkaline phosphatase, and parahormone levels should be drawn. A history of GI disorders, intestinal surgery, or renal disease should also be obtained.

Benign primary bone disease consists of such disorders as unicameral bone cysts, nonossifying fibromas, osteoblastoma, chondroblastoma, and others. On x-ray, these are seen as fractures through a localized defect in the bone. Generally, benign bone processes have what is known as a geographic pattern on x-ray. That is, a confluent defect in the bone occurs with a regular smooth border as opposed to the jagged margin seen in malignant disease. A sclerotic rim of bone around the lesion is also evidence of slow growth and a benign origin. Orthopedic evaluation is done regarding the need for biopsy of the lesion or the need for excision of the lesion to allow bony healing.

Malignant primary bone disease consists of such disorders as osteosarcoma, Ewing's sarcoma, or multiple myeloma. Patients who present with a pathologic fracture from these lesions often have advanced disease. Though these are primarily diseases of younger people, they do occur in elderly patients as well. The radiographic appearance is a fracture through a destructive bony lesion. This can be a geographic lesion that shows a moth-eaten pattern as seen in multiple myeloma or lymphoma, or as a permeative pattern with multiple small punched out lesions around the fracture site. Initial management would be a more detailed history and physical examination for consideration of metastases to other sites, chest x-ray, and admission to the hospital for diagnosis and evaluation of possible treatment of the lesion.

Metastatic disease to bone ranks second to osteoporosis as a cause of pathologic fractures. Thyroid, breast, lung, kidney, and prostate are the most frequent primary sites of disease that metastasizes to bone. The radiographic appearance is usually of a lytic irregular lesion without sclerotic margins. Prostatic disease to bone, however, may lead to an osteoblastic appearance. If the primary source is not known, detailed evaluation will be needed. This includes physical examinations again with attention to thyroid, breast, lung, abdomen, and rectum. Serum and urine protein electrophoresis, calcium, phosphorus, and acid phosphatase levels are determined as well as inpatient diagnostic imaging studies. Patients with a known primary malignancy and bone pain may have metastatic disease without fracture. If the lesion is extensive, this can be considered an impending pathologic fracture. Depending on the patient's prognosis, prophylactic intramedullary rodding or other fixation procedures may be appropriate for both pain control and prevention of the more debilitating fracture in the future. The final miscellaneous category consists of such diseases as a prior irradiation either to bone or adjacent sites or to any old fracture or wound site. Management of pathologic fractures in these sites often is very complicated and should be done by the specialist.

OSTEOPOROSIS AND VERTEBRAL DISEASE

Osteoporosis is the most common of the systemic bone diseases. It is associated with many metabolic diseases; however, in most cases, the etiology is idiopathic. It is characterized by a loss of often up to 50% of the young adulthood mass of bone. Normal mineralization of bone usually remains, as opposed to osteomalacia in which a deficit in bony mineralization occurs. The weakened bones of osteoporosis are susceptible to fracture from minor trauma. All ER physicians who take care of adult patients are familiar with the elderly female with a hip fracture following a "minor" fall. The vertebral column is also susceptible to loss of structural integrity by bony in-

volvement in osteoporosis. The manifestation of this is vertebral compression fractures.[7-10]

Vertebral compression fractures in the elderly can occur from trauma as mild as bending over or coughing or even can occur spontaneously while the patient is sitting still, if the osteoporosis is severe. These fractures occur most commonly in the thoracic and lumbar spine. Radiographically, these take three appearances: 1) an anterior wedging of the vertebral body, which has a similar radiographic appearance to the younger patient with an axial load flexion injury; 2) a fish-mouth appearance of the vertebra, representing a biconcave fracture involving the end plates of the vertebra with compression; and 3) narrowing of the entire vertebra with complete collapse. Clinically, these patients present with acute onset of fairly well-localized pain, and these usually are stable injuries neurologically. Treatment consists of pain control and a short period of bed rest. Surprisingly, very little data exist in regard to neurologic injury with this type of fracture in the elderly patient. If evidence of neurologic deficit exists, the x-ray should be very carefully reviewed. Any disruption of the posterior vertebral body line in combination with either definite or subtle neurologic findings warrants either CT scanning or magnetic resonance imaging of the affected area to reveal retropulsed fragments and cord compression.[8-11]

While osteoporosis is the most common cause of spontaneous skeletal compression fractures, a significant number of these will be from other causes. The second most common etiology behind osteoporosis is metastatic carcinoma. A small number of compression fractures will occur from primary disorders such as multiple myeloma or lymphomatous involvement of the bone. Vertebral osteomyelitis should especially be considered in the differential diagnosis of acute compression fracture.[25]

PAGET'S DISEASE

Paget's disease, also known as osteitis deformans, is a disorder of bone metabolism that has increasing incidence with age. It affects roughly 10% of adults aged 80 or greater. The etiology is not certain, but current thinking suggests the possibility of an intranuclear viral infection of osteoclasts. This leads to proliferation and overactive function of the osteoclasts with resultant excess bone resorption. Compensation by normal osteoblasts leads to deposition of new bone giving a radiographic appearance of areas of bone that show both lytic and sclerotic features.[24-27]

The most common affected sites are the skull, spine, and pelvis. The long bones are less commonly involved. Patients with Paget's disease can present with a myriad of different complaints, though most commonly this disease is asymptomatic and is diagnosed only incidentally through x-rays for other complaints or in the evaluation of a persistently elevated alkaline phosphatase level. Involvement of the skull may cause a headache, which is usually mild and throbbing in nature. Bony hypertrophy in the skull can cause cranial nerve deficits depending on the site, with deafness being the most common cranial nerve finding. This occurs secondary to temporal bone involvement and occlusion of the temporal canal, which the eighth nerve passes through. Involvement of the bone of the skull can also lead to platybasia — a flattening of the base of the skull and subsequent basilar impression.

A rare cause of dementia is a steal syndrome caused by diversion of blood flow into metabolically hyperactive bone away from central nervous system structures. Vertebral disease can present with nondescript back pain. More extensive disease can lead to impingement of neural structures causing radiculopathies, disk syndromes, and, in very advanced disease, cord compression or cauda equina syndrome. This should be kept in mind in elderly patients with progressive lower extremity weakness and development of worsening incontinence. Extremity involvement is usually asymptomatic or a source of chronic low-grade bone pain. A sudden increase in symptoms should be considered pathologic fracture until this can be ruled out by appropriate x-rays.[24,26]

Treatment of Paget's disease is variable. Uncomplicated pain syndromes will usually respond to a mild anti-inflammatory agent. Cranial nerve involvement is more difficult to treat as this often is a fixed defect occurring over a long period of time, and, when detected, lesions are complete. Cord syndromes have traditionally been treated surgically. Recent reports with the use of salmon calcitonin or the use of diphosphonate drugs such as etidronate have shown promise in relieving compression symptoms.[26,27]

CONNECTIVE TISSUE DISORDERS

Connective tissue disease occurs in all age groups. Many are specific for certain age groups, such as the bimodal distribution of polymyositis or the young and middle adulthood onset of systemic lupus. The clinical manifestations of the connective tissue diseases are often protean, and diagnosis in a younger patient can be difficult. In the elderly patient with underlying multiple diseases and organ involvement, accurate diagnosis can be an extreme diagnostic challenge. There are two related diseases, however, that are fairly specific for the geriatric population and that have specific complications and treatment. These are polymyalgia rheumatica and temporal arteritis.[28-30]

Polymyalgia rheumatica is a disorder of the elderly. It is very rare before the age of 50, and by the eighth decade, its incidence is anywhere from 1:100 to 1:1000. It is more common in women than men and more common in Caucasians. No definite pathogenesis for polymyalgia rheumatica has been determined. Of interest, up to half of adults who later develop temporal arteritis have symptoms suggestive of preexisting polymyalgia rheumatica.

Clinically, the patient may present with a history of several weeks of neck, shoulder, and upper back pain. Pain in the pelvic girdle and thigh is also common. The initial pain, however, is often in the neck and shoulders and is usually bilaterally symmetrical. The primary complaint of these patients is extreme stiffness, and the history reveals that it may take several hours for the patient even to loosen up enough to be able to get out of bed in the morning. Fatigue, malaise, weight loss, and low-grade fever are often present and occur early in the course of the disease. Less commonly, the disease may be abrupt over a period of just several hours with fever and marked systemic symptoms making differentiation from an infectious etiology very difficult.[30,31]

Physical examination is usually quite unrevealing. The patient may appear very uncomfortable but not have any definite physical findings. Perhaps mild tenderness may be palpable in the shoulder musculature and the neck, and there should not be any loss of strength. This is in contrast to polymyositis where there may be significant loss of strength of proximal muscle groups. Occasionally, joint effusions may be present in polymyalgia rheumatica. Recent studies with technetium scanning of joints in patients with polymyalgia have suggested that a synovitis, as opposed to an intrinsic muscular pathology, may be the source of the symptoms in this disorder.

There are no diagnostic x-ray findings, and lab tests are not helpful except for the ESR. The ESR in almost all cases of polymyalgia rheumatica is elevated and should be at least 50 mm/hr to be consistent with this disorder. A normal sedimentation rate makes the diagnosis of polymyalgia rheumatica very unlikely.[30-34]

Evaluation in the emergency department should consist of history taking, physical exam, and determination of a sedimentation rate. If fever is present, differentiation with viral myalgias or other underlying infectious disease may be difficult. Differentiation from rheumatoid disease and polymyositis may also be difficult. However, in rheumatoid arthritis, along with the systemic symptoms, there should be symptoms specifically localizable to joints. Treatment of polymyalgia rheumatica is initiation of steroid therapy. Prednisone is given in a dose of 10 to 20 mg/day, and this usually leads, if the diagnosis is correct, to rapid improvement in a matter of 2 to 3 days. In fact, this treatment is so effective that it can be considered as a diagnostic feature of polymyalgia rheumatica.[34]

Giant cell or temporal arteritis is also a disorder almost exclusively of the elderly. The incidence is not certain but may be up to 1% in adults over age 70, and this disorder also has a female preponderance.

The arteritis can affect all vasculature but has a predilection for the facial arteries. Symptoms of giant cell arteritis are usually referable to ischemia of this arterial supply. The most feared complication is rapid onset of visual loss when this disease affects ocular blood supply.

This complication makes a rapid diagnosis and initiation of treatment a true emergency. The etiology is unclear but pathologically granulomatous changes in the intima of the artery and segmental arterial narrowing occur. This diagnosis is not difficult if the patient presents with a unilateral pounding headache and complains of rapid visual loss in one eye. Usually, the diagnosis is not this clear.

A history of polymyalgia rheumatica (PMR) or symptoms of PMR are often present. The symptoms of giant cell arteritis may develop over a long period of time, again with protean manifestations of fever, malaise, and weight loss. Depression and memory loss occur also. Jaw claudication with mastication is a common early symptom of temporal arteritis. This reflects occlusion of the facial artery and ischemia of the muscles of mastication. Unilateral headache and tenderness to palpation of the temporal artery with palpable thickening of the temporal artery are very helpful physical findings but probably occur in less than 50% of the cases. Ulcerations of the scalp, lips, or tongue may also occur. Visual symptoms appear through involvement of the branches of the ophthalmic artery. Initial visual symptoms may be blurring, diplopia, or transient reversible visual loss. Acute visual loss is due to involvement of the short posterior ciliary artery. This artery provides a blood supply for the optic nerve head. Funduscopic findings may show edema of the optic disk and possibly narrowed arterial caliber. This should be differentiated from central retinal artery occlusion, which will show a pale disk and narrow vessels, and central retinal vein occlusion, which will show a characteristic pattern of choked veins, retinal hemorrhage, and often a very dramatic outline of the retinal nerve fibers as they lead back into the optic nerve. A rare presentation of visual loss in temporal arteritis occurs when the long posterior ciliary artery is involved. This supplies the anterior aspect of the eyes and the patient may present with corneal clouding, iritis, and marked visual loss. The differentiation of this should be between more benign causes of iritis and certainly from an acute angle closure glaucoma. This can be done, in the first case, by history of prodromal symptoms suggestive of temporal arteritis and, in the second case, of acute angle closure glaucoma, by determining a normal intraocular pressure by tonometry.[28-30]

The diagnosis rests on history, physical findings if present, and an elevated ESR. The ESR should be elevated into the range of 80 to 120 mm/hour. Unless the patient is on steroids for another disorder, a high sedimentation rate is almost a sine qua non of giant cell arteritis. Steroid therapy should begin with suspicion of the diagnosis. Treatment is in the range of 60 mg of prednisone per day. In an emergency setting, if any visual symptoms are present, either by history or physical exam, the steroid dose should be started IV. Solu-Medrol in the range of 100 to 250 mg would be a reasonable starting dose. A biopsy diagnosis is possible up to 2 to 3 days after initiation of steroids, and withholding of steroids should not be done based on a concern of obscuring the diagnosis. Patients with known temporal arteritis who are already on steroids or patients who are on a steroid taper who present with new symptoms or visual symptoms should be treated as aggressively as the new diagnosis of temporal arteritis.[31-34]

REFERENCES

1. Bergstrom G et al: Prevalence of rheumatoid arthritis, osteoarthritis, chondrocalcinosis, and gouty arthritis at age 79, J Rheumatol 13(3):527–534, 1986.
2. Bergstrom G et al: Joint disorders at ages 70, 75, and 79 years: a cross sectional comparison, Br J Rheumatol 25(4):333–341, 1986.
3. Spiera H: Osteoarthritis as a misdiagnosis in elderly patients, Geriatrics 42(11):37–42, 1987.
4. Stevens MB: Connective tissue disease in the elderly, Clin Rheum Dis 12(1):11–32, 1986.
5. Gamache FW Jr: Cervical spine disease in the elderly, Compr Ther 13(5):26–29, 1987.
6. Kaplan PA, Orton DF, and Asleson RJ: Osteoporosis with vertebral compression fractures, retropulsed fragments, and neurologic compromise, Radiology 165(2):533–535, 1987.
7. MacRae DL: Head and neck pain in the elderly, J Otolaryngol 15(4):224–227, 1986.
8. Murray P: Cervical spondylolytic myelopathy: a cause of gait disturbance and urinary incontinence in older persons, J Am Geriatr Soc 32(4):324–340, 1984.
9. Payne R: Neck pain in the elderly: a management review. I. Geriatrics 42(1):59–62, 1987.
10. Winfield J et al: A prospective study of the radiological changes in the cervical spine in early rheumatoid disease, Ann Rheum Dis 40:109–114, 1981.
11. Calabro JJ: Rheumatoid arthritis: diagnosis and management, Clin Symp 38(2):1–32, 1986.
12. Healey LA: Rheumatoid arthritis in the elderly, Clin Rheum Dis 12(1):173–179, 1986.
13. Malone DE et al: Peptic ulcer in rheumatoid arthritis — intrinsic or related to drug therapy? Br J Rheumatol 25(4):342–344, 1986.
14. Vandenbroucke JP et al: Frequency of infections among rheumatoid arthritis patients, before and after disease onset, Arthritis Rheum 30(7):810–813, 1987.
15. Winfield J et al: Prospective study of the radiologic changes in hands, feet, and cervical spine in adult rheumatoid disease, Ann Rheum Dis 42:613–618, 1983.
16. Evanchich CE, Davis DE, and Harrington TM: Septic arthritis: clinical approach to the "hot joint," Post Grad Med 79(2):11–19, 1986.
16a. Teodori JB and Painter MJ: Basilar impression in children, Pediatrics 74(6):1097–1099, 1984.
17. McGuire NM and Kaufmann CA: Septic arthritis in the elderly, J Am Geriatr Soc 33(3):170–174, 1985.
18. McHenry MC et al: Vertebral osteomyelitis presenting as spinal compression fracture, Arch Intern Med 148:417–423, 1988.
19. Steele K et al: Repeat prescribing of non-steroidal anti-inflammatory drugs excluding aspirin: how careful are we? Br Med J (Clin Res) 295(6604):962–964, 1987.
20. Malchow-Moller A: Treatment of peptide ulcer induced by non-steroidal anti-inflammatory drugs, Scand J Gastroenterol (Suppl) 127:87–91, 1987.
21. Zizic TM et al: The early diagnosis of ischemic necrosis of bone, Arthritis Rheum 29(10):1177–1185, 1986.
22. Schon L and Zuckerman JD: Hip pain in the elderly, Geriatrics 43(1):48–62, 1988.
23. Chang WS, Zuckerman JD, and Ditman MI: Geriatric knee disorders. I. Evaluative techniques, Geriatrics 43(2):73–83, 1988.
24. Jacobs TP: Diagnosis and management of Paget's disease, Compr Ther 12(3):30–34, 1986.
25. Jawad AS and Berry H: Spinal cord compression in Paget's disease of bone treated medically, J R Soc Med 80(5):319–321, 1987.

26. Kattapuram SU and Deluca SA: Paget's disease, Am Fam Physician 35(5):121–126, 1986.

27. Kumar K: Paget's disease of the bone, J Indian Med Assoc 84(10):316–318, 1986.

28. Allen NB and Studendki SA: Polymyalgia rheumatica and temporal arteritis, Med Clin North Am 70(2):369–384, 1986.

29. Branum G, Mussey EW, and Rice J: Erythrocyte sedimentation rate in temporal arteritis, South Med J 80(12):1528–1529, 1987.

30. Espinoza LR, Vidal L, and Pastor C: Diagnosis and managment of polymyalgia rheumatica, Compr Ther 12(9):19–23, 1986.

31. Olhagen B: Polymyalgia rheumatica, Clin Rheum Dis 12(1):33–47, 1986.

32. Periera M and Kaine JL: Polymyalgia rheumatica and temporal arteritis: managing older patients, Geriatrics 41(6):54–66, 1986.

33. Sherard RK and Coleridge ST: Giant cell arteritis, J Emerg Med 4(4):293–299, 1986.

34. Sullivan RJ: Occult temporal arteritis, J Am Geriatr Soc 84:812–813, 1986.

Falls

Falls in the Elderly: Etiology and Prevention

Rein Tideiksaar, Ph.D.

EPIDEMIOLOGY

Falls are a common problem for older people. Approximately 30 to 50% of noninstitutionalized older people report having experienced a fall or a tendancy to fall in the past 12 months.[1-5] Among the institutionalized elderly, up to 20% of hospitalized patients and 45% of those in long-term care facilities will fall.[7] Unfortunately, these figures represent an underestimation of the problem, since the vast majority of falls experienced by older people are underreported.[6,8] Typically, the only falls which are reported are those that lead to physical injury or a significant decline in functional status. In the community, older people may not report a fall because they falsely attribute the event to a "normal" consequence of aging or fear that reporting a fall will lead to restricted activities and placement into a nursing home by family members or health care professionals. As well, the personal embarrassment one suffers from having fallen or having to deny the incident, especially if it is a reminder of increasing frailty and dependency, may be further reasons for fall underreporting by the aged. Within the institutional setting, patients may fail to report their fall if they have an element of cognitive dysfunction, a fear of being placed in physical restraints, or concern over being denied discharge back to the community.

In terms of mortality, falls represent the leading cause of death due to unintentional injury.[9] Fall-related mortality increases with advanced age and more than doubles with each decade of life.[10] While falls are associated with excess mortality, the majority of falls do not end in death.[11] However, the morbidity associated with falling is considerable. A fracture is the most common fall-related injury to occur, with the hip being the most common fracture to result in acute hospitalization.[12] Of the 200,000 hip fractures that occur annually, 84% occur to persons 65 years of age and older.[13] The length of hospital stay for patients with hip fracture is nearly twice the stay for all other causes of hospital admission by the elderly[13]; approximately 40% of older people with hip fractures die within 6 months from the time of injury.[15] In those who survive the hip fracture, 60% have significant mobility problems as a result,[15] and another 25% will become more functionally dependent.[17]

Falls that do not result in physical injury can lead to self-imposed immobility resulting from a fear of falling again.[11,19] Prolonged immobility can lead to the development of joint contractures, pressure sores, urinary tract infections, muscle atrophy, depression, and functional dependency.[11] As a result, falls are a common reason for institutionalization of the elderly. Approximately 25% of hospital admissions of the aged are directly attributable to falling,[21] and 47% of patients admitted to the hospital for falls become long-care stay patients.[21] Those elderly with recurrent falls, declining mobility, and a fear of falling again are often readmitted to a hospital[23] or placed in a nursing home for permanent care.[24]

ETIOLOGY

Falling in itself should not be viewed as a disease state but, rather, as a sign or symptom representative of an underlying problem. For example, the complaint of abdominal pain is usually indicative of underlying peptic ulcer disease, appendicitis, gallbladder disease, diverticulitis, or intestinal obstruction. In similiar fashion, a fall is symptomatic of several intrinsic (i.e., "normal" physiologic aging changes, pathologic and psychologic disease states, and medications) and extrinsic (i.e., environmental hazards) factors. The fall may not be the direct consequence of any single intrinsic or extrinsic factor occurring in isolation but is often representative of several events operating simultaneously. Therefore, just as one would not dismiss a patient with abdominal pain without initiating an investigation into its etiology, a fall patient should not be overlooked without first ruling out a multitude of reversible factors.

NORMAL AGING CHANGES

With advancing age, the visual, neurologic, cardiovascular, and musculoskeletal systems are influenced by several "normal" age-related physiologic changes that place the older person at certain fall risk.

Vision

With increasing age, pupillary response diminishes, resulting in decreased accommodation to varying levels of light and darkness.[25] The result is that older people require more time to adjust to environmental lighting changes in order to ambulate safely. A greater sensitivity of the aging eye to glare, a visual distraction caused by sluggish pupillary reactions, can lead to visual distraction from unshielded light sources and bright lights radiating off highly polished floors.[26] A decrease in lens transparency results in cataract formation, which interferes with the passage of light rays to the retina and leads to diminished vision and increased sensitivity to bright lights. The presence of cataracts may also result in a decreased ability to discriminate between colors of similar intensities, such as blue and green colors.[27] This becomes a problem if older people have difficulty distinguishing a difference between the colors of their medications and risk a fall secondary to inappropriate medication administration. An age-related decline in depth perception can make the visual detection of similarly colored environmental objects, such as grab bars or hand rails of the same color consistency as surrounding walls, undetectable as safety devices. Visual function can be further impaired by a decrease in peripheral vision, a diminished upward gaze, and central field visual deficits caused by macular degeneration.[28]

Balance and Gait

The balancing mechanisms of an older person are affected by changes occurring in the visual, vestibular, and proprioceptive sensory systems. Body sway, the natural motion of the body when standing, normally increases after the sixth decade of life and raises the body's level of instability.[29] Older people with a history of falling have greater sway than those persons without falls.[30] Proprioceptive feedback and vibration sense decline with age,[31,32] which may interfere with proper foot placement while walking. The righting reflex, a vestibular function which signals the body to initiate positional reflexes in an effort to preserve balance, is diminished in older persons.[33]

Changes in gait occur with normal aging and may contribute to falls. Females develop a narrow walking and standing base and ambulate with a pelvic waddle.[34] Older males tend to adopt a wide standing and walking base and a decrease in stride length and steppage height, which results in a small-stepped gait.[35] Both sexes display a decrease in walking speed and spend more time in the support phase of gait.[36]

Cardiovascular Changes

Postural hypotension has been found to be present in relatively healthy people,[37,38] due to a decline in the efficiency of baroreceptor reflexes. The presence of postural hypotension may add to balance dysfunction in older people and contribute to falling.

Reaction Time

Reaction time and the speed at which a task is performed generally decrease with age.[39] As a result, the length of time between perceiving a hazard and taking action to avoid it increases, as does fall risk.

Musculoskeletal Changes

Older people, with age, tend to assume a stooped kyphotic posture, with the head and neck slightly bent forward and the hips and knees flexed. This change, attributable to muscle shrinkage, calcification of tendons and ligaments, and a thinning of the vertebral disks, not only alters the body's balance threshold, but may result in more instability when attempting to stop a fall in progress.

With age, muscular strength and endurance decrease. The proximal muscles of the lower extremities display the greatest decline.[40] This results in older people experiencing difficulty when sitting down or rising from chairs, toilets, and wheelchairs. Joint arthritis, which occurs normally with age due to continuous deterioration and abrasion of articular cartilage, may contribute to transfer difficulties especially if the knee joint is affected. Osteoarthritis of the knees prevents the knee joint from assuming an angle of acute flexion between the lower and upper leg and impairs the ability of the legs to slide underneath a chair to provide leverage when rising. An inability to sufficiently flex the knees may influence the ability to get up from the floor following a fall.

MEDICAL CAUSES

The majority of falls in older persons occur to those with multiple medical problems. The falling episode may be an indication of unstable existing disease or may represent the onset of a new undiagnosed medical condition. In either case, there are a variety of medical factors to consider as causative of falling. Virtually every organ system involved in maintaining homeostatic function can be implicated.[132,133]

Vision

Superimposed on age-related visual changes, dysfunction in sight constitutes a major fall risk.[1,41] Visual impairment may be transient, presenting as a symptom of hypotension, cardiac arrhythmia, temporal arteritis, or vertebrobasilar artery insufficiency. Progressive visual decline is usually due to cataracts, macular degeneration, glaucoma, or nutritional deficiencies, such as vitamin B_{12} and thiamine deficiency.

Dizziness

Older people frequently complain of dizziness.[43] Dizziness results from a dysfunction of at least one of a number of balance control systems. Disturbance of the visual pathway, the vestibular apparatus, or the proprioceptive tracts of the central nervous system or altered homeostasis of systemic circulation can result in vertigo, syncope, or lightheadedness.

Vertigo is usually defined as a sense of rotation of either the patient or his environment and usually indicates vestibular dysfunction. Vertigo is almost always associated with nystagmus, poor balance, and autonomic symptoms and can be caused by peripheral disease (affecting the inner ear or eighth cranial nerve) or central nervous system disease (affecting the brainstem or cerebellum).[44]

Benign Positional Vertigo

This disorder of the peripheral vestibular system is probably the most common form of vertigo experienced by the elderly. Typically, patients will describe a dizzy sensation when they assume a certain position, which subsides when another position is assumed. There is usually a latency period of several seconds between the time of position change and the onset of dizziness. Accompanying symptoms include rotary or horizontal nystagmus and occasionally tinnitus and nausea. Hearing impairments are not usually associated with benign positional vertigo. Recent ear infection or head trauma is a common precipitating factor.

Meniere's Disease

This disease may present as dizziness in the elderly but usually is not seen after the age of 70. Anatomically, the disease represents an impairment of the auditory and labyrinthine portions of the eighth cranial nerve, but the etiology is unknown (although a relationship to endolymphatic hydrops has been suggested). Meniere's disease presents abruptly with severe dizziness and is accompanied by nausea and vomiting. Each episode lasts for a few minutes to several hours, and attacks occur in clusters with long remission periods of weeks or several months between clusters. Attacks may be triggered by emotional upset, fatigue, or excessive sodium or MSG intake.

Acoustic Neuroma

All patients presenting with dizziness or a disturbance of balance accompanied by a progressive unilateral hearing loss or tinnitus must be suspected of having an acoustic neuroma — a benign, enlarging tumor arising from the eighth cranial nerve and located within the auditory canal. Unilateral sensorineural hearing loss will be evident with poor speech discrimination disproportionate to the degree of hearing loss. As the acoustic neuroma enlarges and infiltrates the cerebellopontine angle, neurologic dysfunction becomes more apparent; early signs include a depressed corneal reflex and decreased sensory and motor involvement of the seventh cranial nerve. Patients should have radiographic examinations of the temporal bones and internal auditory canals, including tomography or computerized tomography (CT) scan, to confirm the presence of a tumor. Surgical excision of the tumor is usually curative.

Labyrinthitis

Patients presenting with dizziness associated with positional change and local ear pain should be suspected of having labryinthitis. This disorder has three clinical variants: serous, suppurative, and toxic labyrinthitis.

Serous labyrinthitis results from secondary infection of the ear, such as otitis media. Accumulated cerumen in the affected ear can contribute to an infection as well. A transient sensorineural hearing loss is present, and there is a decreased caloric response. Treatment of the underlying infection or removal of cerumen resolves the problem. Suppurative labyrinthitis is an infection characterized by inflammation of the inner ear. Chronic otitis media, cholesteatoma, or fractures of the inner ear are the common causes. Toxic labyrinthitis is caused by ototoxic drugs such as the aminoglycosides, aspirin, heavy tobacco use, and loop diuretics. The earliest symptoms of drug ototoxicity are tinnitus and hearing loss. After a while, balance problems may develop, indicating inner ear involvement. Patients may develop dizziness and gait ataxia when the vestibular system is active (during ambulation), and symptoms decrease when the vestibular system is inactive (when the patient is lying down). Because toxic labyrinthitis is often irreversible, patients should not be treated with ototoxic drugs unless no alternative medications are available. Also, audiometry and balance tests, administered both before and during treatment with ototoxic drugs, should be standard procedure.

Transient Ischemic Attack

Vascular disease that affects the perfusion of the brain by the vertebral and basilar arteries can cause intermittent dizziness. The drop attack is a particular form of vertebrobasilar insufficiency affecting the elderly.[45] It is estimated that up to 25% of falls are due to drop attacks.[30] The patient will drop to the ground, without a loss of consciousness, state that his legs suddenly gave way, and be unable to get up without assistance. The precise mechanism of these attacks is not known but appears to be associated with cervical abnormalities.[47] Patients should wear cervical collars to prevent backward flexion of the head.

Syncope

Syncope, defined as sudden brief loss of consciousness due to cerebral ischemia, has many underlying responsible causes.[48]

Vasodepressor Syncope

The vasovagal faint is probably the most frequent type of syncope.[49] Characteristically, a few seconds before an attack the patient will have premonitory symptoms, such as nausea, weakness, sweating, and a sensation of impending loss of consciousness. Typically, the attacks occur after emotional upset or injury, during prolonged standing in warm environments, or after prolonged fatigue.

Orthostatic Syncope

In orthostatic hypotension, the autonomic factors responsible for compensation for the upright posture fail. In this sense, orthostatic syncope is similar to vasodepressor syncope. However, it is the effect of posture that is the cardinal feature of orthostatic hypotension. Orthostatic hypotension is demonstrated when there is a drop in systolic pressure of 20 mm Hg or diastolic pressure of 10 mm Hg between the supine and standing positions without a concomitant rise in pulse rate.

Although a small percentage of normal, healthy elderly patients may have orthostatic hypotension of an unknown etiology,[50,51] common causes include factors that deplete body fluids or cause decreased venous return, medications, and diseases with neurologic complications. Antihypertensive drugs, especially those that block or inhibit sympathetic activity, and diuretics, which can cause dehydration, are drugs commonly associated with orthostatic syncope. Neurologic diseases causing orthostatic syncope include disorders of the peripheral nerves, such as diabetic neuropathy,[52] alcoholic neuropathy, and amyloidosis. Postprandial reductions in blood pressure may occur as well. The hypotensive response to eating may be due to splanchnic blood pooling or other local intestinal factors in the presence of inadequate baroreflex compensation. Eating may also affect blood pressure homeostasis through insulin-induced blunting of baroreceptor sensitivity.[53] Patients should be cautioned against sudden rising or activities following meals.

Carotid Sinus Syncope

This syncope occurs frequently in older people, many of whom may have underlying sinus node disease. The responsible mechanism is either carotid sinus hypersensitivity[54] or a mechanical obstruction, which causes interference of the blood supply to the brain.[55] The stimulus for carotid sinus syncope may be turning the head to one side, shaving, or wearing tight collars. Drugs that enhance vagal tone, such as digitalis or propranolol, may also produce carotid hypersensitivity.

Tussive Syncope

This form of syncope is usually encountered in patients with chronic obstructive pulmonary disease or bronchitis.[56] Vigorous coughing, followed by loss of consciousness, is the usual history. A severe Valsalva's maneuver is created by high intrathoracic pressures during coughing episodes, resulting in decreased cardiac output. Treatment is directed toward antitussive medications and care of the underlying disease process.

Micturition Syncope

This syncope is seen primarily in elderly males, presumably because of the upright position for micturition.[56] Patients with bladder outlet obstruction (i.e., BPH) and nocturia are at risk. During or immediately following voiding, a sudden loss of consciousness occurs, related to vagal bradycardia. Having patients sit during micturition is usually helpful.

Arrhythmias

Cardiac arrhythmias are a common cause of syncope.[58] Arrhythmias can occur with either extremely fast or extremely slow heart rates. Supraventricular tachycardias are the most common arrhythmias to cause syncope. The sick-sinus syndrome is also frequently associated with dizziness in older patients, for the sinus typically slows with aging. The 12-lead electrocardiogram (ECG) is essential in the diagnostic evaluation of cardiac syncope. It may reveal evidence of significant first-degree heart block or ventricular irritability as the cause of dizziness. If a cardiac arrhythmia is suspected, then prolonged ECG monitoring is indicated, since it is common for elderly persons without symptoms to exhibit arrhythmias as well.[59] Holter monitoring over 24 or 48 hours that reveals transient bradyarrhythmias or tachyarrhythmias during a dizzy spell is diagnostic. If the Holter (prolonged ECG recording) is negative over a 24- or 48-hour period for arrhythmias, while the patient has symptoms, its value lies in the fact that arrhythmias can be ruled out as a cause of dizziness.

Since rigid definitions of vertigo and syncope do not describe all patients' symptoms, lightheadedness is used to describe symptoms of dizziness without nystagmus or loss of consciousness.

Hypoglycemia

Hypoglycemia can be diabetic or nondiabetic in origin. Although diabetes is always associated with hyperglycemia, the first indication of early diabetes may be a reactive hypoglycemic episode. In these patients, dizziness usually occurs 3 to 5 hours after a meal. Although nondiabetic hypoglycemia is rare, it can arise as a result of organic disease, such as pancreatic tumors or adrenocortical hypofunction.

Hypothyroidism

Although vertigo is not considered a usual symptom of hypothyroidism, balance disturbances occur commonly in the hypothyroid state. Cerebellar ataxia, with the clinical picture of unsteadiness and truncal ataxia, may be noted. Patients may also present with sensorineural hearing loss and tinnitus.

Hyperventilation

Patients who are anxious or under emotional stress may have hyperventilation-induced dizziness.[60] A careful history of underlying psychologic problems will usually pinpoint the diagnosis. Perioral or extremity tingling is a suggestive symptom. Patients with hyperventilation induced dizziness can reproduce their symptoms by hyperventilating for 2 to 3 minutes. Before settling on this diagnosis, however, other causes of dizziness should first be excluded.

Visual Malfunction

Altered visual perception may cause dizziness when the patient is walking. Visual cues relied upon when descending stairs or making turns are often altered during the transition to new glasses or after cataract surgery. In both instances, time, reassurance, and an ophthalmologic checkup should resolve the problem.

Disequilibrium

Dizziness induced by disequilibrium occurs in such common disorders as Parkinson's and Alzheimer's disease and peripheral neuropathy caused by pernicious anemia, alcoholism, or diabetes. Patients will complain of unsteadiness, disturbed balance, a tendency to fall, or a lessened awareness of limb position when walking. Dizziness results from an overreliance on visual and labyrinthine-vestibular responses to achieve a sense of stability. Unless a specific treatable cause is found for the disequilibrium, the patient can be helped to balance with assistive devices for walking or by discontinuing or replacing any medications that exacerbate imbalance.

GAIT DYSFUNCTIONS

A number of studies have attributed falls to gait abnormalities.[61,62]

Senile Gait

The gradual age-related appearance of a broad-based gait, associated with stooped posture, flexion of hips and knees, diminished arm swing, small steps, poor gait initiation, and stiffness in turning, has been described as senile gait.[63] While senile gait is unrelated to clinically detectable neurologic or systemic disease, some have attributed this disorder to early Parkinsonism, with only anecdotal results of improvement with L-dopa.[64] The diagnosis of senile gait disorder as a cause of falling should only be made after other potentially reversible gait disorders are ruled out.

Parkinsonism

Falls are a frequent presentation of parkinsonism.[65,66] Parkinsonism patients undergo a number of gait abnormalities and postural changes that contribute to falling. As the disease progresses, patients may encounter difficulty when rising from a bed or chair. This is due to a failure by the patient to adequately flex his legs closer to his center of gravity.[67] In an effort to rise, patients will initiate small rocking motions and may fall if they don't use their hands to hold themselves in a sitting position. When standing, the ability to maintain an upright posture becomes impaired by a loss of autonomic postural reflexes. To preserve balance, the patient assumes a stooped posture, with the neck, trunk, and limbs held in forward flexion with bent arms and knees. The gait becomes short-stepped and shuffling with patients complaining that their feet feel like they are sticking to the ground. At times, gait initiation becomes difficult, and patients stutter (short, rapid shuffling steps) when they walk. A displaced center of gravity leads to propulsion — an uncontrolled forward motion that can sometimes only be stopped by walking into an immovable object — or retropulsion, falling backward. To offset the risk of falling forward, patients with propulsion may develop a festination or accelerated forward gait to help maintain a center of gravity. Other gait characteristics that may predispose to falls include a "freezing" walk, with the feet suddenly coming to a halt, but the body keeps on moving forward, resulting in a loss of balance. When patients attempt to turn, a loss of ankle movements and associated arm, shoulder, and hip rotation results in turning the body in a fixed unit, which compromises stability.[68]

Hemiplegia

Persons with stroke and mild hemiplegia display poor arm and leg swing, which becomes more obvious during periods of rapid walking. With severe hemiplegia, the knee of the affected limb is held in extension, and the ankle is plantar flexed and slightly inverted as the leg moves in a wide swinging pattern to help with ground clearance. Even so, the hemiplegic foot tends to drag and places the patient at risk for tripping falls. A loss of proprioceptive feedback in the involved limb may lead to uncertain foot placement during ambulation.

Cervical Spondylosis

This condition is a very common degenerative finding in the aged.[69] In most people, cervical spondylosis is a benign condition, but when cervical osteophytes occur posteriorly and impinge on a spinal canal that is narrow, myelopathy may result.[70] The associated myelopathy may lead to nonspecific gait complaints, such as "difficulty climbing stairs," "legs giving away," or "clumsiness of the feet," all of which can cause falls.

Normal Pressure Hydrocephalus

The syndrome of normal pressure hydrocephalus (NPH) includes the triad of dementia, urinary incontinence, and abnormal gait.[71] The gait disturbance, an early manifestation of NPH, is characterized by short steps, a slow unsteady walking speed, and ataxia.[72] Falls related to NPH occur suddenly only while standing and walking, with no warning, and are occasionally accompanied by a brief loss of consciousness.[73]

Ataxia

Patients with ataxia walk with a wide-based gait and frequent side-stepping. Common disorders responsible for ataxia include cerebellar disease, hyponatremia,[74] and vestibular dysfunction.

MUSCULOSKELETAL PROBLEMS
Osteoarthritis

Osteoarthritis can limit the ability to ambulate, climb stairs, and transfer effectively. Arthritis of the knee may interfere with stability and rising from chairs. The locked position of the knee is an important antigravity mechanism for maintaining balance. When the knee is flexed due to arthritis, the body relies to a great extent on the quadriceps for support. Additionally, significant osteoarthritis of the knees may lead to valgus or varus deformity, secondary to involvement of the medial tibiofemoral compartment. This may result in ligamentous weakness and instability, causing the legs to give way or collapse.

Muscle Weakness

Proximal muscle weakness is a leading feature of polymyalgia rheumatica, hyperthyroidism, hypothyroidism, hypokalemia, hyperparathyroidism, osteomalacia, hypophosphatemia, and drugs such as steroids, phenytoin, triamterine, and spironolactone.[75]

Osteomalacia

This common, but often unrecognized, disorder in the elderly is a condition characterized by deficient mineralization of bone.[76,77] Clinically, patients present with ill-defined skeletal pain. Hip involvement results in pain, which is worse during weight-bearing, and proximal muscle weakness, producing an unstable waddling gait.[78]

Paget's Disease

This disease is often a clinically benign condition, but, if symptomatic, several complications may follow that place patients at fall risk. Deformities of the lower extremities, as evidenced by tibial bowing and acetabular protrusion, can alter gait (due to unequal length and change in distribution of mechanical forces in the lower extremities) and predispose a patient to fractures that occur spontaneously or with minimal trauma.

PSYCHOLOGIC PROBLEMS

Cognitive dysfunction appears to be a risk factor for falling.[79-81] Patients with dementia and depression have an excess number of falling episodes.[82] Persons with senile dementia of the Alzheimer's type (SDAT) display certain alterations in gait and vitamin levels that may explain their high fall frequency. SDAT has been demonstrated to result in patients walking more slowly, with shorter steps, increased double support time, and greater step-to-step variability.[83] Serum vitamin B_{12} levels have been found to be low in patients with SDAT, which may lead to proprioceptive loss and increased confusion.[84] Older people with depression are more likely to suffer a loss of concentration, which can lead to judgmental errors, a misperception of environmental hazards, and falls.[85] A loss of friends and family, from either death or relocation, a change in living environments (i.e., entry to a nursing home and giving up one's home), loss of bodily functions (i.e., mobility, cognition, urinary continence), and a decline in performing everyday activities are common reasons for depression. If depression is severe enough, recurrent falling episodes may be a sign of suicidal intent, as persons place themselves in hazardous situations beyond their ability to control.[86]

DRUGS

Although some studies have failed to demonstrate a relationship between falls and drugs,[87-89] it is generally agreed that medications increase the risk of falling in older persons.[90-92] Patients who fall either eat within a few hours of a fall or utilize a large percentage of laxatives,[93] tranquilizers and hypnotics,[94] diuretics, psychotropics, or cardiovascular drugs.[96]

ENVIRONMENTAL FACTORS

The environment in which an older person resides plays an important role in either causing or preventing falls.[95] Within the home environment, the majority of falls occur on stairways,[97,98] in the bedroom,[99] and in the living room.[99] Most falls occur during routine activities, such as transferring from beds and chairs,[21,102] walking and tripping over carpets and door thresholds,[103,104] slipping on wet floors,[105] and descending stairways.[106,107] In the hospital and nursing home environment, the factors related to falling appear to be quite similar to those found in the home. The most common location for falls is the bedroom,[108-110] with the majority occurring during bed transfers.[111,112] Bed rails in the up position appear not to be protective against falling but may actually lead to increased falls, as patients try to climb over the rails when getting out of bed.[113,114] The bathroom is another common fall location,[115,116] with the majority of falls occurring during toilet transfer.[117,118] Chairs and wheelchairs have been found to contribute to falls and occur as a result of poor patient transfer technique.[119,120] A causal relationship between falls and the use of assistive devices (i.e., canes, walkers) has been found by some,[120] while others have found either no relationship[123] or a reduction in falls.[124,125] The use of physical restraints to prevent falls has, in some studies, actually contributed to further falls,[126] presumably due to improper application. The number of staff members present has been discussed as a factor relating to falls. Some have found that falls increase when staff levels are minimum[128] and that falls decrease when staff levels are increased.[125] The peak incidence for institutional falls occurs during the first week of stay.[130,131] While there is lack of sufficient research available on environmental modification and fall reduction, attention towards the assessment of environmental hazards and their correction will minimize fall risk (Table 41–1).

When evaluating the home or institutional environment, many potential fall hazards can be identified, with some presenting more risk to an individual than others. To determine which environmental factors require correction, the environmental assessment should take place in conjunction with an observed functional assessment. Only by watching an older person maneuver and function in his or her living environment can a clear determination be made as to which aspects of the environmental setting are safe or hazardous. Observe the patient ambulating over different floor surfaces (linoleum, ceramic tile, carpets, etc.); climb and descend stairs (if present); transfer on and off chairs, beds, toilets; get in and out of the shower or bathtub; and reach up or bend down to obtain

Table 41–1 Environmental Modification

Obstacle	Modification
Ground surfaces	
Highly polished or wet floors contribute to slipping.	In bathrooms, recommend nonslip glazed ceramic tile; nonslip adhesive strips placed on floor next to tub, sink, and toilet; or indoor-outdoor carpet, which also reduces the risk of fall-related physical injury.
	Linoleum floors can be rendered slip-free with use of slip-resistant floor wax and minimal buffing. Keep a nonskid floor mat by kitchen sink to guard against wet floor.
Thick pile carpets may lead to tripping.	Avoid thick pile or shag carpets. Recommend carpets of uncut, low pile.
Area rugs and mats may lead to sliding falls.	Recommend that all rugs/mats have non-skid backing or line back with double-faced adhesive tape.
Patterned carpets may lead to spatial misjudgment in persons with decreased depth perception.	Recommend plain, unpatterned carpets.
Lighting	
Poor environmental lighting may hide tripping/slipping hazards.	Provide increased lighting in high-risk fall locations (i.e., stairs, bathroom, bedroom).
Distracting glare from sunlight or lights shining on polished floors and unshielded light bulbs may impair vision.	Polarized window glass or application of tinted material to windows will eliminate glare without reducing light. Floor glare can be reduced by placing carpets on floor or repositioning light sources so that they do not shine directly on the floor.
Stairs	
Poor lighting may contribute to stairway tripping.	Place light switches at top and bottom of stairs to avoid traveling darkened stairways, or place night-lights by first and last step to provide visual cuing of steps. Placement of colored, nonslip adhesive strip will help define step edges.
Loss of balance on stairs may lead to serious falls.	Install handrails on both sides of stairs. Handrails should be round and set out far enough from the wall to allow for a good grasp.
Bathroom	
Sink edges and towel bars may be used as assistive devices.	Replace towel bars with nonslip grab bars. Apply nonslip adhesive strips to top of sink to prevent slipping if grasped.
Transfer falls from low toilet seats.	Advise the use of elevated toilet seat and grab bars placed on wall next to toilet.
A slip and loss of balance may occur in the bathtub or shower.	Place nonslip adhesive rubber strips or mat with suction cups on tub floor. Install nonslip grab bars in and around bathtub/shower. Advise use of shower chair and flexible hand-held shower hose for balance-impaired persons.
Beds	
Transfer falls may occur from high/low beds.	A bed height of approximately 18 inches (from top of mattress to floor) will allow for safe transfers. Institutions can achieve a safe transfer height by using height-adjustable beds.
Poor sitting balance may lead to bed falls.	Bed mattress edges should be firm enough to support a seated person without sagging.
Chairs	
Transfer falls from low-seated chairs.	A chair height of 14 to 16 inches (from seat edge to floor) and armrests to provide leverage during rising/sitting will allow for safe transfers.
Shelves	
Reaching or bending to retrieve objects from high or low shelves can lead to imbalance and falling.	Rearrange frequently used kitchen and closet items to avoid excessive reaching/bending. Shelf storage should be between a patient's hip and eye level. Encourage the use of hand-held reacher devices to obtain objects.

objects from closets and kitchen shelves. The functional assessment should be modified according to the environmental setting and the health status of the patient.

HISTORY AND PHYSICAL EVALUATION

In order to obtain as much information as possible about the falling episode, the fall history should include, in addition to a comprehensive review of all medical problems and medications, a precise accounting of the falling (Table 41–2). The physical examination of the fall patient should consist of a comprehensive medical, neurologic, and functional status evaluation to determine the presence of intrinsic problems that may contribute to the fall. Specific emphasis should be placed on examining the cardiovascular, neurologic, and musculoskeletal systems (Table 41–3).

In summary, the majority of falls in older people can be prevented or reduced in frequency if clinicians, first, begin to view the falling event as symptomatic of an underlying problem and, second, perform comprehensive assessments to uncover a multitude of medical, psychologic, and environmental factors that may be causative of falling.

Table 41–2   The Fall History

- A previous history of falling
- Time of fall (hour of day)
- Location
- Symptoms experienced
- Activity engaged in
- Device utilization
- Presence of witness

Table 41–3   Fall Assessment

Evaluation	Rationale
Blood pressure in supine and sitting/standing position	Evaluate presence of orthostatic hypotension
Visual	Evaluate acuity, peripheral and horizontal fields of vision, and color discrimination
Cardiovascular	
Pulse rate	Determine presence of arrhythmia
Neck turning extension	Determine presence of carotid or vertebrobasilar artery involvement
Carotid bulb massage	Determine presence of carotid sinus sensitivity
Gait/balance/musculoskeletal function	
Rise from chair	Observe for proximal muscle weakness
Perform deep knee bend	Observe for quadriceps weakness
Walk 10 feet in a straight line	Observe posture, balance, presence of arm swing, stride length, and steppage height
Climb/descend flight of stairs	Observe balance movements of legs and use of handrails
Tandem walk	Observe for loss of balance
Walk on toes/heels	Observe for plantar/dorsiflexion at ankles and loss of balance
Romberg test	Observe for increased sway/loss of balance
Stand on tiptoes and reach arm upward (as if reaching for an object from a high shelf)	Observe for loss of balance
Bend down and pick up an object from the ground	Observe for loss of position sense, sitting balance, and proximal muscle strength
Check podiatric capabilities	Presence of foot abnormalities that cause gait dysfunction (i.e., corns, bunions, hammer toes, etc.)

REFERENCES

1. Perry BC: Falls among the aged living in a high–rise apartment, J Fam Pract 14:1069–1073, 1982.
2. Waller J: Falls among the elderly: human and environmental factors, Accid Anal Prev 10:21–33, 1978.
3. Prudham D and Evans JG: Factors associated with falls in the elderly: a community study, Age Ageing 10:141–146, 1981.
4. Campbell AJ et al: Falls in old age: a study of frequency and related clinical factors, Age Ageing 10:264–270, 1981.
5. Droller H: Falls among elderly people living at home, Geriatrics 10:239–244, 1955.
6. Swartzbeck EM and Milligan WL: A comparative study of hospital incidents, Nurs Management 13:39–43, 1982.
7. Gryfe CI, Amies A, and Ashley MI: A longitudinal study: I. Incidence and mortality, Age Ageing 6:201–210, 1977.
8. Wild D, Nayak USL, and Isaacs B: Prognosis of falls in old people at home, J Epidemiol Community Health 35:200–204, 1981.
9. Perry BC: Falls among the elderly: a review of the methods and conclusions of epidemiologic studies, J Am Geriatr Soc 30:367–371, 1982.
10. Albanese AA et al: Problems of bone health in the elderly, NY State J Med 75:326–336, 1975.
11. Tideiksaar R and Kay AD: What causes falls? a logical diagnostic procedure, Geriatrics 41:32–50, 1986.
12. Houge CC: Injury in late life. I. Epidemiology, J Am Geriatr Soc 30:183–190, 1982.
13. Haupt BJ and Graves E: Detailed diagnosis and surgical procedures for patients discharged from short stay hospitals, United States, 1979, DHHS Publication Number (PHS) 82-1274-1, US Department of Health and Human Services, Washington, DC, 1982.
14. Reference deleted in proofs.
15. Evans JG, Prudham D, and Wandless I: A prospective study of fractured proximal femur: incidence and outcome, Public Health, London, 93:235–241, 1979.
16. Reference deleted in proofs.
17. Thomas TG and Stevens RS: Social effects of fractures of the neck of the femur, Br Med J 2:456–458, 1974.
18. Reference deleted in proofs.
19. Nickens H: The psychiatric consultant's approach to elderly fallers, Hosp Community Psychiatry 35:1190–1191, 1248, 1984.
20. Reference deleted in proofs.
21. Naylor R and Rosen AJ: Falling as a cause of admission to a geriatric unit, The Practitioner 205:327–330, 1970.
22. Reference deleted in proofs.
23. Andrews K: Relevance of re-admission of elderly patients discharged from a geriatric unit, J Am Geriatr Soc 34:5–11, 1986.
24. Rubenstein LZ: Falls in the elderly: a clinical approach, West J Med 138:273–275, 1983.
25. Kokemen E et al: Neurologic manifestations of aging, J Gerontol 32:411–419, 1977.
26. Wolf E: Glare and age, Arch Ophthalmol 64:502–514, 1960.
27. Andreasen MEK: Color vision defects in the elderly, J Gerontol Nurs 6(7):383–384, 1980.
28. Critchley M: Neurologic changes in the aged, J Chronic Dis 3:459–477, 1956.
29. Murry MP, Seireg A, and Sepic S: Normal postural stability and steadiness: quantitative assessment, J Bone Joint Surg 57A:510–516, 1975.
30. Overstall PW et al: Falls in the elderly related to postural balance, Br Med J 1:261–264, 1977.
31. Skinner HB, Barrack RL, and Cook SD: Age-related decline in proprioception, Clin Orthop 184:208–211, 1984.
32. Steiness I: Vibratory perception in normal subjects, Acta Med Scand 158:315–325, 1957.
33. Cape R: Falling. In Cape R, editor: Aging: its complex management, New York, 1978, Harper and Row.
34. Azar GJ and Lawton AH: Gait and stepping as factors in the frequent falls of elderly women, Gerontologist 4(2):83–84, 103, 1964.
35. Murry MP, Kory RC, and Clarkson BH: Walking patterns in healthy old men, J Gerontol 24:164–178, 1969.
36. Edholm OG: Studies of gait and mobility in the elderly, Age Ageing 10:147–156, 1981.
37. Caird FI, Andrews GR, and Kennedy RD: Effect of posture on blood pressure in the elderly, Br Heart J 35:527–530, 1973.
38. Baker SL: The preventability of falls. In Muir Gray JA, editor: Prevention of disease in the elderly, New York, 1985, Churchill Livingstone.
39. Katzman R: Demography, definitions and problems. In Katzman R and Terry RD, editors: The neurology of aging, Philadelphia, 1983, FA Davis Co.
40. Serratrice G, Roux H, and Aquaron R: Proximal muscle weakness in elderly subjects, J Neurol Sci 7:275–299, 1968.
41. Tinetti ME, Williams TF, and Mayewski R: Risk index for elderly patients based on number of chronic disabilities, Am J Med 80:429–434, 1986.
42. Reference deleted in proofs.
43. Overstall PW, Hazel JPW, and Johnson AL: Vertigo in the elderly, Age Ageing 10:105–109, 1981.
44. Reference deleted in proofs.
45. Lipsitz LA: The drop attack: a common geriatric symptom, J Am Geriatr Soc 31:617–620, 1983.
46. Reference deleted in proofs.
47. Sheehan S, Bauer RB, and Meyer JG: Vertebral artery compression in cervical spondylosis: arteriographic demonstration during life of vertebral artery insufficiency due to rotation and extension of neck, Neurology 10:968–986, 1960.
48. Lipsitz LA: Syncope in the elderly, Ann Intern Med 99:92–105, 1983.
49. Day SC, Cook EF, and Funkenstein H: Evaluation and outcome of emergency room patients with transient loss of consciousness, Am J Med 73:15–23, 1982.
50. Andrews GB and Kennedy RD: Effect of posture on blood pressure in the elderly, Br Heart J 35:527–530, 1973.
51. Rodstein M and Zeman FD: Postural blood pressure changes in the elderly, J Chronic Dis 6:581–588, 1957.
52. Roberts DH: Neurological complications of systemic diseases, Br Med J 1:33–35, 1970.
53. Lipsitz LA et al: Postprandial reduction in blood pressure in the elderly, N Engl J Med 309:81–83, 1983.
54. Heidon GH and McNamara AP: Effect of carotical sinus stimulation on the electrocardiograms of clinically normal individuals, Circulation 19:1104–1113, 1956.
55. Vesu CT, Eisenman JI, and Stemmer EA: The problem of dizziness and syncope in old age: transient ischemic attacks versus hypersensitive carotid sinus reflex, J Am Geriatr Soc 24:126–135, 1976.
56. Johnson RH: Blood pressure and its regulation. In Caird FI, Dall JLC, and Kennedy RD, editors: Cardiology in old age, New York, 1976, Plenum Press.
57. Reference deleted in proofs.
58. Mccarthy ST and Woller L: Cardiac dysrhythmias: treatable causes of transient cerebral dysfunction in the elderly, Lancet 2:202–203, 1977.
59. Rai GS: Cardiac arrhythmias in the elderly, Age Ageing 11:113–115, 1982.
60. Heyman A: Syncope and hyperventilation. In Beeson PB and McDermott, editors: Textbook of medicine, Philadelphia, 1971, WB Saunders Co.
61. Guimaraes RM and Isaacs B: Studies of gait and balance in normal old people and in people who have fallen: characteristics of the gait of old people who fall, Intern Rehab Med 2:177–180, 1980.
62. Wild D, Isaacs B, and Nayak USL: How dangerous are falls in old people at home? Br Med J 282:266–268, 1980.
63. Critchley M: Senile disorders of gait, Geriatrics 3:364–370, 1948.
64. Sabin TD: Biologic aspects of falls and mobility limitations in the elderly, J Am Geriatr Soc 30:51–58, 1982.
65. Lund M: Drop attacks in association with parkinsonism and basilar artery sclerosis, Acta Neurol Scand 39:226–229, 1963.
66. Klawans HL and Topel JL: Parkinsonism as a falling sickness, JAMA 230:1555–1557, 1974.
67. Klawans HL and Topel JL: Parkinsonism as a falling sickness, J Am Med Assoc 230:1555–1557, 1974.
68. Aita JF: Why patients with Parkinson's disease fall, JAMA 247:515–516, 1982.
69. Hunt WE: Cervical spondylosis: natural history and rare indications for surgical decompression. In Congress of Neurological Surgeons: Clinical neurosurgery, Baltimore, 1980, Williams and Wilkins.
70. Murray PK: Cervical spondylotic myelopathy: a cause of gait disturbance and urinary incontinence in older persons, J Am Geriatr Soc 32:324–330, 1984.
71. Adams RD et al: Symptomatic occult hydrocephalus with "normal"

cerebrospinal fluid pressure: a treatable syndrome, N Engl J Med 273:117–126, 1965.

72. Sorensen PS, Jansen C, and Gjerris F: Motor disturbances in normal pressure hydrocephalus: special reference to stance and gait, Arch Neurol 43:34–38, 1986.

73. Botez MI: Falls, Br J Hosp Med 10:494–499, 1982.

74. Kelsey SM, Williams AC, and Corbin D: Hyponatremia as a cause of reversible ataxia, Br Med J 293:1346, 1986.

75. Cook JD and Haller RG: Treatable neuromuscular diseases. In Rosenberg RN, editor: The treatment of neurological disases, New York, 1979, SP Medical and Scientific Books.

76. Exton-Smith AN: Nutrition in the elderly, Br J Hosp Med 5:639–646, 1971.

77. Frame B and Parfitt AM: Osteomalacia: current concepts, Ann Intern Med 89:966–982, 1978.

78. Schlott GD and Wills MR: Muscle weakness in osteomalacia, Lancet 1:626–629, 1976.

79. Prudham D and Evans JG: Factors associated with falls in the elderly: a clinical study, Age Ageing 10:141–146, 1981.

80. Houge CC: Injury in later life. I. Epidemiology, J Am Geriatr Soc 30:183–189, 1982.

81. Berry G, Fisher RH, and Laney S: Detrimental incidents including falls in an elderly institutional population, J Am Geriatr Soc 29:322–324, 1981.

82. Dy DJ: Falling accidents and organic brain syndrome, N Engl J Med 288:1026–1027, 1973.

83. Visser H: Gait and balance in senile dementia of the Alzheimer's type, Age Ageing 12:296–301, 1983.

84. Cole MG and Prachal JF: Low serum vitamin B_{12} in Alzheimer-type dementia, Age Ageing 13:101–105, 1984.

85. Jacobson SB: Accidents in aged, New York State J Med 74:2417–2420, 1974.

86. Lawton AH: Accidental injuries to the aged and their psychological impact, Mayo Clin Proc 42:685–697, 1967.

87. Perry BC: Falls among the elderly living in high-rise apartments, J Fam Pract 14:109–1073, 1982.

88. Morse JM, Tylke SJ, and Dixon HA: The patient who falls and falls again, J Gerontol Nurs 11(11):15–18, 1985.

89. Foerster J: A study of falls: the elderly nursing home resident, J New York State Nurs Assoc 12(2):9–17, 1981.

90. Whitlock FA, Boyce L, and Siskind V: Accidents in old age, Aust Fam Physician 7:389–399, 1978.

91. MacDonald JB: The role of drugs in falls in the elderly. In Radebaugh TS, Hadley E, and Suzman R, editors: Falls in the elderly: biologic and behavioral aspects, Clinics in Geriatrics Medicine, Philadelphia, 1985, WB Saunders Co.

92. Sorock GS: A case control study of falling incidents among the hospitalized elderly, J Safety Res 14:47–52, 1983.

93. Odetunde Z: Fell walking, Nurs Mirror 2:32–35, 1982.

94. Sehested P and Severin-Nielsen T: Falls by hospitalized elderly patients: causes, prevention, Geriatrics 4:101–108, 1977.

95. Barbieri EB: Patient falls are not patient accidents, J Gerontol Nurs 9:165–173, 1983.

96. Morse JM et al: A retrospective analysis of falls, Can J Pub Health 76:116–118, 1985.

97. Sheldon JH: On the natural history of falls in old age, Br Med J 2:1685–1690, 1960.

98. Lucht V: A prospective study of accidental falls and resulting injuries in the home among elderly people, Acta Socio-Med Scand 2:105–120, 1971.

99. Wild D, Nayak USL, and Isaacs B: How dangerous are falls in old people at home? Br Med J 287:266–268, 1981.

100. Reference deleted in proofs.

101. Reference deleted in proofs.

102. Droller H: Falls among elderly people living at home, Geriatrics 10:239–244, 1955.

103. Morfitt JM: Falls in old people at home: intrinsic versus environmental factors in causation, Public Health 97:115–120, 1983.

104. Prudham D and Grimley EJ: Factors associated with falls in the elderly: a community study, Age Ageing 10:141–146, 1981.

105. Gabell A, Simons MA, and Nayak USL: Falls in the healthy elderly: predisposing causes, Ergonomics 28:965–975, 1985.

106. Droller H: Falls among elderly people living at home, Geriatrics 10:239–244, 1955.

107. Svanstrom L: Falls on stairs: an epidemiological accident study, Scand J Soc Med 2:113–120, 1974.

108. Berry G, Fisher RH, and Lang S: Detrimental incidents including falls in an elderly institutional population, J Am Geriatr Soc 29:322–324, 1981.

109. Sehested P and Severin-Nielsen T: Falls by hospitalized elderly patients: causes, prevention, Geriatrics 4:101–108, 1977.

110. Gould G: A survey of incident reports, J Gerontol Nurs 1:23–26, 1975.

111. Parrish HM and Weil TP: Patient accidents occurring in hospitals: epidemiologic study of 614 accidents, New York State J Med 3:838–846, 1958.

112. Kalchthaler T, Bascon RA, and Quintos V: Falls in the institutionalized elderly, J Am Geriatr Soc 26:424–428, 1978.

113. Innes EM and Turman WG: Evaluation of patient falls, Q Rev Bull 2:30–35, 1983.

114. Buehrle R: When, where, how and why of accidents, Hosp Admin Can 11:24–28, 1969.

115. Clark G: A study of falls among elderly hospitalized patients, Aust J Adv Nurs 2(2):34–44, 1985.

116. Pablo RY: Patient accidents in a long-term care facility, Can J Public Health 68:237–247, 1977.

117. Colling J and Park D: Home, safe home, J Gerontol Nurs 9:175–179, 1983.

118. Uden G: Inpatient accidents in hospitals, J Am Geriatr Soc 33:833–841, 1985.

119. Clark G: A study of falls among elderly hospitalized patients, Aust J Adv Nur 2(2):34–44, 1985.

120. Lund CL and Sheafor ML: Is your patient about to fall? J Gerontol Nurs 11(4):37–41, 1985.

121. Reference deleted in proofs.

122. Reference deleted in proofs.

123. Foerster J: A study of falls: the elderly nursing home residents, J New York State Nurs Assoc 2(2):9–17, 1981.

124. Lund CL and Sheafor ML: Is your patient about to fall? Institutionalized elderly, J Am Geriatr Soc 26:424–428, 1978.

125. Kalchthaler T, Bascon RA, and Quintos V: Falls in the institutionalized elderly, J Am Geriatr Soc 26:424–428, 1978.

126. Innes EM and Turman WG: Evaluation of patient falls, Q Rev Bull 2:30–35, 1983.

127. Reference deleted in proofs.

128. Elliott DF: Accidents in nursing homes: implications for patients and administrators. In Miller M, editor: Current issues in clinical geriatrics, New York, 1979, Tiresias Press.

129. Reference deleted in proofs.

130. Feist RR: A survey of accidental falls in a small home for the aged, J Gerontol Nurs 4:15–17, 1978.

131. Manjam NVB and MacKinnon HH: Patient, bed and bathroom: a study of falls occurring in a general hospital, Nova Scotia Med Bull 2:23–25, 1973.

132. Tinetti ME, Speechley M, and Ginter SF: Risk factors for falls among elderly persons living in the community, N Engl J Med 319:26, 1988.

133. Rubenstein LZ et al: Falls and instability in the elderly, J Am Geriatr Soc 36:266, 1988.

Evaluation of Falls and Their Traumatic Consequences

Clark Chipman, M.D., F.A.C.E.P.

EMERGENCY EVALUATION OF FALLS AND THEIR CONSEQUENCES

Persons aged 65 or older comprise 10% of the population of our country but 25% of all fatal injuries or some 28,000 deaths per year. Falls are the single largest cause of accidental death in the elderly and account for over half of all deaths in this age group. Falls are the second leading cause of accidental death in the United States, with almost three quarters of all falls occurring among the aged. The death rate from falls rises significantly for those aged 65 or older.[1] In individuals over age 65, deaths resulting from falls are more common than deaths from all other causes of accidents combined.[2]

However, the majority of elderly patients who fall will not die. The Metropolitan Life Insurance Company states that in the United States 10,000 persons die annually as a result of falls in and around the home, and 7 million are injured.[3] In emergency departments, it is common to treat an elderly person who has fallen. Thus, it behooves both the practitioner of emergency medicine and the physician who cares for aged patients to be familiar with falls and their possible complications. The morbidity from falls is alarming and often forces the older individual to enter a nursing home or make major living changes.[3a] Yet most falls are preventable and require strategies for avoidance.[3b]

It is of interest to note that an elderly individual who has fallen is more likely to be a female. In a study of nursing home patients who fell, most falls (79%) occurred among women.[4] And in a large prospective study of falls occurring in the home, approximately three times as many women as men were involved.[3]

Although it is advisable for the examining physician to follow a systematic approach, ruling out more serious injuries initially, most elderly patients who fall do not present with injuries that are an immediate threat to life. Most patients are all too well aware of what has happened to them and, for them, the fall may be a devastating event. The physician's approach should be gentle and unhurried, and he or she must make every attempt to be aware of, and to administer to, the elderly patients' psychologic needs.

Many elderly patients are partially deaf, and the strange surroundings and turmoil of the emergency department engender confusion, particularly if the patient fails to hear what is said. Great attention must be paid to making sure that patients hear and understand what is to be done.[5] Some elderly patients may become bewildered, frightened, or hostile if treated by the physician in an abrupt or intolerant manner. A sympathetic and cautious response to the patient's questions and needs may make a large difference in allaying fears and gaining cooperation. Patients will be unhappy and distraught by being handicapped and in new surroundings, and while they may not have been disabled prior to hospitalization, they now may well be completely dependent upon others for their care. From the first encounter, every attempt must be made to make the hospital experience one of the greatest possible dignity and comfort.[6]

Why the Elderly Fall

A patient, while walking, may feel her legs give and then falls. She doesn't recall any warning or symptoms; she did not trip or slip, and she did not lose consciousness. When seen in the emergency department, she may say, "I must have slipped" but this means "I don't know what happened, so I must have slipped." These falls should be investigated carefully because a treatable cause may be found. It is particularly important to discover the circumstances of the fall by asking the patient what she was doing at the time of the fall — her exact activity, exactly how she felt, and exactly how she fell.

A recent study has demonstrated that falls in the elderly are often quite serious and may represent a dangerous underlying process that is independent of the trauma caused by the fall.[7] Patients may be labeled "generalized cerebral atherosclerosis," "vertebrobasilar insufficiency," "senility," or "chronic ear disease" in an attempt to define the nature of their disability. Often this occurs without a careful look at potentially treatable conditions. Perhaps this occurs because it is more direct and easier to treat the injury that has occurred, because these patients are very poor historians, or because the possible causes are many.

Causes of falls can be divided into extrinsic or environmental causes resulting in the opportunity to fall, and intrinsic causes resulting in the liability to fall.[8] If the cause of the fall is wholly or partially extrinsic — i.e., something in the patient's environment — of course this should be corrected. Additionally, perhaps, an informed and concerned family member should survey the elderly patient's surroundings for other extrinsic possibilities so that falls may be avoided in the future. Such things as improper hand railings, steep steps, slippery rugs, and slippery bathtub surfaces should be corrected without delay.

The physician must also consider intrinsic causes for falls. If a patient has had a severe fall, and has been fortunate enough not to suffer a fracture or other serious injury, the examining physician should at least consider the possibility of admission to the hospital where a complete workup can be done in an attempt to discover the reason for the fall. On one hand, this might be labeled an "inappropriate admission"; on the other hand, the alternative may be an "appropriate admission" several days later when the same patient returns after sustaining a serious injury from a fall that was potentially preventable. Table 42–1 lists some of the intrinsic causes of falls in the elderly. The scope of this chapter does not allow more than the briefest descriptions for each of these. (Causes are discussed in more detail in Chapter 41.)

Common Changes of Age

The spinal, subcortical, and cortical reflexes that maintain posture are highly susceptible to the changes of aging. As patients become older, the tendency is to assume

Table 42–1   Causes of Falls in the Elderly

1. Common changes of age
2. Orthostatic hypotension
3. Cardiac arrhythmias
4. Poor footwear
5. Vertebrobasilar insufficiency
6. Dizziness
7. Occult blood loss
8. Poor vision
9. Drugs
10. Depression
11. Others (syncope, transient ischemic attack, epilepsy, electrolyte imbalance)

a more stooped posture and a broader-based gait and to propel themselves with shuffling steps as they watch closely in front in an effort to avoid stumbling over obstacles. However, rather than preventing a fall, this "gait of the elderly" seems to ensure it. When one begins to fall, he or she prevents this by reflexly taking a larger step and preventing the fall. But in the elderly patient, not only is the broad-based shuffling gait a poor position from which to stabilize oneself, but slowed reflexes and weaker muscles make prevention of the fall even more unlikely. It has been noted that elderly patients tend to sway more than younger patients when attempting to stand absolutely still with both feet together. The amount of sway can be measured by an instrument attached to the patient's chest that records sway over a period of time. It is thought that the greater the tendency to sway, the greater the tendency to fall. Finally, the mental confusion and faulty judgment of some elderly patients can cause them to fall.[9]

Orthostatic Hypotension

As a person becomes older, he or she usually has decreased muscle mass in the lower extremities. This, along with other changes of aging, leads to diminished vascular tone and increased venous pooling in the lower extremities. A drop of 20 mm Hg or more, either systolic or diastolic, has been reported in between 17 and 25% of apparently healthy older people.[9] If the elderly patient arises suddenly, often vasoactive reflexes are not quick enough to prevent a significant orthostatic drop in blood pressure and a fainting episode. In addition, many of the medications that elderly patients take (diuretics, antihypertensives, and antidepressants) may induce orthostatic hypotension.

Cardiac Arrhythmias

As many as 26% of falls in the elderly may be associated with acute changes in cardiac status. Elderly patients often are not aware of the changes in cardiac rhythm, especially if they are at the same time experiencing temporary cerebral dysfunction. When other causes have been ruled out, Holter monitoring may be helpful.[10]

Poor Footwear

A large percentage of the elderly population has misshapen and poorly functioning feet due to decades of improper footwear. In addition, pedal edema or other disorders may make the patient's current supply of footwear more ill-fitting and encourage the wearing of bedroom slippers. This may seem a mundane problem but certainly can cause falls in the elderly.

Vertebrobasilar Insufficiency

This should be suspected as a cause of the fall if the fall occurred when the patient was reaching overhead or hyperextending his or her head to look at something at a higher elevation.

Dizziness

This in itself has been the topic of numerous lengthy and well-written articles. If the elderly patient is complaining of a recent onset of dizziness for which no cause is readily apparent, he or she should be referred for complete laboratory, neurologic, acoustical, and other appropriate testing. (See also Chapter 41.)

Occult Blood Loss

Any patient who has an unexplained fall should at the very least have postural pulses and blood pressures examined, a rectal exam with stool guaiac, and a hematocrit determined. Occult gastrointestinal bleeding is almost always unrecognized by the elderly patient.

Poor Vision

Often an elderly patient accepts or has lived with a diminution of vision for such a long period of time that he or she seems to forget that it is a fact. However, diminished vision caused by cataracts, diabetes mellitus, or other disorders can predispose an elderly patient to falls.

Drugs

Elderly people on medication fall more often than those in a control group. Drugs given for complaints such as insomnia and mild psychologic disturbances contribute more to accidents than medications prescribed for more specific symptoms. The avoidance of overprescribing in the elderly is one of our most significant contributions to the reduction of falls and fractures in older patients.[11]

Unfortunately, alcohol intoxication is not an infrequent cause of falls in the elderly. It may affect the most in-nocent-appearing of victims. The examining physician must keep this possibility in mind and specifically ask relatives or neighbors if alcohol is a problem.

Depression

This is a common and commonly unrecognized problem of the elderly patient. An episode of depression may cause the patient to take chances that he ordinarily would not, avoid necessary medication, or lead to other behaviors that might promote a fall.

Others

Syncope due to vasovagal attacks (increased carotid sinus sensitivity), cough syncope, micturition syncope, and defecation syncope should be considered. Transient ischemic attacks may be the culprit. Epilepsy has a second peak in incidence in old age due to cerebrovascular disease or occasionally cerebral tumors. Electrolyte imbalance may result from improper diuretic therapy.

The above list is by no means complete. Most readers upon examining it will be able to add two or three other causes for falls in the elderly. What should be remembered is that determining the cause of the fall may in many instances be more important to the patient than caring for the injuries that have occurred. No patient has been treated completely until this question has been asked and answered sufficiently.

Summary

Falls in the elderly are a common problem that the emergency physician or primary care physician must be prepared to manage. Discovering the cause of the fall or initiating investigative efforts to this end may ultimately be more valuable to the patient than treating the injuries suffered as the result of the fall.

TRAUMATIC INJURIES FROM FALLS

Consider yourself for a brief moment in the following circumstances: you are the first physician called to see an 85-year-old female who has been brought to the emergency department following a fall in her home. The emergency medical technicians who have transported the patient do not know the particulars of the fall. They were called by the woman's neighbors who became concerned because they had not seen her for several days and peered in the window of her house, to see her lying on the floor. When you first see the patient she is struggling, terrified, and disoriented as to where she is and how she got there. As you attempt to question her further, it is clear that she is quite confused, somewhat hostile, and she complains bitterly of pain in her hip and in the back of her head.

As you imagine yourself beginning to care for the elderly woman, what are your priorities for treatment? How should you begin your approach to this patient, and what are the most likely possibilities for injury? What other pieces of information are important for this patient's care? What special considerations might be important in managing an elderly, confused, and potentially seriously injured patient?

This chapter will discuss the topic of falls by first reviewing initial considerations and priorities in traumatized patients, emphasizing unique considerations in the elderly patient. It will then discuss specific problems in each of the anatomic areas, with emphasis on the more common orthopedic injuries sustained in falls.

The initial considerations are the same as for any injured patient — airway, breathing, and circulation (Table 42–2). In most emergency departments, as the physician is assessing these "ABCs," the nursing personnel are completely undressing the patient and obtaining the initial vital signs. Along with pulse, blood pressure, and respirations, the initial vital sign in an elderly patient who has fallen that may be of utmost importance is the temperature. A patient who lives alone and falls without being found for several hours may suffer from hypothermia. Hypothermia will not be recognized unless a rectal temperature is taken.[5] The physician should also be aware that in a very elderly patient a fall may herald the onset of serious disease and subsequent death. Often on initial examination the only indication of this may be a drop in blood pressure. This may be followed by rapid deterioration and subsequent manifestations of an acute underlying illness.[12]

Cervical Spine

As he assesses the ABCs in a patient who has fallen, the physician must make every effort to protect the cervical spine. A patient who is alert, complains of no pain in the cervical region, has no tenderness to palpation over the dorsal spinous processes of the cervical spine, and can move his neck with no pain may be reasonably safely presumed to have an intact cervical spine. On the other

Table 42–2 Priorities in the Multiple Trauma Patient

Airway maintenance

Breathing (including control of the cervical spine)

Control of circulation and cardiac dysrhythmias

Control of hemorrhage

Treatment of shock

Splinting of fractures

Evaluation of further injuries

Continuous monitoring

From American College of Surgeons: Advanced trauma life support course provider's manual, American College of Surgeons Committee on Trauma, 1980.

hand, in managing a patient who is comatose, or is alert and has positive findings, the cervical spine must be immobilized with sandbags until a portable cross-table lateral x-ray reveals it to be stable. It should be recalled that a severe injury to the spinal cord can occur without fracture or dislocation of the cervical spine. Hyperextension injuries are especially common in older individuals who fall forward and sustain trauma to the forehead or face. Such hyperextension can "pinch" the spinal cord between the posterior ligamentum flavum (which tends to become thickened with age) and posterior osteophytes, which are especially common in the elderly population.[13]

In a severely injured patient who needs intubation before the status of the cervical spine is determined, this should be accomplished by the blind nasotracheal route if the patient is breathing spontaneously or via the oral route if there are no spontaneous respirations. In both instances intubation should be done with an assistant providing axial traction on the head and preventing any significant amount of extension or flexion of the cervical spine.

Torso Injuries

Any major bleeding point should be controlled with direct pressure, and the physician should auscultate and palpate the chest and abdomen. Elderly patients who fall fairly frequently fracture ribs or the sternum,[3] but during this initial rapid primary survey, the physician is attempting to detect more serious thoracic injuries. Although usually of no major consequence, such injuries to the bony thorax may cause respiratory decompensation in patients with such conditions as chronic obstructive pulmonary disease.

Likewise, in examining the abdomen the physician attempts to diagnose a major intraabdominal injury. In falls, the organs most likely to be injured are the incapsulated ones — specifically the liver, spleen, bladder, and kidneys. If there is any doubt about the possibility of intraperitoneal hemorrhage, a peritoneal lavage should be performed. Surgical recommendations[14] also state that one should perform peritoneal lavage on a patient who has suffered significant injury if he or she is unconscious or intoxicated to a degree where the physician cannot have adequate confidence in the abdominal exam. Finally, although it is of less urgency, it should be mentioned that (particularly with hip fractures) the patient may have a distended bladder with retention. In these circumstances, a catheter should be passed with full aseptic precautions, and the bladder emptied entirely. In either circumstance, a urine specimen should be sent to the laboratory for testing.[5]

In a seriously injured patient, as a physician is performing these initial steps in the primary exam, nursing personnel will be inserting large-bore intravenous lines and placing a nasogastric tube and Foley bladder catheter. The next step the physician will want to perform is to splint all obvious fractures. In turn, the physician's attention will turn to a brief neurologic examination in an attempt to more accurately define the patient's neurologic status.

Head Injuries

While elderly patients who suffer head injuries have relatively fewer severe cerebral contusions than do younger patients, they have a higher incidence of subdural and intraparenchymal hematomas. Subdural hematomas are nearly three times as frequent in the elderly as in younger groups. On the other hand, epidural hematomas are very rare.[15] It should be remembered that a subdural hematoma may produce a rather gradual onset of neurologic decline. In fact, a subdural hematoma resulting from an earlier fall may be the cause of the fall for which the physician is currently examining the patient! This possibility should always be kept in mind.

Orthopedic Injuries: General Considerations

Osteoporosis, which occurs with increasing age, is the condition that most significantly increases the risk of fracture in the elderly skeleton. Osteoporosis should not be viewed as a pathologic process; rather, it is a change of the natural aging process that, unfortunately, makes the skeleton more susceptible to fractures. Compared with a 30-year-old, a 70-year-old woman has lost 25 to 30% of her bone density; a 70-year-old man loses 15 to 20%.[16] These changes can be confirmed both pathologically and radiographically. In a study designed to test osteoporosis by radiographic criteria, it was estimated that the incidence of osteoporosis of the spine of women between the ages of 45 and 79 years was approximately 29%, whereas only 18% of elderly men of a similar age were affected.[17] Perhaps this increased incidence of osteoporosis partially explains the higher incidence of fractures in elderly women.

Osteoporosis does not occur equally throughout the elderly skeleton. The areas most profoundly affected are the distal radius, the lumbosacral spine, and the neck of the femur. This has some interesting correlations in the incidence of sites fractured in elderly patients. If one considers the age distribution of fractures in general, it is noted that fractures of the upper limb have a bimodal age distribution with peaks in the young and the elderly. On the other hand, fractures of the lower limb have a J-shaped distribution, increasing as age increases. The rate of all fractures for both males and females increases progressively as a function of age. At age 35 to 44, the rate is higher in males. At age 45 to 54 the rates are approximately equal. From age 55 on up, the fracture rate in females is progressively higher than that of males.[18] The most common orthopedic injuries from falls are frac-

tures of the neck of the femur, the radius and/or ulna, and the humerus.[3]

Treatment and rehabilitation of the elderly patient with skeletal injuries should start as soon as possible. Sterile dressings should be gently applied to open soft tissue injuries. Too often, fractures are left unsplinted until x-rays are obtained, and such delay only tends to cause more pain and distress.[6]

In the fit adult, conservative treatment of some fractures is often considered a "safe and sure" method. The reverse is often true in the elderly. Morbidity from lying in bed far outweighs the morbidity of properly performed orthopedic surgery. As a rule, if operation is indicated, a reasonable goal is that surgery should take place within 24 hours. If a patient is felt to be unstable from other medical causes (i.e., diabetes mellitus or congestive heart failure), then perhaps 48 hours is a reasonable period for a stabilization.[5]

Finally, the physician must ask about the tetanus immunization status in any patient who has an open wound, however small. Since a majority of older individuals are not adequately protected against diphtheria and tetanus, if there is any question, he or she should receive appropriate immunization.[19]

Specific Sites
Fractures of the Hip

Femoral fractures are the most common type seen in the elderly. Annually 2% of women and 1% of men aged 85 or older have a femoral fracture.[20]

A patient with a fractured hip is, with rare exception, unable to walk. Usually, the patient is unwilling to sit, even partially upright on a gurney, and usually prefers not to be moved at all because this causes excruciating pain. Grossly the affected extremity is externally rotated, abducted, and usually somewhat shortened. The patient usually localizes pain in the area of the greater trochanter or anterior pelvis and is tender to palpation or compression over the area of the greater trochanter. However, a point which must be noted is that, occasionally, a patient with a hip fracture presents only with pain referred to the knee. Particularly in elderly patients this possibility must be considered, and, when suspected, radiograms of the hip on the side of the painful knee should be obtained. Occasionally, a patient with a fractured hip has very little or no pain at the hip but the possibility is considered by the examining physician. In these instances, a test that may be performed is to lift the patient's extended leg off the stretcher and gently "bump" the patient on the plantar surface of the foot. In this instance, the shock wave is transmitted up the tibia through the femur to the affected femoral neck, and the patient will often feel pain in that area. Of course, one would not perform such a test on a patient who had acute pain with any motion of the affected hip. Pulses, sensation, and function should be assessed, compared with the unaffected extremity, and recorded on the patient's chart.

Usually, elderly patients with isolated femoral neck fractures have stable vital signs and are not clinically in shock. However, if there is any doubt about hemodynamic status, an intravenous line should be established before proceeding further.

After completing the total assessment of the patient as described above, and if the physician is assured that no other significant injury has occurred, the patient should be made as comfortable as possible before proceeding further. Meperidine (Demerol) is usually sufficient to control muscle spasm and pain. Pain may also be relieved by proper positioning of the hip in gentle flexion with some support under the knee with pillows and sandbags. However, should severe pain continue, simple traction will be necessary. For emergency care, a Hare traction splint or Thomas half-ring splint is probably the best device to provide the necessary traction. No attempt should be made to try to reduce the fracture by traction and often a very small amount of tension will reduce the patient's pain.[5]

If the patient is otherwise stable, he or she may go to the radiology department for appropriate x-rays. The patient with a suspected hip fracture should have x-rays of the affected hip and pelvis and a routine chest x-ray. The latter, of course, is part of a routine surgical admission; this saves the elderly patient from having to make a second trip to the radiology department. The most helpful radiologic view for the primary practitioner in examining for hip fracture is a straight AP view of the pelvis that includes both femoral necks and trochanters.

There are several facts in interpreting this radiogram that can help the clinician to find what might otherwise be an occult fracture. First, one should be aware that the neck of the femur forms an inferior angle of approximately 135 degrees with the shaft of the femur, and the angle of the affected side should be compared with the non-affected side. These should be very nearly equal if the patient has not been rotated during the radiographic examination. Second, the clinician should follow Shenton's line. This is merely to remind one that in a straight AP view the smooth line formed by the inferior border of the neck of the femur appears to be almost continuous and unbroken with that line formed by the superior margin of the obturator foramen. Third, the physician should look for faint shadows around the neck of the femur superiorly and inferiorly formed by the iliopsoas muscles, bilaterally. These shadows will appear to be distended or bulging if a patient has suffered a fracture that has caused bleeding into the capsule surrounding the neck of the femur. Fourth, and most important, the physician must carefully examine all of the cortex of the femoral neck both superiorly and inferiorly and along both trochanters. If this cortical line appears to be broken or not contiguous in any portion, additional views should be

obtained. Finally, the clinician may wish to note the relative absence or presence of trabecular patterns through the femoral neck. The greater the degree of absence of these trabecular patterns, the more likely that the affected bone is osteoporotic. The greater the amount of osteoporosis, the greater the likelihood there will be a complication with fixation of this particular fracture.[21]

Fractures of the hip in the elderly patient usually occur in one of four areas (Figure 42–1). As one moves from superior to inferior, these fractures are termed subcapital, transcervical, intertrochanteric, and subtrochanteric. Intertrochanteric fractures are most common, followed by transcervical fractures.[22]

One must always seek orthopedic consultation for elderly patients with hip fractures. It is generally agreed that the minimal tests necessary for this patient, other than the aforementioned x-rays, include electrocardiogram, CBC, electrolytes, BUN, blood glucose, and a urinalysis. Any other tests that seem appropriate for the patient's clinical condition or other medical conditions should also be ordered. Since most of these patients will be destined for surgery, it is most important to note the time the last meal was consumed and to withhold anything by mouth except for perhaps an occasional ice chip.

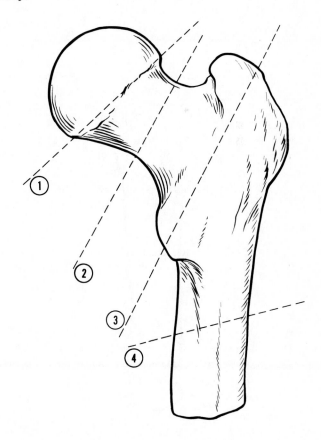

Figure 42–1 Common areas of hip (femoral) fracture in the elderly. *1,* Subcapital. *2,* Transcervical. *3,* Intertrochanteric. *4,* Subtrochanteric.

Fractures of the Humerus

The classic instance for this injury is the elderly person carrying a bag of groceries who slips while crossing a street. Often when an individual falls, particularly if he or she is carrying something and has somewhat slowed reflexes, much of the force of the fall is absorbed on the deltoid area, the "point of the shoulder." In younger patients (this is also a common mechanism of injury in football players) this sort of injuring force usually leads to an acromioclavicular injury. In an elderly patient, the injury that commonly occurs is a fracture of the surgical neck of the humerus (Figure 42–2). Due to force transmitted to the humeral shaft, the same sort of fracture often occurs in the elderly patient even if the force of the fall has been taken on the outstretched hand. In the younger patient a shoulder dislocation is more likely to occur.

The elderly patient with this injury usually presents with pain and tenderness in the shoulder or upper humeral area. Frequently, even early after the injury, there will be a surprisingly large bruise in the area of the fracture. This bruise may later include much of the upper arm, spread into the pectoral area, and may be very alarming in appearance. The nature and spread of this bruise should be explained to the patient to prevent undue concern. After a thorough examination of the neurovascular status of the entire affected arm, radiographs of the painful area should be obtained. The physician should be aware that this injury is not infrequently accompanied by dislocation of the shoulder, and if any suspicion of this accompanying injury is present, additional confirming radiologic views should be obtained. Fracture-dislocations may be very difficult to recognize, especially if the dislocation is posterior.

Once a diagnosis of fracture of the cervical neck of the humerus has been made, the important clinical determination that must be reached is whether or not the fracture is impacted or disimpacted. This is usually very simply done. First, no fracture segment may be displaced more than 1.0 cm or angulated more than 45 degrees. The patient is merely instructed to bend forward from the waist about 20 to 30 degrees and to allow the affected arm to dangle dependently from the shoulder. When a patient has an impacted fracture, the arm can be moved gently while dangling from the shoulder without undue pain: the patient with a disimpacted fracture will have exquisite pain with motion in this position. With impaction, no sense of false motion will be detected by the examiner who palpates the humeral head with one hand and gently rotates the humeral shaft with the other hand at the bent elbow. This determination is important, because a patient with an impacted fracture may be treated with a sling, progressive range of motion, and an orthopedic consultation as an outpatient. On the other hand, a patient with a disimpacted fracture will need to be admitted to the hospital for probable surgery. If there is any question about impaction or disimpaction or appropriate therapy, immediate orthopedic consultation should be sought. In either instance, it is an axiom in the treatment of these fractures that early movement is essential to prevent stiffness of the shoulder. If the patient is so severely incapacitated that this is impossible, it is usually wise to operate.[5]

Colles' Fracture

The usual mechanism for a Colles' fracture is a fall onto the outstretched, dorsiflexed hand. In the elderly patient, this commonly leads to a fracture through the metaphyseal area of the distal radius with dorsal angulation of the distal fracture fragment. Approximately 60% of the time, there will be an accompanying fracture through the base of the ulnar styloid.[23] In most cases, this produces an obvious deformity — the so-called dinner-fork deformity, with a dorsal depression and fullness in the volar aspect of the wrist. Sensation and function of all of the fingers on the affected side should be assessed, and the examiner should be aware that median nerve injury and, less frequently, flexor tendon injury at the wrist may be accompanying findings.

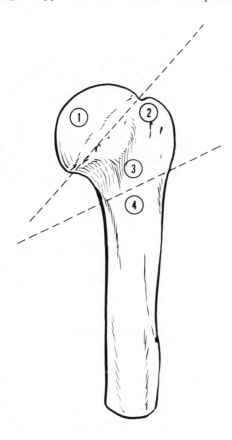

Figure 42–2 Humeral neck fractures occur between two or more segments. *1,* Head. *2,* Lesser tuberosity. *3,* Greater tuberosity. *4,* Shaft.

The minimal x-ray examinations include anteroposterior and lateral views of the affected wrist. The films must also be carefully reviewed to rule out an accompanying carpal fracture. If the fracture line goes either into the distal radioulnar joint or into the radial articular surface, the incidence of complication is higher.[23] If there is any tenderness or swelling at the elbow or if there is severe displacement of the distal radial fracture fragment, accompanying radiograms of the elbow should also be obtained to rule out concomitant elbow fracture.

Perhaps the most important message regarding Colles' fractures in the elderly is that often this is not a simple injury. Various degrees of malunion are not uncommon, patient dissatisfaction with the final result is not unusual, and often it takes a year or more for the injured wrist to reach its final degree of repair. Although some primary care practitioners might think differently, it is a good idea to refer all Colles' fractures in the elderly patient to an orthopedic surgeon. This being the case, no attempts at reduction need be made until the orthopedist arrives. The wrist should merely be splinted in the position of maximum comfort, and an analgesic given as necessary.

Summary

The physician will be more successful in caring for an elderly patient who has fallen if he or she has an understanding of the general priorities of care in an injured patient, the injuries that are most likely to occur in an elderly patient who has fallen, and special considerations in therapy due to the patient's age. The most common significant injuries likely to occur with falls in the elderly are hip fracture, fracture of the surgical neck of the humerus, and Colles' fracture of the distal radius and ulna.

REFERENCES

1. Metropolitan Life Insurance Company: Mortality from leading types of accidents, Statistical Bulletin 59:10, 1978.
2. US Department of Health, Education and Welfare: US Public Health Service Pub No 1459, Vol I:27–28, 1978.
3. Lucht L: A prospective study of accidental falls and resulting injuries in the home among elderly people, Acta Socio Medical Scandinavica 2:105–120, 1971.
3a. Tinetti ME, Speechley M, and Ginter SF: Risk factors for falls among elderly persons living in the community, N Engl J Med 319:1701, 1988.
3b. Tinnetti ME and Speechley M: Geriatrics: prevention of falls among the elderly, N Engl J Med 320:1055, 1989.
4. Kalchthaler T, Bascon RA, and Quintos V: Falls in the institutionalized elderly, J Am Geriatr Soc 26:424, 1978.
5. Devas M: Orthopedics. In Steinberg FU, editor: Care of the geriatric patient: in the tradition of EV Cowdry, ed 6, St Louis, 1983, The CV Mosby Co.
6. Freehafer AA: Injuries to the skeletal system of older persons. In Chinn AB, editor: Working with older people: a guide to practice, Vol IV, US Public Health Service Pub No 1415, Washington, DC, July 1971.
7. Gryfe CI, Amies A, and Ashley MH: A longitudinal study of falls in the elderly population, Age Ageing 6:201, 1977.
8. Stout RW: Falls and disorders of postural balance, Age Ageing 7(suppl):134–136, 1978.
9. Brocklehurst JC: Postural instability in the elderly, Consultant, pp 208–214, June 1980.
10. Bordon M: Occult cardiac arrhythmias associated with falls and dizziness in the elderly: detection by Holter monitoring, J Am Geriatr Soc 26(9):418–423, 1978.
11. Whitlock FA, Boyce L, and Siskind V: Accidents in old age, Aust Fam Physician 7:389–398, 1978.
12. Howell TH: Premonitory falls, Practitioner 206(235):667, 1971.
13. Cloward RB: Acute cervical spine injuries, Clin Symposia 32(1):2–32, 1980.
14. American College of Surgeons: Advanced trauma life support course provider's manual, American College of Surgeons Committee on Trauma, 1980.
15. Kirkpatrick JB and Pearson J: Fatal cerebral injury in the elderly, J Am Geriatr Soc 25(11):489–497, 1978.
16. Witte NS: Why the elderly fall, Am J Nurs, Nov:1959, 1979.
17. Avioli LV: Aging, bone, and osteoporosis. In Steinberg FU, editor: Care of the geriatric patient: in the tradition of EV Cowdry, ed 6, St Louis, 1983, The CV Mosby Co.
18. Garraway WM et al: Limb fractures in a defined population. I. Frequency and distribution, Mayo Clin Proc 54:701–707, 1979.
19. Crossley K et al: Tetanus and diphtheria immunity in urban Minnesota adults, JAMA 242(21):2298, 1979.
20. Brocklehurt JC et al: Fracture of the femur in old age: a two-centre study of associated clinical factors and the cause of the fall, Age Ageing 7:7, 1978.
21. Laros GS: The role of osteoporosis in intertrochanteric fractures, Orthop Clin North Am 11(3):525, 1980.
22. Laskin RS, Gruber MA, and Zimmerman AJ: Intertrochanteric fractures of the hip in the elderly. In Urist MR, editor: Clinical orthopaedics and related research, Philadelphia, 1979, JB Lippincott Co.
23. Dobyns JH and Linscheid RL: Fractures and dislocations of the wrist. In Rockwood CA and Green DP, editors: Fractures, Philadelphia, 1975, JB Lippincott Co.

Ophthalmologic Disorders

A Systematic Approach to Acute Ophthalmologic Disorders in the Geriatric Patient

James Dougherty, M.D., F.A.C.E.P.

Geriatric patients frequently present to the emergency department with such acute ophthalmologic disturbances as ocular pain, visual loss, red eye, or other visual aberrations (i.e., peripheral field cuts, haloes, tunnel vision, etc.). Unfortunately, deciphering the causes and selecting therapy for these conditions are frequently difficult for the nonophthalmologist. Nevertheless, because of the potential for loss of sight in the elderly, many of whom already have compromised vision, such symptoms are usually cause for great concern on the part of most geriatric patients. Consequently, acute ophthalmologic disturbances require diagnostic acumen so that therapy is implemented promptly and consultation, when indicated, is obtained as early as possible. Finally, ophthalmologic emergencies not only can be the first manifestation of underlying systemic disease, but many pharmacotherapeutic agents used to treat ophthalmologic conditions can produce systemic toxicity that is easily overlooked.

THE AGING EYE

The aging eye is associated with a number of characteristic physiologic changes (Figure 43–1).[1-6] Because of the presence of underlying systemic disorders and increased host vulnerability, the geriatric patient represents the largest segment of the population at risk for many common ophthalmologic emergencies. Indeed, acute ocular problems are a source of great concern for this subgroup of patients. Because ocular pain, loss of visual function, and the threat of potential blindness are usually perceived as a medical crisis by the afflicted patient, these symptoms can provoke the patient to seek emergency care.

EVALUATION

As with other acute medical disorders, a thorough symptom-oriented history is invaluable for sorting out

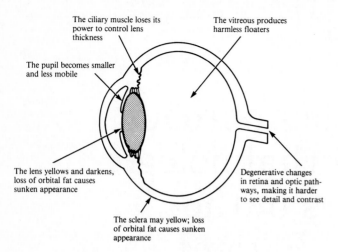

The ciliary muscle loses its power to control lens thickness

The vitreous produces harmless floaters

The pupil becomes smaller and less mobile

The lens yellows and darkens, loss of orbital fat causes sunken appearance

Degenerative changes in retina and optic pathways, making it harder to see detail and contrast

The sclera may yellow; loss of orbital fat causes sunken appearance

Figure 43–1 Aging changes of the eye.[2]

precipitating factors and identifying the most likely diagnosis in acute disorders of the eye.[7] Not surprisingly, there are certain "red flags" that the examining physician should recognize when evaluating elderly patients with ophthalmologic complaints.[6] For example, glaucoma should be suspected in any elderly patient who complains of seeing haloes, even in the absence of ocular pain or other symptoms. On the other hand, a history of significant blunt ocular trauma should lead to a diligent examination of the entire retina for signs of retinal detachment, which may be preceded by such symptoms as flashing lights or drifting shadows across the visual field. In the majority of cases, monocular diplopia is hysterical in origin; it can be caused by retinal detachment, macular edema, subluxation of the lens, or cataracts. Binocular diplopia most often results from dysfunction of the extraocular muscles, ischemic insult to the vertebrobasilar system, or disruption of the orbit as can be seen in retroorbital abscess. Momentary loss of vision (amaurosis fugax) may be the first sign of an impending cerebrovascular accident, spasm of the central retinal artery, or partial occlusion of the internal carotid artery. Quivering or scintillating blind spots (scotomas) may occur transiently as a result of localized constriction of cerebral or retinal arteries.

Visual acuity is to the ophthalmologic exam what routine vital signs are to the general physical exam. In order to be considered complete, the ophthalmologic exam must include a description of visual acuity, whether it is a formal Snellen chart recording or documentation of the patient's ability to count fingers. In general, baseline measurements in the elderly of central acuity at a distance (20 feet) and at close range (comfortable reading distance) must be augmented by the increased physiologic need for additional light. One should obtain the best corrected visual acuity for each eye with the patient's current glasses. Remarkable tolerance by the elderly to spectacle misalignment is common, so it is important that lenses are clean and properly centered.

The lids and the adnexa should be examined closely, noting symmetry, swelling, abnormal discharge, secretions, edema, erythema, or ecchymosis. In addition, if there is suspicion of a foreign body, eversion of the upper and lower lids is mandatory. The tear points (lacrimal puncta) must also be examined. Normally these are directed slightly backward so that the opening is in contact with the bulbar conjunctiva or "lacrimal lake." If lid relaxation has allowed them to rotate forward and open into the air, there will be poor tear siphoning and epiphora. Impairment of lid closure is suggestive of senile or relaxation ectropion of the lower lid. Pupillary light responses should be checked with a flashlight, including the "swinging flashlight test" for a Marcus Gunn afferent pupillary defect.

A number of important conditions, such as glaucoma, are associated with loss of peripheral vision. A simple confrontation test should be performed as a rough test for such gross defects. The physician and patient face each other at arm's length. The patient is then told to hold one hand lightly over the left eye and look with the right eye at the examiner's left eye. The examiner can then use his or her fingers to enter the peripheral fields and ask the patient to recognize when they appear and how many are present. The fullness of the reported field is compared to that of the physician's perception. The test is then repeated for the other eye.

Next, the intraocular pressure of each eye should be estimated by one of several available methods. Finger palpation is useful only when a large difference exists between the intraocular pressure of the two eyes, as in unilateral angle-closure glaucoma. The Schiotz tonometer, although not as accurate as the air puff tonometer or the Goldmann applanation tonometer (used with a slit lamp), is much less expensive than either of these. It relies upon a known quantity of weight to indent the corneal surface after instillation of topical anesthesia. The intraocular pressure (IOP) is generally between 10 and 20 mm Hg.

A slit lamp examination, which should be a routine part of any emergency ophthalmologic exam, is particularly useful for accurate assessment of corneal integrity as well as anterior chamber anatomy. The use of a light source directed horizontally across the cornea is helpful in estimating the depth of the anterior chamber. If there is dangerous shallowing, a shadow will be seen on the opposite side of the anterior chamber. Conversely, broad illumination of the entire chamber signifies adequate depth (Figure 43–2). The presence of a shallow anterior chamber should elicit a thorough evaluation for glaucoma by tonometry and is a contraindication to pupillary dilation.

Ophthalmoscopy can be performed safely using a 2.5% phenylephrine for topical mydriasis.[8] Contraindications to pupillary dilation include: recent head injury, history of angle-closure glaucoma, or the presence of an iris-

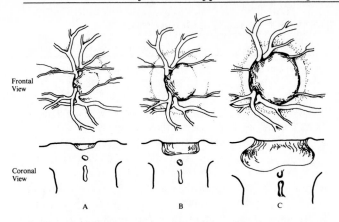

Figure 43–2 Changes in the optic disk with increasing intraocular pressure showing on both the frontal and coronal views: *A*, normal; *B*, early change; *C*, late change. (Reproduced with permission from Kidwell EDR: Glaucoma. In Barker LR, Burton JR, and Zieve PD, editors: Principles of ambulatory medicine, Baltimore, 1986, Williams & Wilkins, p 1376.)

fixated intraocular lens. The optic disk and iris will appear paler with age. Funduscopic exam ordinarily reveals a cup/disk ratio not exceeding 0.3 or 0.4 when measured across the 3 to 9 o'clock diameter of the optic nerve head. If it exceeds this or if there is a difference of 0.2 or greater between the two eyes, the patient should be evaluated for glaucoma. Aging retinal arterioles normally show some physiologic sclerosis with slight yellowing of the arteriolar reflections of light and diffuse narrowing and straightening of arterioles, which tend to obscure venules at crossing points.

Red-free light (a white light with a green filter) allows details of hemorrhages, focal irregularity of blood vessels, and nerve fibers to be seen more clearly.

OPHTHALMOLOGIC MANIFESTATIONS OF SYSTEMIC DISEASE

Although a complete listing of systemic diseases that can cause ocular abnormalities is beyond the scope of this review, some of the more common ocular manifestations of systemic disease found in the geriatric patient are shown in Table 43–1.

Diabetic Changes

Diabetes, for example, should be considered in all elderly patients with cataracts, unexplained retinopathy, optic neuropathy, extraocular muscle palsy, or sudden changes in refractive error. The onset of retinopathy frequently cannot be dated by the elderly diabetic. In most cases, hypertensive or arteriosclerotic vasculopathy is already present and, when combined with diabetes, leads to a maculopathy that is uniquely resistant to therapy. Intraretinal microvascular anomalies occur and result in loss of vascular integrity and leakage of intravascular fluids into the retinal space, especially the macula. Once

Table 43–1   Ocular Manifestations of Systemic Disease

Sign/symptom	Systemic diseases
Retinal hemorrhages	Hypertension, diabetes mellitus, leukemia, polycythemia, acute blood loss, subacute bacterial endocarditis
Uveitis	Toxoplasmosis, sarcoid, rheumatoid arthritis, Behcet's disease, sinusitis, dental disease
Amaurosis fugax	Carotid disease, valvular heart disease, dysrhythmia, anemia, polycythemia, hypotensive or hypertensive episodes, arteritis
Occulusive disease of retinal vessels	Hypertension, atheromatous disease (carotid/vertebral) systems, abnormal blood viscosity syndromes, glaucoma, temporal arteritis
Papilledema	Tumors, benign increased intracranial pressure, hydrocephalus, drugs, trauma, middle ear disease, endocrine abnormalities, blood dyscrasias
Cataracts	Steroid use, diabetes mellitus, uveal disease, retinal detachment, trauma
Optic neuritis	Multiple sclerosis, diabetes mellitus, Graves' disease, toxins (methanol), temporal arteritis
Conjunctivitis	Infections, allergy, chemical exposure
Scleral discoloration	Jaundice, Atabrine (yellow), osteogenesis imperfecta (blue), blacks, alkaptonuria (brown)
Macular degeneration	Senile degeneration, hereditary, traumatic, cystic, histoplasmosis
Dry eye syndrome	Sjögren's syndrome, tranquilizers, other collagen disorders
Angioid streaks	Pseudoxanthoma elasticum, sickle cell disease, Paget's disease, high myopia
Proptosis	Graves' disease, ocular tumors, hemorrhage, orbital cellulitis, carotid-cavernous sinus fistula, leukemia, lymphoma, aneurysms
Oculomotor paralysis	Diabetes mellitus, multiple sclerosis, botulism, Wernicke's encephalopathy, posterior communicating aneurysm, Graves' disease, polyarteritis nodosa
Optic atrophy	Tertiary syphilis, diabetes mellitus, pernicious and other anemias, brain tumor
Diplopia	Myasthenia gravis (worse in the evening), Graves' disease, ptosis, oculomotor palsies
Central retinal vein occlusion	Diabetes mellitus, hypertension, collagen vascular disease, hyperviscosity syndromes

present, macular edema causes structural distortion that can reduce vision to the level of legal blindness (20/200 or less).

Hypertension

Hypertensive retinopathy may be categorized into four groups initially described by Wagner and Keith in 1939. Stages I and II are characterized by mild arteriolar changes with attenuation and an increased light reflex ("copper" or "silver" wiring). Stages III and IV include cotton wool spots, hemorrhages, extensive microvascular changes, and hard exudates. Stage IV is differentiated by the additional features of optic disk edema. The appearance of the fundus in hypertensive retinopathy is determined by the degree of elevation of the blood pressure and the state of the retinal arterioles. Elderly patients with fixed arteriosclerotic vessels are partially protected from the vascular damage associated with accelerated hypertension. Thus, older individuals seldom exhibit signs of florid hypertensive retinopathy.

Arteriosclerosis

Arteriosclerosis is characterized by diffuse fibrosis and hyalinization of the retinal vessels beyond the disk. As the walls of the arterioles become infiltrated with fatty acids and cholesterol, the vessels become sclerotic, and the vessel wall gradually loses its transparency. The blood column appears wider than normal, and the thin light reflex becomes broader. A typical "copper wire" appearance is seen as grayish-yellow, fat products in the vessel wall that blend with the red of the blood column. As sclerosis proceeds from moderate to severe, the vessel wall light reflection resembles a "silver wire," and, at times, even complete occlusion of an arteriolar branch may occur.

Neoplasms

Neoplastic disease may involve the eye and optic pathways by direct spread or by metastatic infiltration. The most frequent tumor metastasizing to the eye is bronchial carcinoma in men and carcinoma of the breast in women, followed by neoplasms of the genitourinary and intestinal tract. Orbital involvement with Hodgkin's disease or lymphosarcoma is not uncommon and usually presents beneath the conjunctiva of the upper cul-de-sac; it may be the only sign of lymphoma.

OCULAR PAIN IN THE ELDERLY

Precise evaluation of the painful eye is an especially difficult and challenging problem in the elderly patient. Potential diagnoses range from minor ocular problems to catastrophic events that may not directly involve the eye, such as a leaking or ruptured internal carotid aneurysm.[9,10] Emergency physicians caring for the aged should be particularly aware of those conditions which are most likely to cause ocular pain in this age group (Table 43–2).

Ocular pain can be defined as gritty irritation or discomfort in the eye and can be especially severe when the trigeminal nerve is involved. The elderly patient complaining of acute pain of the eye or orbit will generally

Table 43–2   Causes of Ocular Pain

Condition	Diagnostic signs
Keratoconjunctivitis sicca	Check tear secretion with Schirmer's tear test, strip and stain for corneal ulceration with rose bengal
Exposure keratopathy	Facial palsy (imperfect lid closure), ulcer in lower third of cornea
Corneal ulcer	Grayish ulcer with crescentic margin; pus in floor of anterior chamber may be seen
Herpetic keratitis	Branching dendritic figures on fluorescein staining
Herpes zoster ophthalmicus	Keratitis or iridocyclitis likely if vesicles on side of nose
Acute iritis	Pupil small, possible irregular; keratic precipitates may be present
Intraocular tumor	Painful blind eye may mask malignancy; eye congested and hard due to secondary glaucoma, does not transilluminate
Angle-closure glaucoma	Pupil semidilated, oval; fixed eye hard to palpate through upper lid

fall into one of two groups: those with signs of external inflammation (i.e., a red eye) and those without such signs. As a rule, pain that occurs in an eye free of inflammation is unlikely to be ocular in origin and is usually of referred origin. Contrary to popular belief, refractive errors are an infrequent source of ocular pain or eye strain.

Dry Eye Syndrome

Dry eye syndrome is quite common in the elderly and results from deficient tear secretion. Patients with dry eyes complain of a burning sensation or sandy feeling. Other common symptoms include itching, excessive mucous secretion, blurred vision, photosensitivity, redness, and difficulty in moving the lids. The eye is usually minimally inflamed with an absent tear meniscus at the lower lid magin. Diagnosis of a dry eye is confirmed most easily by assessing the extent of wetting of a thin strip of litmus paper after 5 minutes (Schirmer's test). In severe cases, there may be signs of keratoconjunctivitis sicca, which is manifested by punctate staining with 1% rose bengal of the cornea and interpalpebral areas of the conjunctiva. Treatment consists of replacement with artificial tears as often as necessary and lubricating ointment at bedtime. For more severe cases, a sustained-release tear insert (Lacrisert, one insert in each eye daily) may be employed.

Exposure keratopathy occurs whenever the cornea is not properly moistened and covered by the eyelids. This can be seen in patients with exophthalmos, ectropion, facial nerve palsies, loss of consciousness, and anesthetic corneas. The two factors at work are the drying of the cornea and its exposure to minor trauma. In addition to conjunctival swelling and hyperemia, the cornea will usually stain abnormally with fluorescein, indicating an epithelial defect or deeper corneal ulceration. The therapeutic objective is to provide protection and moisture for the entire corneal surface. Artificial tears or ointment may be of benefit; treatment requires that the eyelids be taped to maintain closure.

Entropion and ectropion of the lower eyelid cause inflammation of the conjunctiva that is predominantly inferior in location. Loss of posterior support from shrinkage of orbital fat, combined with atony of the tarsoorbital fascia and relaxation of the palpebral skin, are important contributing factors. Trichiasis (turning inward of the lashes so they rub on the cornea) results from senile entropion. It causes corneal irritation and may encourage corneal ulceration. Temporary relief of entropion may be obtained by taping the lower lid to the cheek with tension temporally and inferiorly. Ectropion (sagging and eversion of the lower lid) may precipitate desiccation and hypertrophy of the tarsal conjunctiva of the lid. When this occurs, the eye becomes irritable, watery, and prone to conjunctival infection and exposure keratitis. Marked ectropion is treated by surgical shortening of the lower lid in a horizontal direction.

Corneal Ulcer

A corneal ulcer is a true medical emergency necessitating immediate intervention. Opacification of the cornea with fluorescein staining should alert the physician to this potentially dangerous condition.[11] Hypopyon keratitis is an infective corneal ulcer accompanied by pus in the floor of the anterior chamber. The pus is usually sterile, and the ulcer is grayish with a crescentic advancing edge. Corneal ulcers may result from foreign body injury, but in the elderly, they usually occur spontaneously in debilitated patients with a degenerate cornea or poor hygiene. Swabbing the cornea with the cotton swab supplied in the culture tube and sending it to the laboratory is insufficient to make a bacteriologic diagnosis, with the yield approaching only 10% or less. The ulcer must be scraped with a scalpel blade or platinum spatula and plated directly from the blade onto culture media. The usual bacterial offender is *Staphylococcus aureus*, pneumococcus, or a more virulent organism such as *Pseudomonas*. Any of these can cause corneal perforation and loss of the eye in 12 hours, so any delay in hospitalization or treatment may turn a potentially treatable disease into a blind eye.

Herpes Simplex Keratitis

Dendritic keratitis, or necrotizing herpes simplex keratitis, is the most common cause of corneal ulceration in the United States. It is often painful as a result of con-comitant corneal epithelial edema, uveitis, and secondary glaucoma due to trabecular dysfunction. A branching dendritic figure that stains with fluorescein is characteristic and is composed of small erosions united by branching fissures. Left untreated, the dendrites coalesce to form a shallow geographic ulcer with scalloped margins. Bacterial or fungal keratitis can mimic herpetic keratitis or can occur concomitantly. Appropriate cultures are, therefore, always necessary. Treatment is by topical antiviral agents, such as idoxuridine every 2 hours or vidarabine ointment under the supervision of an ophthalmologist. Topical steroids are contraindicated in the presence of epithelial loss.

Herpes zoster ophthalmicus, a viral infection of the trigeminal ganglion, is usually heralded by pain in the trigeminal nerve distribution. After 3 or 4 days, a vesicular eruption appears in the supra- or infraorbital area, depending on which division of the nerve is involved. Vesicles on the tip of the nose indicating nasociliary involvement should have an ophthalmic evaluation. Ocular complications may involve the cornea, uveal tract, and optic nerve. Topical steroids are indicated, provided there is no coincidental herpes simplex infection; atropine drops are required once or twice a day.

Iritis

Acute iritis and iridocyclitis may produce trigeminal-type pain and ciliary congestion. In contrast to acute angle-closure glaucoma, vision is less severely depressed, the intraocular pressure may be low, and the pupil is small and irregular. Deposits of cells (keratic precipitates) are found on the back of the cornea. Posterior synechiae or adhesions of the iris to the lens occur in untreated cases. Phacoanaphylactic iridocyclitis in the elderly may result from hypersensitivity to lens protein after extracapsular cataract extraction. More often, however, iridocyclitis in this group is secondary to ankylosing spondylitis, diabetes, herpes simplex, herpes zoster, and a focal infection, such as dental root abscesses. Although tuberculosis may occasionally be an etiologic factor in iritis or iridocyclitis in the elderly, as many as 50% of the cases have no known cause.

Pain without Inflammation

Patients who present with a painful eye or orbit, but with no external signs of inflammation, are at high risk for having a number of conditions. Sudden onset of pain combined with an oculomotor palsy (i.e., dilated pupil with or without ophthalmoplegia) should suggest an expanding or leaking internal carotid aneurysm. An aneurysm above the clinoid process may impinge on the optic nerve or chiasm and cause visual field deficits. Temporal arteritis may cause acute pain that is referred to the orbit. Visual loss due to ischemic optic neuropathy is frequent, and a few cases have a central retinal artery occlusion.[12] A painful eye associated with an afferent pupillary deficit (Marcus Gunn pupil) and diminished visual acuity suggests optic neuritis — particularly if associated with painful ocular motion or a tender globe. There may or may not be signs of inflammation of the optic disk depending on whether the process is intraocular or retrobulbar. Finally, migraines and cluster headaches may present as an acutely painful eye or orbit.

GLAUCOMA

Open-Angle Glaucoma

In glaucoma, the intraocular pressure is sufficiently elevated to cause characteristic optic disk changes and visual field defects, eventually leading to blindness in some patients. A pressure greater than 22 mm Hg is considered abnormal but not necessarily an absolute indication for treatment. Glaucoma can be primary or secondary to other disease processes (e.g., trauma or following cataract extraction). Primary glaucoma is further subdivided into open-angle and angle-closure types. The vast majority of affected individuals have chronic open-angle (or "simple") glaucoma. The prevalence of this condition increases with age, rising from a very low level in young adults to as high as 5 to 10% in the eighth decade.

The term "chronic open-angle glaucoma" is used when optic nerve damage and visual field loss result from elevated intraocular pressure in an eye with an open angle (as determined by gonioscopy), and no etiology is found. In the trabecular meshwork there is a poorly understood block to the outflow of the aqueous humor. With continued production of aqueous humor, the intraocular pressure gradually increases. The peripheral field is usually lost first. As the visual fields become progressively constricted later, only a small central island of vision remains and then disappears, causing loss of central visual acuity. Patients are often unaware that there is a problem until the disease is far advanced. A family history, complaints of blurred vision not correctable with lenses, or a halo effect around lights should raise the examiner's level of suspicion. The pupil may be slightly dilated and react sluggishly to light, but otherwise the eye appears perfectly normal externally. Ophthalmoscopic exam may reveal glaucomatous cupping of the disk and atrophy of the optic nerve (Figure 43–2). In glaucomatous cupping, there is a true loss of the substance of the optic nerve head so that it becomes carved out and excavated. A pale, chalk-white nerve head with a large cup/disk ratio (0.5 or greater) is indicative of late open-angle glaucoma.

Treatment

Goals of therapy are to preserve visual function and prevent visual damage in the safest way possible. Because only 5 to 10% of patients with ocular hypertension (pressure greater than 22 mm Hg) develop open-angle glaucoma, most patients with ocular hypertension should be observed without treatment to avoid therapeutic complications. Medications available for open-angled glaucoma are shown in Table 43–3. Medical treatment can lower the intraocular pressure by increasing aqueous outflow with miotics (pilocarpine) or by decreasing aqueous formation with carbonic anhydrase inhibitors (Diamox). Epinephrine may be added to the miotics or used as the primary drug to decrease aqueous production and increase aqueous outflow. Timolol maleate, a beta-adrenergic blocking agent with few side effects, also decreases aqueous production and may increase outflow by an as-yet-unknown mechanism. This drug is used only twice daily and may be extremely effective in responsive patients. When medical therapy has failed to control the intraocular pressure adequately, laser trabeculoplasty or surgical intervention becomes necessary. The operation for open-angle glaucoma creates a fistula between the anterior chamber and the subconjunctival space, allowing an exit for the aqueous humor.

Angle-Closure Glaucoma

Angle-closure glaucoma results from forward displacement of the iris against the cornea and obstruction of flow of the aqueous humor into the chamber angle and the spaces of Fontana (Figure 43–3). The aging eye is more susceptible to this disease as the anterior chamber becomes shallower and the lens increases in size. An attack may be precipitated by the use of mydriatics, sitting in a darkened room, or a sudden increase in the volume of the posterior chamber (e.g., hemorrhage or congestion).

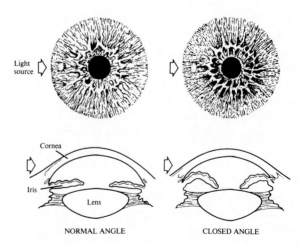

Figure 43–3   Illustration shows a shadow cast on the iris resulting from the bowed iris in angle-closure glaucoma. (Reproduced with permission from Kidwell EDR: Glaucoma. In Barker LR, Burton JR, and Zieve PD, editors: Principles of ambulatory medicine, Baltimore, 1986, Williams & Wilkins, p 1375.)

Table 43–3   Antiglaucoma Medications

Class and name	Dosage	Route	Side effects	Contraindications
I. Miotics (cholinergic)				
Pilocarpine 0.25–10%	1 to 2 drops 4 times/day	Topical	Ciliary muscle spasm, ↓ visual acuity, ↓ dark adaptation, follicular conjunctivitis, headache, nausea, bronchial constriction, ↑ salivation	Hypersensitivity, iritis, asthma, hypertension
Carbachol 0.75–3%	2 drops up to 4 times/day	Topical	As per pilocarpine, transient ciliary, and conjunctival injection	As per pilocarpine
II. Hyperosmotics				
Glycerol 50%	1.0–1.5 g/kg	Oral	Nausea, vomiting, headache, confusion, dehydration, cardiac arrhythmias, ↑ blood sugar, hyperosmotic coma	Hypersensitivity, hypervolemia, congestive heart failure (CHF), confusional states
Mannitol 20%	1.5–2.0 g/kg	Intravenous	Headache, chills, chest pain, diuresis	Hypersensitivity, anuria, pulmonary edema, severe dehydration, intracranial hemorrhage
III. Carbonic Anhydrase Inhibitors (used with miotics)				
Acetazolamide (Diamox)	250 mg tablets 4 times/day	Oral	Paresthesias, anorexia, nausea	Na^+, K^+, abnormalities, marked renal and hepatic disease
	500 mg sequels 2 times/day	Oral	Polyuria, occasional drowsiness, and confusion	Chronic noncongestive angle-closure glaucoma, hypersensitivity, Addison's disease, severe COPD
	250–500 mg 2 times/day	Intravenous	Acidosis (long-term usage), all adverse reactions to sulfonamides	
Dichlorphenamide (Daranide)	100 mg 2 times/day until desired response obtained. Then 25–50 mg 1–3 times/day	Oral	As above	As above
Ethoxzolamide (Ethamide)	125 mg 1–2 times/day	Oral	As above	As above
Methazolamide (Neptazane)	50–100 mg 2–3 times/day	Oral	Anorexia, nausea, vomiting, malaise, fatigue, drowsiness, headache, paresthesias, confusion, vertigo	As above
IV. Adrenergics				
Epinephrine 0.25–2%	1 drop 1–2 times/day	Topical	May cause reversible cystoid macula edema (CME) in aphakics, blurred vision, conjunctival hyperemia, HTN, allergy, pigment deposition in conjunctiva	Narrow-angle glaucoma, use with caution in patients with hypertension, coronary artery disease

Continued

Table 43–3   Antiglaucoma Medications — cont'd

Class and name	Dosage	Route	Side effects	Contraindications
IV. Adrenergics — cont'd				
Dipivefrin HCl (Propine) 0.1%	1 drop 2 times/day	Topical	Aphakic CME, tachycardia, arrhythmias, hypertension, adenochrome deposits, burning, stinging	Narrow-angle glaucoma, hypersensitivity
Timolol (Timoptic) 0.5%	1 drop 2 times/day	Topical	Conjunctivitis, blepharitis, keratitis, visual disturbance, bradyarrhythmia, syncope, hypertension, bronchospasm, rarely confusion, depression, palpitations	Hypersensitivity, bronchospastic disease, bradycardia, first-degree block, CHF, cardiogenic shock, concomitant usage of adrenergic-augmenting psychotropic drugs

In contrast to chronic open-angle glaucoma, acute angle-closure glaucoma is marked by striking and prominent symptoms:

1. Abrupt onset of blurred vision
2. Rainbow-colored haloes around lights
3. Moderate to severe unilateral pain
4. Dramatic loss of vision
5. Nausea, vomiting, and abdominal pain

There may be a family history of angle-closure glaucoma, and the patient may also have a history of previous, less severe attacks. Often, patients find relief in well-lighted rooms or out of doors where daylight causes constriction of the pupil and opening of the angle of the anterior chamber. Examination during an acute attack usually reveals a markedly increased intraocular pressure (50 mm Hg or more), a shallow anterior chamber, an edematous cornea, decreased visual acuity, ciliary injection, and a fixed, semidilated pupil.

Emergency Treatment

Emergency treatment consists of frequent instillation of miotics, parenteral administration of carbonic anhydrase inhibitors, and oral administration of hyperosmotic agents (such as glycerol). If treatment with glycerin is not successful or if the patient is nauseated, intravenous hypertonic mannitol (20%) may be effective. Miotics should be instilled in the other eye, which is also susceptible to acute angle closure. Definitive treatment is surgical. A peripheral iridectomy is performed when the symptoms have diminished and later on the unaffected eye as a prophylactic measure. (See Table 43–3.)

CATARACTS

A cataract is an opacification of the crystalline lens. Cataracts vary markedly in degree of density and may be due to a variety of causes but are usually associated with aging. The crystalline lens is a unique structure: New lens fibers are constantly being formed throughout life, and old lens fibers are not lost but come to lie progressively deeper and more distant from the capsule of the lens. As the lens ages, its nucleus becomes increasingly dark, dense, and relatively opaque with a high refractive index (nuclear sclerosis). Cataracts diminish vision by decreasing the transparency of the lens and by altering the refractive power of the lens. Some degree of cataract formation is to be expected in all persons over the age of 70. Most are bilateral, although the rate of progression in each eye is seldom equal. Traumatic cataract, steroid-induced cataract, and other types are less common.

Visual loss is usually gradual, although occasionally a patient first notices a monocular cataract when the better eye is covered and may interpret this as visual loss of sudden onset. Visual loss is always painless, and the patient may describe a constant fog over the eye. Occasionally, there is annoying diplopia or polyopia due to irregular refraction of the lens. Cataracts that affect the posterior surface of the lens may cause the vision to be much worse for close objects in bright light, because, when the pupil is small, all the light must pass through the area of the cataract.

Cataracts are easily identified by illuminating the lens with a slit lamp, but most emergency practitioners will find that they can see a cataract easily through the plus 4-10 lens of their direct ophthalmoscope. With pupillary dilation, the cataract may be manifested by a general dullness in the red reflex (nuclear sclerosis), peripheral "spokes" (cortical), or a central discrete opacity (posterior subcapsular). The depth of the anterior chamber should be checked, since in some cataracts the lens may swell and reduce the anterior chamber. Likewise, checking the intraocular pressures may identify glaucoma as a complication or cause of the cataract. The clinical degree of cataract formation, assuming that no other eye disease is present, is judged primarily by visual acuity.

There are no medications that have any direct beneficial effect upon cataract formation or progression. Occasionally, dilation of the pupil with mydriatic or cycloplegic drops may enlarge the pupil sufficiently to improve vision by allowing light to enter the eye around the cataract. These drops may improve vision sufficiently to enable elderly patients to function for years without surgery. The decision to remove a cataract is determined by the visual needs of the patient, as well as by the degree of capsular involvement and of any other ocular abnormalities. Surgical intervention, which has a 90 to 95% success rate, is the only definitive treatment.

ACUTE VASCULAR OCCLUSIONS

A number of entities can cause painless monocular visual loss in the elderly: 1) central retinal artery or vein occlusion,[12] 2) temporal arteritis,[13] 3) retinal detachment,[14] 4) macular degeneration,[15] and 5) vitreous hemorrhage resulting from diabetic retinopathy or retinal hole formation. It is imperative that the patient suspected of having retinal artery or venous occlusion be evaluated by an ophthalmologist early in the course of the disease in order to increase the possibility of returning the eye to normal vision.

Emboli or thrombi from the carotid system or cardiac valves may occlude the central retinal artery or one of its branches. When the central retinal artery is affected, the result is sudden, complete or almost complete loss of vision. Total occlusion may be preceded by transient episodes of decreased vision, blindness in the affected eye (amaurosis fugax), or flickering vision. Ophthalmologic examination usually reveals the etiology of the visual loss. The direct pupillary reaction is absent but consensual light reaction is normal. The posterior retina is usually pale and opaque because of ischemic changes in the axons of the nerve fiber layer. Because the fovea lacks this layer, the choroid can be seen as a cherry-red spot. The veins appear dark, and the arteries may be narrowed, with segmentation of the blood column ("boxcar" appearance). Later, the vessel may appear normal, but emboli or plaque is often visible in the arterial tree.

Unfortunately, in most cases, treatment is ineffective. If the patient is seen within 2 hours of the onset of symptoms, one should attempt to restore the blood flow. Treatment is directed toward relief of vasospasm (breathing a mixture of CO_2 and O_2, using a paper bag if necessary) or an attempt to dislodge the embolus by digital massage. The globe is massaged by pressing firmly through the closed lids for 5 seconds and then released for 5 seconds. Acetazolamide, 500 mg given orally, may lower the intraocular pressure to decrease resistance to arterial blood flow. Other methods that may be used by the ophthalmologist are a retrobulbar lidocaine block or anterior chamber paracentesis. The use of thrombolytic agents is recommended by some clinicians, but clinical evidence for effectiveness is lacking.

Retinal vein occlusion is encountered with some frequency in the elderly and also has a poor prognosis for visual recovery. It may occur secondary to diabetes mellitus, hypertension, glaucoma, leukemia, and other conditions that impede venous flow. Arteriosclerosis is the most important systemic condition. External compression of the retinal vein by the rigid arterial wall may severely restrict blood flow, leading to venous stasis and eventual occlusion. Painless loss of vision ensues, although some degree of visual acuity may be preserved in up to 20% of patients. Venous occlusion is often preceded by episodes of transient decrease in vision lasting several hours, in contrast to the brief prodromal episodes associated with central retinal artery occlusion. Ophthalmoscopic examination reveals vascular dilation and tortuosity accompanied by retinal hemorrhage and occasionally retinal edema. When present in its classical form, this hemorrhagic retinopathy is described as "blood and thunder." Emergency medical therapy includes steroids, anticoagulants, vasodilators, and hemodilution, but treatment is even less effective than in central retinal artery occlusion. The natural history of this condition is variable, with spontaneous resolution not uncommon. Patients with branch retinal vein occlusion have a much better prognosis for useful vision, but many will require photocoagulation.

TEMPORAL ARTERITIS

One cause of retinal and ophthalmic artery occlusion that merits separate consideration is temporal or giant cell arteritis.[16] This condition is clearly a disease of the elderly, with a median age of 75 years at diagnosis. It is characterized by giant cell infiltration of the media, progressing to panarteritis and intimal fibrosis. The superficial temporal, ophthalmic, vertebral, and internal carotid arteries are most commonly involved. Patients feel ill and have excruciating pain over the temporal or occipital arteries. Systemic symptoms include fever, malaise, weakness, and altered mentation. The scalp is often tender. Jaw claudication may occur and is sometimes worsened with chewing. The temporal arteries may be pulseless and are usually indurated with overlying erythema. Visual symptoms, such as blurring, diplopia, and transient or permanent visual loss, result when arteritis compromises blood supply to the retina or optic nerve. Approximately 40% of patients with temporal arteritis eventually suffer visual loss secondary to the ischemic optic neuropathy. Ischemic optic neuritis may also result from arteriosclerotic involvement of the small vessels supplying the optic nerve.

Ophthalmoscopy may initially produce unremarkable findings. Commonly, however, there are signs of iritis, extraocular muscle palsies, or manifestations of retinal artery occlusion, including pallor, hemorrhage, or exudates. The sedimentation rate is almost always over 50 mm/hr and frequently over 100 mm/hr. Many patients with active temporal arteritis have a low-grade anemia, leukocytosis, and elevated liver function tests. The definitive diagnosis is accomplished by temporal artery biopsy. Prompt treatment is recommended in suspected cases to prevent further vision loss. Patients with visual symptoms should be hospitalized and treated with high-dose intravenous steroids. Temporal artery biopsy should be done within 3 days. Involvement of the second eye may develop, despite steroid therapy, and usually occurs in the first week following initiation of therapy.

RETINAL DETACHMENT

It is essential that the emergency physician suspect retinal detachment in all cases of visual loss.[14,17] There are 25,000 new cases of retinal detachment annually, many occurring in elderly patients. Surgical repair is often effective if undertaken soon after onset. A complaint of "lightning flashes," cloudy or smoky vision, shower or floaters, or a curtain-like sensation falling over the visual field is an indication for an emergent ophthalmoscopic examination through a dilated pupil to detect the presence of retinal detachment.[18] This is particularly true if the patient has undergone cataract surgery, is myopic, or has sustained recent trauma.

Retinal detachment does not represent true dislocation of the retina from the choroid but, rather, a separation of two retinal layers — the rod and cone layer — from the pigment epithelium. Accumulation of the fluid between these layers causes the detachment. The fluid usually originates in the vitreous, having passed through a hole in the retina. Physical examination will usually demonstrate a relative loss of visual field in the area of the detachment. When the detachment spreads very slowly, the patient may be unaware of any problem until the macula is affected. There may be a disturbance of the red reflex, and, on funduscopic examination, one can observe a grayish mound that appears out of focus or a folding of the retina. The other eye must be examined, since it often has retinal holes or vitreoretinal adhesions that can lead to tears.

It is difficult to make the diagnosis of retinal detachment without indirect ophthalmoscopy and scleral depression to visualize the peripheral retina — the area that is most commonly detached. Thus, the diagnosis should be suspected primarily on the basis of symptoms, confrontation field, and visual acuity, and, if these are abnormal, the patient should be referred immediately for a complete ophthalmologic evaluation. Treatment of retinal detachment requires urgent surgical intervention. Reattachment can be achieved in 95% of cases, and, even with macular involvement, visual restoration to a 20/40 or better acuity level can be accomplished in over half of patients. However, the longer the retina remains detached, the poorer the visual prognosis.

MACULAR DEGENERATION

Macular degeneration affects nearly one third of the geriatric population and is the leading cause of registered blindness in the United States.[15] The risk of senile macular degeneration increases dramatically with age. Unlike cataracts or retinal detachment, macular degeneration is not amenable to surgery and, therefore, constitutes one of the most serious ocular diseases encountered in the geriatric patient. The exact etiology is unknown, although macular degeneration probably results from a decrease in the vascular supply to the macula from the lamina choriocapillaris. The overlying pigment epithelium is disturbed, especially in the macula and at the disk margin. Drusen — discrete hyaline deposits beneath the pigment epithelium — may be present as further evidence of degeneration. Retinal neovascularization may follow formation of the drusen. Disciform scars, macular cysts, and retinal detachment also may develop.

Clinically, senile macular degeneration is marked by a painless, progressive loss of central vision (e.g., close reading) over many months or years. Because retinal involvement is generally limited to the macular region, peripheral vision remains essentially intact. Ophthalmologic examination shows a relative central scotoma and loss of the foveal light reflex. In most patients, a disturbance in the smooth retinal pigment epithelial layer causes a fine stippling or clumping of black pigment associated with varying degrees of depigmentation in the macular region. The neovascularization may hemorrhage, and the patient presents with blood in the vitreous or beneath the retina. A grayish membrane appearing below the retina suggests the existence of neovascularization.

Laser photocoagulation may be useful in some patients who have focal areas of neovascularization identified with fluorescein angiography. However, the vast majority of patients are either never amenable to laser therapy (generalized atrophy) or are diagnosed too late (large disciform scar). Therapy is then confined to prescribing corrective lenses and assuring the patient that total blindness will not result from this disease.

OPHTHALMOLOGIC DRUGS IN THE ELDERLY[8]

It is important to recognize that certain topical ocular medications, in elderly patients, may result in significant systemic reactions, such as cardiac failure (timolol), respiratory distress, myocardial infarction, depression, or suicidal ideation. Systemic side effects of these topical drugs are a result of three basic factors:

1. First-order pass effect
2. Typically high concentrations of the drug
3. Higher concentration of drug retained by the conjunctival sac

With the rapid absorption of medications through the aging conjunctiva, merely one drop of a potent medication may have a marked systemic effect. This occurs because the drug reaches various target organs without first passing through the liver or kidney to be detoxified (first-order pass effect). Because of the variation in dosage forms, the clinician must carefully prescribe the topically applied preparation with the least potential systemic side effects.

Eye medications are often concentrated because their ocular exposure is short. This phenomenon is especially important in the elderly in whom the conjunctival sac retains a greater volume of medication because the eyelids are more lax. When drugs are given in eyedrop form, an estimated 80% of the dose drains rapidly through the nasolacrimal system and is absorbed by the nasal mucosa. Instructing the elderly patients to occlude the punctum by pressing the inner aspect of the lower lid with a finger for several minutes can markedly decrease the amount of systemic dissemination of an eyedrop, enhancing the safe topical use of medication. (See Table 43–4.)

Outlined below are common topical ocular medications and their potential systemic side effects in the elderly.

Corticosteroids. Their use may reduce the facility of aqueous outflow, thereby increasing intraocular pressure. Approximately one third of patients will develop intraocular pressure elevation within 6 weeks of topical steroid therapy. This may induce or aggravate preexisting open-angle glaucoma. Corticosteroid drops may also potentiate herpes simplex or fungal keratitis. In addition, patients with tissue antigen HLA A1 are likely to develop posterior subcapsular cataracts, whether the steroid is given topically or systemically.

Antibiotics. Any of the topical antibiotic drops can cause a local allergic reaction and are capable of causing anaphylaxis in patients with prior histories of hypersensitivity. A skin sensitivity to neomycin — manifested by

Table 43–4 Safe Use of Ocular Drugs in the Elderly

- Prescribe the topically applied preparation with the least potential systemic side effects.
- Instruct the patient to occlude the nasolacrimal punctum for a few minutes after drug application, thereby decreasing systemic absorption.
- Because of the marked variation in "generic equivalents," brand name medications are preferred.
- Use small amounts of ointment rather than drops when possible.
- Use a more dilute concentration.
- Wipe excess solution or ointment from the eye immediately after application.
- Because an informed patient is a better patient, actions as well as undesirable side effects should be discussed with elderly patients.

an erythematous, pruritic scaling dermatitis — may appear in as many as 10 to 15% of patients. Chloramphenicol and Sodium Sulamyd 10% rarely cause local sensitization.

Phenylephrine. Systemic reactions to topical ocular instillation of phenylephrine for dilation of pupils are uncommon but can be serious and even lethal when they occur. Only the 2.5% concentration is recommended for use in the elderly. Blood pressure should be carefully monitored in patients with cardiac disease, hypertension, arteriosclerosis, and aneurysms. Other rare reactions are ventricular arrhythmias, tachycardia, myocardial infarction, and subarachnoid hemorrhage. Tropicamide 0.5% (Mydriacyl) is probably the safest mydriatic, with weak cycloplegic action, for dilation of eyes in the elderly.

Cycloplegics. These sympathomimetic drugs (e.g., atropine, homatropine, scopolamine, and cyclopentolate) blur near vision by interfering with accommodation and are inferior for routine pupil dilation. They should be used with caution in patients with diabetes, hypertension, hyperthyroidism, heart disease, and bronchial asthma. In addition, the pressor response from these drugs may be markedly exaggerated in patients who have received tricyclic antidepressants, MAO inhibitors, propranolol, and anticholinergic drugs.

Epinephrine. The amount of epinephrine absorbed from topical ocular glaucoma therapy is comparable with the amount used systemically for various conditions. Adverse systemic effects include direct cardiovascular toxicity (e.g., hypertension, arrhythmias) and indirect central nervous system (CNS) toxicity (e.g., delusions, psychosis). Local ocular side effects of long-term epinephrine treatment for glaucoma are common. They range from corneal edema to conjunctival scarring, blepharitis, and deposition of pigment in the conjunctiva.

Parasympathomimetic drugs. The miotics are used almost exclusively for the treatment of glaucoma. Pilocarpine is one of the most commonly used and has the lowest reported incidence of systemic side effects. It does produce blurring of vision because of the accommodative spasm, as well as decreased vision due to miosis. This may severely reduce vision in an eye with a cataract. Adverse parasympathetic effects may include nausea, vomiting, diarrhea, headache, bradycardia, muscle cramps, perspiration, and respiratory distress. The anticholinesterase drugs may also be responsible for the development of cataracts, blurred vision, conjunctivitis, and retinal detachment.

Timolol. The adverse effects associated with timolol maleate are more frequent and more severe than those associated with epinephrine and pilocarpine. Systemic side effects of topical ocular timolol are the same as those observed with oral beta-agonists. Cardiovascular, respiratory, CNS, gastrointestinal, and dermatologic reactions can occur. Timolol has been implicated as a causative agent in pulmonary edema, myocardial infarction, respiratory failure, and death and should be used with caution in elderly patients with peripheral vascular disease, asthma, ventricular failure, or bradycardia.

Acetazolamide. Diamox, a carbonic anhydrase inhibitor, markedly reduces the output of aqueous humor by the ciliary body. Its principal use is in the management of acute angle-closure glaucoma not responding to combinations of eyedrops. Diamox is chemically similar to the sulfonamides and may cause potassium depletion, gastric distress, diarrhea, exfoliative dermatitis, renal stone formation, shortness of breath, acidosis, and fatigue. These side effects, although not entirely absent, are less frequent with methazolamide (Neptazane).

REFERENCES

1. Weale R: The eye of the elderly. What is normal aging? Geriatr Med Today 4:29–37, 1985.
2. Abrahamson IA: Eye changes after forty, Am Fam Phys 29:171–181, 1984.
3. Berson FG: The eye in old age. In Rossman I, editor: Clinical geriatrics, Philadelphia, 1986, JB Lippincott Co.
4. Kollarits CR: The aging eye. In Calkins E, Davis PJ, and Ford AB, editors: The practice of geriatrics, Philadelphia, 1986, WB Saunders Co.
5. Leighton DA: Special senses: aging of the eye. In Brocklehurst JC, editor: Textbook of geriatric medicine and gerontology, New York, 1985, Churchill Livingstone.
6. Keeney AH and Keeney VT: A guide to examining the aging eye, Geriatrics 35:81–91, 1980.
7. Eifrig DE and Simons KB: An overview of common geriatric ophthalmologic disorders, Geriatrics 38:55–57, 1983.
8. Fraunfelder FT and Meyer SM: Safe use of ocular drugs in the elderly, Geriatrics 39:97–102, 1984.
9. Stokoe NL: Ocular pain in the elderly: simple symptom or hidden danger? Geriatrics 35:41–50, 1980.
10. Yanofsky NN: The acute painful eye, Emerg Med Clin North Am 6:21–42, 1988.
11. Schlichtemeier WR: Corneal disease: an approach to primary care, Geriatrics 39:56–66, 1984.
12. Hayreth SS and Hayreth MS: Hemicentral retinal vein occlusion: pathogenesis, clinical features and natural history, Arch Ophthalmol 98:1600–1609, 1980.
13. Rosenfield SJ: Treatment of temporal arteritis with ocular involvment, Am J Med 80:143–146, 1986.
14. Sakamoto DK: Retinal detachment: where an early diagnosis is important, Geriatrics 36:87–90, 1981.
15. Ferris FL: Senile macular degeneration: review of epidemiologic features, Am J Epidemiol 118:132–151, 1983.
16. Keltner JL: Giant-cell arteritis: signs and symptoms, Ophthalmology 89:1101–1109, 1982.
17. Zun LS: Acute vision loss, Emerg Med Clin North Am 6:21–42, 1988.
18. Davidorf FH: Retinal breakdown in the aging eye: what are the consequences? Geriatrics 36:103–107, 1981.

SUGGESTED READINGS

Kasper RL: Eye problems of the aged. In Reichel W, editor: Clinical aspects of aging, Baltimore, 1978, Williams & Wilkins.

Vaughan D and Taylor A: General ophthalmology, Los Altos, Calif, 1983, Lange Medical Publishers.

Walshe TM, editor: Manual of clinical problems in geriatric medicine, Boston, 1985, Little, Brown & Co.

Weinstock FJ: Ophthalmic disorders. In Covington TR and Walker JI, editors: Current geriatric therapy, Philadelphia, 1984, WB Saunders Co.

Dermatologic Disorders

Dermatologic Disorders of Aging

Boni E. Elewski, M.D.

As the largest organ in the body, the skin is probably prey to a greater variety of ills than any other system. Cutaneous diseases may represent 10 to 20% of the presenting complaints in emergency medicine departments or urgent care centers. Frequently, the problem is confined to the skin — cellulitis, for example, or atopic dermatitis — and is a source of significant discomfort for the patient. However, there are a number of systemic diseases in which the cutaneous manifestations, although not important themselves, provide a clue to the diagnosis and treatment. And it is often the case that the aged individual is subject to more and different kinds of problems than the younger individual; clinicians can really put their diagnostic acumen to the test as they literally try to decipher the writing on the skin.

The purpose of this chapter is to outline some of the recent advances in our understanding of the skin of the elderly and its special problems, as well as to provide an approach to the diagnosis and treatment of selected common geriatric dermatoses. It concludes with a brief discussion of skin cancer, which is problematic for the elderly, and cutaneous signs of internal malignancy. Less common dermatologic conditions likely to be encountered by the emergency health care provider are not covered here, but information about them is available in a problem-oriented algorithm devised by Lynch.[1,2]

AGING OF THE SKIN

Although no one dies of "old skin," nothing makes us more keenly aware of aging than the associated cutaneous changes. Typically, the skin gradually becomes dry, transparent, and wrinkled in the elderly, with a loss of elasticity, uneven pigmentation, and a variety of benign and malignant proliferative lesions.[3] Functional losses associated with cutaneous aging are listed in Table 44–1.

The most striking and consistent histologic changes are thinning of the epidermal layer and loss of the normal

Table 44-1 Age-Associated Losses in Cutaneous Function

Wound healing	Thermoregulation
Cell proliferation	Pigmentation
Barrier function	Sebum production
Mechanical protection	Sweat production
Skin circulation	Sensory perception
Immune responsiveness	

undulations (rete ridges) at the dermoepidermal junction. This results in a considerably smaller surface area between the two cutaneous compartments and presumably less communication and nutrient transfer. Shearing stress or other minor trauma, therefore, allows easy separation, resulting in torn skin, bruises, and superficial abrasions. It may also contribute to increased prevalence of certain bullous dermatoses in the elderly.[4]

Mitotic activity at all levels of synthesis and turnover gradually decreases with age. This is demonstrated by the slower rate of stratum corneum cell replacement, increased time for epithelization of open wounds, and reduced rate of nail and hair growth.[5] Hard experimental data in humans are limited but do support the contention that wound healing is slow in older persons. Incised wounds gain strength more slowly, and postoperative wound dehiscence is a possible complication.

"Wrinkles," a common feature of aging, probably result from the structural disintegration of elastin and collagen in the dermis. Loss of dermal thickness approaches 20% in elderly individuals and may account for the paper-thin, sometimes nearly transparent, quality of their skin.[4] The remaining tissue is relatively acellular and avascular. The deep dermal vessels and capillary loops diminish in number and take on irregular patterns with areas of dilation. The compromised circulation is thought to underlie many of the physiologic alterations in old skin (e.g., thermoregulation), as well as the graded atrophy and fibrosis of hair follicles, apocrine, eccrine, and sebaceous glands. The loss of sweat glands leads to dry, itchy skin, which is a particular problem in cold weather, when elderly patients tend to overheat and underhumidify their homes. The loss of subcutaneous fat also makes elderly patients less resistant to changes in ambient temperature.

Inflammatory and immunologic age-associated impairments include a decreased number of Langerhans' and mast cells (with a corresponding reduction in histamine release), diminished and delayed hypersensitivity reactions, increased incidence of autoantibodies, and an altered response to ultraviolet light exposure. Clinically, the alterations translate into diminished cutaneous inflammatory response, lower incidence of skin test reactions, increased incidence of pemphigus and pemphigoid, and an increased prevalence of photocarcinogenesis in the elderly.[5]

COMMON DERMATOSES

Xerosis

Xerosis, a dehydration of the stratum corneum, is a very common condition especially prevalent among the elderly. When it is severe enough to be associated with inflammation and pruritus, it has also been termed asteatotic eczema and winter itch.[7] The sequence of events leading to dry skin varies considerably from person to person and in many cases remains obscure. Environmental factors are extremely important and include repeated exposure to soaps or disinfectants, as well as decreasing relative humidity.[7] Dry skin may also develop in 10 to 50% of individuals with such underlying systemic diseases as renal or hepatic failure, lymphoma, hyperthyroidism, and fatty-acid deficiency.[3] On the lower legs, vascular insufficiency may also contribute. The typical patient presents with localized or generalized pruritus and dryness of the lower legs, dorsa of the hands, or forearms. In more severe cases, the skin cracks and becomes fissured with surrounding erythema and lichenification.[7] Nummular or coin-shaped patches of eczema also may be present (Figure 44-1). Secondary bacterial infection is caused by *Streptococcus* or *Staphylococcus*. It is characterized by fragile vesicopustules which break, leaving erythematous oozing erosions that develop thick, honey-colored crusts. Multiple satellite lesions are usually present.

Therapeutic efforts are aimed at replacing the water in the skin and in the immediate environment. Patients should be cautioned to avoid cold, dry winds outdoors and hot, dry air indoors, wool clothing, and excessive use of soaps and hot baths which remove the sebaceous mantle. It is also important to avoid direct forms of heat to the skin such as heating pads and electric blankets. Room temperature should be kept as low as is consistent with comfort; the use of humidifiers is to be encouraged.[7] Bathing should not be excessive (once every 1–2 days) and the bath water should be warm but not hot. A mild, superfatted soap or oil-in-water cleansing emulsion is beneficial. Lubrication with topical emollients and bath oils provides the mainstay of therapy. They are best applied when the skin is moist. Mild topical corticosteroid preparations are the most effective and rapid therapy for symptomatic xerosis with associated eczematous changes. They should be applied in small amounts, but frequently (3 to 6 times/day) and with occlusion if this is tolerated. This will suppress inflammation and stop pruritus, thus interrupting the itch-scratch cycle. Finally, oral antihistamines (i.e., hydroxyzine) will often suppress pruritus, allay anxiety, and permit sleep.

Contact Dermatitis

Four fifths of all cases of contact dermatitis are caused by exposure to universal irritants such as detergents and

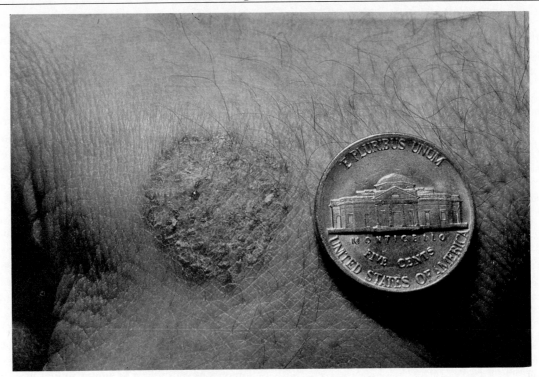

Figure 44–1 Nummular eczema.

organic solvents. An irritant reaction affects most individuals exposed and generally produces discomfort immediately after exposure. Allergic contact dermatitis is a manifestation of delayed hypersensitivity and results from the exposure of sensitized individuals to contact allergens. Most contact allergens produce sensitization in only a small percentage of those exposed. Poison ivy and oak, which induce sensitization in more than 70% of the population, are marked exceptions to this rule. Other common allergens include clothing dyes, such as paraphenylenediamine, formalin in permanent press fabrics, rubber, the dichromates in leather, and nickel compounds. Allergy to topical medications is frequent, probably due to the loss of the protective barrier of inflamed skin. Common culprits include neomycin, anesthetics (e.g., benzocaine), and preservatives in creams (e.g., ethylenediamine). These causes of dermatitis are not limited to the elderly, nor are other exogenous causes such as scabies or lice, which may well occur in institutions or nursing homes.[8]

The diagnosis of contact dermatitis in the elderly may be complicated by a muted inflammatory response and a vague or inaccurate history of local exposure. Pruritus is the primary symptom, accompanied by burning or stinging. Lesions consist of scaling, erythematous macules, papules, vesicles, and, occasionally, large bullae. The distribution and configuration of eruption may suggest the diagnosis. For example, facial involvement may suggest sensitivity to creams, soaps, or shaving materials. A circular irritation on the neck or wrist may indicate a reaction to metals or alloys in jewelry worn by the patient.

The older patient may be more resistant to therapy and heal more slowly that younger patients.

Treatment of contact dermatitis includes application of cool compresses to reduce itching and edema (e.g., Burow's compress — a mild astringent diluted in cool water). If calamine lotion is chosen instead, add 0.25% menthol for relief of pruritus. Soaps are to be avoided as much as possible, and only mild, nonalkaline forms (e.g., Dove) should be used. Topical corticosteroids are useful in reducing inflammation. In order to ensure optimal use of topical steroids, it is necessary to keep in mind the relationship of potency to the drug vehicle and, in turn, to the varying skin permeability that is dependent on the site being treated.[9] In most cases, a medium potency steroid, such as 0.1% betamethasone or 0.1% triamcinolone, should be applied 2 to 3 times per day.[10] Use only nonfluorinated, low potency products, such as hydrocortisone, on the face, axilla, and groin (Table 44–2). To do otherwise leads all too often to the development of a rosacea-like rash on the face and striae formation in the groin. When possible, apply medications to moist skin after bathing or soaking the area in water. If the skin is very dry or fissured, the ointment form is preferred to the cream. Ointments may also be more effective in treatment of palmar and plantar involvement.[9,10]

In the absence of corticosteroid contraindications, very severe cases producing facial edema, extensive bulla formation, or incapacity should be treated with oral prednisone. The starting dose must be individualized according to the patient, coexisting conditions, and the extent and severity of the dermatitis. Begin with 40 to 60 mg of

Table 44-2   Commonly Prescribed Topical Corticosteroids*

High Potency
    Betamethasone dipropionate ointment (Diprosone) 0.05%
    Halcinonide cream, ointment (Halog) 0.1%
    Fluocinonide cream, ointment, gel (Lidex, Topsyn) 0.05%
    Desoximetasone cream, ointment (Topicort) 0.25%

Moderately Strong Potency
    Betamethasone benzoate gel (Benisone, Uticort) 0.025%
    Betamethasone dipropionate cream (Diprosone) 0.05%
    Diflorasone diacetate cream (Florone, Maxiflor) 0.05%
    Triamcinolone acetonide cream (Aristocort) 0.5%

Medium Potency
    Betamethasone valerate cream (Valisone) 0.1%
    Triamcinolone acetonide cream (Aristocort, Kenalog) 0.1%
    Flurandrenolide cream (Cordran) 0.05%
    Fluocinolone acetonide cream (Synalar, Fluonid) 0.025%
    Halcinonide cream (Halog) 0.025%

Low Potency
    Hydrocortisone (Cortaid, Cort-dome) 0.25 to 2.5%
    Methylprednisolone acetate (Medrol) 0.25 to 1%
    Dexamethasone (Decadron) 0.04 to 0.1%
    Prednisolone (Meti-Derm) 0.5%

* Since new agents are continually marketed by the pharmaceutical industry, the examples used are *merely examples.*

prednisone per day, tapering the dose over 3 weeks. Give 60 mg the first week, 40 mg for 1 week, and 20 mg for the last week. Premature discontinuation of treatment may result in return of the skin lesions. The drug should be given as a single daily dose before 8 AM, which helps minimize the cortisol suppression. Severely symptomatic patients may also be treated with an initial intramuscular injection of steroids, such as triamcinolone acetonide, 40 to 80 mg, or possibly with adrenocorticotropic hormone (ACTH). Oral antihistamines, such as hydroxyzine (Atarax) and diphenhydramine (Benadryl) may be beneficial for their antipruritic and sedative effects.[10]

Once the patient has been treated, he or she should be instructed in avoidance. Sometimes the history and distribution of lesions will identify the allergen to be avoided. But if there is any doubt regarding the diagnosis of allergic contact dermatitis, the patient should be referred for patch testing. Pinpointing the allergen with patch testing is also important because there may be cross-reactivity with other substances. For example, chemicals that are very similar to poison ivy may provoke a contact allergy in an individual who is hypersensitive to poison ivy.[11] India ink, cashew nuts, and mango rinds are three common examples.

Seborrheic Dermatitis

This condition steadily increases in incidence after age 50 and is a recurrent chronic disease. Approximately 67% of nursing home patients over the age of 70 suffer from seborrheic dermatitis.[13] It is associated with crusting, scaling, mild redness, and often pruritus of the scalp,

eyebrows, nasolabial folds, postauricular areas, over the sternum, and between the shoulder blades (Figure 44-2). Blepharitis is common, appearing as erythema and scaling of the eyelid margins, and is often associated with a mild conjunctivitis. Seborrheic dermatitis may resemble psoriasis in the flexural creases. However, scales associated with psoriasis tend to be dry and horny, rather than greasy. Microscopic examination of scrapings from the border of a lesion may be quite useful in ruling out a fungal infection. In addition, a history of "dandruff" is helpful in making a diagnosis of seborrheic dermatitis.

The pathophysiology of seborrheic dermatitis is unknown. Sebaceous gland dysfunction is thought to play a role, as is genetic predisposition, hormonal change, nutrition, infection, and emotional stress. There is both increased sebum production and an increased incidence of seborrheic dermatitis in Parkinson's disease and some other neurologic conditions. Chlorpromazine and gold are known to produce a seborrheic dermatitis–like eruption.[10] As the disease runs an unpredictably long course, careful and mild treatment regimens are recommended. Scalp involvement usually responds well to frequent use of shampoos containing selenium sulfide, zinc pyrithione, salicylic acid, or tar. If the scalp lesions are extensive or very inflammatory, use betamethasone valerate (Valisone) 0.1% lotion. Seborrhea of the skin usually responds within a few days to low-potency topical steroid preparations (e.g., 1% hydrocortisone). Creams containing 2 to 3% sulfur (Pragmatar) are good alternatives to topical steroids and should be used for chronic resistant lesions, especially on the face. Ketoconazole cream (Nizoral) may also be beneficial as there are recent data to support the role of *Pityrosporum* yeasts in the pathogenesis of seborrheic dermatitis.

Stasis Dermatitis

Stasis dermatitis is also seen very commonly in the elderly and deserves furthur mention. It is caused by impaired lower extremity circulation, usually as a result of incompetent varicose veins, congestive heart disease, or diabetes. Pruritus, which often accompanies venous stasis, leads to scratching, excoriations, weeping, crusting, and inflammation (see Figure 44-3). The color of the inflamed skin is violaceous rather than bright red because of pooling and deoxygenation of venous blood.[1] Initial skin changes are commonly found on the lower leg, usually just proximal to the medial malleolus. Associated findings are atrophy, mottled pigmentation, ulceration, brawny induration, and onychodystrophy. Superficial venous varicosities may also be present.

Neither stasis dermatitis nor stasis ulcers will heal unless the extremity edema can be reduced — bed rest, elevation of the extremity, supportive stockings, and correction of underlying venous insufficiency when possible. The acute, inflamed, oozing leg requires the application

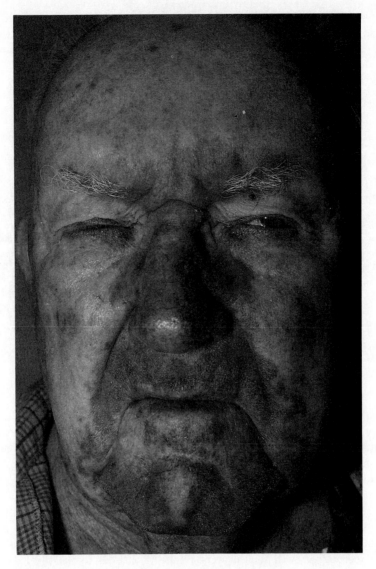

Figure 44–2 Seborrheic dermatitis.

of moist, cool compresses (Burow's solution) for 20 minutes every 3 to 4 hours. Medium-potency corticosteroid creams may be alternated with wet dressings when the acute inflammatory stage subsides.[10] Systemic antibiotics are indicated if cellulitis is present.

Cutaneous Ulcers

Ulcers, particularly of the lower legs, are quite common and represent not only a diagnostic but a therapeutic problem.[8] In the absence of the typical pigmentation and small-vein enlargement of venous insufficiency, the diagnosis of stasis dermatitis is suspect and other causes for ulcers should be considered (Table 44–3). Ulceration due to arteriosclerosis starts as a black pustule which slowly ulcerates to the characteristic "cutaneous infarct." Ischemic ulcerations tend to start on the lateral aspect of the ankle and demonstrate black areas of necrosis surrounded by a zone of cyanosis.[13] Decubitus ulcers are also common in the elderly and result from prolonged immobility and altered perception of pain. They vary in depth and often extend from skin to a bony pressure point such as the greater trochanter or the sacrum.[14] Pyoderma gangrenosum is an indolent ulcer usually on the lower extremities and often associated with ulcerative colitis or regional ileitis. The ulcers in pyoderma gangrenosum have ragged, bluish-red, overhanging margins and a necrotic base.[15] Similar ulcerations have also been described in patients with rheumatoid arthritis. The pathogenesis of these ulcers is not known, but both immunologic and vasculitic factors may be important. Ulcers arising in nodules with inflammation may be seen in sporotrichosis, coccidioidomycosis, histoplasmosis, cryptococcosis, and tertiary syphilis. Several of the atypical mycobacterial infections also result in cutaneous ulcers. The most common of these infections is that due to *Mycobacterium marinum*. Finally, all ulcers of the skin that do not heal within a reasonable period of time must

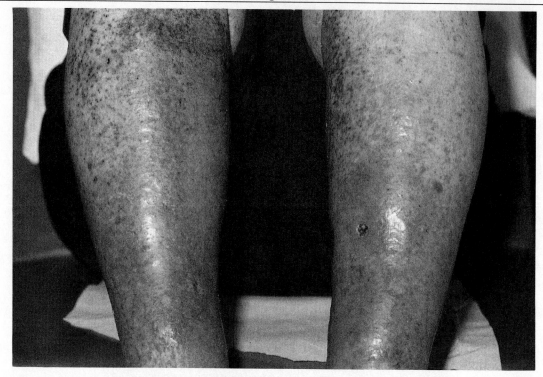

Figure 44–3 Stasis dermatitis with small ulcer.

be assumed to be carcinoma until proven otherwise, and it is essential that a biopsy be obtained.

Impaired wound healing frequently noted in elderly patients may be due to such factors as decreased vascularity, low levels of vitamin C, and decreased epidermal proliferation.[12] Basic ulcer treatment depends on the underlying pathophysiology. Most successful programs are conservative and require the patient to soak the ulcer, treat infections or bacterial overgrowth, debride necrotic tissue, manage associated dermatitis with topical steroids and lubricants, and wait for the ulceration to re-epithelialize. Therapeutic adjuncts useful in improving wound healing are vitamin C, zinc supplements, and hyperbaric oxygen.[3] Finally, foot and heel ulcers are essentially small decubiti and must have pressure removed for healing to take place.

Psoriasis

Psoriasis is the most common papulosquamous disorder, affecting about 3% of the world's population. The average age of onset is in the third decade of life, but psoriasis may make its initial appearance late in life as well. The classic presentation consists of bright red, elevated

Table 44–3   Causes of Skin Ulcers in the Elderly Patient

Infections	Hematologic disorders
Bacterial	Polycythemia vera
Fungal (blastomycosis)	Leukemia
Mycobacterial	Dysproteinemia
Syphilis	Thalassemia
Vascular disorders	Trauma
Arterial insufficiency	Metabolic disorders
Venous stasis	Necrobiosis lipoidica
Lymphatic (lymphedema)	Diabetic ulcer
Vasospastic disease (Sjögren's disease)	Gout
Allergic vasculitis	Porphyria cutanea tarda
Vasculitis	Pyoderma gangrenosum
Lupus erythematosus	Neoplastic
Periarteritis nodosa	Squamous cell, basal cell carcinoma
Rheumatoid arthritis	Lymphoma (mycosis fungoides)
Drug toxicity	Melanoma
Coumadin	Metastatic carcinoma
Bromides, iodides	Prolonged immobility (decubitus ulcers)

plaques covered with silvery scales that peel off easily and bleed. Severe exacerbations do occur and may present emergency situations in the view of patients. During these acute exacerbations, the scales may be absent, and inflamed, beefy-red skin lesions are the presenting sign. Lesions may be widespread or confined to the fingertips and extensor surfaces of the arms and legs.[11] Diverse events such as emotional upsets, steroid withdrawal, certain medications, and streptococcal infections may precede flare-ups of the disease.

Elderly patients with a severe, acute exacerbation require immediate dermatologic consultation. The treatment of psoriasis is quite variable and includes topical coal-tar preparations (Estar), solar or ultraviolet irradiation, fluorinated topical steroids (Lidex, Valisone), and anthralin paste. Psoriasis unresponsive to these approaches may require cytotoxic drugs (methotrexate). A derivative of vitamin A, etretinate (Tigason), has recently been proven to be very effective in this disorder.

Pruritus

Pruritus, or itching, is the most common dermatologic complaint of older people.[12] Senile pruritus is predominantly due to xerosis, but other dermatologic conditions can be responsible (Table 44–4). Because cutaneous inflammatory responses may be muted in the elderly, a careful history and physical examination are necessary before excluding primary disorders of the skin, particularly xerosis, atopic dermatitis, and pediculosis pubis (pubic lice). Proper identification of a causative dermatoses not only leads to effective treatment in most patients but also avoids the workup for unexplained generalized pruritus.[6]

Among patients with pruritus occurring in the absence of skin disease, up to 50% may have an underlying systemic disease.[6] The differential diagnosis must include chronic renal disease, thyroid dysfunction, polycythemia vera, gout, and the results from a variety of drugs. Pruritus is often a prominent, early indication of biliary cirrhosis, but in most other forms of hepatic dysfunction, itching occurs late in the course of the disease. Diabetes may cause pruritus because of neurologic problems or simply because it enhances dryness as the patient loses sugar and water. The itching associated with malignancy can be seen with a wide variety of carcinomas, but the lymphoma-leukemia group ranks highest of all. An outpatient workup of generalized pruritus should include a complete blood count (CBC) with differential; chemical tests of thyroid, hepatic, and renal function; stool for occult blood; and chest x-ray examination.[16]

When the underlying cause cannot be determined or is determined but cannot be eliminated, symptomatic treatment is required. Numerous approaches are available for relief of pruritus:

Table 44–4   Pruritus in the Elderly

Primary skin disorders
  Acute dermatitis (any cause)
  Infestations (scabies, lice)
  Lichen planus
  Lichen simplex chronicus (localized neurodermatitis)
  Infection (varicella, candidiasis)
  Papulosquamous disease (psoriasis)
  Xerosis
  Miliaria (prickly heat)
  Bullous pemphigoid

Drug reactions
  Opiates and derivatives
  Antidepressants
  Aspirin

Psychogenic states

Circulatory
  Stasis dermatitis

Metabolic
  Hepatobiliary disease
  Uremia
  Diabetes mellitus
  Thyroid disease

Hematopoietic
  Iron deficiency anemia
  Polycythemia vera
  Lymphomas, Hodgkin's disease
  Leukemia

Visceral malignancies
  Abdominal cancer
  Central nervous system tumors

Urticaria

- Topical corticosteroids and emollients
- Oral and topical antihistamines (Benadryl)
- Menthol, phenol, or camphor in dilute solution (0.25 to 2%)
- Local anesthetics (benzocaine)
- Salicylic acid (1 to 2%) and coal tar solution
- Ultraviolet phototherapy

It is important to remember that pruritus is a symptom, not a disease or diagnosis. It must be taken as seriously as fever of unknown origin; the implications may be just as grave.

Drug Eruptions

Drug eruptions can mimic virtually all the morphologic expressions in dermatology and must be first on the differential diagnosis in the appearance of a sudden rash. Approximately 3% of elderly, hospitalized patients experience a drug eruption; rates among elderly outpatients are presumed proportional to the number of drug exposures in this population.[6] Almost any drug can produce a cutaneous reaction, and 1 of every 20 courses of drug therapy does just that (Table 44–5). Statistically, allergic reactions are most likely to occur within the first week after initiating therapy, but patients may also be-

Table 44–5 Systemic Drugs Likely to Cause a Cutaneous Reaction

Drug categories	Examples
Antibiotics	Sulfonamides, tetracycline, erythromycin, penicillin and its synthetic derivates
Anticonvulsants	Phenytoin, phenobarbital
Anticoagulants	Warfarin, heparin
Tranquilizers	Lithium, chlordiazepoxide, diazepam
Diuretics	Furosemide, chlorothiazide
NSAIDs	Salicylates, indomethacin, phenylbutazone
Blood products	Whole blood, blood platelets, plasma protein fraction
Preservatives	Phenolphthalein (in many OTC laxatives)

NSAIDs = nonsteroidal antiinflammatory drugs; OTC = over-the-counter.

Table 44–6 Drugs Associated with Characteristic Eruptions

Type of eruption	Common drugs
Acneiform	Lithium, haloperidol, isoniazid, hormones (ACTH, androgens, corticosteroids)
Erythema multiforme	Penicillin, sulfonamides, phenytoin, barbiturates, phenothiazines, NSAIDs, cimetidine, chlorpropamide, carbamazepine
Erythema nodosum	Oral contraceptives, sulfonamides, salicylates, penicillin, halogens
Bullous	Furosemide, bromides, barbiturates, NSAIDs, thiazides, captopril, clonidine
Fixed drug	Barbiturates, phenolphthalein, quinidine, sulfonamides, tetracycline, phenacetin
Photosensitivity	Sulfonamide diuretics and antidiabetics, phenothiazines, tetracycline, nalidixic acid
Lichenoid	Thiazides, gold, phenothiazines, tetracycline, furosemide, captopril, propranolol
Hemorrhagic infarcts	Coumadin, heparin
Exfoliative dermatitis	Lithium, cimetidine, gold, isoniazid
Toxic epidermal necrolysis (TEN)	Sulfonamides, barbiturates, phenytoin, NSAIDs, penicillin, allopurinol, phenolphthalein
Vasculitis	Allopurinol, thiazides, sulfonamides, phenytoin, oral contraceptives, cimetidine, chlordiazepoxide, NSAIDs

NSAIDs = nonsteroidal antiinflammatory drugs.

come sensitized to drugs they have taken for years.[11] This is especially true of the anticonvulsants. Eruptions associated with sporadically used medications, preservatives, and self-prescribed, over-the-counter medications not regarded by the patient as drugs may be particularly difficult to diagnose.[6]

The cutaneous presentation may vary widely, from urticaria and erythema multiforme to vasculitic and exanthematous patterns (Table 44–6). Nearly all drug eruptions will be widespread, asymmetric, and extremely pruritic. Lesions generally appear first on the head and proximal extremities and then on distal areas; palms, soles, and mucous membranes may be involved. Severe eruptions may produce purpuric lesions on the lower extremities without thrombocytopenia; vasculitis or, occasionally, bullae may develop. Routine laboratory analyses show no specific changes and usually are not helpful in the diagnosis of drug eruptions.

Generally, once a drug reaction is suspected, the most likely drugs responsible should be discontinued. Most eruptions resolve in 1 or 2 weeks after withdrawal of the drug. Milder cases usually require only antihistamines, soothing compresses, oatmeal baths (Aveeno), or lubricating antipruritic emollients (0.25% menthol and 1% phenol in Eucerin lotion) to alleviate pruritus. If signs and symptoms are severe, a 2-week course of systemic corticosteroids will usually prevent further progression of the eruption within 48 hours of therapy. Treatment of life-threatening reactions, such as toxic epidermal necrolysis (TEN), is discussed in a later section.

INFECTIOUS DISEASES
Bacterial Infections

Bacterial skin infections in the elderly are not known to differ substantially from those of younger individuals, but certain features are noteworthy. Because of a less responsive immune system, the usual signs of infection are less dramatic, thereby delaying the diagnosis or minimizing the degree of severity. Systemic illnesses, such as diabetes, vascular insufficiency, and peripheral edema, may delay wound healing and make the skin susceptible to a wide variety of aerobic and anaerobic organisms (e.g., clostridial cellulitis). These infections require more sophisticated anaerobic culture techniques and vigorous surgical debridement. The most commonly encountered and potentially serious localized skin infections are cellulitis, furuncles, and necrotizing fasciitis.

Cellulitis is an infection of subcutaneous tissue denoted by erythema, swelling, and local tenderness. Fever and malaise may be present. The lesion differs from erysipelas in that its margin is not as sharply demarcated and is not elevated. Acute cellulitis may arise secondary to minor trauma, a furuncle, or a surgical incision. The most common etiologic agents are *Staphylococcus* and *Streptococcus*. However, drainage or pus should be Gram-stained when available. It is theoretically possible to culture the lesion by way of injection and subsequent aspiration of sterile saline, but most clinicians do not find this helpful or necessary. Management of cellulitis should include the application of moist heat, immobilization and elevation of the extremity, and prompt antibiotic therapy. Severe cases may require hospitalization for the parenteral administration of a penicillinase-resistant penicillin or cephalosporin. This includes patients with extensive lesions, involvement of the face, systemic toxicity, cutaneous necrosis, and/or subcutaneous gas.[17]

A furuncle is an acute, deep-seated, inflammatory nodule which develops about a hair follicle, usually from a more superficial folliculitis. As pus forms in the center of the lesion, the lesion becomes fluctuant, pain increases, and spontaneous drainage of pus ultimately occurs. Large abscesses may form in certain untreated patients. Furuncles are usually caused by *S. aureus* and, occasionally, by gram-negative organisms, especially in patients with other illnesses. Bacteremic spread of infection may occur at any time, in an unpredictable fashion, producing acute endocarditis, osteomyelitis, brain abscess, or other metastatic foci. Treatment consists of systemic antibiotics — penicillinase-resistant penicillin, erythromycin, or cephalosporin — and the application of warm compresses to encourage fluctuance and spontaneous drainage. Cutaneous abscesses resolve most rapidly after they are incised and drained.[18]

Necrotizing fasciitis occurs when cellulitis progresses rapidly to gangrene of the subcutaneous tissue, followed by necrosis of the overlying skin. From 36 to 72 hours after onset of the cellulitis, the characteristic findings of fasciitis appear: the skin color becomes purple, vesicles or bullae develop, and frank cutaneous gangrene ensues. Crepitus may be present on palpation, particularly in patients with diabetes mellitus. The infection most commonly occurs on the lower extremities, abdominal wall, perineum, and about operative wounds.[17] Treatment includes local surgical debridement and administration of parenteral antibiotics that are active against streptococci, gram-negative coliform bacilli, and anaerobic bacteria until cultures provide a rationale for more narrow-spectrum antibiotics.[18] If there is any question as to the adequacy of the initial debridement, a "second-look" procedure is indicated 24 to 48 hours later.

Fungal Infections

Candida albicans, the cause of candidiasis, can be isolated with greater frequency from the skin of older subjects than from younger ones. Predisposing factors include maceration, diabetes mellitus, systemic administration of antibiotics or corticosteroids, malnutrition, and immunosuppression. *Candida* organisms may be responsible for thrush, perlèche (Figure 44–4), vulvovaginitis, balanitis, and paronychia.[7] Intertriginous involvement (inframammary, axillary, groin, interdigital) is classically manifested by bright red, sharply demarcated, tender or pruritic areas surrounded by satellite papules and pustules. This characteristic appearance is often sufficiently diagnostic to warrant treatment with topical antifungal medications. Direct examination with potas-

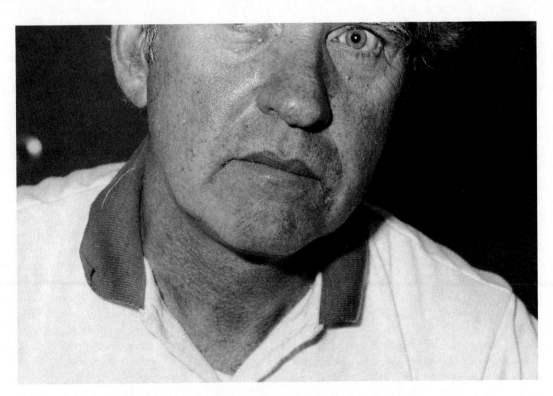

Figure 44–4 Perleche, angular stomatitis due to *Candida* infection.

sium hydroxide (KOH) may reveal blastospores, which are oval budding yeast forms, or pseudohyphae, which have indentations at the septa. Nystatin (Mycostatin), ketoconazole (Nizoral), miconazole (Micatin), and clotrimazole (Lotrimin) applied twice a day are all effective in the treatment of candidiasis. In those patients where inflammation is prominent or where pruritus is severe, the addition of a topically applied steroid such as hydrocortisone reduces the discomfort and shortens the time for healing. Since most *Candida* colonizing the skin come from the gastrointestinal tract, oral nystatin or ketoconazole may also be indicated in recurrent or recalcitrant cases. Conditions leading to moisture and maceration must be eliminated or countered. After lesions subside, continued application of a drying powder or nystatin powder should be emphasized.

The dermatophytoses are superficial fungal (tinea) infections commonly found in the elderly that involve the hair, skin, or nails. They are characterized by intense pruritus and a scaling rash which often assumes an annular or "ring like" configuration. The diagnosis should be based on a positive culture (Sabouraud's agar) or a direct KOH examination. Epilated hairs or scale scraped from skin or nails may be examined in 10 to 20% KOH. Hyphae or, in the case of hair, spores can often be visualized to confirm the diagnosis. Effective broad-spectrum antifungal agents, such as ciclopirox olamine or clotrimazole, should be applied to the affected area twice daily for at least 3 to 4 weeks and for at least 2 weeks after disappearance of the eruption.[6] Thick, hyperkeratotic involvement, as on the palms or soles, may require local therapy with medications containing keratolytic agents such as salicylic acid, which will cause softening and exfoliation of the skin. Good cleansing and careful drying are mandatory. Only very extensive cutaneous involvement warrants use of oral griseofulvin or ketoconazole.

Herpes Zoster

Herpes zoster, or shingles, is an acute, localized infection of the peripheral nerves due to reactivation of latent varicella virus in the dorsal sensory ganglion. Although the disease may be seen in any age group, more than two thirds of reported cases occur in individuals over 50 years of age. It is also seen with increased frequency in illnesses that alter cell-mediated immunity — Hodgkin's disease, other lymphomas, corticosteroid therapy, other types of immunosuppression, and radiation therapy.[19] The reactivated virus spreads antidromically down the sensory nerve, causing neuritis and pain, and to the skin, causing vesicles.

The first symptom of herpes zoster is usually dysesthesia or paresthesia of the involved dermatome. This generally precedes the eruption by 1 to 10 days and varies from superficial itching, tingling, or burning to severe, deep, lancinating pain. A severe prodrome may

mimic pleural or cardiac disease, spinal cord compression, ureteral colic, cholecystitis, or other abdominal catastrophe. Typical skin lesions consist of grouped vesicles or bullae on an erythematous patch involving one or several dermatomes. The area supplied by the trigeminal nerve, particularly the ophthalmic division, and the trunk from T3 to L2 are most frequently affected; the thoracic region alone accounts for more than one half of reported cases.[20] The eruption is nearly always unilateral and sharply demarcated at the midline. However, the earliest lesions will present closest to the ganglia, and the dermatomal distribution may not be obvious.

The diagnosis of a zoster infection can usually be made on the basis of history and physical examination. Laboratory confirmation can be obtained by Tzanck stain of material scraped from the base of an intact vesicle. New lesions continue to appear for 1 to 4 days and evolve into pustules. These dry up and crust in 7 to 10 days. Crusts persist for 3 to 4 weeks and usually heal without complications. Approximately 50% of patients with ophthalmic zoster have eye involvement (conjunctivitis, keratitis, iritis). This is particularly likely to occur if the tip of the nose is involved, representing nasociliary nerve infection (Figure 44–5). In aged and debilitated individuals, the eruption may become locally destructive, ulcerative, or secondarily infected or it may disseminate. Extensive dissemination occurs in 2 to 10% of unselected patients, most of whom have immunologic defects due to underlying malignancy (particularly lymphomas) or immunosuppressive therapy.[1] Postherpetic neuralgia (pain persisting after the lesions have healed) occurs in more than one third of patients over 60 years, especially those with ophthalmic zoster.[20] It may last a number of months and is often refractory to treatment.

Treatment of herpes zoster includes analgesics, application of cool compresses, calamine lotion, antibacterial soaps (Hibiclens) and topical antibotics. Bacterial infection is uncommon and should be treated with systemic antibiotics. If there is any question about ocular involvement and, especially, if the tip of the nose is involved, obtain an ophthalmologic consultation the same day. Herpes zoster keratoconjunctivitis is treated with topical corticosteroids and mydriasis. Antiviral chemotherapy appears to have some benefit for elderly patients. Oral acyclovir (800 mg, 5 times/day for 7 days) initiated within 48 hours of the eruption may shorten the period of virus shedding, accelerate healing, and decrease pain during the acute phase of the infection.[21] However, there appears to be no effect upon the incidence of postherpetic neuralgia. Intravenous acyclovir (5 mg/kg for 5 days) may be necessary in immunosuppressed patients.[22]

Early systemic corticosteroid therapy may reduce the incidence and duration of postherpetic neuralgia in otherwise healthy patients over 60 years of age.[23] If possible, prednisone or its equivalent should be admin-

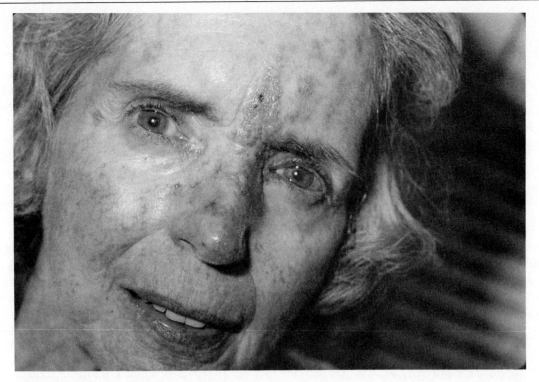

Figure 44–5 Ophthalmic zoster. Note lesions on the tip of the nose representing nasociliary nerve infection.

istered at a dose of 40 mg/day for 10 days, then tapered over 3 weeks. Unless this regimen is started within the first 3 to 5 days of the eruption, however, it is unlikely to help. Already existing postherpetic pain is extremely difficult to treat. Intracutaneously injected triamcinolone, tricyclic antidepressants (amitriptyline), transcutaneous electrical stimulation of nerves, and neurosurgical intervention are possible approaches for those unrelieved by analgesics.[1] Capsaicin (Zostrix) applied topically may be beneficial to some patients.

Scabies

One of the most common infestations of the elderly is by the mite *Sarcoptes scabiei*. It is spread by skin-to-skin contact and is common in nursing homes and hospitals; it is associated with poor living conditions. The severe pruritus is probably caused by an acquired sensitivity to the mite or fecal pellets and is first noted 2 to 4 weeks after the primary infestation. The diagnostic lesion is a short, serpiginous track with a minute vesicle or papule at the end of the burrow. Superimposed excoriations and eczematous dermatitis are common. Lesions are most commonly found in the web spaces of the hands, wrists, elbows, anterior axillary folds, and over the buttocks. Frequent sites of involvement in women are the breasts and in men the shaft and glans of the penis.

Frequent bathing, scratching, and infection can destroy many mites, and typical lesions of scabies may be difficult to detect. In addition, many kinds of hypersensitivity lesions not containing mites are found from head to foot and may be macular, papular, urticarial, vesicular, or nodular. The diagnosis of scabies should be considered in any patient who has a pruritic eruption with excoriated papules, especially if family members or close friends also are experiencing itching. Whenever possible, the diagnosis should be confirmed by microscopic identification of mites' eggs or fecal pellets in scrapings of the burrows.

The most potent topical scabicides contain gamma benzene hexachloride (Kwell, Scabene). Following a warm bath or shower, the lotion should be applied to the entire body from the neck down. The scabicide should be left in place for 8 to 12 hours and then washed off with another bath. Minimal laundering and change of bed clothes and linen are recommended. A second application 1 week later will destroy any recently hatched larvae, as none of the scabicides have been shown to be ovicidal.[7] Following effective therapy, several weeks might be needed before pruritus and erythematous papules disappear. Topical corticosteroid creams and oral antihistamines during this time may hasten resolution of the secondary eczematous dermatitis.[6] Once an epidemic of scabies is established in a nursing home, the infected patients are placed in isolation. Gowns and gloves are worn by employees entering the patients' rooms. Regardless of whether they are symptomatic, everyone in the home, including patients and employees, should be treated. One employee infested with the mite can spread the condition quickly to many patients.[24]

VESICULOBULLOUS DISEASES

Elderly patients who present with large blisters and sloughing skin cannot await elective referral. The patients have cutaneous manifestations of serious systemic problems and are at risk for metabolic complications and sepsis. Most cases will require hospitalization for intravenous hydration and systemic therapy (e.g., antibiotics, corticosteroids).

Erythema Multiforme

Erythema multiforme represents a spectrum of disease that ranges from seemingly trivial cutaneous lesions to severe, sometimes fatal, multisystem illness. The disorder occurs at any age, affects males twice as often as females, and is more common in the spring and the fall.[25] Erythema multiforme, as the name implies, consists of several types of lesions: erythematous or violaceous macules, vesicles, or bullae. Their distribution is often symmetric, most commonly involving the soles and palms, backs of the hands or feet, and the extensor surfaces of the extremities. The presence of lesions on the palms and soles is particularly characteristic (Figure 44–6). The iris or target lesion is seen most often on the hands and consists of a central vesicle or livid erythema surrounded by a concentric pale and then red ring.[7] Blistering and ulceration of the mucous membranes occurs in about a quarter of the cases, and, at times, it represents the sole expression of the disease. Patients often complain of antecedent upper respiratory infections (URIs), fever, fatigue, or arthralgia.

Erythema multiforme usually runs a mild course and subsides within 2 to 3 weeks. The Stevens-Johnson syndrome represents a severe, potentially fatal, variant of erythema multiforme.[26] After a viral prodrome lasting up to 14 days, patients develop a sudden onset of high fever, accompanied by inflammatory bullous lesions, which represent target lesions. Mucosal surfaces of the mouth, eyes, and genitalia are typically involved with widespread, painful erosions. Patients are toxic, dehydrated, and unable to eat.[11] Systemic complications include atypical pneumonia, hepatitis, esophageal strictures, ulcerative colitis, subacute nephritis, and chronic anemia. Mortality varies between 3 to 15%.

Although 80% of cases remain idiopathic, erythema multiforme reflects true hypersensitivity. It has been associated with malignancy, radiation therapy, collagen-vascular diseases, and sarcoidosis. Infection plays an important role, and the syndrome has been directly linked to herpes simplex and *Mycoplasma* pneumonia.[11,25] Drugs account for 10 to 20% of the total number of cases (see Table 44–6). However, in these patients the clinician must consider that the skin eruption may be due to the underlying disease rather than the drug itself.

The clinical features are usually distinctive enough to permit a diagnosis, but a skin biopsy should be obtained in equivocal cases. Appropriate investigative studies should be undertaken to determine the underlying etiology, and all drugs of potential etiologic significance must be stopped. Mild cases require only symptomatic treatment of fever, pain, and myalgias. Bullous lesions should be treated with the application of wet compresses

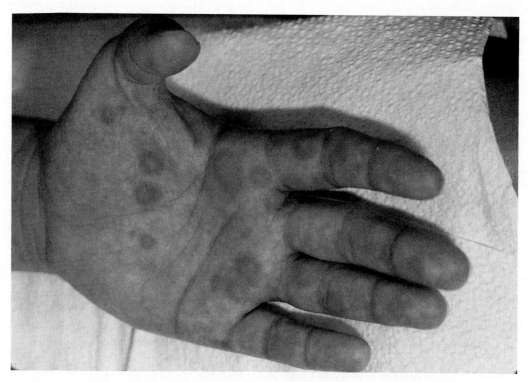

Figure 44–6 Erythema multiforme with characteristic target lesions on the palm.

soaked in a 1:16,000 solution of potassium permanganate or a 0.05% silver nitrate solution several times a day. Oral hygiene is important. Patients with severe mucous membrane involvement require hospitalization and often several days of intravenous fluids. Most clinicians recommend steroids for symptomatic relief in severely ill patients, including those with Stevens-Johnson syndrome (prednisone 50 to 80 mg daily in divided doses).[25,26]

Toxic Epidermal Necrolysis

Toxic epidermal necrolysis (TEN) apparently belongs to the same disease spectrum as erythema multiforme and represents a severe form of the disease. Both conditions share similar pathology, occasional recurrences, inflammation of mucous membranes, and association with drug allergies (Table 44-6).[27] At times, the initial skin lesions of TEN may resemble those of erythema multiforme. However, the macules rapidly coalesce and slough to the dermis, leaving large blisters and exposed areas. Lateral pressure on the erythematous skin causes separation of the epidermis from the dermis (positive Nikolsky's sign). Extensive involvement may lead to a loss of the epidermis from 50% or more of the body surface, resembling generalized scaling. The onset is usually on the face, and mucous membrane involvement is the rule. Involvement of the eyes may be particularly troublesome, even resulting in permanent injury.

Clinically, TEN may be confused with pemphigus vulgaris, thermal or chemical burns, and staphylococcal scaled-skin syndrome. The latter condition usually occurs in children under age 5 and does not involve the mucous membranes. Skin biopsy, which shows epidermal detachment from the dermis and basal layer necrosis, confirms the diagnosis of TEN.

Once exfoliation becomes extensive, the patient encounters problems similar to those of the severely burned individual. High fever, leukocytosis, albuminuria, and loss of body fluids and electrolytes through the skin lead to dehydration, shock, electrolyte imbalance, renal failure, pulmonary edema, and internal hemorrhage.[28] Patients should be admitted to a burn unit or other sterile environment. All drugs should be discontinued, if possible, and skin care such as that for second-degree burns can be lifesaving. Emergency resuscitation includes fluid and electrolyte replacement (Parkland burn protocol or similar formula), hemodynamic monitoring, and high-dose corticosteroids. If the eyes are involved, an ophthalmologist should be consulted. Even with the best of emergency care, the available reports indicate an average mortality of 30 to 50%.[27,28]

Exfoliative Dermatitis

Exfoliative dermatitis, or erythroderma, is an inflammatory disorder in which most or all of the skin surface is involved with a scaly erythematous dermatitis. Approximately 25% of patients have alopecia, and nails become dystrophic early before eventually being totally shed. Palms and soles may be involved; mucous membranes are usually spared. Males are afflicted with the condition twice as often as females, and at least 75% of the patients are over the age of 40. The patient usually has a low-grade fever and complains of intense itching, chills, and tightness of the skin. There is widespread lymphadenopathy and epidermal redness, followed by shedding dry scales or sheets of skin.[29]

Exfoliative dermatitis may result as a sudden exacerbation of preexisting skin disease, such as seborrhea, psoriasis, or atopic dermatitis. It may also be due to a number of drugs (Table 44-6) or to malignancy — Hodgkin's disease, other lymphomas, or visceral malignancy. But in one out of three cases, the etiology is unknown. Regardless of cause, exfoliative dermatitis is often complicated by leukocytosis, anemia, hyperuricemia, hypoalbuminemia, and problems with temperature regulation. Moreover, the vasodilation that accompanies the cutaneous inflammation occasionally leads to high-output cardiac failure.

The elderly patient with a newly diagnosed case of exfoliative dermatitis or one who is experiencing an acute exacerbation should be hospitalized for dermatologic nursing care, supportive treatment, and investigative studies. Rapid clearing of the exfoliation often follows suppression of the underlying dermatosis, discontinuation of the inciting drug, or avoidance of the inciting allergen. Idiopathic exfoliative dermatitis is unpredictable and may continue for 20 years or more. Topical steroids and antipruritic agents may provide relief in many cases, but for more serious disorders, systemic corticosteroids may be necessary.[30]

Pemphigus and Pemphigoid

Bullous pemphigus and pemphigoid are each complex autoimmune disorders, with multiple clinical and laboratory variants described.[31,32] Pemphigus is a rare disease which can start at any age and has predilection for individuals of Jewish or Mediterranean descent. The intraepidermal bullae are associated with a circulating IgG antibody to the intercellular substance of the epidermis. Pemphigoid usually affects adults in the sixth, seventh, and eighth decades. It is a subepidermal process with fixation of IgG and complement to the basement membrane. Differential diagnosis can be a difficult, subtle problem (Table 44-7). Biopsy of the skin and direct immunofluorescence are usually sufficient to confirm a high index of suspicion.

Pemphigus vulgaris is characterized by flaccid bullae arising on normal-appearing or erythematous skin. Because of their location within the epidermis, the bullae rupture easily and may be enlarged by gentle pressure.

Table 44–7   Characteristics of Pemphigus and Pemphigoid

	Pemphigus vulgaris	Bullous pemphigoid
Age	40–60 years	60–80 years
Bullae	Flaccid, fragile	Large, tense
Nikolsky's sign	Positive	Negative
Mucous membrane involvement	Frequent	Rare
Biopsy	Intraepidermal cleavage	Subepidermal cleavage
Immuno-fluorescence	Intercellular	Basement membrane
Course	Mortality high if untreated	Benign, prolonged remissions

Cutaneous areas commonly involved include the scalp, umbilicus, and the intertriginous areas (Figure 44–7). The earliest lesions, which precede cutaneous lesions by days or weeks, usually occur on oral mucous membranes and appear as multiple erosions with irregular borders. The eroded skin heals slowly, often leaving residual hyperpigmentation. Patients often become debilitated and cachectic as the severity and extent of the lesions increase. This disease was once uniformly fatal; however, the use of systemic corticosteroids and immunosuppressive agents (Imuran) has significantly reduced the mortality of this disease. The most common cause of death in these patients is sepsis while on high doses of corticosteroids.

Bullous pemphigoid is the most common blistering disease affecting older patients (Figure 44–8). No racial or sexual prevalence is apparent. The outstanding clinical feature is the presence of large, tense bullae generally with surrounding erythema. Its distribution may differ from pemphigus vulgaris, but that distinction is not diagnostically reliable. Sites of predilection include the medial thighs, flexor surfaces of the forearms, abdomen, and intertriginous areas. Mucous membrane lesions are rarely seen. Bullae may rupture, leaving denuded areas that heal rapidly without scarring. The treatment of bullous pemphigoid is similar to that of pemphigus except that lower doses of corticosteroids and immunosuppressives are required to suppress the disease process. The mortality rate is considered low, even in the absence of steroid therapy. However, reactivation of the disease is common and, for this reason, frequent follow-up is advisable.

CUTANEOUS TUMORS
Benign Lesions

Neoplasia is associated with aging in virtually all organ systems but is especially common in the skin. One or more benign proliferative growths are present in nearly every adult beyond age 65, and most individuals have dozens of lesions.[4] Because the primary-care physician is often the first to confront the myriad skin lesions seen in this population, it is important to recognize the various types and to know when to refer the patient for further evaluation.

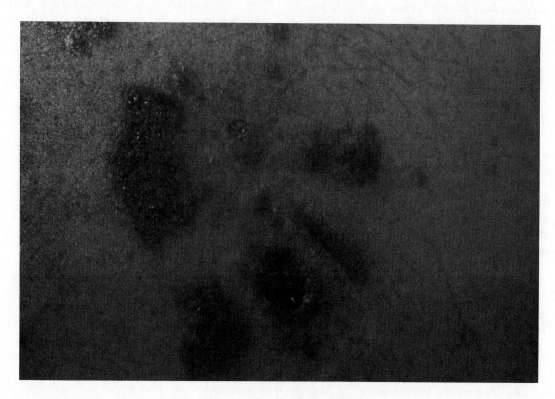

Figure 44–7   Bullous pemphigoid.

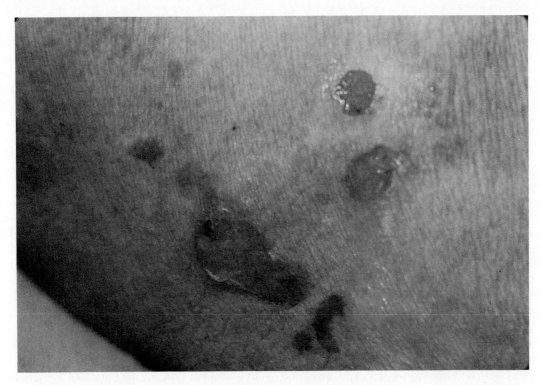

Figure 44–8 Pemphigus vulgaris; bullae have ruptured, leaving erythematous lesions with irregular borders and multiple erosions.

Seborrheic keratosis, or "senile wart," is a common, hereditary, benign tumor that occurs after age 30. These roughly textured "stuck-on" lesions may be intensely pigmented and may crumble when manipulated (Figure 44–9). They represent the proliferation of moderately well-differentiated cells from the epidermis and appear

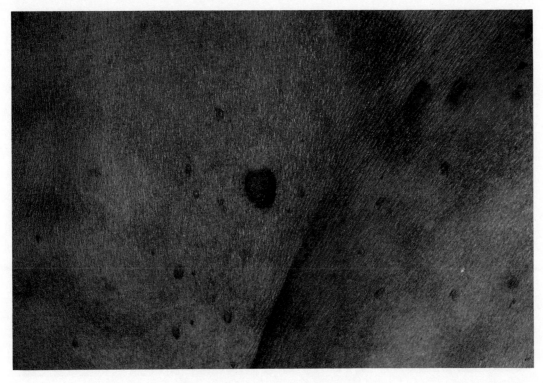

Figure 44–9 Seborrheic keratosis.

almost anywhere on the skin. The development of seborrheic keratoses occurs slowly over decades; the sudden appearance of a shower of new lesions (usually on the trunk) or the rapid growth of existing lesions may be a sign of internal malignancy (Leser-Trélat sign). The skin lesions are easily treated with liquid nitrogen (cryosurgery) or by light electrocautery.

Senile sebaceous hyperplasia usually appears on the face of an elderly individual as small, yellowish papules with a central umbilication. Histopathologically, an increased number of normal-appearing sebaceous gland lobules are present around the sebaceous duct opening to the surface epithelium. Sebaceous hyperplasia may be mistaken for basal cell carcinoma or adnexal tumor. Treatment, if desired by the patient, consists of electrocautery or cryosurgery.[33]

Keratoacanthoma develops as a keratotic crateriform papule or nodule with a predilection for sun-exposed surfaces; when solitary, it occurs most frequently after the fifth decade. Keratoacanthoma is a benign epithelial neoplasm that grows rapidly, achieving a size of 2.5 cm within 6 weeks (Figure 44–10). Ultraviolet radiation, chemical carcinogens, genetic predisposition, and viral infection have been implicated in its etiology. During the active growth phase, a keratoacanthoma closely resembles squamous cell carcinoma. While it is safest to treat a keratoacanthoma by excision, wide excision is usually unnecessary. Left untreated, most heal spontaneously in 4 to 12 months, generally leaving a depressed atrophic scar.

Cherry hemangioma is a bright red, soft, dome-shaped papule only a few millimeters in size. A rather common lesion in the elderly, it often occurs on the trunk as multiple papules (De Morgan's spots).[33] *Spider angiomas* are common on the face or trunk. The lesions consist of a central ascending artery that widens subepidermally, projecting smaller vessels in a radial fashion. They result from chronic sun exposure, liver disease, and prolonged estrogen exposure. Precipitous development of widespread telangiectasis usually signifies internal disease (e.g., Hodgkin's disease, multiple myeloma). *Senile venous lakes* (adult-onset cavernous hemangiomas) also occur on the lips, face, and neck of elderly individuals. They are dark blue, slightly raised, soft, easily compressible nodules. These benign lesions must be differentiated clinically from malignant melanoma.

Lentigines — uniformly pigmented macules, also called "liver spots" — are a completely benign form of melanocytic hyperplasia. Solar lentigo, the most frequently observed lesion, is usually found on the dorsa of the hands of whites beyond 70 years old. It has a medium brown color, completely flat, and without other evidence of epidermal change. The lesions may gradually enlarge to 3 or 4 cm and can be lightened or removed by liquid nitrogen cryotherapy.

Premalignant Lesions

Lentigo maligna, unlike the relatively uniform brown macules of solar lentigo, develops variations of brown

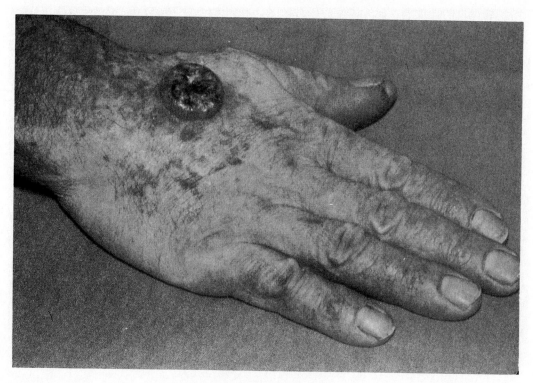

Figure 44–10 Keratoacanthoma.

color and irregularly irregular borders (Figure 44–11). Histopathology shows an increased number of atypical melanocytes and underlying lymphocytic infiltration (melanoma in situ). It is a superficial lesion that grows slowly over a course of years and may reach several centimeters before vertical invasion occurs; it is then called lentigo maligna melanoma. High cure rates have been reported with superficial irradiation, but conservative surgical excision with adequate margins is more reliable.

Leukoplakia is a potentially premalignant keratotic dysplasia of the mucous membranes. A white patch or plaque may be seen on the lips, buccal mucosa, tongue, or vagina. External and internal factors, such as smoking, poor oral hygiene, and infection, may be involved in pathogenesis. Biopsy is necessary to establish the diagnosis and rule out malignant transformation.

Bowen's disease is an in situ epidermoid carcinoma that may occur on covered or sun-exposed areas. It clinically resembles a patch of eczema or psoriasis with a crusty surface. After some time, this epithelial dysplasia has the potential to invade deeply. When Bowen's disease occurs on the glans penis, it is called erythroplasia of Queyrat. Definitive diagnosis is accompanied by skin biopsy, and therapy is instituted via excision or the use of topical 5-fluorouracil (Efudex).

Actinic keratoses are the most common premalignant lesions of the skin. They usually appear on sun-exposed skin as rough-surfaced, scaly patches on an erythematous base. They may appear hyperkeratotic as a result of rubbing or may be atrophic on severely elastotic aged skin.[33] Squamous cell carcinoma should be suspected in the presence of increased nodularity and induration, as well as development of a thick, yellow-crusted ulceration. Individual lesions of actinic keratoses can be treated by electrocautery, cryotherapy, or surgical excision. Multiple lesions are best treated with Efudex, which destroys abnormal keratinocytes. Sunscreens are essential to protect against further solar damage.

Malignant Lesions
Basal Cell Carcinoma

Basal cell carcinoma is the most common cancer seen in the United States. It is a malignant epithelial tumor that rarely metastasizes. Chronic sun exposure and a fair complexion are predisposing factors; hence, these tumors are uncommon in Asiatic races and exceedingly rare in blacks. Most basal cell carcinomas develop in sun-exposed areas. It is seldom seen before age 40 and is more common in men than in women.

Basal cell carcinoma can occur in a variety of morphologic forms. The most common type is the noduloulcerative lesion.[34] This consists of a rolled, telangiectatic, pearly bordered, waxy, transparent nodule measuring 0.5 to 1 cm (Figure 44–12). As the tumor enlarges, it outgrows its blood supply, resulting in central necrosis and the characteristic "rodent ulcer" appearance (Figure 44–13).[33] If left untreated, the lesion will invade deeper to involve the underlying structures. Some nodular basal cell carcinomas may be pigmented and thus confused with

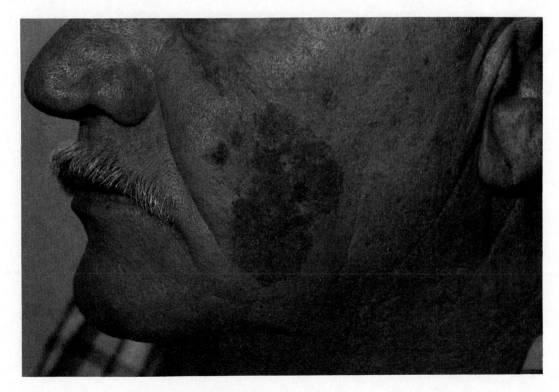

Figure 44–11 Lentigo maligna.

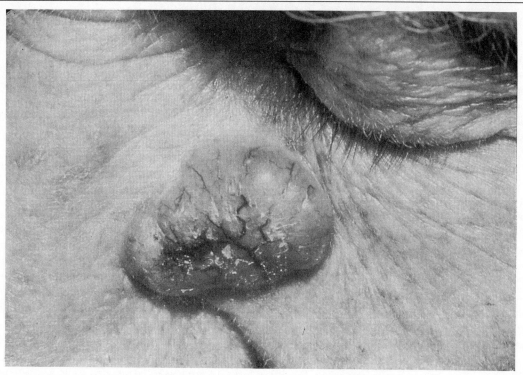

Figure 44–12 Nodular basal cell carcinoma.

malignant melanoma. A general rule of thumb is that if such a pigmented tumor appears in a blue-eyed individual, the diagnosis of malignant melanoma should be considered first; the opposite holds true, however, if the patient has dark eyes.[33] A simple excision will establish the diagnosis. If it is, in fact, a malignant melanoma, a wide reexcision must be done.

A second variant of basal cell carcinoma is the superficial multicentric type. It penetrates only into the superficial parts of the underlying dermis yet may extend

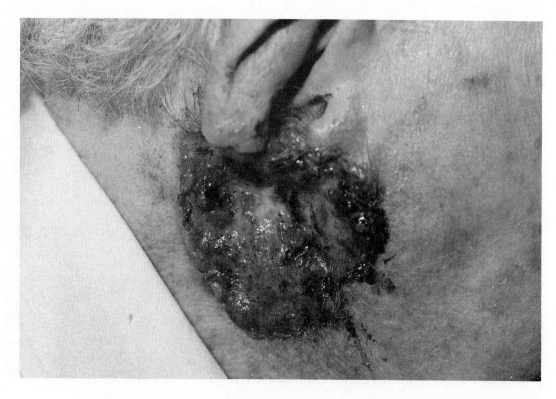

Figure 44–13 Basal cell carcinoma with characteristic "rodent ulcer" appearance.

laterally for several centimeters. This form commonly occurs on the trunk as a scaly erythematous patch, closely simulating a localized plaque of eczema or psoriasis (Figure 44–14). A definitive clinical diagnosis can be made by careful examination of the lesion using a hand lens, which reveals a pathognomonic "threadlike" translucent border.[35]

Morpheaform or fibrosing basal cell carcinoma is an indurated, yellowish plaque with ill-defined borders. In contrast to the noduloulcerative type, the overlying skin remains intact for a long time before ulceration develops. This is an insidious, often widely infiltrating malignant neoplasm whose surface represents only the "tip of the iceberg."[33]

Treatment guidelines have been well reviewed and include electrodesiccation, curettage, excision, ionizing radiation, and treatment of the base with dichloracetic acid (Sherwell's technique).[36] The Mohs' chemosurgical technique, which is removal under microscopic control, is particularly useful for recurrent basal cells or lesions near vital areas.

Squamous Cell Carcinoma

Squamous cell carcinoma, the second most commonly encountered cutaneous cancer, usually occurs in fair-skinned elderly men who live in sunny climates. This lesion originates in sun-damaged skin but may develop in Bowen's disease, radiation dermatitis, chronic stasis ulcers, and scars from injuries such as burns. Chemical carcinogens (e.g., topical hydrocarbons) and exposure to arsenic are also causally associated with squamous cell carcinoma.

The lesions have a variable gross morphology but classically appear as superficial, discrete, firm nodules or reddish-brown verrucous plaques arising from an indurated base (Figure 44–15). Ulceration and crusting are common; those lesions on the mucous membranes are macerated. Their course is variable, but they are fairly rapid-growing tumors, relative to basal cell carcinoma. Metastases may occur early, although they seem less likely with squamous cell carcinoma developing from actinic keratoses than in those that arise de novo.[34] Regional lymph nodes may be enlarged from secondary infection or metastases. The modalities and guidelines for treatment are similar to those used for basal cell carcinomas.[36]

Malignant Melanoma

The incidence of malignant melanoma in the United States is fairly low (9 per 100,000), but these lesions are responsible for two thirds of the deaths attributed to skin cancer. As with most skin cancers, sunlight appears to play a role in the etiology of melanoma. The legs and back are the most comon sites in women, and the back is the most common site in men. All of these areas are exposed to sunlight. Melanoma can also occur in non-exposed sites, such as in the nailbeds, mucous membranes, and the anal canal.

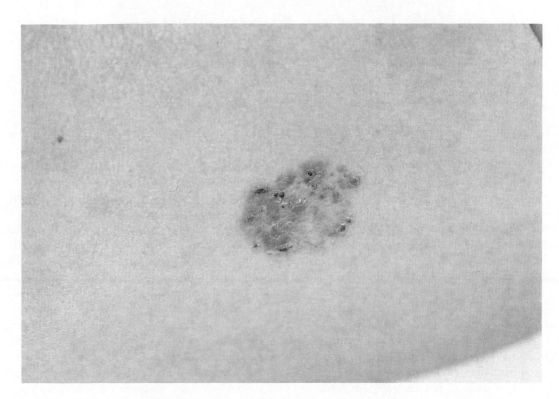

Figure 44–14 Basal cell carcinoma, superficial type.

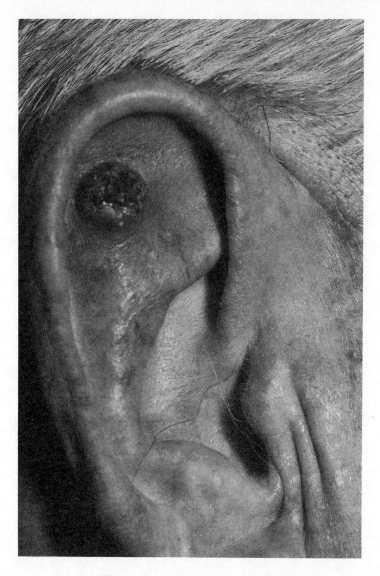

Figure 44–15   Squamous cell carcinoma.

Of the four main types of melanoma, *superficial spreading melanoma* is the most common (70% of all cases). It is a moderately slow-growing (1 to 7 years) plaque with an irregular border and variable shades of color. This tumor spreads horizontally in the skin prior to vertical invasion (Figure 44–16). *Lentigo maligna melanoma* is the least common variety of melanoma and occurs chiefly in the elderly population in sun-exposed areas. Clinically, a palpable, often dark black nodule, which may ulcerate, in seen within a patch of lentigo maligna (Figure 44–17). *Acral lentiginous melanoma* is also macular at onset and occurs on non-sun-exposed skin, especially the palms, soles, terminal phalanges, and genitalia. It is the most common type of melanoma seen in blacks and is manifested by a subtle, irregularly shaped, hyperpigmented macule. *Nodular melanoma* is the fourth type of melanoma, characterized by an early, vertical, invasive phase. It appears as a dome-shaped,

pigmented papule or nodule. As it outgrows its blood supply, the melanoma has a tendency to ulcerate. Coloration may range from dense pigmentation to an absence of melanin pigment (amelanotic melanoma).[33]

Clinicopathologic criteria for the staging and management of malignant melanoma have been extensively reviewed.[37] Therapy is based primarily on tumor thickness. Lesions thinner than 0.75 mm required only wide local resection. Local arterial lymphatic perfusion, systemic immunotherapy, chemotherapy, and palliative radiation therapy may be used to treat advanced disease. Early recognition factors include bleeding, ulceration, pruritus, and enlargement or changes in color, elevation, or surface texture of any skin lesion, particularly a pigmented one. Irregular borders and surfaces, variegate pigmentation and hues, absence of hair follicles, and presence of satellite lesions are features suggestive of a malignant melanoma.[5] .

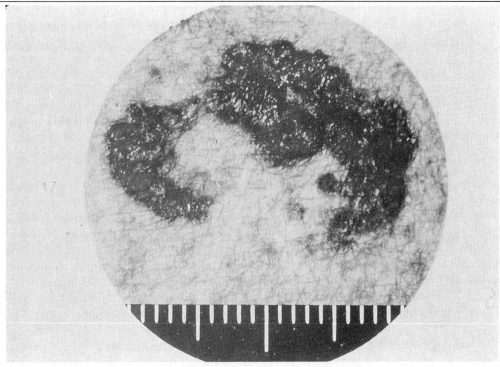

Figure 44–16 Superficial spreading melanoma.

CUTANEOUS SIGNS OF INTERNAL MALIGNANCY

Metastatic Growths

An internal malignant neoplasm may have external manifestations in the skin. Recognition of these cutaneous signs leads to the diagnosis of a previously unknown malignancy. The most specific manifestation, of course, is metastatic deposits from a distant primary tumor.

Such metastases develop in up to 4.5% of cases, depending on the primary site. Approximately half of all metastases to the skin originate from breast cancer;

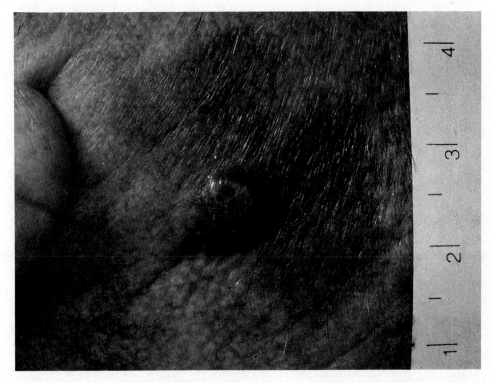

Figure 44–17 Lentigo maligna melanoma.

malignancies of the bowel, lung, uterus, and kidneys account for most of the rest.[38] These metastatic lesions often develop suddenly as rapidly growing intradermal or subcutaneous nodules that tend to be vascular and inflamed (Figure 44–18). Lymphomas and leukemias may involve the skin as erythematous and infiltrative papules, nodules, or plaques.[5] Metastases from malignant melanoma are usually pigmented. Often, there is a bluish tint to the lesion.

Because the lesions often arise via direct invasion from underlying malignant tissue, location is a good clue to the site of the primary cancer. Suspect carcinoma of the breast or lung when metastatic lesions appear on the chest or axilla, and of the gastrointestinal (GI) tract with an abdominal lesion. Metastases from oropharyngeal carcinomas may involve the face and neck. Primary tumors may also metastasize through the lymphatics or blood vessels. Therefore, lung, kidney, and breast cancers may manifest themselves through lesions as distant as the scalp.[38]

Diagnosis is confirmed by excision and biopsy. In general, cutaneous metastases herald a poor prognosis, as evidence of systemic spread to other sites is usually quickly apparent.

Warning Signs

A wide range of dermatoses, both inflammatory and proliferative, raise the possibility of internal cancer. Examples that have already been described include: acute pruritus, erythema multiforme, erythroderma, and seborrheic keratoses (Leser-Trélat sign).

Paget's disease of the nipple is an erythematous scaling eruption that indicates infiltrating ductal carcinoma of the underlying breast. It should be suspected in women with a unilateral "eczema" about the nipple that fails to respond to topical steroids (Figure 44–19). Extramammary Paget's disease, which can occur in perineal and perianal skin, is associated with a carcinoma only 50% of the time.[40] The underlying carcinoma may be of apocrine, eccrine, or other noncutaneous glandular origin (e.g., prostate, bladder, colon).

Mycosis fungoides applies to T-cell lymphoma manifested first in the skin, but, as the neoplastic process involves the entire lymphoreticular system, the lymph nodes and internal organs become involved later in the course of the disease.[35] Early mycosis fungoides may mimic psoriasis in presenting with numerous scaly, erythematous plaques and disappearing with sunlight exposure. Patients with advanced disease develop the characteristic violaceous, boggy, indurated plaques and nodules that may ulcerate as they become larger. Tumors occur in a generalized pattern, usually over the trunk and extremities.[33] Histologic confirmation may not be possible for years despite repeated biopsies. Lymphadenopathy and the detection of abnormal circulating T cells in the blood appear to correlate well with internal organ involvement.[35]

Acquired *ichthyosis* is a disorder of keratinization characterized by rhomboidal-shaped scales ("fish scale") usually localized to the lower legs (Figure 44–20). The disease is clinically identical to the inherited disorder, ichthyosis vulgaris; however, acquired ichthyosis manifests itself in adults. Lymphomas, especially Hodgkin's

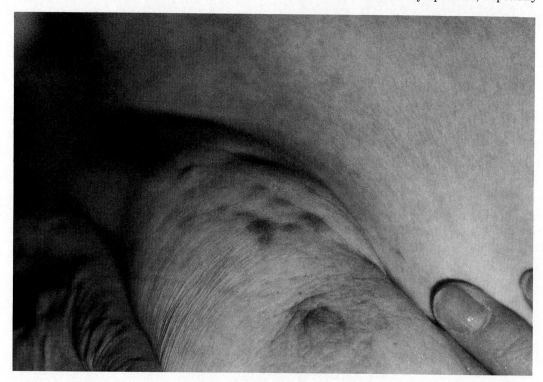

Figure 44–18 Cutaneous metastases from the breast.

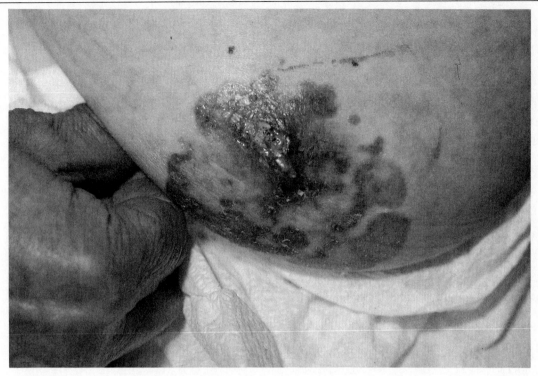

Figure 44–19 Paget's disease of the nipple.

disease, are the most commonly associated neoplasms, but solid tumors have also been reported.[40,41]

Acanthosis nigricans, as the name implies, is a gray-brown thickening of the skin. It is manifested as symmetric, velvety, papulomatous plaques, with increased skin fold markings. The most common sites of involvement are the groin, axilla, base of the neck, and ante-cubital fossa.[39] Although the condition itself is benign, in adults the lesions are strongly associated with internal cancer, especially gastrointestinal. Survival after discovery averages less than one year. Benign causes of acanthosis nigricans include obesity, drug-related complications (glucocorticoids), and endocrinopathies (diabetes).[42]

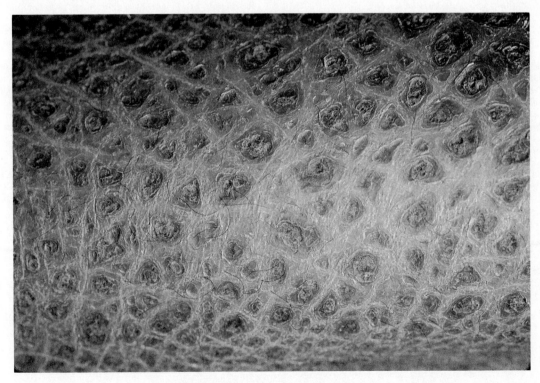

Figure 44–20 Acquired ichthyosis.

The manifestations of *dermatomyositis* — a systemic connective tissue disorder — affect not only the skin but also subcutaneous tissues and muscles. Associated with breast, lung, and GI malignancies, dermatomyositis may first present as periungual telangiectasia, erythema or papules at the joints of the fingers and hands, or distinctive periorbital edema and heliotrope discoloration. Some studies report internal malignancy in over 15% of elderly patients with dermatomyositis. The cancers are usually identifiable by history and physical examination.[43]

Hypertrichosis lanuginosa (malignant down) is represented by the appearance and growth of an excessive number of lanugo hairs. Glossitis and weight loss are additional factors. The presence of this dermatosis in the absence of an endocrinopathy or porphyria strongly suggests the presence of an underlying visceral malignancy (up to 90% of cases).[38] Thus, an awareness of the unusual findings is of value to the primary care physician.[45]

REFERENCES

1. Lynch PJ: Dermatology for the house officer, Baltimore, 1986, Williams & Wilkins Co.
2. Lynch PJ and Edminster SC: Dermatology for the non-dermatologist: a problem oriented system, Ann Emerg Med 13:603–606, 1984.
3. Duvic M: How to treat geriatric dermatoses, Drug Therapy 13:75–84, 1983.
4. Gilchrest BA: Aging of skin. In Fitzpatrick TB et al, editors: Dermatology in general medicine, New York, 1987, McGraw-Hill Book Co, pp 146–153.
5. Orentreich DS and Orentreich N: Alterations in the skin. In Andres R, Bierman EL, and Hazzard WR, editors: Principles of geriatric medicine, New York, 1985, McGraw-Hill Book Co, pp 354–371.
6. Gilchrest BA: Dermatologic disorders in the elderly. In Rossman I, editor: Clinical geriatrics, Philadelphia, 1986, JB Lippincott Co, pp 375–387.
7. Arndt KA: Manual of dermatologic therapeutics: with essentials of diagnosis, Boston, 1983, Little, Brown & Co.
8. Cripps DJ: Skin care and problems in the aged, Hosp Pract 12:119–127, 1977.
9. Weston WL: Topical corticosteroids in dermatologic disorders, Hosp Pract 19:159–178, 1984.
10. Sternbach G and Callen JP: Dermatitis, Emerg Med Clin North Am 3:677–692, 1985.
11. Rosen T and Dwyer BJ: Common dermatologic emergencies and their management, Emerg Med Reports 9:1–8, 1988.
12. Klingman AM: Perspectives and problems in cutaneous gerontology, J Invest Dermatol 73:39–46, 1976.
13. Edwards EA and Coffman JD: Cutaneous changes in peripheral vascular disease. In Fitzpatrick TB et al, editors: Dermatology in general medicine, New York, 1987, McGraw-Hill Book Co, pp 1997–2022.
14. Parish LC and Witkowski JA: The decubitus ulcer: reflections of a decade of concern, Int J Dermatol 26:639–640, 1987.
15. Hickman JG and Lazarus GS: Pyoderma gangrenosum: a reappraisal of associated systemic diseases, Br J Dermatol 102:235–241, 1980.
16. Kantor GR and Lookingbill DP: Generalized pruritus and systemic disease, J Am Acad Dermatol 9:375–382, 1983.
17. Hammar H and Wanger L: Erysipelas and necrotizing fasciitis, Br J Dermatol 96:409–419, 1977.
18. Edminster SC and Lynch PJ: Dermatologic urgencies and emergencies in the elderly. In Judd RL, Warner CG, and Schaffer MA, editors: Geriatric emergencies, Rockville, Md, 1986, Aspen, pp 395–414.
19. Hope-Simpson RE: The nature of herpes zoster: a long-term study and a new hypothesis, Proc R Soc Med 58:9–20, 1965.
20. Bourgoon CF, Burgoon JS, and Baldgridge GD: The natural history of herpes zoster, JAMA 164:265–272, 1957.
21. McKendrick MW et al: Oral acyclovir in acute herpes zoster, Br J Med 293:1529–1532, 1986.
22. Balfour HH and Bean B: Acyclovir halts progression of herpes zoster in immunocompromised patients, N Engl J Med 308:1448–1453, 1983.
23. Diamond S: Postherpetic neuralgia: prevention and treatment, Postgrad Med 81:321–322, 1987.
24. Stawiski MA: Insect bites and stings, Emerg Med Clin North Am 3:785–808, 1985.
25. Tonneson M and Soter NA: Erythema multiforme, J Am Acad Dermatol 1:357–362, 1979.
26. Araujo OE and Flowers FP: Stevens-Johnson syndrome, J Emerg Med 2:129–135, 1984.
27. Rasmussen J: Toxic epidermal necrolysis, Med Clin North Am 64:901–920, 1980.
28. Revuz J, Penso D, and Roujeau JC: Toxic epidermal necrolysis, Arch Dermatol 8:836–840, 1983.
29. Hasan T and Jansen CT: Erythroderma: a follow-up of 50 cases, J Am Acad Dermatol 8:836–840, 1983.
30. Chapel TA: Exfoliative dermatitis. In Tintinalli JE, Rothstein RJ, and Krome RL, editors: Emergency medicine: a comprehensive study guide, New York, 1985, McGraw-Hill, Inc., pp 688–689.
31. Lever WF: Pemphigus and pemphigoid, J Am Acad Dermatol 1:2–31, 1979.
32. Sams WM Jr and Gammon WR: Mechanism of lesion production in pemphigus and pemphigoid, J Am Acad Dermatol 6:431–436, 1982.
33. Proper SA and Fenske NA: Common skin tumors in the geriatric population, Geriatr Med Today 4:17–33, 1985.
34. Lin AN and Carter DM: Skin cancer in the elderly, Dermatol Clin 4:467–471, 1986.
35. Fitzpatrick TB, Polano MK, and Suurmond D: Color atlas and synopsis of clinical dermatology, New York, 1983, McGraw-Hill Book Co.
36. Albright SD: Treatment of skin cancer using multiple modalities, J Am Acad Dermatol 7:143–149, 1982.
37. Sober AJ, Fitzpatrick TB, and Mihm MC: Primary melanoma of the skin: recognition and management, J Am Acad Dermatol 2:179–186, 1980.
38. Kohn SR: Skin signs of internal cancer, Emerg Med 20:66–75, 1988.
39. McLean DI and Haynes HA: Cutaneous aspects of internal malignant disease. In Fitzpatrick TB et al, editors: Dermatology in general medicine, New York, 1987, McGraw-Hill Book Co, pp 1917–1937.
40. Pickard C, Owen LG, and Callen JP: Cutaneous signs of systemic disease, Emerg Med Clin North Am 3:765–783, 1985.
41. Flint GL, Flam M, and Sorter NA: Acquired ichthyosis, Arch Dermatol 111:1446–1449, 1975.
42. Rigel DS and Jacobs MI: Malignant acanthosis nigricans: a review, J Dermatol Surg Oncol 6: 923–929, 1980.
43. Callen JP: The value of malignancy evaluation in patients with dermatomyositis, J Am Acad Dermatol 6:253–258, 1982.

Elderly Abuse

Recognition of Elderly Abuse in the Emergency Department

Gideon Bosker, M.D., F.A.C.E.P.

Elderly abuse is becoming an increasingly recognized entity in the hospital emergency department. Despite the growing recognition of wife abuse and child abuse, the case detection process of elderly abuse has been relatively neglected until recently. Stated simply, elderly abuse is a medical emergency, and the plight of physically abused elderly people reads, at times, like a scenario out of an old Vincent Price movie. The old and infirm arrive in hospital emergency departments, dehydrated, bruised, suffering from welts and cigarette burns or signs of hemorrhaging beneath the scalp because of vigorous hair pulling. Frequently, the abused elderly come by ambulance, and there are no friends or family members to give an account of the findings. Like other forms of intrafamily violence, abuse of the elderly appears to be tied to economics. Joblessness is now matching the highest levels since World War II, and suicide rates and rates of intrafamily abuse have risen with sickening predictability.

Sad as the plight of abused children, wives, and parents is, physical abuse of the elderly poses perhaps an even more difficult problem. The problem is detecting abuse, and it has taken a long time for physicians and social workers to recognize how widespread the problem is. Journalistic documentation of the phenomenon has produced a number of sobriquets for abuse of the elderly, including "battered elder syndrome," "battered parent syndrome," "grandparent abuse," "granny bashing," and "family violence unto elderly." Eloise Rathbone-McCuan, who is presently director of the Social Work Department at the University of Vermont in Burlington, has pioneered work in the field of abuse of the elderly.

According to Rathbone-McCuan, no one is sure of the exact prevalence of the problem, but estimates range from 1:1,000 to 1:10 among the elderly population. In the February 1982 issue of the *American Journal of Psychiatry*, Rathbone-McCuan emphasized that "no matter how objectively the topic is presented, the majority of clinicians who have extensive experience in violence in the form of uncontrolled aggression or sustained anguishing stress within in a family, do not seem to promptly recognize abuse of the elderly. Their current perceptions reflect values that lead to the belief that it is unacceptable to beat a wife and horrible to beat a child, but nobody beats an aged parent."

Unfortunately, this is simply not true. Emergency department physicians have gathered many examples of physical abuse of the elderly in recent years. It is now becoming increasingly recognized that geriatric abuse can refer to anything that endangers the life, health, or financial well-being of an elderly person, and the possibilities include active physical assault, verbal and psychologic assault, denial of adequate nutrition, misuse and abuse of drugs, financial exploitation, and withholding basic life resources.

Abuse of the elderly can be subtle and have insidious ramifications. It may be difficult to separate the normal physical deterioration of aging from bona fide elderly abuse. Physical signs, such as bruises and welts; cigarette, rope, or chain burns caused by involuntary confinement; or lacerations, are suggestive of physical abuse, but neglect can be much more difficult to determine. Experts in the field have emphasized that cases of abuse have been detected in which the elderly person is classified as abused because he or she was ill but forced to remain at home without attention from the proper medical source and was offered no care by the child. While children are frequently the culprits, unrelated caregivers present a special problem because they too are frequently elderly, unemployed, or living on fixed incomes and, thus, may siphon resources away from the abused victim.

Because abused elderly rarely, or only with great trepidation, report acts of violence or aggression against them by family members or caregivers upon whom they depend, the detection of cases of elderly abuse is seriously hampered. Compounding this difficulty is the fact that neglect can masquerade in a myriad of ways. The absence of assistance among those who care for the elderly, especially when there is indifference to the provision of food, bandages, or medications, is one form of elderly neglect that can have serious medical consequences. Cases have been reported from emergency departments in which the elderly caregivers on fixed incomes have used money to purchase food for themselves instead of life-sustaining medications for the elderly for whom they are caring. Some of these substitutions have resulted in death.

Because an adequate history of elderly abuse is frequently not obtainable from the patient, the first and perhaps most important aspect of case detection is understanding the physical signs and symptoms that characterize elderly abuse. Recognition of physical indicators suggestive of elderly abuse is important because emergency department physicians must frequently rely on this evidence to legitimize and facilitate further interventional steps in the elderly. Moreover, as is the case with child and wife abuse, after a case of elderly abuse is confirmed on the basis of physical signs and symptoms, the clinician may have to initiate legal actions that are counter to the wishes of the elderly person and family. This necessitates comprehensive documentation of physical signs and symptoms.

It should also be noted that the conspicuous absence of assisting behaviors can suggest intentionality or indifference to the provision of bandages on injuries, medications, the need for stitches, or the setting of broken bones. Pallor, sunken eyes and cheeks, dry lips, excessive weight loss, and extreme dehydration are complex indicators of malnourishment. While they are common among frail and immobilized elderly, they may also be associated with direct or indirect abuse by the elderly caregiver.

An important aspect in the recognition of elderly abuse is behavioral observation. It may be possible to determine if the elderly patient, for example, seems unusually afraid of the adult caregivers who have brought the patient to medical attention. For instance, in the presence of the caregiver the aged person's eyes may dart continuously. He or she may sit as far from the caregiver as possible or cringe, back off, or dodge as if expecting to be hit by the adult caregiver. Also, the aged patient will huddle when sitting or standing and appear very nervous. Stated simply, the emergency physician should be alerted to cases in which the aged patient seems fearful in a familiar home environment and in the presence of a child or caregiver who is frequently around and presumably offering desired and needed assistance. The unpredictability of the caregiver's responses offers the clinician an opportunity to assess verbal content, communication styles, physical movements, and display of objects that involve threatening gestures.

Another important aspect of the interview is the adult child or caregiver's report of the elderly person's pattern of social contact and the role the child or caregiver assumes in controlling or facilitating that contact outside the home. For example, not allowing the aged person out of the house, preventing outside people, even family members, from making visits and putting locks on doors and phones are a few of the behavior patterns hindering the elderly person's contact with the outside world. These maneuvers discourage kin and other sources of potential help from reaching the elderly person in times of crisis. If the caregiver is attempting to prevent these contacts, he is probably successful. Keeping others out of the home perpetuates the isolation and secrecy of abuse behavior.

Finally, it should be emphasized that although knowledge is lacking about all aspects of this phenomenon, the frequency and cause of elderly abuse must be investigated. Of special importance is the need to recognize that elderly abuse may take a variety of forms and that it represents a complex clinical entity in which many different personalities and potential abuse patterns have been implicated. Chapter 46 covers these areas in some depth and provides an important model framework (Figure 46–1) to assist the acute medical care provider in identifying, assessing, and documenting possible abuse.

SUGGESTED READINGS

Block M and Sinott JP, editors: The battered elder syndrome: an exploratory study, College Park, Md, 1979, Center on Aging, University of Maryland.

Lau EE and Kosberg JI: Abuse of the elderly by informal care providers, Aging 300:10–15, 1979.

Quinn MJ and Tomita SK, editors: Elder abuse and neglect: causes, disagnosis and intervention strategies, New York, 1986, Springer Publishing Co.

Rathbone-McCuen E: Elderly victims of family violence and neglect, Social Casework 61:296–304, 1980.

Taler G and Ansello EF: Elder abuse, Am Fam Pract 32:107–114, 1985.

Geriatric Abuse and Neglect

Jeffrey S. Jones, M.D.

When I was a laddie
I lived with my granny
And many a hiding ma granny di 'ed me
Now I am a man
And I live with my granny
And do to my granny
what she did to me.

— Traditional rhyme[1]

. . . elderly abuse is far from an isolated and localized problem involving a few frail elderly and their pathological offspring. The problem is a full-scale national problem which exists with a frequency that few have dared to imagine. In fact, abuse of the elderly by their loved ones and caretakers exists with a frequency and rate only slightly less than child abuse on the basis of data supplied by the States. (U.S. House Select Committee on Aging, 1981)

Types of abuse

Victim profile

Abuser profile

Causes of abuse

Case detection

   Physical indicators

   X-ray and laboratory studies

Intervention

Abuse of the elderly has occurred throughout the ages, as can be determined by historical and literary sources. Until recently, however, research on domestic violence has focused primarily on child and spouse abuse. In 1981, the U.S. House of Representatives Select Committee on Aging held extensive hearings and published a report entitled *Elder Abuse: An Examination of a Hidden Problem*. In that report, the committee estimated that 4% of the nation's elderly population, or approximately 1 million persons, are victims of abuse or neglect.[2] This maltreatment is becoming more prevalent, with an increase of 100,000 moderate to severe abuse cases annually since 1981.[3]

Geriatric abuse may be more difficult to identify than other forms of domestic violence because of professional and public unawareness, relative isolation of the victims, and their reluctance to report abuse. Many of these cases involve only subtle signs, such as poor hygiene or dehydration, and have a great potential to pass undetected. Because of these factors, it is estimated that only one in six cases of elder abuse comes to the attention of authorities.[2]

Compounding the problem of identifying the abused elder is the general lack of consensus on a definition of elder abuse and the ambiguity of many definitions used in state reporting laws. Earlier studies coined terms such as the "battered parent syndrome" or flip phrases like "granny bashing." In March 1985, the Elder Abuse Prevention, Identification and Treatment Act (H.R. 1674) was introduced in Congress. Among other provisions, this legislation serves to clarify and standardize the language relating to elder abuse. Abuse and neglect are defined as follows:

abuse — the willful infliction of injury, unreasonable confinement, intimidation or cruel punishment with resulting physical harm, pain, or mental anguish; or the willful deprivation by a caretaker of goods or services that are necessary to avoid physical harm, anguish, or mental illness

neglect — the failure of a caretaker to provide the goods or services that are necessary to avoid physical harm, mental anguish, or mental illness

TYPES OF ABUSE

Abuse and neglect range from actual beatings to total ignorance of needed care. Many different types of abuse have been defined in various studies, but all can be condensed into four primary types: physical abuse, neglect, psychologic abuse, and material abuse (Table 46–1).[4] Physical abuse, or battery, is the least common type of maltreatment.[4,5] This includes direct beatings, deliberate burns, sexual assault, and unreasonable physical restraint. Aged parents may be battered to control their behavior or merely to vent unchecked frustration.

Physical neglect. Physical neglect as a subtype of abuse seems far more common than deliberate injury.[4] This occurs in situations in which the well-intentioned caregiver is not capable of meeting the needs of the elder or involve maliciousness. Examples include withholding personal care, medical therapy, or food. Nonambulatory patients may be left unattended for long periods, resulting in vermin infestation and decubitus ulcers.[5] Neglect may entail deliberate misuse of medications, such as oversedation to control behavior, or withholding pre-

scribed medicines to hasten death.[6] The study by Kimsey and colleagues[7] cites anecdotal evidence expanding these observations.

Psychologic abuse. Psychologic abuse occurs on a more subtle level but is not necessarily less damaging that physical abuse.[5] Infantilization; derogation; social isolation; and threats of institutionalization, abandonment, and homicide come under this heading. Fear may be provoked when family members, who are aware of their power over the aged, use subtle or obvious pressures and threats to force the elderly to conform.

Financial abuse. Financial abuse typically occurs in one of two forms.[6] It may be the misuse of the elderly person's funds by another person, usually a caretaker or close relative, or a caretaker may withhold medical attention or refrain from making necessary expenditures for the elderly person's benefit. Money saved to provide for retirement needs may be used by the family for other purposes, sometimes with the result of depriving the aged person of basic needs.[8]

The majority of victims suffer from more than one type of abuse or neglect.[6,8] Not only does one incident lead to another, but the occurrence of one form of abuse or neglect appears to provoke other forms.[6]

VICTIM PROFILE

Although the profile of an at-risk elder may include any older person, there are specific characteristics that emerge in the literature (Table 46–2). The vast majority of the victims are women; typically, they are over age 75, widowed, and socially isolated.[9] Dependency is an important factor because it limits the victim's ability to resist abuse and often dissuades the victim from reporting maltreatment for fear of a worse alternative care setting.[6] Pillemer and Wolf[10] examined the role of dependency in a comparative study of 64 elderly persons who were physically abused by their caretakers. Control cases were also used. They found that the abused group had less physical impairment than their nonabused counterparts but that they had significantly greater degrees of mental impairment. The increase in dependency had usually occurred recently and was associated with problematic behavior, such as shouting, paranoia, and incontinence. Strong dependency resulting from the elder's

Table 46–1 Types of Geriatric Abuse

Physical abuse
  Assault
  Rough handling
  Burns
  Sexual abuse
  Unreasonable physical confinement

Physical neglect
  Dehydration
  Malnutrition
  Poor hygiene
  Inappropriate or soiled clothing
  Medications given improperly
  Lack of medical care

Psychologic abuse
  Verbal or emotional abuse
  Threats
  Isolation/confinement

Material abuse
  Withholding finances
  Misuse of funds
  Theft
  Withholding means for daily living

Table 46–2 Characteristics of Abused Victims

- Age over 75 years
- Female
- White
- Widowed
- Severe cognitive and/or physical impairment
- Dependent on caretaker for most daily care needs
- Exhibits problematic behavior: incontinence, shouting, paranoia, nighttime shouting
- Socially isolated
- Psychosomatic or functional complaints

disability places a heavier burden on the caretaker, in terms of both the work demanded to care for the patient and the psychologic toll on the caretaker's sense of responsibility. The fact that abused elders tend to be older than 75 is consistent with the greater dependency that occurs as mental and physical processes deteriorate.

Having outlined a "typical" picture of the elder abused person, it is important to realize that we must not think solely in terms of a profile. Practitioners working with frail elders know that being in good health does not necessarily exempt the elderly from being abused. Geriatric abuse crosses all racial, socioeconomic, and ethnic backgrounds.[9] No specific social criterion has been found to identify segments of the population at high risk of elder abuse.

ABUSER PROFILE

As with the victims of elder abuse, no universal traits are shared by all abusers. Nonetheless, the literature strongly identifies family members or a significant caretaker as the most frequent perpetrators of abuse (Table 46–3). Daughters and sons were the most likely abusers, followed by grandchildren, spouse, and siblings.[4] Daughters are involved more frequently in psychologic abuse and neglect. Adult sons are more frequently involved in physical abuse and assault.[11] Wolf and Pillemer found that 64% of the abusers were dependent on the victim for financial support and 55% were dependent on the victim for housing.[10]

The majority of principal caretakers are over age 50 and nearly 20% are over age 70.[9] Studies suggest that the least socially integrated child (e.g., unmarried, unemployed) is likely to be given the responsibility for caretaking. These abusers frequently suffer from some form of stress, such as alcoholism, inadequate housing, lack of support from other family members, marital discord, illness, or a general lack of awareness that services are available to help cope with these stresses.[12] These environmental stressors may create an explosive situation for the abuser.

CAUSES OF ABUSE

A number of factors contribute to the problem of elder abuse. These include demographic shifts toward longer

Table 46–3   Characteristics of Caretaker/Abuser

- Age over 50 years
- Family member (usually daughter)
- Dependent on the victim for financial support and housing
- Alcohol or drug abuse
- Ill-prepared or reluctant to provide care
- Severe external stress (loss of job, illness, marital discord)
- Demonstrates poor impulse control
- History of domestic violence (spouse, child abuse)

survival, inadequate economic or family support for care of the elderly, inadequate community-based social services for informal care of the elderly, and negative attitudes toward old and disabled persons.[6] O'Malley and coworkers[13] reviewed case reports and research studies of elder abuse/neglect and developed some preliminary hypotheses regarding the causes. These hypotheses can be grouped into four categories:

1. Impairment and physical dependency of the elderly
2. The effect of situational stress on the abuser
3. Abuse as a learned behavior in violent families
4. Individual pathology of the abuser

Theories of impairment and consequent dependency underlie much of the analysis of child abuse.[13] The inability of the elderly person to do some activities of daily living leads to dependency and consequent vulnerability to abuse and neglect by a caretaker. In one sample of 240 elderly clients referred for intensive home supports because of significant unmet needs, 17% were reported to have been abused or severely neglected.[14]

The situational stress category is probably the most understandable of the theories as to why elder abuse occurs. Many duties and responsibilities that are associated with providing care for elderly parents may place overwhelming demands on adult child caretakers. They may have to give up previous life-styles, social relationships, and possibly jobs to be home to care for the elderly parent.[5] These stressors may cause the abuser to lash out in a burst of anger or slowly transfer personal enmities to an elder scapegoat.[6]

The third theory suggests that abusive adults were abused as children. Domestic violence is a learned behavior and normative in some families.[13] In a Detroit study of 77 cases of elder abuse, 10.4% of the documented cases showed clear evidence of mutual abuse between family members.[15] In this vicious cycle, family members alternately reinforce the abusive behavior of one another.

The pathologic abuser may have personality traits or character disorders that cause him or her to be abusive. A care provider who is mentally retarded, has a psychiatric disorder, or is a substance abuser may not have the decision-making capacity to make appropriate judgments regarding the older person's needs.[16]

CASE DETECTION

To intervene effectively and prevent cases of geriatric abuse within the family, two major barriers must be overcome. First, clinicians must be aware that the problem exists and that, in the face of present economic conditions, its prevalence may be increasing. Second, the physician must realize that the detection of elderly abuse requires a high index of suspicion. In some cases, the victim reports the battering and requests some form of assistance. More often, the presentation is covert, requiring physicians to take an active role in identifying the problem. Currently, there are few professional or legal guidelines to determine what information is necessary to assess and report cases of geriatric abuse accurately.[4] A practitioner is more likely to inquire about an elderly patient's bruises if he has training in detecting abuse and feels comfortable with a protocol for identifying and reporting suspected victims.[1,16]

The accompanying model (Figure 46–1) provides a framework to aid the emergency physician in the crucial first steps of identification, assessment, and documentation of both abusive and high-risk families. The criteria suggested are based on a review of the available literature on the abused elder, child and spouse abuse models, and demographic data from the medical records of abused elderly victims.[4] Although originally created for

use in emergency department settings, it may assist practitioners in family practice or outpatient clinics.

The protocol is a four-page form consisting of sections for obtaining patient consent and history, interviewing the potential abuser, recording the physical examination, and disposition. Informed consent should be obtained with regard to several aspects of the evaluation including taking photographs and the release of medical records to authorities.

During the medical history, the patient should be examined alone, without the caretaker. Medically ill patients constitute the largest portion of abused elderly presenting to the emergency department.[4,17] Therefore, besides querying patients about the circumstances surrounding their injuries and asking psychiatric patients about their domestic situation, medical complaints

**AKRON GENERAL MEDICAL CENTER
GERIATRIC ABUSE PROTOCOL**

Account No.	EMD No.
Full Name of Patient	Date

AUTHORIZATION FOR EXAMINATION AND FOR RELEASE OF INFORMATION

I hereby authorize physicians of AKRON GENERAL MEDICAL CENTER to:

☐ Perform a medical examination including pelvic (internal) examination if necessary

☐ Take necessary photographs by examining physician

☐ Report to law enforcement authorities that an alleged assault/neglect has been committed

☐ Record and maintain a file of the examination

☐ Collect and analyze necessary specimens

☐ Administer treatment indicated

The procedures outlined above, all other procedures to be performed, and the purpose for performing such procedures have been clearly explained to the undersigned. The undersigned hereby authorizes their performance and the release of copies of all medical reports, including any laboratory reports, to the police department, the office of the District Attorney, or prosecutor having jurisdiction.

Patient: _____

Witnesses: _____ R.N. _____ M.D.

Date: _____ Brought to EMD by: _____

If authorization to report has been granted, then the nurse in charge must notify the law enforcement authorities.

_____ Police Department notified at _____ a.m./p.m.

_____ Adult Protective Services notified at _____ a.m./p.m.

_____ Private physician notified at _____ a.m./p.m.

A

Figure 46–1 Geriatric abuse protocol form.

**AKRON GENERAL MEDICAL CENTER
GERIATRIC ABUSE PROTOCOL**

Account No.	EMD No.
Full Name of Patient	Date

MEDICAL & PSYCHOSOCIAL HISTORY: (Quote Where Possible)

1. **History of present illness/injury.** If patient, caregiver, or other informants (EMS, police) give different histories, document what is said by each.

   _____
   _____
   _____

2. **Past medical history.** Other current problems, severe cognitive and/or physical impairment requiring extended care, history of abuse or neglect, repetitive admissions because of injuries or poor health. _____

   _____
   _____

3. **Dependence on caregiver.** Financial, physical, and or emotional support. Social isolation.

   _____
   _____
   _____

4. **Recent household crises or conflicts.** Inadequate housing, financial difficulties, dysfunctional relationships. _____

   _____
   _____
   _____

5. **Can the patient relate to instances of:**
   - rough handling
   - sexual abuse
   - alcohol or drug abuse by family
   - verbal or emotional abuse
   - isolation and/or confinement
   - misuse of property or theft
   - threatened
   - gross neglect (fluids, food, hygiene)

   _____
   _____
   _____

6. **Interview with caregiver:**
   - recent household conflicts
   - knowledge of patient's medical condition; care and medicine required
   - mental health of caregiver - abuse as a child, poor self-image, history of violent behavior
   - willingness and ability to meet elder needs
   - commission of any threatening or abusive acts
   - demonstration of poor self-control - blaming the patient for being old or ill, denial, exaggerated defensiveness

   _____
   _____
   _____

B

Figure 46–1 — cont'd.

**AKRON GENERAL MEDICAL CENTER
GERIATRIC ABUSE PROTOCOL**

Account No.	EMD No.
Full Name of Patient	Date

PHYSICAL ASSESSMENT:

Temp_____ Pulse _____ Resp _____ B.P. _____ Weight _____

1. **General appearance** (include condition of clothing).

   _____

   _____

2. **Current mental/emotional status.** Mental status exam; behavior during exam - extremely fearful or agitated, overly quiet and passive, depressed. _____

   _____

3. **Physical neglect.** Dehydration and/or malnutrition, inappropriate or soiled clothing, poor hygiene, injury that has not received proper care, evidence of inappropriate care (eg, neglected gross decubiti).

   _____

   _____

4. **Evidence of sexual abuse.** Torn, stained, or bloody underclothing; bruises or bleeding of genitalia, anal areas; signs of STD. _____

   _____

5. **Physical abuse findings** (also mark on pictures below):

   _____

   _____

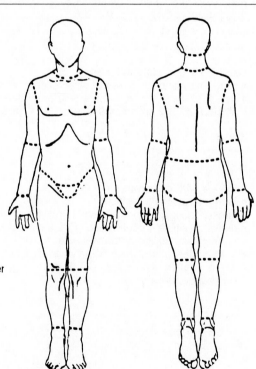

Indicators

Head injuries
   Absence of hair
   Hemorrhaging below scalp
   Broken teeth
   Eye injuries
Unexplained bruises:
   Face, lips, mouth
   Torso, back, buttocks
   Bilaterally on upper arms
   Clustered, forming patterns
   Morphologically similiar to
      striking object
   In various stages of healing
Unexplained burns:
   Cigar or cigarette burns
   Immersion burns
   Friction from ropes or chains
   Patterned like electric iron, burner
Sprains/dislocations
Lacerations or abrasions:
   Mouth, lips, gums
   Bite marks

C

Figure 46–1 — cont'd.

**AKRON GENERAL MEDICAL CENTER
GERIATRIC ABUSE PROTOCOL**

Account No.	EMD No.
Full Name of Patient	Date

DIAGNOSTICS

1. **Color photos** - labeled with name of patient, date, photographer, witness. Include picture with ruler in plane or lesions and picture of patient's face.

2. **Laboratory confirmation** (depending on type of injury/neglect present):
   - complete blood count
   - Partial thromboplastin time, prothrombin time, platelet count (easy bleeding)
   - Urinalysis, electrolyte panel (dehydration)
   - GC and chlamydia cultures, wet mount, VDRL (sexual abuse)
   - Radiologic screening for fractures
   - Metabolic screening for nutritional or endocrine abnormalities
   - Serum drug levels or toxicologic screens (over - or undermedication)

3. **Computerized axial tomogram** (CAT scan) - major changes in neurological status or head trauma that could result in subdural hematoma.

ASSESSMENT

1. No form of abuse is evident
2. Psychological abuse-verbal assault, threats, isolation
3. Material abuse or theft
4. Physical abuse - deliberate inappropriate care, direct beatings, sexual abuse
5. Physical neglect; determine causes:
   - age or frailty of caregiver
   - caregiver's lack of knowledge of patient's condition; care or medicine needed
   - physical or mental illness of caregiver
   - lack of support systems for the caregiver
   - financial difficulties

In my opinion, the medical findings are consistent with:

_____

_____

_____

FINAL DISPOSITION: _____

_____

SIGNED: _____

      Attending Physician   Date

_____

      Nurse   Date

_____

D   House Officer   Date

Figure 46–1 — cont'd.

should be explored as a screening device for domestic violence. While giving attention to the presenting complaint, the model protocol includes specific questions about the nature of the abusive situation. Many abuse victims could be identified simply by asking patients if they can relate instances of rough handling, confinement, or verbal or emotional abuse. The clinician should narrow the focus of the interview to the specific incident or incidents mentioned and obtain more detail, such as the precipitating factors for the abuse and how often the abuser repeats these incidents. In addition, the patient should be asked whether she is given enough to eat and drink and whether her medications are being given on time. The history should be explicitly described and quotations used to record the patient's verbatim statements.

In assessing the primary caretaker (when available), the physician should ask about life-style, family structure, personality, and caretaking skills. Whether or not the family understands the patient's medical condition and the necessity of care and medication may be crucial in determining whether inadvertent or willful neglect is involved. Other factors in the caretaker's history include excessive use of alcohol or drugs, mental illness in the residence, alienation, social isolation, poor self-image, and behavior that reveals unmet dependency needs or senility. The caretaker may resist an interview with the treating physician; however, if a protocol is introduced as a standard part of the exam and read by the interviewer, he or she may be less defensive or less likely to feel unjustly accused of wrongdoing.

An important aspect of the initial interview is the interaction between the elderly patient and caretaker. The elder may exhibit abnormal or fearful behavior in the presence of the adult "child." For instance, she may sit as far away from the caretaker as possible or cringe as if expecting to be struck. In addition, a family member may be overconcerned with correcting the patient's "bad behavior" or demonstrate poor self-control.[18] Suspicion should be aroused if the patient's version of how she was injured is different from the caretaker's. Other findings which may be suspicious for abuse or neglect are listed in Table 46–4. Any patient with a suspicious history, such

Table 46–4 Indicators of Possible Abuse or Neglect

- Conflicting or implausible accounts regarding how injuries or incidents occur
- Elder brought to the ED by someone other than caretaker
- Patient or caretaker has a history of "doctor shopping"
- The patient is not given the opportunity to speak for herself or see others without the caretaker being present
- There has been a prolonged interval between the trauma or illness and presentation for medical care
- Inadequate housing is available or unsafe conditions are present in the home
- There is a history of similar episodes or of other suspicious injuries in the past

as doctor "shopping," may be a candidate for further probing. Emergency medical service (EMS) personnel who routinely transport elderly patients may provide valuable information regarding the setting in which the patient lives. The lack of necessary appliances such as walkers, canes, and bedside commodes; lack of necessities such as heat, food, and water; or unsafe conditions in the home may indicate abuse. Further study remains to be done to identify with precision the highest risk groups and to identify marker conditions for geriatric abuse.

Physical Indicators

Because an adequate history of elderly abuse is frequently not obtainable from the patient, one of the most important aspects of case detection is understanding physical indicators. Clinicians need to be aware of these because of the potential urgency of treating a patient's injury and the necessity of gathering hard evidence to legitimize and facilitate further interventional steps. The classic symptoms of child abuse do not always pertain to elder abuse cases. For example, improper skin hygiene or bruises in infants indicate abuse; in the case of the elderly, diagnosis must be more circumspect. Because of decreased skin elasticity, minor trauma may result in significant bruises, falsely implying abuse.

Physical indicators of abuse range from signs of obvious injury to physical neglect. Physical injury is the most obvious type of abuse and has been cited in 44 to 50% of the elderly victims.[4,13] The accompanying protocol calls for the notation of any bruises or burns. The physician should look for unusual patterns that might reflect the use of an instrument (i.e., electrical cord, belt buckle), human bite marks, or confinement with ropes or chains. Injuries that appear in different stages of resolution must have multiple explanations to account for them. Contusions of soft tissue can be staged according to age:

Color of Lesion	Approximate Age
Swollen, tender	0–2 days
Red-blue	0–5 days
Green-yellow	5–7 days
Yellow-brown	10 days
Normal tint	3 weeks

Thermal injuries, both burns and cold injuries, can also be suspicious because of their shape and location. The injury may take the shape of common hot objects, such as pressing or curling irons, cigarette tips, and heating grills.[1]

Head injuries, lacerations and abrasions to the face, and trauma to the eyes are frequently encountered in geriatric abuse and should be treated with a high index of suspicion.[18] Ambulation must be observed when possible; painful or unusual gait may be symptoms of sexual assault and other "hidden" injuries. All findings should be recorded on a sketch sheet or photographed.

Physical neglect as a subtype of abuse seems far more common than deliberate injury.[4] Neglect may be suspected if the physical examination shows the aged patient is malnourished or dehydrated or demonstrates wasting of subcutaneous tissue. However, these problems are common among frail and immobile elderly and, therefore, difficult to associate with abuse by the caretaker. Improper care of medical problems, untreated injuries, poor hygiene, and inappropriate dress for the weather require care to discriminate, if possible, the effects of poverty from those of neglect. Either case necessitates involvement of social services.

Psychosocial indicators of abuse may include extreme withdrawal or agitation, infantile behavior, depression, and expression of ambivalent feelings toward family. A mental status exam should be conducted at some point during the interview to add credibility to the patient's report of abuse. Evaluation tools such as the Mini Mental State Exam[19] or the Short Portable Mental Status Questionnaire[20] are easy to administer and score. If patients score poorly, it may indicate that they are incapable of caring for themselves or of giving consent for intervention.

X-Ray and Laboratory Studies

Radiologic studies appropriate for the short-term management of the elderly patient must be obtained. X-ray films can be invaluable in identifying previously undetected fractures or physical injuries and may indicate the "age" of the trauma. All elders with suspected abuse plus any patient with documented radiologic injuries should have survey films taken. Special signs to look for include periosteal thickening and transverse or oblique fractures of the midshafts of long bones and fingers. Radiologic findings noted on examinations for intercurrent illnesses may identify previously unsuspected cases. A computerized tomography (CT) scan may be necessary if there has been a major change in neurologic status or head trauma.

Laboratory tests should be done as individually indicated. Hematologic screening for a coagulation defect is important when abnormal bleeding or bruising is documented. The workup may also include metabolic screening for nutritional, electrolyte, or endocrine abnormalities; a urinalysis to rule out urinary system trauma; and a toxicologic or drug-level screen to determine overmedication or undermedication. Finally, the laboratory evaluation of the elderly patient suspected of having been sexually abused may include serology and cultures for sexually transmitted disease (STD); saline preps to look for sperm (if 72 hours since last assault); and laboratory specimens such as fingernail scrapings, pubic hair, and torn clothing.

INTERVENTION

If an emergency physician suspects elder abuse, the proper course of action will depend on the type of abuse present, severity, and the caretaker's interest in improving the home environment. The first step is to explore the situation to see if there are possibilities, such as respite care, homemaker services, home nursing, day programs, or accessible transportation. Although the family is often the source of abuse, it is still potentially the most nurturing source of long-term care for the elderly person.[13] Efforts should be directed toward assisting the stressed caregiver to cope with the role and to prevent the occurrence of situations that might lead to abuse. Clinicians must take the responsibility of educating themselves about various local community social and health services available. The trend toward encouraging earlier hospital discharge of the ill and injured elderly has resulted in an increased need for medical care among people in nursing homes and those receiving home health care. As a result, caretakers are required to devote more effort and perform more patient care tasks. The stressed caregiver thus needs more assistance than before.[13a]

Immediate action is needed in cases where the magnitude of abuse or neglect may lead to permanent physical or mental damage. Hospitalization is warranted in these high-risk situations and is more likely to be accepted by the elder and family as treatment for a specific problem (i.e., dehydration, decubiti) rather than as protection from further harm. Hospitalization then provides adequate time and opportunity to define the actual care needs of the patient and arrange for necessary services. In a retrospective study of abused patient served by a chronic illness center, Lau and Kosberg[8] found that patients were subsequently institutionalized in 46% of the cases. Support services were provided in 28% of cases, but intervention was refused in 26% of situations. I have similarly noted that institutionalization is the most common intervention reported (58% of cases).[4]

The elderly person has the right to refuse protective services. Unless a court issues a finding of incompetence and appoints a guardian, the elder is assumed to be able to judge his or her own needs. This differs from child abuse, in which the government assumes the right to intervene, if necessary, without regard to the parents. Upon discharge from the emergency department (ED), follow-up arrangements must be made immediately, with the guarantee of a home visit by someone (i.e., visiting nurse, social worker).

Because of increased awareness of elder abuse, most states now have legislation providing for a system of protective services.[9] These statutes vary widely in different states. Typical provisions of an adult protective statute include a statewide system with the capability for immediate investigation and emergency services, including evaluation, counseling, and relocation. Intervention without the caretaker's consent is protected when there is probable cause of suspected abuse and the elderly victim either consents or is incapable of giving informed consent.[9] In larger cities, the emergency physician should first contact the adult protective services division of the social service agency.[5] Depending on the state statute, this division may have the authority to request a court order. In smaller communities, the physician should contact the local law enforcement agency or state attorney's office to determine the proper procedure.[6]

A final intervention is research. It has previously been acknowledged that geriatric abuse as a social problem is in its infancy. Research, investigation, and the systematic collection of data are needed in all areas. There is also a need for study and research focusing on the frequency, causes, and most effective techniques of intervention. Coexistent with data collection systems is the need for efficient and effective laws to protect both the abused elderly and informants.

To summarize, the emergency department staff has an important role in the initial management of suspected cases of abuse, neglect, or inadequate care for any reason. Awareness that the problem exists and improved detection and intervention procedures are needed to prevent abuse of elderly persons from becoming more widespread. As mentioned in Ephesians 6:2, "Honor thy father and mother [which is the first commandment with promise]; That it may be well with thee, and thou mayest live long on the earth."

REFERENCES

1. Quinn MJ and Tomita SK, editors: Elder abuse and neglect: causes, diagnosis and intervention strategies, New York, 1986, Springer Publishing Co.
2. U.S. House of Representatives Select Committee on Aging: Elder abuse: an examination of a hidden problem. 97th Congress (Comm. Pub. No. 97-277), Washington, DC, !981, Government Printing Office.
3. Pepper C: Opening statement: Elder abuse: a national disgrace. Hearing before the U.S. House Select Committee on Aging, Subcommittee on Health and Long-Term Care. May 10, 1985, Washington, DC.
4. Jones J, Dougherty J, and Schelble D: Emergency department protocol for the diagnosis and evaluation of geriatric abuse, Paper presented at the 17th Annual Meeting of the University Association for Emergency Medicine, Philadelphia, 1987.
5. Steuer J and Austin E: Family abuse of the elderly, J Am Geriatr Soc 28:372–376, 1980.
6. Palincsar J and Cobb DC: The physician's role in detecting and reporting elder abuse, J Leg Med 3:413–441, 1982.
7. Kimsey LR, Tarbox AR, and Bragg DF: Abuse of the elderly—the hidden agenda. I. The caretakers and the categories of abuse, J Am Geriatr Soc 29:465–472, 1981.
8. Lau EE and Kosberg JI: Abuse of the elderly by informal care providers, Aging 300:10–15, 1979.
9. Taler G and Ansello EF: Elder abuse, Am Fam Pract 32:107–114, 1985.
10. Wolf RS and Pillemer KA: Working with abused elders: assessment, advocacy, and intervention, Worcester, Mass, 1984, University of Massachusetts Medical Center.
11. Block M and Sinott JP, editors: The battered elder syndrome: an exploratory study, College Park, Md, 1979, Center on Aging, University of Maryland.
12. Douglass R: Domestic neglect and abuse of the elderly: implications for research and service, Family Relations 32:395–402, 1983.
13. O'Malley TA et al: Identifying and preventing family-mediated abuse and neglect of elderly persons, Ann Intern Med 98:998–1005, 1983.
13a. Shaughnessy PW and Kramer AM: The increased needs of patients in nursing homes and patients receiving home health care, N Engl J Med 322:21–27, 1990.
14. Hageboeck H and Brandt K: A summary report of rural urban abuse of the elderly in Scott County, Iowa: Iowa Gerontology Model Project, Iowa City, 1981, University of Iowa.
15. Sengstock M and Liang J: Identifying and characterizing elder abuse, Final Report Submitted to the NRTA-AARP Andrus Foundation, Institute of Gerontology, Wayne State University, Detroit, February, 1982.
16. Fulmer T, Street S, and Carr K: Abuse of the elderly: screening and detection, J Emerg Nurs 10:131–140, 1984.
17. Goldberg WG and Tomlanovich MC: Domestic violence victims in the emergency department: new findings, JAMA 251:3259–3264, 1984.
18. Rathbone-McCuan E: Elderly victims of family violence and neglect, Social Casework 61:296–304, 1980.
19. Folstein MF, Folstein SE, and McHugh PR: Mini-mental stste: a practical method of grading the cognitive state of residents for the clinician, J Psychiatr Res 12:189–198, 1975.
20. Pfeiffer E: A short portable mental status questionnaire for the assessment of organic brain deficit in elderly patients, J Am Geriatr Soc 23:433–441, 1975.

Acute Geriatric Nursing

The Approach of the Emergency Department Nurse to the Geriatric Patient

Marjorie Chevrier, R.N., C.E.N., and Jeffrey S. Jones, M.D.

As most elderly people will freely tell you, it isn't easy to be old. As most emergency nurses would just as freely add, treating the elderly isn't easy either. It's not only that they may be extremely frustrating to manage or that their prognosis is inherently limited. The difficulty is also clinical, because of important differences from younger adults in the character, specificity, and significance of signs and symptoms.[1]

To reduce problems in evaluating acute and other complaints of the elderly, the emergency nurse must understand how aging alters both normal and abnormal physiology. She has to know how classic signs and symptoms of disease may change, be masked or subdued, or be absent altogether. And she must understand the needs

and expectations of the older patient. Only then can emergency personnel focus on the whole patient and approach evaluation and management of his or her complaints both thoughtfully and rationally.[1]

This chapter provides an approach to evaluating the elderly patient in the emergency setting. It gives some background in the physiology of aging and highlights the more common problems in dealing with the geriatric population. Details relevant to particular diseases are left to other chapters.

PHYSIOLOGY OF AGING

With aging, physiologic changes occur in many organ systems that will influence the patient's presentation of illness and the response to pharmacologic and surgical intervention.[2] Virtually no organ system escapes change, with the process starting at about age 30.[3] After this time, the body's ability to exert homeostatic control and to respond to the stress of illness wanes. From the clinical perspective, it is the weakening of the renal, hepatic, immunologic, cardiac, pulmonary, and intellectual functions which cause the greatest concern.[4]

In the kidney, both structural and functional changes occur. Renal mass, for example, declines an average of 20% between the ages of 40 and 80.[1] As the decades pass, significant impairment develops in the renal concentrating function, diuresis, sodium conservation, filtration, and renal plasma flow. Hepatic blood flow also decreases, making liver metabolism less efficient. These decreases in renal and hepatic function, combined with changes in lean body mass and body water, make it more likely that the elderly patient will accumulate toxic levels of drugs.[5]

Immunologically, aging causes a decrease in primary response and cellular immunity, as well as elevations in the amount of abnormal immunoglobulins. These changes create an increased risk for infection, auto-immunity, and, perhaps, cancer.[4]

Normal changes in cardiac function cause the heart to work harder yet achieve less. Cardiac output decreases by almost 50%. Valves become more rigid, and blood vessels lose their elasticity. There may be significant increase in systolic pressure, due to the increased peripheral resistance; diastolic pressure should increase only slightly. Baroreceptor sensitivity also decreases, frequently resulting in postural hypotension.[6] Coronary artery disease is reported to affect some 40 to 50% of the elderly.[4] In addition, there is diminished circulation to all parts of the body, especially to the brain and other organs, as well as increased irritability of the cardiac muscle.

The pulmonary system, too, deteriorates with reduced elastic recoil, vital capacity, and expiratory muscle strength. This leads to "senile" emphysema.[6] There is up to a 33% decrease in blood flow to the pulmonary circulation; hence, oxygen and carbon dioxide diffusion is decreased. Pulmonary defenses are compromised due to a diminished cough reflex and lessened effectiveness of the ciliary mechanism.

Finally, the neurologic system may show some mild memory deficits with age, but significant cognitive dysfunction and behavioral or personality changes are not due to the aging process. Learning capabilities often relate more to decreased visual or auditory acuity, pace, and presence of central nervous disease than to age itself.

Aside from its influence on symptomatology, the altered physiology of age has some direct effects on drug treatment, and these are discussed in another chapter.

CLINICAL PRESENTATION IN THE ELDERLY

Compared to younger patients visiting the emergency department (ED), older patients more often have life-threatening or urgent medical conditions. At the same time, the most frequent "chief complaint" among the elderly, especially those older than 75, is not a classical medical emergency but rather a problem of self-care, falling, or dehydration (19% of diagnoses). Other common diagnoses among elderly ED patients are acute dyspnea or chest pain (10%), abdominal complaints (10%), changes in mentation (7%), minor trauma (6%), and respiratory infections and musculoskeletal pain (5% each).[7] This is by no means a complete list, and the specific conditions seen in a particular ED will depend on how it is used by the aged population near it.

The challenge of geriatric medicine is the unusual and diverse presentation of illness in the older patient. Geriatric illness is often atypical because of the diminished reserve of many systems. The most vulnerable system is attacked or decompensates and manifests as illness, although that may not be the primary problem.[8] For example, myocardial infarction, acute abdominal conditions,

pneumonia, hypothyroidism and hyperthyroidism, and urinary tract infections may present with a change in mental status as the dominant clinical sign. Conversely, emotional problems, such as depression, may manifest as a physical complaint. Even those older patients who are functioning well may have a variety of health problems, including one or more chronic ailments, that complicate whatever acute illnesses or flare-ups are the current focus. Finally, given the increased sensitivity of the elderly to drug therapy and the likelihood of multiple drug usage, as well as drug-nutrient interactions,[8a] the ED nurse may be further bewildered in the attempt to differentiate an organic entity from an adverse drug reaction. It's important, then, to bear in mind a number of clinical realities that influence nursing assessment and triage (Table 47–1).

NURSING ASSESSMENT
Person to Person

Sir William Osler's aphorism — "Listen to the patient, he'll give you the diagnosis" — is as true in the elderly as it is in the young. In the elderly, however, the quality of information you obtain is strongly influenced by the hospital environment, your attitude, and that of other health care personnel.

The interview of an elderly person often takes longer and may be complicated by barriers to communication, such as hearing loss, visual impairment, distraction, and fatigue, that can be anticipated and minimized (Table 47–2). Every effort should be made to eliminate as many potential distractions as possible, for example, telephone calls and coming and going of personnel. The room should be well lighted and warm, with bathroom facilities nearby. The interviewer should speak slowly and clearly in deep tones while facing the patient; this is best accomplished by sitting at the patient's eye level, rather than by looming over the patient or speaking from the foot of the bed.[9]

Keep a magic slate on hand for the person with severe deafness. Unless he or she is unable to give an adequate history because of obtundation or severe dementia, a patient should be interviewed alone. Family members can be interviewed separately in terms of their perceptions and related problems in daily living.

Table 47–1   Characteristics of Aging Patients[1,4]

- Because the elderly have little physical reserve, seemingly minor illness can progress rapidly to serious disease.
- "Classical" signs and symptoms of disease are possibly absent, delayed, or altered.
- Physical disease may present as a psychiatric syndrome.
- Social or psychologic difficulties may present as a medical complaint.
- Many older people have more than one illness, so symptoms of one condition may mask or exacerbate symptoms of another.
- Drug effects are more pronounced and adverse reactions more common.

Table 47-2 The Interview: Special Considerations With the Elderly Client[12,13]

- The triage area should allow privacy; interview family members separately.
- Eliminate distractions and extraneous noises in the environment.
- Address the patient by title and last name.
- Sit close to the patient to optimize eye contact and hearing.
- Phrase questions simply and clearly.
- Touch can be especially reassuring to elderly clients and can assist in gaining cooperation.
- Careful use of leading questions may help to obtain a sufficient history for initial ED intervention.
- Explain all nursing procedures and interventions carefully to the patient.
- Respect an older person's concern about modesty during the physical examination.

To obtain correct and precise information from your patient, you must establish a proper rapport. Demonstrate respect for the elder by addressing him or her by title (e.g., Mr., Miss) and last name — unless specifically requested to do otherwise. In emergency medicine, we are often reminded of the "golden hour" in assessing our patients. However, unless our patient is emergent, we should take a few minutes to introduce ourselves. As with most individuals, the geriatric patient responds to a caring, compassionate approach. Touch your patients; hold their hand or rest a hand on their shoulders. Convey an unhurried, interested demeanor.

Patience is a necessary virtue when obtaining a history, as response times and speech are often slower in the elderly. Data are lost when the interviewer fails to listen or does not allow adequate time for the person to process the question or make a request for information. Ask simple questions. Don't run together ideas or ask multiple questions at one time. This will only confuse some geriatric patients. Careful use of leading questions may assist in obtaining a sufficient history for initial intervention in the ED setting.

It is of utmost importance to explain everything you are going to do to the elderly patient, if he is somewhat confused. The apprehension your patient feels toward medical care can then be greatly lessened. During the physical examination, the ED nurse must remember that older people may be more sensitive to cold and are especially concerned about modesty. Removal of clothing and cosmetic or function devices (e.g., false teeth, wigs) may cause embarrassment, and modesty should be respected as long as health is not compromised.

One of the first questions you will need answered while taking the patient's history is the chief complaint. Obtain a statement in the patient's own words on the problem that brought him or her to the ED. The occurrence of multiple, chronic, nonspecific, chief complaints is frequent in the elderly. However, you must clarify what has made the problem different now — what warrants medical intervention at this moment. All facts believed associated with the complaint should be brought out, and the patient should be encouraged to give his or her feelings about the symptoms. This may be the hardest information to obtain from the geriatric patient. A patient may consider the symptoms to be a consequence of aging or is fearful because he or she perceives them as very serious. Altered physical and physiologic responses to disease processes can result in the absence of symptoms. For example, some older people generally do not perceive pain as intensely, and they may be unable to pinpoint its location. Thus, discomfort and pain may be absent, even in situations where one would expect severe pain (e.g., myocardial infarction). The absence of pain could delay diagnosis and treatment. Do not get caught in the trap: "No pain, no problem."[6]

The purpose of isolating certain symptoms as chief complaints is twofold. They often serve as important clues with which to begin making a differential diagnosis. The other purpose is to present a prominent list that serves to remind the physician that these symptoms brought the patient for treatment; they require therapy or an explanation of why therapy is not given.

Health History

Before your history-taking begins, make note of the way the patient walks into the room and sits down, the nature of his or her handshake, manner of dress, and other similar observations. Be alert to any incongruity between the patient's age, amount of functional decline, and magnitude of suspected illness. This is also the ideal time to assess hearing, visual acuity, ability to articulate ideas, and mental orientation.[1]

After having afforded the patient the opportunity to describe his or her **present illness**, the ED nurse should then proceed to analyze each complaint within the following framework[11]:

- Mode of onset and chronology
- Location and radiation
- Character (or quality)
- Intensity (or quantity)
- Precipitating, aggravating, and relieving factors
- Accompanying symptoms

Focusing on the chief complaint throughout the assessment may neglect the **social and environmental factors** that caused the problems in the elderly. For example, changes in the environment may intensify confusion or even bring on incontinence in a minimally demented individual. Ascertain whether the patient has suffered a loss of spouse or other significant persons. Determine previous employment and retirement status, economic status, living arrangements, and use of community and social services.

When obtaining either present or past history of illness, make note of special considerations or problems that might need the attention of a social worker, dietitian, or visiting nurse.

Unlike younger patients, elderly patients have often had multiple prior illnesses. The **past medical history** is, therefore, important in putting the patient's current problems in perspective; this can also be diagnostically important.[12] For example, vomiting in an elderly patient who has had previous intraabdominal surgery should raise the suspicion of intestinal obstruction from adhesions. Nonspecific constitutional symptoms (such as fatigue, weight loss, and anorexia) in a patient with a history of depression should prompt consideration of a relapse.[12]

Medication is an important component of your assessment of the geriatric patient. Polypharmacy and altered pharmacokinetics place the elderly at special risk for drug misuse, side effects, and interactions that may have precipitated emergency admission.[13] It is prudent to ask particularly about a number of medications, including digoxin, nitroglycerin, diuretics, insulin, corticosteroids, aspirin, and warfarin. Your geriatric patient may be taking multiple nonprescription medications in conjunction with his prescribed drugs. This can cause a variety of problems. The patient may not consider nonprescription items to be "medicine," and you must be quite clear when questioning the patient. Many medications can provide clues as to the health problems the patient has. Serious drug allergies should also be recorded on the problem list or triage note, and these patients should be encouraged to wear a Medic-Alert bracelet or necklace.

Most familial diseases have manifestations in earlier adulthood and do not pertain to elderly patients. It may be valuable to inquire about contact with tuberculosis in family members, Alzheimer's disease, and some malignant diseases that have a genetic predisposition that is manifested in later years.[14] A **family history** can provide information relevant to nurse-patient rapport. For example, experience with previous illness of significant others may explain the patient's attitudes toward his or her own health problems.

A complete **systems review** is designed to survey the problems that are known to be occult but nevertheless common in the elderly population (Table 47–3). The complexities of interpreting these symptoms in elderly patients should be reemphasized. A disinterest in life, weight loss, anorexia, and agitated behavior may be subtle manifestations of a thyroid disease, chronic infection, malignancy, uremia, dementia, drug side effect, congestive heart failure, or depression.[14] Even relatively specific symptoms can have multiple causes in the elderly. For example, back pain can result from degenerative arthritis, osteoporosis and vertebral compression fractures, metastatic cancer, or several other processes. A thorough review of systems requires time and patience, especially with a slowly responsive, partially deaf patient. In an emergency setting, it may be neccessary to perform a limited but detailed review of body systems depending upon the specific diseases under consideration (Figure 47–1).

Table 47–3   Review of Symptoms in the Elderly[12,14]

System	Key symptom
General	Anorexia, fatigue, fever, malaise, weight loss
Skin	Bruising, pressure sores
Eye, ear, nose, and throat	Dizziness, hearing loss, visual disturbances
Cardiovascular	Chest pain, claudication, diaphoresis, edema, orthopnea, palpitations, syncope
Respiratory	Cough and expectorations, hemoptysis, increasing dyspnea
Digestive	Abdominal pain, change in bowel habits, dyspepsia, dysphagia, melena, nausea and vomiting
Genitourinary	Dysuria, frequency, incontinence, hematuria, retention, vaginal bleeding
Musculoskeletal	Focal or diffuse pain, inability to ambulate, weakness
Neurologic	Confusion, headache, seizures, sleep disorders, transient focal symptoms, unsteadiness
Psychologic	Anxiety and/or agitation, depression, paranoia

When an older person cannot give an adequate history, then the majority of the patient's history must come from **secondary sources of information**. If a patient arrives in the ED by ambulance, paramedics may supply information concerning the present illness, current medications, and the environment from which the patient was received. Was everything neat and clean or dirty and cluttered? Is the home adequately cooled or heated? Does the patient live alone? The more information available about the home situation, the easier it will be to arrange discharge planning.[10] The major problem may not be a concern of a patient but rather a problem that is observed by the caregivers (spouse, family, friends). Interviewing family and friends can be critical to the patient's assessment. In addition, their assistance may be necessary in ensuring the patient's compliance with evaluation and treatment. Old medical records are an invaluable source of information to provide the details of past illnesses and surgeries. Even mentally intact individuals often have gross misunderstandings about their past history and treatments.

Physical Examination

When the medical history has been completed, the focus of the physical examination is established. The decision to perform either a baseline total examination or a limited but detailed examination of specific body systems will depend on the priority of the patient. Begin by diagnosing and treating those problems of a life-threatening nature, i.e., follow the ABCs — maintain airway management, monitor breathing rate, and check circulatory system functioning. An ECG may be necessary

NURSING ASSESSMENT SHEET

EMERGENT	URGENT	NON-URGENT	TIME	EDM#
DATE		PHYSICIAN		

PATIENT NAME: _____

DATE OF BIRTH: _____

PERSON ACCOMPANYING PT.: _____

CHIEF COMPLAINT:

PERTINENT HISTORY RELATED TO ILLNESS:

MEDICATIONS:

ALLERGIES: ☐ NONE KNOWN

TETANUS TOXOID	< 5 YRS. AGO	> 10 YEARS AGO
	> 5 YEARS. AGO	UNKNOWN

RELEVANT REVIEW OF SYSTEMS

MENTAL STATUS	YES	NO
A + 0 × 3		

EENT	YES	NO
BLURRING		
PHOTOPHOBIA		

VISUAL ACUITY: GLASSES

	OD	OS	OU
< S			
> C			

GU	YES	NO
RETENTION		
FREQUENCY		
DYSURIA		
HEMATURIA		
INCONTINENCE		

LACERATION	YES	NO
LOCATION		
DESCRIPTION		
NEURO INTACT		
ICRC. ADEQUATE		

NEURO	YES	NO
HEADACHE		
LOC		
NAUSEA		
VOMITING		
SENSORY INTACT		
MOTOR INTACT		
PERRL		

ORTHO	YES	NO
☐ UPPER EXTREMITY ☐ LOWER EXTREMITY		
LOCATION		
NEURO INTACT		
CIRC. ADEQUATE		
DEFORMITY		
ROM		

NECK, BACK, SPINE	YES	NO
LOCATION		
DURATION		
RADIATION		
FULL ROM		
SPINE POINT TENDER		
SUBJECTIVE NUMBNESS AND TINGLING		

GYN	YES	NO
VAG. DISCHARGE		
LMP		
NORMAL		
POSS. PREGNANT		

HEART & LUNGS	YES	NO
BREATH SOUNDS		
DYSPNIC		
COUGH:		
SKIN COLOR		
NAUSEA/VOMITING		
DIAPHORETIC		
PAIN		
LOCATION		
DURATION		
RADIATION		
QUALITY		

VITAL SIGNS	
T	P
R	BP

ABD	YES	NO
PAIN		
LOCATION		
DURATION		
RADIATION		
NAUSEA		
VOMITING		
SKIN COLOR		
ANOREXIA		
DIARRHEA		
BOWEL SOUNDS		
B.M.		

PLAN OF CARE:

COMMENTS:

RN SIGNATURE

Figure 47–1 Nursing assessment sheet.

to record the heart's function. Vital signs should be closely followed to verify the patient's status and note progress or deterioration.

Examination of the older person doesn't differ substantially from that of a younger person, although the type and nature of the abnormalities sought are often different.

Vital signs. The vital signs may not accurately reflect an underlying illness. For example, temperature frequently remains normal in elderly patients, even when they have a serious infection. If fever is present, it should never be taken lightly. Fever in people over 60 may be one of the few clues to the presence of serious infection. Hypothermia is also associated with many severe illnesses in the elderly (e.g., hypothyroidism, stroke, alcoholism) but is frequently missed. If the oral temperature is 35°C (95°F), which is as low as most thermometers read, take the temperature rectally with a low-reading thermometer. If the temperature falls below 32°C (90°F), urgent treatment is required. Keep in mind that elderly persons are at risk for hyperthermia and hypothermia during the extremes of summer and winter weather.

The American Heart Association defines hypertension as that blood pressure in which the systolic pressure is greater than 160 mm Hg and diastolic is usually greater than 90 mm Hg.[14] A series of at least three readings must be taken to accurately establish the baseline blood pressure. Obtain readings with the patient lying down, sitting, and/or standing. A decline of greater than 20 mm Hg in systolic pressure with standing is seen in elderly patients who have symptomatic postural hypotension. If it is accompanied by tachycardia, the cause may be volume depletion due to dehydration or blood loss.

Pulse rates may vary between 60 to 100, regular or irregular, depending upon the patient's past history of cardiac disease and current medications. Tachycardia may indicate a systemic problem with thyrotoxicosis or occult blood loss and may be the only significant abnormal finding on an examination. When you note any pulse irregularity, use the stethoscope to listen to the apical heartbeat while, at the same time, palpating the radial pulse to determine the pulse deficit. These patients should be placed on a heart monitor to identify the arrhythmia.

Finally, note the quality of respirations as well as their rate, depth, and pattern. Use the following terms to describe changes in respiratory rate[15]:

Tachypnea — increased respiratory rate (>20 per minute) seen in fever, for example, as the body tries to rid itself of excess heat; respirations increase about 4 breaths per minute for every 1°F rise in temperature

Bradypnea — decreased respiratory rate (<12 per minute), such as the depression of the CNS by opiate narcotics or intracranial pressure

Apnea — total absence of breathing may be periodic

Cheyne-Stokes — a cycle where respirations gradually increase in rate and depth and decrease over a cycle of 30 to 45 seconds; periods of apnea (20 seconds) alternate the cycles; caused by increased intracranial pressure, renal failure, meningitis, drug overdose, and severe CHF

Biot's — similar to Cheyne-Stokes except that each breath is of the same depth; may be seen with spinal meningitis or other CNS conditions

Kussmaul's — increased rate (>20 per minute) and increased depth; a panting, labored kind of respiration seen in metabolic acidosis or renal failure

Skin. The skin of an older person is notably thin and dry, with a loss of elasticity. These changes make an evaluation of dehydration less reliable.[14] Ulcerations, moles, rashes, and other new skin lesions should be carefully noted, as well as any stated changes in their appearance. An increased capillary fragility may result in reddish-purple spots that appear on the hands and forearms (senile purpura). Bruisability, however, also may reflect fragile skin, vitamin deficiency, coagulopathy, liver disease, and/or elder abuse.[14] Patients who have been confined to a wheelchair or bed for long periods of time should be turned to note any pressure sores. There is a predilection for these to occur over bony prominences, such as heels or sacrum.

Eyes. Although visual impairment may be normal and gradual, it should not be overlooked, especially when it hampers the patient's ability to function. Visual acuity should be checked via the use of the Snellen chart and a newspaper or book. Careful observation of the conjunctiva may uncover early icterus, and attention to the pupillary reaction and the extraocular movements may reflect abnormalities of the nervous system. Wrinkling and loosening of the skin around the eyelids produces an eversion or ectropion of the eyelids with exposure of the conjunctiva. Entropion, or inversion of the eyelids, may irritate the conjunctiva by the eyelashes.

Ears, nose, and throat. Wax accumulation is a common cause of hearing loss. Patients reported as senile may simply have become hard of hearing. Presbycusis (loss of auditory acuity from nerve degeneration) may cause loss of ability to hear high-pitched sounds, progressing to loss of ability to hear normal speech sounds. Olfactory nerve degeneration is also common and leads to a diminished sense of smell. The gums and teeth should be checked for infection, caries, and intraoral lesions. Remove dentures before examining the oral cavity for leukoplakia (white mucosal lesions) or carcinoma.

Neck. Examine for abnormal lymph nodes and thyroid enlargement. Note should be made of the carotid artery pulsation and the presence or absence of bruits, but be careful not to confuse them with murmurs from the heart. Careful study of the neck veins may reveal heart failure, rhythm disturbance, or even cardiac tamponade.

Thorax. An examination should determine the ability to generate a cough, the pattern of respiration, expansion of the chest, and auscultation of the lung fields. Rales at the base of the chest are normal in the elderly. Older patients tend to have stasis of blood and lung secretions due to weakness of respiratory muscles, changes in lung mechanics, and diminished cough reflexes. Dullness at the base of the lung may be a very early sign of consolidation in the toxic-appearing elderly patient without other signs of pneumonia, and wheezing may represent incipient pulmonary edema. Examination of the breasts in elderly women is usually made easier by the loss of breast tissue which occurs with aging. Irreversible retraction or discharge from the nipple may indicate a tumor.

Cardiovascular. Atypical presentation of cardiac disease must always be in the mind of the ED nurse. Findings in the elderly may include increased incidence of murmurs, increased systolic and diastolic blood pressure, and irregular cardiac rhythms, including ectopic beats or arrhythmia from degeneration of the conduction system. Lower extremity edema is also not unusual and may be caused by heart failure on one hand or by venous insufficiency on the other. If swelling is not the same in both legs, look for local causes. Check the pulses, starting from the feet and working up. If more than one pulse is absent on one side, note the temperature of both limbs. Clubbing of the fingers or cyanosis indicates circulatory impairment.

Gastrointestinal. With the abdominal wall often thin, examining this area is simplified. A palpable, abdominal aortic aneurysm should be carefully distinguished from a simple tortuous aorta, which is less than 3 cm wide and seldom has an associated bruit.[14] Be sure to palpate for possible hernias, which are often more localized in older people. It's especially easy to miss femoral hernias.[1] Acute abdominal emergencies may also mislead you because local or general systemic signs may well be absent. Perforation of a viscus and gangrene of the bowel may be marked by nothing more than sudden confusion.[1]

Genitourinary. Vaginal and urethral atrophy predisposes older women to infection and superficial bleeding. A thorough pelvic examination by the physician must be done on symptomatic patients. Tumors of the uterus, an organ which is normally atrophic at this age, may produce enlargement or noteworthy bleeding at the cervical os, and ovarian tumors easily noted by the pelvic approach may not be palpable at all on the routine abdominal examination. A rectal examination may be necessary in select patients to check for colorectal masses, constipation or impaction, or occult blood.

Nervous system. Neurologic disease is a major cause of disability in old age, often producing significant functional impairment. Formal testing of the cranial nerves is accomplished by the usual means, a great part of which may already have been accomplished while examining the eyes and ears. Cerebellar function is noted by watching the gait and noting fine movements of the extremities. A senile tremor, which occurs at a rate of three to seven per second, is coarser than a parkinsonian tremor and involves the head, jaw, and hands. The tremor occurs with movement and doesn't involve limb rigidity. Muscle strength and reflexes should generally be equal on both sides. Loss of vibratory or position sense in the lower extremities may be the stimulus for considering pernicious anemia or even some degree of glucose intolerance.[16]

A screening mental status examination should also be performed as part of the standard evaluation, since patients with mild organic brain disease often camouflage their illness by restricting comments as much as possible. A series of simple questions will help you determine more precisely the condition of the patient's memory, orientation, intellectual functioning, judgment, and affect. The ED nurse can gauge orientation, for example, by asking about date, time, and place; recent recall by asking what he had for breakfast that morning; distant recall by having the patient name the presidents since Roosevelt; reasoning by asking him to subtract one number from another serially; and abstract function by having him interpret an aphorism (e.g., "Don't throw stones if you live in a glass house").

Functional Ability

How well people function in their daily lives can tell you a great deal about their physical and mental status. For example, elderly people may be septic without having a fever. Instead, they may lose the ability to dress themselves. Establishing what patients could do in the recent past, as a baseline, is an important part of this evaluation.[1]

In addition to the mental status exam, your functional assessment should include the patient's emotional state, socialization, mobility, and ability to carry out the activities of daily living (Table 47–4). Be alert for signs of emotional lability and indicators of anxiety, depression, or paranoia, or recent personality changes. Knowledge of an individual's social circumstances is often essential to

Table 47–4 Evaluation of Functional Ability in the Elderly Patient[1,13]

Category	Assessment areas
Cognitive status	Memory, orientation, intellectual functioning and judgment
Emotional state	Affect, indicators of anxiety, depression, or paranoia, personality changes
Socialization	Personal activities (hobbies), use of community and social services, living arrangements, social activities (neighbors, church)
Activities of daily living	Performs household duties and personal hygiene, prepares meals, shops, manages money, drives or uses public transportation
Mobility	Ambulates independently, climbs stairs, maintains balance, appears stiff, uses aids (e.g., walker)

outpatient management. Although more than 75% of people over 65 are engaged in relatively normal activities and only 5% reside in nursing homes, this balance is precarious.[17] The loss of a spouse, changes in economic status, relocation of grown children to other cities, retirement, and change of living quarters all have a profound influence on the patient's well-being and, thus, on the potential need for medical attention.

Mobility is the cornerstone of physical ability — assess gait, balance, stiffness, and the use of aids.[13] Your questions should cover such basics as the patient's ability to dress himself, use the toilet, bathe, feed himself, and communicate. And, finally, you should be concerned about the patient's ability to perform the slightly more complex tasks that are necessary to function in our society. These include using the telephone, cooking, cleaning the house, shopping for groceries, managing money, adhering to prescribed drug regimens, or using public transportation.[1,12] Any sudden change in the patient's normal functioning is as likely to herald serious illness as a physical symptom would be.

A combination of data from the social, physical, and mental areas will thus provide a complete assessment and allow the correct nursing diagnosis to be made. In addition, this information will also help the ED team identify those outpatient services (e.g., home nursing, Meals-on-Wheels) necessary to maintain the older person's ability to function and be self-reliant.

NURSING DIAGNOSIS

A nursing diagnosis is a statement of the patient's needs, problems, or concerns which can be modified by nursing actions. Nursing diagnoses have been made throughout the history of modern nursing; however, formal effort toward their identification and classification is recent.[18,19]

Nursing diagnoses are written in two parts. The first part identifies the patient's problem, e.g., airway obstruction. The second part states the probable cause of the problem, e.g., thick tracheal secretions. The two phrases are connected by either "related to" or "associated with." This completed nursing diagnosis would read, "airway obstruction related to thick tracheal secretions." If the problem is a potential one, use the words "potential for" or "at risk for" before the problem ("potential for airway obstruction related to thick tracheal secretions"). Selected diagnoses that have relevance for the elderly in an emergency setting are listed below:

- Dehydration associated with fever
- Abdominal pain related to flatus and constipation
- Potential for physical injury related to noncompliance with walker
- Anxiety related to lack of knowledge about condition and separation from family

Each nursing diagnosis, when correctly written, can accomplish two things. By identifying the patient's problem or need, it tells you exactly what should change. This change is what the patient goals in your care plan will describe. And, by identifying the probable cause of the problem, it tells you what to do to effect the change. What you should do is what the nursing interventions in your care plan will describe.[20] The use of nursing diagnosis saves time in the ED by improving communication among staff members and ensuring consistent care. Each nurse who cares for a particular patient will know exactly what his problems and goals are and what must be done to solve those problems.

INTERVENTION

Triage

In many institutions where emergently ill adults are treated, the nurse is the first professional to encounter the sick or injured elderly patient. The responsibility of sorting out or "triaging" the sick adults from the well adults falls initially on the nurse, unless an effective prehospitalization system has initiated this process. The nurse must act on observations and assessments and thus plays a pivotal role in this initial stage.

The ED nurse must look beyond just taking vital signs. The "typical" geriatric patient often arrives with nonspecific and vague complaints, and the nurse must develop skills to identify elders with life-threatening and high-risk problems. Rapid deterioration is common, and early intervention is crucial.

Many approaches to triage have been used. Both nursing and nonprofessional systems have been developed, and they must be modified and restructured for individual patient care settings. The three major triage categories include emergent, life-threatening conditions requiring immediate medical attention; urgent conditions, requiring medical attention within a few hours; and nonurgent minor illnesses or injuries. Table 47–5 provides a foundation for triage and effective screening that may serve as a basis for formalization of geriatric triage protocols. If none of these emergent or urgent conditions are present, the patient should be appropriately screened and treated according to normal facility flow patterns unless there is a complicating condition.

Emotional Support

The ED nurse should consider herself a therapeutic tool, providing comfort by manner, approach, interest, and kindness. Sensitive communication is one of the most valuable skills a nurse can offer. As noted earlier, touching is extremely useful in imparting a sense of security and caring. Ongoing verbal reassurance and comfort builds confidence between patient and caretaker. A stroke patient, for example, might be acutely aware of what is being said and happening around him although he is unable to speak. The ED nurse's touch and communication are the only reassuring link the patient has. Observe the following guidelines[21]:

Table 47-5   Major Geriatric Triage Categories

Emergent	Urgent*
Abnormal vital signs	Behavioral alteration
Blood pressure	Bite, poisonous snake
Hypertensive (diastolic > 130)	Bleeding, moderate
Hypotensive (systolic < 90)	Dehydration
Respirations	Diabetic complication
Irregular	Drowning (near)
Apneic	Fever ≥ 40°C
Labored	Headache
Pulse	Acute
Irregular	Severe
Arrhythmic	Hyperthemia
Bleeding	Hypothermia
Acute	Pain
Significant	Acute
Chest pain	Severe
Coma	Poisoning
Cyanosis	Sexual assault
Eye	
Alkali, acid,	
or chemical burns	
Major burn	
Multiple or major trauma	
Status epilepticus	
Stroke syndromes	
Syncope	

*May be emergent, depending on patient's condition.

- Reduce anxiety by explaining procedures thoroughly
- When you leave your patient, let him or her know when you'll return
- Pay special attention to nonverbal communication
- Respect your patient's privacy
- Allow family members and possessions to stay with the patient, whenever feasible

The Family in the ED

With geriatric patients, the presence of the family in the ED is of enormous assistance to the staff. As a matter of policy, the family should be encouraged to be with the patient as an active member of the treatment team. By providing a history and emotional support, the family feels involved in the care of the loved ones. This model of patient care is effectively used in pediatrics and would be of benefit in geriatric care.[22]

If the patient is in a crisis situation — myocardial infarction, stroke, or major accident — it is imperative that staff be able to treat the patient's needs without interference. Therefore, the family must be separated from the patient for a time and taken to a private waiting area. Here an ED nurse or social worker should be available to explain procedures to the family and work as liaison with staff personnel. Emotional support and counseling for the patient's family reduces the stress of the ED experience and may defuse a potentially hostile situation. If life support efforts are later required, attention should be given to preservation of the integrity of patient and family and to ethical considerations in decision making for resuscitation of elderly clients.

If death occurs, the ED nurse must be prepared for a variety of emotional responses from the family. A member of the clergy should be available to attend to the family if requested. The sudden shock might cause denial, an ongoing pattern used to soften the pain of acceptance.[9] As shock recedes, the family should be allowed to view the body. A staff member may accompany the family to help them identify the loss and vent feelings about it. The ED nurse should recognize the abnormal or excessive response that requires referral.

Patient Education

Education of patient and family about the treatment plan, medications, and diagnosis helps prevent unnecessary complications and subsequent ED visits.[13] Each patient who is discharged from the ED should be given a copy of written home care instructions if reading and cognitive levels permit. These instructions should include referral for adequate follow-up and reinforcement. Instructions are reviewed verbally with each patient and the family or other support person, when available. It is not at all difficult to teach some caring relatives to give general nursing care of a high order, including hypodermic injections, irrigations, tube feedings, and oxygen administration. If your patient needs help remembering when to take medications, make a chart listing all drugs, their purposes, and how and when to take them.

Noncompliance with medical treatment and follow-up referral is a problem in emergency medicine that has been well documented. A telephone follow-up system may be a practical tool for extending emergency care into the postvisit phase. Calls may be made by an ED nurse, physician, or social worker on the day following the patient's visit. The purpose of these calls is to question patients about changes in clinical status, reinforce discharge instructions/referral, and demonstrate concern and interest in the patient. Experience has shown that many of these patients (42%) need further direction at the time of the call.[22]

A final area of concern is ensuring a safe home environment for prevention of falls, burns, hyperthermia, and hypothermia. For example, you can teach the elderly how to adapt their homes for safety and comfort and how to make use of services available in the community.

Community Resources

Emergency care intervention with the elderly client should be viewed as only a beginning in the health management plan. These patients frequently need referral to social services for linkage into a long-term care system for follow-up by appropriate inpatient and community resources. Examples include respite care, homemaker services, home nursing, day programs, and accessible transportation. Emergency department staff must take the responsibility of educating themselves about various local community social and health services available.

Hospitalization may be warranted in high-risk situations (i.e., malnutrition, depression) to provide adequate time and opportunity to define the actual care needs of the patient and arrange for necessary services. The elderly patient has a right to refuse home nursing or community services. However, if the patient's home is known to be a poor resource (i.e., lack of heat, food), it should be reported to the appropriate authorities, such as adult protective services of the social service agency.

STROKES FROM OLD FOLKS

Too often elderly patients are viewed as burdensome and difficult. Yet, diagnosing and treating them offers a unique challenge that demands ED nurses to utilize all of their training and diagnostic skills to properly assess and handle the situation. Special features of the presentation of illness in the elderly have been reviewed, and the need for a comprehensive approach has been emphasized.[2] Providing high-quality care for the elderly requires that ED nurses be aware of:

- The altered physiology, presentation of illness, and, in some cases, physical examination that occurs in the elderly
- Techniques necessary for accurate assessment of the elderly with their slowed responses and physical impairments
- Some assessment of function status (mobility, self-care capacities, mental status) as a routine part of the evaluation process
- Various local community social and health services available to the elderly client
- Education of patient and family about the treatment plan, medications, and diagnosis to prevent unnecessary complications and subsequent ED visits

Old folks have "strokes" to give as well as experience. It is up to us to rid ourselves of stereotypic thinking and defeatist attitudes in regard to the elderly. Let me leave you with a poem that was found among the possessions of an elderly woman who died in the geriatric ward of Ashludie Hospital, near Dundee, England. There is no information as to her name, when she died, or who she was.

What do you see, nurses, what do you see?
Are you thinking when you are looking at
    me —
A crabbit old woman, not very wise.
Uncertain of habit, with far-away eyes,
Who dribbles her food and makes no reply
When you say in a loud voice, "I do wish
    you'd try."
Who seems not to notice the things that
    you do,
And forever is losing a stocking or shoe.
Who unresisting or not, lets you do as
    you will,
With bathing and feeding, the long day to
    fill.
Is that what you're thinking, is that what you see?
Then open your eyes, nurses, you're not
    looking at me.
I'll tell you who I am as I sit here so still;
As I rise at your bidding, as I eat at
    your will,
I'm a small child of ten with a father and
    mother,
Brothers and sisters, who love one another
A young girl of sixteen with wings on her
    feet,
Dreaming that soon now a lover she'll meet
A bride soon at twenty — my heart gives a
    leap,
Remembering the vows that I promised to
    keep;
At twenty-five now I have young of my own,
Who need me to build a secure happy home;
A woman of thirty, my young now grow fast
Bound to each other with ties that should last;

At forty, my young sons have grown and
    are gone,
But my man's beside me to see I don't
    mourn;
At fifty once more babies play around my
    knee,
Again, we know children, my loved one and
    me.
Dark days are upon me, my husband is
    dead,
I look at the future, I shudder with dread,
For my young are all rearing young of
    their own
And I think of the years and the love that
    I've known.
I'm an old woman now and nature is
    cruel —
'Tis her jest to make old age look like a
    fool.
The body is crumbled, grace and vigor depart,
There is now a stone where I once had a heart.
But inside this old carcass a young girl
    still dwells,
And now and again my battered heart
    swells,
I remember the years, I remember the
    pain,
And I'm loving and living life over again.
I think of the years all too few – gone
    too fast,
And accept the stark fact that nothing
    can last.
So open your eyes, nurses, open and see
Not a crabbit old woman, look closer
    — see ME.

REFERENCES

1. Aged patient, altered signs, Acute Care Med 2:47–63, 1985.
2. Johnson JC: Evaluation of the geriatric emergency patient. In Wilson LB, Simson SP, and Baxter CR, editors: Handbook of geriatric emergency care, Baltimore, 1984, University Park Press, pp 7–11.
3. Fries JF: Aging, natural death and the compression of morbidity, N Engl J Med 303:130–133, 1980.
4. Freedman ML: Problems in detecting acute disease in the elderly, ER Reports 3:49–54, 1982.
5. Vestal RE: Drug use in the elderly, a review of problems and special considerations, Drugs 16:358–362, 1978.
6. Duncan LB: Treating the elderly, Emerg Med Services 16(25):80–81, 1987.
7. Lowenstein SR et al: Care of the elderly in the emergency department, Ann Emerg Med 15:528–535,1986.
8. Chillag SA: Recognizing atypical geriatric illness, Geriatr Consultant 4:25–27, 1985.
8a. Schifferdecker C, Driscoll DF, and Bistrian BR: Management guidelines when drugs and nutrients interact, J Crit Illness 5(1):34, 1990.
9. Dunne ML and Strauss RW: Approach to the elderly patient. In Judd RL, Warner CG and Shaffer MA, editors: Geriatric emergencies, Rockville, MD, 1986, Aspen Publishers, pp1–11.
10. Taylor BW: Altered factors in the assessment of the geriatric patient, Emerg Med Services 14:26–30, 1985.
11. Kraytman M: The complete patient history, New York, 1979, McGraw-Hill Book Co.
12. Kane RL: Essentials of clinical geriatrics, New York, 1984, McGraw-Hill Book Co., pp. 37–55.
13. Lloyd M: The role of the emergency department nurse in geriatric emergency care. In Wilson LB, Simson SP, and Baxter CR, editors: Handbook of geriatric emergency care, Baltimore, 1984, University Park Press, pp 227–233.
14. Cassel CK and Walsh JR, editors: Geriatric medicine. Vol 1, Medical, psychiatric and pharmacological topics, New York, 1984, Springer-Verlag.
15. Heine E, editor: Assessing vital functions accurately, Horshman, Penn, 1977, Intermed Communications, p 27.
16. Steel K: Evaluation of the geriatric patient. In Reichel W, editor: Clinical aspects of aging, Baltimore,1978, Williams & Wilkins Co., pp 3–12.
17. Cohen HJ: The elderly patient: a challenge to the art and science of medicine, Drug Therapy 13:41–43, 1983.
18. Gordon M: Manual of nursing diagnosis, New York, 1982, McGraw-Hill.
19. Gordon M: Nursing diagnosis: process and application, New York, 1982, McGraw-Hill.
20. Tartaglia MJ: Nursing diagnosis: keystone of your care plans, Nursing 85 15:34–37, 1985.
21. Lawson PK, editor: Helping geriatric patients, Springhouse, Penn, 1982, Intermed Communications, Inc.
22. Jones J et al: Efficacy of a telephone follow-up system in the emergency department, J Emerg Med (in press).

Assessment and Initial Management of Acute Medical Problems in a Nursing Home

Sally E. Martin, M.A.S.N., R.N.C., G.N.P.,
Carole L. Turner, M.N., R.N.C., G.N.P.,
Sue Mendelsohn, M.N., R.N.C., G.N.P., **and Joseph G. Ouslander,** M.D.

Every day a growing number of frail elderly are admitted to the 20,000 nursing homes in this country. These nursing homes provide care for over 1.5 million Americans of whom 90% are over age 65. The proportion of the very old is growing. It is expected that by the year 2000, one half of nursing home patients will be 85 years old and over.[1] It can safely be predicted that the 2.2 million patients in nursing homes at that time will be frailer and sicker.[1a,1b] It is a common fallacy that individuals admitted to a nursing home require minimal medical supervision. In reality, nursing home patients have a propensity for problems requiring ongoing medical assessment and treatment as well as episodic acute hospitalizations. These problems arise from multiple medical diagnoses, complex medication regimes, and functional and cognitive deficits which place individuals at risk for iatrogenic complications.

Of all patients who are designated as discharged from nursing homes, 30% are actually transferred to an acute care facility because they require management of acute problems.[3,14] In 1980, 340,000 nursing home patients were transferred to acute hospitals.[3] This number has increased since 1983 when the Social Security Reform Act mandated the prospective payment system for Medicare. As a result of this diagnosis-related group (DRG) reimbursement system, elderly patients, who previously remained in the hospital longer, are being admitted to nursing homes with subacute illnesses that many facilities are not equipped or staffed to care for.

In order to ensure quality care to these patients, nursing homes must improve clinical services within the facility and strengthen linkages with the acute care medical system. This chapter will describe a model of care which was developed and implemented at the Academic Nursing Home of Sepulveda Veterans Administration Medical Center for managing acute medical problems in a nursing home. The model combines a "teaching nursing home" philosophy with the expertise of gerontological nursing home practitioners who are prepared to assess, manage, and triage acute medical conditions with the aid of standardized procedures. Nine such standardized procedures, or protocols, will be presented.

THE NURSING HOME DILEMMA

Nursing homes, as referred to in this chapter, are one of two major types: skilled nursing facilities (SNFs) or intermediate care facilities (ICFs). Differences in these facilities are defined by detailed sets of standards and reimbursement systems. Primary differences are seen in staffing guidelines and physician visit requirements. SNFs must be staffed with a registered nurse (RN) at all times and provide three nursing hours per patient day. A physician is required to visit each patient once a month. ICFs are only required to staff an RN or licensed vocational nurse (LVN) at least one shift per day and provide two nursing hours per patient day. Physicians need only visit patients in an ICF once every 3 months.[9] Using the guidelines for an SNF, a 100-bed facility could be acceptably staffed with one RN, two or three LVNs, and seven to ten certified nursing assistants (NAs) for an 8-hour period.[23]

There is no requirement that RNs employed in a nursing home have expertise in geriatrics or skills in physical assessment. Even if they do have these skills, they often remain unused because RNs usually assume a supervisory role and have minimal patient contact. NAs provide over 90% of the hands-on care. Most have a limited education, and some may not speak English. The job of NA shows a high turnover rate.[25]

Most nursing homes have limited involvement by other health care professionals, such as social workers and physical, occupational, and recreational therapists.[18]

Relatively few physicians are prepared by medical school or postgraduate medical education to treat, or are willing to treat, nursing home patients.[1a] Several factors encourage this unwillingness: reimbursement rates which are too low to offset time and travel costs, general dislike for nursing home patients, the nursing home environment, minimum visitation requirements, and Medicare and Medicaid red tape. Only 20% of physicians attend patients in nursing homes and when they do visit they do so very briefly — about 2 hours per month per patient.[17,18,20] When physicians are notified of changes in patients' conditions, treatment decisions are often based on a telephone assessment rather than a visit.[18]

There is a large and growing disparity between the minimal requirements for professional staff involvement and the complexity of the problems and needs of patients residing in nursing homes. The nursing home population is far from homogenous by either diagnosis or length of stay. At the time of admission, two distinct categories of patients can be identified: "short stayers" and "long stayers."[12]

"Short stayers," for the most part, are those patients admitted from acute care hospitals who need a period of convalescence following an acute episode, such as a fractured hip, stroke, pneumonia, congestive heart failure, or patients with end-stage or terminal disease, such as cancer, severe brain injury, or chronic lung disease. These patients either are discharged or die within 6 months of their admission.

"Long stayers" are usually of advanced age and suffer from cognitive impairment, physical impairment, or both, which renders them unable to live outside of an institu-

tion. This subpopulation in nursing homes may live there 6 months or 2 or more years.[18]

The well-being of both of these subpopulations is in a delicate balance because they have fewer resources than the younger, healthier person. The most frequent conditions that have been found to require medical assessment and acute intervention at Sepulveda VAMC Academic Nursing Home are listed in Table 48–1. These problems are considered comparable to other nursing home populations. Infection alone is a frequent cause of acute illness requiring hospitalization among nursing home patients.[7] The absence of qualified health professionals in nursing homes seriously jeopardizes the appropriateness and quality of care a patient will receive when an imbalance in his or her condition occurs. Failure to identify problems or a delay in initiation of therapy can result in remedial problems developing into life-threatening episodes necessitating transfer to an acute care facility.[20]

The presence of highly trained RNs who have knowledge of each patient's normal status and the authority to adjust the treatment regimen to restore balance can dramatically improve care to the nursing home patient. Gerontologic nurse practitioners (GNPs) fill this role well because they are prepared to combine physical assessment skills and medical decision making with an interest in the psychosocial aspects of patient care.[10] Unfortunately, of the 23,600 nursing homes in the United States, only approximately 250 employ a GNP.[4]

THE GERONTOLOGIC NURSE PRACTITIONER

A nurse practitioner is defined in the state of California as a registered nurse with additional preparation and skills in physical diagnosis, psychosocial assessment, and

Table 48–1 Acute Conditions Commonly Requiring Assessment and Intervention*

Fever/infection	Psychiatric
Cardiovascular	agitation/aggression
chest pain	altered mental status
heart failure	wandering
hypotension	depression
hypertension	General geriatric problem
pacemaker malfunction	falls and other trauma
arrhythmia	medication problems
phlebitis	pressure sores
cardiac arrest	Neurologic
Gastrointestinal	transient ischemia
bleeding	seizures
ileus	Musculoskeletal
abdominal pain	arthritic pain
diarrhea	Genitourinary
	hematuria
	complications from
	indwelling catheters

*Based on unpublished data from the Sepulveda VAMC Academic Nursing Home program.

management of health care, who has been prepared in a program conforming to the Board of Registered Nursing Standards.[2] The GNP has these advanced skills plus a broad knowledge of the unique needs and problems of the elderly person. Approximately 26 institutions of higher learning in the United States offer GNP programs. These programs are either at a master's degree level or are continuing education programs within universities.[5] The continuing education programs are being supplanted by graduate programs as recommended by the American Nurses' Association (ANA). The ANA offers certification by exam for GNPs and, effective in 1992, will require an earned graduate degree related to an area of nursing for certification eligibility.[27]

The GNP has much to offer in a nursing home setting and is an attractive alternative to the sole reliance on physicians for the clinical management of patients. Being first and foremost a nurse, the GNP is able to identify and relate to problems from both the patient's and the nurse's perspective. For example, when a patient has a primary diagnosis of diabetes mellitus, the GNP can focus care not only on the medical issue of controlling the blood glucose but also on the nursing diagnoses of impairment of skin integrity and alteration in comfort. The GNP combines both the nursing and medical models of care to develop patient-centered goals and interventions.

Nurses have always been comfortable with the team care concept. Working with an interdisciplinary team is essential to quality care in a nursing home. To ensure that all of the problems of an elderly person are managed appropriately, collaboration with a variety of health professionals including social workers, rehabilitation therapists, and spiritual advisors is necessary. The GNP is comfortable and well prepared to utilize team input in designing treatment plans and is also prepared to provide patient education for specific health problems and positive health practices. The GNP is almost always in a position as a role model for nursing skills and interactions with physicians. Oftentimes, the GNP can act as a liaison person between nurses and physicians by better defining patient problems and developing realistic treatment plans.

The GNP has expertise in assessing for overmedication, drug interactions, and drug/diet interactions and can prevent iatrogenesis, which is common in the nursing home due to the complexity of medical problems and treatment regimens in the older person. Other benefits of the GNP in a nursing home are listed in Table 48-2.

When a GNP is present in a nursing home, acute medical problems and potential acute problems can be identified early and interventions can be initiated to either prevent or appropriately expedite a transfer to an acute care facility. In California, nurses can legally implement or change a treatment regimen and initiate emergency procedures in accordance with standardized procedures. The scope of nursing practice which includes these

Table 48-2   Potential Benefits of the Gerontologic Nurse Practitioner in a Nursing Home

Integration of nursing and medical models of care for elderly and chronically ill
Reduced turnover among nursing staff
Higher occupancy rate
Reduced medical expenses per patient
Higher patient and family satisfaction
Lower drug utilization and cost
Cost and liability avoidance potential
Positive change in public perception of institutional quality
Improved image of facility among community physicians

Modified from Smith A, Dickey W, and Wrenschel D: Institutional perspectives, J Long Term Care Administration 11(3):23–24, 1983.

functions is outlined in the California Business and Professions Code.[2]

STANDARDIZED PROCEDURES

Standardized procedures are policies and protocols developed by a health facility through the collaboration of administrators and health professionals, including nurses and physicians. Well-developed protocols that are mutually agreed upon by nursing, medicine, and administration serve as guidelines for how the GNP performs tasks within the scope of practice as a registered nurse. They not only ensure uniformity of health care delivery but serve as a delineation of the GNP role in a specific setting. A completed protocol should ideally contain elements of history taking, physical examination, laboratory workup, specific treatment, who should manage, and when to refer.[11,22] Protocols in a nursing home should address the common chronic conditions that are prevalent in this population. However, given the frailty of this population, the specter of sudden acute episodes and exacerbation of existing conditions is ever present. These acute episodes warrant an early and aggressive approach if the patient is to be spared the disruption of transfer to an acute hospital. The use of protocols can be an efficient means for rapid assessment and initial management of acute problems prior to the arrival of a physician.[16]

THE TEACHING NURSING HOME MODEL

The GNPs at the Academic Nursing Home of Sepulveda VAMC found the need for clear, concise guidelines for the assessment and management of the frequent acute medical problems they encountered. This 200-bed skilled nursing care facility adopted a teaching nursing home philosophy in 1984. One of the primary objectives of this program is to prepare physicians and other health professionals to provide high-quality care to nursing home patients at Sepulveda and in their future practices.

Medical residents in the UCLA–San Fernando Valley Residency Training Program are primary physicians for five to seven nursing home patients during their second- and third-year residency program. The program is designed to provide the residents with a longitudinal view of patient care in a nursing home. The residents are not in the nursing home on a daily basis but are responsible for visiting their patients at least every 30 days and communicating regularly with the GNPs. Attending physicians, who are full-time faculty members of the Division of Geriatric Medicine, make monthly rounds with each resident and GNP. GNPs provide day-to-day clinical management of sudden acute medical problems. The nursing home is located about 300 yards from the acute hospital and has readily accessible laboratory, x-ray, and physician services on a 24-hour basis. The Academic Nursing Home is also a training site for students of nursing (LVN, RN, and graduate nurses specializing in geriatrics), social work, psychology, speech pathology, audiology, pharmacy, gerodentistry, and occupational therapy. The nursing staff has an approximate ratio of 50:50 of licensed nurses (RN, LVN) to NAs. This nursing home selectively admits patients with unstable medical problems, and because of the shift of the acute hospital to the DRG-based reimbursement system there is a high incidence (approximately 6 to 10 per week) of acute medical conditions.[16,26]

This frequent need for acute medical intervention spurred the development of nine protocols for the most common acute medical conditions encountered. These were developed as a collaborative effort by GNPs and physicians. These protocols were designed as flow-chart algorithms because this format seemed to lend itself to more rapid decision making. The following acute conditions are addressed by these protocols: fever, seizures, acute dyspnea, chest pain, abdominal pain, gastrointestinal bleeding, loss of consciousness, sudden mental status change, and focal neurologic deficits. The implementation of four of these protocols will be described by case histories, and the other five protocols can be reviewed in Figure 48–1.

SELECTED CASE PRESENTATIONS
Fever

Mrs. D, an 85-year-old woman, was transferred from the acute hospital after being treated for a fractured hip. During her hospitalization, she developed urinary incontinence, and an indwelling catheter was inserted. On admission to the nursing home, she was alert, but the nurses noted that she was disoriented at times. She had experienced three relocations during the last month: one from her home, a move from one ward to another in the hospital, and, finally, her admission to the nursing home.

Two days after admission, the nursing staff reported that Mrs. D's disorientation had increased, and she was trying to pull out her catheter. When vital signs were taken, she was found to have a temperature elevation of 103.2°F rectally. Her blood pressure and respirations were stable. The GNP did a rapid physical exam at the bedside. A short mental status questionnaire revealed significant deterioration of her mental status. It was also

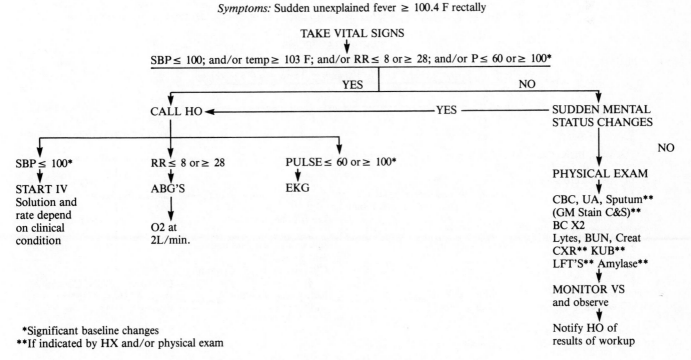

Figure 48–1   Acute onset of fever.

observed that her urine was cloudy with heavy sedimentation. Her lungs were clear, the incision was without inflammation, and there were no other skin lesions. Her abdomen was not tender. The GNP ordered and drew stat blood work, which included a complete blood count (CBC), electrolytes, two sets of blood cultures, blood urea nitrogen (BUN), and creatinine. A urine sample was sent for culture and sensitivity and urinalysis. An intravenous (IV) line of 5% dextrose in 0.45% normal saline was started in anticipation that IV antibiotics would be initiated. Since Mrs. D showed no signs of dehydration, a rate of TKO was considered adequate. At this point, the physician was notified of her condition. The physician responded, saw the patient, and reviewed the laboratory results, which were significant for an elevated white blood count (WBC) of 20,000, pyuria, and bacteriuria. IV antibiotics were given, and within 24 hours Mrs. D was afebrile, and her mental status had cleared considerably. After another 24 hours, she was switched to oral antibiotics. As soon as her acute episode had resolved, the catheter was removed; physical therapy was initiated to improve her functional status. With increased mobility and improved mental status, she was able to regain bladder control. Mrs. D was effectively treated in the nursing home, thus avoiding another relocation that may have resulted in unwanted complications.

Abdominal Pain (Figure 48–2)

Mr. J, a 78-year-old widower with a mild dementia, had been a patient in the nursing home for 2 months. He was placed by a niece who lives in another state because he was no longer able to care for himself at his own home. After admission, he was diagnosed as being depressed and was prescribed a trial of antidepressant medication. The nurses also identified him as a chronic laxative abuser. The staff reported that Mr. J was complaining of cramping abdominal pain and was not going to the dining room for meals due to anorexia. He denied vomiting and was unsure of when his last bowel movement had been. His vital signs were unchanged from baseline, and he was afebrile.

The GNP performed a bedside physical exam. The abdominal exam was significant for hyperactive, high-pitched bowel sounds, mild distention, and dullness to percussion over the sigmoid area. The patient had no rebound tenderness. His bladder was not distended, and no organomegaly was present. A rectal exam revealed hard stool which was guiaic negative, and no masses were palpated.

Stat laboratory work included a CBC, electrolytes, BUN, creatinine, and amylase. A urinalysis was obtained as well as a kidney, ureter, and bladder (KUB) exam and upright chest x-ray. The abdominal x-ray revealed an extensive fecal impaction in the transverse and descending colon. The blood work was within normal limits except for a mild anemia.

The findings were reported to the physician who agreed with prompt, aggressive treatment to remove the impaction. An oil-retention enema was ordered with manual removal of stool if necessary followed by isotonic saline solution enemas to avoid electrolyte imbalance. A stool softener and a bowel-stimulating laxative were added until the entire impaction was relieved.

Symptoms: Sudden onset of diffuse or localized abdominal pain with or without nausea/vomiting/diarrhea.

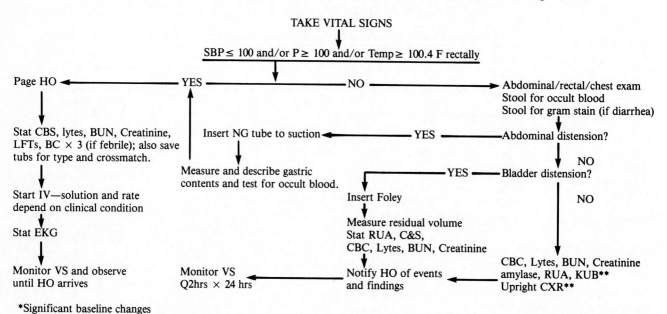

Figure 48–2 Acute abdominal pain.

Additional plans were to work up the anemia, which included a barium enema and proctosigmoidoscopy, and repeat stool for occult blood. Thyroid function tests, evaluation of medications, and further evaluation of Mr. J's psychosocial status were also warranted to rule out hypothyroidism. Although the problem of constipation may seem mundane to some practitioners, this was hardly the case from the patient's perspective. Mr. J's mood and sense of well-being improved dramatically. He is currently being evaluated for placement in a board and care home.

Not all problems seen in nursing homes are as clear-cut and easily resolved as the previous case of constipation. Sometimes acute problems present with atypical symptoms and represent a therapeutic dilemma. Such was the case of Mrs. C.

Chest Pain (Figure 48–3)

Mrs. C, an 83-year-old widow, had been a patient of the nursing home for 2 years. She had a history of hypertension, obesity, and congestive heart failure. Her blood pressure and cardiac status had been well controlled with digoxin, a thiazide diuretic, and a low-salt diet. She

was very active in the arts and crafts classes and often helped the other patients with their projects.

An NA notified the nurse practitioner that Mrs. C was complaining of chest pain. When interviewed, Mrs. C stated that she was too tired to get out of bed. She was confused as to the day of the week and month. The staff related that she had been up wandering during the night and had one episode of urinary incontinence. This history represented a drastic change in behavior and mentation.

On physical exam, she was agitated and uncooperative. She was afebrile; her blood pressure was at a baseline, and her pulse was 88. Mrs. C's respirations were shallow and rapid at 40 per minute. She was given nitroglycerin 1/150 SL, which seemed to resolve her chest pain.

The GNP, realizing that chest pain, dyspnea, confusion, and fatigue could be the manifestation of a number of acute conditions, arranged to have a call made to the physician at once. On continuation of the physical exam, the GNP found an irregular apical pulse, S3 gallop, and 2+ ankle edema. Rales were auscultated in the lung bases. Pulses were full and equal bilaterally. There was no jaundice or pallor, and the abdominal exam was benign. Mrs. C was given oxygen via nasal cannula, and a stat ECG was ordered. The GNP drew blood for CBC,

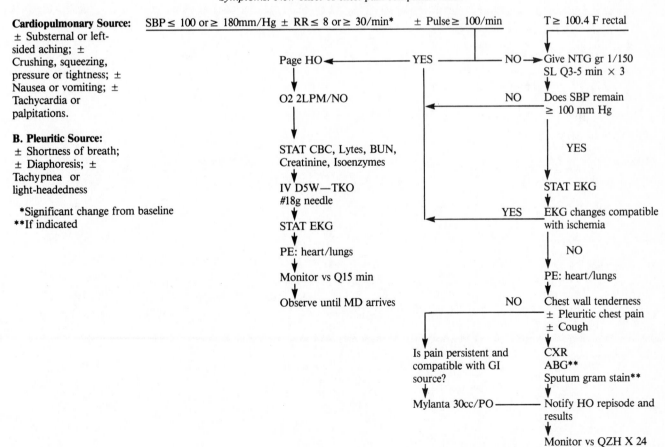

Symptoms: New onset of chest pain compatible with—

Figure 48–3   Chest pain.

electrolytes, BUN, creatinine, isoenzymes, and a digoxin level. An IV of 5% dextrose in water was started at a rate of TKO. The physician returned the GNP's call and decided to transfer Mrs. C to the acute hospital immediately. At the hospital a more complete exam and chest x-ray were done which confirmed the diagnosis of congestive heart failure. Mrs. C responded well to treatment and was soon back in the nursing home, alert and oriented, and participating in the arts and crafts class. Early intervention was instrumental to a shortened hospital stay and the avoidance of complications that might have occurred had her symptoms been treated superficially.

Seizures (Figure 48–4)

Mr. T, a 76-year-old male, was admitted to the nursing home approximately 4 months after the death of his wife. His daughter sought medical attention for him because she had become concerned about his weight loss and lack of interest in friends and his usual activities. He was requiring almost constant supervision to ensure that he

ate, bathed himself, and complied with his complicated medicine regimen. His daughter was unable to supervise him to this extent.

He was admitted to the nursing home with a diagnosis of depression and a history of multiple medical problems which included the following: coronary artery disease, hypertensive cardiovascular disease, compensated congestive heart failure, adult-onset diabetes with visual impairments due to senile macular degeneration, and degenerative joint disease. His medical treatment plan included nortriptyline, Sorbitrate Chewables, Cardizem, Diabeta, digoxin, Motrin, Lasix, potassium supplements, and PRN Tylenol, milk of magnesia, nitroglycerin, and Mylanta. Three months after his admission, the nurses observed that he remained socially withdrawn and sad. The nortriptyline dosage was increased from 50 mg per day to 75 mg per day.

Three days thereafter, the nursing staff noted some subtle mental status changes when Mr. T began forgetting familiar faces and routines. His appetite was poor; he wasn't sleeping well at night but was drowsy during the day. One morning, as he was getting out of his bed,

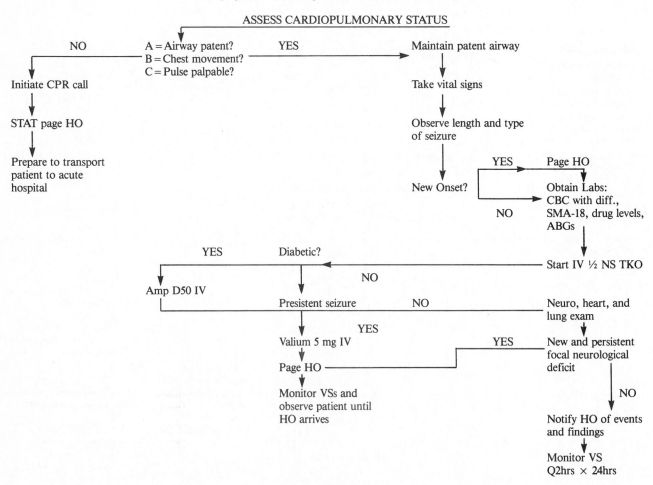

Figure 48–4 Seizures.

"his knees buckled," and he fell. No evidence of injury was found on a physical exam, and his vital signs were at baseline. Two days later while in the bathroom, he felt "faint" and called for help. An NA found him on the floor having generalized body contractions, shallow respirations, generalized cyanosis, oral drooling, and urinary incontinence. Mr. T was beginning to respond when the GNP arrived. His blood pressure was 198/110, pulse — 104, respirations — 28, and rectal temperature — 99.8°F. The physician was paged. The seizure protocol was initiated. Arterial blood gases, CBC, creatinine, glucose, and digoxin levels were drawn. An IV of 0.045 normal saline was started, and 50 cc of 50% glucose was given IV push.

The physician returned the call and asked the GNP to maintain the IV, complete the seizure protocol workup, have Valium on hand, and page her stat if Mr. T had another seizure. The physical exam was significant for slurred speech, orientation to self only, decreased strength on the right side, hyperactive deep-tendon reflexes, both big toes upgoing, regular heart rhythm, and bilateral nonpitting ankle edema. A rectal exam was positive for occult blood. His vital signs lying were: blood pressure — 170/98, pulse — 94, and respirations — 26. His vital signs sitting were: blood pressure — 130/90, pulse — 110, and respirations 28. Laboratory results were significant for a BUN — 48, creatinine — 1.8, glucose — 510, Hgb — 9.2, and Hct — 29%. The GNP phoned the physician to report the physical findings and

laboratory results. Mr. T was transferred immediately to the hospital.

Three days after his admission to the hospital, Mr. T underwent a craniotomy for the removal of bilateral subdural hematomas. The GNP pieced together the events that had occurred prior to the seizure and determined that Mr. T had become orthostatic and fallen after taking increased nortriptyline. The anemia, related to medication gastritis, contributed to his weakness and falling. He returned to the nursing home 10 days after his surgery on reduced doses of nortriptyline and Cardizem. The Motrin was discontinued and he had been started on Tegretol prophylactically. Remarkably, he returned to his baseline mental and functional status.

These protocols, as well as those for other conditions (see Figures 48–5 thru 48–9) were written as decision support maps and are intended to be guidelines to foster appropriate management of acute situations. When implementing the protocols, the GNP must be prepared to exercise independent judgment. Modification of the approach is dictated by each individual patient.

For example, in the fever case the GNP determined that Mrs. D was in no imminent danger. Therefore, she was able to do a more thorough physical exam and draw blood to collect additional data prior to calling the physician. In the chest pain example, the GNP, in collaboration with the physician, quickly transferred Mrs. C to the acute hospital where an additional diagnosis workup was done. In the abdominal pain case, the GNP

Symptoms: Patient unresponsive to verbal stimuli

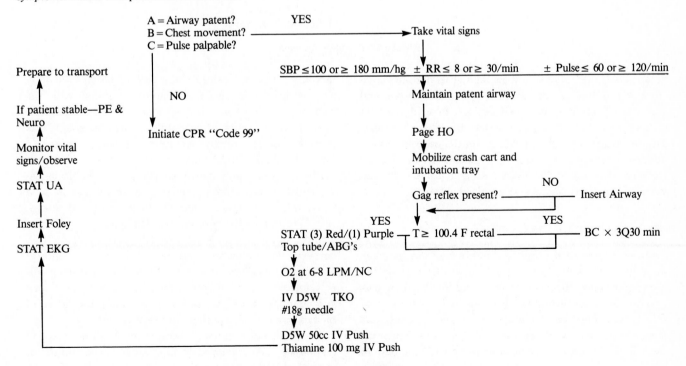

Figure 48–5   Loss of consciousness.

Symptoms: Sudden ONSET OF S.O.B. with or without cough/wheezes/anxiety/cyanosis

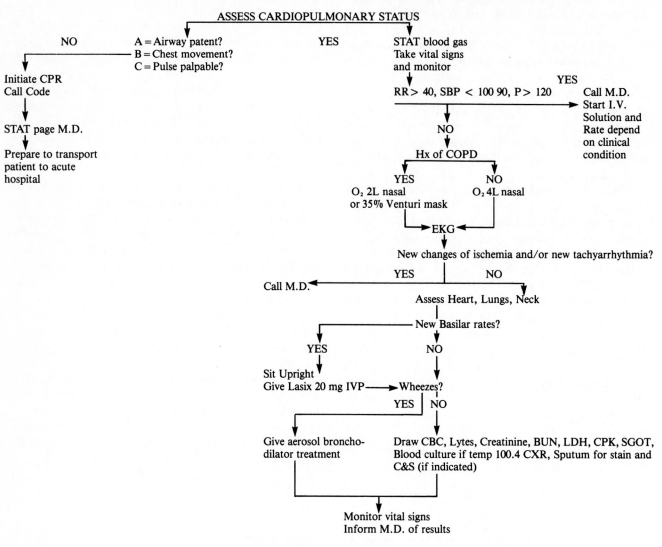

Figure 48–6   Acute dyspnea.

determined that a nasogastric tube was not indicated since Mr. J had no epigastric distress or nausea and vomiting. Therefore, the GNP decided to wait and not subject the patient to an unnecessary invasive procedure. The seizure protocol does not indicate the need for an abdominal examination; however, due to Mr. T's medication regimen, which included Motrin, an abdominal examination was done and stool for occult blood obtained.

TREATMENT DECISIONS

Protocols for rapid decision making during the management of acute medical conditions are vital to the GNP in a nursing home. However, prior to and during their use, several factors, including medical and nursing considerations, emotional, clinical, economic, ethical, and legal issues, must be considered.[18] The physician must assume the responsibility for discussing with the patient or the legally authorized representative the degree of in-

tervention that is desired if the patient becomes acutely or critically ill. Physicians should be familiar with the various guidelines and the concept of limited resuscitation in hospital and prehospital settings, although this partial approach is opposed by the Hastings center (a medical ethics think tank).[18a] The patient's decision-making capacity and treatment preference should be established either before or shortly after admission to a nursing home. The physician should identify and specifically document the procedures the patient would or would not want — for example: CPR, treatment in ICU, surgery, hospitalization but no CPR or ICU, enteral feedings, or comfort measures only without specific medical interventions.[18] Some facilities have developed guidelines to assist the staff in determining the extent of medical treatment a patient will receive.[13,24]

At a Baltimore geriatric center and hospital a set of guidelines was developed to individualize the treatment of critically and terminally ill patients. In this facility,

Symptoms: Altered state of consciousness, disorientation, lethargy, psychomotor agitation, psychosis (hallucinations, delusions)

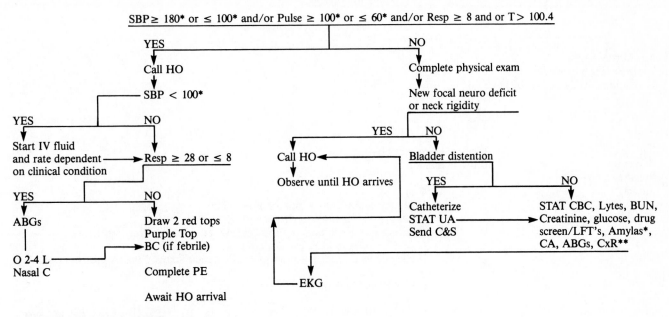

*Significant change from baseline
**If indicated by Hx and/or Physical Exam

Figure 48–7 Acute mental status changes.

Symptoms: Patient/staff report episode of blood loss compatible with GI source: Hematemesis; Tarry stools; BRB per rectum

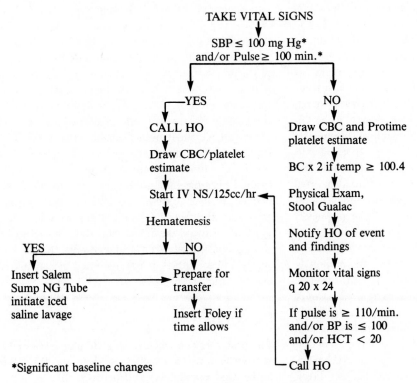

Figure 48–8 Gastrointestinal bleeding.

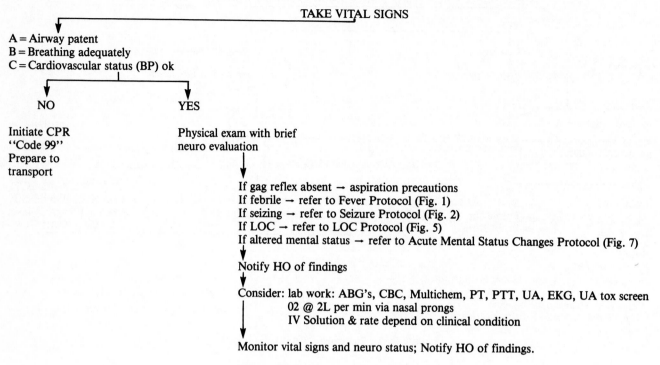

Symptoms: New onset of hemiparesis, hemiplegia, cranial nerve deficit, visual field loss, dysarthria, dysesthesia, agnosia, apraxia, ataxia, mental status change.

TAKE VITAL SIGNS

A = Airway patent
B = Breathing adequately
C = Cardiovascular status (BP) ok

NO   YES

Initiate CPR   Physical exam with brief
"Code 99"   neuro evaluation
Prepare to
transport

If gag reflex absent → aspiration precautions
If febrile → refer to Fever Protocol (Fig. 1)
If seizing → refer to Seizure Protocol (Fig. 2)
If LOC → refer to LOC Protocol (Fig. 5)
If altered mental status → refer to Acute Mental Status Changes Protocol (Fig. 7)

Notify HO of findings

Consider: lab work: ABG's, CBC, Multichem, PT, PTT, UA, EKG, UA tox screen
02 @ 2L per min via nasal prongs
IV Solution & rate depend on clinical condition

Monitor vital signs and neuro status; Notify HO of findings.

Figure 48–9   New neurologic deficit.

four separate designations are made for each long-term patient: 1) treatment in the event of critical illness, 2) treatment in the event of terminal illness, 3) plan in the event of need for resuscitation, witnessed, and 4) plan in the event of need for resuscitation, unwitnessed. During the period after admission, an interdisciplinary team assesses the patient's overall condition and capacity for decison making as well as the family's capacity to speak on the patient's behalf. The team arrives at one of the following treatment classifications: 1) maximum therapeutic effort, which includes transfer to an acute hospital and ICU if needed, 2) maximum therapeutic efforts within the limits of the institution, 3) limited therapeutic measures, and 4) no therapeutic measures.[18] These categories of treatment can be useful as guidelines for the physician when treatment preferences are discussed. The final decision with respect to the care he or she is to receive, however, rests with the patient, if competent. If the patient is not competent, the legally authorized representative has the responsibility for making these decisions. Court decisions repeatedly uphold the right of a competent person to decide on the degree of treatment interventions.[13] More and more patients and families are taking an active part in the decision-making process. As the public becomes more aware of "living wills" and "right-to-die" laws, they are relying less on others to make these decisions.

If a patient does request treatment in the event of acute illness, several factors must still be considered. The

GNP and physician must at the time make a thorough assessment of the patient's clinical needs and the nursing home's capability to meet these needs. Protocols, like those discussed, can assist the GNP in determining the stability of the patients. The GNP can provide the physician with objective data and assist in the decision making as to whether or not the patient should be admitted to an acute hospital. If it is determined that the patient could be treated safely in the nursing home, the GNP and physician must consider the staffing, the skill level of staff, and the acuity level of other patients. The impact of numerous acutely ill patients can influence a limited nursing staff's ability to provide the level of care needed by each patient. Several patients requiring frequent monitoring, IVs, and other complex treatments place an unusual burden on the staff as well as other patients. The acuity level of all patients that the staff can safely and comfortably manage must be considered in the decision-making process.

CONCLUSION

The protocols described in this chapter have proven to be straightforward and efficient tools for the assessment and initial management of acute problems in a nursing home.[16] Protocols similar to these but with modifications to reflect the skill level of the nurse using them and the diagnostic resources (e.g., laboratory, x-ray) available can be developed in any nursing home. It should be remembered that a nurse does not have to be a nurse practitioner to legally implement or change a treatment regimen and initiate emergency procedures in accordance with standardized procedures. The primary reason for establishing and utilizing protocols is to develop a systematic and standardized approach to the evaluation of clinical emergencies.

The protocols presented here have done much more than fulfill a mandate by state law. They have proven to be beneficial not only to the GNPs but to the patient, nursing staff, physicians, and acute care hospital. The protocols ensure rapid, standardized, and appropriate care to the patients in the nursing home. Fewer patients are unnecessarily transferred to the acute hospital, and more can receive care in the nursing home environment with the advantage of familiar personnel and surroundings. Avoiding inappropriate hospitalization reduces the risk of iatrogenic illnesses, especially adverse drug reactions, and complications of immobility.[6] Also, the cost of caring for patients in a nursing home is less than in the hospital.

The protocols have also been an effective tool for increasing the knowledge and expertise of all the nursing staff. The nurses have become more aware of signs and symptoms of acute medical problems and potential problems, and they have learned what is expected of them when each protocol is used. They can anticipate the GNP's needs, thus adding to the efficiency of managing acute problems.[16]

The physician has the assurance that early assessment and appropriate intervention will take place prior to his notification or arrival. He can then make sound clinical decisions for ongoing management of the acute problem. The acute care facility will be less resistant to admitting patients from nursing homes because they will not receive inappropriate admissions.

The major obstacles that nursing homes face in improving the management of acute medical problems are 1) current reimbursement policies for caring for subacutely ill patients, 2) minimal standards for staffing and consultation, 3) ineligibility for third-party payments or the absence of any reimbursement mechanism that would remunerate nurse practitioners, and 4) inaccessibility to immediate laboratory and x-ray services.[14,15,19,20]

Major policy changes must be made so that the growing numbers of elderly in nursing homes are guaranteed quality and appropriate care when they become acutely ill.[1a,1b] But until those changes are made, each nursing home must explore ways to improve their services. The nursing home care model described in this chapter is not feasible for implementation in all nursing home settings. The Sepulveda VAMC Academic Nursing Home has the luxury of an acute care facility in close proximity and on-call physicians as well as laboratory and x-ray services on a 24-hour basis. The reimbursement of nurse prac-

titioners is also not an issue. However, each facility can extrapolate aspects of this model after exploring their available resources and can adapt similar procedures. Strengthening linkages with acute hospitals whereby acute hospitals assist with provision of service education, consultation, and medical coverage is becoming an absolute necessity. Encouraging physicians to form joint practices with nurse practitioners and encouraging physicians and nurses to collaborate to develop standardized procedures, such as the ones described here, can improve the standard of care now for managing acute medical problems in nursing homes.

The movement toward certifying geriatrics as a specialty has been slow, although internists and family physicians have awarded certificates of special competence. The standard of care in nursing homes and for the elderly in general requires all physicians and nurses to have basic competence in geriatrics. Bortz[28] makes the argument well and points out how the lack of attention given to geriatric medicine has resulted in a frustrating and illogical system, including Medicare, which is "not only fiscally, but philosophically bankrupt." He believes we have reached the time when attention to our system of care for the elderly is critical.

REFERENCES

1. Aging America: trends and projections, Prepared by the US Senate Special Committee on Aging, 1984.
1a. Portnoi VA: Care of the nursing home patient, N Engl J Med 322:135, 1990.
1b. Shaughnessy PW and Kramer AM: The increased needs of patients in nursing homes and patients receiving home health care, N Engl J Med 322:21, 1990.
2. Board of Registered Nursing: Nursing Practice Act. Sections 1470, 1480–1485 (Amendments through October 1984), California Department of Consumer Affairs, Sacramento, 1985.
3. Butler RN: Principles of care in the nursing home. In Calkins E, Davis PG, and Ford AB, editors: The practice of geriatrics, Philadelphia, 1986, WB Saunders Co.
4. Ebersole P: Gerontological nurse practitioners past and present, Geriatric Nursing 219–222, July/August, 1985.
5. Enloe C: Curriculum and training, Journal of Long Term Care Admin 11(3):5–9, 1983.
6. Harron J and Schaeffer J: DRGs and the intensity of skilled nursing, Geriatric Nursing 31–33, Jan/Feb, 1986.
7. Irvine P, Van Buren N, and Crossley K: Causes for hospitalization of nursing home residents: the role of infection, J Am Geriatr Soc 32(2):103–107, 1984.
8. Kane RL: Long term care: policy and reimbursement. In Cassel C and Walsh J, editors: Geriatric medicine, Vol 2, New York, 1984, Springer-Verlag.
9. Kane RL, Hammer D, and Byrnes N: Getting care to nursing home patients: a problem and a proposal, Medical Care 15(2):174–180, 1977.
10. Kane RL, Jorgensen LA, Teteberg B, and Kuwahara J: Is good nursing home care feasible, JAMA 235:516–519, 1976.
11. Kane RL, Ouslander JG, and Abrass IB: Essentials of clinical geriatrics, New York, 1984, McGraw-Hill Book Co..
12. Keeler EB, Kane RL, and Solomon DH: Short and long term residents of nursing homes, Med Care 19:363–369, 1981.
13. Levenson SA, List ND, and Saw-Win B: Ethical considerations in critical and terminal illness in the elderly, J Am Geriatr Soc 29:563–567, 1981.
14. Lewis MA, Cretin S, and Kane RL: The natural history of nursing home patients, Gerontologist 25(4):382–388, 1985.

15. Lewis MA, et al: Immediate and subsequent outcomes of nursing home care, AJPH 75(7):758–762, 1985.

16. Mendelsohn S et al: Assessment protocols for acute medical conditions, J Gerontol Nurs 12(7):176–21, 1986.

17. Mitchell JB: Physician visits to nursing homes, Gerontologist 22(1):45–48, 1982.

18. Ouslander JG and Martin S: Assessment in the nursing home, Clin Geriatr Med 3(1):155–174, 1987.

18a. Ayres RJ: Current controversies in prehospital resuscitation of the terminally ill patient, Prehospital and Disaster Medicine 5:49, 1990.

19. Panicucci C, Ingman S, and Alyea B: The nurse practitioner–physician team in nursing home practice, Gerontol Geriatr Educ 5(2):55–64, 1985.

20. Position paper on patient care in long term care facilities, Board of Registered Nursing, Sacramento, Calif, Oct 1983, California Department of Consumer Affairs.

21. Smith A, Dickey W, and Wrenschel D: Institutional perspectives, J Long Term Care Admin 11(3):23–24, 1983.

22. Steel K et al: Iatrogenic illness on a general medical service at a university hospital, N Engl J Med 304:638–642, 1981.

23. Tennenhouse DJ: California health care law, Danville, Calif, Contemporary Forums, 1985.

24. Vilicer L et al: Hospice approach to the treatment of patients with advanced dementia of the Alzheimer type, JAMA 258(16):2210, 1986.

25. Waxman HM, Carner EA, and Berkenstock G: Job turnover and job satisfaction among nursing home aides, Gerontologist 24(5):503–509, 1984.

26. Wieland D et al: Organizing an academic nursing home, JAMA 255(19):2622–2627, 1986.

27. Woodson A: Nurse practitioners emerge with impact, Provider 30–33, August, 1986.

28. Bortz WM: Geriatrics: through the looking glass, Med Times 117:85, 1989.

Ethical Issues in the Care of the Elderly in Long-Term Care Facilities

Wendy Levinson, M.D.

Policy development

Increasing responsibilities of nursing homes

CPR in nursing homes

Documenting "no-CPR" instructions

Ethical dilemmas with antibiotics, nutrition, and life-sustaining treatments

Transfer of patients to acute care facilities

Future directions

POLICY DEVELOPMENT

Significant developments have been made in the definition and implementation of hospital policies for withholding or withdrawing life support for terminally ill patients.[1-10] Many acute care hospitals have developed policies pertaining to decisions regarding cardiopulmonary resuscitation (CPR). Institutional ethics committees have been formed in order to advise health care workers regarding difficult ethical issues pertaining to use of life-sustaining treatments, including antibiotics and nutrition. These newly developed policies and institutional ethics committees are designed to increase patient, family, and hospital staff comfort and to improve the quality of patient care. They are particularly pertinent to needs of elderly patients.

INCREASING RESPONSIBILITIES OF NURSING HOMES

To date, however, long-term care facilities have focused little attention on these issues.[11-13] A survey of long-term care facilities in Minnesota conducted in 1984 found that only 10% had CPR policies.[14] It has become increasingly important in recent years for nursing homes to address issues related to life support and develop appropriate policies. One impetus for increased attention to these issues has come from the shorter hospital stays and resultant increased number of patients transferred to nursing homes for convalescent or rehabilitative care. A preliminary report by the U.S. Special Committee on Aging in February 1985 evaluated the impact of the Medicare prospective payment system (diagnosis-related groups — DRGs) on long-term care services. The report stated that, "Patients are being discharged from hospitals after shorter lengths of stay and in poorer states of health than prior to DRGs," and that, "It is not clear that post-hospital providers — including nursing homes . . . are equipped to deal with these sicker patients."[15] One recent study showed that after Medicare's prospective payment system was put into use, there was an increase in transferral of terminally ill patients to nursing homes.[22] As a result of the change in patient population, nursing home personnel are increasingly faced with the issues of withholding or withdrawing life support.

A survey on these issues was conducted in Portland, Oregon, in 1984 in 76 licensed nursing home facilities.[16] Fifty-seven facilities completed the questionnaire; less than half (41%) of the nursing homes reported having a policy regarding limitation of resuscitation. In those facilities where no policy existed, 70% felt one was needed. Less than half of the facilities indicated that resuscitation decisions were routinely discussed with patients or families. Those institutions that did have an existing "no-CPR" policy were significantly more likely to conduct routine discussions of these issues with patients or families (Table 49–1). Usually, these discussions were initiated by the attending physician or registered nurse. When an attending physician did classify a patient as

Table 49–1 Presence of Written No-CPR Policy by Discussion of Resuscitation Orders in Nursing Homes, Portland, Oregon

Presence of written no-CPR policy	Routinely discuss resuscitation orders		
	Yes	No	Total
Yes	14	9	23 (41%)
No	9	23	32 (59%)
Total	23 (41%)	32 (59%)	56

$\chi^2 = 5.90, p = .008$

Reprinted with the permission of the *Journal of the American Geriatrics Society.*

"no-CPR," a majority of the designations were recorded as a written order and displayed in the patient's chart or information cards.

CPR IN NURSING HOMES

This survey also inquired about the ability of the nursing home staff to perform CPR effectively. Thirty percent of nursing homes reported having an emergency cart; 58% reported having some resuscitation equipment, usually oxygen and suction machines (Table 49–2). Only five nursing homes had endotracheal tubes; three had electrocardiogram machines; and none had defibrillators. Furthermore, although CPR certification was required by approximately two thirds of the institutions for registered nurses (RNs) and licensed practical nurses (LPNs), only one half had a recertification policy. Hence, even if a policy was in place, many of the nursing homes surveyed would have difficulty in performing adequate CPR until appropriate paramedical support was available. This is an extremely hazardous situation — medically and legally.

This study points out the present lack of appropriate CPR policies in nursing homes. In order to be better equipped to provide high-quality care for the increasing number of elderly patients transferred to long-term care facilities, nursing homes need to develop policies. These

Table 49–2 Resuscitation Equipment at Nursing Homes, Portland, Oregon (n = 57)

Equipment	No. with item (%)
Emergency cart	17 (30.4)
Available equipment	
Oxygen	28 (49.1)
Suction	27 (47.4)
Hand-held ventilation	
equipment (Ambu bag)	19 (33.3)
IV equipment	17 (29.8)
Endotracheal tube	5 (8.8)
ECG	3 (5.3)
None/no answer	24 (42.1)

NOTE. Multiple answers were possible. Reprinted with the permission of the *Journal of the American Geriatrics Society.*

policies allow nursing home personnel to deal more appropriately with difficult decisions with advance directives from patients and families. These types of policies are both in the best interest of patients and staff. Nursing homes are increasingly aware of the importance of developing appropriate guidelines.

An example of how a specific nursing home facility attempts to ensure adequate direction regarding CPR is provided here. This nursing home requires that the attending physician complete a standard form at the time of admission of a patient. The form includes questions regarding the degree of intervention in the event of a cardiopulmonary arrest and asks the physician to indicate specifically if a "full CPR" procedure should be undertaken. Completion of this form ensures that the physician, under the guidance of the patient and/or family, provides specific individualized guidelines in advance of a problem. The physician order form used is shown in Figure 49–1. Furthermore, in order to keep this decision current with any change in the patient's condition, this order is updated monthly along with all other medical orders.

DOCUMENTING "NO-CPR" INSTRUCTIONS

In addition to developing policies, long-term care facilities must ensure adequate communication between physicians and nurses in order to implement policies effectively and to follow the directives of individual patients. Several studies have pointed out an existing communication gap between health care providers. The study in Oregon demonstrated significant disagreement between the medical director of the nursing home and the director of nursing services regarding whether a "no-CPR" policy existed and regarding discussions of resuscitation with patients. The responses of the medical director and nurse were compared for 24 long-term care facilities. The physicians were more likely than the nurses to report that their facilities had a "no-CPR" policy. The nurses were more likely than the doctor to report that "no-CPR" status was discussed with patients.[17] Similarly, in a study conducted in a community hospital in Rochester, New York, nurses were found more willing than physicians to limit care efforts for patients.[18] This study found that attending physicians thought they had communicated with the nursing staff regarding aggressiveness of care in 34% of patients, but the nurses thought communication had occurred in only 3% of patients. These studies conclude that in order to remedy this communication gap, guidelines must be developed to ensure that appropriate personnel are informed about the wishes of the patient and family. On an individual basis, doctors and nurses must try to communicate clearly with each other. Furthermore, documentation of these discussions must be readily available to all the

NAME:

MEDICAL RECORD NO.

PHYSICIAN:

The decision has been made to limit or not perform resuscitation of this patient. The orders are as follows:

CODE 99 LIMITATION

☐ Cardiopulmonary resuscitation but no endotracheal intubation.

☐ Cardiopulmonary resuscitation but no electrical stimulation.

☐ Other (specify) _____

_____

_____

_____

*Orders such as "partial code, slow code and chemical code" are invalid orders and are not acceptable.

☐ No cardiopulmonary resuscitation, place "NO CPR" designation on the front of the medical record.

Verbal order from DR. _____

                                 Date   Time

_____
RN or Resident   Date   Time

_____
Witness   Date   Time

I certify that discussion of the "Limited" or "No CPR" decision has been discussed with the family or guardian and has been documented in the medical record.

_____
Signature of Attending/Coodinating M.D.   Date   Time

☐ FULL CODE

_____
Signature of Attending/Coordinating M.D.   Date   Time

Figure 49–1 Medical record sheet for CPR.

personnel who may be called during the middle of the night to implement or withhold treatments.

In previous years, health care providers have been reticent to document in patient charts decisions to withhold aggressive treatments. Fears of legal liability have deterred physicians from adequately documenting these decisions. The Presidential Commission for the Study of Ethical Problems in Medical and Biomedical Research[19] recommended that no-CPR orders be made part of the medical record with documentation supporting the decision. This written documentation is essential for adequate communication of these important patient decisions. The Presidential Commission report has helped providers to feel more comfortable about writing appropriate notes without fears. In addition, many state governments are attempting to lessen the liability associated with no-CPR orders through legislation.

ETHICAL DILEMMAS WITH ANTIBIOTICS, NUTRITION, AND LIFE-SUSTAINING TREATMENTS

Difficult decisions in long-term care facilities are not just limited to those pertaining to CPR. Decisions about use of antibiotics and nutrition pose difficult ethical dilemmas in long-term care. Though the administration of drugs or provision of nutrition may seem simple and basic to health care providers, patients may have different ideas. Some patients who are terminally ill or debilitated may consider that these treatments will only prolong their pain and suffering. The Hastings Center has recently published a set of practical guidelines on the termination of life-sustaining treatment in the care of the dying.[20] These guidelines are highly pertinent to the care of the elderly in long-term care facilities. They provide an approach to consideration of life-sustaining treatment and include delineation of the ethical values, evaluation and discussion with the patient and family, decision and documentation making, and implementation of the decision. Underscored in this document is the importance of the discussions with the patient or family regarding all potentially life-sustaining treatments, including nutrition and antibiotics.[27] The benefits and burdens of any treatment may be weighed differently by each individual, and, hence, it is imperative for health care professionals to seek direction from patients in advance anticipating the decisions. The report specifically addresses the concerns of long-term care facilities. It states, "Because nursing homes are long-term residential institutions, patients who have not developed advance directives before admission should be encouraged to do so. Patients should be asked in particular under what circumstances they would desire transfer to a hospital, because of the common use of life sustaining treatments in that setting." When the nursing home develops a treatment plan for a patient, the patient should participate in this process.[20]

The report encourages nursing homes to establish clear guidelines for transfer within the nursing home to more intensive care areas or to acute care hospitals.

TRANSFER OF PATIENTS TO ACUTE CARE FACILITIES

The decisions regarding the transfer of patients to acute care facilities are challenging to the staff of nursing homes. Usually, when a patient experiences an acute deterioration in his condition, the physician transfers the patient to a location for more intensive therapy. Frequently, the nursing staff believe that a nonaggressive approach would be more appropriate for the patient. A study of nursing home head nurses reported that nurses believed that 37% of the patients in their facility should not be hospitalized, even under the most compelling circumstances. Yet, 76% of that group had in fact been hospitalized in the previous 12 months.[21] Of 174 instances of illness requiring referral to an acute care facility for diagnosis or treatment, a decision to keep the patient in the nursing home was made in only one instance. In general, unless the staff of the nursing home have anticipated this situation and have specific instructions from the patient or family to refrain from transferring, it is likely that a physician or nurse will initiate a transfer to settings where more intensive therapy is provided.[23]

FUTURE DIRECTIONS

In the last decade, increased attention has been paid to the process of decision making in the seriously ill and elderly population.[24,25] Health care workers and institutions have shifted from an approach that automatically provides life-sustaining treatments in an acute medical situation to a more reflective and systematic approach that considers when these treatments are appropriate. Advance directives from patients and families allow thoughtful planning of medical decisions. Long-term care facilities, including nursing homes, are just beginning to grapple with these issues. Clearly, work is needed to develop new policies and guidelines for implementation, to educate health care professionals, and to ensure adequate communication between patient, family, and health care providers. This requires an expanded approach and one in which the role of the nursing home is viewed with the importance it is beginning to occupy.[27]

REFERENCES

1. Lee MA and Cassel CK: The ethical and legal framework for the decision not to resuscitate, West J Med 140:117–122, 1984.
2. Jonsen AR: Orders not to resuscitate, West J Med 40:91–92, 1984.
3. Hirsch HL: Guidelines for withholding treatment in the terminally ill, Nursing Homes 32:25–26, 1983.
4. Farber NJ, et al: Cardiopulmonary resuscitation (CPR); patient factors and decision making, Arch Intern Med 44:2229–2232, 1984.
5. Miles SH, Cranford R, and Schultz AL: The do-not-resuscitate order

in a teaching hospital: considerations and a suggested policy, Ann Intern Med 295:364–366, 1976.

6. Rabkin MT, Gillerman G, and Rice NR: Orders not to resuscitate, N Engl J Med 295:364–366, 1976.

7. Gordon M and Hurowitz E: Cardiopulmonary resuscitation of the elderly, J Am Geriatr Soc 32:930–934, 1984.

8. Lo B et al: Do not resuscitate decisions: a prospective study at three teaching hospitals, Arch Intern Med 145:1115–1117, 1985.

9. Uhlmann RF, McDonald WJ, and Inui TS: Epidemiology of no-code orders in an academic hospital, West J Med 140:114–116, 1984.

10. Levy MR, Lambe ME, and Shear CL: Do-not-resuscitate orders in a county hospital, West J Med 140:111–113, 1984.

11. Besdine RW: Decisions to withhold treatment from nursing home residents, J Am Geriatr Soc 31:602–606, 1983.

12. Greenlaw J: Orders not to resuscitate: dilemma for acute care as well as long-term care facilities, Law Med Health Care 10:29–32, 1982.

13. Levenson SA, List ND, and Saw-Win B: Ethical considerations in critical and terminal illness in the elderly, J Am Geriatr Soc 29:563–567, 1981.

14. Miles SH and Ryden MS: Limited-treatment policies in long-term care facilities, J Am Geriatr Soc 33:707–711, 1985.

15. Newsletter of the US Senate Special Committee on Aging, February 25, 1985. Washington, DC, 1985, US Government Printing Office.

16. Levinson W, et al: Cardiopulmonary resuscitation in long-term care facilities: a survey of do-not-resuscitate orders in nursing homes, J Am Geriatr Soc 35:1059–1062, 1987.

17. Dunn PM and Levinson W: Letter. The "No-CPR" policy and physician-nurse communication, J Gen Intern Med 3(2):209, 1988.

18. Frampton MN and Mayewski RJ: Physicians' and nurses' attitudes toward withholding treatment in a community hospital, J Gen Intern Med 2:394–399, 1987.

19. President's Commission for the Study of Ethical Problems in Medicine and Biomedical and Behavioral Research: Deciding to forego life-sustaining treatment: a report on the ethical, medical and legal issues in treatment decisions, Washington, DC, 1983, US Government Printing Office, p. 249.

20. Guidelines on the termination of life-sustaining treatment and the care of dying. A report of the Hastings Center, 1987, Indiana University Press.

21. Wolff ML, Smolen S, and Ferrara L: Treatment decisions in a skilled-nursing facility: discordance with nurses' preference, J Am Geriatr Soc 33:440–445, 1985.

22. Sager MA et al: Changes in location of death after passage of Medicare's prospective payment system, N Engl J Med 320:433, 1989.

23. Mott PD and Barker WH: Hospital and medical care used by nursing home patients: the effect of patient care plans, J Am Geriatr Soc 36(1):47–53, 1988.

24. Uhlmann RF et al: Medical management decisions in nursing home patients, Ann Intern Med 106(6):879–885, 1987.

25. Cassel CK, Meier DE, and Traines ML: Selected bibliography of recent articles in ethics and geriatrics, J Am Geriatr Soc 34(5):399–409, 1986.

26. Mott PD and Barker WH: Treatment decisions for infections occurring in nursing home residents, J Am Geriatr Soc 36(9):820–824, 1988.

27. Wanzer SH: The physician's responsibility toward hopelessly ill patients, N Engl J Med 320:844, 1989.

Family Dynamics in Geriatric Crises

George R. Schwartz, M.D., F.A.C.E.P., and Sally Shaw Garrigan, M.S.W.

GENERAL CONSIDERATIONS

Under stressful conditions, such as acute illness and injury, family members tend to regress to earlier behavior, reawaken authority conflicts, and renew long-buried sibling rivalries. The Talmud says, "Do not judge a man (or woman) in his time of grief," which is wise counsel.

Looking at family dynamics one must be as non-judgmental as possible. Conflicting human emotions are part of the human condition. Physicians must encourage children of the elderly to openly discuss questions and concerns. Support for family members is often needed and, occasionally, outside counseling can be of benefit, although not as a rule. The acute care physician or nurse can often be the most helpful of the medical team. Family consultations/conferences with total freedom of expression can be helpful in dealing with the emotions and feelings of hopelessness and despair involved in caring for the elderly patient. On the other hand, their professional concern and advice can give hope in these difficult times.[1] This involvement is in keeping with the "Family

Sensitivity Concept"[2,3] or the family epidemiologic model. This context model is an attempt to rekindle the flame of broader perspective that has been partly extinguished through extensive subspecialization. Cultural differences must also be recognized.

Scheduled follow-ups for a surviving spouse should be mandatory to address the changes in eating and sleeping habits, as well as the depression that frequently occurs. *Such changes may occur while the spouse is in an acute care hospital or nursing unit as well as following a spouse's death.* Most studies, though not all, show an increased risk of mortality among bereaved spouses.[4]

Levav and his colleagues discuss the elderly patient and his or her spouse's reactions. They contrast the increased mortality in the elderly spouse with their findings that loss of a child was not associated with increased short- or long-term mortality in married parents.[5]

Though one may not get full agreement as to increased mortality, there is unanimity as to increased morbidity and disturbance in vegetative functions (e.g., eating, sleeping) associated with illness or death of an elderly spouse. However, the oft-suspected increase in cancer risk associated with bereavement has been recently questioned.[6]

The reasons, of course, for the increased morbidity and probably mortality may involve more than the feelings of grief and dissolution. The reason can include exposure to similar environmental risks and possible increases in suicide and life-endangering behaviors. Regardless, these studies clearly indicate that acute illness and death in an elderly person sometimes has marked effects on the family and the survivors.

Severe illness in a loved family member brings every member closer to facing his or her own mortality and carries to a personal level the time-limited nature of our physical life and our relative helplessness against aging. Certain emotional dynamics are particularly common: grief, guilt, fear, and anger. By understanding some of the dynamics discussed here as well as being sensitive to other family dynamics in individual cases, the acute geriatric care team can help maintain family cohesiveness.

GRIEF

Even when the elderly person is acutely ill or injured and has not died, severe illness reinforces this as a possibility and can cause a sudden, acute sense of loss. Grieving within the family may begin with an acute illness. In some cases, when the person who is not expected to survive makes a dramatic recovery, family members who have started grieving find themselves emotionally confused.

If the person does not survive the health crisis, the survivors usually go through a grieving process, which in the acute care setting often begins with denial. Emotional blunting is common in these circumstances and can lead to family misperception (e.g., he or she "didn't care" because he or she didn't cry).

In some instances family members are directly involved in decision making about matters such as withholding of life support and "do not resuscitate" orders.[6a] In such instances intrafamilial conflicts may be awakened as well. Physicians involved in caring for such patients need to recognize the frequently conflicting emotions experienced in such decision making.

GUILT

Regardless of the medical condition, there are some family members who retrospectively berate themselves for not seeing early signs or symptoms and for not bringing the patient to the hospital sooner or not visiting more or being more attentive. These retrospective feelings of guilt tend to be greater when there have been mixed feelings about the ill person.

For example, in Case 1, a 76-year-old man was admitted into the hospital in a comatose state. Though cerebrovascular accident (CVA) was the initial working diagnosis, eventually a Doriden overdose was found to be the cause.

The children knew of their father's depression after the loss of their mother several years before and had seen his deterioration for several months before he attempted suicide. Despite their attempts to comfort him, the children had great guilt that they had not earlier recognized the seriousness of the situation.

In this case, the self-inflicted damage brought the severity of his problems rapidly into medical awareness while complicating the treatment. On the other hand, the elderly tend not to seek medical assistance, partly due to fear (of cost, of hospital, and diagnostic tests). Also, this delay in seeking care is due to an expectation of and an increased tolerance for symptoms as just part of aging, as

well as the frequent lethargy and depression that are too often considered part of "normal aging." Underreporting of illness or serious symptoms in elderly persons can be dangerous when coupled with our primarily passive health care system.[7]

FEAR

This stage includes both the fear that the parent or family member might die and also concern about the care the patient might need in the future. While the acute care is, of course, hospital based, impaired elderly patients most frequently receive care from other family members when they leave the hospital.[8] While the care might require a relatively minor commitment (e.g., a 70-year-old woman after a mild "stroke"), in some cases the care required can be all-encompassing (e.g., a 73-year-old man with rapidly progressive amyotrophic lateral sclerosis).

Added to this, also, is an element of fear about financial arrangements for the care of the elderly patient. The elderly patient with an acute illness may manifest great fear of hospitalization, often equating it with pain, suffering, or death, as well as fear about becoming ill and dependent and being forced to relocate.

ANGER

Often, family members who see their elderly parent or sibling with a serious acute illness may become very angry at the person for their contributions to the illness. For example, in Case 1, the children were feeling both guilty and angry at their father for this act of his own doing. Other manifestations can be seen in Case 2. In this situation, a 66-year-old woman had a 40-year history of smoking two packs of cigarettes per day. She was admitted into intensive care after suffering an acute myocardial infarction. The family members expressed great anger because they had repeatedly told her of the dangers of smoking. This anger may be employed to help relieve feelings of guilt.

Other forms of anger might relate to the deteriorating medical course and the patient's eccentricity, stubbornness, and personality change. For example, Case 3 illustrates personality change in an elderly woman that created feelings of anger and hurt in her spouse. This case also illustrates other aspects of the family's dynamics.

After years of struggling with hypertension, Mrs. Y, 82 years old, began suddenly to lose her vision. Her 83-year-old husband drove her to the nearest medical facility for testing. After one hospital admission of several days, and intensive testing, Mrs. Y checked herself out against the advice of her physician. Questionable masses had been found in a CT scan, and a biopsy had been done of her lungs and her arteries, both of which were negative.

Refusing to be readmitted to the hospital for further testing, Mrs. Y returned, with her husband, to their home in a small town. Their two sons, both living with their families out-of-state, were upset. The oldest son and his wife visited frequently and tried to convince Mrs. Y to return for more diagnostic testing. Her husband said the choice was her own to make, and although he would prefer she return to the hospital, he would not make her go against her will. The younger son, very religious, said she should do as she wished and let God's will decide her course.

Mrs. Y steadily declined over the next few months, gradually losing all of her vision. She lost large amounts of weight and was bedridden. She became terribly angry and unreasonable with her spouse and, finally, demanded to be placed in a nursing home. Although demanding to be hand fed, she refused to eat for anyone except one nurse. When family visited, she would not respond to their questions and often told them to "go away."

The spouse was terribly hurt and angry and, eventually, visited her only twice a day for a few minutes at a time. Mrs. Y died without her husband at her bedside. The older brother immediately went to help his father. The younger brother and wife arrived several days later. Their purpose was to attend the funeral and retrieve the jewelry that was to be left to them by prior agreement. (Mrs. Y kept a well-known list of who would receive her jewelry.)

The husband refused to view the body at the funeral home. He did attend the funeral, although he confided to a granddaughter that he would never again go to the cemetery to visit the grave site. He became unable to sleep due to nightmares and removed all of his wife's personal belongings.

The spouse in this case was reacting to his wife's illness and behavior induced by her condition as if she were in a preillness state; the resultant anger, hurt, and probably guilt prevented a suitable grief reaction.

It becomes the physician's and the nurse's responsibility to help the family to cope when the illness, or possibly the treatment, results in marked personality or mental changes.

GREED AND MATERIAL CONCERNS

The elderly are different from younger people in their concerns. For example, frequent topics may be wills, living trusts, and inheritance patterns. The 82-year-old lady in Case 3 began keeping a list of all her possessions, with the name of a relative after each one. This sort of behavior may possibly contribute to the avarice and material concerns of family members that often surface when an elderly person becomes acutely ill.

Regardless of the cause, it is apparent that some family members have enormous concern about what they will inherit and will "jockey" themselves to secure their position.

Occasionally, this behavior may cloud medical judgment. In Case 1, for example, there was pressure from the family members to remove artificial life support systems when the patient did not rapidly respond. In retrospect, the patient's wealth appeared to be a factor in this situation.

In general, the range of family dynamics is rarely openly explored, and often family members are left with hostility against each other, reawakening sibling rivalries and feelings of insufficient love and abandonment if their inheritance is not up to their expectations.

The increased longevity of our population is more and more accompanied by chronic disease, frailty, and dependency. These problems pose an urgent challenge to the health care professionals working with the acutely ill patient in the context of his or her family.

A critical element of sensitivity and judgment is to know when to intervene and when the most intelligent and compassionate course is that of minimal interference as the family finds their own support, care, and social arrangements. Even when the patient is receiving the finest medical attention and home care, attention must still be focused upon the caregiver(s) who may be experiencing too great a burden or signs of distress. Sensitivity to caregiver distress has been the subject of recent reports[9-11] as well as increased attention to concepts and attitudes of filial obligation toward aging parents and siblings.[12,13] The greater stress on caregivers today has multiple roots. A recent study[14] has clearly demonstrated that because of changing governmental guidelines and payments, elderly patients are being discharged earlier and sicker, still requiring treatment that previously would have been provided in a hospital. These conditions, coupled with frequently inadequate home health care assistance, result in families having to take up the slack. The increased role may strain the coping abilities of caregivers, lead to family bitterness, and increase the risk of elderly abuse. It is the responsibility of the geriatric emergency medicine team to be aware of all available community resources, so that maximum care and assistance can be provided to the patient and family after discharge.

Attention to family dynamics in acute illness and injury will be an increased focus of concern as our society slowly learns how to effectively care for and interact with our growing elderly population. Some specific considerations are explored in the remainder of this chapter.

EMERGENCY GERIATRIC INTERVENTION

While gathering information about the presenting illness, it is usually helpful to include any accompanying family members in the interview. Skillful questioning can help determine who the family spokesperson is and, more importantly, who the decision maker is. Discovering how the family has coped with prior problems gives clues as to whether this family system has closed or open boundaries. A closed family system is going to be resistant to a plan that includes outside help. The decision to accept outside help is something with which families eventually have to struggle, since their willingness and capacity to provide care at home usually erodes over time. The family's capacity to provide home care depends upon such resources as time, health, availability, and, most importantly, the pattern of reciprocity established over the years. Many elderly whom we assess as having no support system have alienated their biologic families.[14] It is helpful to keep in mind that the trip to the emergency department may be viewed by the family as a crisis, a crisis, in fact, that may reawaken many old family issues.

Crisis can also be a catalyst for new issues and feelings. Elderly spouses, in particular, may feel guilty for being healthy. Children can make unwise decisions in order to avoid feeling guilty. Guilt may also be related to events that occurred years ago. Spouses may be enraged by the loss of a partner and unfulfilled plans. Children may feel hostile toward a parent they remember as being abusive or neglectful. Old feelings of sibling rivalry may also erupt as one family member accuses others of being unresponsive to the present crisis. Relatives, on the other hand, may be too responsive. They may be overprotective and exaggerate limitations and underestimate capabilities of elderly family members. Some adult children, who may themselves be in their sixties or seventies, are unable to respond appropriately because of their own health and physical limitations. It is often difficult for elderly parents to accept that their children cannot care for them, as they frequently perceive those children as still being young and ageless.[15]

Few people understand their Medicare benefits, and many have inadequate insurance coverage. For some partners, there is despair as savings reserved for retirement are depleted.[16] Few individuals or families make concrete plans for caregiving, and many elderly arrive in the emergency department in a state of crisis because of their inability to care for themselves.

Cultural Considerations

Because of the broad range of elderly patients using emergency care, an awareness is needed of the impact of cultural heritage on some families. None of these examples are absolute givens but rather possibilities to consider.

Southeast Asian families, for example, may struggle with the concept of filial piety (honoring their elders) versus the reality of the demands of life in today's society. For these people, family business is a private affair, and the process of seeking information for an assessment will be invasive. Family business is so private that acceptance of outside help may be accompanied by shame.

Crisis may precipitate family role changes; a black or Mexican or Native American male may not perceive himself to be a provider of personal care to a parent or spouse. The elderly patient may possibly be homosexual, in which case the family may try to exclude his or her life partner from long-term care decisions.

Crisis Intervention

It is important to be aware that, in the emergency department, most patients perceive themselves to be in a state of crisis. Simply put, a crisis is a perturbation in the patient's steady state, not a pathologic state. It may occur to anyone at any stage of life. Not only do roles change in crisis but behaviors and attitudes change as well. Adult children who are very close to their parents when things are going well may feel overwhelmed at times of illness, and people who are warm and caring may be neutral or even hostile when tired and faced with a crisis. The intensity of the crisis will determine how long it takes for a person to reorganize.

It is helpful for emergency staff to be aware of the stages of crisis and to recognize that not all people go through it in the same manner. The first stage is *shock,* followed by a *defensive retreat,* a period during which the elderly patient and/or the family will attempt to keep things the same and in balance. Help is not seen as beneficial and an attempt to maintain control is made by refusing assistance. The reality of the situation is accepted during the *acknowledgment* stage, and only at the point of *adaptation* will new responses and coping patterns be formed.[17]

Crisis resolution and intervention is designed to offer immediate emotional-environmental first aid, utilizing reassurance and encouragement. While allowing some time for the patient and family to ventilate, crisis intervention in an emergency department setting is no time for psychologic interpretation but, rather, a time for mobilizing significant others, creating action, and accomplishing practical things.[18] It is during this process of mobilization that one of the most detrimental of family dynamics occurs: Families and staff in their attempt to respond to the present situation may exclude the patient from any decision making.

Self-Determination Issues

The legal and civil rights of older people are not always considered or respected. When a memory-impaired relative can no longer make rational decisions, families may act on their behalf, but they must be legally empowered to do so.[19]

In addition to the legal aspects, self-esteem issues come into play. Assistance must be compensatory in nature but also contribute to the maintenance of self-worth. Assistance and decisions about providing assistance must be balanced between doing what is needed and doing more than what is actually required. Professionals, especially, fall into the trap of taking over which, in fact, infantilizes aged persons. Professionals also have the added problem of meeting institutional needs. Value conflicts arise when obligation to the hospital conflicts with needs of the patient and family. Tight guidelines for admission criteria and length of hospital stay contribute to the conflict. Complicating the issue is a paucity of community resources. Having few alternatives erodes self-determination and limits patient decision making.[20] Patient advocacy, assistance with access to community resources, as well as family assessment are areas where an emergency department social worker may be especially helpful.

Medical social workers operate in consultative, collaborative roles. They are enablers assessing the situation and enhancing the problem solving and coping capacities of families. They are brokers who link patients with a number of systems. Finally, they are patient advocates, never losing sight of the patient's decision-making rights.

CONCLUSION

Few elderly and their families prepare for a crisis. When crisis, either physical or social, occurs, they present to the emergency department and bring with them a history of family interactions and influence. Those who work in this setting do not have the advantage of a detailed history or the luxury of time to obtain one. Some general knowledge about family dynamics and families in crisis, however, may enable us to better understand, accept, and serve our geriatric clients.

REFERENCES

1. Medalie JH, Kitson GC, and Zyzanski ST: A family epidemiologic model, J Fam Pract 12:79, 1981.
2. Culpepper L, Murphy J, and Fretwell B: Biology, primary care and community: a basis for rational geriatric care, Clin Geriatr Med 2:1, 1986.
3. Maddox GL: Families as context and resource in chronic illness. In Sherwood S, editor: Long term care, New York, 1975, Spectrum Publishers.
4. Kaprio J, Koskenvvo M, and Rita H: Mortality after bereavement, Am J Pub Health 77:283, 1987.
5. Levav I et al: An epidemiologic study of mortality among bereaved parents, N Engl J Med 319:457, 1988.
6. Jones DR, Goldblatt PO, and Leon DA: Bereavement and cancer, Br Med J 289:461,1984.
6a. Smedira NG et al: Withholding and withdrawal of life support from the critically ill, N Engl J Med 322:309, 1990.
7. Rowe JW: Health care of the elderly, N Engl J Med 13:827, 1985.
8. Ouslander JG and Beck JC: Defining the health problems of the elderly, Annu Rev Pub Health 3:55, 1982.
9. Pearson J, Verma S, and Nellett C: Elderly psychiatric patient status and caregiver perceptions and predictors of caregiver burden, Gerontologist 28:79, 1988.
10. Gilhooly ML: The impact of caregiving on caregivers, Br J Med Psychol 57:35, 1984.
11. Sanford JFA: Tolerance of debility in elderly dependents by supports at home: its significance for hospital practice, Br Med J 3:471, 1985.
12. Finely NJ, Roberts MD, and Banahan BF: Motivators and inhibitors of attitudes of filial obligation toward aging parents, Gerontologist 28:73, 1988.
13. Houser BB, Berkman SL, and Bardsley P: Sex and birth order differences in filial behavior, Sex Roles 13:641, 1985.
14. Silverstone B and Weiss A: Social work practice with the frail elderly and their families, Springfield, Ill, 1983, Charles C Thomas, Publisher.
15. Hancock B: Social work with older people, Englewood Cliffs, NJ, 1987, Prentice-Hall, Inc.
16. Pilisuk M and Parks SH: Caregiving: where families need help, Social Work 33(5):436–440, 1980.
17. Hubschman L: Hospital social work practice, New York, 1983, Praeger Publishers.
18. Dougherty AB: Emergency room: fighting a stage of crisis, Nurs Management 15(6):11–13, 1984.
19. Powell LS and Courtice K: Alzheimer's disease: a guide for families, Reading, Mass, 1983, Addison-Wesley.
20. Blayzk S and Canavan MM: Therapeutic aspects of discharge planning, Social Work 489–494, 1985.

SUGGESTED READINGS

Cox EO, Parsons RJ, and Kimboko PJ: Social service and intergenerational caregivers, Soc Work 33(5):430–434, 1988.
Golan N: Treatment in crisis situations, New York, 1978, The Free Press.
Hepworth DH, and Larson JA: Direct social work practice, Chicago, IL, 1986, The Dorsey Press.

A Comprehensive Emergency Care Program for the Elderly

Pam Wheeler, R.N.

During the past few years, departments of emergency medicine have increasingly become focal points for primary medical care as well as emergency care. Between 1954 and 1974, emergency room visits increased approximately 600%. A significant number of the more than 80 million annual visits made to emergency departments were by individuals seeking primary, not emergency, medical care. This pattern has been true for rural and suburban areas, as well as for cities.

The emergency department is viewed as a site for primary care by older adults (those 65 years of age and above). Some studies point out that utilization of emergency services by older adults for medical care is equal to or less than the percentage of this group as represented in the general population. However, many older adults with multiple, complex physical, psychologic, and socioeconomic needs seek medical care, on a continuing basis, in emergency departments. Some of these individuals will follow the recommendations made by emergency department staff to receive subsequent care from primary care physicians. Others return to emergency departments for nonemergency care, without being seen outside the emergency department system. (This pattern of emergency services utilization may be more commonly seen in urban elderly populations, where no primary physicians are available or identified.) Nursing homes frequently use emergency facilities and can also be sites for linkage.

Emergency department staff are not only in the position of providing specialized care to this population but also serve the function of referring patients to appropriate resources for follow-up care in the community, if hospitalization is not warranted. The emergency department initially serves as an access point for older adults to medical and nursing care by staff who have clinical expertise related to the needs of this population as well as knowledge about such conditions as patient abuse. In addition, emergency department staff serve as resources for linking patients with appropriate follow-up care. For those individuals with multiple physical, psychologic, and socioeconomic needs, this "linking" function, if done thoroughly, can mean the difference between an individual's securing comprehensive care or "falling through the cracks" — only to be seen in the emergency department when nonemergency medical attention is again necessary.

It has become increasingly apparent and more generally acknowledged that in the elderly population, a review of the medical, psychologic, and social aspects of the individual's life must be evaluated thoroughly. Any attempt to isolate and alleviate the individual's medical problems without an equal effort at coping with relevant psychosocial and environmental problems would not be in his or her best interests.

With the knowledge that older adults do have different health care needs, a movement to establish a specialized geriatric assessment unit was initiated in Great Britain during the late 1930s by Dr. Marjorie Warren. At that time, she was working in a large London workhouse infirmary, with older adults who had been neglected and were bedridden. In an effort to provide comprehensive care to these patients, she began a program that incorporated both a systematic evaluation process and a rehabilitation component. This assessment and rehabilitation program was completed prior to admitting a patient to a long-term care facility.

Although specific aspects of geriatric assessment units vary from region to region, in Great Britain and other countries, two basic concepts remain constant: 1) that elderly patients need a special, more broadly based, and interdisciplinary approach to their care than do younger patients and 2) that no patient should be admitted to a long-term care facility without a careful medical and psychosocial assessment and at least a trial of rehabilitation.

In the United States, geriatric assessment units have taken on many forms. Some are based on acute hospital wards, some are found in outpatient settings, while others are located in long-term care facilities. Some programs offer comprehensive diagnostic assessments only, some provide a minimal assessment but extensive rehabilitation, while others combine the extensive assessment with therapy and rehabilitative services. In general, these specialized assessment units support the contention that major improvements can be made in the delivery of health care services through comprehensive assessment, delivery of care by interdisciplinary teams, rehabilitation efforts, planning for optimal placements, and arranging for long-term follow-up.

In an effort to provide comprehensive care, a Gerontology Program was established between the Department of Emergency Medicine and the Senior Health Services Program at Good Samaritan Hospital & Medical Center. Planning for this linkage occurred over the course of a few months and involved staff from both programs. Planning meetings resulted in development of the following:

1. Specific criteria for referral of older adults from the Department of Emergency Medicine to the Senior Health Services Program with an accompanying guide to assist staff in clarifying appropriate referrals (Table 51–1, parts A and B)
2. A patient/physician flow diagram noting under which circumstances patients with or without primary care physicians would be directed to the Senior Health Services Program
3. Specific guidelines as to who should be contacted in the Senior Health Services Program regarding referrals and under what circumstances
4. A checklist to accompany referral information and provide additional psychosocial information (Table 51–2)

Table 51–1 (Part A). Criteria for Referral from Good Samaritan Hospital and Medical Center Emergency Room Department to the Senior Health Services Program

1. 65 or older
2. Medical, psychologic, social, and functional
   Problems (i.e., multiproblem) associated with aging, requiring a multidisciplinary evaluation. (This includes patients who exhibit evidence of cognitive and/or behavioral disorders.) Please see attached Guideline for Gerontology Program Referral.
3. Patient consents to a multidisciplinary assessment, which includes an assessment by a nurse in the home.
4. No primary care physician can be identified and/or the patient did not follow through with recommended ED physician referral.
5. Identified primary physician requests referral to the Gerontology Program.

Table 51–1 (Part B). Guideline for Senior Health Services Program Referral*

The following statements may serve as a guide in determining if a referral to the Gerontology Program is appropriate. If an individual ranks as a number 2 or 3 consistently, he/she may be in need of a multidisciplinary assessment.

During the last week, the patient:

A. ACTIVITY
1. Has been working or studying full time, or nearly so, in usual occupation, managing own household, or participating in unpaid or voluntary activities, whether retired or not
2. Has been working or studying in usual occupation, managing own household, or participating in unpaid or voluntary activities but requires major assistance or a significant reduction in hours worked (voluntary or paid)
3. Has not been working (on a voluntary or paid basis), studying in any capacity, or managing own household

B. DAILY LIVING
1. Has been self-reliant in eating, washing, toilet, and dressing; uses public transport or drives own car
2. Has been requiring assistance (another person or special equipment) for daily activities and transport but performing light tasks
3. Has not been managing personal care or light tasks and/or not leaving own home

C. HEALTH
1. Has been appearing to feel well or reporting feeling "great" most of the time
2. Has been lacking energy or not feeling entirely "up to par" more than just occasionally
3. Has been feeling very ill or "lousy," seeming weak and washed out most of the time

D. SUPPORT
1. Has been having good relationships with others and receiving strong support from at least one family member and/or friend.
2. Support received or perceived has been limited from family and friends and/or by the patient's condition
3. Support from family and friends occurred infrequently or only when absolutely necessary

E. OUTLOOK
1. Has usually appeared calm and positive in outlook, accepting and in control of personal circumstances, including surroundings
2. Has sometimes been troubled because not fully in control of personal circumstances or has been having periods of obvious anxiety or depression
3. Has been seriously confused or very frightened or consistently anxious and depressed.

*Quality of Life Index adapted from Spitzer WO et al: Measuring the quality of life of cancer patients: a concise QL-index for use by physicians, J Chronic Dis 34(12):585–597, 1981.

Table 51–2   Checklist for Gerontology Referral From the Emergency Department

Patient's name: _____   Date _____

Please check those items which best describe the patient. Feel free to add written comments when necessary. This information will be useful to gerontology staff when contact is made with the patient and/or family:

1. Living arrangement:

   a. alone _____   b. house _____
      with spouse _____   apartment _____
      with friend _____   mobile home _____
      with family _____   other _____
      other _____

2. Activities of daily living:

   needs help with bath _____   has access to transportation
   walks safely alone _____   and uses appropriately:
   able to prepare own meals _____   a. bus _____
   b. car _____
   c. other _____

3. Social contact — is contacted
   by friend/family by phone or
   in person: 7. Known to other community agencies (please list):

   a. daily _____
   b. 3–4 times each week _____
   c. once/week _____
   d. every 2–3 weeks _____   8. Last seen by physician (other
   than ED physician):

4. Mental status: a. Date _____
   b. Name _____
   recent memory intact _____
   oriented to time, place,
     person _____
   reports visual and/or   **Additional Comments**
     auditory hallucinations _____
   delusional _____
   paranoid _____
   symptoms/signs of
     depression present _____

5. Economic status:

   a. income per month _____
   b. does the patient perceive
      this as adequate? _____

6. Family/friend to contact:

Once the planning phase was completed, in-service programs about the Senior Health Services Program and its linkage with the Department of Emergency Medicine were provided to the medical and nursing staff from the Department of Emergency Medicine.

Implementation of the linkage began in January of 1983.

It was anticipated that those patients who would be referred to the Gerontology Program would have multiple medical, psychologic, and socioeconomic problems, would live within the Medical Center's general geographic area, would probably be living alone, frequently would either not have an identified primary physician or if one was

identified, the patient was not, by history, consistent in following through with recommendations by staff to see the primary physician, and could be identified as a patient, who, without follow-up in the community, could "fall through the cracks," and consequently not receive appropriate health care.

For example, one patient referred from the Department of Emergency Medicine was an 88-year-old woman who had come by ambulance from her hotel apartment after experiencing a seizure. She had a chronic seizure disorder which was controlled by 300 mg of Dilantin daily. However, there was a question about compliance in taking the drug. When discharged from the emergency department, she was instructed to continue the Dilantin and to contact her primary physician. In addition, a referral was made to the Senior Health Services Program for follow-up.

The patient was seen by a nurse within 2 days. She found that the patient had seen her primary physician the day after her emergency department visit. The patient's friend, who had been with her during the seizure episode, was also present during the home visit. As the nurse was asking the patient if she was taking the medicine as prescribed, the friend volunteered that when the patient took the Dilantin upon arising in the morning, she became nauseated. Consequently, she had reduced her Dilantin to 100 mg every morning. The patient said the medicine did not bother her if she had food in her stomach and asked if she could eat breakfast first. She was instructed to eat first and then take the prescribed amount of medicine, which she said she would do. She had forgotten to ask her primary doctor about this when she had seen him in his office.

Following the home visit, the patient's primary physician was contacted and informed of the follow-up visit and outcome. In addition, a dictated report was sent to the Department of Emergency Medicine as well as to the Medical Records Department so that, should the patient come into the emergency department again, the follow-up visit would be noted.

Other cases have involved elderly individuals in their eighties who lived alone in hotel apartments. One, who exhibited symptoms/signs of dementia and had been hospitalized for psychiatric problems in the past, was to be seen on an outpatient basis for a thorough workup. He was in danger of being evicted from his present living environment and had a daughter who lived 50 miles away, who was concerned and willing to assist her father as needed.

Another patient had marked cardiovascular problems but was uncomfortable with physicians and was usually seen in the emergency department only when others insist she get medical assistance. It was anticipated that the development of trust and rapport via in-home con-

tacts and telephone calls would take some time. However, the goal would be to have her secure a thorough medical assessment at some point in the future.

The ability to refer elderly patients in need of follow-up care through home visits and/or multidisciplinary assessments via a gerontology program enhances the service capability of emergency departments and offers a broader range of care for older patients. Further linkages with nursing homes can help to ensure emergency department capabilities to deal with particular needs of the old and very old.

Demographic data reveal that more than 25 million Americans are 65 years of age or older. Although by the year 2000 this number will increase to 31 million, the percentage of older adults in the population then, as now, will be approximately 11%. By the year 2030, however, almost one of every five Americans will be 65 or older. The importance of planning, formulating policies, and developing programs that provide comprehensive health care for this population cannot be overstated. The development of specialized programs for older adults and concomitant linkages with other components of care, such as departments of emergency medicine, is a first step in developing a range of programs capable of meeting the diversity of needs found in the older population.

SUGGESTED READINGS

Gerson L and Skvarck L: Emergency medical service utilization by the elderly, Ann Emerg Med 11:610–612, 1982.

Leonard L and Kelly A: The development of a community-based program for evaluating the impaired older adult, Gerontologist 15:114–118, 1975.

Libow LS and Starer P: Care of the nursing home patient, N Engl J Med 321:93, 1989.

Rubenstein L: Specialized geriatric assessment units and their clinical implications, West J Med 135:497–502, 1981.

Rubenstein L: Geriatric assessment programs in the United States: their growing role and impact, Clin Geriatr Med 2:99, 1986.

Rubenstein L and Rhee L: The role of geriatric assessment units in caring for the elderly: an analytic review, J Gerontol 37(5):521, 1982.

Straus J, Orr ST, and Charney E: Referrals from an emergency room to primary care practices at an urban hospital, Am J Pub Health 73:57–61, 1983.

Walker L: Inpatient and emergency department utilization: the effect of distance, social class, age, sex, and marital status, J Am Coll Emerg Phys 5:105–110, 1976.

Prehospital Care

Prehospital Geriatric Emergency Care

Diana Koin, M.D., and Knut Eie, EMT-IV

Care of the elderly is often characterized by a sense of incompleteness for many physicians. This sense of incompleteness can best be characterized by instances in which diagnoses seem to fit in a haphazard fashion, prescriptions often cause more side effects than beneficial outcomes, or recommendations for home care fail to be met with compliance on the part of the patient or the patient's family. There are many reasons for this disarray in attempting to care for elderly patients. One additional maneuver in the health care plan for older people can often help the physician avoid this problem. Prehospital care for the elderly will allow for more efficient and enlightened care of this particular population. It provides a missing link to meet the frustration and disenchantment which many health care providers experience in attempting to offer good care. This is particularly true in the emergency situation where health care providers lack the insight and knowledge obtained over time that primary care providers have available to them.

THE BRITISH STRATEGY: DOMICILIARY VISITS

The national health system in Britain initiated geriatric medicine as a specific entity at the time of its inception. Since that time, those responsible for the care of elderly patients have developed several strategies for enhancing health care despite strictly limited health care dollars. One of the most effective procedures has been the visitation of the patient in his or her own home prior to possible admission to a geriatric medicine unit in the hospital. This is possible in the British system because primary care is provided by general practitioners who will have seen the elderly patients first. The general practitioner will then contact the consultant in geriatric medicine requesting expertise for this patient. In Britain, there is a shortage of institutional beds for people no longer able to live independently; thus any triage that can be accomplished prior to hospitalization is of the utmost help. The domiciliary visit by a British geriatrician will usually be initiated to address specific problems (e.g., pneumonia, stroke). The general practitioner will meet at the patient's home with the patient and the geriatrician to decide the proper course of action. The patient will then be treated at home or admitted into the hospital. In the latter instance, the physician in charge of the patient will have access to many guidelines that will aid in diagnosis and treatment of this patient.

PREHOSPITAL CARE DEFINED

Prehospital care is that part of the spectrum of health care delivery which includes meticulous assessment of the patient's physical, psychologic, and social status prior to admission to an acute care hospital.

THE ICEBERG PHENOMENON

Williamson and colleagues described one of the distinguishing hallmarks of geriatric medicine: the Iceberg Phenomenon. This classical study emphasizes that most health care providers are well aware of their elderly patient's cardiac, pulmonary, and neurologic diseases.

However, there are specific problems common to an elderly population that are frequently overlooked. These include impaired mobility, incontinence, dementia, and anemia. Impaired mobility and dementia are the most important reasons why prehospital care of the elderly has a major role in determining a given patient's outcome. For example, if prehospital care providers find that a patient is able to walk independently, this stands in sharp contrast to the patient who is found to be able to only shuffle a few steps from his bed to his chair. Thus, if the patient smells of urine, his "incontinence" is likely to be a phenomenon of his inability to reach the bathroom rather than other more insidious causes.

More important is the determination of a patient's baseline mental status prior to hospitalization. Careful work by many investigators has shown that mental status evaluation in the acute hospital setting is of less valid reproducibility than is mental status evaluation in the patient's own environment; family and neighbors will often provide information regarding the onset of the mental status change. Acute onset implies reversibility, chronic onset often has a more insidious outcome. However, the knowledge that an acute change in mental status has occurred is indeed a true emergency in geriatric medicine.

PILLS AND POTIONS, OR WHAT YOUR PATIENT NEVER TELLS YOU

In the days of the house call, seasoned practitioners had access to a much clearer appreciation of the way in which patients took or failed to take their medications. Prehospital evaluation can often implicate poor compliance as a major cause of a current illness. In addition to noncompliance, additional compliance (i.e., medications purchased over-the-counter, borrowed from neighbors, or hoarded over decades) may be contributing to a current illness. Home health nurses are very knowledgeable in understanding how seldom patients are able to comprehend the logic of pharmacokinetics and be able to translate that into a sound therapeutic regimen.

PARAMETERS FOR PREHOSPITAL CARE

1. Environmental status
   a. Safety from falls (rugs, extension cords, stairs, pets)
   b. Temperature
   c. Physical safety/care providers
2. Functional capability
   a. Bathing and toileting
   b. Dressing
   c. Shopping
   d. Cooking
   e. Financial management
3. Cognitive function
4. Medications

PERSONNEL PROVIDING PREHOSPITAL CARE

Many health care providers have a potential for effectiveness in the arena of prehospital care. Elderly patients bemoan the demise of the house call because they intuitively recognize the significance of the information their physician was able to collect in a home visit. However, in today's world of technologic medicine, seldom is a physician's visit a possibility. Home health nurses provide extensive home evaluation. (See Chapter 51.) Rehabilitation experts (physical therapists, occupational therapists, and speech and language specialists) are able to provide assessment in a prehospital fashion in many communities.

THE ROLE OF THE PARAMEDIC

The term prehospital emergency care (PHEC) is often used interchangeably with out-of-hospital emergency care (OHEC). This is confusing, and perhaps incorrect, because the term prehospital care implies that all patients seen by paramedics will be transported for additional in-hospital treatment. When paramedics care for the older person, this is very often not the case. However, the term prehospital emergency care has gained widest usage, despite the occasional inaccuracy.

While in some countries physicians ride in ambulances to render care personally to patients at the scenes of medical emergencies, in the United States economic and logistic realities have led to staffing ambulances with emergency medical technicians (EMTs) and paramedics.

The Western civilian world was exposed to out-of-hospital advanced life support (ALS) in the mid-sixties. The organized Emergency Medical Services Systems (EMSS) did not become a reality in this country until the late sixties and early seventies. At first, emergency treatment in the field was limited to basic and advanced cardiac and respiratory resuscitation. It was soon recognized that the public used emergency services for other than cardiac problems. The need for more extensive paramedic education became evident. In 1977, the first National Standard Curriculum for the EMT-Paramedic was developed at the University of Pittsburgh with funds from the United States Department of Transportation. This "15-Module D.O.T. curriculum" included educational objectives in the following general areas:

1. The role of the paramedic
2. Human systems and patient assessment
3. Fluids and shock
4. General pharmacology
5. Respiratory system

6. Cardiovascular system
7. Central nervous system
8. Soft tissue injuries
9. Musculoskeletal system
10. Medical emergencies
11. Obstetric and gynecologic emergencies
12. Pediatric emergencies
13. Management of the emotionally disturbed
14. Telemetry and communications
15. Multiple injuries, multiple casualties, and triage

Unfortunately, there was no module on geriatrics and gerontology. When asked why not, a medical director of one nationally renowned paramedic training institute stated, "Paramedics trained by the Paramedic Training Institute are instructed in pre-hospital care of pediatric emergencies as well as adult medical and trauma emergencies. There are no specific lectures geared to the geriatric patient. We do not feel it is the paramedic's role to deal with the psycho-social problems of the geriatric patient." A nurse coordinator of a paramedic training program on the East Coast felt differently: "Just as children have traits characteristic to their age group, so do older people. It is imperative that we and the paramedics understand the loneliness, disease process and change they go through."

USE OF THE PREHOSPITAL CARE SYSTEM BY THE ELDERLY

After one and one-half decades of explosive growth of EMS, thousands of PHEC systems have been implemented nationwide. Today, there are over 300 paramedic training programs in the United States. Over 300,000 EMTs and 40,000 paramedics respond to more than 10 million emergencies across the nation. As a retrospective surprise to EMS designers, administrators, politicians, educators, and practitioners, there are indications that approximately 34% of these calls or 3.4 million emergency responses involve patients over the age of 60. Further, L.W. Gershon, Ph.D., has shown that in Akron, Ohio, patients over 65 account for 22% of EMS or paramedic utilization (*Annals of Emergency Medicine*, November, 1982). In addition, data collected by the Oregon State Health Division in 1980 indicated that 40% of ambulance "transports" in Portland were geriatric.

The older person frequently uses PHEC. Most of these services are rendered by paramedic personnel. Providing health care to the older person has become a major paramedic function and responsibility. Before we investigate how paramedics can assist in improving the quality of health care provided to the older person in the community, it may be helpful to consider why older persons utilize paramedic service as much as they do.

When the older person suffers from "aches and pains," or what others may call illness or injury, there is often a hesitance on their part to ask anyone for help. Older people often don't like to bother anybody, don't want to be a burden. Many like independence, self-determination, and things "their way." The reluctance to seek prompt assistance from family, friends, or health service agencies when having a medical problem may, with time, cause the patient's condition to reach a point of crisis or a state of emergency. Now, the patient or a friend dials 911, and the community responds by dispatching the "closest paramedic unit." Sometimes an older person may recognize a particular symptom but could fail to understand its medical significance. As a result, a subtle discomfort, although possibly a sign of significant disease, may be written off as a "normal" result of aging and something you "just have to live with" — in other words, just part of growing old.

Institutionalization, or involuntary relocation, may create a major disruption in the lives of elderly people and may in itself be the cause of a major crisis. Therefore, the older person may, in fear of losing independence to institutionalization, decide not to seek help at all even when the medical problem in question is one that could have been managed at home or in an outpatient clinic. The older person's hesitation to seek help may also stem from a lack of awareness of the various health and social service programs available, as well as what these programs can offer. Many times, when an older person does use the system due to what appears to be a nonurgent problem, it may prove difficult to receive timely and appropriate assistance. Finding the most appropriate health/social service for a particular medical, psychosocial, or financial problem can also be difficult. At times, the maneuvering of the bureaucracy is time consuming, confusing, and even intimidating to old people. A call to a physician's office or medical clinic may result in: "I'm sorry, Dr. X will not be taking any new patients until after the first of the year. Please let me take your name and number, and I will call you back as soon as I have an opening or a cancellation."

To the older person with limited mobility or chronic disease and no transportation, the emergency departments are not easily accessible unless the patient is transported by ambulance.

The Akron study alluded to another reason why the older person was a frequent user of paramedic services: 57% of the geriatric patients who were seen by paramedics used their EMS systems between 3:30 PM and 7:30 AM. This represented the time of the day when the older person may have the most difficulty getting a doctor's appointment.

Of those patients who succeeded in getting help in a timely manner, many had experiences that were bad enough to make them suffer through almost anything to avoid a similar experience. The idea of spending a couple of hours in a smoke-filled emergency waiting room with the intoxicated and obnoxious "Friday night crowd" is not very enticing to a 75-year-old woman with nausea and abdominal pain. Being stripped of clothes and dignity on a cold stretcher with a horde of strangers peering eagerly to "take a stab" at this case of nonspecific altered mental status is no better . . . "Hold still! . . . I can't get this darned subclavian in if you keep moving . . ."

Elderly victims of abuse represent another category of patients who avoid making outside contact with the health care system in fear of reprisals. The situation these patients are in may not be recognized until there is a life-threatening problem. A neighbor or friend may recognize the situation and notify the paramedics — the patient then receives treatment.

Finally, the fear of not being able to pay the medical bills may be another reason why the person avoids seeking medical help promptly, or unless it is "absolutely necessary."

The reality is that older persons frequently are not willing to use, may not benefit from, or may not be capable of using the traditional health care network. As a result, they wait and wait, just hoping that they can carry on a little longer on their own and in their own homes. Then there is the question of pride: Who wants to bother anyone?

As time passes . . . perhaps a fall, and then another one — no bones broken, just bruises . . . not walking so well anymore. No friends. Becoming bored. Lonesome. Don't feel like cooking anything. Dizzy in the morning . . . just a little fuzz . . . orthostatic; and then the fainting spells! "Mom, Mom, come here. I think Gram has passed out. Come — call the ambulance!"

"Care 82, respond to 2237 N.W. Northrup. There is an elderly lady there who keeps passing out. Code 3!" "82 en route."

For increasing numbers of older people in our society the paramedic is the only health care worker, outside the hospital ED, who is immediately available to assist the older person in crisis, 24 hours a day, 7 days a week, anywhere in the community.

When 911 is activated and paramedics respond, there is usually some sort of crisis. The older persons, their family, or friends may be overwhelmed by events that have left the individual helpless and unable to cope effectively by usual methods. This disruption of harmonious life may be psychosocial, physiologic, financial, or any combination of these in origin. The specific problem that triggered the crisis could range anywhere from loneliness and depression to dehydration, shortness of breath, coma of unknown cause, or being penniless. To the person who is crying for immediate and outside help, the crisis represents an **emergency.**

What can paramedics do to help the older person, their neighbors, family, and friends when these situations arise? The outline below is a general description of the type of services that a paramedic should be capable of providing. (Keep in mind that the objective is to do what is best for the patient — not the system.)

1. Reassurance
2. Primary assessment and emergency stabilization
3. Crisis intervention
4. Secondary assessment and emergency treatment
5. Information gathering and holistic assessment
6. Provide access to private clinician (M.D., R.N., etc.)
7. Patient education
8. Education of family, friends, neighbors
9. Information and referral service
10. Counseling
11. Transportation
12. Verbal/written medical reporting
13. Patient and family follow-up

If the older patient is conscious, communication and reassurance is the first step. Without a reassured and trusting patient, it is impossible to obtain an accurate history and to perform a worthwhile physical exam. Of course, without both, the proper tentative working diagnosis may not be made and improper treatment or disposition may result, causing increased instead of decreased morbidity and mortality. Communication with an older person may be extremely difficult for the clinician who has little interaction with older people or who has not developed professional skills in this area. Speaking slowly, being a good listener, and not asking "yes–no" questions are important points to remember when interviewing the older person.

If the patient is physiologically unstable, the approach must change and be very aggressive. In the older patient, vital organ function may be significantly reduced as a result of normal aging or chronic illness. The highly specialized tissues of cardiopulmonary, central nervous, and renal organs may be damaged so that there is no reserve capacity. Therefore, any delay in providing vital organ (life) support or reversal of a potentially life-threatening problem may have irreversible and devastating consequences.

For example, in the older person with acute gastrointestinal (GI) bleeding who is hemodynamically unstable, the administration of oxygen and crystalloids in the field may help decrease the work load of the heart, improve oxygenation, decrease the possibility of cardiac irritability and life-threatening arrhythmias, increase stroke volume, and maintain normal perfusion until the bleeding can be controlled in the hospital. Without this support in the field, perfusion of vital tissues may have gone below the tolerable threshold for this particular patient and essential vital organ function may be lost.

Likewise, the overdose victim with a depressed gag reflex and hypoventilation needs endotracheal intubation and positive pressure ventilation in the field before the patient is transported, not after the patient arrives in the ED with vomitus in the lungs and irreversible brain damage.

Another important assistance the paramedic can offer the medical team is in the home assessment of the older patient with altered mental status. This category of patients is often the most difficult for the hospital team to diagnose and treat. The total picture is often confusing because of the limited information at first available. Because of insufficient information, the correct diagnosis may be delayed, and the appropriate definitive care may be withheld. By the time the correct diagnosis is made, irreversible damage may have occurred. To complicate matters, the older person often does not see a physician or any health practitioner on a regular basis. The patient's chart, if there is one, may therefore not contain a lot of helpful information. The only useful information available about a patient's past medical history, environment, recent changes in life-style, etc., may be what the paramedics can gather at the scene. Talking with neighbors, friends, and family as well as carefully inspecting the patient's home environment may provide information that is necessary to make the diagnosis. Paramedics must look for medications, poisons, signs of violent acts or repetitive physical abuse, and indications of a person's inability to care for himself or to take medications as prescribed. Without the best observation and recording of the older person's life-style and recent changes in behavior, the differential diagnosis becomes difficult for the hospital team caring for the patient. A simple observation such as recognizing that a patient is receiving prescriptions from two or three different physicians may in context be the only clue needed to understand that the cause of coma in the older person was drug interaction. This would be impossible to ascertain if the paramedics had not realized the significance of finding all the patient's medications and bringing them to the ED.

When the older person is a victim of trauma, the clinical presentation is often misleading. For example, the older person who is hypovolemic may present with a normal blood pressure in the supine position. The heart rate may also be normal because of preexisting cardiac pathology. A detailed description of the mechanism of injury from the paramedic is therefore important and may influence the ED physician or surgeon in deciding whether to place the patient in the ICU or on the ward for observation.

Most of the time, a diagnosis can be made based on the history alone. Often, in caring for the older person, the only history available to the medical team is the one obtained by the paramedic. It is, therefore, of utmost importance that the nurse or physician who receives the patient in the hospital take the time to solicit a detailed report from the paramedic team who transported the patient. A paramedic's detailed report on a patient's home environment could also assist hospital personnel in discharge planning from the ward or from the ED. A patient's private physician could also prescribe follow-up visits after a patient is transported from the hospital by the paramedic team who initially responded to the patient's emergency.

EMTs and paramedics transport a lot of cancer patients. Many of these patients are taking large doses of pain medications. An ambulance ride could be tolerable for many of these patients if there were a way for physicians and paramedics to coordinate the time of transport with the time that pain medications were administered.

Sometimes patients call their physicians with a complaint or a problem that is difficult to assess over the phone. For example, "I am just not feeling well today," or "I have had a weird feeling in my chest all morning." What can a physician do in this situation? The waiting room is filled with patients who are waiting to be seen. Whether physicians are called by their patients at home or in the office, at the hospital, or through their answering services, it is often difficult to determine from a remote location what the severity and/or the urgency of a particular complaint is. It may also be impossible to determine over the phone what disposition is the most appropriate. Under these circumstances, it may be helpful for the physician, and reassuring and beneficial to the patient, if a paramedic unit was dispatched for more detailed home evaluation. After a primary and secondary survey, the paramedic team could report back to the private physician and answer the physician's questions. Based on the paramedic's assessment, it may be easier for the physician to dictate what therapy and disposition would be most beneficial to the patient.

For the past decade, paramedics have played a major role in providing health care to the older person, and will continue to do so. As the average life expectancy continues to increase and the older population continues to grow in numbers, an increase in utilization of paramedic services by older persons should be expected. Paramedics in general have learned to care for the older person through on-the-job training. With formal didactic and clinical training in geriatrics and gerontology, paramedics can make a more complete assessment and provide more appropriate treatment and disposition. Because of the complexity of the older person's medical problems and the frequent utilization of EMS by this group, it is imperative that extensive training in geriatrics and gerontology be made part of the National Standard Curriculum for EMT-Paramedics.

With an educational background, it is easier for the paramedic to understand the feelings, beliefs, attitudes, and, therefore, the total needs of the older person. This promotes more extensive assessment of the older person in the field, which in turn facilitates a better interaction between paramedics and other members of the health care team. From this, the most appropriate treatment and disposition follows.

Assessment and information gathering are two important functions of the out-of-hospital emergency care team. Another important paramedic function is to provide screening and referral services for the older person. Contact with the patient's primary physician is a vital early step.

We are finally beginning to realize and accept that one of the main responsibilities of EMS is to provide care for the older person. In fact, paramedics may provide the only immediate and practical access to emergency health care for the elderly. Originally, EMS was designed with the goal in mind of meeting the physiologic needs of patients who suffer from cardiac arrest and trauma. As a result, a *medical emergency* has traditionally been defined as *a condition which poses an immediate threat to life or limb.* This definition is dangerously narrow and may inappropriately exclude many emergent problems of the older person. The probability of the EMS system's meeting the common needs of the older person is thus significantly reduced. We must be open minded and flexible enough to change this attitude. It should be the needs and decision of the individual older person that determine what condition constitutes a crisis or an emergency.

The Spectrum of Prehospital Care for the Elderly

Elizabeth Hatfield Keller, R.N., B.S.N., C.E.N., EMT-P

Prehospital care is one of the newest aspects of medicine and, if used to its full potential, can become one of its greatest resources. The first advanced life support ambulances — mobile coronory care units — were developed in the late 1960s by Pantridge in Belfast, Ireland, and Grace in New York. It was not until the mid-1970s that widespread education and the deployment of ambulances staffed by trained advanced life support technicians — paramedics — occurred in many large cities in the United States. This was in large part due to a large grant sponsored by the Department of Health, Education and Welfare (EMS act of 1973) subsidizing the development of emergency medical systems in communities nationwide.

The discipline of prehospital medicine has appropriately grown since its inception, as have the skills and knowledge of paramedics. Many practitioners, however, have little knowledge not only of the skills, training, capabilities, and limitations of emergency medical technicians and paramedics but also of such concepts as the legal basis of prehospital medicine, medical control, and physician supervisors. In addition, practitioners need to know how best to access this care not only to be most cost effective but to provide the most beneficial and medically safe treatment and transport of their patients.

The transfer legislation of the Congressional Omnibus Reconciliation Act of 1986 has now made physicians' knowledge of prehospital care mandatory. According to this act, physicians are, among other things, responsible for ensuring that the *mode* of patient transfer is appropriate. This certainly includes the choice of the correct type of ambulance.

Yet daily, physicians can still be seen calling for an ambulance for the transport of an unstable patient and telling skilled paramedics to "do nothing except transport this patient" — severely endangering their patient in the process or interrupting paramedics on the scene of a medical or traumatic emergency and giving orders that are either inappropriate for the skills and scope of practice of the paramedic or are outright wrong. Or physicians will call for "just an ambulance" without consideration of the skill of the ambulance or its cost. These are just a few examples of physician misuse of prehospital care, and this is largely because they have never learned the specifics of what prehospital care is all about.

This chapter will hopefully bring much of this into focus by describing the elements of an emergency medical system; defining the types, levels, skills, training, and general abilities of emergency medical technicians and paramedics; and giving the practitioner the level of knowledge of making the most of this valuable resource and exploring its potential uses.

Transportation of patients to hospitals where physicians and nurses are available to give medical assistance must frequently be done by ambulance for comfort or convenience. Occasionally, there is a need for more immediate care which is given by emergency medical technicians and paramedics while en route to the emergency department, intensive care unit, or hospital ward. These personnel may also be the only direct link the physician has with the elderly person's home environment and can provide valuable information, which will facilitate the diagnosis, treatment, and disposition of the patient. This chapter will explain the role, background, and capabilities of emergency medical technicians and the method of accessing and making optimal use of the emergency medical services system (EMSS).

DEFINITIONS

The EMSS delivers prehospital emergency care and transportation to ill and injured persons. There is frequently an EMS director or coordinator who is responsible for developing and enforcing regulations and policies governing all aspects of this service. The boundaries of an EMS system, based on county, municipal, or arbitrary lines, are determined by each state. Legal authority exists for the EMS system to function, and the EMS director answers to the governing body of the district. There are physicians, nurses, emergency medical technicians, and citizens who may sit on advisory boards to provide information and opinions when policies are being formulated.

Emergency Medical Technician (EMT). This is a generic term used to refer to persons trained and certified at the basic (EMT-A or EMT-1), intermediate (EMT-I, EMT-2, or EMT-3), or advanced (EMT-P or EMT-4) level. Only those EMTs certified at the advanced level are called paramedics.

Each EMS system has the right to test and certify persons at whatever level designations are used by that area. Many states use a national certification exam and may certify EMTs by reciprocity who come from other states also using the national registry exam. Some states, such as California, administer certification exams on a county by county basis, while other states, such as Oregon, design their own state-wide exam and administer it, offering limited or no reciprocity. Exams consist of written, practical, and oral testing stations and are administered and evaluated by physicians, nurses, and other EMTs. Applicants pay testing fees and must provide proof of successful completion of a program of education that meets the topic and contact hours criteria determined by each EMS system for didactic, clinical rotation, and internship experience.

Supervising Physician. EMTs may practice under one or more supervising physicians. All legal and medical accountability rests with this physician or committee of physicians. EMTs may not operate unless they have this authorization to practice granted formally. Statutes may exist defining the necessary qualifications, responsibilities, and limitations of this physician's authority. The American College of Emergency Physicians issues policy statements about the role of supervising physicians.

Some EMS systems may use the term "physician advisor" although the role is that of a medical authority, not merely an advisor.

Medical Resources or Medical Control. This designated hospital provides EMTs with immediate accessible consultation via radio or phone with physicians or specially trained registered nurses, who have physician backup. Advice and medical direction are given and must be followed. Mandatory contact on all patient encounters or on certain types of patients or when certain therapies are indicated is determined by each EMS.

Ambulance, Rescue, Mobile Intensive Care Unit (MICU), or Medic Unit. All of these terms refer to specially outfitted and equipped vehicles which, if used for transporting patients, must conform to the U.S. Department of Transportation specifications. Sometimes the term used indicates the staffing level, but this varies greatly between EMS systems.

HISTORICAL PERSPECTIVE

The days of "scoop and run" ambulance drivers and attendants dressed in milkman uniforms and racing through streets with sirens blaring and lights flashing are over. The EMS systems of the current decade have developed into structured, accountable, professional teams of highly skilled and well-trained personnel able to rapidly access and give medical care to the ill and injured.

Advanced life support, out-of-hospital care originated from the need to provide cardiac and respiratory support to victims of myocardial infarction. Studies in the 1950s and 1960s showed a decreased mortality rate for victims of cardiac arrest who received interventions (especially cardioversion of ventricular fibrillation rhythms) prior to arrival at the hospital. The first mobile intensive care units were staffed by physicians, but this soon proved to be too costly. Emergency medical technicians, who would act as physician extensions and who would follow radio orders of hospital physicians, were thus developed and trained to provide cardiac and also trauma care using armed services medics as role models.

TRAINING AND CERTIFICATION LEVELS

EMT-A. This basic level training includes approximately 120 hours of classroom lecture, skill labs, emergency department observation rotation, and ambulance ride-along time. The material covered includes basic anatomy and physiology, recognition and management of common medical and traumatic injuries, and triage techniques for disaster management. The skills taught are cardiopulmonary resuscitation (CPR), the use of simple airway devices, administration of oxygen, suctioning, splinting of the spine and extremities, extrication of victims from vehicles, and application of pressurized antishock garments (PASG). In some areas, EMT-As are being taught to administer oral glucose for diabetic patients and subcutaneous epinephrine for anaphylaxis and to cardiovert ventricular fibrillation (although they may not treat other rhythms).

EMT-I. In addition to the above, training of an EMT-I includes recognition and treatment of shock with intravenous fluids, more aggressive airway management (this may include endotracheal intubation), cardiac rhythm recognition and therapies, and a more in-depth study of anatomy and physiology.

EMT-P. As a result of the U.S. Department of Transportation funding and support, the first national paramedic curriculum was developed in 1977. The latest revision in 1985 means paramedic students now receive a minimum of 212 hours of didactic clinical experience in hospitals and clinics, and 100 patient care hours in a preceptored field internship on MICU. Most training programs greatly exceed these requirements. These students receive education in the following:

- Roles of the paramedic and EMS systems
- Medicolegal issues
- Human systems, pathophysiology, and patient assessment
- Shock recognition, differentiation, and management
- General pharmacology, toxicology, and drug/alcohol abuse
- Respiratory section with advanced airway management
- Cardiovascular emergencies and treatment
- Nervous system events
- Musculoskeletal and soft tissue injuries
- Medical emergencies and infectious diseases
- Trauma and burn management
- Obstetrics/gynecology/neonatal care
- Pediatrics
- Geriatrics
- Behavioral emergencies
- EMS communications
- Rescue and extrication techniques
- Major incident response and management

To date, fewer than 10 paramedic training programs have added a formal track on geriatric emergencies. Oregon is one of the few states to actually include geriatric-specific questions on its certification exam. This continues to be a significant problem that physicians involved with geriatric care must address and, hopefully, resolve.

Paramedics may use cardiac monitors/defibrillators, administer medications by any appropriate route, initiate and maintain intravenous lines (peripheral and central), and perform endotracheal intubation, pericardiocentesis, and thoracic decompression of tension pneumothorax. They do history and physical examinations, handle mental health crises, and extricate patients from automo-

biles, hazardous environments, and buildings. All EMTs must also be aware of the issues involved in transporting a patient, including patient comfort and safe driving techniques, and be able to perform most of their skills and interventions in a moving MICU. At mass-casualty incidents, paramedics triage and direct patient care and transportation.

MEDICAL CONTROL AND ACCOUNTABILITY

Regulations governing the scope of an EMT's practice vary. Although EMTs are trained and certified to perform the skills previously listed, a supervising physician must still authorize such practice. He or she may issue the permission in the form of written patient care protocols or through case by case decision. This on-line medical control is when a physician or specially trained registered nurse is in voice contact with the prehospital team via radio or phone and gives direction for patient care. Specific hospitals are usually designated as base station hospitals so that EMTs are dealing with a consistent group of medical staff who know the EMTs' capabilities and are trained to communicate over radios. This also prevents "shopping around" for a physician who will give the desired orders.

Whether they practice under standing orders or direct medical control, all EMTs must use their best clinical judgment when doing patient care. They answer always to the physician under whose license they practice. In turn, the physician is responsible for all decisions made and care given by the EMTs. Quality assurance is done by physicians, nurses, peers, and various county and state committees and agents who audit charts and conduct oral case reviews. All aspects of an EMS system are measured to community and national standards of appropriate medical practice and are subject to internal and external review and evaluation.

CONTINUING EDUCATION REQUIREMENTS

The nature of emergency medicine necessitates a constant formal review and upgrading of knowledge and skills and is a mandatory part of the EMT's job. Continuing education requirements for paramedics include contact hours in each of the areas of original training, Basic and Advanced Cardiac Life Support (BCLS and ACLS) recertification, participation in case review sessions conducted by physicians, literature review, and further supervised clinical practice opportunities. Currently, many EMS systems are requiring EMTs to become certified in Prehospital Trauma Life Support (PHTLS), a course designed by the American College of Surgeons, or Basic Trauma Support (BTLS), a similar course designed by the American College of Emergency Physicians. New courses in advanced care for pediatric patients are being designed and taught for certification also. Additionally, a great deal of informal learning occurs as nurses and physicians in the emergency departments share their expertise and allow paramedics to observe and participate in the continuation of patient care.

The responsibility for having a group of currently trained personnel rests with supervising physicians. They may delegate the tasks of setting up in-service time to a training coordinator and may assign a quality assurance coordinator to conduct chart audits. They may also institute a peer review committee to assist with accountability and professionalism issues. Nurses may teach many of the continuing education classes and evaluate at skill labs. However, the supervising physician has the duty to ensure that the continuing education and quality assurance is relevant to the prehospital setting and yet maintain the highest possible level of education and expectations of practice for the EMTs.

INFORMATION AVAILABLE FROM EMTS

Emergency department physicians and nurses have the most frequent contact with EMTs and quickly learn their capabilities. Besides evaluating the patient, EMTs are taught to be careful observers and reporters of the environment in which they encounter the patient. Sometimes the information about the home or accident scene is only obtainable from the EMTs and may be critical in the physician's decisions about the patient. The temperature and sanitation conditions may preclude sending an elderly patient back home and may require intervention by a home health agency. Many elderly persons living at home may be unable to perform or afford routine maintenance and repairs, which may lead to the presence of hazardous conditions.

Food may be discovered spoiled or of little nutritional value. Prescription bottles are sometimes found full because they are in childproof containers, and the geriatric patient with arthritis cannot open the lid. Illicit drugs and bottles of alcohol about the residence may indicate a substance abuse problem or an explanation for an altered mental status in an otherwise healthy elderly person. Falls are occurring because the patient cannot use his/her prostheses: a walker that is too wide for the available cramped hall space, a commode too high for the patient to get up on, or a pair of glasses that has dropped behind the bed and is out of reach. The rest of the medical team may never know about these conditions without a home visit, for which many institutions do not have the available staff. Yet the EMTs called to such a home routinely report this information to the emergency department personnel when delivering the patient.

Frequently, the EMTs provide information about the level of care the patient receives. This may not be synonymous with either what is needed or what is expected from the arrangements made by the social service or home health agency. For example, an elderly person living alone may be unable to do simple housekeeping and cooking chores and has hired a companion arranged by social workers at the hospital following the last admission. The EMTs report that at noon the caregiver smells strongly of alcohol and has not yet made breakfast or changed the incontinent patient's clothing. Out of fear of losing his or her last bit of independent living or available care, this geriatric patient may never tell the physician why, in spite of the best efforts at medication and nutrition advice, the patient's condition continues to deteriorate. Discharge plans will need to include modifications in the home care provided.

ELDERLY ABUSE

Neglect and abuse of the elderly, whether in their own homes, foster care, or nursing facilities, continues to occur at alarming rates. Many families attempt to keep aged parents at home but find the physical and mental deterioration too stressful. Sometimes lacking funds, elderly patients are forced to remain in their children's home instead of being placed in a nursing home. This may be when physical and emotional violence against the geriatric person occurs. As a routine part of the environmental assessment, EMTs learn the clues to observe. This information is given to medical staff members and is reported to legal authorities as mandated by state statutes. EMTs, nurses, and physicians do not make the final judgment on elderly abuse and neglect but are legally and ethically obligated to report their suspicions.

"DO NOT RESUSCITATE" ORDERS

Paramedics respond to homes and care centers where they are told to "just take this person to the hospital." The EMTs must follow the standing orders of their supervising physician or medical resource and provide appropriate intervention and care to each patient. Any deviation from standard medical practice must be cleared with the medical control authority unless such orders are written and signed by the attending physician. When told a patient is a "no code" or "do not resuscitate" (DNR) by family or nurses without appropriate documentation, the paramedic may have to begin resuscitating the patient until orders to stop come from medical control. Attempts to contact the attending physician while performing basic life support will usually be made and his or her wishes followed. However, to protect a patient's right to die, written "no code" or DNR orders should be immediately available and with the patient at all times.

In most communities, DNR means that no resuscitation will occur in the event of cardiopulmonary arrest but that all care and comfort measures will be done prior to that point. If it is decided to extend the DNR to include withholding fluids, medication, oxygen, etc., the physician must completely document this on the order sheet. Families caring for dying patients at home often panic and call 911 when death is imminent. The EMTs must interpret this call as implied consent for treatment and give medical care and resuscitation unless a written "no code" order is found. In all cases, the patient's and family's wishes will be followed if they now choose to rescind the order.

SPECIAL CONSIDERATIONS IN THE ELDERLY

Paramedic level EMTs must receive training in recognizing signs and symptoms of medical conditions that present differently in the geriatric patient. For example, subtle changes in functioning can indicate impending catastrophic events that might otherwise be unsuspected. When sent to an elderly person who has fallen, paramedics need to immediately assess the patient's cardiovascular status, since nearly one half of these falls result from intrinsic causes. A stumble in the garden may result in a hip or spine injury. Cervical spine precautions will be taken and the patient immobilized because of the greater potential for fractures from osteoporosis. A decreased pain perception makes the older person more susceptible to occult injuries, and the paramedic must protect the patient from further harm.

Paramedics need to know that cardiac ischemia often presents as dyspnea and exercise intolerance, not as classical chest pain. Syncope and weakness frequently accompany seizures, strokes, and myocardial infarctions. An infection can precipitate shock in an elderly person who has a decreased reserve capacity and so is unable to compensate for the rapid progression of disease. Fluid resuscitation must be started immediately but carries with it special risks as aging causes changes in physiologic responses to medications and other therapies. Paramedics often need to consult with medical resources for information about the side effects and potentiation caused by the multiple pharmaceuticals prescribed for a geriatric person.

ACCESSING THE EMS SYSTEM

The procedure for obtaining medical assistance and transport differs in each community, but the same general principles apply in each EMS system. Dispatching an ambulance may be done by fire, police, or public or private ambulance dispatch centers. Some communities have direct dial numbers for emergency and nonemergency requests while others take all medical calls through 911. A prioritization of both code response and appropriate personnel response is done by the dispatchers, sometimes regardless of what the caller, including a physician, requests. Again, this is determined by local policies designed to provide the most rapid, appropriate level of care and minimize the liability risk. The public and medical profession may not be aware of what terms to use and what services are available so dispatchers are trained to ask a series of questions that assist them in sending the correct unit to the call.

TYPES OF RESPONSE

A code 1 or nonemergency response brings a transporting unit without lights and sirens. A code 2 response, which is not a legal response in some states, brings an ambulance that may use its lights but not siren. A code 3 or emergency response is with lights and sirens on. A fire department engine, truck, or rescue squad may respond along with a transporting ambulance, medic unit, or MICU. This tiered response is designed to provide additional personnel and specialized equipment when certain triage criteria exist. Even when medical professionals are on a scene, this multilevel dispatch may occur because of local guidelines.

Considerations are given to the patient's symptoms and to the location and traffic conditions when dispatching an ambulance. A stable patient who has only a possible hip fracture from a mechanical fall in a nursing home would tolerate the extra few minutes a code 1 ambulance might take to arrive. However, this same patient lying on the sidewalk at night would probably require a code 3 response because of the added hazards of the environment. Even though lights and sirens may be embarrassing to the family or care center, the unstable patient needs rapid help. A request made to the dispatcher for a quiet approach allows the ambulance to proceed rapidly to the scene, shutting down the warning devices when within a few blocks. This request is usually honored, although for safety, the flashing lights may be left on when the ambulance is parked in the roadway.

ADVANCED LIFE SUPPORT VS. BASIC LIFE SUPPORT

Often more than one type of unit is available to send on a call. Advanced life support (ALS) units are staffed with at least one and sometimes two paramedics and carry cardiac and respiratory equipment and drugs. Basic life support (BLS) units have at least one EMT trained at the basic or intermediate level. In general, ALS units cost two to three times what a BLS unit costs. Both ALS and BLS units provide another team member, usually an EMT, to drive. Regulations differ as to whether BLS units respond or transport with lights and sirens. The patient is always monitored by the most qualified EMT who rides in the back of the ambulance. Sometimes a physician, nurse, or respiratory therapist accompanies an unstable patient during interhospital transfers when care may be required that is beyond the scope of the paramedic's training.

The practitioner must not use cost as the only basis of his/her decision for choosing an ambulance for the patient. He/she must be aware of the critical difference between these two units (ALS vs. BLS). Practitioners will certainly do their patients a disservice by ordering a BLS ambulance for a patient who might very well become unstable.

This has become even more important since the passage of the Transfer Legislation in the Congressional Omnibus Reconciliation Act (COBRA) of 1986, which stipulates that the *method* of transportation in transferring a patient must be appropriate. This *method* specifically relates to the choices of private car, BLS ambulance, or ALS ambulance.

It must be remembered that the BLS ambulance cannot *by law* do more than their scope of practice. Therefore, practitioners can not only endanger their patients but also incur financial and legal risk if they do not select the right ambulance.

CONCLUSION

EMTs can provide valuable data about the patient and the home setting necessary for making treatment and disposition decisions by the rest of the health care team. This information is retrievable from written patient care report forms which are kept as part of the hospital medical record. Paramedics are capable of performing complete patient assessments with limited diagnostic tools and initiating advanced procedures and therapies in an uncontrolled environment. They safely transport patients to hospitals and return them to residences. They are always accountable to their supervising physician and must maintain the highest possible level of professionalism. The specialized training that EMTs receive and the unique role they have as extensions of physicians should be appreciated so that optional use of this very valuable resource can be made by practitioners.

Index